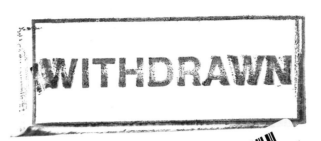

Histopathology
of the Skin

Histopathology
of the Skin

WALTER F. LEVER, M.D.

Professor of Dermatology and Chairman of the Department, Tufts University School of Medicine; Lecturer on Dermatology, Harvard Medical School; Chief, Dermatology Service, New England Medical Center; Physician, Dermatology Service, Boston City Hospital; Member of the Board of Consultation, Massachusetts General Hospital; Consultant in Dermatology, Robert Breck Brigham Hospital

GUNDULA SCHAUMBURG-LEVER, M.D.

Assistant Professor of Dermatology, Tufts University School of Medicine; Associate in Dermatology, New England Medical Center

FIFTH EDITION

386 Light Microscopic Illustrations
With 8 in Color, and
50 Electron Microscopic Plates

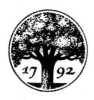

J. B. Lippincott Company
Philadelphia • Toronto

Fifth Edition

Copyright © 1975, by J. B. Lippincott Company

Copyright © 1967, 1961, by J. B. Lippincott Company
Copyright 1954, 1949, by J. B. Lippincott Company

ISBN–0–397–52069–7

Library of Congress Catalog Card No. 75–5729

PRINTED IN THE UNITED STATES OF AMERICA

1   3   5   4   2

Library of Congress Cataloging in Publication Data

Lever, Walter F.
  Histopathology of the skin.
  Includes bibliographies.
  1. Skin—Diseases. 2. Histology, Pathological.

I. Schaumburg-Lever, Gundula, joint author.
II. Title.
RL95.L48 1975   616.5'07   75–5729
ISBN 0–397–52069–7

In Memory of My Father

Dr. Alexander Lever

1877-1946

My First Teacher in Dermatology

Preface to the Fifth Edition

In the eight years that have passed since publication of the fourth edition so much new information has become available on nearly every major dermatosis that the book had to be entirely rewritten. The greatest changes were required in the description of the lymphomas because they have been reclassified in recent years. Many changes have been made also in the description of the bullous dermatoses and of the metabolic diseases, especially of amyloidosis, colloid milium, hyalinosis cutis et mucosae, and porphyria. Also the division of malignant melanoma in situ into two types with different prognosis has been given due consideration.

More than 20 diseases not mentioned in the fourth edition are described in this edition. Some of them are newly recognized entities, such as disseminated superficial actinic porokeratosis, perforating folliculitis, reactive perforating collagenosis, angiolymphoid hyperplasia with eosinophilia, infantile digital fibromatosis, trichilemmoma, and malignant eccrine poroma. Also several previously known diseases because of their increased interest for the dermatologist have been incorporated, among them regional enteritis (Crohn's disease), Tangier disease, lipogranulomatosis (Farber's disease), and generalized eruptive histiocytoma.

The greatest change in the present edition in comparison with the preceding fourth edition lies, however, not in the histologic descriptions but in the much more detailed discussion of the histogenesis of the various diseases. The allotment of more space to histogenesis seemed justified because of the many significant findings in histochemistry, immunology, and especially electron microscopy that have greatly contributed to the understanding of disease processes. The discussions of the histogenesis have been set in small print, as in the previous edition, in order to separate them clearly from the histologic descriptions.

In the electron microscopic presentations my wife Dr. Gundula Schaumburg-Lever has collaborated. Since electron microscopy is very useful in explaining disease processes, 50 plates of electron microscopic illustrations were produced by Dr. Schaumburg-Lever. The electron micrographs have been placed at the end of the book as an appendix. Thus, someone interested in the electron microscopic aspects may study the electron micrographs together.

The bibliography following each chapter has been brought up to date, and, as in previous editions, articles written in English have been given preference. Forty-four photomicrographs have been added. Most of them were produced by Mr. Richard W. St. Clair with the same great skill as for the previous editions.

I wish to thank Mr. Lewis Reines, Editor of Medical Books, J. B. Lippincott Company, for his help and constructive suggestions.

WALTER F. LEVER

Preface to the First Edition

This book is based on the courses of dermatopathology which I have been giving in recent years to graduate students of dermatology enrolled at Harvard Medical School and Massachusetts General Hospital. The book is written primarily for dermatologists; I hope, however, that it may be useful also to pathologists, since dermatopathology is given little consideration in most textbooks of pathology.

I have attempted to keep this book short. Emphasis has been placed on the essential histologic features. Minor details and rare aberrations from the typical histologic picture have been omitted. I have allotted more space to the cutaneous diseases in which histologic examination is of diagnostic value than to those in which the histologic picture is not characteristic. In spite of my striving for brevity I have discussed the histogenesis of several dermatoses, because knowledge of the histogenesis often is of great value for the understanding of the pathologic process.

Primarily for the benefit of pathologists who usually are not too familiar with dermatologic diseases, I have preceded the histologic discussion of each disease with a short description of the clinical features.

A fairly extensive bibliography has been supplied for readers who are interested in obtaining additional information. In the selection of articles for the bibliography preference has been given, whenever possible, to those written in English.

I wish to express my deep gratitude to Dr. Tracy B. Mallory and Dr. Benjamin Castleman of the Pathology Laboratory at the Massachusetts General Hospital for the training in pathology they have given me. It has been invaluable to me. Their teaching is reflected in this book. Furthermore, I wish to thank Mr. Richard W. St. Clair, who with great skill and patience produced all the photomicrographs in this book.

WALTER F. LEVER

Contents

Histopathology
of the Skin

1

Introduction

TECHNIC FOR BIOPSY

It is important to select a proper site for biopsy. In most instances histologic examination of a fully developed lesion will give more information than examination of an early or an involuting lesion. Vesicular, bullous, and pustular lesions represent exceptions to this rule. For their histologic examination a very early lesion is required; otherwise, secondary changes (such as regeneration, degeneration, or secondary infection) may obscure essential features and make recognition of their mode of formation impossible. Generally, it is inadvisable to include normal tissue in the biopsy specimen, unless a large specimen is taken, or the physician personally supervises the processing of the specimen, because improper sectioning by the technician may result in only normal skin being seen in the section. If the submitted specimen is supposed to contain tumor tissue but the sections do not show it, it is advisable that, before a final report of absence of tumor tissue is rendered, deeper sections into the tissue block be carried out in the laboratory; and if the laboratory fails to do this, the physician who submitted the specimen should request it.

Whenever possible, the biopsy specimen should include subcutaneous fat, because in many dermatoses characteristic histologic features are found in the lower dermis or in the subcutaneous fat. If several lesions are present, and the diagnosis hinges on the histologic findings, much time may be saved by taking specimens for biopsy from more than one lesion.

In the author's experience a specimen obtained with a 6-mm biopsy punch nearly always has proved to be adequate for histologic study. In many instances a specimen obtained with even a 3- or a 4-mm punch is adequate. After use of the 3-mm punch, usually no suturing is required, except on the face, an adhesive plaster to approximate the wound edges being sufficient; after use of the 4-mm punch, one suture is adequate to close the wound; and after use of the 6-mm punch, two sutures are recommended.

Tissue obtained by means of curettage rarely is fully satisfactory for histologic examination because the submitted material usually is scanty and superficial in location, and has lost its architecture. However, the procedure may be condoned because of its convenience if it is carried out prior to electrodesiccation of lesions that are regarded as benign or of low malignancy, as in the case of solar keratoses, seborrheic keratoses, verrucae, or small basal cell epitheliomas. Curettings obviously are inadequate for ruling out malignant melanoma or for differentiating between squamous cell carcinoma and keratoacanthoma.

As fixative, 10 per cent formalin in aqueous solution can be used in nearly all instances (see p. 46). However, if the specimen is to be mailed during the winter period, 10 per cent aqueous formalin which freezes at −11° C. may allow the formation of ice crystals in the specimen, resulting in damage and distortion in the specimen, particularly in the epithelial cells, and thus preventing adequate histologic evaluation. It is then preferable to use Lillie's AAF, a fixative containing 40 per cent formaldehyde, 10 parts; glacial acetic acid, 5 parts; and absolute ethyl alcohol, 85 parts, since its freezing point is below −30° C. (Okun et al.).

If any special stains are desired, this should be indicated on the requisition sheet that is being sent to the laboratory with the specimen. If, for instance, a stain for lipids is to be carried out, the specimen must not be processed in the Autotechnicon (see Table 4-1, p. 47).

LIMITATIONS OF HISTOLOGIC DIAGNOSIS

Although histologic study is one of the most valuable means of diagnosis in dermatology, it has its limitations. Often no definitive diagnosis can be made. The reason for this is that few dermatoses, aside from the tumors, are associated regularly with a diagnostic histologic picture. Instead, the histologic features may be merely suggestive of a diagnosis or may be entirely nonspecific. Even in the case of tumors, difficulties in diagnosis may arise. For instance, distinction of squamous cell carcinoma from pseudocarcinomatous hyperplasia or from keratoacanthoma is not always possible. In cases of infectious granulomas, such as syphilis, tuberculosis, and the deep mycoses, a specific diagnosis often cannot be made

unless the causative organism can be demonstrated. Great difficulties may also be encountered in the histologic study of the large group of noninfectious inflammatory dermatoses. In some diseases of this group, such as lichen planus and lupus erythematosus, the histologic picture, although diagnostic in most instances, may be merely suggestive, especially in cases in which the clinical picture is not typical. In other noninfectious inflammatory dermatoses, such as psoriasis, the histologic picture is rarely diagnostic. Similarly, in subacute and chronic dermatitis the histologic findings generally are nonspecific and resemble those seen also in other dermatoses, for instance, in pityriasis rosea, prurigo simplex, and parapsoriasis en plaques. Nevertheless, frequently, when the histologic picture is not diagnostic, correlation of the histologic with the clinical findings will make a diagnosis possible.

In many instances the chief value of histopathologic study lies in corroborating the clinical diagnosis or in ruling out possible diseases that are being considered on the basis of clinical appearance. It is obvious that the histopathologist can give the clinician a maximum amount of information only if every specimen submitted for histologic diagnosis is accompanied by detailed clinical information, including a differential diagnosis.

BIBLIOGRAPHY

Okun, M. R., Ellerin, P., and Piotrowicz, M. A.: Prevention of ice crystal damage in biopsy specimens in transport. Arch. Derm., *105*: 458, 1972.

2

Embryology of the Skin

THE EPIDERMIS

Keratinocytes. The epidermis at the earliest time at which it has been examined so far, at an age of 6 weeks, when the crown-to-rump length of the embryo is 14 mm, consists in some areas of only a single layer of ectodermal cells; but in most areas there already are two layers: a basal germinative layer and an outside layer of periderm cells (Breathnach and Robins). At an age of 9 weeks, through upward movement of cells of the germinative layer, another row of cells between the two layers becomes apparent: the stratum intermedium. The cells of the stratum intermedium are large and, because of the presence of glycogen, possess a clear cytoplasm. In embryos 12 weeks old and 6 cm long, the stratum intermedium varies from one to three layers in thickness; and at an age of 14 to 16 weeks (8 to 12 cm length) keratinization of the cells of the periderm takes place (Fig. 2-1). Small keratohyaline granules may then be seen in the subjacent cells (Hashimoto et al., 1966). In embryos 17 weeks old and older the epidermis appears similar to that of an adult.

HISTOGENESIS. On electron microscopic examination, embryos 6 to 7 weeks of age show immature desmosomes between the epidermal cells but no tonofilaments are as yet attached to them; and, although a distinct basal lamina is seen, half-desmosomes either are absent or just begin to appear (Hashimoto et al., 1966; Matsunaka and Mishima). The surface of the cells of the periderm shows indentations and numer-ous microvilli, providing a large area of exposure to the amniotic fluid. This, together with the presence of numerous cytoplasmic vesicles within the periderm cells, suggests an active exchange between the periderm cells and the amniotic fluid (Breathnach). At 10 weeks of age, embryos show well developed desmosome-tonofilament complexes (Matsunaka and Mishima). At 16 weeks of age the cells of the periderm become flattened, and show a purely filamentous internal structure and a thickened plasma membrane characteristic of keratinized cells (Breathnach).

Melanocytes. The colonization of the skin by melanocytes is closely related to the development of the cutaneous nerves, since both are derived from the neural crest. The appearance of both nerves and melanocytes in the skin takes place in a cranio-caudal direction (Leopold and Richards). Using light microscopy on sections either treated with impregnation by ammoniated silver nitrate or exposed to the dopa reaction, melanocytes are first seen in the dermis of Negro fetuses 10 weeks old. By the eleventh week the first melanocytes have migrated into the epidermis. Between the twelfth and fourteenth weeks the number of melanocytes in the epidermis increases greatly. At birth melanocytes remain in only a few areas of the dermis, especially in the sacral region Zimmermann and Becker).

HISTOGENESIS. Electron microscopy has led to an earlier recognition of melanocytes in the epidermis than had been possible by light microscopy, namely at 8 to 10 weeks, rather than at 11 to 14 weeks (Sagebiel and Odland). The reason for the earlier detection by electron microscopy lies, of course, in the fact that recognition of melanocytes by electron microscopy is made through identification of melanosomes rather than through the presence of melanin or of enzymatic activity in the melanocytes. Beginning of melanin deposition on the melanosomes was noted at 10 weeks of age. The observation of melanocytes in the epidermis at 8 weeks of age correlates well with the time when the neural crest from which they are derived has completed its differentiation. Langerhans cells recognizable by the presence of Langerhans granules are first observed by electron microscopy in the embryonal epidermis at an age of 14 weeks (Breathnach and Wyllie).

THE EPIDERMAL APPENDAGES

The embryonal stratum germinativum differentiates not only into basal cells, giving rise to the keratinizing epidermis, but also into primary epithelial germs, also called hair germs, giving rise to the hair, sebaceous glands, and apocrine glands, and into eccrine gland germs, giving rise to the eccrine glands (Chart 1).

Hair. Primary epithelial germs, or hair germs, are first observed in embryos in the eyebrow region and the scalp during the third month (Hashimoto, 1970, I). The general development of hair begins in the fourth fetal month in the face and scalp and gradually extends in a cephalocaudal direction. Thus, during the fourth month, while some hair follicles on the head are already well matured and are producing hair, most of those on the trunk are barely differentiated (Serri et al.). In addition, new primary epithelial germs keep developing between earlier ones so that, in any section obtained from the beginning of the fifth month up to birth, hair structures in different stages of development are found (Mishima and Widlan).

The development of hair begins with the formation of primary epithelial germs which in their earliest stage consist of an area of crowding of deeply basophilic cells in the basal layer of the epidermis. Subsequently the areas of crowding develop into buds that protrude into the dermis (Fig. 2-1). Beneath each bud lies a group of mesenchymal

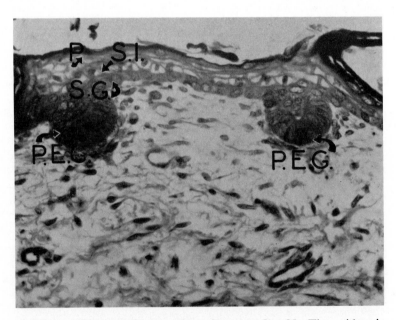

Fig. 2-1. **The skin of an embryo four months old.** The epidermis consists of three layers: the stratum germinativum (S.G.), the stratum intermedium (S.I.), and the periderm (P.). Two primary epithelial germs (P.E.G.) are shown. The fetal dermis shows many more fibroblasts than the adult dermis. (×400)

cells from which later the hair papilla is formed. As the primary epithelial germ grows deeper into the dermis under induction by the underlying mesenchymal cells it forms first the hair peg, and, as the hair matrix cells and the dermal hair papilla develop, the bulbous hair peg (Pinkus, 1958).

As the bulbous peg stage is reached, differentiation occurs in the lower and upper portions of the hair follicle as well as in the overlying epidermis. Differentiation in the lower portion of the follicle leads to the formation of the hair cone and subsequently to the formation of the hair, the cuticle, and the two inner root sheaths. The intradermal hair canal is formed by premature death of the core cells in the upper portion of the hair follicle before full keratinization has occurred. In contrast, the intraepidermal hair canal is produced by complete keratinization, desquamation, and self-destruction of the matrix cells of the hair canal which previously had organized themselves in a cordlike fashion in the epidermis. By the time the hair cone has reached the upper portion of the hair follicle the hair canal is already open (Hashimoto, 1970, III).

The hair follicles grow at a slant and develop on their undersurface two or three bulges while in the late hair peg or early bulbous stage. The lowest of the three bulges develops into the attachment for the arrector pili muscle, while the middle bulge differentiates into the sebaceous gland. The uppermost bulge develops into the apocrine gland; however, the apocrine bud does not develop on all hair follicles but only on those located in certain regions (see p. 25) (Hurley and Shelley).

Melanocytes, in sections treated with the dopa oxidase reaction or stained with ammoniated silver nitrate, are distributed at random in primary epithelial germs and in hair pegs. During the bulbous peg stage the melanocytes concentrate in the so-called pigment matrix region, i.e., in the basal cell layer lying on top of the hair papilla, and to a lesser degree in the lower hair bulb located peripheral to the dermal hair papilla (Mishima and Widlan).

HISTOGENESIS. Electron microscopic examination of primary epithelial germ buds and hair pegs of the embryo has revealed that relatively large cytoplasmic processes extend like pseudopodia from their basal cells through breaks in the basal lamina into the dermal mesenchyme. The mesenchymal cells that are concentrated beneath the hair germs are in contact with the basal lamina of the hair germs, either directly, or indirectly through various types of fibrils. Also, the mesenchymal cells are connected to each other through desmosomelike cell-to-cell contacts (Hashimoto, 1970, I). These morphologic findings suggest that the "hair germ mesenchymal cells" provide a force pulling down the hair germ as they move deeper in the dermal mesenchyme.

The formation of the intraepidermal portion of the hair canal through cellular destruction, on electron microscopy, is found to be associated with the presence of lysosomelike dense bodies.

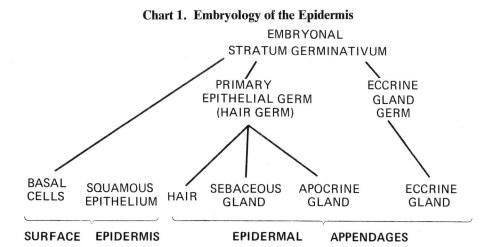

Chart 1. Embryology of the Epidermis

Thus, the intraepidermal portion of the hair canal seems to form by lysosomal digestion of cellular cytoplasm analogous to the formation of the intraepidermal eccrine duct and of the intrafollicular apocrine duct (see below) (Hashimoto, 1970, III).

Sebaceous Glands. The development of the sebaceous gland from the middle bulge of the hair follicle begins on the scalp and face in the fourth month of fetal life. Their development, like that of the hairs, spreads caudad. By the time of birth the sebaceous glands are well developed and contribute their secretion to the vernix caseosa (Montagna).

Apocrine Glands. Apocrine glands develop only in certain areas (see p. 25). Wherever they form, they develop from the upper bulge of hair follicles that are either in the late hair peg stage or in the early bulbous peg stage and show a hair cone. The formation of the apocrine glands thus begins late in the fourth month and continues until late in embryonic life as long as new hair follicles develop. In the earliest stage a solid epithelial cord projects into the perifollicular mesenchyme at a right angle to the long axis of the hair follicle and then grows downward past the developing sebaceous gland and arrector pili bulge. By the time the tip of the epithelial cord has reached the level of the sebaceous gland anlage the intradermal ductal lumen begins to form and simultaneously also the intrafollicular lumen (Hashimoto, 1970, II). Prior to adolescence, only short ducts are found in the skin, having a wall composed of two rows of cells like that of the eccrine duct. The secretory coil forms only after adolescence has been reached (Pinkus, 1972).

HISTOGENESIS. Electron microscopic examination shows that the apocrine dermal duct forms through separation of apposing luminal cells. In contrast, the intrafollicular lumen forms through lysosomal formation of intracytoplasmic vacuoles in neighboring cells and subsequent extracytoplasmic coalescence of these vacuoles (Hashimoto, 1970, II). The formation of the intrafollicular portion of the apocrine duct is analogous to the formation of the intraepidermal portion of the eccrine duct (See below for a more detailed description.)

Eccrine Glands. Eccrine glands are present in mammals, with exception of the anthropoid apes, only on the soles. Their presence in other parts of the skin in humans thus is a late development from the phylogenetic point of view. Accordingly, the eccrine glands develop in man earlier on the palms and soles than elsewhere. On the palms and soles eccrine gland germs are first seen in 12- to 13-week-old embryos, i.e., early in the fourth month (Hashimoto et al., 1965). In the early part of the fifth fetal month they develop in the axillae, and from the later part of the fifth month on they begin to appear elsewhere (Horstmann). The eccrine gland germs begin as areas of crowding of deeply basophilic cells in the basal layer of the epidermis. They differ from primary epithelial germs by being narrower and by showing fewer mesenchymal cells at their base. As in the case of the hair follicles, eccrine glands are seen in different stages of development. Thus, in embryos 16 weeks old some eccrine glands on the palms and soles are already beginning to form coils, while at the same time new eccrine gland germs are still forming in the epidermis (Hashimoto et al., 1966). At an age of 16 weeks both intraepidermal and intradermal lumens begin to form on the palms and soles.

At the time of lumen formation the intradermal duct as well as the secretory segment show a wall composed of two layers of cells, an inner layer of luminal cells and an outer layer of basal cells. Whereas the dermal duct continues to consist of these two layers of cells throughout life, in the secretory segment the two layers undergo differentiation: The luminal cells differentiate into tall, columnar secretory cells extending from the basement membrane to the luminal border; and the basal cells differentiate either into secretory cells or into myoepithelial cells which appear as pyramidal, relatively small cells wedged at the base between secretory cells (Hashimoto et al., 1966). The differentiation into secretory and myoepithelial cells in the secretory segment is well advanced on the palms and soles in embryos 22 weeks old. At the time of birth the appearance of the eccrine glands resembles that of adult eccrine glands.

HISTOGENESIS. On electron microscopic examination the embryonic lumen formation occurring in the eccrine dermal duct and in the secretory segment differs from the lumen formation occurring in the intraepidermal portion of the eccrine duct. (This difference exists also in the apocrine gland, in regard to which it was mentioned briefly, see p. 6.)

In the eccrine dermal duct the lumen formation results from a separation of desmosomes between apposing luminal cells and subsequent formation of microvilli at the luminal surfaces. In the secretory portion the lumen formation also begins with the separation of luminal cells from one another and is followed by the appearance of numerous small secretory vesicles and dense secretory granules in the secretory cells (Hashimoto et al., 1966).

In the intraepidermal portion of the eccrine duct intracytoplasmic vacuoles form through lysosomal action within the inner cells of the intraepidermal eccrine duct units. These vacuoles enlarge, coalesce and break through the plasma membrane. Through the coalescence with similarly produced vacuoles from adjoining inner cells a patent extracellular lumen is formed. After formation of the lumen the intraepidermal eccrine duct unit undergoes keratinization, the outer cells at the level of the stratum granulosum, and the inner cells at the level of the stratum corneum (Hashimoto et al., 1965).

THE DERMIS

The dermis of a 2-month-old embryo consists of loosely arranged mesenchymal cells that are embedded in ground substance. During the third month argyrophilic reticulum fibers appear. As these fibers increase in number and in thickness, they arrange themselves in bundles that no longer can be impregnated with silver and, instead, stain with the methods for collagen (Montagna). Simultaneously, the mesenchymal cells develop into fibroblasts.

Elastic fibers appear in the dermis much later than the collagenous fibers, usually in the sixth month (Lynch). Most elastic fibers are formed after birth (Montagna).

Fat cells begin to develop in the subcutaneous tissue toward the end of the fifth month. Histologic examination at that time shows (1) lipid-free mesenchymal cells as precursor cells; (2) immature fat cells containing multiple lipid droplets, so-called mul-

berry cells; and (3) mature fat cells possessing one large central lipid droplet and a peripherally located nucleus, so-called signet-ring cells (Fujita et al).

BIBLIOGRAPHY

The Epidermis

Breathnach, A. S.: Embryology of human skin. J. Invest. Derm., *57*:133, 1971.

Breathnach, A. S., and Robins, J.: Ultrastructural features of epidermis of a 14 mm. (6 weeks) human embryo. Brit. J. Derm., *81*: 504, 1969.

Breathnach, A. S., and Wyllie, L. M.: Electron microscopy of melanocytes and Langerhans cells in human fetal epidermis at fourteen weeks. J. Invest. Derm., *44*:51, 1965.

Hashimoto, K., Gross, B. G., DiBella, R. J., and Lever, W. F.: The ultrastructure of the skin of human embryos. IV. The epidermis. J. Invest. Derm., *47*:317, 1966.

Leopold, J. G., and Richards, D. B.: The interrelationship of blue and common naevi. J. Path., *95*:37, 1968.

Matsunaka, M., and Mishima, Y.: Electron microscopy of embryonic human epidermis at seven and ten weeks. Acta dermatoven., *49*: 241, 1969.

Sagebiel, R. W., and Odland, G. F.: Ultrastructural identification of melanocytes in early human embryos. J. Invest. Derm., *54*:96, 1970.

Zimmermann, A. A., and Becker, S. W., Jr.: Melanoblasts and melanocytes in fetal Negro skin. Illinois Monographs in Medical Science. Vol. 6, no. 3, p. 1. Urbana, Ill., Univ. of Illinois Press, 1959.

The Epidermal Appendages

Hashimoto, K.: The ultrastructure of the skin of human embryos. V. The hair germ and perifollicular mesenchymal cells. Brit. J. Derm., *83*:167, 1970, (I).

————: The ultrastructure of the skin of human embryos. VII. Formation of the apocrine gland. Acta dermatoven., *50*:241, 1970, (II).

————: The ultrastructure of the skin of human embryos. IX. Formation of the hair cone and intraepidermal hair canal. Arch. klin. exp. Derm., *238*:333, 1970, (III).

Hashimoto, K., Gross, B. G., and Lever W. F.: The ultrastructure of the skin of human embryos. I. The intraepidermal eccrine sweat duct. J. Invest. Derm., *45*:139, 1965.

————: The ultrastructure of human embryo skin. II. The formation of intradermal portion of the eccrine sweat duct and of the secretory segment during the first half of embryonic life. J. Invest. Derm., *46*:513, 1966.

Horstmann, E.: Die Haut. *In* von Möllendorf, W. (ed.): Handbuch der mikroskopischen Anatomie des Menschen. Vol. 3, p. 1. Berlin, Springer, 1957.

Hurley, H. J., and Shelley, W. B.: The human apocrine sweat gland in health and disease. Springfield, Charles C Thomas, 1960.

Mishima, Y., and Widlan, S.: Embryonic development of melanocytes in human hair and epidermis. J. Invest. Derm., *46*:263, 1966.

Pinkus, H.: Embryology of hair. *In* Montagna, W., and Ellis, R. A. (eds.): The Biology of Hair Growth. p. 1. New York, Academic Press, 1958.

————: Anatomy and histology of skin. *In* Graham, J. H., Johnson, W. C., and Helwig, E. B. (eds.): Dermal Pathology. p. 1. Hagerstown, Md., Harper and Row, 1972.

Serri, F., Montagna, W., and Mescon, H.: Studies of the skin of the fetus and the child. J. Invest. Derm., *39*:199, 1962.

The Dermis

Fujita, H., Asagami, C., Oda, Y., *et al.*: Electron microscopic studies of the differentiation of fat cells in human fetal skin. J. Invest. Derm., *53*:122, 1969.

Lynch, F. W.: Elastic tissue in fetal skin. Arch. Derm. Syph., *29*:57, 1934.

Montagna, W.: The structure and function of skin. Ed. 2. New York, Academic Press, 1962.

3

Histology of the Skin

In histologic sections of normal skin the border between the epidermis and the dermis is irregular because numerous cone-shaped dermal papillae extend upward into the epidermis. The ridges of epidermis separating the papillae, even though they appear as pegs in histologic sections, should be called rete ridges, and not rete pegs.

KERATINOCYTES OF THE EPIDERMIS

Two types of cells constitute the epidermis: keratinocytes, and dendritic cells. The keratinocytes differ from the dendritic cells, or clear cells, by possessing intercellular bridges and ample amounts of stainable cytoplasm. The keratinocytes as they differentiate into horny cells are arranged in four layers: (1) the basal cell layer, (2) the squamous cell layer, (3) the granular layer, and (4) the horny layer (Fig. 3-1). The terms *stratum malpighii* or *rete malpighii* are often applied to the three lower layers that contain the basal, squamous and granular cells and comprise the nucleated epidermis. An additional layer, the stratum lucidum, can be recognized in some sections as forming the lowest portion of the horny layer, especially on the palms and soles.

The Basal Cell Layer. The basal cells form a single layer, are columnar in shape and lie with their long axis perpendicular to the dividing line between the epidermis and the dermis. They have a deeply basophilic cytoplasm and a dark-staining oval or elongated nucleus. They are connected with each other and with the overlying squamous cells by intercellular bridges or desmosomes. These desmosomes are less distinct than those in the squamous cell layer. At their base the basal cells are attached to the subepidermal basement zone which, however, can be demonstrated only with special stains, such as the PAS stain (see below). The amount of melanin present in the basal cells parallels the skin color. In light-skinned Caucasoids the basal cells contain only a few small melanin granules that are hardly visible with a routine hematoxylin-eosin stain, whereas in Caucasoids with sun-tanned skin or dark complexion and in Mongoloids and Negroids numerous distinct melanin granules are present, often with a predominant localization as supranuclear caps. (Concerning the transfer of melanin from the melanocytes to the basal cells and the autophagocytosis of melanin in basal cells, see p. 19.)

MITOTIC ACTIVITY. Mitoses denoting nuclear and cellular division are found in the normal human epidermis largely in the basal cell layer. Even mitoses that appear to be located at a level above the basal cell layer, on serial sectioning often are found to be in juxtaposition with a dermal papilla and thus to represent basal cells (Van Scott and Ekel). A more efficient method of determining the location of proliferating cells in the human epidermis consists of either the intradermal injection of tritiated thymidine in vivo or the incubation of skin slices with tritiated thymidine in vitro. This method labels all cells in the S-phase of DNA synthesis which is approximately 7 times longer than the mitotic or M-phase. Thus many more tritiated-thymidine–labeled cells can be visualized than mitoses. With the labeling method 45 per cent of the labeled cells in normal human epidermis were found to be suprabasal in location; but after the study of tracings of serial sections the corrected value was 32 per cent (Penneys et al.). Accordingly, the germinative cell population in normal human epidermis can be considered to consist of 1½ cell layers.

REPRODUCTION OF CELLS AND TRANSIT THROUGH THE EPIDERMIS. On the basis of a germinative layer 1½ cell layers thick and on the basis of data obtained by Weinstein and Frost indicating that the average normal epidermal germinative cell with a DNA synthesis time of 16 hours takes approximately 19 days to reproduce, it was concluded by Halprin that, once a cell has been formed, the time required for it to travel from the basal cell layer to the surface of the granular layer is probably between 26 and 42 days in normal human skin. The passage of the horny cells through the normal horny layer has been calculated to require about 14

days, both on the basis of autoradiographs with radioactive glycine (Frost et al.) and on the basis of disappearance of fluorescence from the stratum corneum after it has been permeated by a fluorescent dye (Baker and Kligman). The total epidermal renewal time thus is 59 to 75 days, if the reproduction time of germinal cells is presumed to be 19 days, the transit time through the stratum malpighii 26 to 42 days, and the transit time through the stratum corneum 14 days (Halprin). In psoriasis in particular, but also in other diseases involving the epidermis, the total epidermal renewal time is greatly reduced, and may be only 8 to 10 days, with a germinative reproduction time of 1.5 days, a transit time through the stratum malpighii of 4 to 6 days, and a transit time through the stratum corneum of 2 days.

The transit time of epidermal cells through the stratum malpighii varies greatly for individual cells. Epstein and Maibach, on labeling the nuclei of the normal epidermis by the intradermal injection of tritiated thymidine, found that the labeled nuclei migrated at differing speeds, so that some of the labeled nuclei reached the granular layer within 1 week, whereas others required 6 weeks. From this they

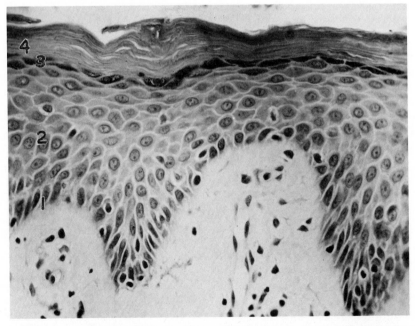

FIG. 3-1. **Normal epidermis, dorsum of the hand.** Four layers can be recognized: (1) basal layer, (2) squamous cell layer, (3) granular layer, and (4) horny layer. Note the presence of intercellular bridges between the basal cells. Several clear cells (melanocytes) are present in the basal layer. They possess a small dark nucleus and clear cytoplasm. (×400)

concluded that the intercellular bridges are not permanent fixtures but can open up and form anew, a characteristic that allows the epidermal cells to alter their size, shape and movement. Unlike the situation in the viable epidermis, where cells are released to pass upward in a random fashion, once they get to the stratum corneum they are tightly attached to one another and travel in unison, as seen in autoradiographs published by Weinstein and by Frost et al., which show a band of radioactive protein moving up through the stratum corneum.

Subepidermal Basement Zone. A subepidermal basement zone, not visible in sections stained with hematoxylin and eosin, is seen on staining with the periodic acid-Schiff stain (PAS stain; see p. 48). It appears as a homogeneous band, 0.5 to 1.0 μm thick, at the epidermal-dermal junction (Fig. 3-2) (Bourlond and Vandooren-Deflorenne). Its positive staining with the PAS reaction indi-

cates the presence of a relatively large amount of neutral mucopolysaccharides in this zone (Stoughton and Wells). Furthermore, impregnation with silver nitrate reveals in the uppermost dermis a meshwork of reticulum fibers (Fig. 3-2). Staining with alcian blue, which stains the band of polysaccharides as well as the reticulum meshwork, reveals that the band of polysaccharides is located above the reticulum layer (Cooper). The light microscopic PAS-positive subepidermal basement zone appears heterogeneous on electron microscopy (see under Electron Microscopy of the Epidermis, p. 14). It must be differentiated from the electron microscopic basal lamina, which is a true membrane and, being only 35 to 45 nm thick, is submicroscopic. Thus, the light microscopic PAS-positive basement zone is, on the average, 20 times thicker than the electron micro-

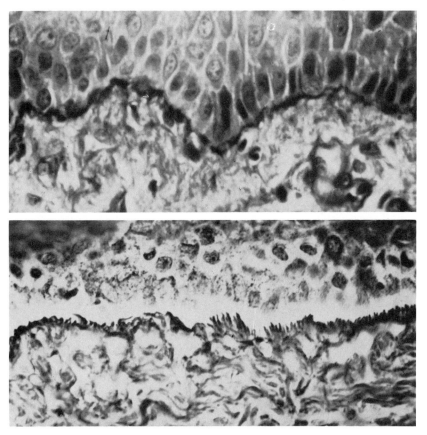

FIG. 3-2. **Subepidermal basement zone.** (*Top*) Periodic acid-Schiff stain shows a homogeneous band. ($\times$400) (*Bottom*) Impregnation with silver nitrate shows a meshwork of reticulum fibers in the uppermost dermis. ($\times$400)

scopic basal lamina (Bourlond and Vandooren-Deflorenne). (The factors causing
the firm attachment of the epidermis to the
dermis are discussed under Electron Microscopy of the Epidermis; see p. 14.) A similar
basement zone as seen at the epidermal-
dermal border is present also around the cutaneous appendages.

The Squamous Cell Layer. The cells of
the squamous cell layer are polygonal and
form a mosaic of cells, usually from 5 to 10
layers thick. They become flattened toward
the surface, with their long axis arranged
parallel to the skin surface (Fig. 3-1). The
cells are separated by spaces that are tra-
versed by intercellular bridges.

Examination of the epidermis with the
polarizing microscope reveals in the cytoplasm of the cells composing the stratum
malpighii numerous doubly refractile tonofibrils forming a tridimensional network
around the nucleus and radiating out to the
cell border (Nieuwmeijer). The tonofibrils
contain sulfhydryl and disulfide groups
(Montagna et al.) and in x-ray diffraction
patterns show the pattern of keratin (Nelemans et al.), indicating that tonofibrils are
precursors of keratin.

X Chromatin. The so-called X chromatin,
also called sex chromatin or Barr body, can be
found in the nuclei of epidermal cells. However,
as a rule buccal scrapings are used for
X-chromatin determinations. The X chromatin
can be seen in sections stained with hematoxylin
and eosin, although it is preferable to use the
Feulgen stain (Goldman and Goldman). The
X chromatin appears as a basophilic, Feulgen-
positive, planoconvex body about 1 μm in
diameter, flattened against the nuclear membrane. It is found in the epidermal nuclei of
skin biopsy specimens in 25 to 54 per cent of
females, and in 0 to 9 per cent of males (Emery
and McMillan). The observation of X chromatin
in the cells of normal males is based on artifacts
resembling the X chromatin; and the observation
of X chromatin in less than 100 per cent of the
cells of normal females is explained by its location on the nuclear border at points other than
the plane of sectioning (Platt and Kailin). The
presence of the X chromatin is due to the fact
that female cells possess 2 X chromosomes, in
contrast to male cells having only one. Since
only one X chromosome is utilized during
mitosis, the other is inactivated and is deposited
as X chromatin during the interphase.

The Granular Cell Layer. The cells of the
granular layer are diamond-shaped or flattened and filled with keratohyaline granules
that are deeply basophilic and irregular in
size and shape (Fig. 3-1). The thickness of
the granular layer in normal skin is proportional to the thickness of the horny layer: It
is only one to three cell layers thick in areas
where the horny layer is thin but measures
up to 10 layers in thickness in areas with a
thick horny layer, such as the palms and
soles.

In the process of keratinization the keratohyaline granules form the interfibrillary
substance that cements the keratin fibrils, or
tonofibrils, together. Keratohyaline granules,
in contrast to the tonofibrils, do not contain
sulfhydryl groups. The presence of considerable amounts of keratohyaline cement in
the epidermal horny layer accounts for its
relatively low sulfur content in comparison
with the sulfur content of hair and nails
(Matoltsy and Matoltsy). The epidermal
horny layer because of its content of keratohyaline cement is referred to as soft keratin; whereas the hair and the nails being free
of keratohyaline cement represent hard
keratin.

The granular cell layer represents the
keratogenous zone of the epidermis in which
the dissolution of the nucleus and other cell
organelles is being prepared. In contrast
with the basal and squamous cell layers in
which lysosomal enzymes, such as acid phosphatase and aryl sulfatase, are present as only
a few granular aggregates, there is diffuse
staining for lysosomal enzymes in the granular cell layer (Rees; Johnson and Daniels)
(see also under Electron Microscopy of the
Epidermis).

The Horny Layer. As the result of their
abrupt and complete keratinization the cells
of the horny layer are anuclear. The horny
layer stains eosinophilic in contrast with the
underlying stratum malpighii. The thickness
of the horny layer is often difficult to ascertain in formalin-fixed specimens because frequently some of the outer cell layers have
detached themselves. Most of the horny
layer is apt to show a basket-weave pattern
in formalin-fixed specimens because of the
presence of large intercellular and intracellular spaces. These spaces are the result

of an inadequate fixation of soluble constituents within the horny cells by the formalin and the subsequent removal of these constituents by water, ethanol, and xylene during histologic processing. Thus, the keratinized portion of the cytoplasm which contains disulfide bonds of cystine has shrunk to form a shell along the cell membrane (Spearman). In contrast, osmium tetroxide or glutaraldehyde fixation, as used for electron microscopy, causes precipitation of the formalin-soluble substances within the horny cells and stains the horny layer uniformly black.

Stratum Lucidum. In many sections fixed with formalin the lowest portion of the horny layer, after processing and staining, appears as a thin homogeneous eosinophilic zone, referred to as stratum lucidum. This zone is most pronounced in areas where the horny layer is thick, especially on the palms and soles. The stratum lucidum differs histochemically from the rest of the horny layer by being rich in protein-bound phospholipids. It is likely that the stratum lucidum through its content of hydrophobic phospholipids acts as the physiologic barrier to water penetration (Blank and Scheuplein).

As such it has been referred to also as stratum conjunctum, in contrast to the overlying stratum disjunctum with its basketweave pattern (Spearman).

The Oral Mucosa. The mucous membrane of the mouth, with the exception of the dorsum of the tongue and the hard palate, possesses neither a granular nor a horny layer. Where these layers are absent the epithelial cells in their migration from the basal layer to the surface first appear vacuolated, largely as the result of their glycogen content, then shrink, and finally desquamate (Fig. 3-3).

Electron Microscopy of Keratinocytes. A characteristic electron microscopic feature of keratinocytes, in contrast with the dendritic cells in the epidermis, is the presence of desmosome-tonofilament complexes (E.M. No. 1).

Desmosome-Tonofilament Complexes. The tonofilaments within the cytoplasm of the keratinocytes of the stratum malpighii are loose bundles of electron-dense filaments (E.M. No. 2), each filament measuring 7 to 8 nm in diameter. The tonofilaments at one end are attached to the attachment plaque of a desmosome, while the other end lies free in the cytoplasm near the nucleus. The desmosomes represent the intercellular bridges (E.M. No. 3). Even though

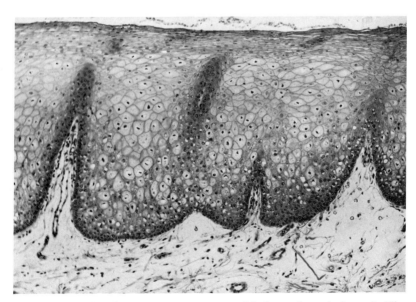

FIG. 3-3. **Epithelium of the oral mucosa.** No horny layer is formed. The epithelial cells in their migration from the basal layer to the surface become vacuolated, then shrink, and finally desquamate. (×200)

desmosomes show minor variations depending on whether osmium tetroxide or glutaraldehyde is used as fixative and whether uranyl acetate or lead citrate is used as stain (Komura and Ofuji), generally each desmosome consists of an electron-dense attachment plaque at each end, located in the cytoplasm of the two keratinocytes connected by the desmosome (E.M. No. 3, *inset*). Centrally to each attachment plaque lies the trilaminar plasma membrane of the two keratinocytes. Each plasma membrane is 8 nm thick and consists of two electron-dense lines separated by an electron-lucent line (E.M. No. 3, *inset*). In the center of the desmosome lies the intercellular cement substance (E.M. No. 3, *inset*), showing greater electron density in the portion directly adjoining the outer leaflet of the trilaminar plasma membrane, the so-called cell surface coat (Hashimoto and Lever, 1970, II). The cell surface coat often cannot be separated visually from the outer leaflet and thus the two components were referred to as the intermediate dense layer by Odland. The remaining central portion of the intercellular cement appears electron-lucent except for a thin electron-dense line exactly in the center of the intercellular cement and thus also of the desmosome, named by Odland the intercellular contact layer (E.M. No. 3, *inset*). The irregular location of desmosomes shows that the plasma membrane of keratinocytes is remarkably convoluted.

Intercellular Cement Substance. The intercellular cement substance between adjoining keratinocytes contains glycoproteins, which are stainable with ruthenium red, and lipoproteins, stainable with lanthanum. In vitro staining with either ruthenium red or lanthanum often results in greater electron density along the cell surface than in the center of the intercellular space because of a higher concentration of the cement substance there as cell surface coat. Both substances stain the intradesmosomal cement substance but do not penetrate into the space between basal cells and basal lamina (see below). Both dyes may be seen within pinocytotic vesicles that are continuous with the intercellular space but do not penetrate the trilaminar plasma membrane of keratinocytes (Wolff and Schreiner, 1968).

Attachment of Basal Cells to the Dermis. The plasma membrane at the undersurface of basal cells shows half-desmosomes possessing only one intracytoplasmic attachment plaque to which tonofilaments from the interior of the basal cell are attached (E.M. No. 2, *inset*). Beneath the plasma membrane of the basal cells a rather electron-lucent zone, 35 to 40 nm wide, separates the trilaminar plasma membrane, about 8 nm wide, from the medium electron-dense basal lamina, 35 to 45 nm wide (Bourlond and Vandooren-Deflorenne). Within the electron-lucent zone one observes beneath each half-desmosome attachment plaque and extending parallel to it, a line 7 to 9 nm thick, the sub-basal cell dense plaque (E.M. No. 2, *inset*), lying about 10 nm from the outer leaflet of the basal cell plasma membrane (Hashimoto and Lever, 1970, I; Tarnowski). Filaments, 5 to 7 nm thick and called anchoring filaments, extend from the basal cell plasma membrane to the basal lamina (E.M. No. 2, *inset*). Filaments arising from the plasma membrane beneath the attachment plaque of a half-desmosome extend vertically to the underlying sub-basal cell dense plaque and from there to the basal lamina, whereas filaments not attached to sub-basal cell dense plaques show an irregular "criss-crossing" course from the basal cell plasma membrane to the basal lamina.

The basal lamina, 35 to 45 nm thick, consists of a feltwork of very fine filaments (E.M. No. 2, *inset*). Extending from the basal lamina downward into the dermis one observes anchoring fibrils of a thickness varying from 20 to 60 nm (E.M. No. 2, *inset*). They thus approach the thickness of collagen fibrils but differ from the latter by showing nonperiodic striation (Susi et al.) rather than a regular periodicity of 68 nm (see p. 34). The dermal end of the anchoring fibrils is difficult to determine. Some fibrils seem to split up into microfibrils at a depth of 150 to 200 nm beneath the basal lamina (Bourlond and Vandooren-Deflorenne); while others loop back to the basal lamina, forming a sling through which solitary collagen fibrils course (Swanson and Helwig). The anchoring fibrils are derived from fibroblasts, whereas the basal lamina is thought to be of epidermal origin (Briggaman et al.).

Keratinization of Keratinocytes. The number of tonofilaments and the thickness of the tonofilaments increase in the upper portions of the squamous cell layer. However, the decisive changes initiating keratinization occur in the granular cells characterized by the appearance of keratohyaline granules and of Odland bodies, or keratinosomes (E.M. No. 4).

The earliest formation of keratohyaline granules consists of the aggregation of electron-dense ribonucleoprotein particles largely along tonofilaments. The keratohyaline granules increase in size through further peripheral aggregation of ribonucleoprotein particles (Bell and Kellum). As the keratohyaline granules increase in size, more and more tonofilaments are seen within them, and by extending along numerous tonofilaments, the keratohyaline granules assume an irregular, often star-shaped outline (E.M. No. 4). They may reach a size of 1 or 2 μm. After ultimately ensheathing all tonofilaments they form in the horny cells the electron-dense interfilamentous protein matrix of mature keratin.

Odland bodies, also referred to as membrane-coating granules and keratinosomes, are small organelles, from 100 to 300 nm in diameter (E.M. No. 4), that originate in the granular cells and have some function in relation to the physiologic water barrier. They are round to oval, and possess a trilaminar membrane and a laminated interior (E.M. No. 4, *insets*). They contain acid phosphatase, just as do lysosomes. They also contain phospholipids that are demonstrable with osmium zinc iodide fixation (Niebauer) and are susceptible to digestion with phospholipase C (Hashimoto, 1971). The Odland bodies arise in the Golgi area, like lysosomes, and are extruded into the intercellular space (E.M. No. 4, *right inset*) where they form densely packed lamellar masses before they disintegrate (Wolff and Holubar). The discharged contents of the Odland bodies, particularly their phospholipids, provide a significant amount of the intercellular material at just the level where the physiologic barrier to water penetration is located, namely in the lowermost horny layer, the stratum conjunctum (Orfanos) (see also p. 13). It is of interest in this connection that when a solution of horseradish peroxidase used as an electron microscopic tracer protein is injected intradermally in vivo, it penetrates the basal lamina and the intercellular spaces of the epidermis up to the upper portion of the granular layer where remnants of the Odland bodies lie (Schreiner and Wolff). It is thus likely that the phospholipids of the Odland bodies contribute materially to the physiologic barrier. Possibly, also the abundance of Odland bodies in the upper layers of the oral mucosa (Hashimoto et al.), where keratinization is highly inadequate, favors the function of the Odland bodies as an essential part of the physiologic barrier.

Horny Cells. The transformation of granular cells into horny cells usually is abrupt. Glutaraldehyde fixation, as used for electron microscopy, like osmium tetroxide fixation, preserves the internal structure of horny cells (E.M. No. 5), in contrast to formalin fixation for light microscopy (see p. 13). In the lower portions of the horny layer the cytoplasm of the cells consists of relatively electron-lucent filaments, about 8 nm thick, embedded in an interfilamentous substance having the same high degree of electron density as the keratohyaline granules

(Brody, 1970). In the upper portions of the horny layers the cells lose their filamentous structure. Together with the sudden keratinization an electron-dense, homogeneous marginal band forms in the peripheral cytoplasm in close approximation to the trilaminar plasma membrane. When fully developed the marginal band measures 16 nm in thickness, as compared with 8 nm for the trilaminar plasma membrane. The marginal band has the same location, thickness, and ultrastructure as the desmosomal attachment plaques in the nonkeratinized epidermis (Brody, 1969). Whereas in the lowermost horny layer the trilaminar plasma membrane is still preserved, in the midportion of the horny layer it becomes discontinuous and then desquamates so that the marginal band serves as the real cell membrane (Hashimoto, 1969). In the uppermost portion of the horny layer even the marginal band often disappears concomitant with the degeneration and desquamation of the horny cell. Desmosomal contacts are at first still present in the horny layer, but prior to desquamation of the horny cells they disappear.

Lysosomes in Keratinocytes. Primary lysosomes that are membrane-bound and contain a variety of hydrolytic enzymes, such as acid phosphatase, aryl sulfatase, and beta galactosidase, are seen in small numbers within keratinocytes, largely but not exclusively in the basal cell layer and lower squamous cell layer (Wolff and Schreiner, 1970). These primary lysosomes are seen in the Golgi area, where they arise, and elsewhere in the cytoplasm. A great amount of lysosomal enzymes is demonstrable also in the granular layer and in the lowermost horny layer, as already mentioned in the light microscopic description (see p. 12). However, on electron microscopic examination, only a very small proportion of these lysosomal enzymes is seen inside of primary lysosomes; most of the lysosomal enzymes are found free in the cytoplasm as irregularly shaped aggregates that are not membrane-bound (Braun-Falco and Rupec). As already discussed, lysosomal enzymes are found also in the so-called Odland bodies, not only while they are within granular cells but also after their discharge into the intercellular space (Wolff and Schreiner, 1970).

In addition to primary lysosomes, secondary lysosomes, also called phagolysosomes, are present in the lower epidermis, especially in the basal cells. They digest phagocytized melanosomes usually as melanosome complexes. (For a detailed description see p. 19.) In cases of epidermal injury, such as sunburn or contact dermatitis, numerous phagosomes containing cellular organelles are present in the keratinocytes which, as the result of the influx of lysosomal enzymes from primary lysosomes, have become phago-lysosomes (Wolff and Schreiner, 1970).

Oral Mucosa. Electron microscopic examination reveals in the keratinocytes of the oral mucosa, in comparison with those of the epidermis, a poor development of tonofilaments. Instead of increasing, the tonofilaments diminish in number in the upper layers and become dispersed. The keratinocytes of the oral mucosa, furthermore, show rather few well-developed desmosomes. Instead, these cells show numerous microvilli at their border. Large aggregates of glycogen are present in the cells. In the upper layers numerous small Odland bodies, or kera-tinosomes, are present both within the cells and in the intercellular spaces. Although the cells of the upper layers do not keratinize, they nevertheless develop a marginal band. Also, they appear cemented to each other by an amorphous, moderately electron-dense material which forms an efficient barrier. The resolution of this cement causes the detachment of the uppermost cells (Hashimoto et al., 1966). It seems likely that the numerous Odland bodies contribute significantly to the increased intercellular cement substance present in the upper oral mucosa and thus to the barrier existing at that level.

DENDRITIC CELLS OF THE EPIDERMIS

Of the three types of dendritic cells present in the epidermis only one type, the melanocyte, can easily be identified in histologic sections stained with hematoxylin and eosin. The second type, the Langerhans cell, can be identified with certainty only with histochemical methods or by electron microscopy. The third type, the indeterminate dendritic cell, can be identified only with the electron microscope.

Melanocytes. In sections stained with hematoxylin and eosin melanocytes appear as clear cells having a small, dark-staining nucleus and, largely as the result of shrinkage, a clear cytoplasm. They are found wedged in between the basal cells of the epidermis. Although the number of melanocytes in relation to the basal cells varies with the body region and increases with repeated exposures to ultraviolet light (see p. 18), the average number of clear cells in hematoxylin and eosin stained vertical sections is one cell out of 10 cells in the basal layer (Cochran). However, not all clear cells seen in routine sections necessarily are

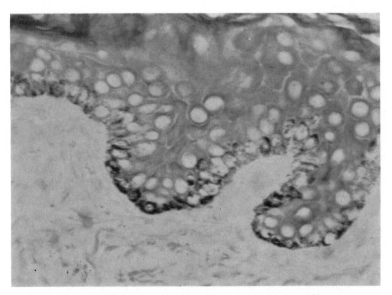

FIG. 3-4. **Moderately pigmented epidermis of Caucasoid skin.** Masson-Fontana stain. Melanin is present in melanocytes as well as basal keratinocytes. In melanocytes it extends into the dendritic processes. (×400)

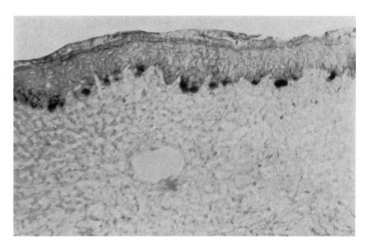

FIG. 3-5. **Melanocytes stained with dopa.** On incubation in a solution of 3,4-dihydroxyphenylalanine, called dopa for short, melanocytes stain blackish because the melanogenic enzyme that they contain oxidizes dopa to dopa-melanin. (×300) (Milton R. Okun, M.D.)

melanocytes, since occasionally basal keratinocytes may show the same shrinkage artifact and then are indistinguishable from melanocytes (Clark et al.). As a rule, melanocytes stain with Bloch's dopa reaction because they possess the ability to form melanin, and they stain with silver stains because they contain melanin. (For details see p. 18.) The dendritic processes of the melanocytes can be recognized with the dopa reaction; and usually they also can be seen on staining with silver, provided that they contain a sufficient amount of melanin (Fig. 3-4). From the melanocytes the melanin is transferred by means of the dendritic processes to the basal keratinocytes where it is stored at first and later degraded. As a rule, a greater amount of melanin is present in the basal keratinocytes than in the melanocytes. Since only about 10 per cent of the cells in the basal layer are melanocytes each melanocyte supplies several keratinocytes with melanin, forming with them an epidermal melanin unit (Fitzpatrick et al., 1967).

In individuals with a light skin color, on staining with silver nitrate, melanin granules are seen only in the basal layer. In individuals with a dark skin color, especially in Negroids, melanin granules, even though present predominantly in the basal layer, are found throughout the epidermis, including the horny layer, and in some instances also in the upper dermis within macrophages, called melanophages.

Staining Reactions. The dopa reaction,

originated by Bloch in 1917 and improved by Becker et al, and Furuya and Ikeda, requires that fresh unfixed tissue be submitted to the laboratory. It consists of the incubation of sections of skin in a 0.1 per cent solution of 3,4-dihydroxyphenylalanine (called "dopa" for short). Melanocytes stain blackish because the melanogenic enzyme that they contain (see p. 18) changes the colorless dopa of the staining solution through oxidation into "dopa-melanin" at sites where the enzyme is located (Fig. 3-5). Dopa melanin generally is easily distinguished from naturally formed melanin by light microscopy, since dopa-melanin appears black and homogeneous rather than brown and granular (Okun). The dopa reaction imitates the physiologic melanin formation which begins with the enzymatic hydroxylation of tyrosine to dopa and the oxidation of dopa to dopa quinone. The latter through nonenzymatic oxidation is polymerized into melanin, and melanin then combines with protein to melanoprotein (Fitzpatrick et al., 1967). (For more details about Enzymatic Melanogenesis, see p. 18.)

Silver stains indicate the presence of melanin, which is both argyrophilic and argentaffin. Because melanin is argyrophilic, it can be impregnated with silver nitrate solutions and, by subsequent reduction to silver, it stains black. Because melanin is argentaffin, the Masson-Fontana stain with ammoniated silver nitrate may be used. With this staining method the phenolic groups present in melanin reduce the silver salt to free black silver. Impregnation with silver nitrate is not specific for melanin but demonstrates also nerve fibers and reticulum fibers. Bleaching of melanin by strong oxidizing agents, such as hydrogen peroxide or potassium permanganate, is of value as a specific identifying measure (Pearse).

DENSITY OF DISTRIBUTION OF MELANOCYTES. The density of melanocytes has been determined either by correlating the number of clear cells or dopa-reactive cells to that of basal cells in vertical sections (Cochran) or by counting the number of melanocytes per square millimeter in epidermal sheets that have been separated from the dermis and stained by the dopa reaction (Staricco and Pinkus; Fitzpatrick and Szabo; Quevedo et al.). It has thus been determined that the concentration of melanocytes varies in different areas, being highest in exposed areas, and in the genital region. On the other hand, the concentration is quite constant for any particular region. No significant difference in the density of distribution of the melanocytes for any given area of the skin exists between Negroid and Caucasoid skin. However, whereas in Negroid skin the melanocytes are uniformly highly reactive, the melanocytes of Caucasoids, when not exposed to sunlight, are highly variable in dopa-reactivity (Quevedo et al.). In addition, Negroid skin contains larger and more highly dendritic melanocytes than Caucasoid skin (Staricco and Pinkus; Fitzpatrick and Szabo) (see also under Electron Microscopy of Melanocytes).

EXPOSURE TO ULTRAVIOLET LIGHT. After a single exposure to ultraviolet light in vivo, the skin of Caucasoids, when examined with the dopa reaction, shows no increase in the density of melanocyte population but an increase in the size and in the functional activity of the existing melanocytes (Pathak et al.). Repeated exposure to ultraviolet light, however, causes, in addition to an increase in the size and in the functional activity, also an increase in the concentration of dopa-positive melanocytes (Quevedo et al.; Mishima and Tanay). Quevedo et al. assume that the increase in melanocytes resulted from previously amelanotic melanocytes becoming melanogenic in response to ultraviolet light.

ENZYMATIC MELANOGENESIS IN MELANO-CYTES. The traditional view of enzymatic melanogenesis, as expressed by Lerner and Fitzpatrick in 1950 and subsequently by Fitzpatrick and Szabo in 1959 and by Lerner in 1971, holds that tyrosinase is the melanogenic enzyme. According to this view, tyrosinase, a copper-containing enzyme, catalyzes the hydroxylation of tyrosine to dihydroxyphenylalanine (dopa) and the oxidation of dopa to dopa quinone. However, before tyrosinase can act on tyrosine two cupric atoms present in tyrosinase must be reduced to cuprous atoms. It is believed that dopa activates this reduction so that dopa, in addition to being a substrate, also acts as a cofactor in the reaction. The conversion of tyrosine to melanin by tyrosinase is characterized by a variable "lag" period. In the presence of low concentrations of tyrosinase, such as exist in epidermal melanocytes of nonirradiated skin, this lag period is markedly prolonged and no utilization of tyrosine by tyrosinase is detectable. On the other hand, in skin exposed in vivo to ultraviolet light (Fitzpatrick), as well as in epidermal sheets (Szabo) and in hair bulbs (Fitzpatrick and Szabo), tyrosinase activity is detectable utilizing tyrosine as substrate. Since there is no lag period with dopa as substrate, tyrosinase in epidermal melanocytes can be readily demonstrated even in nonirradiated skin when skin sections are incubated in dopa rather than in tyrosine. The enzyme acting on dopa thus is thought to be tyrosinase, rather than dopa oxidase, as Bloch had originally assumed in 1917.

The role of tyrosinase as the enzyme causing the hydroxylation of tyrosine to dopa has been questioned by Okun et al. They believe that peroxidase, rather than copper-dependent tyrosinase, mediates the conversion of tyrosine to melanin, in the presence of dopa as cofactor. They found no conclusive evidence that tyrosinase was capable of oxidizing tyrosine to melanin. Since tyrosinase has strong dopa oxidase activity, they assume that tyrosinase functions as a dopa oxidase, as conceived by Bloch.

ELECTRON MICROSCOPY OF MELANOCYTES. Melanocytes differ from keratinocytes by possessing no tonofilaments or desmosomes (E.M. No. 6). However, at their base where they lie in close apposition to the basal lamina melanocytes show structures resembling the half-desmosomes of basal keratinocytes (Tarnowski). This structure consists of a cytoplasmic dense plate attached to the inner leaflet of the trilaminar plasma membrane and, except for being slightly smaller, has the same appearance as the attachment plaque of a half-desmosome. Anchoring filaments extend from the outer leaflet of the plasma membrane to the basal lamina. However, there is no sub-basal cell dense plaque, as in the case of basal keratinocytes. Also, fewer anchoring fibrils extend from the basal lamina into the dermis in conjunction with melanocytes than with basal keratinocytes.

The melanogenic enzyme, usually referred to as tyrosinase but thought to be peroxidase by

Okun et al. (see above), is synthesized in ribosomes, as established by ultracentrifugal separation of cell particles, density gradient centrifugation and electron microscopic monitoring (Seiji et al.). Melanogenesis can be observed by electron microscopy in epidermal melanocytes after in vivo ultraviolet irradiation, using either dopa or tyrosine as substrate (Hunter et al.). In sections obtained 24 to 72 hours after irradiation the melanogenic enzyme is present in linear arrangement in (1) smooth endoplasmic reticulum not clearly associated with the Golgi complex, (2) smooth endoplasmic reticulum associated with the Golgi complex, and (3) Golgi saccules. In sections obtained 5 days after irradiation the linear reaction product has become divided up in the Golgi complex into discrete small, round vesicles, each surrounded by a membrane, representing Stage I melanosomes (Hunter et al.).

Melanosomes in their development from Stage I to Stage IV (E.M. No. 6, *insets*) gradually move from the Golgi area through the cytoplasm of the melanocyte into the dendritic processes. However, even in the dendritic processes Stage II melanosomes may be seen. As melanosomes mature, their concentration of melanogenic enzyme, as measured by the electron microscopic dopa reaction, decreases while their content of melanin increases (Fitzpatrick et al.; Toda et al.).

Stage I melanosomes are round, measure about 0.3 μm in size, and possess very intense enzyme activity concentrated along the membrane. They contain a granular material but no melanin (Toshima et al.).

Stage II melanosomes are ellipsoid and measure approximately 0.5 μm in length, as do also the melanosomes of Stages III and IV. They contain longitudinal filaments that are cross-linked with one another (E.M. No. 6, *upper inset*). Enzyme activity is present both on the enveloping membrane and on the filaments. Melanin deposition on the cross-linked filaments is beginning.

Stage III melanosomes show very little enzyme activity but show continued melanin deposition (E.M. No. 6, *middle inset*), partially through nonenzymatic polymerization.

Stage IV melanosomes no longer possess enzyme activity. Melanin, which now is formed entirely by nonenzymatic polymerization, fills the entire organelle and obscures its internal structure (E.M. No. 6, *lower inset*).

Transfer of Melanosomes to Keratinocytes. The transfer of melanosomes from melanocytes to epidermal keratinocytes and to hair cortex cells is the result of an active phagocytosis of the tips of melanocytic dendrites by keratinocytes

and hair cortex cells, as demonstrated in tissue cultures (Cruickshank and Harcourt). With electron microscopy one can observe that pseudopodlike cytoplasmic projections of keratinocytes or hair cortex cells are wrapped around the tip of dendrites. After these projections have been completely enveloped the tip of the dendrite is pinched off. At first the melanosomes in the pinched-off dendrite are separated from the cytoplasm of the keratinocyte by the plasma membrane of the dendrite and that of the keratinocyte (Mottaz and Zelickson). After the breakdown of these two plasma membranes the melanosomes are dispersed throughout the cytoplasm of the keratinocyte.

Melanosomes in Keratinocytes. In the nonexposed skin of Caucasoids, especially those with light skin, the melanosomes are found almost exclusively in the basal cell layer and to a slight degree only in the adjacent layer of keratinocytes. In Negroids, however, even though melanosomes also are principally seen in the basal cell layer, moderate quantities of melanosomes are found throughout the epidermis, including the stratum corneum (Olsen et al.).

In addition to this difference in the distribution of melanosomes, already known through light microscopy, the following important difference exists: In all Caucasoids and Mongoloids, the melanosomes present in keratinocytes lie largely aggregated within membrane-bound melanosome complexes containing 2 or 3 melanosomes, and only a small proportion of melanosomes are seen to be singly dispersed. The melanosomes present within complexes often show signs of degeneration (Olsen et al.; Szabo et al.). On the other hand, in Negroids and Australian Aborigines the great majority of melanosomes lie singly dispersed and rather few melanosome complexes are found (Olsen et al.; Szabo et al.; Mitchell).

The reason for the lack of aggregation of melanosomes in Negroids seems to be their larger size. Whereas in Caucasoids individual melanosomes range from 0.3 to 0.5 μm in length, in Negroids they range in length from 0.5 to 0.8 μm (Flaxman et al.). Since the membrane-bound melanosome complexes show considerable acid phosphatase activity they represent phagolysosomes in which the melanosomes are being degraded (Wolff and Schreiner, 1971). Thus, melanosomes are removed more rapidly in Caucasoids than in Negroids. It may be concluded that the difference in skin color between Caucasoids and Negroids has the following reasons: In Negroid skin, (1) there is a greater production of melanosomes per melanocyte; (2) the individual melanosomes show a higher degree of melanization, and (3) they are larger in size. As a consequence of their larger size, there is (4) a higher degree of dispersion in the keratinocytes and (5) a slower rate of degradation (Flaxman et al.).

Langerhans Cells. The second type of dendritic cells in the epidermis, the Langerhans cells, are seen in histologic sections stained with hematoxylin and eosin as "high level clear cells" in the upper epidermis. Even though in hematoxylin and eosin stained sections they resemble the "basal layer clear cells" or melanocytes, being completely surrounded by keratinocytes they are more difficult to distinguish from keratinocytes than the basal layer clear cells.

Staining Reactions. Langerhans cells appear as dendritic cells in sections impregnated with gold chloride, a stain that is specific for Langerhans cells (Zelickson and Mottaz, 1968, II). Fixation with osmium zinc iodide, on the other hand, demonstrates both melanocytes and Langerhans cells as dendritic cells (Niebauer et al., 1969). Both Langerhans cells and melanocytes are argyrophilic, i.e., impregnable with silver nitrate; but, in contrast with melanocytes, Langerhans cells are not argentaffin and thus do not stain with the Masson-Fontana stain (see p. 17).

Several enzyme-histochemical stains may be used for identifying Langerhans cells and differentiating them from melanocytes. Among them are adenosine triphosphatase and aminopeptidase (Wolff and Winkelmann, 1967, III). In contrast with melanocytes Langerhans cells are dopa-negative.

Functions of Langerhans Cells. Nothing definite is known about the functions of Langerhans cells. A relationship to the melanocytes, formerly widely accepted (Masson), is now denied by most present authors (Wolff; Bleehen et al.; Breathnach et al.), although a few authors still believe that such a relationship exists, possibly via the indeterminate cell (see p. 21). A relationship to keratinization has been postulated, since the keratinizing oral mucosa, as found on the dorsum of the tongue and the hard palate, contains significantly more Langerhans cells than the nonkeratinizing oral mucosa on the buccal mucosa and on the undersurface of the tongue (Hutchens et al.). On the other hand, fewer Langerhans cells are found in hyperkeratotic verrucae than in parakeratotic verrucae (Fritsch).

Electron Microscopy of Langerhans Cells. On electron microscopic examination, Langerhans cells show a markedly folded nucleus, and absence of tonofilaments and desmosomes (E.M. No. 7). Melanosomes are only rarely found in them, and if they are, they are always located within lysosomes (E.M. No. 7), indicating that they have been phagocytized (Breathnach and Wyllie).

Of great interest is the regular presence of an organelle in the cytoplasm of Langerhans cells, referred to as the Langerhans granule (E.M. No. 7). The size of these granules varies from 100 nm to 1 μm (Niebauer et al., 1970). The granule is disk-shaped and often shows a vesicle at one end, and occasionally at both ends. Cross-sections of the central disk have the appearance of a rod and, if a vesicle is attached to the rod at one side, the Langerhans granule has the highly characteristic appearance of a tennis racquet (E.M. No. 7, *inset*). The central rod-shaped disk has a central lamella showing cross striation with a periodicity of 6 nm (Niebauer et al., 1969; 1970). On fixation with osmium zinc iodide the cross striations of the central lamella and also the vesicles of the "tennis racquets" are deeply stained, whereas the limiting membrane of the organelle does not stain. The nuclear membrane and the Golgi complex of the Langerhans cell are also stained, but its plasma membrane is not.

There is as yet no full agreement whether the Langerhans granules arise in the Golgi area and migrate to the plasma membrane (Niebauer et al., 1969; Wolff and Schreiner, 1970), or arise from the plasma membrane by endocytosis and migrate to the Golgi region (Hashimoto). Niebauer et al. (1969) point out that the failure of the plasma membrane to stain with osmium zinc iodide, in contrast with the Langerhans granules and the Golgi region, makes an origin of the Langerhans granules from the plasma membrane unlikely. In addition, they have observed a discharge of the osmium-zinc-iodide-positive contents of the granules into the intercellular space. Furthermore, Wolff and Schreiner (1970) and Sagebiel, after an intradermal injection in vivo of peroxidase or ferritin as electron microscopic tracer, observed no tracer substance within intracytoplasmic Langerhans granules, even though the Langerhans cells phagocytized the tracer substance by endocytosis and stored it within phagolysosomes. On the other hand, Hashimoto observed the ingestion of peroxidase by Langerhans granules at the cell periphery and the migration of such labeled granules into the interior of Langerhans cells.

Origin of Langerhans Cells. Two theories exist at present about the origin of the Langerhans cell. Some regard it as dermal in derivation, and others as epidermal.

The theory of a *dermal* origin of the Langerhans cell seemed to receive considerable support from the observation that the histiocytes present in the cutaneous and visceral lesions of histiocytosis contain Langerhans granules (see p. 376). However, whether the Langerhans granules in the histiocytes of histiocytosis are identical with those seen in true Langerhans cells is doubtful, since the Langerhans granules seen in the histiocytes of histiocytosis do not stain with osmium zinc iodide fixation and also are larger than true Langerhans granules (Niebauer et al., 1970). Also, the epidermal Langerhans cells are not macrophages like the histiocytes of histiocytosis. Although they are capable of phagocytizing small amounts of melanin, of peroxidase or of ferritin, in cases of epidermal damage keratinocytes are capable of much more phagocytosis than Langerhans cells (Wolff and Schreiner, 1970).

Even though it is not a macrophage, there are many reasons to regard the Langerhans cell as being a mesodermal cell (Wolff and Schreiner, 1970). The presence of Langerhans cells in the dermis, especially in the dermal papillae and in the subpapillary region, has been described in several electron microscopic studies (Zelickson, 1965; Hashimoto and Tarnowski, 1968; Kiistala and Mustakallio). Also, Langerhans cells have been seen in electron micrographs to cross the basal lamina, presumably from the dermis into the epidermis (Hashimoto and Tarnowski), and to undergo mitosis in the epidermis (Konrad and Hönigsmann). In addition, Langerhans cells have been found in the dermis by electron microscopy in various dermatoses, as, for instance, in pityriasis rosea (Hashimoto and Tarnowski), in Ehlers-Danlos disease (Ebner), and in necrobiosis lipoidica and granuloma annulare (Carrington and Winkelmann).

The theory of an *epidermal* origin of the Langerhans cell is based on the assumption that they are related to either the melanocytes or the indeterminate cells. Zelickson and Mottaz (1970) believe that a quantitative relationship exists between melanocytes and Langerhans cells. By direct counting and linear scanning of electron micrographs they determined the number of melanocytes, Langerhans cells, and indeterminate cells before and following two weeks of daily ultraviolet radiation, and found a marked increase in the concentration of melanocytes, together with a marked decrease in Langerhans cells, and no significant change in the concentration of indeterminate cells. It should be mentioned, however, that other authors in similar experiments observed an increase in the concentration of melanocytes, whereas the Langerhans cell population remained constant (Wolff and Winkelmann). The relationship between Langerhans cells and indeterminate cells is discussed briefly in the next section.

Indeterminate Cells. Indeterminate dendritic cells are identifiable only by electron microscopy and are characterized by the absence of both melanosomes and Langerhans granules. The indeterminate cells are usually located in the lowermost levels of the epidermis (Zelickson and Mottaz, 1968, II).

Two views have been expressed concerning the nature of the indeterminate cells: They may be undifferentiated cells capable of differentiation into either a Langerhans cell or a melanocyte (Zelickson and Mottaz, 1968, II); or they may be precursors of melanocytes, since electron microscopic histochemistry with dopa as substrate has revealed precursors of melanosomes with melanogenic activity within indeterminate cells (Fitzpatrick, 1968). The observation made by Konrad and Hönigsmann that a Langerhans cell undergoing mitosis contains numerous Langerhans granules speaks against the view that indeterminate cells may represent young Langerhans cells which as yet have not formed any granules.

NERVES OF THE EPIDERMIS

Intraepidermal nerve endings are present as Merkel-cell–neurite complexes (see below). It is doubtful whether or not, in addition, free nerve endings exist in the human epidermis. Light microscopic examinations are not decisive because the staining methods used for the demonstration of nerves are not sufficiently specific. Thus, in sections impregnated with silver nitrate (Montagna and Ford) or stained with methylene blue (Arthur and Shelley) not only nerves but also the melanocytes and their dendrites are stained (Fitzpatrick et al.); and in thick sections stained for cholinesterase (Montagna) it is impossible to decide whether a nerve is located within a papilla or intraepidermally. In any case, electron microscopic examinations have failed so far to prove conclusively the presence of free nerve endings in human epidermis (Orfanos and Mahrle).

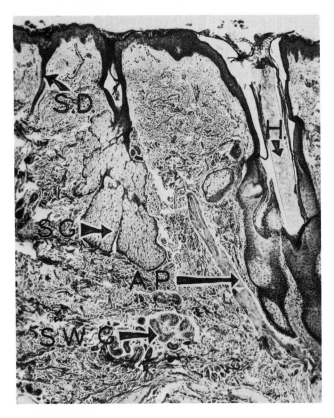

FIG. 3-6. **Normal skin, back of neck.** On the left side of the illustration, a sweat duct (S.D.) enters the epidermis. In the center, a large sebaceous gland (S.G.) leads into a follicle containing a lanugo hair. On the right side, a large hair (H.) lies within a follicle surrounded by sebaceous lobules. An arrector pili muscle (A.P.) is situated in the obtuse angle of the hair. Beneath the large sebaceous gland, a coiled-up eccrine sweat gland (S.W.G.) is present. (×50)

Merkel-Cell–Neurite Complexes. The Merkel cell as such cannot be recognized in light microscopic sections, although in silver-impregnated sections the meniscoid neural terminal that covers the basal portion of each Merkel cell can be seen as Merkel's disk (Smith). A sensory nerve fiber terminates at the disk. Merkel cells are located at the undersurface of the epidermis. They are quite scarce, are irregularly distributed and occasionally are arranged in groups (Hashimoto). It is assumed that the Merkel cell is a touch receptor (Kidd et al.).

Histogenesis. On electron microscopic examination Merkel cells usually are located directly above the basal lamina (E.M. No. 8). They are quite easily recognized by electron microscopy since they possess electron-dense granules, strands of filaments, and occasional desmosomes (E.M. No. 8) (Kidd et al.). The electron-dense granules vary in size between 80 and 200 nm and are membrane-bound (E.M. No. 8, *inset*). They are identical to the norepinephrine containing granules of the adrenal medulla and other chromaffin cells (Hashimoto). The filaments re-

semble tonofilaments and, similar to tonofilaments, are seen in some areas to converge upon desmosomes. In some sections the Merkel disk can be seen above the basal lamina as a "cushion" on which the Merkel cell rests. It consists of a mitochondria-rich, nonmyelinated axon terminal (Hashimoto). In other sections the nonmyelinated neurite is located below the basal lamina (Kidd et al.). Melanosome complexes are present in some Merkel cells.

Since Merkel cells migrate with the peripheral nerves during fetal life, they are neuroectodermal cells (Hashimoto).

ECCRINE GLANDS

Eccrine glands are present everywhere in the human skin; but they are absent in areas of modified skin that lack all cutaneous appendages, i.e., the vermilion border of the lips, the nail beds, the labia minora, the glans penis, and the inner aspect of the prepuce. They are found in greatest abundance on the palms and soles and in the axillae. They are tubular glands whose secretory cells under appropriate stimulation, especially heat, can produce large amounts of sweat. The secretory cells during the process of secretion do not change their size and shape. Eccrine sweat is not visible in the lumen on staining with hematoxylin and eosin. Schiefferdecker called the sweat glands eccrine glands because, as merocrine glands, their secretory cells simply excrete.

Eccrine glands possess a basal coil and lead through the dermis directly into the epidermis (Fig. 3-6). They are composed of three segments: the secretory portion, the intradermal duct, and the intraepidermal duct. The secretory portion makes up about one half of the basal coil, the other half being composed of duct. The basal coil lies either at the border between the dermis and the subcutaneous fat, or in the lower third of the dermis (Fig. 3-6). When located in the lower dermis, it is surrounded by fatty tissue that connects with the subcutaneous fat.

The *secretory portion* of the eccrine gland shows only one distinct layer composed of secretory cells (Fig. 3-7). The reason that there is only one distinct layer lies in the fact that the outer layer of epithelial cells has become differentiated either into secretory or into myoepithelial cells during the sixth to the eighth month of embryonic life. The secretory cells lining the lumen consist of two types: clear cells and dark cells. They are present in about equal numbers. The clear cells generally are broader at the base than they are near the lumen, appear somewhat larger than the dark cells, and contain very faint, small granules. The dark cells, on the other hand, are broadest near the lumen, and contain numerous basophilic granules (Montagna et al.). The clear cells contain glycogen, and the dark cells contain PAS-positive, diastase-resistant neutral mucopolysaccharides. The clear cells secrete abundant amounts of aqueous material together with glycogen, whereas the dark cells

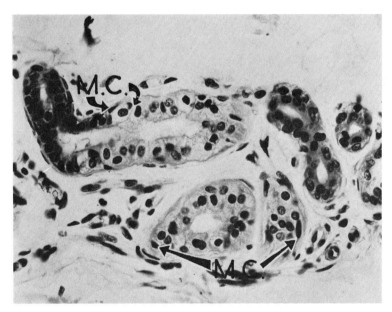

FIG. 3-7. **Eccrine glands.** A basal coil is shown. In the center, three secretory tubules, and on the right side three ductal tubules are seen. On the left side, the secretory portion changes into the duct. The wall of the secretory portion is composed of only one layer of secretory cells. Here and there small myoepithelial cells are wedged in at their bases (M.C.). The wall of the duct is composed of two layers of small cuboidal dark-staining cells. The lumen of the duct is lined with a homogeneous cuticle. (×400)

secrete a mucoid substance (O'Hara and Bensch). Prolonged sweating leads to a depletion of glycogen in the clear cells (Dobson et al.). The myoepithelial cells possess a small spindle-shaped nucleus and long contractile fibrils. The fibrils run in a spiral fashion, their long axis aligned obliquely to the direction of the secretory tubule. Delivery of the sweat to the skin surface is greatly aided by myoepithelial contraction (Hurley and Witkowski). Peripheral to the myoepithelial cells lies a hyaline basement zone composed of collagen fibers and containing fibroblasts whose nuclei greatly resemble the nuclei of the myoepithelial cells. The transition from the secretory to the ductal epithelium is abrupt (Fig. 3-7).

The *intradermal eccrine duct* is composed of two layers of small, cuboidal, deeply basophilic epithelial cells. The eccrine duct, in contrast with the secretory portion of the eccrine gland, has no peripheral hyaline basement zone, but the lumen of the duct is lined with a deeply eosinophilic, homogeneous cuticle, which is PAS-positive and diastase-resistant.

The *intraepidermal eccrine duct* extends from the base of a rete ridge to the surface and follows a spiral course. The cells composing the duct are different from the cells of the surrounding epidermis so that the intraepidermal eccrine duct has been referred to as acrosyringium or the epidermal sweat duct unit. The intraepidermal eccrine duct consists of a single layer of inner or luminal cells and several rows of outer cells. The ductal cells undergo partial keratinization, as evidenced by the presence of keratohyaline granules, at a lower level than the cells of the surrounding epidermis and are fully keratinized at the level of the stratum granulosum of the surrounding epidermis (Hashimoto et al.). Prior to keratinization the intraepidermal lumen is lined by an eosinophilic cuticle.

The lumen of the secretory portion of the eccrine gland, measuring approximately 20 μm in diameter, is small in comparison with that of the apocrine gland (see p. 26). The lumen of the eccrine duct measures about 15 μm across.

Histogenesis. By electron microscopy the clear cells contain numerous small aggregates of electron-dense glycogen granules (E.M. No. 9). The most striking feature is the presence of numerous villous folds wherever two clear cells lie side by side. The villous folds of adjacent clear cells interdigitate with one another (Ellis). In addition, intercellular canaliculi are present between adjoining clear cells (E.M. No. 9). The luminal surface of clear cells is generally small, since dark cells occupy most of the luminal border. Only a few short microvilli are seen at the luminal surface of the clear cells. Nearly all their aqueous secretion reaches the secretory lumen via the intercellular canaliculi (Dobson and Sato). The dark cells contain, particularly in their luminal portion, large electron-dense granules (E.M. No. 9) containing a mucoid substance (Ellis; O'Hara and Bensch). After the granules have dissolved in the apical cytoplasm the mucoid material is excreted into the lumen. The luminal surface of the dark cells, like that of the clear cells, shows only short microvilli.

The intradermal duct shows an outer layer of basal cells and an inner layer of luminal cells. The cells of both layers show pronounced folding of their lateral borders and, in addition, well developed desmosomes. The luminal cells show a periluminal filamentous zone composed of tonofilaments, giving a certain rigidity to the periluminal region and thus assuring patency of the ductal lumen. Their luminal border possesses numerous tortuous microvilli covered with amorphous material which together form the eosinophilic cuticle seen by light microscopy (Hashimoto et al.). It is likely that the PAS-positive, diastase-resistant granules of the dark cells contribute to the PAS-positive, diastase-resistant cuticle.

The intraepidermal duct has luminal cells that until they keratinize also have tortuous microvilli coated with amorphous material, resulting in the eosinophilic cuticle seen by light microscopy.

APOCRINE GLANDS

The apocrine glands differ from eccrine glands in origin, distribution, size, and mode of secretion. Whereas the eccrine glands primarily serve in the regulation of heat, the apocrine glands represent scent glands.

Apocrine glands, together with hair and sebaceous glands, originate from the primary epithelial germ (see p. 5). Accordingly, the duct of an apocrine gland usually leads into a pilosebaceous follicle, entering it above the entrance of the sebaceous duct in the infundibulum. An occasional apocrine duct, however, opens directly on the skin surface close to a pilosebaceous follicle.

Apocrine glands are encountered in only a few areas: in the axillae, in the anogenital region, and as modified glands in the external ear canal (ceruminous glands), in the eyelids (Moll's glands), and in the breast (mammary glands). Occasionally, a few apocrine glands are found on the face, in the scalp and on the abdomen; they usually are small and nonfunctional (Hurley and Shelley). The glands of Montgomery, present in the areola of the female breast as small elevations, are regarded by many as apocrine glands (Ellis; Braun-Falco and Rupec). However, Montagna and Yun regard them as mammary glands, since they are often functional during lactation. Apocrine glands develop their secretory portion and thus become functional only at puberty (Pinkus).

Apocrine glands are tubular glands whose secretory cells pass through various stages. Schiefferdecker, who in 1917 first described these glands, observed that during the process of secretion part of the cell was pinched off and released into the lumen. He referred to this process as decapitation secretion. He chose the name apocrine for these glands to indicate that part of the cytoplasm of the secretory cells was pinched off (apo = off).

Apocrine glands, like eccrine glands, are composed of three segments: the secretory portion, the intradermal duct, and the intraepidermal duct. In contrast to the eccrine glands, the basal coil located in the subcutaneous fat is composed entirely of secretory cells and contains no ductal cells.

The *secretory portion* of the apocrine gland shows a single layer of secretory cells, since the outer layer of cells consists, just as in the eccrine gland, of myoepithelial cells. The secretory cells vary greatly in height, depending on the stage of secretion. However, the secretory cells lining the lumen of one gland always show the same stage of secretion (Hashimoto et al.). The secretory cells possess an eosinophilic cytoplasm. They contain in their cytoplasm, except in their apical portion, fairly large PAS-positive, diastase-resistant granules which appear much larger than similar granules seen in the dark secretory cells of eccrine glands. In addition, the apocrine granules frequently contain iron (Soltermann). The lumen of

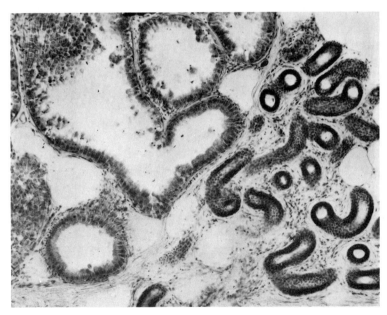

Fɪɢ. 3-8. **Apocrine glands and eccrine glands in the axilla.** Note the great difference in the size of the lumina of the apocrine glands (*left*) and of the eccrine glands (*right*). (×100)

the secretory portion of the apocrine glands is large, measuring up to 200 μm in diameter. This is 10 times the average diameter of the lumen of the eccrine glands (Fig. 3-8). The myoepithelial cells contain numerous contractile fibers extending in a spiral fashion around the secretory tubules (Pinkus). A hyaline basement membrane containing scattered fibroblasts is seen peripheral to the myoepithelium.

The type of secretion occurring in apocrine glands, referred to as decapitation secretion by Schiefferdecker, consists of a release of portions of cytoplasm into the lumen (Fig. 3-9). Because of the presence of portions of cytoplasm in the secretion, apocrine secretion, in contrast with eccrine secretion, is visible in histologic sections stained with hematoxylin and eosin. (For details of the apocrine secretion, see under Histogenesis.) It should be kept in mind, however, that some of the large cytoplasmic globules that in histologic sections appear to be located in the lumen in reality are dome-shaped projections attached to subjacent cells (Montagna). The apocrine secretion contains amorphous PAS-positive, diastase-resistant material originating from the granules that have dissolved in the apical portion of the secretory cells (Montes et al.).

A fairly common event is the occurrence of mucinous metaplasia in some of the axillary apocrine glands. The secretory portion of the involved glands shows considerable cystic dilatation with flattening of the secretory cells and the presence of mucinous material in the lumen, which is PAS-positive and diastase-resistant and stains orthochromatically with toluidine blue. Since these changes can be found at any age, they cannot be regarded as abnormal (Winkelmann and Hultin).

The *ductal portion* of the apocrine glands has the same histologic appearance as the eccrine duct, showing a double layer of basophilic cells and a periluminal eosinophilic cuticle. The intraepidermal portion of the apocrine duct is straight and not spiral in appearance, as is the intraepidermal eccrine duct (Hurley and Shelley).

Histogenesis. Electron microscopic examination reveals an abundant amount of large gran-

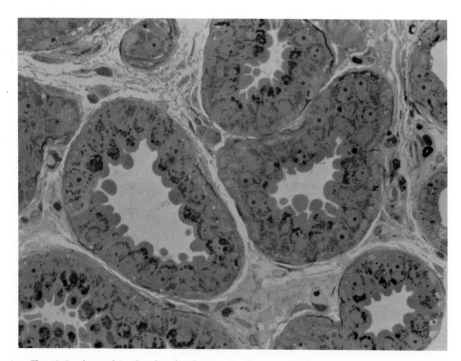

FIG. 3-9. **Apocrine glands.** On fixation in Karnowsky's solution semithin sections, ½ μm thick, show decapitation secretion of the apocrine secretory cells. The secretory granules are deeply stained with methylene blue. (×120)

ules surrounding the nucleus of the secretory cells. Two types of granules are readily distinguished: dark, and light granules (E.M. No. 10, *insets*) (Hashimoto et al.). The dark granules initially consist of a dense protein substance within a small membrane-bound vesicle. By growth and coalescence large dark granules form, up to 5 μm in diameter, that contain, in addition to the dense protein substance, lipid globules (E.M. No. 10, *left inset*), ferritin particles, and myelin figures. The strong reaction of the dark granules for acid phosphatase and beta-glucuronidase indicates that the dark granules are lysosomes. The second type of granules, the light granules, are derived from mitochondria, since they possess, like mitochondria, cristae and a double-layered membrane (E.M. No. 10, *right inset*).

Maturation of the secretory cells is indicated by the formation of a dome-shaped apical cap. The apical cap is nearly free of large granules but contains numerous small smooth vesicles, about 50 nm in diameter. Beneath the apical cap, however, numerous large granules, both of the dark and of the light type, are seen. The luminal plasma membrane shows a moderate number of microvilli.

No agreement has been reached as yet among electron microscopists about the mode of secretion in apocrine secretory cells. Several authors have denied the existence of an apocrine type of secretion, since they found no cellular debris in the secretory lumen, and have concluded that secretion takes place as merocrine secretion as in eccrine glands through excretion of small smooth vesicles present in the apical cap (Munger; Biempica and Montes; Ellis). Other authors observed, in addition to merocrine secretion, the discharge of cellular contents into the lumen through small discontinuities in the luminal plasma membrane of secretory cells (Hibbs; Hashimoto et al.; Braun-Falco and Rupec). In addition, Braun-Falco and Rupec observed in a few instances dissolution of entire secretory cells suggestive of holocrine secretion.

Decapitation secretion, comparable to that seen by light microscopy, has been found on electron microscopic examination by Kurosumi et al., Hashimoto et al., and Schaumburg-Lever and Lever. Although Kurosumi et al. did not actually observe decapitation to take place, they found detached apical caps. Hashimoto et al. believed that the apical portion of secretory cells escaped into the lumen through a defect in the luminal plasma membrane.

Schaumburg-Lever and Lever found three types of secretion: merocrine, apocrine and holocrine secretion. In the apocrine type of secretion three stages were observed: (1) formation of an apical cap; (2) formation of a dividing membrane at the base of the apical cap; and (3) formation of tubules above and parallel to the dividing membrane, bringing about the decapitation of the apical cap by supplying the plasma membrane for both the undersurface of the apical cap and the top of the secretory cell (E.M. No. 10).

SEBACEOUS GLANDS

Sebaceous glands are present everywhere on the skin except on the palms and soles. On the skin they are found in association with hair structures. In addition, free sebaceous glands that are not associated with hair structures may occur in some areas of modified skin, such as the areola of the female breast, the labia minora, and the inner aspect of the prepuce. However, sebaceous glands do not occur on the corona or the glans of the penis (Hyman and Brownstein). The not infrequent presence of free sebaceous glands on the vermilion border of the lips and on the buccal mucosa is known as Fordyce's condition (see p. 503). The meibomian glands of the eyelids are modified sebaceous glands.

A sebaceous gland may consist of only one lobule but often has several lobules leading into a common excretory duct composed of stratified squamous epithelium (Fig. 3-6). Sebaceous glands, being holocrine glands, form their secretion by decomposition of their cells. In sebaceous glands of the skin the pilosebaceous follicle into which the sebaceous duct leads may possess a large hair or a vellus hair that may be too small to reach the skin surface. There is no relationship between the size of the sebaceous gland and the size of the associated hair. For example, in the center of the face and on the forehead, where the sebaceous glands are very large, the associated hairs are of the vellus type.

Each sebaceous lobule possesses a peripheral layer of cuboidal, deeply basophilic cells that usually contain no lipid droplets. The more centrally located cells contain lipid droplets if lipid stains are used on frozen or formalin-fixed sections; but in routine sections in which the lipid has been extracted the cytoplasm of these cells appears as a delicate network. The nucleus is centrally

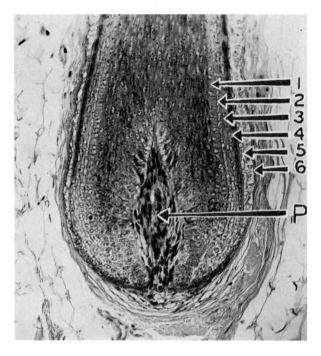

FIG. 3-10. **Lower part of a hair.** The dermal hair papilla (P), composed of connective tissue, protrudes into the hair bulb. The various linings of the hair can be recognized. They are, from the inside to the outside: (1) the hair cuticle, (2) the inner-root-sheath cuticle, (3) the Huxley layer, (4) the Henle layer (which stains dark because of the presence of trichohyaline granules), (5) the outer root sheath, and (6) the glassy or vitreous layer. (×200)

located. In the portion of the lobule located closest to the duct the cells disintegrate. In lipid stains one sees coalesced lipid droplets in the excretory duct, and in routine stains amorphous material.

Histogenesis. The composition of lipids in the sebaceous glands is not uniform. Thus, under polarized light doubly refractile lipids may be present in small to moderate amounts or may be absent (Suskind). Histochemical examination reveals the presence of triglycerides and of small amounts of phospholipids. Esterfied cholesterol is present but no free cholesterol. There also are waxes present, but they are not identifiable by histochemical means (Suskind). Surface sebum contains, in addition, free fatty acids formed through the action of a lipase on the sebum triglycerides. This lipase is produced by bacteria, such as *Corynebacterium acnes* (see p. 180).

Electron microscopic studies have confirmed that the cells of the peripheral layer usually contain no lipid vacuoles (E.M. No. 11). Analogous to the basal cells of the epidermis they are attached to a basal lamina by half-desmosomes (Cashion et al.). In the cells located farther inside one can observe a marked increase in the volume of cytoplasm and, at the same time, the appearance of smooth endoplasmic reticulum and the formation of fine lipid material within the cisterns of the smooth endoplasmic reticu-

lum (E.M. No. 11). This indicates that the smooth endoplasmic reticulum synthesizes the lipid (Cashion et al.; Rupec). In the Golgi region the synthesized lipid material aggregates as lipid vacuoles. Toward the center of the sebaceous lobules the cells, as a result of continued lipid synthesis, are almost completely filled with lipid vacuoles.

Lysosomal enzymes bring about the physiologic autolysis that occurs in the holocrine secretion. Histochemical staining of electron microscopic sections for lysosomal enzymes, such as acid phosphatase and aryl sulfatase, reveals an increasing number of lysosomes as the sebaceous cells are becoming more lipidized. In the disintegrating cells located in the preductal region the acid phosphatase and aryl sulfatase activity is most pronounced, but this activity is present largely outside of lysosomes, since the lysosomes have released their contents in their function as "suicide bags" (Rowden; Rupec and Braun-Falco).

HAIR

The hair follicle is composed of five major portions: the dermal hair papilla, the hair matrix, the hair, the inner root sheath, and the outer root sheath. The histologic appearance of the hair follicle changes considerably during the hair cycle that causes the hair to turn, from an anagen hair into a catagen hair and, further, into a telogen hair, which is followed by a new anagen hair (see below, under Histogenesis). Since the anagen phase persists for years, in contrast with the catagen phase that lasts from two to three weeks and the telogen phase that lasts a few months, anagen hairs comprise more than 80 per cent of the hair present in the normal scalp (Van Scott et al.).

During its growing or anagen stage the hair follicle shows at its lower pole a knob-like expansion, the hair bulb, composed of matrix cells and melanocytes. A small, egg-shaped dermal structure, the *dermal hair papilla,* protrudes into the hair bulb (Fig. 3-10). The papilla induces and maintains the growth of the hair follicle (Kollar). Because of the presence of large amounts of acid mucopolysaccharides in its ground substance, the dermal hair papilla stains positively with alcian blue and metachromatically with toluidine blue. Since positive staining with alcian blue takes place not only at pH 2.5 but also at pH 0.5, it can be concluded that the ground substance of the hair papilla contains not only nonsulfated acid mucopolysaccharides, such as hyaluronic acid, but also sulfated acid mucopolysaccharides, such as chondroitin sulfate (Johnson and Helwig). In addition, considerable alkaline phosphatase activity is found in the hair papilla during the anagen stage as a result of the presence of large numbers of capillary loops (Kopf and Orentreich; Cormia). In individuals with dark hair large amounts of melanin can be seen in the dermal hair papilla situated within melanophages.

The pluripotential cells of the *hair matrix* present in the hair bulb give rise to the hair and to the inner root sheath. The outer root sheath, on the other hand, represents a downward extension of the epidermis. The cells of the hair matrix have large vesicular nuclei and a deeply basophilic cytoplasm. Dopa-positive melanocytes are interspersed mainly between the basal cells of the hair matrix lying on top of the hair papilla and to a lesser degree between the basal cells of the lower hair bulb that is located peripheral to the dermal hair papilla (Mishima and Widlan). Melanin, varying in quantity in accordance with the color of the hair, is produced in these melanocytes and is incorporated into the future cortical cells of the hair through phagocytosis of the distal portion of dendritic processes by the future cortical cells. This transfer of melanin is analogous to that observed from epidermal melanocytes to keratinocytes (see p. 19).

The cells arising from the hair matrix differentiate into six different types of cells as they move upward. These different types of cells keratinize at different levels. The outermost layer of the inner root sheath, the Henle layer, keratinizes first, thus establishing a firm coat around the soft central parts. The two apposed cuticles covering the inside of the inner root sheath and the outside of the hair keratinize next, followed by Huxley's layer. The hair cortex then follows and the medulla is last (Pinkus). (For keratinization of the outer root sheath as the seventh follicular structure to keratinize, see below.)

The *hair medulla* of human hair is often difficult to find by routine light microscopy, but it is easily seen not only by electron microscopy (Mahrle and Orfanos) (see below) but also by polariscopic examination, since the only partially keratinized medulla, in contrast with the cortex, contains hardly any doubly refractile structures (Garn). If the medulla is seen by light microscopy in human hairs it appears amorphous after its partial keratinization.

The *hair cortex* consists of cells that during their upward growth from the hair matrix keratinize gradually by losing their nuclei and becoming filled with keratin fibrils. The process of keratinization takes place without the formation of keratohyaline granules, as seen in the keratinizing epidermis, or of trichohyaline granules, as seen in the inner root sheath.

The *hair cuticle* (1 in Fig. 3-10) located peripheral to the hair cortex consists of overlapping cells arranged like shingles and pointing upward with their peripheral portion. The cells of the hair cuticle are tightly interlocked with the cells of the inner root sheath cuticle (see below), resulting in a firm attachment of the hair to its inner root sheath. In contrast with the cortex cells, the cells of the hair cuticle contain no melanin.

The *inner root sheath* is composed of three concentric layers; from the inside to outside, these are: the inner-root-sheath cuticle (2 in Fig. 3-10), the Huxley layer (3 in Fig. 3-10), and the Henle layer (4 in Fig. 3-10). None of these three layers contains melanin. All three layers keratinize, in contrast with the cells of the hair cortex and of the hair cuticle, by means of trichohyaline granules, which in many respects resemble the keratohyaline granules of the epidermis. Closest to the hair is the single-layered inner-root-sheath cuticle, consisting of flattened overlapping cells that point downward in the direction of the hair and thus, by following the same direction as the cells of the hair cuticle, interlock tightly with them. Trichohyaline granules are few in the inner-root-sheath cuticle cells. The Huxley layer usually consists of two layers of cells and develops numerous trichohyaline granules at the level of the keratogenous zone of the hair. The Henle layer, the first layer to undergo keratinization, already shows numerous trichohyaline granules at its emergence from the hair matrix (Montagna). The cells of all three layers composing the inner root sheath, after having become fully keratinized, disintegrate when they reach the isthmus of the hair follicle which extends from the area of attachment of the arrector pili muscle to the entrance of the sebaceous duct. The cells of the inner root sheath thus do not contribute to the emerging hair (Parakkal and Matoltsy).

The *outer root sheath* (5 in Fig. 3-10) extends from the epidermis downward to the sides of the hair bulb, where it ends. It is thickest near the epidermis and gradually decreases in thickness toward the hair bulb. In its lower portion, i.e., from the isthmus of the hair follicle downward, the outer root sheath is covered by the inner root sheath and does not undergo keratinization, and its cells have a clear, vacuolated cytoplasm because of the presence of considerable amounts of glycogen in their cytoplasm. Although active, melanin-producing melanocytes are present in the basal layer of the outer root sheath above the entrance of the sebaceous duct, only inactive amelanotic melanocytes, demonstrable with toluidine blue, are present below the entrance of the

sebaceous duct. These inactive melanocytes, however, can become melanin-producing cells after skin injuries, such as dermabrasion, when they increase in number and migrate upward into the regenerating upper portion of the outer root sheath and into the regenerating epidermis (Staricco).

In the middle portion of the hair follicle, the so-called isthmus, extending from the attachment of the arrector pili muscle to the entrance of the sebaceous duct, the outer root sheath no longer is covered by the inner root sheath which by then has keratinized and disintegrated. The outer root sheath, therefore, undergoes keratinization. This type of keratinization, referred to as trichilemmal keratinization by Pinkus (1969), produces large homogeneous keratinized cells without the formation of keratohyaline granules. Trichilemmal keratinization is found also in the catagen hair, and in pilar cysts and pilar tumors (see pp. 462 and 521).

In the upper portion of the hair follicle, above the entrance of the sebaceous duct, the outer root sheath, just like the sebaceous duct, undergoes keratinization in the same fashion as the surface epidermis, with formation of keratohyaline granules. This upper portion of the hair follicle often is referred to as infundibulum or as pilosebaceous follicle.

The *glassy* or *vitreous layer* (6 in Fig. 3-10) forms a homogeneous, eosinophilic zone peripheral to the outer root sheath. Like the subepidermal basement zone it is PAS-positive and diastase-resistant; but it differs from the subepidermal basement zone by being thicker and visible with routine stains. It is thickest around the lower third of the hair follicle. Peripheral to the vitreous layer lies the fibrous root sheath, composed of thick collagen bundles.

Histogenesis. The *hair cycle* consists of the involutionary stage (catagen) and the end stage (telogen) of the old hair and its replacement by a young new hair (early anagen). At the onset of the catagen stage, mitotic activity and melanin production in the hair bulb cease. Next, the bulb shrinks, setting the dermal hair papilla free (Montagna). As the hair moves upward, the entire lower follicle collapses, with its epithelial part becoming a thin cord and the fibrous root sheath becoming wrinkled in thick folds. Also, as the hair moves upward, growth of the inner root sheath ceases before that of the hair cortex, so that the lower end of the hair shaft becomes surrounded by dense keratin that is formed by the outer root sheath and has been referred to as trichilemmal keratin by Pinkus (1969). This then represents the club hair of the *catagen stage*.

Next, the thin cord of epithelial cells retracts upward, faithfully followed by the dermal hair papilla, which thus also moves upward. The cord of epithelial cells shortens until it forms only a small downward protrusion from the club hair, called the secondary hair germ. Under it lies the dermal hair papilla. With the hair follicle decreased to about one third of its former length, the lowest portion of the hair follicle lies at the level of the attachment of the arrector pili. The hair is surrounded by a sac of trichilemmal keratin. Folds of the fibrous root sheath extend downward from the hair follicle. At this stage the hair has reached the *telogen stage* (Pinkus and Mehregan).

When regrowth of the hair begins, the secondary hair germ begins to elongate by cell division and grows down as an epithelial column together with the dermal hair papilla inside of the old, collapsed fibrous root sheath of the previous hair. As it is growing down, the lower end of the epithelial column becomes invaginated by the dermal hair papilla. A new hair bulb thus is formed, representing the *early anagen stage*. By subsequent differentiation a new hair arises. As Kligman has pointed out, the formation of an active hair follicle from the secondary germ recapitulates the embryonic pattern of development of the hair from the primary epithelial germ.

Electron microscopic examination of a hair follicle during its anagen stage shows the *hair medulla* to be composed of an irregular network of immature keratin containing in its spaces large irregular vacuoles and a homogeneous electron-dense material. The latter is analogous to the interfibrillary material of the hair cortex but is present in much greater amount than in the hair cortex. Melanosomes are present in both components of the hair medulla (Mahrle and Orfanos, 1971). The *hair cortex* consists of closely packed keratinized spindle cells. Their keratin consists of filaments arranged in fibrils that are separated by small amounts of electron-dense interfibrillary material. The melanosomes of the hair cortex are larger than those of the epidermis. They lie singly or in groups but not within lysosomes. They are located usually in the interfibrillary matrix within the cells and only rarely in the intercellular space.

Three types of melanosomes occur in hair: Polymorphous erythromelanin granules are seen in red hair. In contrast, homogeneous eumelanin granules and lamellated pheomelanin granules are round to oval; they are found in varying proportions in blond and dark hair. Dark hair contains more melanosomes than light hair and the melanosomes are largely of the homogeneous eumelanin type, whereas in light hair lamellated pheomelanin predominates (Mahrle and Orfanos, 1973).

In grey and white hair the melanocytes in the hair bulb are greatly reduced in number or absent. The melanocytes that are present show degenerative changes, especially of their melanosomes (Herzberg and Gusek). The hair shafts contain only detritus of melanin or none at all (Mahrle and Orfanos, 1973).

NAIL

The nail plate is composed of keratinized cells. They originate in the nail matrix, formerly referred to as the ventral nail matrix, and keratinize without the formation of keratohyaline granules (Zaias). The proximal nail fold, formerly referred to as dorsal nail matrix, merely forms the nail cuticle which keratinizes with the formation of keratohyaline granules. Neither the proximal nail fold nor the nail bed contribute to the nail plate (Zaias and Alvarez). The rete ridges of the nail bed are oriented not as a network of anastomosing ridges, as elsewhere in the skin, but as parallel longitudinal ridges.

Histogenesis. The conclusion reached by Zaias and Alvarez that only the nail matrix was responsible for the formation of the nail plate was based on their in vivo experiments on monkeys with tritiated glycine. An additional observation made by Norton on human volunteers with tritiated thymidine or glycine was that, even though the main stream of labeled cells was from the nail matrix into the nail plate, there was some cellular progression distally from the nail plate into the nail bed, indicating that some of the nail bed cells have their origin in the nail matrix. Norton assumes that the migration of nail matrix cells into the nail bed allows for the distal movement of the nail bed together with the attached nail plate. He points out that in the experiments conducted by Zaias and Alvarez the labeling of the nail bed was obscured by the abundance of melanin present in the primate nail bed.

Electron microscopic examination has confirmed that nail cells, analogous to hair cortex cells, keratinize by accretion of tonofilaments without the formation of keratohyaline granules. The cellular envelope of the horny cells of the nail, similar to the horny cells of the epidermis, becomes thickened through the cytoplasmic formation of a marginal band (see p. 15) (Hashimoto).

CONNECTIVE TISSUE OF THE DERMIS

The connective tissue of the dermis consists of collagenous and elastic fibers embedded into ground substance. All three components are formed by fibroblasts. Reticulum fibers, being merely thin collagen fibers, are not a separate entity.

Collagenous Fibers. Collagen represents by far the most abundant constituent of the connective tissue of the dermis. On light microscopy, collagen consists of fibers. They are united into bundles in the normal dermis except in the vicinity of the epidermis, of the epidermal appendages, and of the blood vessels. The diameter of collagen fibers is quite variable, varying from 2 to 15 μm. The collagen bundles in histologic sections are thickest in the lower portion of the dermis. In the uppermost dermis, the so-called papillary dermis, consisting of the papillae and the subpapillary layer, the collagen bundles are thin, extend in an apparently haphazard manner, and do not interlace. In the midportion and the lower dermis, which together form the reticular dermis, the collagen bundles are arranged nearly parallel to the surface of the skin and interlace. Nevertheless, they extend in various directions horizontally, and thus some are cut lengthwise and others across in histologic sections. As a rule, collagen bundles that are cut lengthwise appear slightly wavy. A small number of fibroblasts are interspersed between the collagen bundles. Their nuclei are rather pale-staining. When cut lengthwise these nuclei appear spindle-shaped. The cytoplasmic border of the fibroblasts cannot be recognized with routine stains. The only other cell type present in the normal dermis is the mast cell, seen generally in small numbers in perivascular arrangement. Usually, they can be recognized only with special stains, such as the Giemsa stain which stains the mast cell granules metachromatically purple (see pp. 56 and 84), although occasionally, their cytoplasmic membrane and their very pale-staining cytoplasm can be recognized even in routine stains.

Reticulum Fibers. Reticulum fibers are not recognizable with routine stains; but, being argyrophilic, can be impregnated with silver nitrate solutions and, by subsequent reduction to silver, they stain black. Reticulum fibers represent thin collagen fibers that measure from 0.2 to 1.0 μm in diameter rather than 2 to 15 μm, which is the diameter of collagen fibers (Schmidt). The argyrophilia shown by reticulum fibers, in contrast with collagen fibers, probably represents a surface phenomenon based on the fact that reticulum fibers have a greater amount of ground substance associated with them than do collagen fibers. (For details see Histogenesis.)

Reticulum fibers, representing small collagen fibers, are the first-formed fibers during embryonic life (see p. 7), during wound healing, and in various pathologic conditions associated with increased fibroblastic activity (see below).

In the normal skin, even though collagen is being continuously replaced, the formation of new collagen is not preceded by an argyrophilic phase. Rather, all newly formed collagen consists of large fibers, except in a few areas where normally small collagen fibers occur as reticulum fibers. These areas are located around the eccrine glands, the sebaceous glands, the hair follicles and the capillaries (Rehtijärvi). Reticulum fibers are present also as a meshwork in the subepidermal region (Fig. 3-3). Furthermore, reticulum fibers form a basketlike capsule around each fat cell.

In contrast with the sparsity of reticulum fibers in normal skin is the abundance of reticulum fibers in pathologic conditions in which active fibroblasts form new collagen. Thus, large numbers of reticulum fibers are present in granulomas, such as tuberculosis and sarcoidosis, in fibroblastic tumors, such as dermatofibroma and fibrosarcoma, and in healing wounds. In all these conditions histologic sections, when impregnated with silver nitrate, show that in areas where the reticulum fibers are densest they tend to aggregate into collagen fibers and bundles, and in doing so, they lose their argyrophilia (Fig. 12-3).

Ground Substance. The ground substance, an amorphous substance that fills the spaces between collagen fibers and collagen bundles, is present in normal skin in such small amounts that usually it cannot be demonstrated with either routine or special histologic staining methods, except in the hair papilla of anagen hair which contains both nonsulfated and sulfated acid mucopolysaccharides (see p. 29). Only rarely, small amounts of nonsulfated acid mucopolysaccharides can be demonstrated in the subepidermal papillae, around the epidermal appendages, and around capillaries (Montagna). Still, through the study of tissues with an active growth of fibroblasts, as seen in the papillary dermis in dermatofibroma and in the connective tissue around the tumor islands of basal cell epithelioma, it is known that the dermal ground substance consists largely of nonsulfated acid mucopolysaccharides, such as hyaluronic acid (Johnson and Helwig). In healing wounds, however, in which new collagen is being laid down, the ground substance contains, in addition to nonsulfated, also sulfated acid mucopolysaccharides and neutral mucopolysaccharides (Jacques and Cameron). The *nonsulfated acid* mucopolysaccharides consist largely of hyaluronic acid and are stainable with alcian blue at pH 2.5 but not at pH 0.5, and show metachromasia with toluidine blue at pH 3.0 but not at pH 1.5. The *sulfated acid* mucopolysaccharides consist largely of chondroitin sulfate and are stainable with alcian blue also at pH 0.5, and show metachromasia with toluidine blue also at pH 1.5. Both nonsulfated and sulfated acid mucopolysaccharides stain with colloidal iron and are extractable with testicular hyaluronidase. The *neutral* mucopolysaccharides show a positive PAS-reaction that is also diastase-resistant. Both the acid and the neutral mucopolysaccharides are covalently linked to peptide chains to form high molecular weight complexes. These protein-polysaccharide complexes are called proteoglycans (Winand).

Elastic Fibers. In light microscopic sections that are routinely stained elastic fibers are not visible. With special elastic tissue stains, such as orcein or resorcin-fuchsin, they are found entwined among the collagen bundles. Since elastic fibers are rather thin in comparison with collagen bundles, measuring from 1 to 3 μm in diameter, and are wavy, only a small portion of any fiber is seen in histologic sections, giving even normal elastic fibers a "fragmented" appearance. The elastic fibers are thickest in the lower portion of the dermis, where they are arranged, like the collagen bundles, chiefly parallel to the surface of the skin. In the subepidermal papillae, however, thin elastic fibers ascend almost vertically toward the epidermis and end free just below the dermal-epidermal border (Pinkus, 1970).

Histogenesis. In regard to the *function of the collagenous and elastic fibers,* it is generally agreed that collagen is not extensible, although its wavy arrangement in the dermis allows for skin to stretch somewhat. The elastic fibers, on the other hand, are extensible like rubber and return to their original shape after stretching (Jansen; Smith). As has been pointed out by Jansen, the bovine ligamentum nuchae is very extensible, and its elastic fibers, though coarser, are of the same type as the elastic fibers of the human skin.

Electron Microscopy of Fibroblasts. Fibroblasts that actively synthesize collagen have a prominent rough endoplasmic reticulum composed of many membrane-lined cisternae with large numbers of attached ribosomes (E.M. No. 12). The dilated cisternae are filled with an amorphous material produced by the ribosomes lining the cisternae (Scarpelli and Goodman). The amorphous material is presently believed to consist of triple helical procollagen molecules, with each molecule composed of three pro-alpha chains (see below, under Biosynthesis). Conversion of procollagen molecules into collagen molecules composed of three alpha chains then occurs outside the cell (Nigra et al.). While some of the procollagen molecules are excreted directly from the cisternae into the extracellular space through intercommunications of the cisternae with the extracellular space, others are first transferred to the Golgi area where the mucopolysaccharides of the ground substance are formed. From there the procollagen molecules are excreted into the extracellular space together with the mucopolysaccharides by means of secretory vesicles (Ross and Benditt).

The *biosynthesis of collagen* begins within the fibroblast by the assembly of 3 pro-alpha polypeptide chains into a triple helical procollagen molecule (Nigra et al.). The assembly of the 3 pro-alpha polypeptide chains is mediated by coordination peptides located at the N terminal end of the polypeptide chains. After excretion into the extracellular space the 3 pro-alpha chains of each procollagen molecule are shortened by 10 to 20 per cent through the enzymatic removal of the coordination peptides, changing them into the alpha chains of the collagen molecule, also called tropocollagen (Lapière, 1972). The specific enzyme splitting off the coordination peptides in the extracellular space is called procollagen peptidase (Lapière, 1973). It is produced by the fibroblast (Lapière and Piérard). Whereas the additional peptides present in procollagen inhibit its intracellular polymerization, collagen molecules polymerize readily. The collagen molecule is a rigid rod in which each of the three coiled alpha chains consists of about 1,000 amino acids (Nigra et al.). The collagen molecule is about 300 nm long and 1.5 nm wide (Lapière, 1972; Lazarus). Collagen fibrils form through polymerization of collagen molecules side by side as well as head to tail. Collagen fibrils show varying degrees of polymerization of collagen molecules and therefore vary in diameter, with younger collagen fibrils being thinner than older fibrils. In the normal dermis the thickness of collagen fibrils varies between 70 and 140 nm, with most of the fibrils being around 100 nm thick (E.M. Nos. 2, 6, 8 and 13) (Hayes and Rodnan).

Collagen fibrils possess characteristic cross striations with a periodicity of 68 nm. The periodicity of the cross striations in the collagen fibrils can be explained as follows: Each collagen molecule has 5 charged regions, 68 nm apart, and collagen molecules lying in parallel arrangement have charged regions side by side (Grant and Prockop). Neighboring collagen molecules, however, are displaced longitudinally with respect to one another by a distance of 68 nm, and two consecutive collagen molecules are separated by a gap of about 40 nm (Grant and Prockop; Lapière, 1972).

Electron microscopy of reticulum fibrils reveals them to possess the same 68-nm periodicity of their cross striations as collagen fibrils but to have a smaller diameter than collagen fibrils, varying between 40 and 65 nm, rather than between 70 and 140 nm. In this respect, reticulum fibrils are analogous to young collagen fibrils, which also have a smaller diameter than mature collagen fibrils. Reticulum and collagen furthermore differ in the number of fibrils and

the content in ground substance within each fiber. Although the ground substance cannot be visualized either by light microscopy or electron microscopy, quantitative determination of the content of mucopolysaccharides has revealed it to amount to 4.5 per cent in reticulum fibers, in comparison to 1 per cent in collagen fibers (Schmidt). The amount and the distribution of ground substance around the fibrils and on the surface of the fiber may explain the presence of argyrophilia in reticulum fibers, and its absence in collagen fibers (Schmidt).

Electron Microscopy of Elastic Fibers. Elastic fibers form much later than collagen during the repair of skin wounds. When they begin to form, they are seen in close proximity to fibroblasts (Williams). Elastic fibers are found, on electron microscopy, to consist of two components: an amorphous substance, and filaments (E.M. No. 13). The amorphous substance, the elastin, is moderately electron-dense. Embedded in it are electron-dense fine filaments, 5 to 15 nm in diameter. They have been referred to by different names, such as protofilaments (Hashimoto and DiBella), elastic fibrils (Kobayasi), and microfibrils (Breathnach). Generally, the filaments are present as strands, 15 to 80 nm in diameter. These strands have been referred to by Hashimoto and DiBella as skeleton fibrils. The skeleton fibrils, in addition to being present throughout the elastic fiber, are aggregated at the periphery of the elastic fiber, giving the fiber its characteristic frayed appearance (E.M. No. 13) (Breathnach). The amorphous substance, the elastin, is removable by elastase. It appears likely that the skeleton fibrils are the elastic resilient component of the elastic fiber (Hashimoto and DiBella).

NERVES AND NERVE END-ORGANS OF THE DERMIS

In sections stained with routine methods one can recognize only the large nerve bundles and the Meissner and Vater-Pacini end organs. The finer nerves require special staining. Among the staining methods are: impregnation with silver salts as, for example, with the Bodian stain (Bodian); vital staining with methylene blue (Woollard et al.); and in-vitro staining of thick sections with methylene blue (Arthur and Shelley).

The skin is supplied with sensory nerves as well as autonomic nerves, both of which permeate the entire dermis with nerve fibers showing frequent branching. Sensory and autonomic nerves differ in that sensory nerves possess a myelin sheath up to their terminal ramifications, whereas autonomic nerves do not. The autonomic nerves, derived from the sympathetic nervous system, supply the blood vessels, the arrectores pilorum, and the eccrine and apocrine glands. The sebaceous glands possess no autonomic innervation, and their functioning depends on endocrine stimuli.

All autonomic nerves end in fine arborizations. Similarly do the sensory nerves, except in a few areas in which there are, in addition to fine arborizations, special nerve end-organs (see below). Also hair follicles, but especially large hair follicles, are surrounded below the entry of the sebaceous duct by a network of sensory nerves that lose their myelin sheath near the outer root sheath and end in numerous arborizations of fine nonmyelinated fibers.

Histogenesis. Electron microscopic examination reveals that all sensory nerves not connected with specialized receptor organs, such as the Merkel cells in the epidermal basal layer (see p. 22) or the Meissner corpuscles in the dermal papillae (see below), are in contact with the epidermis or the outer root sheath epithelium. No free dermal nerve endings seem to occur. The contact zones show contact between the epi-dermal or epithelial basal lamina and the basal lamina of the Schwann cell covering the sensory nerve axon (Orfanos and Mahrle).

Special Nerve End-Organs. In the areas of hairless skin on the palms and the soles and in the areas of modified hairless skin at the mucocutaneous junctions some of the sensory nerves end in special nerve end-organs. They are of three types: mucocutaneous end-organs, Meissner corpuscles, and Vater-Pacini corpuscles. Although it is customary to speak of them as "end organs," they actually represent "starting organs" in a functional sense, since the nerve impulse starts there and is transmitted to the sensory cells of the spinal cord (Orfanos and Mahrle).

MUCOCUTANEOUS END-ORGANS. The mucocutaneous end-organs, on the average 50 μm in diameter, are found in the modified hairless skin at the mucocutaneous junctions, namely, the glans, the prepuce, the clitoris, the labia minora, the perianal region, and the vermilion border of the lip. Although located chiefly in the subpapillary layer, they extend into the dermal papilla. They possess no capsule, in contrast with the Meissner and the Vater-Pacini corpuscles. From 2 to 6 myelinated nerve fibers enter

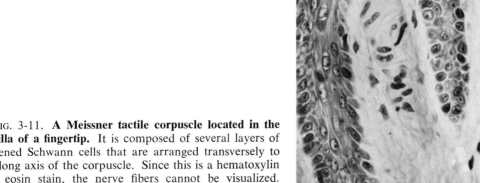

FIG. 3-11. **A Meissner tactile corpuscle located in the papilla of a fingertip.** It is composed of several layers of flattened Schwann cells that are arranged transversely to the long axis of the corpuscle. Since this is a hematoxylin and eosin stain, the nerve fibers cannot be visualized. ($\times$400)

a mucocutaneous end-organ and, after losing their myelin sheath, form many loops of nerve fibers, resembling an irregularly wound ball of yarn (Winkelmann).

MEISSNER CORPUSCLES. The Meissner corpuscles are located in dermal papillae (Fig. 3-11) and mediate a sense of touch. They occur exclusively on the ventral aspect of the hands and feet, with their number increasing distally. Also, their number is greater on the hands than on the feet. At the site of their greatest concentration, the fingertips, approximately every fourth papilla contains a Meissner corpuscle (Winkelmann). The size of the Meissner corpuscles averages 30 by 80 μm in diameter. On account of their size and their elongated shape, resembling that of a pine cone, they occupy the greater part of the papilla in which they are located. They possess a capsule composed of several layers of flattened Schwann cells that are arranged transversely to the long axis of the corpuscle. Impregnation with silver salts reveals that several myelinated nerves, as they approach the base or the side of the corpuscle, lose

their myelin sheath and then enter it. Within the corpuscle the nerves take a meandering course upward.

HISTOGENESIS. Electron microscopic studies reveal that the principal part of the Meissner corpuscle is made up of irregular layers of flattened, greatly elongated laminar cells. The nuclei of the laminar cells are located largely at the periphery of the corpuscle. The axons terminate within the Meissner corpuscle with bulbous swellings that are surrounded by slender processes of laminar cells. This enveloping of axons by laminar cells or their processes is analogous to the enveloping of axons by infolding of the plasma membrane of Schwann cells and indicates that the laminar cells are modified Schwann cells (Cauna and Ross).

Some Meissner corpuscles show a few areas of direct contact of either axons or laminar cells with epidermal basal cells without interposition of a basal lamina (Hashimoto).

VATER-PACINI CORPUSCLES. These very large nerve end organs are located in the subcutis and measure up to 1 mm in diameter and thus are detected easily by light microscopy (Fig. 3-12). They mediate a sense of pressure. They are found most commonly below

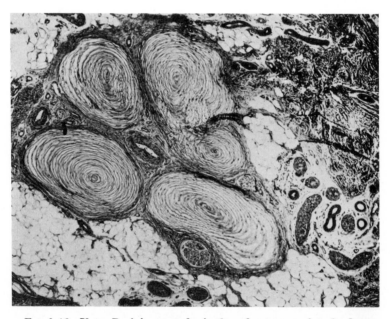

FIG. 3-12. **Vater-Pacini corpuscles in the subcutaneous fat of a fingertip.** Their largeness becomes apparent if one compares their size with that of the eccrine sweat glands and their ducts, which are located on the right side of the field. ($\times$50)

the skin of the volar aspects of the palms and soles, showing their greatest concentration at the tips of the fingers and toes. In addition, a few Vater-Pacini corpuscles occur in the subcutis of the nipple and of the anogenital region (Winkelmann). The Vater-Pacini corpuscles vary in shape. Some are ovoid, others have the appearance of a flattened sphere, and still others have an irregular shape (Winkelmann and Osment). They consist of a stalk and of the body proper, the latter having a small core and a thick capsule. In the stalk the single thick nerve supplying the Vater-Pacini corpuscle makes several turns. Just before entering the core, the nerve loses its myelin sheath. The core shows a granular substance surrounding the ascending meandering nerve. The thick capsule consists of 30 or more concentric, loosely arranged lamellae.

HISTOGENESIS. On electron microscopic examination the single nerve fiber present in the inner portion of the core retains its Schwann cell cytoplasmic covering for a short distance. The outer portion of the core shows closely packed, greatly elongated laminar cells. The thick capsule consists of at least 30 layers of flattened laminar cells separated from one another by fluid-filled spaces. Between the core and the capsule lies in the newborn the intermediate growth zone composed of laminated cells with relatively numerous nuclei. These laminated cells contribute cytoplasmic laminae to both the outer core and the capsule. In the fully developed Vater-Pacini corpuscle the intermediate growth zone is no longer an obvious feature, since most of its cells have become incorporated either into the outer core or into the capsule (Pease and Quilliam). The laminated cells of the Vater-Pacini corpuscle, analogous to those of the Meissner corpuscle, are modified Schwann cells.

BLOOD VESSELS AND LYMPH VESSELS

Dermal Blood Vessels. The arrangement of the cutaneous blood vessels consists of a subdermal plexus of small arteries from which arterioles ascend into the dermis and are interconnected. Some arterioles lead into a subpapillary capillary plexus from which individual capillary loops branch off at a right angle (Davis and Lawler); others divide in a treelike fashion, forming a capillary "candelabra" each of which gives rise to several capillary loops (Cormia; Copeman and Ryan). Generally, each subepidermal dermal papilla possesses one capillary loop, consisting of an ascending arterial limb and a descending venous limb. The venous portion empties into the subpapillary plexus of postcapillary venules, and further through larger venules into the subdermal plexus of small veins.

Histologically, the small arteries of the subdermal plexus and the arterioles of the dermis possess three layers: (1) an intima, composed of endothelial cells and an internal elastic lamina; (2) a media, containing two or more layers of muscle cells in the small arteries, a single layer of muscle cells in the arterioles of the lower dermis, and a discontinuous layer of muscle cells in the arterioles of the upper dermis; and (3) an adventitia of connective tissue (Moretti). The capillaries that are present throughout the dermis and in the papillary dermis are composed of a layer of endothelial cells surrounded by an incomplete layer of pericytes. Reticulum fibers representing the basement membrane are present peripheral to the endothelial cells and surround the pericytes. Alkaline phosphatase activity is present in the endothelial cells of the ascending arterial limb of the capillary loops in the papillary dermis (Kopf; Klingmüller).

The walls of veins generally are thinner than those of arteries and are less clearly divided into the three classical layers. The postcapillary venules resemble capillaries, since they consist of endothelial cells, pericytes and a basement membrane. In larger venules muscle cells appear and also elastic fibers, but the latter are diffusely arranged and do not form an internal elastic lamina. Large venules and veins, on the other hand, show an internal elastic lamina but differ from arteries by possessing valves (Moretti).

HISTOGENESIS. On electron microscopy, the endothelial cells of capillaries show a well developed endoplasmic reticulum, bundles of fairly thick cytoplasmic filaments with a diameter of 5 to 10 nm, and many pinocytotic vesicles at their luminal surface (E.M. No. 14). Peripheral to the endothelium lies a basal lamina. The peripheral row of cells, the pericytes (E.M. No.

14), have long cytoplasmic processes and form a discontinuous layer. They are completely surrounded by the basal lamina. They contain, like smooth muscle cells, fine cytoplasmic filaments, about 5 nm in diameter; but, in contrast to smooth muscle cells, these filaments are few in number and do not form dense bodies (Kuhn and Rosai). In larger capillaries more than one layer of pericytes may be present and transitional forms between pericytes and smooth muscle cells (see p. 39) may be seen (Weber and Braun-Falco).

The capillary loops at the tips of papillae show a relatively wide lumen and a very thin endothelium with areas of fenestration between the endothelial cells, allowing a maximal exchange between capillaries and tissue (Seifert and Klingmüller). Aside from the loops, the capillaries of both the arterial and the venous limb show a thick endothelium and a narrow, slitlike lumen. The endothelial cells of the arterial limb of the capillaries show alkaline phosphatase activity. This activity is present within pinocytotic vesicles and therefore is seen intracellularly near the capillary lumina and occasionally also within capillary lumina (Seifert and Klingmüller).

The Glomus. A special vascular structure, the glomus, is located within the dermis in certain areas. Glomus formations occur most abundantly in the pads and the nailbeds of the fingers and toes, but also elsewhere on the volar aspect of the hands and feet, in the skin of the ears, and in the center of the face. The glomus is concerned with temperature regulation and represents a special arteriovenous shunt that connects, without the interposition of capillaries, an arteriole with a venule. When open, these shunts cause a great increase in blood flow in the area. Each glomus consists of an arterial and a venous segment. The arterial segment, called the Suquet-Hoyer canal, branches from an arteriole and has a narrow lumen and a thick wall, measuring 20 to 40 μm in diameter. The wall shows a single layer of endothelium, surrounded by reticulum fibers but not by an internal elastic lamina, and a media that is densely packed with 4 to 6 layers of glomus cells. These are large cells with a clear cytoplasm resembling epithelioid cells. Although myofibrils cannot be recognized within the glomus cells with light microscopic staining methods, these cells have generally been regarded as smooth muscle cells (Mescon et al.). Peripheral to

the glomus cells there is a zone of loose connective tissue. Staining with silver salts shows within this zone many nerve fibers extending to the glomus cells. These nerve fibers are nonmyelinated, and stain positive for specific acetylcholinesterase (Mescon et al.). The venous segment of the glomus is thin-walled and has a wide lumen. This wide collecting venule functions as a reservoir. It drains either into a subpapillary or a dermal venule.

HISTOGENESIS. Electron microscopic study of the Suquet-Hoyer canal reveals the glomus cells to be vascular smooth muscle cells. As such each glomus cell is surrounded by a basal lamina. The cytoplasm of the glomus cells is filled with filaments having a diameter of about 5 nm. Cytoplasmic as well as peripheral dense bodies, 300 by 400 nm in diameter, are present in the glomus cells, as a result of condensations of the myofilaments. Numerous nonmyelinated nerves and Schwann cells are present peripheral to the glomus cells. Most nerves are ensheathed by Schwann cells (Goodman).

Lymph Vessels. Lymph vessels are difficult to recognize in histologic sections because of their resemblance to blood vessels. The lymph vessels can be divided into lymph capillaries, postcapillary lymph vessels, and deep lymph vessels (Pfleger).

The lymph capillaries are not recognizable in histologic sections of normal skin, even by means of lymphangiography. However, in areas of lymph stasis they can be recognized in the subpapillary and deeper dermis as lumina lined only by endothelial cells. In contrast to blood capillaries, they lack pericytes and do not possess a basement membrane composed of reticulum fibers (Seifert and Klingmüller). The lumina are surrounded by loosely arranged collagen fibers and elastic fibers.

The postcapillary lymph vessels located in the deep layers of the dermis, at the border between the dermis and the subcutis, and in the subcutaneous septa are stained by lymphangiography, as a rule (Pfleger). They have a wider lumen and a thicker connective tissue wall than the lymph capillaries. Also, a few smooth muscle cells are present in the wall. The postcapillary lymph vessels possess valves lined by endothelium.

The deep lymph vessels located at the

border between the dermis and subcutis and in the subcutaneous septa possess 3 layers and valves, similar to veins. An internal elastic lamina between the intima and media is regularly present (Pfleger).

MUSCLES OF THE SKIN

Smooth Muscle. Smooth or involuntary muscle of the skin occurs as arrectores pilorum, as tunica dartos of the external genitals, and also in the areola of the nipples. The muscle fibers of the arrectores pilorum arise in the connective tissue of the upper dermis and are attached to the hair follicle below the sebaceous glands. They are situated in the obtuse angle of the hair follicle (Fig. 3-6). Thus, on contracting they pull the hair follicle into a vertical position and produce the perifollicular elevations of "gooseflesh."

HISTOPATHOLOGY. Smooth muscle is characterized by the absence of striation and by the location of the nuclei in the center of the muscle cells. Argyrophilic reticulum fibers surround each muscle cell.

HISTOGENESIS. Electron microscopic examination reveals the smooth muscle cells to possess a basal lamina peripheral to the plasma membrane. The cytoplasm of the cells is filled with myofilaments, 5 nm in diameter, that form cytoplasmic and peripheral dense bodies as a result of condensations, just as the myofilaments do in myoepithelial cells, in vascular smooth muscle cells, and in glomus cells (Breathnach) (see p. 38). The rather narrow spaces between the muscle cells are occupied by collagen fibrils, and by Schwann cells with associated nonmyelinated axons (Orfanos).

Striated Muscle. Striated or voluntary muscle is found in the skin of the neck as platysma, and of the face as muscles of expression.

HISTOPATHOLOGY. The striated muscle bundles take their origin either from a fascia or from the periosteum, or they form a closed ring, as in the musculus sphincter oris. They extend through the subcutaneous tissue into the lower dermis (Schmidt). The muscle fibers, like skeletal muscle, show cross striation and a location of their nuclei at the periphery of the fibers, immediately beneath the sarcolemma, the limiting membrane of the fibers.

BIBLIOGRAPHY

Keratinocytes of the Epidermis

Baker, H., and Kligman, A. M.: Technique for estimating turnover time of human stratum corneum. Arch. Derm., *95*:408, 1967.

Bell, R. F., and Kellum, R. E.: Early formation of keratohyalin granules in rat epidermis. Acta dermatoven., *47*:350, 1967.

Blank, I. H., and Scheuplein, R. J.: The epidermal barrier. *In* Rook, A., and Champion, R. H. (eds.): London, Cambridge University Press, Progress in the Biologic Sciences in Relation to Dermatology. Vol. 2, p. 245, 1964.

Bourlond, A., and Vandooren-Deflorenne, R.: La membrane basale sous-epidermique: sa structure et son ultrastructure. Arch. belg. derm. syph., *24*:119, 1968.

Braun-Falco, O., and Rupec, M.: Die Verteilung der sauren Phosphatase bei normaler und psoriatischer Verhornung. Dermatologica, *134*:225, 1967.

Briggaman, R. A., Dalldorf, F. G., and Wheeler, C. E.: Formation and origin of basal lamina and anchoring fibrils in adult human skin. J. Cell Biol., *51*:384, 1971.

Brody, I.: The modified plasma membranes of the transition and horny cells in normal human epidermis as revealed by electron microscopy. Acta dermatoven., *49*:128, 1969.

————: An electron microscopic study of the fibrillar density in the normal human stratum corneum. J. Ultrastruct. Res., *30*:209, 1970.

Cooper, J. H.: Microanatomical and histochemical observations on the dermal-epidermal junction. Arch. Derm., *77*:18, 1958.

Emery, J. L., and McMillan, M.: Observations on the female sex chromatin in human epidermis and on the value of skin biopsy in determining sex. J. Path. Bact., *68*:17, 1954.

Epstein, W. L., and Maibach, H. I.: Cell renewal in human epidermis. Arch. Derm., *92*:462, 1965.

Frost, P., Weinstein, G. D., and Van Scott, E. J.: The ichthyosiform dermatoses. II. Autoradiographic studies of epidermal proliferation. J. Invest. Derm., *47*:561, 1966.

Goldman, L., and Goldman, J.: Some studies of sex chromatin in dermatology. Dermatologica, *127*:445, 1963.

Halprin, K. M.: Epidermal "turnover time"—a reexamination. Brit. J. Derm., *86*:14, 1972.

Hashimoto, K.: Cellular envelopes of keratinized cells of the human epidermis. Arch. klin. exp. Derm., *235*:374, 1969.

————: Cementsome, a new interpretation of

the membrane-coating granule. Arch. Derm. Forsch., *240*:349, 1971.

Hashimoto, K., DiBella, R. J., and Shklar, G.: Electron microscopic studies of the normal human buccal mucosa. J. Invest. Derm., *47*: 512, 1966.

Hashimoto, K., and Lever, W. F.: An ultrastructural study of cell junctions in pemphigus vulgaris. Arch. Derm., *101*:287, 1970 (I).

————: The cell surface coat of normal keratinocytes and of acantholytic keratinocytes in pemphigus. Brit. J. Derm., *83*:282, 1970 (II).

Johnson, B. E., and Daniels, F., Jr.: Lysosomes and the reactions of skin to ultraviolet radiation. J. Invest. Derm., *53*:85, 1969.

Komura, J., and Ofuji, S.: Ultrastructure of half-desmosomes fixed only in glutaraldehyde. Dermatologica, *144*:35, 1972.

Matoltsy, A. G., and Matoltsy, M.: A study of morphological and chemical properties of keratohyalin granules. J. Invest. Derm., *38*: 237, 1962.

Montagna, W., Eisen, A. Z., Rademacher, A. H., and Chase, H. B.: Histology and cytochemistry of the skin. VI. The distribution of sulfhydryl and disulfide groups. J. Invest. Derm., *23*:23, 1954.

Nelemans, T. G., Keuning, F. J., van Rijssel, T. G., and Ruiter, M.: Histologic changes in the tonofibrils in vesicular and bullous diseases of the skin. Brit. J. Derm., *64*:177, 1952.

Nieuwmeijer, A. H.: Tonofibrils in bullous dermatoses: A histo- and cyto-pathologic study. Dermatologica, *106*:379, 1953.

Odland, G. F.: The fine structure of the inter-relationship of cells in the human epidermis. J. Biophys. Biochem. Cytol., *4*:529, 1958.

Orfanos, C. E.: Feinstrukturelle Morphologie und Histopathologie der verhornenden Epidermis. p. 36. Stuttgart, Thieme Verlag, 1972.

Penneys, N. S., Fulton, J. E., Jr., Weinstein, G. D., and Frost, P.: Location of proliferating cells in human epidermis. Arch. Derm., *101*: 323, 1970.

Platt, L. I., and Kailin, E. W.: Sex chromatin frequency. J.A.M.A., *187*:182, 1964.

Rees, K. R.: Lysosomes and skin injury. Trans. St. John's Hosp. Derm. Soc., *53*:107, 1967.

Schreiner, E., and Wolff, K.: Die Permeabilität des epidermalen Intercellularraums für kleinmolekulares Protein. Arch. klin. exp. Derm., *235*:78, 1969.

Spearman, R. I. C.: Some light microscopical observations on the stratum corneum of the guinea-pig, man and common seal. Brit. J. Derm., *83*:582, 1970.

Stoughton, R., and Wells, G.: A histochemical study on polysaccharides in normal and diseased skin. J. Invest. Derm., *14*:37, 1950.

Susi, F. R., Belt, W. D., and Kelly, J. W.: Fine structure of fibrillar complexes associated with the basement membrane in human oral mucosa. J. Cell Biol., *34*:686, 1967.

Swanson, J. L., and Helwig, E. B.: Special fibrils of human dermis. J. Invest. Derm., *50*:195, 1968.

Tarnowski, W. M.: Ultrastructure of the epidermal melanocyte dense plate. J. Invest. Derm., *55*:265, 1970.

Van Scott, E. J., and Ekel, T. M.: Kinetics of hyperplasia in psoriasis. Arch. Derm., *88*: 373, 1963.

Weinstein, G. D.: Autoradiographic studies of turnover time and protein synthesis in pig epidermis. J. Invest. Derm., *44*:413, 1965.

Weinstein, G. D., and Frost, P.: Methotrexate for psoriasis. Arch. Derm., *103*:33, 1971.

Wolff, K., and Holubar, K.: Odland Körper (Membrane Coating Granules, Keratinosomen) als epidermale Lysosomen. Arch. klin. exp. Derm., *231*:1, 1967.

Wolff, K., and Schreiner, E.: An electron microscopic study on the extraneous coat of keratinocytes and the intercellular space of the epidermis. J. Invest. Derm., *51*:418, 1968.

————: Epidermal lysosomes. Electron microscopic cytochemical studies. Arch. Derm., *101*:276, 1970.

Dendritic Cells of the Epidermis

Becker, S. W., Praver, L. L., and Thatcher, H.: An improved (paraffin section) method for the dopa reaction. Arch. Derm. Syph., *31*: 190, 1935.

Bleehen, S. S., Pathak, M. A., Hori, Y., and Fitzpatrick, T. B.: Depigmentation of skin with 4-isoproplycatechol, mercaptoamines, and other compounds. J. Invest. Derm., *50*:103, 1968.

Bloch, B.: Das Problem der Pigmentbildung in der Haut. Arch. f. Derm. u. Syph., *124*:129, 1917.

Breathnach, A. S., Silvers, W. K., Smith, J., and Heyner, S.: Langerhans cells in mouse skin experimentally deprived of its neural crest component. J. Invest. Derm., *50*:147, 1968.

Breathnach, A. S., and Wyllie, L. M. A.: Melanin in Langerhans cells. J. Invest. Derm., *45*:401, 1965.

Carrington, S. G., and Winkelmann, R. K.: Ultrastructure of histiocytes in cutaneous pathology. J. Invest. Derm., *52*:372, 1969.

Clark, W. H., Jr., Watson, M. C., and Watson, B. E. M.: Two kinds of "clear" cells in the human epidermis. Am. J. Path., *39*:333, 1961.

Cochran, A. J.: The incidence of melanocytes in normal skin. J. Invest. Derm., *55*:65, 1970.

Cruickshank, C. N. D., and Harcourt, S. A.: Pigment donation in vitro. J. Invest. Derm., *42*:183, 1964.

Ebner, H.: Beitrag zum Ehlers-Danlos Syndrom. Z. Haut, *43*:177, 1968.

Fitzpatrick, T. B.: Human melanogenesis. Arch. Derm. Syph., *65*:379, 1952.

————: In discussion of: Zelickson, A. S., and Mottaz, J. H.: Epidermal dendritic cells. Arch. Derm., *98*:652, 1968.

Fitzpatrick, T. B., Miyomato, M., and Ishikawa, K.: The evolution of concepts of melanin biology. Arch. Derm., *96*:305, 1967.

Fitzpatrick, T. B., and Szabo, G.: The melanocytes: cytology and cytochemistry. J. Invest. Derm., *32*:197, 1959.

Flaxman, B. A., Sosio, A. C., and Van Scott, E. J.: Changes in melanosome distribution in Caucasoid skin following topical application of N mustard. J. Invest. Derm., *60*:321, 1973.

Fritsch, P.: Langerhanszellen in Viruswarzen. Arch. Derm. Forsch., *242*:70, 1971.

Furuya, T. and Ikeda, S.: Studies on DOPA reaction (stain). Jap. J. Derm., series B, *81*:259, 1971.

Hashimoto, K.: Langerhans' cell granule. An endocytic organelle. Arch. Derm., *104*:148, 1971.

Hashimoto, K., and Tarnowski, W. M.: Some new aspects of the Langerhans cell. Arch. Derm., *97*:450, 1968.

Hunter, J. A. A., Mottaz, J. H., and Zelickson, A. S.: Melanogenesis: ultrastructural histochemical observations on ultraviolet irradiated human melanocytes. J. Invest. Derm., *54*:213, 1970.

Hutchens, L. H., Sagebiel, R. W., and Clarke, M. A.: Oral epithelial dendritic cells of the Rhesus monkey, histologic demonstration, fine structure and quantitative distribution. J. Invest. Derm., *56*:325, 1971.

Kiistala, U., and Mustakallio, K. K.: The presence of Langerhans cells in human dermis with special reference to their potential mesenchymal origin. Acta dermatoven., *48*:115, 1968.

Konrad, K., and Hönigsmann, H.: Elektronenmikroskopischer Nachweis einer mitotischen Langerhans-Zelle in normaler menschlicher Epidermis. Arch. Derm. Forsch., *246*:70, 1973.

Lerner, A. B.: On the etiology of vitiligo and gray hair. Am. J. Med., *51*:141, 1971.

Lerner, A. B., and Fitzpatrick, T. B.: Biochemistry of melanin formation. Physiol. Rev., *30*:91, 1950.

Masson, P.: Pigment Cells in Man. Spec. Publ. N. Y. Acad. Sci., *4*:15, 1948.

Mishima, Y., and Tanay, A.: The effect of alpha-methyldopa and ultraviolet irradiation on melanogenesis. Dermatologica, *136*:105, 1968.

Mitchell, R. E.: Melanocytes in Australian Aboriginal skin. J. Invest. Derm., *94*:93, 1970.

Mottaz, J. H., and Zelickson, A. S.: Melanin transfer; a possible phagocytic process. J. Invest. Derm., *49*:605, 1967.

Niebauer, G., Krawczyk, W. S., Kidd, R. L., and Wilgram, G. F.: Osmium zinc iodide reactive sites in the epidermal Langerhans cell. J. Cell Biol., *43*:80, 1969.

Niebauer, G., Krawczyk, W. S., and Wilgram, G. F.: Über die Langerhans-Zellorganelle bei Morbus Letterer-Siwe. Arch. klin. exp. Derm., *239*:125, 1970.

Okun, M. R.: Dermal dopa-positive cells in lichen planus. Arch. Derm., *106*:422, 1972.

Okun, M. R., Edelstein, L. M., Or, N., Hamada, G., and Donnellan, B.: The role of peroxidase vs. the role of tyrosinase in enzymatic conversion of tyrosine to melanin in melanocytes, mast cells and eosinophils. J. Invest. Derm., *55*:1, 1970.

Olson, R. L., Nordquist, J., and Everett, M. A.: The role of epidermal lysosomes in melanin physiology. Brit. J. Derm., *83*:189, 1970.

Pathak, M. A., Sinesi, S. J., and Szabo, G.: The effect of a single dose of ultraviolet radiation on epidermal melanocytes. J. Invest. Derm., *45*:520, 1965.

Pearse, A. G. E.: Histochemistry: Theoretical and Applied. ed. 3, p. 1056. Edinburgh, Churchill Livingstone, 1972.

Quevedo, W. C., Jr., Szabo, G., Virks, J., and Sinesi, S. J. P.: Melanocyte populations in UV-radiated human skin. J. Invest. Derm., *45*:295, 1965.

Sagebiel, R. W.: In vivo and in vitro uptake of ferritin by Langerhans cells of the epidermis. J. Invest. Derm., *58*:47, 1972.

Seiji, M., Shimao, K., Fitzpatrick, T. B., and Birbeck, M. S. C.: The site of biosynthesis of mammalian tyrosinase. J. Invest. Derm., *37*:359, 1961.

Staricco, R. J., and Pinkus, H.: Quantitative and qualitative data on the pigment cells of adult human epidermis. J. Invest. Derm., *28*:33, 1957.

Szabo, G.: Tyrosinase in the epidermal melanocytes of white human skin. Arch. Derm., *76*:324, 1967.

Szabo, G., Gerald, A. B., Pathak, M. A., and Fitzpatrick, T. B.: The ultrastructure of racial color differences in man. Abstract, VII. Internat. Pigment Cell Conference. J. Invest. Derm., *54*:98, 1970.

Tarnowski, W. M.: Ultrastructure of the epidermal melanocyte dense plate. J. Invest. Derm., *55*:265, 1970.

Toda, K., Hori, Y., and Fitzpatrick, T. B.: The site of tyrosinase activity within the melanosome. J. Invest. Derm., *52*:380, 1969. (abstr.)

Toshima, S., Moore, G. E., and Sandberg, A. A.: Ultrastructure of human melanoma in cell culture. Electron microscopic studies. Cancer, *21*:202, 1968.

Wolff, K.: Die Langerhans-Zelle. Arch. klin. exp. Derm., *229*:54, 76, 1967.

Wolff, K., and Schreiner, E.: Uptake, intracellular transport and degradation of exogenous protein by Langerhans cells. J. Invest. Derm., *54*:37, 1970.

————: Melanosomal acid phosphatase. Arch. Derm. Forsch., *241*:255, 1971.

Wolff, K., and Winkelmann, R. K.: The influence of ultraviolet light on the Langerhans cell population and its hydrolytic enzymes in guinea pigs. J. Invest. Derm., *48*:531, 1967.

Zelickson, A. S.: The Langerhans cell. J. Invest. Derm., *44*:201, 1965.

Zelickson, A. S., and Mottaz, J. H.: Localization of gold chloride and adenosine triphosphatase in human Langerhans cells. J. Invest. Derm., *51*:365, 1968 (I).

————: Epidermal dendritic cells. Arch. Derm., *98*:652, 1968 (II).

————: The effect of sunlight on human epidermis. Arch. Derm., *101*:312, 1970.

Nerves of the Epidermis

Arthur, R. P., and Shelley, W. B.: The innervation of human epidermis. J. Invest. Derm., *32*:397, 1959.

Fitzpatrick, T. B., Seiji, M., and McGugan, A. D.: Melanin pigmentation. New Eng. J. Med., *265*:328, 1961.

Hashimoto, K.: Fine structure of Merkel cell in human oral mucosa. J. Invest. Derm., *58*: 381, 1972.

Kidd, R. L., Krawczyk, W. S., and Wilgram, G. F.: The Merkel cell in human epidermis: Its differentiation from other dendritic cells. Arch. Derm. Forsch., *241*:374, 1971.

Montagna, W.: Histology and cytochemistry of human skin. XXXIV. The eyebrows. Arch. Derm., *101*:257, 1970.

Montagna, W., and Ford, D. M.: Histology and cytochemistry of human skin. XXXIII. The eyelid. Arch. Derm., *100*:328, 1969.

Orfanos, C. E., and Mahrle, G.: Ultrastructure and cytochemistry of human cutaneous nerve. J. Invest. Derm., *61*:108, 1973.

Smith, K. R., Jr.: The ultrastructure of the human Haarscheibe and Merkel cells. J. Invest. Derm., *54*:150, 1970.

Eccrine Glands

Dobson, R. L., Formisano, V., Lobitz, W. C., Jr., and Brophy, D.: Some histochemical observations on the human eccrine sweat gland. III. The effect of profuse sweating. J. Invest. Derm., *31*:147, 1958.

Dobson, R. L., and Sato, K.: The secretion of salt and water by the eccrine sweat gland. Arch. Derm., *105*:366, 1972.

Ellis, R. A.: Eccrine, sebaceous and apocrine glands. *In* Zelickson, A. S. (ed.): Ultrastructure of Normal and Abnormal Skin. p. 132. Philadelphia, Lea and Febiger, 1967.

Hashimoto, K., Gross, B. G., and Lever, W. F.: Electron microscopic study of the human adult eccrine gland. I. The duct. J. Invest. Derm., *46*:172, 1966.

Hurley, H. J., and Witkowski, J. A.: The dynamics of eccrine sweating in man. J. Invest. Derm., *39*:329, 1962.

Montagna, W., Chase, H. B., and Lobitz, W. C., Jr.: Histology and cytochemistry of human skin. IV. The eccrine sweat glands. J. Invest. Derm., *20*:415, 1953.

O'Hara, J. M., and Bensch, K. G.: Fine structure of eccrine sweat gland adenoma, clear cell type. J. Invest. Derm., *49*:261, 1967.

Schiefferdecker, P.: Die Hautdrüsen des Menschen und der Säugetiere, ihre biologische und rassenanatomische Bedeutung, sowie die Muscularis sexualis. Zentralbl. Biolog., *37*: 534, 1917. Also Stuttgart, F. Enke, 1922.

Apocrine Glands

Biempica, L., and Montes, L. F.: Secretory epithelium of the large axillary sweat glands. Am. J. Anat., *117*:47, 1965.

Braun-Falco, O., and Rupec, M.: Apokrine Schweissdrüsen. *In* Marchionini, A. (ed.): Handbuch der Haut- und Geschlechtskrankheiten, Ergänzungswerk. Vol. 1, part 1, p. 267. Berlin, Springer, 1968.

Ellis, R. A.: Eccrine, sebaceous and apocrine glands. *In* Zelickson, A. S. (ed.): Ultrastructure of Normal and Abnormal Skin, p. 132. Philadelphia, Lea and Febiger, 1967.

Hashimoto, K., Gross, B. G., and Lever, W. F.: Electron microscopic study of apocrine secretion. J. Invest. Derm., *46*:378, 1966.

Hibbs, R. G.: Electron microscopy of human apocrine sweat glands. J. Invest. Derm., *38*: 77, 1962.

Hurley, H. J., and Shelley, W. B.: The Human Apocrine Sweat Gland in Health and Disease. Springfield, Charles C Thomas, 1960.

Kurosumi, K., Yamagishi, M., and Sekine, M.: Mitochondrial deformation and apocrine secretory mechanism in the rabbit submandibular organ as revealed by electron microscopy. Z. Zellforsch., *55*:297, 1967.

Montagna, W.: The Structure and Function of Skin. ed. 2. New York, Academic Press, 1962.

Montagna, W., and Yun, J. S.: The glands of Montgomery. Brit. J. Derm., *86*:126, 1972.

Montes, L. F., Baker, B. L., and Curtis, A. C.: The cytology of the large axillary sweat glands in man. J. Invest. Derm., *35*:273, 1960.

Munger, B. L.: The cytology of apocrine sweat glands. II. Human. Z. Zellforsch., *68*:837, 1965.

Pinkus, H.: Anatomy and histology of skin. *In* Graham, J. H., Johnson, W. C., and Helwig, E. B. (eds.): Dermal Pathology, p. 1. Hagerstown, Harper and Row, 1972.

Schaumburg-Lever, G., and Lever, W. F.: Secretion from human apocrine glands. J. Invest. Derm., *64*:38, 1975.

Schiefferdecker, P.: Die Hautdrüsen des Menschen und der Säugetiere, ihre biologische und rassenanatomische Bedeutung, sowie die Muscularis sexualis. Zentralbl. Biolog., *37*: 534, 1917. Also Stuttgart, F. Enke, 1922.

Soltermann, W.: Die Bedeutung des Eisennachweises in der Haut für die Diagnose einer Hämochromatose unter besonderer Berücksichtigung der Axillargegend und der apokrinen Schweissdrüsen. Dermatologica, *112*: 335, 1956.

Winkelmann, R. K., and Hultin, J. V.: Mucinous metaplasia in normal apocrine glands. Arch. Derm., *78*:309, 1958.

Sebaceous Glands

Cashion, P. D., Skobe, Z., and Nalbandian, J.: Ultrastructural observations on sebaceous glands of the human oral mucosa (Fordyce's disease). J. Invest. Derm., *53*:208, 1969.

Hyman, A. B., and Brownstein, M. H.: Tyson's glands. Arch. Derm., *99*:31, 1969.

Rowden, G.: Aryl sulfatase in the sebaceous glands of mouse skin. J. Invest. Derm., *51*: 41, 1968.

Rupec, M.: Zur Ultrastruktur der Talgdrüsenzelle. Arch. klin. exp. Derm., *234*:273, 1969.

Rupec, M., and Braun-Falco, O.: Zur Frage lysosomaler Aktivität in normalen menschlichen Talgdrüsen. Arch. klin. exp. Derm., *232*:312, 1968.

Suskind, R. R.: The chemistry of the human sebaceous gland. I. Histochemical observations. J. Invest. Derm., *17*:37, 1951.

Hair

Cormia, F.: Vasculature of the normal scalp. Arch. Derm., *88*:692, 1963.

Garn, S. M.: The examination of hair under the polarizing microscope. Ann. N. Y. Acad. Sci., *53*:649, 1951.

Herzberg, J., and Gusek, W.: Das Ergrauen des Kopfhaares. Arch. klin. exp. Derm., *236*:368, 1970.

Johnson, W. C., and Helwig, E. B.: Histochemistry of the acid mucopolysaccharides of skin in normal and in certain pathologic conditions. Am. J. Clin. Path., *40*:123, 1963.

Kligman, A. M.: The human hair cycle. J. Invest. Derm., *33*:307, 1959.

Kollar, E. J.: The induction of hair follicles by embryonic dermal papillae. J. Invest. Derm., *55*:374, 1970.

Kopf, A. W., and Orentreich, N.: Alkaline phosphatase in alopecia areata. Arch. Derm., *76*: 288, 1957.

Mahrle, G., and Orfanos, C. E.: Das spongiöse Keratin und die Marksubstanz des menschlichen Kopfhaares. Arch. Derm. Forsch., *241*:305, 1971.

———: Haarfarbe und Haarpigment. Arch. Derm. Forsch., *248*:109, 1973.

Mishima, Y., and Widlan, S.: Embryonic development of melanocytes in human hair and epidermis. J. Invest. Derm., *46*:263, 1966.

Montagna, W.: The Structure and Function of Skin. ed. 2, p. 174. New York, Academic Press, 1962.

Parakkal, P. F., and Matoltsy, A. G.: A study of the differentiation products of the hair follicle cells with the electron microscope. J. Invest. Derm., *43*:23, 1964.

Orfanos, C., and Ruska, H.: Die Feinstruktur des menschlichen Haares. II. Der Haar-Cortex. III. Das Haarpigment. Arch. klin. exp. Derm., *231*:264, 279, 1968

Pinkus, H.: "Sebaceous cysts" are trichilemmal cysts. Arch. Derm., *99*:544, 1969.

———: Anatomy and histology of skin. *In* Graham, J. H., Johnson, W. C., and Helwig, E. B. (eds.): Dermal Pathology, p. 1. Hagerstown, Harper and Row, 1972.

Staricco, R. G.: The melanocytes and the hair follicle. J. Invest. Derm., *35*:185, 1960.

Van Scott, E. J., Reinertson, R. P., and Steinmuller, R.: The growing hair roots of the human scalp and morphologic changes therein following amethopterin therapy. J. Invest. Derm., *29*:197, 1957.

Nail

Hashimoto, K.: The marginal band. A demonstration of the thickened cellular envelope of the human nail cell with the aid of lanthanum staining. Arch. Derm., *103*:387, 1971.

Norton, L. A.: Incorporation of thymidine-methyl-H[3] and glycine-2-H[3] in the nail matrix and bed of humans. J. Invest. Derm., *56*:61, 1971.

Zaias, N.: The movement of the nail bed. J. Invest. Derm., *48*:402, 1967.

Zaias, N., and Alvarez, J.: The formation of the primate nail plate. An autoradiographic study in squirrel monkey. J. Invest. Derm., *51*:120, 1968.

Connective Tissue of the Dermis

Breathnach, A. S.: An Atlas of the Ultrastructure of Human Skin. p. 174. London, Churchill, 1971.

Grant, M. E., and Prockop, D. J.: The biosynthesis of collagen. New Eng. J. Med., *286*: 194, 1972.

Hashimoto, K., and DiBella, R. J.: Electron microscopic studies of normal and abnormal elastic fibers of the skin. J. Invest. Derm., *48*:405, 1967.

Hayes, R. L., and Rodnan, G. P.: The ultrastructure of skin in progressive sclerosis (scleroderma). Am. J. Path., *63*:433, 1971.

Jacques, J., and Cameron, H. C. S.: Changes in the ground-substance of healing wounds. J. Path., *99*:337, 1969.

Jansen, L. H.: The structure of the connective tissue, an explanation of the symptoms of the Ehlers-Danlos syndrome. Dermatologica, *110*:108, 1955.

Johnson, W. C., and Helwig, E. B.: Histochemistry of the acid mucopolysaccharides of the skin in normal and in certain pathologic conditions. Am. J. Clin. Path., *40*:123, 1963.

Kobayasi, T.: Electron microscopy of the elastic fibers and the dermal membrane in normal human skin. Acta dermatoven., *48*:303, 1968.

Lapière, C. M.: Biology and pathology at the molecular level of connective tissue fibrous proteins. Arch. belg. derm. syph., *28*:15, 1972.

————: The molecular basis of connective tissue pathology. Brit. J. Derm., *89*:87, 1973.

Lapière, C. M., and Piérard, G.: Skin procollagen peptidase in normal and pathologic conditions. J. Invest. Derm., *62*:582, 1974.

Lazarus, G. S.: Collagen, collagenase and clinicians. Brit. J. Derm., *86*:193, 1972.

Montagna, W.: The Structure and Function of Skin. ed. 2, p. 126. New York, Academic Press, 1962.

Nigra, T. P., Friedland, M., and Martin, G. R.: Controls of connective tissue synthesis: collagen metabolism. J. Invest. Derm., *59*:44, 1972.

Pinkus, H.: The direction of growth of human epidermis. Brit. J. Derm., *83*:556, 1970.

Rehtijärvi, K.: Reticular network and karyometric properties of lymphomas of the skin. Acta dermatoven., *43,* Suppl. 53, 1963.

Ross, R., and Benditt, E. P.: Wound healing and collagen formation. V. Quantitative electron microscopic radioautographic observations of proline-H[3] utilization by fibroblasts. J. Cell Biol., *27*:83, 1965.

Scarpelli, D. G., and Goodman, R. M.: Observations on the fine structure of the fibroblast from a case of Ehlers-Danlos syndrome with the Marfan syndrome. J. Invest. Derm., *50*: 214, 1968.

Schmidt, W.: Die normale Histologie von Corium und Subcutis. *In* Marchionini, A. (ed.): Handbuch der Haut- und Geschlechtskrankheiten, Ergänzungswerk. Vol. 1, part 1, p. 430. Berlin, Springer, 1968.

Smith, J. G., Jr.: The dermal elastoses. Arch. Derm., *88*:382, 1963.

Williams, G.: The late phases of wound healing: histologic and ultrastructural of collagen and elastic-tissue formation. J. Path., *102*:61, 1970.

Winand, R.: Biosynthesis, organization and degradation of mucopolysaccharides. Arch. belg. derm. syph., *28*:35, 1972.

Nerves and Nerve End-Organs of the Dermis

Arthur, R. P., and Shelley, W. B.: The innervation of human epidermis. J. Invest. Derm., *32*:397, 1959.

Bodian, D.: A new method for staining nerve fibers and nerve endings in mounted paraffin section. Anat. Rec., *65*:89, 1936.

Cauna, N., and Ross, L. L.: The fine structure of Meissner's touch corpuscles of human fingers. J. Biophys. Biochem. Cytol., *8*:467, 1960.

Hashimoto, K.: Fine structure of the Meissner corpuscle of human palmar skin. J. Invest. Derm., *60*:20, 1973.

Orfanos, C. E., and Mahrle, G.: Ultrastructure and cytochemistry of human cutaneous nerves. J. Invest. Derm., *61*:108, 1973.

Pease, D. C., and Quilliam, T. A.: Electron

microscopy of the Pacinian corpuscle. J. Biophys. Biochem. Cytol., *3*:331, 1957.

Winkelmann, R. K.: Nerve Endings in Normal and Pathologic Skin. Springfield, Charles C Thomas, 1960.

Winkelmann, R. K., and Osment, L. S.: The Vater-Pacinian corpuscle in the skin of the human finger tip. Arch. Derm., *73*:116, 1956.

Woollard, H. H., Weddell, G., and Harpman, J. A.: Observations on neuro-histological basis of cutaneous pain. J. Anat., *74*:413, 1940.

Blood Vessels and Lymph Vessels

Copeman, P. W. M., and Ryan, T. J.: Cutaneous angiitis. Brit. J. Derm., *85*:205, 1971

Cormia, F. E.: Vasculature of the normal scalp. Arch. Derm., *88*:692, 1963.

Davis, M. J., and Lawler, J. C.: The capillary circulation of the skin. Arch. Derm., *77*:690, 1958.

Goodman, T. F.: Fine structure of the cells of the Suquet-Hoyer canal. J. Invest. Derm., *59*:363, 1972.

Klingmüller, G.: Die Darstellung alkalischer Phosphatase in Capillaren. Hautarzt, *9*:84, 1958.

Kopf, A. W.: The distribution of alkaline phosphatase in normal and pathologic human skin. Arch. Derm., *75*:1, 1957.

Kuhn, C., III, and Rosai, J.: Tumors arising from pericytes. Arch. Path., *88*:653, 1969.

Mescon, H., Hurley, H. J., and Moretti, G.: The anatomy and histochemistry of the arteriovenous anastomosis in human digital skin. J. Invest. Derm., *27*:133, 1956.

Moretti, G.: The blood vessels of the skin. *In* Marchionini, A. (ed.): Handbuch der Haut- und Geschlechtskrankheiten, Ergänzungswerk. Vol. 1, part 1, p. 491. Berlin, Springer, 1968.

Pfleger, L.: Histologie und Histopathologie cutaner Lymphgefässe der unteren Extremitäten. Arch. klin. exp. Derm., *221*:1, 1964.

Seifert, H. W., and Klingmüller, G.: Elektronenmikroskopische Struktur normaler Kapillaren und das Verhalten alkalischer Phosphatase. Arch. Derm. Forsch., *242*:97, 1972.

Weber, K., and Braun-Falco, O.: Ultrastructure of blood vessels in human granulation tissue. Arch. Derm. Forsch., *248*:29, 1973.

Muscles of the Skin

Breathnach, A. S.: An Atlas of the Ultrastructure of Human Skin. p. 330. London, Churchill, 1971.

Orfanos, C.: Elektronenmikroskopische Untersuchung glatter Hautmuskelfasern und ihrer Innervation. Dermatologica, *132*:445, 1966.

Schmidt, W.: Die normale Histologie von Corium und Subcutis. *In* Marchionini, A. (ed.): Handbuch der Haut- und Geschlechtskrankheiten, Ergänzungswerk. Vol. 1, part 1, p. 430. Berlin, Springer, 1968.

4

Laboratory Methods

FIXATION, PROCESSING, AND STAINING

Fixation. As already stated in Chapter 1, the fixative of choice is a 10 per cent aqueous solution of formalin, except during the winter months when, in order to prevent freezing of the specimen, it is preferable to use Lillie's AAF solution (acetic acid, alcohol, and formalin) as fixative (see p. 2).

It is important that adequate time be allowed for fixation. The minimum period for specimens 4 mm thick is 8 hours, and for specimens 6 mm thick, 24 hours.

Large specimens, such as excised tumors, should be cut in the laboratory into slices, 4 to 5 mm thick, for further fixation. It is important that such specimens be cut not lengthwise but across so that, after the histologic examination, information can be provided as to whether or not an adequate margin of normal skin is present between the tumor and the border of the specimen.

For the demonstration of *enzyme activities* specimens should not be placed into formalin. Instead, it is recommended that the specimen be delivered to the laboratory wrapped in water-moistened gauze and placed in a plastic bag, since, for enzyme staining, frozen sections cut on a cryostat are generally used. It should be kept in mind that staining for enzyme activities is not routinely done in all pathology laboratories and, therefore, should not be requested without prior checking with the laboratory. Actually, staining for enzymes is necessary only in very rare instances for purposes of diagnosis.

Two enzyme stains are occasionally of value: those demonstrating the presence of "dopa oxidase" and of peroxidase, respectively. Demonstration of "dopa oxidase" activity in melanocytes may aid in distinguishing a malignant melanoma from tumors not composed of melanocytes (see p. 18 and p. 673). Demonstration of peroxidase activity in granulocytes may aid in the distinction between myeloblastomas and lymphomas, especially when the circulating blood contains no immature cells (see pp. 50 and 706).

In two diseases, namely, scleredema of Buschke and amyloidosis, unfixed frozen sections may show a more conclusive reaction to specific staining methods than are obtainable with formalin-fixed material. It is recommended therefore that in these two diseases only part of the tissue be fixed in formalin and the remainder be used for frozen sections. In scleredema demonstration of hyaluronic acid with toluidine blue at pH 7.0 may be more intense in unfixed, frozen sections than in formalin-fixed sections (see p. 407); and in amyloidosis the reactions of the amyloid with crystal violet or Congo red may be conclusive only in unfixed, frozen sections (see p. 386).

Processing. All routine specimens, after having been fixed for a sufficient length of time in formalin, are processed in an automatic processor, such as an Autotechnicon, with the exception of those specimens that are to be stained for lipids. Since lipids are extracted by the xylene used in the Autotechicon for the processing of the specimens, formalin-fixed, frozen sections are used for lipid staining.

The Autotechnicon, regulated by clockwork, automatically controls overnight the duration of the processing in a succession of beakers. The specimens pass first through increasing concentrations of ethanol for dehydration, then through xylene for lipid extraction, and finally through several changes of hot, melted paraffin or Paraplast. The next morning the specimens are embedded with the epidermis upward in the still liquid paraffin or Paraplast which then is allowed to harden. The specimens are cut on a rotary microtome into sections 5 to 7 μm thick.

Staining. All routine sections are stained with hematoxylin and eosin, the most widely used routine stain. With this staining method nuclei stain blue, whereas collagen, muscles and nerves stain red. Special stains are employed only when needed for the demonstration of particular structures (Table 4-1). (For details see the Manual of Histologic Staining Methods of the Armed Forces Institute of Pathology.)

HISTOCHEMICAL STAINING

Histochemistry, especially enzyme histochemistry both at the light microscopic and electron microscopic level, has gained increasing importance in recent years and has

TABLE 4-1. Survey of Commonly Used Staining Methods

Stain	Purpose of Stain	Results
Hematoxylin and eosin	Routine	Nuclei: blue; collagen, muscles, nerves: red
Masson's trichrome	Collagen	Collagen: green; nuclei, muscles, nerves: dark red
Verhoeff-van Gieson	Elastic fibers	Elastic fibers: black; collagen: red; nuclei, muscles, nerves: yellow
Silver nitrate impregnation	Melanin, reticulum fibers, nerves (argyrophilic)	Melanin, reticulum fibers, nerves: black
Fontana-Masson (ammoniated silver nitrate)	Melanin (argentaffin)	Melanin: black
Methenamine silver	Fungi, Donovan bodies, Frisch bacilli	Fungus walls, Donovan bodies, Frisch bacilli: black
PAS (periodic acid-Schiff) and diastase	Glycogen, neutral mucopolysaccharides, fungi	Glycogen: diastase-labile; Neutral MPS, fungus walls: diastase-resistant
Alcian blue	Acid mucopolysaccharides	Acid MPS: blue
Toluidine blue	Acid mucopolysaccharides	Acid MPS: metachromatically purple
Giemsa's	Mast cell granules, acid mucopolysaccharides, eosinophils, *Leishmania*	Mast cell granules, acid MPS: metachromatically purple; eosinophil granules, *Leishmania*: red
Fite's	Acid-fast bacilli	Acid-fast bacilli: red
Perl's potassium ferrocyanide	Hemosiderin	Hemosiderin: blue
Alkaline Congo red	Amyloid	Amyloid: green birefringence in polarized light
Von Kossa's	Calcium	Calcium: black
Scarlet red	Lipids	Lipids: red

Note: All stains, except the stain for lipids, can be carried out on formalin-fixed specimens that have been processed in the Autotechnicon. The stain for lipids requires formalin-fixed, frozen sections.

been largely responsible for the expansion of histopathology from a purely descriptive science to one that is dynamic and functional (Pearse). Most enzyme histochemical methods are used only for research, and, as already pointed out, have the limitation of requiring fresh tissue in place of formalin-fixed tissue (see p. 46).

Two histochemical stains that stain chemical substrates rather than enzymes and thus can be carried out on formalin-fixed, Auto-technicon-processed material have attained considerable diagnostic importance: the periodic acid-Schiff reaction (Kligman et al.), and the alcian blue reaction (Cawley et al.).

The *periodic acid-Schiff reaction,* or PAS stain, demonstrates the presence of certain polysaccharides, particularly of glycogen and of mucoproteins containing neutral muco-polysaccharides, by staining them red. The PAS reaction is of value also in the study of fibrinoid degeneration (see p. 429), since the fibrin deposits in such areas are PAS-positive. Furthermore, since the cell walls of fungi are composed of a mixture of cellulose and chitin and thus contain polysaccharides, all fungi stain a bright red with the PAS reaction.

The PAS reaction consists of the oxidation of adjacent hydroxyl groups in 1,2 glycols to aldehydes, and the staining of the aldehydes with fuchsin-sulfuric acid (Stoughton and Wells).

For the distinction of neutral mucopoly-saccharides and fungi from glycogen deposits it is necessary to compare two serial sections, one exposed to diastase prior to staining, and the other not. Since glycogen is diastase-labile, i.e., digested by the diastase and thus no longer colored red by the PAS reaction, it can be easily distinguished from neutral mucopolysaccharides and fungi that are diastase-resistant. Since glycogen is present in outer root sheath cells and in eccrine gland cells, and neutral polysaccharides are found in eccrine and apocrine gland cells, demonstration of the presence of glycogen often is of diagnostic value in pilar tumor (see p. 521), in trichilemmoma (see p. 522), in clear cell hidradenoma (see p. 528), and in eccrine poroma (see p. 531); and demonstration of the presence of neutral mucopoly-saccharides is of value in Paget's disease of the breast (see p. 487) and extramammary Paget's disease (see p. 490), in clear cell hidradenoma (see p. 528), and intraluminally in eccrine spiradenoma (see p. 534) and eccrine poroma (see p. 531).

The *alcian blue reaction* demonstrates the presence of acid mucopolysaccharides by staining them blue. Acid mucopolysaccharides are present in the dermal ground substance, but in amounts too small to be demonstrable in normal skin. However, in the dermal mucinoses one finds a great increase in the nonsulfated acid mucopolysaccharides, mainly hyaluronic acid, so that the mucin stains with alcian blue (see p. 404). In extramammary Paget's disease of the anus with rectal carcinoma (see p. 490) and also in cutaneous metastases of carcinomas of the gastrointestinal tract containing goblet cells (see p. 566), the tumor cells in the skin, like the parent cells, secrete sialomucin containing neutral mucopolysaccharides, that are PAS-positive, as well as nonsulfated acid mucopolysaccharides. Whereas sulfated acid mucopolysaccharides, present for instance in mast cell granules and in cartilage, stain with alcian blue both at pH 4.5 and at pH 0.5, nonsulfated acid mucopolysaccharides found in the dermal mucinoses, in perianal Paget's disease, and in the cutaneous metastases of gastrointestinal carcinoma stain with alcian blue only at pH 4.5 but not at pH 0.5 (Johnson and Helwig; Helwig and Graham).

POLARISCOPIC EXAMINATION

Polariscopic examination is the examination of histologic sections under the microscope with polarized light, i.e., with light from which all rays except those vibrating in one plane are excluded.

For the polariscopic examination two disks made of polarizing plastics are inserted in the microscope. One disk is placed below the condenser of the microscope and acts as the polarizer. The second disk is placed in the eyepiece of the microscope and acts as the analyzer. When the eyepiece containing the analyzing disk is rotated so that the path of the light through the two disks is broken at a right angle, the field is dark. However, when doubly refractile substances are introduced between the two disks, they break the polarization and are visible as bright white bodies in the dark field.

Polariscopic examination is useful in evaluating lipid deposits, certain foreign bodies, gout, and amyloid.

In regard to lipids, it is not fully known why certain lipids are doubly refractile and others are not. In general, however, cholesterol esters are doubly refractile, whereas free cholesterol, phospholipids, and neutral fat are not. It should be remembered that only formalin-fixed, frozen sections can be used for a polariscopic examination for lipids.

Doubly refractile lipids are present regularly: (1) in the tuberous and plane xanthomas and xanthelasmata (but not always in the eruptive xanthomas) of hyperlipoproteinemia (see p. 366); (2) in the cutaneous lesions of diffuse normolipemic plane xanthoma (see p. 378); and (3) in the vascular walls of angiokeratoma corporis diffusum (Fabry's disease) (see p. 370).

Doubly refractile lipids are present, provided that the cutaneous lesions contain a sufficient amount of lipid: (1) in histiocytosis (Hand-Schüller-Christian type) (see p. 375); (2) in juvenile xanthogranuloma, or nevoxantho-endothelioma (see p. 378); (3) in erythema elevatum diutinum (extracellular cholesterosis type) (see p. 168); and (4) in dermatofibroma (lipidized "histiocytoma") (see p. 572).

Doubly refractile lipids are absent in the lipid-containing lesions, as a rule: (1) in necrobiosis lipoidica (see p. 220); (2) in hyalinosis cutis et mucosae, or lipoid proteinosis (see p. 395), and (3) in multicentric reticulohistiocytosis and solitary reticulohistiocytic granuloma (see p. 380).

Among foreign bodies, silica causes granulomas showing doubly refractile spicules. Such granulomas are caused either by particles of soil or glass (silicon dioxide) or by talcum powder (magnesium silicate) (see p. 204).

Gout tophi show double refraction of the urate crystals present within them, provided that the crystals are sufficiently preserved. This is accomplished by using alcohol rather than formalin for fixation (see p. 402).

Amyloid shows a characteristic green birefringence in polarized light after staining with alkaline Congo red (see p. 386).

BIBLIOGRAPHY

Cawley, E. P., Lupton, C. H., Jr., Wheeler, C. E., and McManus, J. F. A.: Examination of normal and myxedematous skin. Use of Mowry's Alcian blue periodic acid-Schiff technique. Arch. Derm., *76*:537, 1957.

Helwig, E. B., and Graham, J. H.: Anogenital (extramammary) Paget's disease; a clinicopathological study. Cancer, *16*:387, 1963.

Johnson, W. C., and Helwig, E. B.: Histochemistry of the acid mucopolysaccharides of the skin in normal and in certain pathologic conditions. Am. J. Clin. Path., *40*:123, 1963.

Kligman, A. M., Mescon, H., and DeLamater, E. D.: The Hotchkiss-McManus stain for the histopathologic diagnosis of fungus diseases. Am. J. Clin. Path., *21*:86, 1951.

Luna, L. G. (ed.): Manual of Histologic Staining Methods of the Armed Forces Institute of Pathology. ed. 3. New York, McGraw-Hill, 1968.

Pearse, A. G. E.: Histochemistry, Theoretical and Applied. ed. 3. Boston, Little, Brown and Co., 1972.

Stoughton, R., and Wells, G.: A histochemical study on polysaccharides in normal and diseased skin. J. Invest. Derm., *14*:37, 1950.

5

Morphology of the Cells
in the Dermal Infiltrate

Various types of cells, largely derived from the bone marrow, infiltrate the dermis and occasionally also the epidermis in the inflammatory and the granulomatous dermatoses. It is important for diagnostic purposes to identify the cell types. Three groups of cells are derived from the bone-marrow: (1) the granulocytic group; (2) the lymphocytic group, including the plasma cell; and (3) the monocytic or macrophagic group. In addition there are two types of cells present as such in the dermis that may participate in the cellular proliferation occurring in the inflammatory and granulomatous dermatoses: the mast cell and the fibroblast. (For discussion of the fibroblast and its functions, see p. 33.)

GRANULOCYTIC GROUP

Neutrophilic and eosinophilic granulocytes are found in the skin in various dermatoses. Basophilic granulocytes are seen in the skin in delayed hypersensitivity reactions, such as contact dermatitis (Dvorak and Mihm).

Neutrophilic Granulocyte. This cell, also called neutrophil or polymorphonuclear leukocyte, has a lobated nucleus consisting of several segments that are connected only by narrow bridges of nucleoplasm. The slightly basophilic cytoplasm contains numerous neutrophilic to slightly eosinophilic granules that measure from 0.1 to 0.3 μm in diameter (Macher). On histochemical examination, the granules contain, in addition to peroxi-

dase, lysosomal enzymes and thus represent primary lysosomes.

Neutrophilic granulocytes play an important role (1) in the early phase of some inflammatory responses; (2) in the phagocytosis of microorganisms; and (3) in the immobilization and attempted phagocytosis of antigen-antibody complexes in the presence of compliment (Wilkinson). The phagocytosis of microorganisms and of antigen-antibody complexes is accompanied by partial to complete degranulation of the neutrophils (Parish, 1969).

Examples of the participation of neutrophils in the early phase of inflammation is their presence in primary irritant dermatitis, and in the early phase of nodular nonsuppurative perniculitis and of erythema nodosum. Phagocytosis of microorganisms is seen in the subcorneal pustules of impetigo and candidiasis, in staphylococcal folliculitis, in erysipelas, and in cellulitis. Association of neutrophils with immune complexes occurs in allergic vasculitis (anaphylactoid purpura) and possibly also in its variants: erythema elevatum diutinum and acute febrile neutrophilic dermatosis of Sweet, as well as in the neutrophilic vasculitis and papillary microabscesses of dermatitis herpetiformis. The reason for the presence of neutrophils in the spongiform pustule of Kogoj observed in psoriasis and its variants, and in the subcorneal pustule of subcorneal pustular dermatosis is not known.

Histogenesis. Neutrophils phagocytize and kill microorganisms by incorporating the microorganisms into their cytoplasm through endocytosis, resulting in a phagocytic vacuole or phagosome that is lined by the invaginated plasma membrane. Into this phagosome many neutrophilic granules discharge their lysosomal enzymes, making it a phagolysosome. Among the lysosomal enzymes are acid phosphatase, beta-glucuronidase and nonspecific esterase, as well as phagocytin and myeloperoxidase. Phagocytin degrades and lyses bacterial cell walls; and myeloperoxidase mediates the formation of hydrogen peroxide within the phagolysosome. Hydrogen peroxide is essential for the killing of many bacteria (Klebanoff and White). (The inability of the neutrophils in "chronic granulomatous disease of childhood" to generate hydrogen peroxide, according to Klebanoff and White, is the cause of the frequent severe infections that ultimately cause death in this disease.)

Immune complexes, when activated by complement, induce the accumulation of neutrophils, possibly by chemotaxis. The immune complexes may be phagocytized by neutrophils which then discharge lysosomal enzymes into the phagosome; or, if the complexes are attached to the basal lamina located either around a blood vessel or at the epidermal-dermal border, the neutrophils may release their lysosomal constituents by direct exocytosis of granules (Henson). Since the granules also contain a collagenase and an elastase, considerable damage can ensue to the basal lamina and even the walls of blood vessels through the exocytosis of neutrophilic granules (Lazarus et al.).

Eosinophilic Granulocyte. The eosinophil is characterized by the presence of numerous large, eosinophilic granules that nearly fill the cytoplasm. They are considerably larger than the granules of neutrophils, measuring up to 1 μm in diameter (Poole). The granules are visible with routine stains but stand out more clearly in brilliant red color when Giemsa's stain is used. The nucleus of eosinophils, in contrast to that of neutrophils, usually is bilobed, rather than segmented (Macher).

Since eosinophils can phagocytize mast cell granules and certain antigen-antibody complexes, tissue eosinophilia in the skin occurs: (1) as the result of anaphylactic or atopic hypersensitivity; (2) subsequent to the degranulation of mast cells; and (3) in certain diseases associated with deposits of antigen-antibody complexes in the skin.

The tissue eosinophilia appearing in anaphylactic reactions and other forms of "immediate" allergy such as atopy is based on the attachment of antibodies of the IgE type to the surface of mast cells. The anaphylactic reaction occurs following the binding of the specific antigen to the specific antibody on the surface of the mast cells. This leads to a degranulation of mast cells, and to the release of the histamine present in their granules. Wherever degranulation of mast cells occurs eosinophils appear, and the eosinophils phagocytize the released mast cell granules (Parish, 1970).

Degranulation of mast cells as the cause of tissue eosinophilia occurs also in urticaria pigmentosa after stroking the lesions. Diseases in which deposition of antigen-antibody complexes are the cause of eosinophilia include pemphigus vulgaris, particularly pemphigus vegetans, pemphigus foliaceus, bullous pemphigoid, and granuloma faciale. The reasons for the occasional presence of tissue eosinophilia in histiocytosis, in Hodgkin's disease, and in mycosis fungoides are not fully apparent.

Histogenesis. The granules of eosinophils, on electron microscopic examination, are oval or boat-shaped. In the center of each granule is a crystal having a rectangular or rhomboidal outline. In electron microscopic sections stained with lead compounds the crystal is more darkly stained than the rest of the granule (Poole). The eosinophilic granules, because of their specific structure, cannot actually be called lysosomes, even though they do contain lysosomal enzymes, e.g., a peroxidase in the crystals, and acid phosphatase in the granule envelope (Poole). The phagocytic potential of eosinophils seems to be limited to immune complexes and mast cell granules. It is doubted that eosinophils are attracted by histamine as such, but rather by the mast cell granules containing the histamine (Mann). Also microorganisms generally are not phagocytized by eosinophils. (For phagocytosis of mast cell granules, see p. 57.)

LYMPHOCYTIC GROUP

Histogenesis. There are two types of peripheral lymphocytes: T and B lymphocytes. Both types of cells arise in the bone marrow, from which one type migrates to the thymus, where it differentiates to a lymphocyte, and then proceeds to the peripheral lymphoid tissues as thymus-derived or T lymphocyte. In lymph nodes T lymphocytes are located predominantly in the paracortical areas. The other type of lymphocyte, the B lymphocyte, differentiates without passing through the thymus. It may differentiate in the gut-associated lymphoid tissue, such as the tonsils, the appendix and the Peyer patches. In lymph nodes B lymphocytes occupy largely the medullary cords and the lymphoid follicles including their germinal centers (Alonso et al.). The term B lymphocytes, meaning bursa-derived lymphocytes, was given to them because in birds this type of lymphocyte differentiates in the bursa of Fabricius. In humans, the term B lymphocyte is used to mean bone-marrow-derived lymphocyte (Raff). Although T and B cells are indistinguishable by light microscopy, they can be differentiated by in vitro tests and by scanning electron microscopy. Human T lymphocytes have receptors for sheep red blood cells so that sheep red blood cells form rosettes around T lymphocytes. In contrast, human B lymphocytes generally have receptors for the third component of complement bound to human red blood cells so that complement-coated human red blood cells form rosettes around B lymphocytes. By scanning electron microscopy, T rosetting lymphocytes usually are smaller than B rosetting lymphocytes and have fewer and shorter microvilli (Lin et al.). The percentage of B cells among lymphocytes in normal human blood is approximately 25 per cent (Wybran and Fudenberg).

The T lymphocytes, on stimulation by an antigen, change in lymph nodes into pyroninophilic lymphoblasts or blast cells that produce antibodies built into their cell membrane. After a few days the blast cells change back into small lymphocytes and circulate. These antibody-carrying "committed" lymphocytes evoke a delayed or "cell-mediated" hypersensitivity on re-exposure to the antigen to which they have become sensitized. (See also p. 100.)

The B lymphocytes, on antigenic stimulation, become plasma cells which produce immunoglobulins, either IgA, IgD, IgE, IgG, or IgM. These immunoglobulins circulate in the peripheral blood as "humoral" antibodies which, on encountering the appropriate antigen, produce humoral hypersensitivity (Nowell and Wilson). (For further discussion on humoral antibodies, see below, under Plasma Cells.)

Of interest is the prevalence of B lymphocytes and T lymphocytes, respectively, in various lymphoid proliferations. Most examples of chronic lymphocytic leukemia and of nodular lymphoma represent B cell proliferations (Jaffe et al.); whereas the Sézary syndrome and mycosis fungoides represent T cell proliferations (Seligmann).

Histology of Lymphocytes. Lymphocytes possess a relatively small, round nucleus that appears deeply basophilic because of the presence of numerous chromatin particles. It is usually impossible by light microscopy to distinguish lymphocytes from monocytes in routinely stained histologic sections; and in several instances where it was once assumed that lymphocytes were an important constituent of the dermal infiltrate it has been shown through demonstrating the presence of lysosomal enzymes within the cells and through electron microscopy that many of the cells are monocytes rather than lymphocytes, for instance, in contact dermatitis and in sarcoidosis. It is, therefore, preferable to refer to cells with a histologic appearance of lymphocytes as lymphoid cells.

Lymphocytes in Delayed Hypersensitivity. Delayed hypersensitivity can be evoked by a variety of agents, such as contact allergens and many microorganisms, such as mycobacteria, virus and fungi. In addition, the rejection of tissue homografts represents a delayed hypersensitivity reaction. The number of specifically sensitized or "committed" lymphocytes, which carry the antibody to the antigen and thus induce the delayed hypersensitivity reaction, generally is small so that they do not dominate the histologic picture. Thus, in contact dermatitis monocytes or macrophages predominate. They phagocytize the damaged cells at the site of the antigen-antibody reaction (Macher). Their number is increased by a factor released by the committed lymphocytes called macrophage migration inhibiting factor (MIF). (For further details see under Histogenesis of contact dermatitis, p. 100.) In many instances, the delayed hypersensitivity reaction to microorganisms is granulomatous in nature, for instance in tuberculosis and many deep fungal infections, such as blastomycosis.

Nonsensitized Lymphocytes. Lymphocytes are the predominant cell in most chronic inflammations of the skin. They predominate, for instance, in psoriasis, lichen planus, and lupus erythematosus. They also predominate in lymphocytic vasculitis, as seen in pityriasis lichenoides et varioliformis acuta.

PLASMA CELL

The plasma cell has abundant cytoplasm that is deeply basophilic, homogeneous, and sharply defined. The round nucleus is eccentrically placed and shows along its membrane coarse, deeply basophilic, regularly distributed chromatin particles. This gives the nucleus a cartwheel appearance. The fact that patients with agammaglobulinemia lack plasma cells has been responsible for an early recognition of the fact that the plasma cell is the site of formation of all immunoglobulins that circulate as humoral antibodies. The synthesis of immunoglobulins takes place in plasma cells located mainly in the lymph nodes, the spleen, and the bone marrow. Since plasma cells are tissue cells and are not seen in the peripheral circulation, it can be assumed that, if they are present in the dermis, they have developed in the dermis from B lymphocytes (see p. 52 and under Histogenesis).

Plasma cells are apt to be present in conspicuous numbers in several infectious diseases, e.g., in early syphilis, rhinoscleroma and granuloma inguinale, as well as in chronic deep folliculitis and in balanitis chronica plasmacellularis. It is not clear why in some instances the chronic inflammatory infiltrate of mycosis fungoides, solar keratosis, or other diseases, contains numerous plasma cells, whereas in most instances the infiltrate contains few plasma cells or even none.

In the presence of many plasma cells, but especially in rhinoscleroma and multiple myeloma, round, hyaline, eosinophilic bodies, called Russell bodies, may be found within and outside of plasma cells. They form within plasma cells as the result of a disturbance in their protein synthesis and are ultimately expelled (Pearse). They may possess a size twice that of normal plasma cells, measuring up to 20 μm in diameter. They contain varying amounts of glycoproteins and are as a rule gram-positive as well as PAS-positive and diastase-resistant (Tappeiner et al.).

Histogenesis. On electron microscopy plasma cells are characterized by the presence in their cytoplasm of an extensive system of cisternae lined by a rough endoplasmic reticulum. The cisternae usually are flat but may be irregularly dilated. Numerous ribosomes not only line the membranes of the endoplasmic reticulum but are present also in the cytoplasm. The abundant ribosomes and the highly developed endoplasmic reticulum are involved in the synthesis of immunoglobulins. Thus, the cisternae are often filled with a homogeneous to granular substance which is released into the extracellular space. Also, the Russell bodies form within the rough endoplasmic reticulum. It is likely that these bodies represent accumulated light chains that are not utilized in the biosynthesis of the complete immunoglobulin molecule (Fisher and Zawadzki).

The development of plasma cells from B lymphocytes in lymph nodes can be observed following a secondary challenge with horseradish peroxidase. The lymphocytes in their development into plasma cells change into blast cells, in which a system of antibody-secreting rough endoplasmic reticulum then appears (Murphy et al.).

MONOCYTIC OR MACROPHAGIC GROUP

Macrophages, also called histiocytes, are of bone marrow origin. They circulate in the blood and enter the tissue as monocytes (Carr; Spector). Upon proper stimulation monocytes develop into macrophages and may develop further into epithelioid cells and foreign body giant cells, thus forming granulomas. The stimulation of monocytes to become macrophages can come (1) from microorganisms; (2) from damaged tissue and cells; or (3) from metabolic by-products or foreign material. In the process of phagocytosis of pyogenic microorganisms macrophages follow the neutrophils, since neutrophils constitute the "first line of defense" in combatting pyogenic infection (Stossel). However, in other infections macrophages phagocytize the microorganisms from the beginning, e.g., bacteria, such as lepra bacilli, Frisch bacilli, and Donovan bodies; fungi, such as *Histoplasma capsulatum;* and protozoa, such as *Leishmania tropica.* In the phagocytosis of damaged tissue and cells after the development of delayed hypersensitivity the effectiveness of the macrophages is increased through various factors secreted by the specifically sensitized lymphocytes. One of these factors is the macrophage migration inhibiting factor (MIF) (see p. 52 and p. 101). Among the metabolic by-products and foreign substances that may be ingested by macrophages are lipids, changing the macrophages into foam cells; melanin, changing them into melanophages; and hemosiderin.

Histologically, monocytes are indistinguishable from lymphocytes, since both cells have a small, dark, rounded nucleus and very scanty cytoplasm that cannot be recognized in routine sections. The only means by which monocytes can be differentiated from lymphocytes in histologic sections is through staining for lysosomal enzymes, such as acid phosphatase, since they are present in monocytes and absent in lymphocytes. Thus, it has been possible through enzymatic staining and electron microscopy to identify as monocytes most of the cells with small, dark nuclei present in contact dermatitis and at the periphery of sarcoidal granulomas (see pp. 101 and 213).

Macrophages, or histiocytes, since they are activated monocytes, are larger cells than monocytes and usually have a lightly staining, elongated nucleus with a clearly visible nuclear membrane. Their cytoplasm cannot be recognized in routine stains. Often, it is impossible in routinely stained sections to distinguish macrophages from fibroblasts or from endothelial cells, except through their respective locations or activities, but this is not always a reliable criterion. Histochemical staining for enzymes often is helpful in their distinction, although it must be kept in mind that in some pathologic conditions fibroblasts may also contain many lysosomes and then stain positive for lysosomal enzymes, for instance in dermatofibroma and Kaposi's sarcoma (see pp. 573 and 608).

Epithelioid Cell. Epithelioid cells arise from macrophages (1) when there is nothing to phagocytize, as in sarcoidosis; (2) after the macrophages have completed phagocytosis of a digestible product such as bacteria; or (3) after the macrophages have eliminated by exocytosis an indigestible product, as, for instance, certain foreign materials of metabolic by-products (Papadimitriou and Spector, 1971). It seems likely that the majority of epithelioid cells in lesions of tuberculosis and tuberculoid leprosy are derived from macrophages that have never digested bacilli because more macrophages entered the area than were needed to engulf the organisms present (Papadimitriou and Spector, 1972) (see below under Electron microscopic examination). Epithelioid cells thus form in infections that already have evoked an immunologic reaction (see p. 53), as it occurs in instances of tuberculosis with little necrosis, in tuberculoid leprosy, in tertiary syphilis, and in deep fungus infections. Foreign body reactions in which epithelioid-cell granulomas are apt to be seen include systemic berylliosis, zirconium granulomas, and tattoo granulomas, all of which are associated with a delayed hypersensitivity reaction. The cause for the formation of epithelioid-cell granulomas in sarcoidosis, in which delayed hypersensitivity reactions are depressed, is not known.

Histologically, epithelioid cells lie, similar to epithelial cells, in groups, either as "naked" epithelioid-cell tubercles or intermingled with monocytes, macrophages, and often also foreign body giant cells. (Formerly, the monocytes were misinterpreted as lymphocytes; see p. 52.) Epithelioid cells possess a large, usually oval, pale, vesicular nucleus with a clearly visible nuclear membrane. The nucleus thus does not differ from that of macrophages, except that it is on the average slightly larger. The two cells, however, differ in their cytoplasm. Whereas the cytoplasm of macrophages is difficult to recognize in routine stains, epithelioid cells have abundant, ill defined, slightly eosinophilic cytoplasm. Pseudopodic elongations of the cytoplasm usually are present, and the cytoplasm of adjoining epithelioid cells often has coalesced.

Foreign Body Giant Cells. As macrophages mature they show less tendency to divide and a greater tendency to fuse into multinucleated giant cells (Carter and Roberts). Thus, foreign body giant cells, like epithelioid cells, no longer are phagocytizing cells. It has been customary to distinguish between multinucleated giant cells of the Langhans type occurring with epithelioid cells in delayed hypersensitivity granulomas and multinucleated giant cells of the foreign body type: Whereas in giant cells of the Langhans type the nuclei are located along the periphery of the giant cell in a semicircular fashion, they lie in giant cells of the foreign body type either irregularly distributed or in clusters. However, transitions between the two forms occur and they often occur together, both in delayed hypersensitivity granulomas and in foreign body granulomas so that their morphologic distinction often is impossible. Multinucleated foreign body giant cells are seen: (1) in a number of foreign body reactions, as in paraffinomas and silica reactions; (2) in the vicinity of metabolic by-products, as in gout and calcinosis; (3) in areas where keratin is in direct contact with the dermis, as in calcifying epithelioma of Malherbe, in ruptured hair follicles, as seen in acne vulgaris and Trichophyton rubrum granuloma, and in ruptured epidermal cysts or milia, and (4) in areas of tissue necrosis, as in necrobiosis lipoidica.

Histologically, both types of multinucleated giant cells usually show a well demarcated cytoplasm. The number of nuclei may exceed 100. The occasional presence of asteroid bodies and of Schaumann bodies within them is not specific for any disease. (For their discussion, see pp. 212 and 213.)

Histogenesis. The origin of the tissue monocytes in human skin from blood monocytes has been established in healthy probands through transfusion of tritiated-thymidine-labeled monocytes which were observed 3 hours later in skin window exudates (Meuret et al.). On the other hand, the dermal infiltrate of monocytes and macrophages in patients with chronic dermatitis is largely self-renewing, since the monocyte recruitment rate is low in these patients following the autotransfusion of labeled monocytes (Meuret et al.).

The derivation of the macrophages present in cutaneous granulomas from the circulating blood has been proved also in animals. In rats, fairly persistent cutaneous granulomas can be produced by the intradermal injection of bovine serum albumin, provided that the rats have a high antibody titer against the bovine serum albumin (Spector and Heesom). In rats in whom granulomas have thus been produced labeling of the circulating neutrophils and monocytes with tritiated thymidine shows that during the first week more labeled neutrophils than monocytes invade the granulomas. In subsequent weeks considerably more labeled monocytes than labeled neutrophils emigrate from the capillaries into the granulomas. In the final weeks, however, of the 12-week life span of the granulomas fresh emigration of labeled monocytes makes only a minor contribution to the granulomas in comparison with the mitotic division of the macrophages in the granulomas (Spector et al.).

Electron microscopic examination reveals monocytes to possess scattered through their cytoplasm many primary lysosomes as small dense bodies (Papadimitriou and Spector, 1971). Macrophages, which represent stimulated monocytes, differ from monocytes by being larger, by showing longer processes, and by containing a greater number of lysosomes (Carr). Many macrophages contain phagocytized material within phagosomes that through the influx of the contents of primary lysosomes have become phagolysosomes. If in experimental infections the bacteria kill the macrophages, other macrophages take over (Papadimitriou and Spector, 1972). Most epithelioid cells appear to evolve from macrophages that have never ingested any bacteria or antigen-antibody complexes. Such epithelioid cells are characterized by the presence of many primary lysosomes. Only a small percentage of the epithelioid cells show some evidence of past phagocytosis in the form of small residual bodies or of phagolysosomes. In general, it seems therefore that persistence of active phagolysosomes is an effective deterrent to epithelioid cell formation (Papadimitriou and Spector, 1971).

Multinucleated foreign body giant cells are formed by the fusion of nonproliferating macrophages. Active phagocytosis by macrophages and giant cell formation are mutually exclusive (Papadimitriou et al.). As evidence that the macrophages that form the multinucleated giant cells are nondividing cells, on labeling with tritiated thymidine, the macrophages in the vicinity of the giant cells show no DNA-synthesis (Carter and Roberts). Similarly, there is no DNA-synthesis in the nuclei of giant cells (Black and Epstein).

MAST CELL

Mast cells occur in the normal dermis in small numbers as spindle-shaped cells with an oval nucleus. They contain in their cytoplasm numerous granules which do not stain with routine stains such as hematoxylin and eosin. Mast cells, therefore, in normal skin usually are indistinguishable from fibroblasts, although occasionally one can recognize in mast cells, in contrast with fibroblasts, the cell membrane. The granules stain with methylene blue, which is present in Giemsa's stain, with toluidine blue, and with alcian blue. The granules stain metachromatically with methylene blue or toluidine blue, i.e., they stain in a color different from that possessed by the dye. In this sense methylene blue and toluidine blue stain the granules purplish-red rather than blue. The granules measure up to 0.8 μm in diameter (Hashimoto et al., 1967).

Mast cell granules produce and store two substances, heparin and histamine. On degranulation of the mast cell these two substances are released into the tissue, whereby histamine increases the permeability of the capillaries and, if released in sufficient amounts, may produce a histamine shock. The surface of the mast cells carries in "anaphylactically" sensitized individuals specific antibodies of the IgE type. When the specific antigen combines with these antibodies and anaphylactic reaction is elicited through the degranulation of mast cells and the release of histamine from the mast cell granules (Mota; Macher).

The normal dermis contains mast cells mainly in the vicinity of capillaries. Since the greatest number of capillaries is present in the subpapillary region and in the vicinity of the cutaneous appendages, most mast cells are observed in these areas (Okonkwo et al.). The number of mast cells in the dermis is increased in many inflammatory conditions, where they are found intermingled with various "inflammatory" cells, for instance, in the granulation tissue of healing wounds and in atopic dermatitis, lichen planus, lupus erythematosus, and pemphigus vulgaris (Mikhail and Miller-Milinska). The dermal infiltrate in these conditions is, as a rule, easily differentiated from that of urticaria pigmentosa in which the infiltrate, even though it may be fairly slight, consists exclusively of mast cells, except for the presence of a slight admixture

of eosinophils as a result of the degranulation of some of the mast cells (see below under Histogenesis, and on p. 84 under Urticaria Pigmentosa). Also in many tumors, particularly in benign tumors, the stroma contains an increased number of mast cells (Cawley and Hoch-Ligeti). The number of mast cells in neurofibromas is particularly large (Crowe et al.).

Histogenesis. The fact that mast cell granules produce and store heparin and histamine was first established on the basis of the good correlation between the amounts of extractable heparin and histamine on the one side and the mast cell count of certain tissues on the other (Jorpes; Riley and West). The synthesis of histamine and heparin in mast cells has been proved with the aid of radioactive compounds. Thus, Schayer demonstrated that mast cell suspensions decarboxylate ^{14}C-L-histidine and bind the resulting histamine; and Korn proved the synthesis of heparin in mast cells, by showing that incubation of slices of mouse mast cell tumors with either radioactive glucose or sulfate resulted in the incorporation of this radioactive material into the heparin extractable from the tumor slices.

Basophilic leukocytes possess slightly larger granules than mast cells (Dvorak and Mihm) but with the same physiologic functions (Rorsman et al.) and the same electron microscopic appearance (Poole) (see below). However, basophilic leukocytes differ from mast cells in their genesis and the appearance of their nuclei. Whereas mast cells arise from undifferentiated mesenchymal cells in the perivascular areas of connective tissue (Asboe-Hansen), basophilic leukocytes are of myeloid origin; and, in contrast to the oval nucleus of mast cells, the nucleus of basophilic leukocytes is segmented. Mast cells show a certain relationship to melanocytes, as pointed out by Okun and Zook (see p. 85).

Electron microscopic examination of mast cells reveals numerous large and long villi at their periphery (E.M. No. 18, see under Urticaria Pigmentosa). The mast cell granules appear as rounded structures of varying electron density. They seem to arise in the Golgi zone (Kobayasi and Asboe-Hansen). Three major components can be seen within the mast cell granules: (a) moderately electron-dense fine filaments in parallel arrangement often containing crystalloid structures; (b) very dense, finely granular material; and (c) thick curved parallel lamellae suggesting finger prints in their configuration (E.M. No. 18, see under Urticaria Pigmentosa) (Hashimoto et al., 1967; Lagunoff). Each granule is surrounded by a trilaminar membrane.

Degranulation of the human mast cells following stroking of a lesion of urticaria pigmentosa is maximal after one minute (Kobayasi and Asboe-Hansen). However, in vitro degranulation of peritoneal mast cells of rats induced by the histamine liberator Compound 48/80 requires 4 minutes; and the degranulation brought about by horse serum in sensitized animals is maximal only after an incubation period of 20 minutes (Mann, 1969, II). Degranulation usually consists of the extrusion of entire granules, but some of the granules may undergo intracellular disintegration (Hashimoto et al; Kobayasi and Asboe-Hansen). Extrusion of granules takes place through extensive membrane fusion between the plasma membrane and perigranular membranes, and between adjacent perigranular membranes, resulting in extensive labyrinthine channels in the cell, through which the granules are released from their intracellular sacs (Lagunoff).

Concomitant with their release into the extracellular space the granules release histamine and heparin and lose much of their electron density. Many granules are phagocytized by eosinophils. The granules are taken into the eosinophil by endocytosis in a membrane-lined vacuole. Once within the eosinophil the phagosomal membrane surrounding the mast cell granule breaks down and the mast cell granule is digested by the eosinophil not through lysosomal activity but by intracytoplasmic enzymes. It has been shown that it is the mast cell granule and not just the histamine to which the eosinophil is attracted. The eosinophil, in phagocytizing the mast cell granules, reduces the severity of histamine shock (Mann, 1969, I).

BIBLIOGRAPHY

Granulocytic Group

Dvorak, H. F., and Mihm, M. C., Jr.: Basophilic leukocytes in a case of poison ivy. New Eng. J. Med., *285*:54, 1971.

Henson, P. M.: Pathologic mechanisms in neutrophil-mediated injury. Am. J. Path., *68*:593, 1972.

Klebanoff, S. J., and White, L. R.: Iodination defect in the leukocytes of a patient with chronic granulomatous disease of childhood. New Eng. J. Med., *280*:460, 1969.

Lazarus, G. S., Daniels, J. R., Lian, J., and Burleigh, M. C.: Role of granulocyte collagenase in collagen degradation. Am. J. Path., *68*:565, 1972.

Litt, M.: Studies in experimental eosinophilia. VI. Uptake of immune complexes by eosinophils. J. Cell Biol., *23*:355, 1964.

Macher, E.: Das entzündliche Haut-Infiltrat. *In* Marchionini, A. (ed.): Handbuch der Haut- und Geschlechtskrankheiten, Ergänzungswerk. Vol. 1, part 2, p. 473. Berlin, Springer, 1964.

Mann, P. R.: An electron-microscope study of the relations between mast cells and eosinophil leukocytes. J. Path., *98*:183, 1969.

Parish, W. E.: Effects of neutrophils on tissues. Brit. J. Derm., *81*(suppl. 3):28, 1969.

————: Investigations on eosinophila. Brit. J. Derm., *82*:42, 1970.

Poole, J. C. F.: Electron microscopy of polymorphonuclear leukocytes. Brit. J. Derm., *81* (suppl. 3):11, 1969.

Wilkinson, D. S.: Pustular dermatoses. Brit. J. Derm., *81*(suppl. 3):38, 1969.

Lymphocytic Group

Alonso, K., Dew, J. M., and Starke, W. R.: Thymic alymphoplasia and congenital aleukocytosis (reticular dysgenesis). Arch. Path., *94*:179, 1972.

Fisher, E. R., and Zawadzki, Z. A.: Ultrastructural features of plasma cells in patients with paraproteinemia. Am. J. Clin. Path., *54*:779, 1970.

Jaffe, E. S., Shevack, E. M., Frank, M. M., *et al.*: Nodular lymphoma—evidence for origin from follicular B lymphocytes. New Eng. J. Med., *290*:813, 1974.

Lin, P. S., Cooper, A. G., and Wortis, H. H.: Scanning electron microscopy of human T-cell and B-cell rosettes. New Eng. J. Med., *289*:548, 1973.

Macher, E.: Das entzündliche Haut-Infiltrat. *In* Marchionini, A. (ed.): Handbuch der Haut- und Geschlechtskrankheiten, Ergänzungswerk. Vol. 1, part 1, p. 473. Berlin, Springer, 1964.

Murphy, M. J., Hay, J. B., Morris, B., and Bessis, M. C.: Ultrastructural analysis of antibody synthesis in cells from lymph and lymph nodes. Am. J. Path., *66*:25, 1972.

Nowell, P. C., and Wilson, D. B.: Lymphocytes and hemic stem cells. Am. J. Path., *65*:641, 1971.

Pearse, A. G. E.: The nature of Russell bodies and Karloff bodies. J. Clin. Path., *2*:81, 1949.

Raff, M. C.: T and B lymphocytes in mice studied by using antisera against surface antigenic markers. Am. J. Path., *65*:467, 1971.

Seligmann, M.: B-cell and T-cell markers in lymphoid proliferations. New Eng. J. Med., *290*:1483, 1974.

Tappeiner, J., Pfleger, L., and Wolff, K.: Das Vorkommen und histochemische Verhalten von Russellschen Körperchen bei plasmacellulären Hautinfiltraten. Arch. klin. exp. Derm., *222*:71, 1965.

Wybran, J., and Fudenberg, H.: How clinically useful is T and B cell quantitation? (Editorial) Ann. Intern. Med., *80*:765, 1974.

Monocytic or Macrophagic Group

Black, M. M., and Epstein, W. L.: Formation of multinucleate giant cells in organized epithelioid cell granulomas. Am. J. Path., *74*:263, 1974.

Carr, I.: The cellular basis of reticulo-endothelial stimulation. J. Path., *94*:323, 1967.

Carter, R. L., and Roberts, J. D. B.: Macrophages and multinucleate giant cells in nitrosoquinoline-induced granulomata in rats: An autoradiographic study. J. Path., *105*:285, 1971.

Meuret, G., Marwendel, A., and Brand, E. T.: Makrophagenrekrutierung aus Blutmonocyten bei Entzündungsreaktionen der Haut. Arch. Derm. Forsch., *245*:254, 1972.

Papadimitriou, J. M., Sforsina, D., and Papaelias, L.: Kinetics of multinucleate giant cell formation and their modifications by various agents in foreign body reactions. Am. J. Path., *73*:349, 1973.

Papadimitriou, J. M., and Spector, W. G.: The origin, properties and fate of epithelioid cells. J. Path., *105*:187, 1971.

———: The ultrastructure of high- and low-turnover inflammatory granulomata. J. Path., *106*:37, 1972.

Spector, W. G.: Recent advances in the study of leukocyte emigration. Brit. J. Derm., *81* (suppl. 3):19, 1969.

Spector, W. G., and Heesom, N.: The production of granulomata by antigen-antibody complexes. J. Path., *98*:31, 1969.

Spector, W. G., Lykke, A. W. J., and Willoughby, D. A.: A quantitative study of leukocyte emigration in chronic inflammatory granulomata. J. Path., *93*:101, 1967.

Stossel, T. P.: Phagocytosis: The department of defense. New Eng. J. Med., *286*:776, 1972.

Mast Cell

Asboe-Hansen, G.: The mast cell in health and disease. Acta dermatoven., *53* (suppl. 73): 139, 1973.

Cawley, E. P., and Hoch-Ligeti, C.: Association of tissue mast cells and skin tumors. Arch. Derm., *83*:92, 1961.

Crowe, F. W., Schull, W. J., and Neel, J. V.: Multiple Neurofibromatosis. Springfield, Ill., Charles C Thomas, 1955.

Dvorak, H. F., and Mihm, M. C., Jr.: Basophilic leukocytes in a case of poison ivy. New Eng. J. Med., *285*:55, 1971.

Hashimoto, K., Gross, B. G., and Lever, W. F.: An electron microscopic study of the degranulation of mast cell granules in urticaria pigmentosa. J. Invest. Derm., *46*:139, 1966.

Hashimoto, K., Tarnowski, W. M., and Lever, W. F.: Reifung und Degranulierung der Mastzellen in der menschlichen Haut. Hautarzt, *18*:318, 1967.

Jorpes, E. J.: Heparin. p. 30. London, Oxford University Press, 1939.

Kobayasi, T., and Asboe-Hansen, G.: Degranulation and regranulation of human mast cells. Acta dermatoven., *49*:369, 1969.

Korn, E. D.: The synthesis of heparin by slices of mouse mast cell tumor. J. Biol. Chem., *234*:1321, 1959.

Lagunoff, D.: Contributions of electron microscopy to the study of mast cells. J. Invest. Derm., *58*:296, 1972.

Macher, E.: Immunologische Mechanismen der Allergie. Z. Haut, *47*:307, 1972.

Mann, P. R.: An electron-microscope study of the relations between mast cells and eosinophilic leukocytes. J. Path., *98*:183, 1969 (I).

———: An electron microscope study of the degranulation of rat peritoneal mast cells brought about by four different agents. Brit. J. Derm., *81*:926, 1969 (II).

Mikhail, G. R., and Miller-Milinska, A.: Mast cell population in human skin. J. Invest. Derm., *43*:249, 1964.

Mota, I.: Mast cells and anaphylaxis. Ann. N.Y. Acad. Sci., *103*:264, 1963.

Okonkwo, B., Rust, S., and Steigleder, G. K.: Die Verteilung der Mastzellen in der gesunden menschlichen Haut. Arch. klin. exp. Derm., *223*:99, 1965.

Okun, M. R., and Zook, B. C.: Histologic parallels between mastocytoma and melanoma. Arch. Derm., *95*:275, 1967.

Poole, J. C. F.: Electron microscopy of polymorphonuclear leukocytes. Brit. J. Derm., *81*(suppl. 3):11, 1969.

Riley, J. F., and West, G. B.: Skin histamine; its location in the tissue mast cells. Arch. Derm., *74*:471, 1956.

Rorsman, H., Slatkin, M. W., Harber, L. C., and Baer, R. L.: The basophil leukocyte in urticarial hypersensitivity to physical agents. J. Invest. Derm. *39*:493, 1962.

Schayer, R. W.: Formation and binding of histamine by free mast cells of rat peritoneal fluid. Am. J. Physiol., *186*:199, 1956.

6

Congenital Diseases (Genodermatoses)

ICHTHYOSIS

A classification of ichthyosis includes four major forms: (1) dominantly inherited ichthyosis vulgaris; (2) sex-linked ichthyosis; (3) dominantly inherited congenital ichthyosiform erythroderma, with a diagnostic histologic picture referred to either as epidermolytic hyperkeratosis or granular degeneration; and (4) recessively inherited congenital ichthyosiform erythroderma, also referred to as lamellar ichthyosis.

In addition, there are two rare forms of ichthyosis, namely: (5) dominantly inherited erythrokeratodermia variabilis and (6) recessively inherited ichthyosis linearis circumflexa; and at least four syndromes associated with ichthyosis (Tay). All four syndromes are recessively inherited. They are: (7) Rud's syndrome in which ichthyosis vulgaris is associated with infantilism and epilepsy; (8) Refsum's syndrome, showing ichthyosis vulgaris in association with ataxia, progressive paresis of the extremities, and retinitis pigmentosa; it is caused by a metabolic error consisting of an inability to degrade exogenous phytanic acid (Steinberg et al.); (9) Sjögren-Larsson syndrome, showing congenital ichthyosiform erythroderma in association with mental retardation and spastic paresis (Heijer and Reed); and (10) Netherton's syndrome, consisting of a combination of either congenital ichthyosiform erythrodema or ichthyosis linearis circumflexa with anomalies of the scalp hair (see p. 183).

DOMINANT ICHTHYOSIS VULGARIS

Dominantly inherited ichthyosis vulgaris, a common disorder, develops a few months after birth. The skin shows scales that on the extensor surfaces of the extremities are large and adherent, resembling fish scales, and elsewhere are small, resulting in fine branny scaling. The flexural creases are spared. Follicular hyperkeratosis is often present and the palms and soles may show hyperkeratosis. A significant percentage of the patients have atopic dermatitis. A non-inherited form of the disease may appear in patients with lymphoma, especially Hodgkin's disease (Stevanovic).

Histopathology. The characteristic finding is an association of a moderate degree of hyperkeratosis with a thin or absent granular layer (Fig. 6-1). The hyperkeratosis often extends into the hair follicles, resulting in large keratotic follicular plugs. The dermis is normal.

Histogenesis. Labeling with tritiated thymidine shows a normal rate of epidermal proliferation (Frost et al.). The hyperkeratosis is regarded as a retention keratosis resulting from an increased adhesiveness of the stratum corneum (Frost and Van Scott). The reason for this is, as seen by electron microscopy, a delay in the dissolution of the desmosomal disks in the horny layer (Anton-Lamprecht, 1973). The thinness or even absence of the granular layer is the result of a defective synthesis of keratohyaline granules which, by electron microscopy, appear small, crumbly or spongy (Schnyder). The sparsity of keratohyaline matrix in the horn cells makes the horny layer less flexible than it normally is (Anton-Lamprecht, 1973).

SEX-LINKED ICHTHYOSIS

This form of ichthyosis occurs only in males. It may start shortly after birth and, in contrast to dominant ichthyosis vulgaris, may involve the flexural creases.

Histopathology. There is hyperkeratosis, with the granular layer being normal or slightly thickened but not thinned as in dominant ichthyosis vulgaris. The epidermis may be slightly thickened (Feinstein et al.).

Histogenesis. Sex-linked ichthyosis, like dominant ichthyosis vulgaris, shows a normal rate of epidermal proliferation. It is a retention hyperkeratosis resulting from a delayed dissolution of the desmosomal disks in the horny layer. In contrast with dominant ichthyosis vulgaris the synthesis of keratohyaline granules is normal and slightly increased (Anton-Lamprecht, 1974).

DOMINANT CONGENITAL ICHTHYOSIFORM ERYTHRODERMA

A generalized bullous form and a localized nonbullous form exist. The generalized bullous form is also called dominant ichthyosis congenita and, because of the histologic changes it presents, epidermolytic hyperkeratosis (Frost and Van Scott). It shows from the time of birth generalized erythema and thick, brown verrucous scaling. The flexural surfaces of the extremities show marked involvement, often consisting of furrowed hyperkeratosis. Vesicles and bullae are encountered usually only during the first few years.

The histologic findings in the localized nonbullous form of dominant congenital ichthyosiform erythroderma are similar to those of the generalized bullous form. Clinically, however, the nonbullous form resembles systematized linear epidermal nevus and is therefore discussed under that heading (see p. 452).

Histopathology. A characteristic histologic picture is seen in the epidermis (Fig. 6-2). It is referred to as granular degeneration (Ishibashi and Klingmüller) or, not quite justifiedly, as epidermolytic hyperkeratosis (Frost and Van Scott). Although it is most pronounced in bullous areas, it is present also in nonbullous areas (Salamon and Lazovic; Ackerman). One observes: (a) variously sized clear spaces around the nuclei in the upper stratum spinosum and in the stratum granulosum; (b) peripheral to

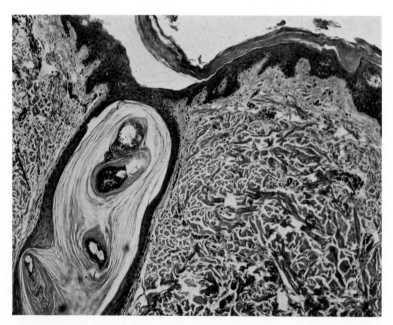

FIG. 6-1. **Dominant ichthyosis vulgaris.** There is a moderate degree of hyperkeratosis in the absence of a granular layer. A large keratotic plug is located within a hair follicle. (×100)

the clear spaces indistinct cellular boundaries formed either by lightly staining material or by keratohyaline granules; (c) a markedly thickened granular layer containing an increased number of irregularly shaped keratohyaline granules; and (d) compact hyperkeratosis (Ackerman). When bullae form they arise intraepidermally, through separation of edematous cells from one another (McCurdy and Beare). The upper dermis shows a moderately severe, chronic inflammatory infiltrate. Mitotic figures are five times more numerous than in normal epidermis (Frost and Van Scott).

Histogenesis. Examination of cryostat and electron microscopic sections from nonbullous areas has revealed that the intracellular clear spaces in the upper epidermis, as seen in routine paraffin sections, are artifacts of shrinkage (Braun-Falco et al.; see p. 453). The essential electron microscopic features are excessive production of tonofilaments and excessive and premature formation of keratohyaline granules so that around the nucleus of the cells numerous keratohyaline granules are embedded in thick shells of irregularly clumped tonofilaments (Ishibashi and Klingmüller; Schnyder). The desmosomes appear normal, but the association of the tonofilaments and desmosomes is disturbed so that many desmosomes are attached to only one keratinocyte, instead of connecting two neighboring keratinocytes. Blister formation takes place because of this disturbance of desmosomal attachment; hence, real acantholysis occurs (Anton-Lamprecht and Schnyder). Labeling with tritiated thymidine reveals greatly increased proliferative activity in the epidermis of dominant congenital ichthyosiform erythroderma (Frost et al.). It can thus be concluded that keratinization is both excessive and abnormal.

RECESSIVE CONGENITAL ICHTHYOSIFORM ERYTHRODERMA

This disorder, also called recessive ichthyosis congenita and lamellar ichthyosis, never shows bullae. It usually is present at birth. In its severest form, the newly born child has the appearance of the "harlequin fetus,"

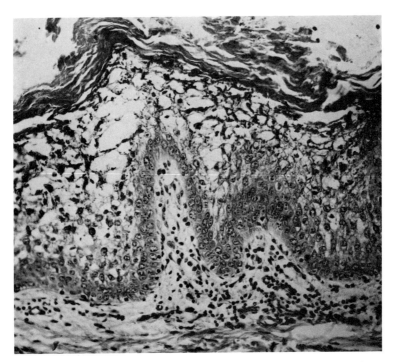

FIG. 6-2. **Dominant congenital ichthyosiform erythroderma.** There is pronounced vacuolization of the cells in the middle and upper portions of the stratum malpighii. These cells show indistinct cellular boundaries. The keratohyaline granules are large and irregularly shaped. (×400)

whereby the skin consists of a thick, horny cuirass with deep fissures, and death usually occurs within two days (Craig et al.). In the less severe "lamellar" type the enveloping horny layer is thin, like collodion, and after its detachment the entire skin, including the flexural surfaces, appears red and scaling. This appearance may persist through life; but in milder cases the erythroderma may gradually subside (Bloom and Goodfried).

Histopathology. In contrast to dominant congenital ichthyosiform erythroderma, the histologic findings in the recessive form are nonspecific. There is moderate hyperkeratosis, with focal parakeratosis in some cases. A granular layer is present and it often is thickened in some areas. In addition, there are moderate acanthosis and a chronic inflammatory infiltrate in the upper dermis (Schnyder and Konrad).

Histogenesis. Labeling with tritiated thymidine has revealed greatly increased numbers of labeled cells per unit surface line in recessive, just as in dominant, congenital ichthyosiform erythroderma, indicative of an increased proliferative activity (Frost et al.). Accordingly, there is an increased number of keratinosomes. An increased amount of intercellular cement substance in the stratum corneum is indicative of an increased adherence of the horny cells (Vandersteen and Muller, 1972).

ERYTHROKERATODERMIA VARIABILIS

This rare, dominantly inherited disorder starts in infancy rather than at birth. It has two morphologic components: (1) discrete configurate patches of erythema that differ in size, location and number and are transient ("variable") but may develop into fixed hyperkeratotic plaques and (2) fixed discrete configurate hyperkeratotic plaques arising as such on normal skin.

Histopathology. The changes are nonspecific and consist of hyperkeratosis with moderate papillomatosis and acanthosis. The granular layer is of normal thickness.

Histogenesis. Labeling with tritiated thymidine shows a normal rate of proliferation (Schellender and Fritsch). The reduction of keratinosomes on electron microscopic examination also

suggests a retention type of hyperkeratosis, since in states of rapid epidermopoiesis they would be increased (Vandersteen and Muller, 1971).

ICHTHYOSIS LINEARIS CIRCUMFLEXA

This recessive disorder is present at birth or starts shortly thereafter and shows extensive migratory polycyclic lesions of erythema and scaling having at the periphery a distinctive "double-edged" scale. The presence of extensive erythema causes a resemblance to psoriasis. The dermatosis persists through life.

Histopathology. The nonspecific changes resemble psoriasis since they include acanthosis, elongation of the rete ridges, and parakeratosis at the periphery of the lesions. However, the center of the lesions shows hyperkeratosis with a well developed granular layer (Altman and Stroud).

KERATOSIS PALMARIS ET PLANTARIS

Four major dominant forms and two recessive forms exist. The four dominant forms are: (1) keratosis palmo-plantaris circumscripta of Unna-Thost, in which there is diffuse palmar and plantar hyperkeratosis without extension to other parts, except occasionally to the volar aspects of the wrists and to the dorsal aspects of the fingers and toes (Schirren and Dinger); (2) keratosis palmo-plantaris linearis, which in some families may alternate with keratosis palmo-plantaris circumscripta (Bologa); (3) keratosis palmo-plantaris punctata (or papulosa), with multiple keratotic papules (Buchanan); and (4) dominant keratosis palmo-plantaris progrediens, showing gradual extension throughout life to the dorsa of the hands and feet, to the ankles and wrists, and to the elbows and knees (Greither, 1952; Meyer-Rohn). The two recessively transmitted forms are: (5) recessive keratosis palmo-plantaris progrediens, also known as the Meleda type, clinically identical with dominantly inherited keratosis palmo-plantaris progrediens (Salamon et al.); and (6) the Papillon-Lefèvre syndrome showing the clinical characteristics of keratosis palmo-plantaris progrediens in association with periodontosis resulting in the loss of first the deciduous teeth and later of the permanent teeth (Bach and Levan).

Histopathology. In all forms, except keratosis palmo-plantaris punctata, the usual histologic picture is nonspecific and consists of considerable hyperkeratosis, hypergranulosis, acanthosis and a mild inflammatory infiltrate in the upper dermis (Salamon et al.; Callan). However, in 6 families with keratosis palmo-plantaris circumscripta of Unna-Thost the histologic examination showed the same type of granular degeneration in the middle and upper malpighian layers seen in dominant congenital ichthyosiform erythroderma and in some lesions of nevus verrucosus (Klaus et al.; Orbaneja et al.). The relative incidence of this change is difficult to determine from the literature, since most reports of cases with keratosis palmo-plantaris do not include a biopsy report.

In keratosis palmo-plantaris punctata there is massive hyperkeratosis over a sharply limited area, with depression of the underlying malpighian layer below the general level of the epidermis. There is increase in thickness of the granular layer. The dermis is free of any inflammatory infiltrate (Buchanan). In two cases reported by Brown and by Herman a cornoid lamella was seen in the center of the hyperkeratotic plug, so that it is possible that these cases represented porokeratosis with the lesions limited to the palms and soles, rather than keratosis palmo-plantaris punctata.

PACHYONYCHIA CONGENITA

In this dominantly inherited disorder hard, keratinous material accumulates at the distal portion of the nails, lifting the nails from their nail bed. In association with the nail changes one frequently sees (a) keratosis palmo-plantaris; (b) areas of follicular hyperkeratosis; and (c) thick whitish areas on the oral mucosa that resemble those seen in white sponge nevus and possess no tendency to malignant degeneration (Kelly and Pinkus).

Histopathology. The nail bed shows marked hyperkeratosis. As in a normal nail bed, there is no granular layer (Kelly and

Pinkus). The oral lesions show thickening of the oral epithelium with extensive intracellular vacuolization, exactly as seen in white sponge nevus (see p. 453), and without evidence of dyskeratosis (Witkop and Gorlin).

DYSKERATOSIS CONGENITA

This rare disorder usually has a sex-linked recessive inheritance. Thus, with the exception of one patient reported by Sorrow and Hitch, it has been observed only in males. It is characterized by the following triad: (1) dystrophy of the nails, with failure of the nails to form a nail plate; (2) whitish thickening (leukokeratosis) of the oral and occasionally also of the anal mucosa; and (3) extensive areas of netlike pigmentation of the skin suggestive of poikiloderma atrophicans vasculare but with less atrophy and telangiectasia. Carcinoma may develop in the areas of buccal and anal leukokeratosis (Garb). Quite frequently, Fanconi's syndrome, consisting of pancytopenia due to bone marrow hypoplasia, has been observed in patients with dyskeratosis congenita (Cole et al.; Garb).

Histopathology. The areas of netlike pigmentation show, as the only constant feature, melanophages in the upper dermis (Bryan and Nixon). In contrast to poikiloderma atrophicans vasculare, atrophy of the epidermis, vacuolization of basal cells and inflammatory infiltration of the upper dermis are either absent (Costello and Buncke) or are mild and thus not diagnostic (Bryan and Nixon). Oral biopsies may show leukoplakia or squamous cell carcinoma (Garb).

POROKERATOSIS (MIBELLI)

This dominantly inherited dermatosis is characterized by lesions showing an atrophic center surrounded by a raised wall having on its top a furrow filled with keratotic material. The lesions have a tendency to peripheral extension. Four different forms may be distinguished (Mikhail and Wertheimer): (1) the plaque type showing usually a single large lesion; (2) a superficial disseminated form, often widely distributed, including the trunk and occasionally also the palms, soles and oral mucosa, in which the lesions are small and surrounded by only a narrow, slightly raised, hyperkeratotic ridge showing no distinct furrow clinically; (3) disseminated superficial actinic porokeratosis, recently described by Chernosky and Freeman, and resembling the last described form, except that the lesions are distributed symmetrically over sun-exposed areas, especially the extensor surfaces of the extremities and can be elicited by prolonged exposure to the sun; and (4) a linear unilateral type (Goldner; Rahbari et al.). Development of a squamous cell carcinoma within lesions of porokeratosis has been repeatedly reported in patients with solitary lesions (Oberste-Lehn and Moll), as well as in those with disseminated lesions (Guss et al.), or a linear unilateral lesion (Swint and Klaus).

Histopathology. The specimen for biopsy is best taken from the peripheral, raised wall with its central furrow. The furrow then appears as a keratin-filled invagination of the epidermis extending downward at an

angle the apex of which points away from the central portion of the lesion. In the center of this keratin-filled invagination rises a parakeratotic column, the so-called cornoid lamella, representing the most characteristic feature of porokeratosis Mibelli (Fig. 6-3). The parakeratotic column shows at its base irregularly arranged epidermal cells having pyknotic nuclei with perinuclear edema (Braun-Falco and Balsa). No granular layer is found at the site where the parakeratotic column arises, whereas elsewhere the keratin-filled invagination of the epidermis has a well-developed granular layer. The histologic changes in disseminated superficial actinic porokeratosis are similar to those seen in the other forms of porokeratosis, but they are much less pronounced, with the central furrows being rather shallow (Fig. 6-4). Since the peripheral, raised wall slowly moves centrifugally, it stands to reason that the furrow is not bound to a definite structure, such as the sweat pore, as originally assumed by Mi-

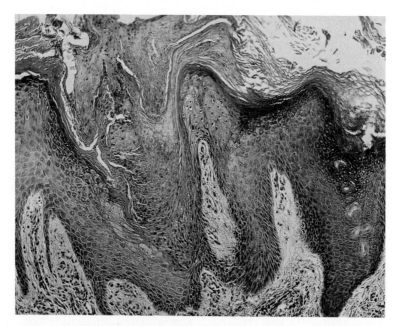

FIG. 6-3. **Porokeratosis Mibelli.** The section is taken from the peripheral raised wall, showing in its center a keratin-filled furrow. In the center of the furrow rises a parakeratotic column, the so-called cornoid lamella. The parakeratotic column shows at its base epidermal cells having pyknotic nuclei with perinuclear edema. On the right side is a normal sweat duct. ($\times 100$)

Fig. 6-4. **Disseminated superficial actinic porokeratosis.** In this type of porokeratosis, because of its superficial location, the central furrow from which the parakeratotic column arises is often very shallow. (×100)

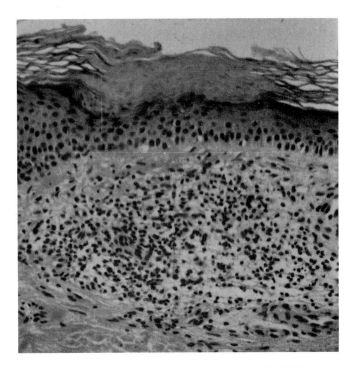

belli. Thus, even though the furrow occasionally may be seen within a sweat pore or pilosebaceous follicle, most commonly it is found in the epidermis independently of these cutaneous appendages (Reed and Leone).

The epidermis overlying the central portion of a lesion of porokeratosis may be either flattened or normal in thickness or, rarely, acanthotic. A nonspecific perivascular infiltrate of chronic inflammatory cells is present in the dermis.

Histogenesis. It appears likely that the clone of abnormal epidermal cells located at the base of the parakeratotic column explains the lesions of porokeratosis. As a result of a gradual centrifugal movement of this clone the furrow is slanted, with its apex pointing away from the center of the lesion (Reed and Leone).

On electron microscopic examination the abnormal cells at the base of the parakeratotic column show degeneration of their cytoplasmic organelles, vacuolization of their cytoplasm, and only very few small keratohyaline granules. Within the parakeratotic column the cells appear rounded rather than flattened and contain only little keratinlike material at their periphery, but they show severe vacuolar degeneration of their cytoplasm and an electron-dense pyknotic nucleus (Mann et al.).

XERODERMA PIGMENTOSUM

This autosomal recessive disorder is caused by a marked hypersensitivity to sunlight. Consequently, the lesions occur chiefly in areas of the skin habitually exposed to sunlight. Three stages are recognized (Hadida et al.): In the first stage one observes slight diffuse erythema associated with scaling and small areas of hyperpigmentation resembling freckles. In the second stage atrophy of the skin, mottled pigmentation, and telangiectases are present, giving the skin an appearance similar to that of a chronic radiodermatitis. In the third stage, usually starting in adolescence, various types of malignant tumors of the skin appear, often causing premature death. They include squamous cell carcinoma, basal cell epithelioma, and, rarely, fibrosarcoma (Bell and Rothnem; Hadida et al.). In about 3 per cent of the patients with xeroderma pigmentosum malignant melanomas arise (Lynch et al.). In some patients they show no tendency to metastasize (Ronchese), but in others they metastasize rapidly (McGovern). In addition to the skin, the eyes are affected, showing conjunctivitis and often also keratitis with corneal opacities (El-Hefnawi and Mortada).

Histopathology. In the first stage the histopathologic appearance is not specific, but the diagnosis is suggested by a combination of changes that normally are not seen in the skin of young individuals. They are: (1) hyperkeratosis, (2) thinning of the stratum malpighii with atrophy of some of the rete ridges and elongation of others, (3) a chronic inflammatory infiltrate in the upper dermis, and (4) irregular accumulations of melanin in the basal cell layer, either with or without an increase in the number of melanocytes (Lynch et al.).

In the second stage the hyperkeratosis and irregular hyperpigmentation already present in the first stage are more pronounced. The epidermis shows atrophy in some areas and acanthosis in others. There may be disorder in the arrangement of the epidermal nuclei and in some areas the epidermis may show atypical downward growth, so that the histologic picture in such areas is identical with that of solar keratosis (see p. 468). The upper dermis shows the same changes as seen in solar degeneration, namely, basophilic degeneration of the collagen and solar elastosis (see p. 249).

In the third, or tumor, stage, histologic evidence of the various malignant tumors mentioned above is found.

Histogenesis. In most patients with xeroderma pigmentosum, as first shown by Cleaver (1970), the fibroblasts when cultured are extremely sensitive to ultraviolet light and perform reduced amounts of repair replication during the repair of damage to DNA. Cleaver found that the main biochemical defect in the fibroblasts occurred at an early step in DNA repair as the result of a deficiency of an ultraviolet light specific endonuclease. Jung, however, on studying two patients with onset of their xeroderma pigmentosum in adult life, rather than in early childhood, found the defect not during the early phase in the excision repair system but at a later stage, in the recovery process during recombination. Furthermore, Cleaver (1972) encountered instances of xeroderma pigmentosum in which the fibroblasts in vitro showed a normal sensitivity to ultraviolet light and performed normal amounts of repair replication. Thus, there are at least 3 varients of xeroderma pigmentosum. Cleaver concluded that any possible relationship between DNA repair and carcinogenesis required cautious evaluation.

Electron microscopic examination of the epidermis has revealed in pigmented areas a definite increase in the number of melanosomes as well as pleomorphism of the melanosomes (Rasheed et al.). In some cases very large melanosomes, referred to as giant melanosomes, are present in both melanocytes and keratinocytes (Guerrier).

ECTODERMAL DYSPLASIA

Two forms of ectodermal dysplasia are recognized: a hidrotic and an anhidrotic. The hidrotic form has an autosomal dominant inheritance and primarily is a disorder of keratinization, with dystrophy of the hair, nails and teeth but without a deficiency in the sweat glands. Not infrequently, one finds, as an additional finding, keratosis palmaris et plantaris (Bolck and Barth). The anhidrotic, or hypohidrotic, form of ectodermal dysplasia is a sex-linked recessive disorder occurring in its full form only in males. Females as heterozygotes may be mildly affected, with reduced sweating and faulty dentition.

Males affected with anhidrotic ectodermal dysplasia show greatly reduced or no function of their eccrine sweat glands, resulting in intolerance to heat. Other epidermal appendages also are incompletely developed or absent: hair, nails, teeth and sebaceous glands. In addition, the mucous glands of the mouth and respiratory tract may be absent (Reed et al.). The facies is typical: it shows prominent frontal bosses and a depressed nasal bridge.

Histopathology. Both the hidrotic and the anhidrotic form show hypoplasia of the hair and sebaceous glands with decreased maturation of the sebaceous cells (Korting and Salfeld). In the anhidrotic form there is, in addition, either a total absence or hypoplasia of the eccrine sweat glands. In the case of hypoplasia the secretory cells may be small and flat so that they resemble endothelial rather than epithelial cells; and the excretory ducts may be composed of a single instead of a double layer of epithelial cells (Malagon and Taveras). In the anhidrotic form the apocrine glands of the axillae are present in some patients (Sunderman), whereas in others they are hypoplastic and cannot be distinguished from hypoplastic eccrine glands (Dominok and Rönisch), and in still others they are absent (Upshaw and Montgomery).

FOCAL DERMAL
HYPOPLASIA SYNDROME

The focal dermal hypoplasia syndrome is seen predominantly in females. It is characterized by a widespread dysplasia of mesodermal and ectodermal structures. Although it occurs in some instances as a mutation, in others it is an autosomal dominant trait with sex-limited inheritance, since the syndrome in its full expression is lethal in males, resulting in abortion (Ishibashi and Kurihara). The mode of inheritance thus is similar to that of incontinentia pigmenti (see p. 86).

The cutaneous manifestations include: (1) widely distributed linear areas of hypoplasia of the skin resembling striae distensae;

(2) soft yellowish nodules, often in linear arrangement, representing herniation of fat through an underdeveloped dermis (Goltz et al.); and (3) large ulcers due to congenital absence of skin, which gradually heal with atrophy. Frequent additional abnormalities include: (4) lack of a digit which may be associated with syndactyly, resulting in the very characteristic "lobster-claw deformity"; (5) colobomata of the eyes, or microphthalmia, or agenesis of an eye (Lever); and (6) hypoplasia of hair, nails and teeth.

Histopathology. The linear areas of hypoplasia of the skin and soft yellowish nodules both show a marked diminution in the thickness of the dermis, with the collagen present as thin fibers not united into bundles (Howell). In some areas very little dermis is present so that the subcutaneous fat extends upward to the epidermis (Fig. 6-5) (Goltz et al.; Lever). Remnants of collagen

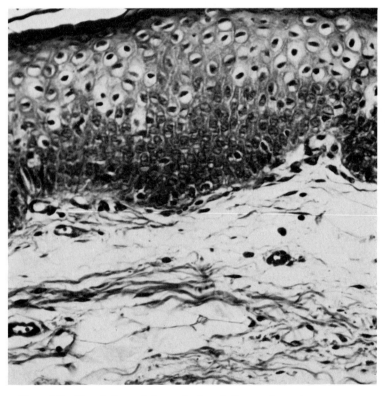

Fig. 6-5. **Focal dermal hypoplasia.** Adipose tissue is present very near to the epidermis, being separated from the epidermis by only a few collagen fibers. (×200)

may be found between the subepidermal adipose tissue and the subcutaneous fat (Howell).

Differential Diagnosis. Fat cells are seen in the dermis also in nevus lipomatosus of Hoffmann and Zurhelle (see p. 618); but the extreme attenuation of the collagen occurring in some areas of the skin in patients with focal dermal hypoplasia syndrome has not been observed in nevus lipomatosus.

POIKILODERMA CONGENITALE (ROTHMUND-THOMSON)

Poikiloderma congenitale is recessively inherited. It begins, a few months after birth, with erythema on the face and subsequently extends to the dorsa of the hands and feet and occasionally also to the arms, legs and buttocks. Later on, slight atrophy develops with telangiectases and mottled hyper- and hypopigmentation, so that the appearance is that of poikiloderma atrophicans vasculare.

Exposure to light aggravates the lesions. Most patients show dwarfism and hypogonadism. In about 40 per cent of the cases cataracts develop between the ages of 4 to 7 (Rook et al.).

Histopathology. During the early phase, occurring in infancy and early childhood, one observes hydropic degeneration of the basal layer leading to "pigmentary incontinence" with presence of melanophages in the upper dermis (Tritsch and Lischka). A mild chronic inflammatory infiltrate is intermingled with the melanophages and may show a bandlike arrangement close to the flattened epidermis (Fig. 6-6) (Rook et al.). The histologic changes thus may be identical with those seen in the early stage of poikiloderma atrophicans vasculare (see p. 439). In later childhood and adult life the epidermis is flattened, and dilated capillaries as well as melanophages are present in the upper dermis; but there no longer is any inflammatory infiltrate (Thannhauser).

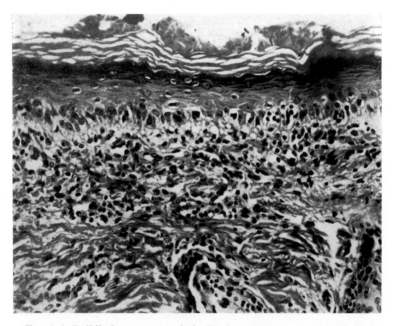

FIG. 6-6. **Poikiloderma congenitale (Rothmund-Thomson), early stage.** This section, obtained from a young child, shows flattening of the epidermis, hydropic degeneration of the basal layer, and a bandlike inflammatory infiltrate in the upper dermis. (×200)

BLOOM'S SYNDROME: CONGENITAL TELANGIECTATIC ERYTHEMA

Bloom's syndrome, also recessively inherited, resembles poikiloderma congenitale by showing: (1) telangiectatic erythema of the face starting in infancy and often extending to the forearms and dorsa of the hands; (2) sensitivity to sunlight; and (3) growth retardation. It differs from poikiloderma congenitale by (1) lacking the netlike hyper- and hypopigmentation (Braun-Falco and Marghescu); (2) absence of hypogonadism and cataracts; (3) low IgA and IgM fractions (Landau et al.; Bloom and German); (4) a high incidence of nonspecific chromosomal breakage (Landau et al.); and (5) occasional occurrence of acute leukemia (Sawitzky et al.).

Histopathology. The epidermis is flattened but lacks the hydropic degeneration of the basal cell layer and pigmentary incontinence seen in poikiloderma congenitale. There is dilatation of the capillaries in the upper dermis. This may be associated with a mild perivascular infiltrate (Katzenellenbogen and Laron); but there may not be any infiltrate (Braun-Falco and Marghescu).

Histogenesis. Bloom's syndrome shares with ataxia-telangiectasia certain immunologic deficiencies, such as low values for IgA, absence of delayed hypersensitivity (Bloom and German), and a tendency to develop lymphoreticular malignancies. However, the immunologic defects are much more pronounced in ataxia-telangiectasia, which is characterized by scleral and diffuse facial telangiectasia (Reed et al.) and by progressive ataxia. Still, both Bloom's syndrome and ataxia telangiectasia show impairment of cellular and humoral immunity. Impairment of the thymic lymphoid system mediating cellular immunity results in decrease or absence of delayed hypersensitivity; and impairment of the bone-marrow-derived lymphoid system mediating humoral immunity results in a decrease in immunoglobulins, especially of IgA. However, only ataxia-telangiectasia shows great susceptibility to infections, particularly to sinopulmonary infections (Scott; McFarlin et al.), causing the death of the patient, usually in the second decade of life.

PROGERIA OF THE ADULT (WERNER'S SYNDROME)

Werner's syndrome recessively inherited, does not manifest itself until the second or third decade of life. The subcutaneous fat and the musculature of the extremities undergo atrophy, so that the patient exhibits thin arms and legs. The skin of the extremities gradually becomes taut and ulcers may develop on the legs. As signs of premature senility the patients show early graying of the hair, cataracts, and atherosclerosis in early adult life. Diabetes of the "late-onset" type (Epstein et al.) and hypogonadism due to interstitial fibrosis of the testes (Tritsch and Lischka) are common. Death usually occurs in the fifth decade of life because of atherosclerosis.

Histopathology. On the arms and legs where the skin is taut, the epidermis is thin and devoid of rete ridges, and the dermis is thickened and shows fibrosis with or without hyalinization of the collagen, together with disappearance of the pilosebaceous structures and atrophy of the sweat glands. The subcutaneous fat is atrophic (Epstein et al.; Tritsch and Lischka).

Differential Diagnosis. Differentiation from a late lesion of scleroderma may be difficult, because in its late stage scleroderma, too, may show no inflammatory infiltrate, so that the differentiation has to be made on the basis of the patient's history and clinical manifestations.

EPIDERMOLYSIS BULLOSA

The following forms of the disease exist: (1) epidermolysis bullosa simplex (dominant); (2) epidermolysis bullosa of Cockayne, of the hands and feet (dominant); (3) dominant-dystrophic epidermolysis bullosa; (4) recessive-dystrophic epidermolysis bullosa; and (5) epidermolysis bullosa letalis (recessive). In addition, there is a form of epidermolysis bullosa that is not inherited but acquired. In all forms the blisters usually form as the result of minor trauma.

In epidermolysis bullosa simplex the bullae heal without scarring, and the mucous membranes and the nails are rarely affected. In the Cockayne form of epidermolysis bullosa the bullae are limited to the hands and feet. In the dominant-dystrophic form mild scarring ensues; occasionally the oral mucosa is affected, and often the nails are thickened or lost. In the recessive-dystrophic form extensive erosions resulting in ulcerations and scarring are seen; the oral mucosa is affected nearly always, the nails are rudimentary, and esophageal stenoses can occur (Bergenholtz et al.). The ulcers and scars may give rise to squamous cell carcinomas that often metastasize (Wechsler). In especially severe cases death may ensue. In epidermolysis bullosa letalis death usually occurs within the first three months of life. The bullae show little tendency to healing; but when they heal, no scars remain. Oral lesions and dystrophic changes of the nails usually are present. A few patients survive to adult life without scarring (Ridley and Levy), whereas others later on have shown some scarring (Eberhartinger and Niebauer), making it difficult to separate such cases from the recessive-dystrophic form. Acquired epidermolysis bullosa starts in adult life. In most instances the bullae leave atrophic scars (Roenigk et al.).

Histopathology. Histopathologic observations on the various forms of epidermolysis bullosa have been somewhat contradictory, and one of the reasons for this is the fact that the site of cleavage may vary in bullae of different duration. This is true particularly of epidermolysis bullosa simplex where the bullae often persist without breaking for several days. Thus, the cleavage in old bullae of epidermolysis bullosa simplex may be found subcorneally (Johnson and Test). However, in experimentally produced or early lesions of *epidermolysis bullosa simplex* there is vacuolization and degeneration of basal cells and the primary separation occurs either within the basal cell layer (Lowe; Pearson, 1971) or, as the result of complete disintegration of the basal cell layer, subepidermally (Pearson, 1971).

In *epidermolysis bullosa of the hands and feet* a cytolytic process takes place in the cells of the upper stratum malpighii associated with some dyskeratosis so that the blisters form in the mid-epidermis, just as seen in friction blisters (Pearson, 1971) (see p. 127).

In *epidermolysis bullosa letalis* the separation occurs between epidermis and dermis, with the PAS-positive basement zone remaining with dermis (Pearson et al.). In some instances the basal cells show vacuolization but they detach from the dermis in their entirety (Bergenholtz and Olsson).

In *dominant-dystrophic* and in *recessive-dystrophic epidermolysis bullosa* the bullae form through dermal-epidermal separation and the underlying papillary dermis often shows fragmentation (Pearson, 1971). A PAS stain is of little help in ascertaining the exact level of cleavage, since the PAS-positive basement zone generally is poorly developed and the papillary dermis shows diffuse positive staining (Pearson, 1971). This might explain why, according to some authors, the PAS-positive basement zone is split or found in contact with the detached epidermis (Lowe) and, according to others, it is still attached to the dermis (Vogel and Schnyder).

In *acquired epidermolysis bullosa,* in which healing usually takes place with scarring, the histologic picture is analogous to dystrophic epidermolysis bullosa. The bulla forms by means of dermal-epidermal separation (Roenigk et al.; Purdy and Fairbrother).

Histogenesis. Electron microscopic examination of spontaneously as well as experimentally formed blisters has resulted in somewhat contradictory findings in regard to the site of bulla formation, especially in regard to the location of the basal lamina in recessive-dystrophic epidermolysis bullosa. However, most commonly the primary defect, as seen by electron microscopy, occurs from top to bottom: within the basal cell layer, in epidermolysis bullosa simplex; between the basal cell layer and basal lamina, in epidermolysis bullosa letalis; between the basal lamina and anchoring fibrils, in dominant-dystrophic epidermolysis bullosa; and in the upper layers of the dermis, in recessive-dystrophic epidermolysis bullosa (Pearson, 1971; Pearson et al.; Anton-Lamprecht and Schnyder).

In epidermolysis bullosa simplex the cleavage is the result of degenerative changes in the basal cells (Pearson, 1962). In epidermolysis bullosa letalis the basal lamina generally is found at the floor of the bulla, probably because of the action of lytic enzymes at the junction between basal cells and basal lamina (Pearson et al.). In dominant-dystrophic epidermolysis bullosa the basal lamina is found on top of the blister, probably as the result of a defect in the anchoring fibrils, since they are absent or rudimentary even in areas without blisters (Anton-Lamprecht and Schnyder). Electron microscopic findings obtained in recessive-dystrophic epidermolysis bullosa have varied. On the one hand, Pearson (1962, 1971) always found the basal lamina detached from the dermis. On the other hand, Vogel and Schnyder and also Kobayashi found in some instances of recessive-dystrophic epidermolysis bullosa the basal lamina attached to the dermis (E.M. No. 15). Still, it is agreed that in such instances of recessive-dystrophic epidermolysis bullosa in which the basal lamina is detached from the dermis this is accompanied by degeneration of the underlying collagen, particularly by a loss of the anchoring fibrils (Pearson; Vogel and Schnyder).

Collagenase activity is elevated in the dermis of patients with recessive-dystrophic epidermolysis bullosa, according to Eisen et al.; but Lazarus regards this as a secondary tissue reaction. Still, he assumes that in recessive-dystrophic epidermolysis bullosa there is a primary abnormality of the connective tissue.

KERATOSIS FOLLICULARIS (DARIER'S DISEASE)

Darier's disease, although often dominantly transmitted, may occur as a mutation. It is characterized usually by a more or less extensive, slowly progressive eruption consisting of hyperkeratotic or crusted papules often showing a follicular distribution. By coalescence verrucous, crusted areas may form. Occasionally, hypertrophic lesions are present with elevated, papillomatous formations. In a few cases the occurrence of vesicles, in addition to papules, has been described (Piérard et al.). The so-called seborrheic areas are the sites of predilection. The oral mucosa is involved occasionally (Weathers et al.). In rare instances Darier's disease may manifest itself

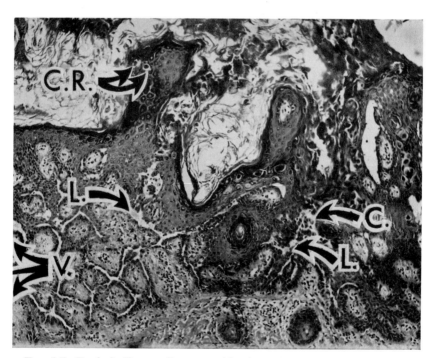

FIG. 6-7. **Darier's disease.** Low magnification. One observes hyperkeratosis and papillomatosis. Numerous lacunae (L.) are present. On the left are elongated papillae lined by a single layer of cells, so-called villi (V.). Corps ronds (C.R.) are present in the granular layer, and grains in the horny layer. The lacunae contain desquamated acantholytic cells (C.). (×100)

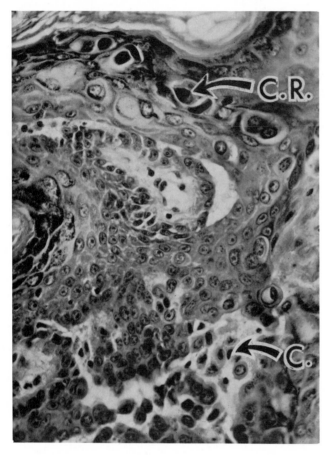

Fig. 6-8. **Darier's disease.** High magnification of Figure 6-7. In the upper third of the illustration, within the granular layer, are several corps ronds (C.R.), showing a central large, round, homogeneous, basophilic, dyskeratotic mass surrounded by a clear halo. In the lower third, within a lacuna, are acantholytic cells which on account of premature partial keratinization have a shrunken appearance (C.). (×400)

as a unilateral localized linear lesion in later life without a family history (Kellum and Haserick; Leeming). Occasionally the characteristic histologic features of Darier's disease are found in clinically nonspecific, solitary papular or nodular lesions. The term *focal acantholytic dyskeratosis* has been applied to such lesions (Ackerman). For a discussion of the relationship of warty dyskeratoma to Darier's disease, see p. 467.

Histopathology. The characteristic changes in Darier's disease are (1) a peculiar form of dyskeratosis resulting in the formation of corps ronds and grains, (2) suprabasal acantholysis leading to the formation of suprabasal clefts or lacunae, and (3) irregular upward prolifertion into the lacunae of papillae lined with a single layer of basal cells, so-called villi (Fig. 6-7). There also are papillomatosis, acanthosis and hyperkeratosis. The dermis shows a chronic inflammatory infiltrate. In some cases there is downward proliferation of epidermal cells into the dermis.

The corps ronds occur in the upper stratum malpighii, particularly in the granular and horny layers; grains are found in the horny layer and as acantholytic cells within the lacunae. Corps ronds possess a central large, round, homogeneous, basophilic mass that is surrounded by a clear halo. By virtue of their size and conspicuous halo, corps ronds stand out clearly (Fig. 6-8). The central basophilic mass consists either of the pyknotic nucleus or of dyskeratotic material or both. Peripheral to the halo lies additional basophilic dyskeratotic material as a shell. The nonstaining halo may be partially replaced by homogeneous, eosinophilic dyskeratotic material. In contrast to the corps ronds, the grains are much less conspicuous. They resemble parakeratotic cells, except that they are somewhat larger. The nucleus of grains is elongated, often grain-shaped and is surrounded by homogeneous dyskeratotic material that usually stains basophilic but may stain eosinophilic.

The lacunae represent small, slitlike intra-epidermal vesicles located most commonly directly above the basal layer. They contain acantholytic cells that are devoid of inter-cellular bridges and show premature partial keratinization. Some of them because of shrinkage are elongated, and then appear identical with the grains in the horny layer.

The villi projecting into the lacunae may be quite tortuous, so that on histologic examination some of the villi appear in cross section as rounded dermal structures lined by a solitary row of basal cells (Fig. 6-7).

Hyperkeratosis and papillomatosis may cause the formation of keratotic plugs. Often they fill the pilosebaceous follicles, but they are found also outside of follicles. Therefore, Darier's disease is not exclusively a follicular disorder. Proof of this is the fact that areas devoid of follicles, such as palms, soles, and oral mucosa, may be affected (Ellis).

In hypertrophic lesions of Darier's disease one occasionally can observe considerable downward proliferation of the epidermis, either as a proliferation of basal cells or as pseudocarcinomatous hyperplasia. The pro-liferations of basal cells consist of long, nar-row cords composed of two rows of basal cells separated by a narrow lacunar space (Beerman; Krinitz).

The vesicles, which occur in rare in-stances, differ from lacunae merely in size; they contain numerous shrunken cells with the appearance of grains (Jablonska and Chorzelski; Piérard et al.).

The lesions on the oral mucosa are anal-ogous in appearance to those observed on the skin and thus show lacunae and dyskera-tosis, although definite well-formed corps ronds generally are absent (Weathers et al.).

Histogenesis. The occurrence of suprabasal acantholysis represents a genetic defect. There is, however, no agreement as yet about the nature of this defect on study by electron microscopy. Some authors believe that the primary defect lies in the desmosomes which either fail to form

(Charles) or separate into two halves by dis-appearance of the desmosomal contact layer (Mann and Haye). On the other hand, Caulfield and Wilgram as well as Piérard and Kint believe that separation of tonofilaments from their at-tachment at the desmosomes is the first change to occur, and that this is followed by a loss of desmosomes. It would seem that a primary defect of the tonofilaments would best explain the "dyskeratotic" nature of Darier's disease. In any case, tonofilaments without attachment to desmosomes aggregate around the nucleus of epidermal cells and increase rapidly in number. Thus, in association with large keratohyaline granules, the bundles of tonofilaments form large aggregates of homogenized dyskeratotic material.

The corps ronds, on electron microscopic ex-amination, are characterized by extensive cyto-plasmic vacuolization (Gottlieb and Lutzner). They may show in their center a pyknotic nucleus surrounded by a halo of autolyzed elec-tron-lucid cytoplasm and at their periphery a shell of homogenized tonofilaments (E.M. No. 16) (Mann and Haye; Forssmann et al.). In other instances, corps ronds contain in their center both a nucleus and dyskeratotic material (Piérard and Kint); and in still others the center no longer shows a nucleus but only dyskeratotic material (Caulfield and Wilgram). The presence of a nucleus in some corps ronds and its absence in others is supported by the observation that the center of corps ronds is Feulgen-positive at first, but in the higher layers of the epidermis becomes Feulgen-negative (Douwes). The grains, on electron miscroscopic examination, consist of nuclear remnants surrounded by dyskeratotic bundles of tonofilaments.

Differential Diagnosis. Corps ronds are highly characteristic of Darier's disease. The only other disease in which they regularly occur is warty dyskeratoma (see p. 466). Occasionally, a few corps ronds are seen also in familial benign pemphigus (see be-low).

FAMILIAL BENIGN PEMPHIGUS (HAILEY AND HAILEY)

This disease is dominantly inherited, with a family history obtainable in about two thirds of the patients (Palmer and Perry). It is characterized by a localized, recurrent eruption of vesicles. By peripheral extension the lesions may assume a circinate configura-tion. The sites of predilection are the intertriginous areas, especially the axillae and the groins. Only two instances of involvement of the oral mucosa have been reported (Schneider et al.; Botvinick), and one instance of esophageal involvement (Kahn and Hutchinson).

Histopathology. Although early lesions may show, as in Dariers' disease, small suprabasal separations, so-called lacunae, fully developed lesions show large separations, namely vesicles and even bullae in predominantly suprabasal position (Fig. 6-9). Villi, i.e., elongated papillae lined by a single layer of basal cells, protrude upward into the bulla; and in some cases narrow strands of epidermal cells proliferate downward into the dermis. Many cells of the detached stratum malpighii show loss of their intercellular bridges, so that acantholysis affects large portions of the epidermis. Individual cells as well as groups of cells are seen in large numbers in the bulla cavity. In spite of the extensive loss of intercellular bridges, in many places the cells of the detached epidermis show only slight separation from one another because a few surviving intercellular bridges still hold them loosely together. This quite typical feature gives the detached epidermis the appearance of a "dilapidated brick wall" (Haber and Russell).

Many of the cells of the stratum malpighii that have lost all or most of their intercellular bridges show a fairly normal cytoplasm and a normal nucleus in which even mitotic activity has been observed (Winer and Leeb; Herzberg). Some of the cells, however, have a homogenized cytoplasm, suggesting premature partial keratinization. Some of the acantholytic cells with premature keratinization resemble the grains of Darier's disease. Occasionally, a few corps ronds are present in the granular layer (Fig. 6-9) (Ellis; Winer and Leeb; Herzberg; Gönczöl and Szodoray).

Histogenesis. Based on electron microscopic findings there are two schools of thought about the primary event in the suprabasal acantholysis seen in familial benign pemphigus. One group of authors (Nürnberger and Müller; Gottlieb and Lutzner; Thies et al.) believes that acantholysis results from an insufficiency of cellular adhesion.

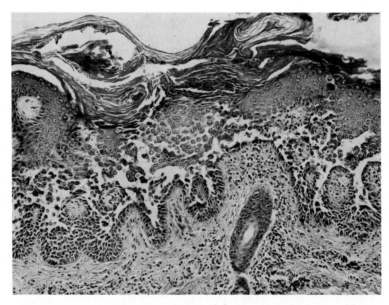

FIG. 6-9. **Familial benign chronic pemphigus (Hailey and Hailey).** The bulla is largely in suprabasal position. The extensive loss of intercellular bridges with partial coherence of cells gives the detached epidermis the appearance of a dilapidated brick wall. On the right side, within the granular layer, a corps rond can be seen. (×200)

Plate 1

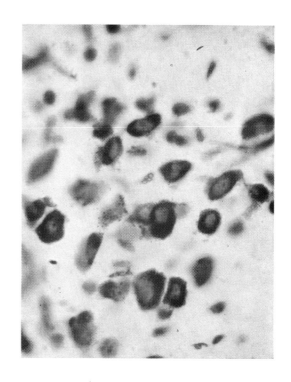

Urticaria pigmentosa.
Methylene blue stain. Numerous basophilic granules are present in the cytoplasm of the mast cells. (×800)

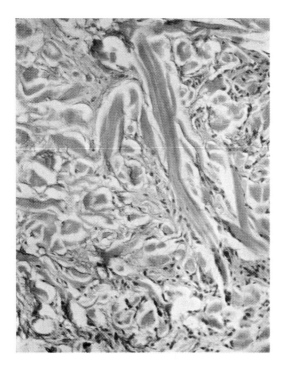

Granuloma annulare.
Foci of incomplete degeneration of collagen show partially degenerated and partially normal collagen bundles. Fine threads and granules of mucinous material are located at the sites of collagen degeneration. (×150)

This may manifest itself either by primary dissolution of many desmosomes (Thies et al.) or by the formation of numerous elongated and branching microvilli at the periphery of the keratinocytes, such as may be seen also in early lesions of pemphigus vulgaris (Braun-Falco and Vogell). It is assumed that the microvilli form as the result of a faulty synthesis of either the intercellular substance (Nürnberger and Müller) or the plasma membrane (Gottlieb and Lutzner). The microvillar changes are associated with disappearance of many desmosomes, leading to acantholysis. On the other hand, Wilgram et al. and Piérard and Kint believe that the same basic defect in the tonofilament-desmosome complex observed by them in Darier's disease exists also in familial benign pemphigus, resulting in a detachment of the tonofilaments from the desmosomes and followed by the disappearance of many desmosomes and by acantholysis. It is generally agreed that subsequent to the loss of desmosomes excessive amounts of tonofilaments form within the keratinocytes and aggregate around the nucleus as thick, electron-dense bundles, often in a whorling configuration. Thus even though dyskeratosis is present, it is less pronounced than in Darier's disease, and most of the keratinocytes keratinize normally and only a few, as the result of dyskeratotic degeneration, become grains or corps ronds.

Intradermal injection of tritiated thymidine in vivo into lesions of familial benign pemphigus and those of Darier's disease has revealed in familial benign pemphigus labeling of many acantholytic epidermal cells. This suggests that such cells participate in the renewal of the epidermis. On the other hand, in Darier's disease no labeling of acantholytic epidermal cells was seen, probably because they are undergoing keratinization (Lachapelle et al.).

Differential Diagnosis. Histologically, familial benign pemphigus shares certain features with both Darier's disease and pemphigus vulgaris. In all three diseases one finds (1) predominantly suprabasal separation of the epidermis caused by acantholysis, and (2) upward proliferation of papillae as so-called villi into the lacunae or bullae resulting from the separation.

Differentiation from Darier's disease as a rule is not too difficult because in Darier's disease (1) the suprabasal separations usually are smaller, thus appearing as lacunae rather than as bullae; (2) acantholysis is less pronounced, being limited to the lower epidermis, especially the suprabasal region;

and (3) dyskeratosis consisting of the formation of corps ronds and grains is much more evident.

Pemphigus vulgaris often resembles familial benign pemphigus to a striking degree, and in some specimens histologic differentiation of these two diseases may be impossible. As a rule, however, one observes in pemphigus vulgaris (1) less extensive acantholysis, limited largely to the suprabasal region so that the detached epidermis appears normal and lacks the appearance of a "dilapidated brick wall"; and (2) more severe degeneration of the acantholytic cells within and near the bulla cavity, so that in pemphigus vulgaris the acantholytic cells as a result of degeneration show peripheral condensation of their cytoplasm and no evidence of keratinization (Dupont). The presence of eosinophils in the bulla points toward a diagnosis of pemphigus vulgaris, but their absence does not rule it out.

In the past, there has been much discussion as to whether or not familial benign pemphigus represented a bullous variant of Darier's disease. Two points in favor of a basic unity of the two diseases were stressed: the alleged simultaneous presence of both diseases in the same patient and the occurrence of corps ronds in both diseases. However it has since become apparent that patients having allegedly both diseases either had Darier's disease with vesicular lesions, such as the cases described by Niordson and Sylvest and by Ganor and Sagher; or had familial benign pemphigus with the presence of corps ronds, such as the case described by Finnerud and Szymanski. Against a relationship between these two dominantly inherited diseases is also the fact that in affected families always only one of the two diseases occurs (Raaschou-Nielsen and Reymann).

ACROKERATOSIS VERRUCIFORMIS (HOPF)

Numerous flat, hyperkeratotic, occasionally verrucous papules are present in this disorder on the distal part of the extremities, predominantly on the dorsa of the hands and feet. Frequently, this dominantly inherited disorder occurs in patients with Darier's disease (Waisman; Penrod et al.). Also, it may occur in patients who later on develop lesions of Darier's disease (Jordan and Spier), or in patients who have in their family instances of Darier's disease (Herndon and Wilson). Thus the two disorders represent variants of a single underlying genetic defect in keratinization. Nevertheless, acrokeratosis verruciformis may occur as a familial disease in families without Darier's disease (Niedelman and McKusick) and in individuals without a family history of either acrokeratosis verruciformis or Darier's disease (Schueller).

Histopathology. The papules show considerable hyperkeratosis, increase in thickness of the granular layer, and acanthosis. In addition, there is slight papillomatosis, which frequently, but not always, is associated with circumscribed elevations of the epidermis resembling church spires (Fig. 6-10) (Waisman; Schueller). The rete ridges are slightly elongated and extend to a uniform level.

Occasionally, patients having both acrokeratosis verruciformis and Darier's disease show in some of their lesions with the clinical appearance of acrokeratosis verruciformis, instead of hyperkeratosis, the histologic features of Darier's disease (Waisman; Krause and Ehlers).

Differential Diagnosis. Although the "church spire" type of elevations of the epidermis are quite typical of acrokeratosis verruciformis, they may be absent in that disease. On the other hand, they are present in the hyperkeratotic type of seborrheic keratosis (see p. 455). Thus, even though seborrheic keratoses usually are larger than the lesions of acrokeratosis verruciformis, clinical data may be necessary for the differentiation of these two conditions. Also, acrokeratosis verruciformis may resemble verrucae clinically, but it differs from verruca plana by the absence of vacuolization in the cells of the upper epidermis, and from verruca vulgaris by the absence of parakeratosis.

PSEUDOXANTHOMA ELASTICUM

In this recessively inherited disorder, genetically abnormal elastic fibers with a tendency to calcification occur not only in the skin but frequently also in the oral mucosa and the eyes. In addition, calcification is often found within the walls of gastric mucosal arteries, coronary arteries, and large peripheral arteries (Goodman et al.).

The cutaneous lesions consist of soft, yellowish, coalescing papules, and the affected

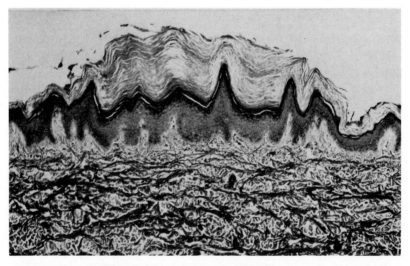

Fig. 6-10. **Acrokeratosis verruciformis (Hopf).** A well circumscribed lesion shows hyperkeratosis and papillomatosis. The latter is associated with elevations of the epidermis resembling church spires. (×100)

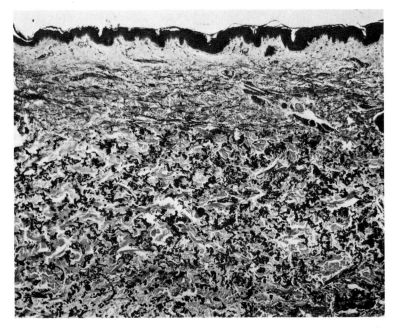

FIG. 6-11. **Pseudoxanthoma elasticum.** Low magnification, elastic tissue stain. In the middle and the lower layers of the dermis the elastic fibers are increased in number. They appear swollen and irregularly clumped. (×50)

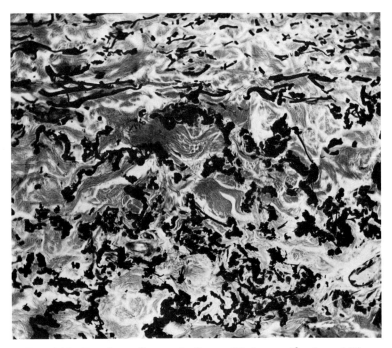

FIG. 6-12. **Pseudoxanthoma elasticum.** High magnification of Figure 6-11, elastic tissue stain. The elastic fibers in the upper fourth of the illustration have a normal appearance; those in the lower three fourths show marked degeneration. (×200)

skin appears loose and wrinkled. The sides of the neck, the axillae and the groin are the most common sites of lesions. In the eyes so-called angioid streaks of the fundi often cause progressive impairment of vision. Involvement of the arteries of the gastric mucosa may lead to gastric hemorrhages; involvement of coronary arteries may result in coronary occlusion; and involvement of the large peripheral arteries may cause weak peripheral pulses but only rarely causes ischemic manifestations because of the presence of good collateral circulation. Radiologic examination in such cases reveals extensive calcification of the affected peripheral arteries (Eddy and Farber).

Histopathology. Histologic examination of the involved skin reveals in the middle and lower thirds of the dermis considerable accumulations of swollen and irregularly clumped fibers staining like elastic fibers; i.e., they stain deeply black with orcein or the Verhoeff stain (Figs. 6-11 and 6-12). Although normally elastic fibers do not stain with routine stains, such as hematoxylin and eosin, the altered elastic fibers in pseudoxanthoma elasticum stain faintly basophilic because of their calcium imbibition. Staining for calcium with von Kossa's method also shows them well. In the vicinity of the altered elastic fibers one finds accumulations of a slightly basophilic mucoid material, staining strongly positive with the colloidal iron reaction or with alcian blue (Huang et al.). In addition, the amount of collagen bundles is reduced in such areas and numerous reticulum fibers are seen on impregnation with silver (Danielsen et al.). In cases of pronounced elastic tissue degeneration a macrophage and giant cell reaction may be present (Goodman et al.).

The angioid streaks occur in Bruch's membrane, which is located between the retina and the choroid and possesses numerous elastic fibers in its outer portion, the lamina elastica. Calcification of these fibers causes fissures to form in the lamina elastica of Bruch's membrane. These fissures result in repeated hemorrhages and exudates; and they in turn cause degenerative changes in the retina, consisting of scar formation and pigment shifting (Goodman et al.; Kreysel et al.).

The gastric bleeding is the result of calcification of elastic fibers in the arteries immediately beneath the gastric mucosa. The elastic fibers of the internal elastic lamella are particularly affected (Flatley et al.). In contrast, the calcification in the coronary arteries and in the large peripheral arteries occurs predominantly in the media, probably as a result of calcification of the elastic fibers located in both the external and internal elastic lamellae and in the media (Goodman et al.).

Histogenesis. Electron microscopic examination of the skin lesions shows an increase in the number of elastic fibers. In young patients only some of the elastic fibers are calcified, and the calcification is variable in degree. In adult patients, on the other hand, most elastic fibers show considerable calcification and, as a result of this, degeneration. Early calcification of elastic fibers consists either of diffuse granular deposits throughout the elastic fiber, or of dense aggregates that may be located in the center or near the margin of the fiber (E.M. No. 17). With progression of the calcification the elastic fibers ultimately become fully calcified, resulting in marked swelling and bizarre distortions of the affected elastic fibers. In addition, heavy calcium deposits may be seen in the ground substance adjacent to elastic fibers and also free in the ground substance. In the latter case it is likely that an elastic fiber has been completely replaced by calcium deposits (Hashimoto and DiBella; Danielsen et al.).

Besides varying numbers of normal collagen fibrils, irregularly twisted collagen fibrils and, in addition, granulofilamentous aggregates are present. Whereas Huang et al. have expressed the view that the process of calcification began in the granulofilamentous material which they regarded as an abnormal elastic precursor, most authors regard the granulofilamentous material as arising secondary to the calcification of the elastic fibers and to be composed of immature collagen and of elastic microfibrils (Danielsen et al.). Even though the granulofilamentous material contains areas of calcification it is likely that in such calcified areas pre-existing elastic fibers have been completely replaced by calcium deposits (Danielsen and Kobayasi).

Differential Diagnosis. Solar elastosis, like pseudoxanthoma elasticum, shows a great increase in material taking elastic tissue stains. However, in solar elastosis this material is located in the upper third of the

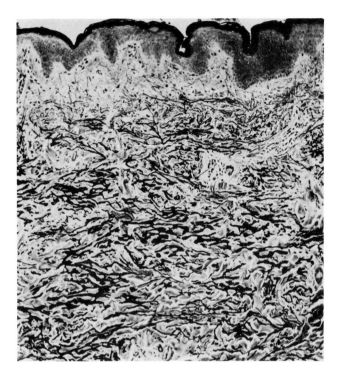

FIG. 6-13. **Connective tissue nevus (nevus elasticus).** The elastic fibers are markedly increased in number and size without showing signs of degeneration. (×100)

dermis and is present as dense masses rather than as individual curls. Furthermore, the staining of this material for calcium is always negative in solar elastosis. For differential diagnosis from connective tissue nevus with increase in elastic tissue, see below.

CONNECTIVE TISSUE NEVUS

The connective tissue nevus represents a hamartoma in which the amount of collagen is increased whereas the amount of elastic tissue may be decreased, normal or increased. The lesions consist of slightly elevated, slightly indurated nodules that may be grouped together in one or several plaques or may be widely disseminated. The connective tissue nevus can occur (a) without alterations in other organs, (b) with tuberous sclerosis, and (c) with osteopoikilosis (Raque and Wood).

In tuberous sclerosis the connective tissue nevus is apt to consist of nodules that are asymmetrically distributed over the trunk and may be grouped together in one or several plaques referred to as shagreen patches. The latter are seen most commonly in the lumbosacral region (see p. 575).

In osteopoikilosis the nodules usually show a widespread symmetrical distribution referred to as dermatofibrosis lenticularis disseminata (Danielsen et al.); but occasionally they are grouped as isolated plaques in asymmetric distribution just as in tuberous sclerosis (Raque and Wood). The associated bone lesions are asymptomatic and, on x-ray examination, consist of round or oval densities, from 2 to 10 millimeters in diameter, located in the long bones, the pelvis, and the bones of the hands and feet.

Histopathology. The classification of connective tissue nevi into different categories, such as nevus elasticus, nevus anelasticus and collagenoma, has been generally abandoned since it became apparent that variations in the histologic composition occur not only in different patients but also in different lesions from the same patient, and even within an individual lesion (Raque and Wood).

Since the lesions are nodular, the amount of collagen obviously is always increased, although this may be difficult to ascertain if the collagen bundles are normal in appearance (Smith and Waisman). In some lesions, however, the collagen bundles are thickened and appear homogeneous (Rocha and Winkelmann; Schorr et al.).

The elastic fibers may appear normal or may be sparse or absent (Schorr et al.). In other lesions they show a marked increase in number and size without showing signs of degeneration (Fig. 6-13) (de Graciansky and Leclercq; Staricco and Mehregan). Frequently, however, when there is an increase in the amount of elastic tissue, the elastic fibers show coalescence into irregular clusters (Smith and Waisman; Danielsen et al.).

Differential Diagnosis. In connective tissue nevi with increase in elastic tissue the elastic fibers show, in contrast to pseudo-xanthoma elasticum, no breaking up into individual curls and no depositions of calcium.

CUTIS HYPERELASTICA (EHLERS-DANLOS SYNDROME)

Ehlers-Danlos syndrome, dominantly inherited with variable penetrance, occurs in three types (Barabas). The classical type shows pronounced involvement of the skin and joints and is characterized by (a) hyperextensibility of the skin, (b) hypermobility of the joints, and (c) fragility of the skin with impaired wound healing, resulting in the formation of atrophic scars. Occasionally, raisinlike pseudotumors form at the site of traumatic hematomas. They are raised and soft and have a wrinkled surface. In some cases hard subcutaneous nodules form at points of traumatic fat necrosis. The second type of Ehlers-Danlos syndrome is called the varicose type, with mild skin and joint manifestations but with varicose veins. The third or arterial type also has only mild hyperextensibility of the skin, and the hypermobility of the joints usually is limited to the hands; but the prognosis is serious because of potentially fatal ruptures of arteries which may or may not be preceded by the formation of aneurysm. Ruptures have been reported, among others, of the aorta (Lynch et al.), of the subclavian and popliteal arteries (McFarland and Fuller) and of the splenic artery (Imahori et al.). In addition, arteriovenous fistulae have been described, such as a carotid-cavernous fistula (Imahori et al.). A fourth type, recently described by Pinnell et al., is characterized by severe scoliosis, recurrent joint dislocation and hyperextensibility of skin and joints.

Histopathology. Aside from areas of the skin that have been altered secondarily by trauma, there are no obvious abnormalities either in the collagen or in the elastic fibers. Since the dermis is thinner than normal, the amount of collagen is decreased. The amount of elastic fibers appears increased; but this increase is only relative, being due to the decrease in the amount of collagen (Wechsler and Fisher).

The raisinlike pseudotumors at the site of hematomas consist of a proliferation of connective tissue and of numerous capillaries; they may also show accumulations of foreign-body giant cells (Ronchese). The hard subcutaneous nodules contain calcified necrotic fat surrounded by thick fibrous tissue (Johnson and Falls).

Examination of ruptured arteries reveals a decrease in collagen and muscle fibers in the media, and the collagen fibers appear loosely and irregularly arranged (McFarland and Fuller; Imahori et al.).

Histogenesis. A basic disturbance in Ehlers-Danlos syndrome appears to be an insufficient production of collagen by the dermal fibroblasts during the healing of wounds. Contrary to experimental wounds in control persons which in the healing phase contain large, elongated fibroblasts with enlarged and intensely basophilic nuclei and moderate amounts of extracellular fibrillar material, the experimental wound in a patient with Ehlers-Danlos syndrome showed fibroblasts with small, rounded and less basophilic nuclei and only little extracellular material (Scarpelli and Goodman). On electron microscopy, the healing wounds of control persons contain fibroblasts that appear highly active with a well organized rough endoplasmic reticulum and a conspicuous Golgi complex and, furthermore, show large bundles of collagen fibrils in the extracellular space. In contrast, the healing wound of the patient with Ehlers-Danlos syndrome showed in many fibroblasts only little rough endoplasmic reticulum and an inconspicuous Golgi complex and in the extracellular space inadequate collagen consisting of sparse bundles of collagen fibrils and, in addition, finely fibrillar material (Scarpelli and Goodman). It is of interest in this connection that in the uninjured skin of patients with Ehlers-Danlos syndrome the fibroblasts appear normal on electron microscopy (Wechsler and Fisher). Thus, the defect becomes manifest only in fibroblasts that have been stimulated to proliferate and to synthesize collagen.

An explanation for the hyperextensibility of the skin was offered by Jansen in 1955. On finding the collagen fibrils to be normal by electron microscopy, he regarded the hyperextensibility as the result of insufficient weaving together of the collagen fibrils. This, however, has remained an unproved theory. Since then a chemical abnormality of the collagen has been found by Pinnell et al. in the type of Ehlers-Danlos syndrome described by them (see above). They found a deficiency of hydroxylysine in dermal collagen, probably due to a deficiency of enzymatic hydroxylation of lysine in collagen. Since hydroxylysine participates in the cross-linking between collagen molecules within the collagen fibril, the collagen fibrils are defective.

CUTIS LAXA (DERMATOMEGALY)

Cutis laxa is characterized by loose, pendulous skin. There are two types, a congenital and an acquired type. In the congenital type, severe cases usually show recessive transmission (Goltz et al.), whereas less severe cases with a tendency to spontaneous improvement may show dominant transmission (Schreiber and Tilley). The acquired type has no genetic background (Reed et al.).

In severe cases of both the congenital and the acquired type internal organs are involved, in addition to the skin. There may be pulmonary emphysema leading to heart failure and death, in infancy in some of the congenital cases (Goltz et al.), or later in life in some of the acquired cases (Reed et al.). In addition, there may be diverticula in the gastrointestinal tract or in the bladder. Also, rectal prolapse and inguinal, umbilical and hiatal hernias have been observed (Goltz et al.), as well as congenital dislocation of the hips (Chadfield and North).

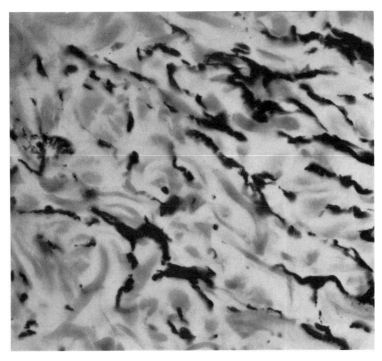

FIG. 6-14. **Cutis laxa.** Elastic tissue stain. The elastic fibers show granular degeneration and have an indistinct border. (×400) (Robert W. Goltz, M.D.)

Some of the cases of acquired cutis laxa are accompanied by a cutaneous eruption resembling erythema multiforme (Reed et al.) or a nonspecific dermatitis (Jablonska).

Histopathology. The elastic fibers of the dermis not only appear diminished, but also show granular degeneration, leading to their dissolution (Fig. 6-14) (Goltz et al.). The elastic fibers, prior to their dissolution, no longer appear sharply demarcated but have an indistinct and hazy border. Some fibers appear thickened in their midportion, tapering to a point at both ends.

In patients with involvement of internal organs the lungs and the gastrointestinal tract show the same granular degeneration of elastic fibers as seen in the skin (Goltz et al.; Reed et al.).

Histogenesis. Cutis laxa represents a degenerative disease of elastic fibers. In congenital cases the elastic fibers are digested by bacterial elastase more rapidly than normal elastic fibers (Goltz et al.). In acquired cases of cutis laxa accompanied by a cutaneous eruption it is likely that the inflammatory infiltrate contributes to the destruction of the elastic fibers (Jablonska). Electron micrographs also show the granular degeneration of the elastic fibers. Not only the granular fragments but also the relatively intact portions of elastic fibers show greatly increased electron density (Hult et al.). No calcification of elastic fibers is seen.

PACHYDERMOPERIOSTOSIS

An idiopathic and an acquired form exist, the latter being secondary to carcinoma of the lung. The idiopathic form is transmitted as a sex-linked dominant trait, occurring only in males (Hambrick and Carter). The manifestations include: (1) clubbing of the digits with periosteal proliferation of the bones of the hands and feet; (2) hyperplasia of the soft parts of the forearms and legs with periosteal proliferation of the corresponding bones; and (3) thickening and furrowing of the skin of the face and scalp (cutis verticis gyrata). In abortive forms there may be only clubbing of the fingers with periosteal proliferation of the bones of the hands and forearm (Curth et al.).

Histopathology. The skin of the face shows thickening of the dermis, with thick

fibrous bands extending into the subcutaneous tissue (Vogl and Goldfischer). In addition to an increase in the amount and size of the collagen bundles in the dermis, there is an increase in the number of fibroblasts and in the amount of ground substance, particularly hyaluronic acid, staining with alcian blue-PAS stain at pH 2.5, but not at pH 0.45, and with colloidal iron-PAS (Hambrick and Carter).

URTICARIA PIGMENTOSA

Urticaria pigmentosa, although occasionally occurring as a dominantly transmitted disease (Shaw; Bazex et al.), in most instances occurs without a family history. It can be divided into three forms: (1) urticaria pigmentosa arising in infancy or early childhood without significant systemic lesions; (2) urticaria pigmentosa arising in adolescence or adult life without significant systemic lesions; and (3) systemic mast cell disease. In the first form the cutaneous lesions often improve or even clear at puberty (Klaus and Winkelmann). Visceral lesions are absent as a rule and, if present, they usually are few in number. In the second form, urticaria pigmentosa arising in adolescence or adult life, systemic lesions are often present, but as a rule their course is rather static (Caplan). However, spontaneous regression has never been documented in adults, in contrast to children (Roberts et al.). In only very few patients is there progression to systemic mast cell disease with a fatal outcome (Asboe-Hansen). In the third form, systemic mast cell disease, there is progressive involvement of many organs, including the liver, spleen, intestinal tract, meninges, bones and bone marrow, with release of mast cells into the blood, occasionally reaching the proportions of mast cell leukemia (Efrati et al.; Friedman; Brinkmann). Of a total of 29 cases of systemic mast cell disease reviewed by Mutter et al. in 1963, 11 had died at the time of reporting. In 5 of the 29 patients cutaneous lesions were absent. Although most cases of fatal systemic mast cell disease have been reported in adults, a fatal outcome may occur in children (Ellis; Waters and Lacson).

Five types of cutaneous lesions are seen in urticaria pigmentosa (Klaus and Winkelmann, 1965). Two types can occur in both the infantile and the adult form. They are: (a) the maculopapular type, consisting usually of dozens or even hundreds of brownish lesions that urticate on stroking, and (b) multiple nodules or plaques, also brownish in color and, on stroking, showing always urtication and occasionally also blister formation. The third type is seen almost exclusively in infants, namely, (c) the type characterized by a solitary large cutaneous nodule which often on stroking shows not only urtication but also large bullae. In rare instances, such a solitary nodule has been described as arising in adults but without giving rise to bullae (Baraf and Shapiro). The fourth type (d) the diffuse erythrodermic type always starts in early infancy and shows generalized brownish-red, soft infiltration of the skin, with urtication on stroking and formation of multiple blisters during the first two years of life not only on stroking but also spontaneously (Burgoon et al.; Orkin et al.). Although visceral lesions are common in the diffuse erythrodermic type they usually improve (Robinson et al.) and only very rarely progress into fatal systemic mast cell disease (Waters and Lacson). In a few instances, death occurred in early infancy, apparently as a result of histamine shock without any or with only insignificant mast-cell infiltration in visceral organs (Yasuda and Kukita; Allison). The fifth type of lesion occurs only in adults, namely, (e) telangiectasia macularis eruptiva perstans, consisting of an extensive eruption of brownish-red macules showing fine telangiectasias, with little or no urtication on stroking. Minor visceral involvement may occur in this type, especially bone lesions (Sagher et al.).

Histopathology. The histologic picture

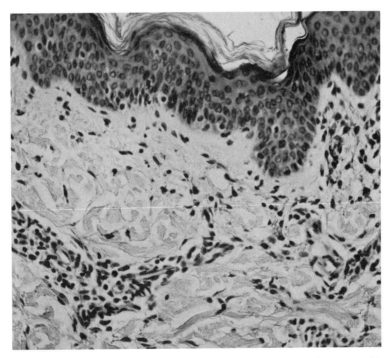

FIG. 6-15. **Urticaria pigmentosa, maculopapular type.** The mast cells are present only in small numbers and are predominantly spindle-shaped and perivascular in location. Since in routinely stained sections the mast cells resemble fibroblasts, the diagnosis may be missed. Giemsa stain will demonstrate the mast cell granules (see Plate 1, facing p. 74). ($\times 100$)

shows in all five types of lesions an infiltrate composed chiefly of mast cells. Although mast cells are characterized by the presence of metachromatic granules in their cytoplasm, these granules are not visible with routine stains (see p. 56); but they can be seen well after staining with Giemsa's stain or with toluidine blue (Plate 1, facing p. 74).

In the maculopapular type and in telangiectasia macularis eruptiva perstans the mast cells are limited to the upper third of the dermis and are located especially around capillaries. In some of the mast cells the nuclei may be round or oval, but in most mast cells the nuclei are spindle-shaped (Fig. 6-15). Since the mast cells may be present only in small numbers and since in sections stained with hematoxylin and eosin their nuclei resemble those of fibroblasts or pericytes, the diagnosis may be missed unless special staining is employed (Cramer).

In cases with multiple nodules or plaques or with a solitary large nodule, the mast cells lie closely packed in tumorlike aggregates (Figs. 6-16 and 6-17). The infiltrate may extend through the entire dermis and even into the subcutaneous fat (Johnson and Helwig). Whenever the mast cells lie in dense aggregates, their nuclei are cuboidal rather than spindle-shaped and they show ample and well defined eosinophilic cytoplasm. Because of the shape of their nuclei and distinct cytoplasm they have a rather distinctive appearance, so that the diagnosis usually can be made even before special staining has been carried out.

In the diffuse, erythrodermic type, one observes in the upper dermis a dense bandlike infiltrate of mast cells having a rather uniform appearance, showing round to oval nuclei and a distinctly outlined cytoplasm (Degos; Braun-Falco and Jung; Robinson et al.; Burgoon et al.).

All types of lesions, with the exception of telangiectasia macularis eruptiva perstans, may contain eosinophils in small numbers. If a biopsy is taken shortly after the lesion has been stroked, one observes an increased number of eosinophils and also extracellular mast cell granules as an indication that granules have been released by the cells (Drennan).

The bullae that may occur in infants with multiple or solitary nodules or with the diffuse erythrodermic type arise subepidermally

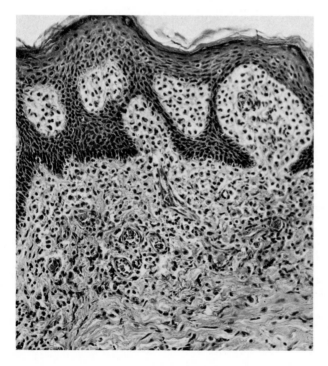

FIG. 6-16. **Urticaria pigmentosa, nodular type.** Low magnification, hematoxylin-eosin stain. Mast cells lie closely packed in the upper dermis. They are cuboidal in shape. Because of staining with hematoxylin-eosin, the granules in the mast cells are not visible. (×200)

(Miller and Shapiro). Older bullae, because of regeneration of the epidermis at the base of the bulla, may be located intraepidermally. The bullous cavity often contains mast cells and, in addition, eosinophils (Dewar and Milne). The pigmentation of lesions of urticaria pigmentosa is due to the presence of increased amounts of melanin in the basal cell layer and, occasionally, also of melanophages in the upper dermis.

Systemic Lesions. Mast cell aggregates to a slight degree may be present in internal organs in the diffuse erythrodermic type of infantile urticaria pigmentosa and in urticaria pigmentosa arising in adult life. Extensive aggregates of mast cells occur in systemic mast cell disease, with diffuse infiltration especially of lymph nodes, spleen, liver, intestinal tract, bones and bone marrow (Mutter et al.; Roberts et al.). Whereas mild infiltration of the bones with mast cells causes asymptomatic osteoporotic and osteosclerotic changes (Sagher et al.), massive infiltration, as it occurs in systemic mast cell disease, can cause collapse of several vertebrae (Mutter et al.).

Histogenesis. Both by light microscopy and by electron microscopy the mast cells of urticaria pigmentosa do not differ from normal mast cells either in structure or in the mode of degranulation (E.M. No. 18) (Freeman). Since mast cells contain histamine and release it during degranulation, chemical analysis of cutaneous lesions of urticaria pigmentosa reveals, in comparison with normal skin, a considerable increase in histamine (Davis et al.). Also, in patients with extensive lesions irritation of the involved skin by a hot bath and brushing may lead to flushing and a markedly increased excretion of histamine in the urine (Cramer).

The increased melanin pigmentation in lesions of urticaria pigmentosa is the result of stimulation of the epidermal melanocytes by the mast cells. Thus, the pigmentation is not caused by any substance present within the mast cells, even though there is evidence of a relationship between mast cells and melanocytes, according to Okun, who observed in lesions of urticaria pigmentosa mast cells with dual granulation containing both mast cell granules and melanosomes. Also, mast cells possess the enzymatic potential to form in vitro melanin from tyrosine, with peroxidase mediating the conversion in the presence of dopa as cofactor (Okun et al.) (see also p. 18).

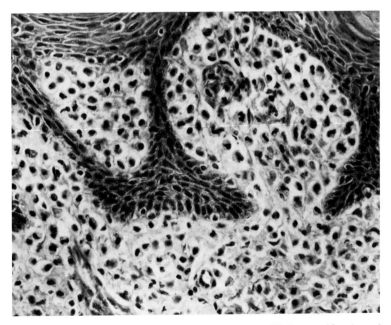

Fig. 6-17. **Urticaria pigmentosa, nodular type.** High magnification of Figure 6-16, hematoxylin-eosin stain. The mast cells appear as large cuboidal cells. (×400)

Differential Diagnosis. An absolutely reliable diagnosis of urticaria pigmentosa requires the demonstration of the mast cell-granules with the Giemsa stain. On routine staining the mast cells in macular lesions may resemble fibroblasts or pericytes, whereas those in nodular or erythrodermic lesions may resemble the histiocytes seen in Letterer-Siwe disease or in eosinophilic granuloma. Differentiation of urticaria pigmentosa from these two diseases on routine staining can be particularly difficult, because in all three diseases the infiltrate contains eosinophils. However, in contrast with Letterer-Siwe disease, the cells of urticaria pigmentosa have no tendency to invade the epidermis. Also occasionally the cuboidal mast cells in nodular urticaria pigmentosa resemble nevus cells, but they show no tendency to nesting and no junction activity.

Histologic differentiation between the lesions of urticaria pigmentosa and those of systemic mast cell disease is often possible, since in systemic mast cell disease the mast cells, including those present in the skin, are immature and have a larger, more pleomorphic nucleus. Also mitotic figures are present, and there may be decreased metachromatic staining of the granules (Lennert).

INCONTINENTIA PIGMENTI

Incontinentia pigmenti is an X-linked dominantly inherited disorder. Females with the abnormal gene on only one of their two X chromosomes are heterozygous for this condition and not severely affected; whereas males with the abnormal gene on their single X chromosome are homozygous for this condition and hence they are so severely affected that they usually die in utero. This theory explains the predominance of female patients (Lenz; Gordon and Gordon). Of 231 reported cases only 13 have been boys (Pallisgaard).

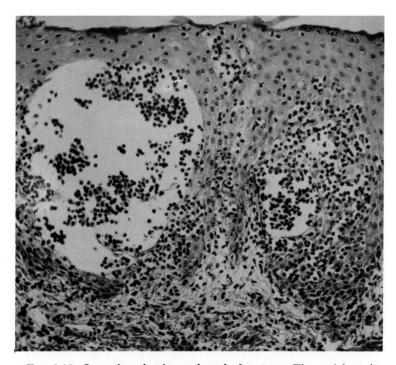

FIG. 6-18. **Incontinentia pigmenti, vesicular stage.** The vesicles arise within the epidermis and are associated with spongiosis. Numerous eosinophils and also mononuclear cells are present in the vesicles as well as in the epidermis and the dermis. ($\times$200)

The disease has three stages. The first stage, consisting of erythema and bullae arranged in lines, either is present at birth or starts shortly after birth. The extremities are predominantly affected. After about two months, the vesicular lesions gradually are superseded in the second stage by linear, verrucous lesions which persist for about two months. Either during the verrucous stage, or within a few months thereafter, widely disseminated areas of irregular, spattered or whorled pigmentation develop. This pigmentation, representing the third stage, is most pronounced on the trunk. It diminishes gradually after several years and may even clear completely. During the first stage there is marked blood eosinophilia.

Not infrequently, incontinentia pigmenti is associated with certain congenital anomalies, particularly inadequate dentition, partial alopecia at the vertex, strabismus and microphthalmia (Wodniansky; Carney and Carney).

Histopathology. The vesicles seen during the first stage arise within the epidermis and are associated with spongiosis. Thus they are of the type seen in dermatitis (see p. 98) (Epstein et al.; Wodniansky). They differ, however, from the vesicles of dermatitis by the presence of numerous eosinophils within the vesicles as well as around the vesicles in the epidermis (Fig. 6-18). The epidermis between the vesicles often contains small whorls of epidermal cells (Epstein et al.) and scattered, large dyskeratotic cells with eosinophilic hyaline cytoplasm (Grüneberg). The dermis shows an infiltrate containing, like the epidermis, many eosinophils and also mononuclear cells.

The alterations in the second stage consist of acanthosis, irregular papillomatosis and hyperkeratosis. Intraepidermal keratinization, consisting of whorls of keratinocytes and of scattered dyskeratotic cells, is often present (Epstein et al.). The dermis shows a rather mild, chronic inflammatory infiltrate that often contains a few melanophages. This infiltrate is seen to extend into the epidermis in many places.

The areas of pigmentation seen in the third stage show extensive deposits of melanin within melanophages located in the upper dermis. Usually, this dermal hyper-pigmentation is found in association with a diminution of pigment in the basal layer, the cells of which show vacuolization and degeneration (Sulzberger; Doornink). In some cases, however, the cells of the basal layer contain abundant amounts of melanin (Vilanova and Aguade; Rubin and Becker).

Histogenesis. The fact that the first two stages of incontinentia pigmenti are seen predominantly on the extremities and the third stage mainly on the trunk led to the assumption that the pigmentary changes of the third stage occurred independently of the bullous and verrucous lesions of the first two stages and were not postinflammatory in nature (Carney and Carney). Rather, it was thought that the dermal pigmentation in cases with diminished amounts of melanin in the basal cell layer occurred as the result of pigmentary incontinence of the basal cells (Sulzberger; Doornink); and that in cases with increased amounts of melanin in the basal cell layer exhaustion and death of the melanocytes led them to release their melanin into the dermis (Rubin and Becker). Electron microscopic studies, however, have revealed common features, although to varying extent, in all three stages of incontinentia pigmenti and thus suggest that all three stages are related to each other (Schaumburg-Lever and Lever). Even in the first stage many keratinocytes and melanocytes show degenerative changes resulting in a migration of macrophages into the epidermis where they phagocytize dyskeratotic keratinocytes and melanosomes. Subsequently the macrophages return to the dermis (E.M. No. 19). The macrophages in the second and third stages contain abundant melanosome complexes and thus are easily recognizable as melanophages even by light microscopy, whereas the macrophages in the first stage contain only few melanosome complexes and therefore can be identified as melanophages only in the electron microscope.

INCONTINENTIA PIGMENTI ACHROMIANS

This dominantly inherited pigmentary disorder at first was described as occurring among Japanese (Hamada et al.) but lately has been observed also in Europe (Grosshans et al.) and in the United States (Rubin). It begins early in life and persists for many years. Linear depigmented areas are seen on the trunk and extremities in a bizarre pattern. The pattern of the depigmented areas is similar to a negative picture of the pigmented areas in incontinentia pigmenti.

Histopathology. In the depigmented areas the amount of melanin granules in the basal cell layer is reduced irregularly so that in some areas melanin is completely absent (Grosshans et al.). The melanocytes stain more weakly with the dopa reaction and are smaller in size than in the adjacent normal skin, and their dendrites are shorter (Hamada et al.).

No inflammatory cells or melanophages are found in the dermis (Rubin).

BIBLIOGRAPHY

Ichthyosis

Ackerman, A. B.: Histopathologic concept of epidermolytic hyperkeratosis. Arch. Derm., *102*:253, 1970.

Altman, J., and Stroud, J.: Netherton's syndrome and ichthyosis linearis circumflexa. Psoriasiform ichthyosis. Arch. Derm., *100*:550, 1969.

Anton-Lamprecht, I.: Zur Ultrastruktur hereditärer Verhornungsstörungen. III. Autosomal-dominante Ichthyosis vulgaris. Arch. Derm. Forsch., *248*:144, 1973.

———, I.: Zur Ultrastruktur hereditärer Verhornungsstörungen. IV. X-chromosomal-recessive Ichthyosis. Arch. Derm. Forsch., *248*: 361, 1974.

Anton-Lamprecht, I., and Schnyder, U. W.: Ultrastructure in inborn errors of keratinization. Arch. Derm. Forsch., *250*:207, 1974.

Bloom, D., and Goodfried, M. S.: Lamellar ichthyosis of the newborn. Arch. Derm., *86*:336, 1962.

Braun-Falco, O., Petzoldt, D., Christophers, E., and Wolff, H. H.: Die granulöse Degeneration bei Naevus verrucosus bilateralis. Arch. klin. exp. Derm., *235*:115, 1969.

Craig, J. M., Goldsmith, L. A., and Baden, H. A.: On abnormality of keratin in the harlequin fetus. Pediatrics, *46*:437, 1970.

Feinstein, A., Ackerman, A. B., and Ziprkowski, L.: Histology of autosomal dominant ichthyosis vulgaris and X-linked ichthyosis. Arch. Derm., *101*:524, 1970.

Frost, P., and Van Scott, E. J.: Ichthyosiform dermatoses. Arch. Derm., *94*:113, 1966.

Frost, P., Weinstein, G. D., and Van Scott, E. J.: The ichthyosiform dermatoses. II. Autoradiographic studies of epidermal proliferation. J. Invest. Derm., *47*:561, 1966.

Heijer, A., and Reed, W. B.: Sjögren-Larsson syndrome. Arch. Derm., *92*:545, 1965.

Ishibashi, Y., and Klingmüller, G.: Erythrodermia ichthyosiformis congenita bullosa Brocq. Arch. klin. exp. Derm., *232*:205, 1968.

McCurdy, J., and Beare, J. M.: Congenital bullous ichthyosiform erythroderma. Brit. J. Derm., *79*:294, 1967.

Salamon, T., and Lazovic, O.: Über einen Fall von Erythrodermia ichthyosiformis congenita bullosa (Brocq, 1902). Arch. klin. exp. Derm., *210*:547, 1960.

Schellander, F. G., and Fritsch, P. O.: Variable erythrokeratoderma. Arch. Derm., *100*:744, 1969.

Schnyder, U. W.: Inherited ichthyoses. Arch. Derm., *102*:240, 1970.

Schnyder, U. W., and Konrad, B.: Zur Histogenetik der Ichthyosen. Hautarzt, *18*:445, 1967.

Steinberg, D., Mize, C. E., Herndon, J. H., Jr., et al.: Phytanic acid in patients with Refsum's syndrome and response to dietary treatment. Arch. Int. Med., *125*:75, 1970.

Stevanovic, D. V.: Hodgkin's disease of the skin. Arch. Derm., *82*:96, 1960.

Tay, C. H.: Ichthyosiform erythroderma, hair shaft anomalies, and mental and growth retardation. Arch. Derm., *104*:4, 1971.

Vandersteen, P. R., and Muller, S. A.: Erythrokeratodermia variabilis. Arch. Derm., *103*: 362, 1971.

———: Lamellar ichthyosis. Arch. Derm., *106*: 694, 1972.

Keratosis Palmaris et Plantaris

Bach, J. N., and Levan, N. E.: Papillon-Lefèvre syndrome. Arch. Derm., *97*:154, 1968.

Bologa, E. I.: Dominant vererbliche, durch vier Generationen geschlechtsgebundene Keratosis palmaris striata (linearis). Derm. Wschr., *152*: 446, 1966.

Brown, F. C.: Punctate keratoderma. Arch. Derm., *104*:682, 1971.

Buchanan, R. N., Jr.: Keratosis punctata palmaris et plantaris. Arch. Derm., *88*:644, 1963.

Callan, N. J.: Circumscribed palmoplantar keratoderma. Austral. J. Derm., *11*:76, 1970.

Greither, A.: Keratosis extremitatum hereditaria progrediens mit dominantem Erbgang. Hautarzt, *3*:198, 1952.

Herman, P. S.: Punctate porokeratotic keratoderma. Dermatologica, *147*:206, 1973.

Klaus, S., Weinstein, G. D., and Frost, P.: Localized epidermolytic hyperkeratosis. A form of keratoderma of the palms and soles. Arch. Derm., *101*:272, 1970.

Meyer-Rohn, J.: Keratoderma hereditarium palmare et plantare Unna-Thost und Meledakrankheit. Derm. Wschr., *129*:49, 1954.

Orbaneja, J. G., Lozano de Sosa, J. L. S., and Huarte, P. S.: Hiperqueratosis palmoplantar diffusa y circunscrita (tipo Thost-Unna) con degeneracion reticular del cuerpo mucoso. Intern. J. Derm., *11*:96, 1972.

Salamon, T., Bogdanovic, B., and Lazovic-Tepavac, O.: Die Krankheit von Mljet. Dermatologica, *138*:433, 1969.

Schirren, C., and Dinger, R.: Untersuchungen bei Keratosis hereditaria palmo-plantaris diffusa. Arch. klin. exp. Derm., *220*:266, 1964.

Pachyonychia Congenita

Kelly, E. W., Jr., and Pinkus, H.: Report of a case of pachyonychia congenita. Arch. Derm., *77*:724, 1958.

Witkop, C. J., and Gorlin, R. J.: Four hereditary mucosal syndromes. Arch. Derm., *84*:762, 1961.

Dyskeratosis Congenita

Bryan, H. G., and Nixon, R. K.: Dyskeratosis congenita and familial pancytopenia. J.A.M.A., *192*:203, 1965.

Cole, H. N., Cole, H. N., Jr., and Lascheid, W. P.: Dyskeratosis congenita. Arch. Derm., *76*: 712, 1957.

Costello, M. J., and Buncke, C. M.: Dyskeratosis congenita. Arch. Derm., *73*:123, 1956.

Garb, J.: Dyskeratosis congenita with pigmentation, dystrophia ungium, and leukokeratosis oris. Arch. Derm., *77*:704, 1958.

Sorrow, J. M., Jr., and Hitch, J. M.: Dyskeratosis congenita. Arch. Derm., *88*:340, 1963.

Porokeratosis (Mibelli)

Braun-Falco, O., and Balsa, R. E.: Zur Histochemie der cornoiden Lamelle. Hautarzt, *20*: 543, 1969.

Chernosky, M. E., and Freeman, R. G.: Disseminated superficial actinic porokeratosis (DSAP). Arch. Derm., *96*:611, 1967.

Goldner, R.: Zosteriform porokeratosis of Mibelli. Arch. Derm., *104*:425, 1971.

Guss, S. B., Osbourn, R. A., and Lutzner, M. A.: Porokeratosis plantaris, palmaris et disseminata. Arch. Derm., *104*:366, 1971.

Mann, P. R., Cort, D. F., Fairburn, E. A., and Abdel-Aziz, A.: Ultrastructural studies on two cases of porokeratosis of Mibelli. Brit. J. Derm., *90*:607, 1974.

Mikhail, G. H., and Wertheimer, F. W.: Clinical variants of porokeratosis (Mibelli). Arch. Derm., *98*:124, 1968.

Oberste-Lehn, H., and Moll, B.: Porokeratosis Mibelli und Stachelzellencarcinom. Hautarzt, 20:543, 1969.

Rahbari, H., Cordero, A. A., and Mehregan, A. H.: Linear porokeratosis. Arch. Derm., *109*:526, 1974.

Reed, R. J., and Leone, P.: Porokeratosis, a mutant clonal keratosis of the epidermis. Arch. Derm., *101*:340, 1970.

Swint, R. B., and Klaus, S. N.: Malignant degeneration of an epithelial nevus. Arch. Derm., *101*:56, 1970.

Xeroderma Pigmentosum

Bell, E. T., and Rothnem, T. P.: Xeroderma pigmentosum with carcinoma of the lower lip in two brothers aged 16 and 13 years. Am J. Cancer, *30*:574, 1937.

Cleaver, J. E.: DNA damage and repair in light-sensitive human skin disease. J. Invest. Derm., *54*:181, 1970.

———: Xeroderma pigmentosum: variants with normal DNA repair and normal sensitivity to ultraviolet light. J. Invest. Derm., *58*:124, 1972.

El-Hefnawi, H., and Mortada, A.: Ocular manifestations of xeroderma pigmentosum. Brit. J. Derm., *77*:261, 1965.

Guerrier, C. J., Lutzner, M. A., Devico, V., and Pruniéras, M.: An electron microscopical study of the skin in 18 cases of xeroderma pigmentosum. Dermatologica, *146*:211, 1973.

Hadida, E., Marill, F. G., and Sayag, J.: Xeroderma pigmentosum. Ann. derm. syph., *90*: 467, 1963.

Jung, E. G.: Das pigmentierte Xerodermoid. Arch. Derm. Forsch., *241*:33, 1971.

Lynch, H. T., Anderson, D. E., Smith, J. L., Jr., *et al.*: Xeroderma pigmentosum, malignant melanoma and congenital ichthyosis. Arch. Derm., *96*:625, 1967.

McGovern, V. J.: Melanoblastoma, with particular reference to its incidence in childhood. Austral. J. Derm., *6*:190, 1962.

Rasheed, A., El-Hefnawi, H., Nagy, G., and Wiskemann, A.: Elektronenmikroskopische Untersuchungen bei Xeroderma pigmentosum. Arch. klin. exp. Derm., *234*:321, 1969.

Ronchese, F.: Melanomata pathologically malignant, clinically nonmalignant, in a case of xeroderma pigmentosum. Arch. Derm. Syph., *68*:335, 1953.

Ectodermal Dysplasia

Bolck, F., and Barth, C.: Ein Beitrag zur hidrotischen Form der ektodermalen Dysplasie. Z. Haut, *48*:1041, 1973.

Dominok, G. W., and Rönisch, F.: Histologische Hautbefunde bei ektodermaler Dysplasie vom anhidrotischen Typ. Derm. Wschr., *154*:774, 1968.

Korting, G. W., and Salfeld, K.: Zur weiteren Kenntnis der Anhidrosis hypotrichica und der dabei vorkommenden Ekzemreaktion. Derm. Wschr., *144*:1141, 1961.

Malagon, V., and Taveras, J. E.: Congenital anhidrotic ectodermal and mesodermal dysplasia. Arch. Derm., *74*:253, 1956.

Reed, W. B., Lopez, D. A., and Landing, B.: Clinical spectrum of anhidrotic ectodermal dysplasia. Arch. Derm., *102*:134, 1970.

Sunderman, F. W.: Persons lacking sweat glands. Arch. Intern. Med., *67*:846, 1941.

Upshaw, B. Y., and Montgomery, H.: Hereditary anhidrotic ectodermal dysplasia. Arch. Derm. Syph., *60*:1170, 1949.

Focal Dermal Hypoplasia Syndrome

Goltz, R. W., Henderson, R. R., Hitch, J. M., and Ott, J. E.: Focal dermal hypoplasia syndrome. Arch. Derm., *101*:1, 1970.

Howell, J. B.: Nevus angiolipomatosus versus focal dermal hypoplasia. Arch. Derm., *92*:238, 1965.

Ishibashi, A., and Kurihara, Y.: Goltz's syndrome: focal dermal hypoplasia syndrome (focal dermal hypoplasia). Dermatologica, *144*:156, 1972.

Lever, W. F.: Hypoplasia cutis congenita. Arch. Derm., *90*:340, 1964.

Poikiloderma Congenitale (Rothmund-Thomson)

Rook, A., Davis, R., and Stevanovic, D.: Poikiloderma congenitale. Rothmund-Thomson syndrome. Acta dermatoven., *39*:392, 1959 (review).

Thannhauser, S. J.: Werner's syndrome (Progeria of the adult) and Rothmund's syndrome: two types of closely related heredofamilial atrophic dermatoses with juvenile cataracts and endocrine features. Ann. Intern. Med., *23*:559, 1945.

Tritsch, H., and Lischka, G.: Zur Histopathologie der kongenitalen Poikilodermie Thomson. Z. Haut, *43*:(155), 1968.

Bloom's Syndrome: Congenital Telangiectatic Erythema

Bloom, D., and German, J.: The syndrome of congenital telangiectatic erythema and stunted growth. Arch. Derm., *103*:545, 1971.

Braun-Falco, O., and Marghescu, S.: Kongenitales telangiektatisches Erythem (Bloom-Syndrom) mit Diabetes insipidus. Hautarzt, *17*:155, 1966.

Katzenellenbogen, I., and Laron, Z.: A contribution to Bloom's syndrome. Arch. Derm., *82*:609, 1960.

Landau, I. W., Sasaki, M. S., Newcomer, V. D., and Norman, A.: Bloom's syndrome. Arch. Derm., *94*:687, 1966.

McFarlin, D. E., Strober, W., and Waldman, T. A.: Ataxia-telangiectasia. Medicine, *51*:281, 1972.

Reed, W. B., Epstein, W. L., Boder, E., and Sedgwick, R.: Cutaneous manifestations of ataxia-telangiectasia. J.A.M.A., *195*:746, 1966.

Sawitsky, A., Bloom, D., and German, J.: Chromosomal breakage and acute leukemia in congenital telangiectatic erythema and stunted growth. Ann. Int. Med., *65*:487, 1966.

Scott, R. E.: Ataxia-telangiectasia. Arch. Path., *88*:78, 1969.

Progeria of the Adult (Werner's Syndrome)

Epstein, C. J., Martin, G. M., Schultz, A. L., and Motulsky, A. G.: Werner's syndrome. Medicine, *45*:177, 1966.

Tritsch, H., and Lischka, G.: Werner Syndrom, kombiniert mit Pseudo-Klinefelter-Syndrom. Hautarzt, *19*:547, 1968.

Epidermolysis Bullosa

Anton-Lamprecht, I., and Schnyder, U. W.: Epidermolysis bullosa dystrophica dominans—ein Defekt der anchoring fibrils? Dermatologica, *147*:289, 1973.

Bergenholtz, A., and Olsson, O.: Epidermolysis bullosa hereditaria. I. Epidermolysis bullosa hereditaria letalis. Acta dermatoven., *48*:220, 1968.

Bergenholtz, A., Olsson O., Arwill, T., and Lundström, N. R.: Die Epidermolysis bullosa hereditaria dystrophica mit Oesophagusveränderungen. Arch. klin. exp. Derm., *217*:518, 1963.

Eberhartinger, C., and Niebauer, G.: Zur Herlitzschen Sonderform von Epidermolysis bullosa. Z. Kinderheilk., *82*:227, 1959.

Eisen, A. Z., Bauer, E. A., and Jeffrey, J. J.: Animal and human collagenases. J. Invest. Derm., *55*:359, 1970.

Johnson, S. A. M., and Test, A. R.: Epidermolysis bullosa simplex of the hands and feet. Arch. Derm. Syph., *53*:610, 1946.

Kobayashi, T.: Dermo-epidermal junction in the recessive type of epidermolysis bullosa. Acta dermatoven., *47*:57, 1967.

Lazarus, G. S.: Collagenase and connective tissue metabolism in epidermolysis bullosa. J. Invest. Derm., *58*:242, 1972.

Lowe, L. B.: Hereditary epidermolysis bullosa. Arch. Derm., *95*:587, 1967.

Pearson, R. W.: Studies on the pathogenesis of epidermolysis bullosa. J. Invest. Derm., *39*: 551, 1962.

————: The mechanobullous diseases. *In* Fitzpatrick, T. B., *et al.* (eds.). Dermatology in General Medicine. p. 621. New York, McGraw-Hill, 1971.

Pearson, R. W., Potter, B., and Strauss, F.: Epidermolysis bullosa hereditaria letalis. Arch. Derm., *109*:349, 1974.

Purdy, M. J., and Fairbrother, G. E.: Case report: Epidermolysis bullosa acquisita. Austral. J. Derm., *13*:27, 1972.

Ridley, C. M., and Levy, I. S.: Epidermolysis bullosa and amyloidosis. Trans. St. John's Hosp. Derm. Soc., *54*:75, 1968.

Roenigk, H. H., Jr., Ryan, J. G., and Bergfeld, W. F.: Epidermolysis bullosa acquisita. Arch. Derm., *103*:1, 1971.

Vogel, A., and Schnyder, U. W.: Feinstrukturelle Untersuchungen an rezessiv-dystrophischer Epidermolysis bullosa hereditaria. Dermatologica, *135*:149, 1967.

Wechsler, H. L., Krugh, F. J., Domonkos, A. N., *et al.*: Polydysplastic epidermolysis bullosa and development of epidermal neoplasms. Arch. Derm., *102*:374, 1970.

Keratosis Follicularis

Ackerman, A. B.: Focal acantholytic dyskeratosis. Arch. Derm., *106*:702, 1972.

Beerman, H.: Hypertrophic Darier's disease and nevus syringocystadenomatosus papilliferus. Arch. Derm. Syph., *60*:500, 1949.

Caulfield, J. B., and Wilgram, G. F.: An electron-microscope study of dyskeratosis and acantholysis in Darier's disease. J. Invest. Derm., *41*:57, 1963.

Charles, A.: An electron microscope study of Darier's disease. Dermatologica, *122*:107, 1961.

Douwes, F. R.: Zur Histologie und Histochemie des Morbus Darier. Arch. klin. exp. Derm., *233*:309, 1968.

Ellis, F. A.: Keratosis follicularis is not primarily a follicular disease. Arch. Derm. Syph., *50*:27, 1944.

Forssmann, W. G., Holzmann, H., and Hoede, N.: Elektronenmikroskopische Untersuchungen der Haut bein Morbus Darier. Z. Haut, *42*:211, 1967.

Gottlieb, S. K., and Lutzner, M. A.: Darier's disease. Arch. Derm., *107*:225, 1973.

Jablonska, S., and Chorzelski, T.: Zur Klassifikation des Pemphigus Hailey-Hailey. Dermatologica, *117*:24, 1958.

Kellum, R. E., and Haserick, J. R.: Localized linear keratosis follicularis. Arch. Derm., *86*: 450, 1962.

Krinitz, K.: Tumoröse Veränderungen bei Morbus Darier. Hautarzt, *17*:445, 1966.

Leeming, J. A. L.: Acquired linear naevus showing histological features of keratosis follicularis. Brit. J. Derm., *81*:128, 1969.

Mann, P. R., and Haye, K. R.: An electron microscope study on the acantholytic and dyskeratotic processes in Darier's disease. Brit. J. Derm., *82*:561, 1970.

Piérard, J., Geerts, M. L., Vandeputte, H., and Fontaine, A.: A propos de quelques cas de dyskeratose folliculaire. Arch. belg. derm., *24*:381, 1968.

Piérard, J., and Kint, A.: Die Dariersche Krankheit. Arch. klin. exp. Derm., *231*:382, 1968.

Weathers, D. R., Olansky, S., and Sharpe, L. O.: Darier's disease with mucous membrane involvement. Arch. Derm., *100*:50, 1969.

Familial Benign Pemphigus

Botvinick, I.: Familial benign pemphigus with oral mucous membrane lesions. Cutis, *12*: 371, 1973.

Braun-Falco, O., and Vogell, W.: Elektronenmikroskopische Untersuchungen zur Dynamik der Acantholyse bei Pemphigus vulgaris. Arch. klin. exp. Derm., *223*:328, 1965.

Dupont, A.: Note sur l'histologie du pemphigus familial héréditaire bénin (Maladie de Gougerot-Hailey). Ann. derm. syph., *78*:703, 1951.

Ellis, F. A.: Vesicular Darier's disease (so-called benign familial pemphigus). Arch. Derm. Syph., *61*:715, 1950.

Finnerud, C. W., and Szymanski, F. J.: Chronic benign familial pemphigus, a possible vesicular variant of keratosis follicularis. Arch. Derm. Syph., *61*:737, 1950.

Ganor, S., and Sagher, F.: Keratosis follicularis (Darier) and familial benign chronic pemphigus (Hailey-Hailey) in the same patient. Brit. J. Derm., *77*:24, 1965.

Gönczöl, I., and Szodoray, L.: Hailey-Hailey'sche Pemphigusfälle bei Grossvater und Enkel. Dermatologica, *120*:214, 1960.

Gottlieb, S. K., and Lutzner, M. A.: Hailey-Hailey disease, an electron microscopic study. J. Invest. Derm., *54*:368, 1970.

Haber, H., and Russell, B.: Sisters with familial benign chronic pemphigus (Gougerot, Hailey and Hailey). Brit. J. Derm., *62*:458, 1950.

Herzberg, J. J.: Pemphigus Gougerot/Hailey-Hailey. Arch. klin. exp. Derm., *202*:21, 1955 (review).

Kahn, D., and Hutchinson, E.: Esophageal involvement in familial benign chronic pemphigus. Arch. Derm., *109*:719, 1974.

Lachapelle, J. M., de la Brassinne, M., and Geerts, M. L.: Maladies de Darier et de Hailey-Hailey: Etude comparative de l'incorporation de thymidine tritiée dans les cellules épidermiques. Arch. belges derm., *29*:241, 1973.

Niordson, A. M., and Sylvest, B.: Bullous dyskeratosis follicularis and acrokeratosis verruciformis. Arch. Derm., *92*:166, 1965.

Nürnberger, F., and Müller, G.: Electronenmikroskopische Untersuchungen über die Akantholyse bei Pemphigus familiaris benignus. Arch. klin. exp. Derm., *228*:208, 1967.

Palmer, D. D., and Perry, H. O.: Benign familial chronic pemphigus. Arch. Derm., *86*:493, 1962.

Piérard, J., and Kint, A.: Pemphigus familial bénin chronique (maladie de Hailey-Hailey). Dermatologica, *139*:1, 1969.

Raaschou-Nielsen, W., and Reymann, F.: Familial benign chronic pemphigus. Acta dermatoven., *39*:280, 1959.

Schneider, W., Fischer, H., and Wiehl, R.: Zur Frage der Schleimhautbeteiligung beim Pemphigus benignus familiaris chronicus. Arch. klin. exp. Derm., *225*:74, 1966.

Thies, W., Merker, H. J., and Fassbinder, K.: Zur Kasuistik des Pemphigus chronicus benignus (Hailey-Hailey) unter Berücksichtigung elektronenmikroskopischer Befunde. Hautarzt, *23*:244, 1972.

Wilgram, G. F., Caulfield, J. B., and Lever, W. F.: An electron microscopic study of acantholysis and dyskeratosis in Hailey and Hailey's disease. J. Invest. Derm., *39*:373, 1962.

Winer, L. H., and Leeb, A. J.: Benign familial pemphigus. Arch. Derm., *67*:77, 1953.

Acrokeratosis Verruciformis

Herndon, J. H., Jr., and Wilson, J. D.: Acrokeratosis verruciformis (Hopf) and Darier's disease. Arch. Derm., *93*:305, 1966.

Jordan, P., and Spier, H. W.: Morbus Darier-Veränderungen als Späterscheinungen bei Akrokeratosis verruciformis. Arch. Derm. Syph., *189*:441, 1949.

Krause, W., and Ehlers, G.: Über die Beziehung zwischen Akrokeratosis verruciformis Hopf und Dyskeratosis follicularis vegetans Darier. Hautarzt, *20*:397, 1969.

Niedelman, M. L., and McKusick, V. A.: Acrokeratosis verruciformis (Hopf). Arch. Derm., *86*:779, 1962.

Penrod, J. N., Everett, M. A., and McCreight, W. G.: Observations on keratosis follicularis. Arch. Derm. Syph., *82*:367, 1960.

Schueller, W. A.: Acrokeratosis verruciformis of Hopf. Arch. Derm., *106*:81, 1972.

Waisman, M.: Verruciform manifestations of keratosis follicularis. Arch. Derm., *81*:1, 1960.

Pseudoxanthoma Elasticum

Danielsen, L., and Kobayasi, T.: Pseudoxanthoma elasticum. Acta dermatoven., *54*:121, 1974.

Danielsen, L., Kobayasi, T., Larsen, H. W., et al.: Pseudoxanthoma elasticum. Acta dermatoven., *50*:355, 1970.

Eddy, D. D., and Farber, E. M.: Pseudoxanthoma elasticum. Arch. Derm., *86*:729, 1962.

Flatley, F. J., Atwell, M. E., and McEvoy, R. K.: Pseudoxanthoma elasticum with gastric hemorrhage. Arch. Intern. Med., *112*:352, 1963.

Goodman, R. M., et al.: Pseudoxanthoma elasticum, a clinical and histopathological study. Medicine, *42*:297, 1963 (review).

Hashimoto, K., and DiBella, R. J.: Electron microscopic studies of normal and abnormal elastic fibers of the skin. J. Invest. Derm., *48*:405, 1967.

Huang, S. N., Steele, H. D., Kumar, G., and Parker, J. O.: Ultrastructural changes of elastic fibers in pseudoxanthoma elasticum. Arch. Path., *83*:108, 1967.

Kreysel, H. W., Lerche, W., and Jänner, M.: Beobachtungen zum Grönblad-Strandberg-Syndrom (Angioid streaks, Pseudoxanthoma elasticum). Hautarzt, *18*:25, 1967.

Connective Tissue Nevus

Danielsen, L., Midtgaard, K., and Christensen, H. E.: Osteopoikilosis associated with dermatofibrosis lenticularis disseminata. Arch. Derm., *100*:465, 1969.

de Graciansky, P., and Leclercq, R.: Le "naevus elasticus" en tumeurs disséminées. Ann. derm. syph., *87*:5, 1960.

Raque, C. J., and Wood, M. G.: Connective-tissue nevus. Arch. Derm., *102*:390, 1970.

Rocha, G., and Winkelmann, R. K.: Connective tissue nevus. Arch. Derm., *85*:722, 1962.

Schorr, W. F., Optiz, J. M., and Reyes, C. N.: The connective tissue nevus–osteopoikilosis syndrome. Arch. Derm., *106*:208, 1972.

Smith, A. D., and Waisman, M.: Connective tissue nevi. Arch. Derm., *81*:249, 1960.

Staricco, R. G., and Mehregan, A. H.: Nevus elasticus and nevus elasticus vascularis. Arch. Derm., *84*:943, 1961.

Cutis Hyperelastica

Barabas, A. P.: Heterogeneity of the Ehlers-Danlos syndrome: Description of three clinical types and a hypothesis to explain the basic defects. Brit. Med. J., *2*:612, 1967.

Imahori, S., Bannerman, R. M., Graf, C. J., and Brennan, J. C.: Ehlers-Danlos syndrome with multiple arterial lesions. Am. J. Med., *47*: 967, 1969.

Jansen, L. H.: The structure of the connective tissue, an explanation of the symptoms of the Ehlers-Danlos syndrome. Dermatologica, *110*:108, 1955.

Johnson, S. A. M., and Falls, H. F.: Ehlers-Danlos syndrome. Arch. Derm. Syph., *60*: 82, 1949.

Lynch, H. T., Larsen, A. L., Wilson, R., and Magnuson, C. L.: Ehlers-Danlos syndrome and "congenital" arteriovenous fistulae. J.A.M.A., *194*:1011, 1965.

McFarland, W., and Fuller, D. E.: Mortality in Ehlers-Danlos syndrome due to spontaneous rupture of large arteries. New Eng. J. Med., *271*:1309, 1964.

Pinnell, S. R., Krane, S. M., Kenzora, J. E., and Glimcher, M. J.: A heritable disorder of connective tissue. New Eng. J. Med., *286*:1011, 1972.

Ronchese, F.: Dermatorrhexis. Am. J. Dis. Child., *51*:1403, 1936.

Scarpelli, D. G., and Goodman, R. M.: Observations on the fine structure of the fibroblast from a case of Ehlers-Danlos syndrome with the Marfan syndrome. J. Invest. Derm., *50*: 214, 1968.

Wechsler, H. L., and Fisher, E. R.: Ehlers-Danlos syndrome. Arch. Path., *77*:613, 1964.

Cutis Laxa

Chadfield, H. W., and North, J. F.: Cutis laxa. Trans. St. John's Hosp. Derm. Soc., *57*:181, 1971.

Goltz, R. W., Hult, A. M., Goldfarb, M., and Gorlin, R. J.: Cutis laxa. Arch. Derm., *92*: 373, 1965.

Hult, A. M., Goltz, R. W., and Midtgaard, K.: The dermal elastic fibers in cutis hyperelastica (Ehlers-Danlos syndrome) and in cutis laxa (generalized elastolysis). Acta dermatoven., *44*:415, 1964.

Jablonska, S.: Inflammatorische Hautveränderungen, die einer erworbenen Cutis laxa vorausgehen. Hautarzt, *17*:341, 1966.

Reed, W. B., Horowitz, R. E., and Beighton, P.: Acquired cutis laxa. Arch. Derm., *103*:661, 1971.

Schreiber, M. M., and Tilley, J. C.: Cutis laxa. Arch. Derm., *84*:266, 1961.

Pachydermoperiostosis

Curth, H. O., Firschein, I. L., and Alpert, M.: Familial clubbed fingers. Arch. Derm., *83*: 828, 1961.

Hambrick, G. W., and Carter, D. M.: Pachydermoperiostosis. Arch. Derm., *94*:594, 1966.

Vogl, A., and Goldfischer, S.: Pachydermoperiostosis. Am. J. Med., *33*:166, 1962.

Urticaria Pigmentosa

Allison, J.: Skin mastocytosis presenting as a neonatal bullous eruption. Austral. J. Derm., *9*:83, 1967.

Asboe-Hansen, G.: Urticaria pigmentosa with generalized tissue mastocytosis and blood basophilia. Arch. Derm., *81*:198, 1960.

Baraf, C. S., and Shapiro, L.: Solitary mastocytoma. Arch. Derm., *99*:589, 1969.

Bazex, A., Dupré, A., Christol, B., and Andrieu, H.: Les mastocytoses familiales. Ann. derm. syph., *98*:241, 1971.

Braun-Falco, O., and Jung, J.: Über klinische und experimentelle Beobachtungen bei einem Fall von diffuser Haut-Mastocytose. Arch. klin. exp. Derm., *213*:639, 1961.

Brinkmann, E.: Mastzellenreticulose (Gewebsbasophiliom) mit histaminbedingtem Flush und Übergang in Gewebsbasophilen-Leukämie. Schweiz. med. Wschr., *89*:1046, 1959.

Burgoon, C. F., Graham, J. H., and McCaffree, D. L.: Mast cell disease. Arch. Derm., *98*: 590, 1968.

Caplan, R. M.: The natural course of urticaria pigmentosa. Arch. Derm., *87*:146, 1963.

Cramer, H. J.: Telangiectasia macularis eruptiva perstans, eine Sonderform der Urticaria pigmentosa. Hautarzt, *15*:370, 1964.

Davis, M. J., Lawler, J. C., and Higdon, R. S.: Studies on an adult with urticaria pigmentosa. Arch. Derm., *77*:224, 1958.

Degos, R.: Mastocytoses en dehors de l'urticaire pigmentaire, réticuloses mastocytaires diffuses. Arch. belg. derm. syph., *11*:10, 1955.

Dewar, W. A., and Milne, J. A.: Bullous urticaria pigmentosa. Arch. Derm., *71*:717, 1955.

Drennan, J. M.: The mast cells in urticaria pigmentosa. J. Path. Bact., *63*:513, 1951.

Efrati, P., Klajman, A., and Spitz, H.: Mast cell leukemia? Malignant mastocytosis with leukemia-like manifestations. Blood, *12*:869, 1957.

Ellis, J. M.: Urticaria pigmentosa. Arch. Path., *48*:426, 1949.

Freeman, R. G.: Diffuse urticaria pigmentosa. Am. J. Clin. Path., *48*:187, 1967.

Friedman, B. I., Will, J. J., Freiman, D. G., and Braunstein, H.: Tissue mast cell leukemia. Blood, *13*:70, 1958.

Johnson, W. C., and Helwig, E. B.: Solitary mastocytosis (urticaria pigmentosa). Arch. Derm., *84*:806, 1961.

Klaus, S. N., and Winkelmann, R. K.: Course of urticaria pigmentosa in children. Arch. Derm., *86*:68, 1962.

————: The clinical spectrum of urticaria pigmentosa. Proc. Mayo Clin., *40*:923, 1965.

Lennert, K.: Zur pathologischen Anatomie von Urticaria pigmentosa und Mastzellenreticulose. Klin. Wschr., *40*:61, 1962.

Miller, R. C., and Shapiro, L.: Bullous urticaria pigmentosa in infancy. Arch. Derm., *91*:595, 1965.

Mutter, R. D., Tannenbaum, M., and Ultmann, J. E.: Systemic mast cell disease. Ann. Int. Med., *57*:887, 1963.

Okun, M. R.: Histogenesis of melanocytes. J. Invest. Derm., *44*:285, 1965.

Okun, M. R., Edelstein, L. M., Or, N., Hamada, G., and Donnellan, B.: The role of peroxidase vs. the role of tyrosinase in enzymatic conversion of tyrosine to melanin in melanocytes, mast cells, and eosinophils. J. Invest. Derm., *55*:1, 1970.

Orkin, M., Good, R. A., Clawson, C. C., *et al.*: Bullous mastocytosis. Arch. Derm., *101*:547, 1970.

Roberts, P. L., McDonald, H. B., and Wells, R. F.: Systemic mast cell disease in a patient with unusual gastrointestinal and pulmonary abnormalities. Am. J. Med., *45*:638, 1968.

Robinson, H. M., Jr., Kile, R. L., Hitch, J. M., *et al.*: Bullous urticaria pigmentosa. Arch. Derm., *85*:346, 1962.

Sagher, F., Cohen, C., and Schorr, S.: Concomitant bone changes in urticaria pigmentosa. J. Invest. Derm., *18*:425, 1952.

Shaw, J. M.: Genetic aspects of urticaria pigmentosa. Arch. Derm., *97*:137, 1968.

Waters, W. J., and Lacson, P. S.: Mast cell leukemia presenting as urticaria pigmentosa. Pediatrics, *19*:1033, 1957.

Yasuda, T., and Kukita, A.: A fatal case of purely cutaneous form of diffuse mastocytosis. Proc. XIIth Internat. Congress Derm. Vol. 2, p. 1558. Washington, D.C., 1962.

Incontinentia Pigmenti

Carney, R. G., and Carney, R. G., Jr.: Incontinentia pigmenti. Arch. Derm., *102*:157, 1970.

Doornink, F. J.: Über Incontinentia pigmenti und über die Siemens-Bloch'sche Pigmentdermatose. Dermatologica, *102*:63, 1951.

Epstein, S., Vedder, J. S., and Pinkus, H.: Bullous variety of incontinentia pigmenti (Bloch-Sulzberger). Arch. Derm. Syph., *65*:557, 1952.

Gordon, H., and Gordon, W.: Incontinentia pigmenti: Clinical and genetical studies of two familial cases. Dermatologica, *140*:150, 1970.

Grüneberg, T.: Zur Frage der Incontinentia pigmenti (Bloch-Sulzberger). Arch. klin. exp. Derm., *201*:218, 1955.

Lenz, W.: Zur Genetik der Incontinentia pigmenti. Ann. paediat., *196*:149, 1961.

Pallisgaard, G.: Incontinentia pigmenti in a newborn boy. Acta dermatoven., *49*.197, 1969.

Rubin, L., and Becker, S. W., Jr.: Pigmentation in the Bloch-Sulzberger syndrome (incontinentia pigmenti). Arch. Derm., *74*:263, 1956.

Wodniansky, P.: Das Syndrom der Incontinentia pigmenti. Arch. klin. exp. Derm., *201*:49, 1955 (review).

Schaumburg-Lever, G., and Lever, W. F.: Electron microscopy of incontinentia pigmenti. J. Invest. Derm., *61*:151, 1973.

Sulzberger, M. F.: Incontinentia pigmenti (Bloch-Sulzberger). Arch. Derm. Syph., *38*:57, 1958.

Vilanova, X., and Aguade, J. P.: Incontinentia pigmenti. Ann. Derm. Syph., *86*:247, 1959.

Wodniansky, P.: Das Syndrom der Incontinentia pigmenti. Arch. klin. exp. Derm., *201*:49, 1955 (review).

Incontinentia Pigmenti Achromians

Grosshans, E. M., Stoebner, P., Bergoend, H., and Stoll, C.: Incontinentia pigmenti achromians (Ito). Dermatologica, *142*:65, 1971.

Hamada, T., Saito, T., Sugai, T., and Morita, Y.: Incontinentia pigmenti achromians (Ito). Arch. Derm., *96*:673, 1967.

Rubin, M. B.: Incontinentia pigmenti achromians. Arch. Derm., *105*:424, 1972.

7

Noninfectious Vesicular and Bullous Diseases

CLASSIFICATION OF BLISTERS

Before discussing individual vesicular and bullous diseases it seems appropriate to present a classification of the different types of vesicles and bullae and to outline briefly their mode of formation. (Since from a histologic or histogenetic point of view it is immaterial whether a lesion is a vesicle or bulla, only the term blister will be used in the classification.)

Seven types of blisters can be recognized (Table 7-1).

1. Subcorneal Blister. Detachment of the horny layer occurs. (For a detailed description see p. 125.)

2. Blister Due to Intracellular Degeneration. Pronounced intracellular degeneration leads to intraepidermal bulla formation below the granular layer. (For detailed descriptions see pp. 61 and 127.)

3. Spongiotic Blister. Intercellular edema (spongiosis) is an early and characteristic feature of this type of bulla. It is accompanied by intracellular edema and a mononuclear cell infiltrate extending from the upper dermis into the epidermis (exocytosis). Pronounced intercellular edema stretches the intercellular bridges (desmosomes) until they disappear, and pronounced intracellular edema leads to reticular degeneration of the epidermis. (For a detailed description see p. 98.)

4. Acantholytic Blister. As a result of dissolution of the intercellular cement substance, including the intradesmosomal sub-stance, epidermal cells lose their coherence, leading to rifts between them that can enlarge into bullae. Detached (acantholytic) cells are present in the bulla cavity. Acantholysis takes place predominantly in the suprabasal region in some diseases, and predominantly in the subcorneal region in others (see Table 7-1). (For detailed descriptions see pp. 74 and 112.)

5. Viral Blister. Invasion of epidermal cells by certain viruses causes two types of degenerative changes in epidermal cells: ballooning and reticular degeneration. The ballooning degeneration leads to extensive "secondary" acantholysis, affecting even the basal layer. (For a detailed description see p. 338.)

6. Blister Due to Degeneration of Basal Cells. Degenerative changes in the basal cells lead to the formation of subepidermal bullae in several diseases (see Table 7-1). (For a detailed description see pp. 70, 149, and 426.)

7. Blister Due to Degeneration of the Basement Zone. Degenerative changes in one or several of the structures causing the coherence of the basal cells with the dermis lead to the formation of subepidermal bullae. There may be on light microscopic examination splitting, thinning or absence of the PAS-positive basement zone, and on electron microscopic examination damage to the half-desmosomes, the basal lamina, or the anchoring fibrils. (For detailed descriptions see pp. 115 and 119.)

Table 7-1. Classification of Blisters

Type of Blister	Mode of Formation	Site of Formation	Disease
1. Subcorneal blister	Detachment of horny layer	Subcorneal	Miliaria crystallina Erythema toxicum neonatorum Subcorneal pustular dermatosis Impetigo
2. Blister due to intracellular degeneration	Separation of cells from one another	Upper epidermis	Bullous congenital ichthyosiform erythroderma Epidermolysis bullosa of hands and feet Friction blisters
3. Spongiotic blister	Intercellular edema	Intraepidermal	Dermatitis (eczema) Incontinentia pigmenti Miliaria rubra
4. Acantholytic blister	Dissolution of intercellular cement substance	Intraepidermal (a) Suprabasal	Pemphigus vulgaris Familial benign pemphigus Darier's disease Transient acantholytic dermatosis Solar keratosis
		(b) Subcorneal	Pemphigus foliaceus
5. Viral blister	Ballooning degeneration leading to acantholysis	Intraepidermal	Variola Herpes simplex Varicella-herpes zoster
6. Blister due to degeneration of basal cells	Damaged basal cells lose contact with dermis	Subepidermal	Epidermolysis bullosa simplex Erythema multiforme, epidermal type Herpes gestationis Lichen planus Lichen sclerosus et atrophicus Lupus erythematosus
7. Blister due to degeneration of basement zone	Damage in the structures causing coherence of basal cells	Subepidermal	Epidermolysis bullosa, dystrophic type Urticaria pigmentosa Bullous pemphigoid Benign mucosal pemphigoid Dermatitis herpetiformis Erythema multiforme, dermal type Porphyria cutanea tarda

DERMATITIS (ECZEMA)

The terms *dermatitis* and *eczema* are used by many dermatologists as synonyms. They refer to an inflammation of the skin that often represents an allergic response of the skin to a variety of agents, such as chemicals, proteins, bacteria and fungi. They may act on the skin from either the outside or the inside. In many types of dermatitis, however, the cause is obscure.

Dermatitis may be acute, subacute, or chronic. The clinical picture is characterized by polymorphism of the eruption. Among the primary lesions that may be observed are macules, papules and vesicles. If macules coalesce they form patches of erythema that may be edematous; and if papules coalesce they form plaques. Among the secondary lesions are oozing, crusting, scaling, lichenification and fissuring. Usually, the lesions of dermatitis are not sharply demarcated but merge gradually into the surrounding normal skin. Itching is common in all types of dermatitis.

No generally accepted classification of dermatitis exists, and many cases defy assignment to any definite type. In this section the following types of dermatitis will be discussed: (1) contact dermatitis, (2) nummular dermatitis, (3) atopic dermatitis, (4) lichen simplex chronicus, (5) seborrheic dermatitis, (6) stasis dermatitis, and (7) generalized exfoliative dermatitis. In addition, lesions of dermatitis may occur in superficial fungal infections, as drug eruptions, and in lymphoma. The last three types will be discussed when the respective diseases are described.

Contact dermatitis is caused by contact of the skin with an agent that acts either as a specific allergic sensitizer or as a primary irritant. Contact dermatitis may be acute, subacute, or chronic. In the acute and subacute forms, diffuse erythema, edema, oozing and crusting predominate; in addition, often vesicles and bullae are present, particularly if a specific allergic sensitizer is the cause. In the chronic form, erythema, scaling and lichenification prevail.

Nummular dermatitis presents as the most characteristic lesion fairly sharply demarcated patches of erythema studded with "pinpoint vesicles" or "pinpoint erosions." In addition, there are scattered papulovesicles with a tendency to coalescence. On the palms and soles, where the tendency to coalesce is often lacking, the terms *dyshidrotic eruption* or *pompholyx* have been often used; but it seems best to discontinue the use of these terms (Calnan).

Atopic dermatitis, a genetically determined disorder that may occur in association with asthma and hay fever in the same patient or family, shows erythematous, scaling and lichenified areas, which, when active, also show oozing and crusting but no vesicles.

Lichen simplex chronicus shows one or several areas of erythema, scaling and lichenification. Oozing may be present but vesiculation is absent. The designation *neurodermatitis* for this eruption is misleading and should be avoided.

Seborrheic dermatitis shows fairly sharply demarcated, brownish-red areas that exhibit only slight infiltration and often have on their surface fine scaling, causing some resemblance to psoriasis. Oozing may be present, but there are no vesicles. Generalized seborrheic dermatitis may occur in infants as a self-limited disorder and is often referred to as Leiner's disease.

Stasis dermatitis occurs only on the lower portions of the legs as the result of venous stasis. It presents erythema, edema, scaling, and occasionally oozing and crusting. It differs from other forms of dermatitis, first, by showing brownish pigmentation and, second, by resulting in some instances in ulceration and atrophic scarring.

Generalized exfoliative dermatitis or *generalized erythroderma* shows involvement of the entire skin with erythema, scaling, and, in severe cases, oozing. It represents a peak reaction to which several types of dermatitis may lead, namely contact dermatitis, atopic dermatitis, seborrheic dermatitis, stasis dermatitis, drug dermatitis and lymphoma dermatitis. In addition, it may occur as a chronic idiopathic disease. When occurring as an apparently idiopathic disease, especially in older persons, and in association with peripheral lymphadenopathy, mainly of inguinal and axillary lymph nodes, it often represents Sézary's syndrome, a form of mycosis fungoides (see p. 703). A generalized erythroderma also may be seen in several diseases not belonging to the dermatitis group, namely in psoriasis, pemphigus foliaceus, and congenital ichthyosiform erythroderma. However, in psoriasis the erythroderma has a more uniform appearance because of the absence of oozing; in pemphigus foliaceus the Nikolsky sign is positive and on histologic examination acantholysis is present; and in congenital ichthyosiform erythroderma the eruption has been present since birth.

Histopathology. In all clinical types of dermatitis there are both epidermal and dermal changes. The various types of dermatitis rarely present a histologic picture sufficiently diagnostic to allow their differentiation, because similar histologic reactions occur in all forms of dermatitis: spongiotic microvesicles or macrovesicles with oozing in acute dermatitis; acanthosis with parakeratosis in chronic dermatitis; and a combination of these two reaction patterns in subacute dermatitis. Since as a rule no diagnosis more specific than acute, subacute, or chronic dermatitis can be made, the histologic picture as presented by an acute, a subacute, and a chronic dermatitis will be described first. Thereafter, the more or less distinctive features occasionally presented by the various types of dermatitis will be listed.

In *acute dermatitis* intraepidermally located vesicles or bullae dominate the histologic picture. Considerable intercellular edema (spongiosis) and intracellular edema may be present in the epidermis surrounding the vesicles. If the number of vesicles is great, and the intracellular edema is pronounced, the histologic picture of reticular degeneration of the epidermis results. The vesicles then are separated from one another only by thin septa formed by the resisting walls of edematous epidermal cells and thus

form a multilocular bulla (Fig. 7-1). The vesicles and bullae as well as the edematous portions of the epidermis may be permeated by an inflammatory infiltrate composed mainly of mononuclear cells formerly regarded as lymphocytes but now known to be largely monocytes and histiocytes or macrophages, with lymphocytes in the minority. (See under Histogenesis of Contact Dermatitis, p. 101.) Lesions more than a few days old may also contain neutrophils, particularly in the stratum corneum. The stratum corneum may be parakeratotic and contain aggregates of coagulated plasma, the substrate of crusts. The upper dermis shows vascular dilatation, edema and a mononuclear cellular infiltrate around the superficial capillaries extending from there into the epidermis (exocytosis).

In *subacute dermatitis* one observes spongiosis, intracellular edema and, usually, vesicles. The vesicles, although smaller in size, arise, like those of an acute dermatitis, at sites of spongiosis and intracellular edema and enlarge through reticular degeneration of epidermal cells (Fig. 7-2). The vesicles

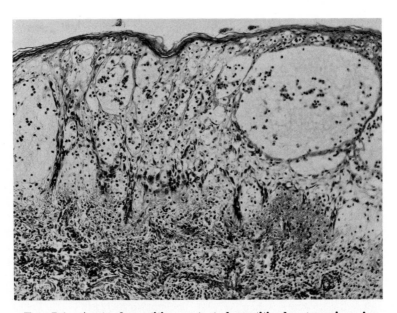

FIG. 7-1. **Acute dermatitis: contact dermatitis due to poison ivy.** Numerous intraepidermal vesicles and pronounced intracellular edema are present, so that the histologic picture of reticular degeneration of the epidermis results. The vesicles are separated from one another only by thin septa formed by the resisting walls of edematous epidermal cells and thus form a multilocular bulla. ($\times$100)

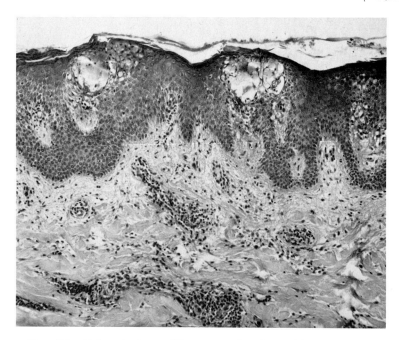

FIG. 7-2. **Subacute dermatitis: nummular dermatitis.** The vesicles arise at sites of spongiosis and intracellular edema and enlarge through reticular degeneration of epidermal cells. The epidermis shows moderate acanthosis. The dermis contains a perivascular infiltrate. (×100)

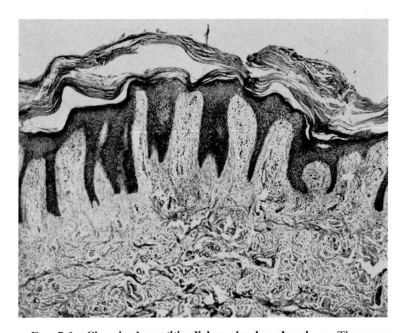

FIG. 7-3. **Chronic dermatitis: lichen simplex chronicus.** There are hyperkeratosis, acanthosis, elongation of the rete ridges, and elongation and broadening of the papillae. The dermis shows a chronic inflammatory infiltrate and fibrosis. (×50)

are seen at various levels of the epidermis. Even though they probably form in the lower epidermis, the rapid proliferation of the epidermis causes vesicles that are a few days old and are still increasing in size to be located in the upper stratum malpighii. One finds moderate acanthosis and, in the stratum corneum, varying degrees of parakeratosis and crusting. The inflammatory infiltrate is similar to that seen in acute dermatitis.

In *chronic dermatitis* one encounters moderate to marked acanthosis with elongation of the rete ridges. There also is hyperkeratosis with areas of parakeratosis (Fig. 7-3). Slight spongiosis may be present, but vesicles are absent. Intracellular vacuolization, if present, may be the result not of edema but of glycogen accumulation (Neumann and Winter). The inflammatory infiltrate generally has a perivascular distribution in the upper dermis, and exocytosis, i.e., extension of the infiltrate into the epidermis, is absent, as a rule. The number of capillaries is increased, and their walls may be thickened. There also may be some increase of collagen, manifesting itself as fibrosis, in the upper dermis, including the papillae.

A few words about the histologic aspects of the various types of dermatitis are now in order.

Contact Dermatitis. Contact dermatitis may be acute, subacute, or chronic. The histologic descriptions given above for acute, subacute and chronic dermatitis apply in general to contact dermatitis. Usually, it is not possible to distinguish histologically between an allergic contact dermatitis and a primary irritant, or toxic, contact dermatitis. This is due to the fact that a biopsy usually is carried out days or weeks after appearance of the dermatitis. By that time, regenerative processes, complications, etc., have altered the original picture of the dermatitis and the findings are those of a nonspecific subacute or chronic dermatitis. However, the patch testing of sensitized individuals with the specific sensitizing substance and of nonsensitized individuals with a primary irritant or toxic substance results in different histologic responses. Similarly, it often is not possible to distinguish histologically between a photo-

allergic and a phototoxic contact dermatitis, although such distinction may be important, since some drugs like chlorpromazine are capable of producing either. However, differentiation of a photoallergic from a phototoxic reaction usually is possible through the histologic examination of photopatch tests, since the histologic responses differ in a manner similar to that of the patch test results in allergic and toxic contact dermatitis (see below) (Epstein).

Patch Testing. Patch tests with the allergen in allergic contact dermatitis show in humans, on light microscopic examination, about 3 hours after application of the patch test, the first alteration, consisting of vasodilatation and extravasation of mononuclear cells from the papillary and subpapillary capillaries into the dermis (Miescher). The mononuclear cells migrate toward the epidermis and, on entering it, produce basal spongiosis about 8 hours after application of the test; and, as they migrate upward between the epidermal cells, spongiosis develops also in the upper epidermis, after 12 to 24 hours (Bandmann, 1960). The areas of spongiosis soon develop into spongiotic vesicles.

In contrast to patch tests with allergens, those with primary irritants induce damage to the epidermal cells usually within very few hours, although the speed with which the damage occurs and the degree of damage depend on the type and the concentration of the primary irritant (Hall et al.). With moderately strong primary irritants, such as 10 per cent dinitrochlorobenzene, both intracellular and intercellular edema throughout the epidermis is evident after 3 to 6 hours. Within 24 hours epidermal necrosis characterized by cellular vacuolation and nuclear pyknosis occurs (Epstein). This may result in subepidermal blister formation (Kerl et al.). There is less of a dermal infiltrate and less exocytosis than on patch testing with allergens, and neutrophils, usually absent in patch tests with allergens, make up a significant proportion of the infiltrate (Epstein).

Histogenesis. A substance capable of inducing a contact dermatitis is called a hapten; but, after its application to the skin, in order to act as an allergen or antigen, it must be conjugated with epidermal proteins. In persons in whom sensitization takes place this hapten-protein conjugate is phagocytized by macrophages. These antigen-carrying macrophages "inform" lymphocytes. Subsequently the "informed" lymphocytes aggregate in the paracortical areas of the regional lymph nodes, where they transform into lymphoblasts, or blast cells. From the 5th day on after the application of the hapten to the skin the lymphoblasts divide and form clones of "sensitized" lymphocytes in the paracortical areas of regional lymph nodes. Such sensitized lymphocytes, since they form in the paracortical areas, are thymus-derived or T lymphocytes. They have on their surface a receptor capable of recognizing the specific antigen to which they have become sensitized. The sensitized lymphocytes circulate in the peripheral blood as "memory cells" or "committed" lymphocytes in rather small numbers, carrying the specific antibody (Macher, 1962; Achten and Delescluse).

If subsequently the skin is re-exposed to the specific hapten, the hapten again is rapidly conjugated with epidermal proteins to form the allergen or antigen. The antigen now attracts circulating committed antibody-carrying lymphocytes to the site of contact. Because of the relatively small number of committed lymphocytes present in the circulation, several hours pass before sufficient antibody-carrying lymphocytes have gathered at the site of contact for the antigen-antibody reaction to take place. This lag period has given this reaction the name *delayed hypersensitivity reaction*. As this reaction takes place, the antibody-carrying lymphocytes release a number of factors or "lymphokines" (Macher, 1972; Achten and Delescluse). Among these factors are: (a) a cytotoxic factor, causing damage at the site of the antigen-antibody reaction and leading to spongiosis in the epidermis; (b) a chemotactic factor, or permeability-increasing factor, causing vasodilatation and the migration of monocytes through the walls of capillaries to the site of the reaction (Inderbitzin et al.); (c) a mitogenic factor, activating the multiplication of monocytes, which by their phagocytic activity become macrophages; (d) a migration inhibiting factor (MIF), preventing macrophages from leaving the reaction site so that they can phagocytize the damaged tissue (Nordquist and Rorsman); (e) a mediator attracting basophils to the reaction site (Dvorak et al.), and (f) a factor causing the formation of additional committed lymphocytes in the paracortical areas of the regional lymph nodes.

The committed lymphocytes of a sensitized individual, when exposed in vitro to the specific antigen, are stimulated to transform into lymphoblasts, or blast cells, that synthesize DNA, demonstrable by labeling with tritiated thymidine, and subsequently undergo mitosis. This is the so-called lymphocyte transformation test.

Since the number of committed lymphocytes at the site of the antigen-antibody reaction is small at all times, usually amounting to only 5 to 8 per cent of the cellular infiltrate, the great majority of aggregating cells are monocytes which change into macrophages whose purpose it is to phagocytize antigen and debris. Bandmann, in 1967, first discovered that monocytes were the prevailing cell in the cellular infiltrate in contact dermatitis, rather than lymphocytes, as had been assumed until then. He recognized the monocytes as such by their content of peroxidase.

Electron Microscopy. The histologic and immunologic findings just described have been confirmed by electron microscopic studies. Wolff and Braun-Falco, on examining human skin 44 hours after application of allergic patch tests, found in the dermis an infiltrate composed predominantly of monocytes containing only a few lysosomes and of macrophages with numerous organelles, including lysosomes, and pseudopodic processes. In addition, lymphocytes were present, occasionally in close contact with the pseudopods of macrophages. Eosinophils were rare and neutrophils and plasma cells were absent. The epidermis, according to Braun-Falco and Wolff, showed as the most striking feature intercellular edema in the lower epidermis with a marked diminution in the number of desmosomes, referred to by them as microacantholysis. Lymphocytes and macrophages were present in the dilated intercellular spaces of the epidermis. Metz confirmed the existence of microacantholysis in similar experiments and stated that intradesmosomal separation preceded the disappearance of the desmosomes. He believes that intradesmosomal separation was present only in the initial phase of contact dermatitis and was the result of the proteolytic activity of lymphocytes as they invaded the epidermis.

On the basis of the immunologic findings it would seem unlikely that epidermal spongiosis precedes the appearance of a dermal and epidermal cellular infiltrate, as claimed by Carr et al. in an electron microscopic study of human skin after the induction of poison ivy contact dermatitis.

Medenica and Rostenberg, on studying by electron microscope the course of patch test reactions in guinea pigs that had been sensitized to DNCB, noted a dermal infiltrate within 3 hours after application of the patch test. After 6 hours lymphocytes and monocytes were seen in the lower epidermis together with early spongiosis, and after 12 hours the entire epidermis showed exocytosis and spongiosis.

In contrast to the electron microscopic studies cited so far, all of which are investigations of the early phase of experimentally induced contact dermatitis, Frichot and Zelickson studied spontaneously arisen contact dermatitis of several days duration by electron microscope. They found as the most striking finding in the keratinocytes large clear perinuclear vacuoles, which were interpreted by them as lysosomes because of a positive acid phosphatase reaction. Most of these lysosomes had either a broken or no limiting membrane. In a case of contact dermatitis 10 days old lysosomal vacuoles occupied most of the cytoplasm, with the rest of the cell appearing shrunken, including the nucleus. This was interpreted by them as the beginning of cellular destruction in which lysosomes acted as autophagosomes ("suicide bags").

Nummular Dermatitis. This eruption, characterized clinically by "pinpoint vesicles," usually shows the histologic picture of a subacute dermatitis (Fig. 7-2). In a moderately acanthotic epidermis one finds scattered intraepidermal vesicles at various levels of the epidermis surrounded by spongiosis (Braun-Falco and Petry).

Histogenesis. In an electron microscopic study of nummular dermatitis Braun-Falco and Petry found that the intercellular edema had led to a reduction in the number of desmosomes between the cells of the basal layer (so-called microacantholysis, see above under contact dermatitis). In the stratum spinosum, however, the desmosomes were largely preserved and appeared stretched, with thick tonofilament bundles within them extending through the intercellular space. When the desmosomes tore they did so near one of the cellular borders, rather than in the central intradesmosomal area.

Atopic Dermatitis. The histologic picture usually is that of a chronic dermatitis showing acanthosis with varying degrees of spongiosis. Rarely, small intraepidermal spongiotic vesicles are seen (Prose and Sedlis). In cases with marked spongiosis parakeratosis is pronounced. In cases of long standing the rete ridges may be greatly elongated. The dermal infiltrate consists, on the basis of enzyme determinations, mainly of lymphocytes, but it also contains fairly numerous monocytes. Mast cells are present in increased number, but eosinophils are found only rarely (Braun-Falco and Burg).

Histogenesis. A correlation exists between the severity of atopic dermatitis and the serum level of IgE, the reaginic antibody (Ogawa et al.). Electron microscopic examination has revealed in atopic dermatitis associated with either parakeratosis (Prose et al.) or crusting (Frichot and Zelickson) the presence of rather numerous lysosomes in the keratinocytes of the uppermost portion of the epidermis. It can be assumed that the lysosomes form as a response to cellular damage (Prose et al.).

Lichen Simplex Chronicus. The histologic appearance is essentially that of a chronic dermatitis (Fig. 7-3). One observes hyperkeratosis interspersed with small areas of parakeratosis, acanthosis with rather regular elongation of the rete ridges, and elongation and broadening of the papillae. There may be some spongiosis, but vesiculation does not occur. In addition to a chronic inflammatory infiltrate, often the dermis shows a fair number of fibroblasts and some fibrosis even in the papillae.

Seborrheic Dermatitis. The histologic picture is not diagnostic. It may be said to be halfway between psoriasis and chronic dermatitis. The horny layer shows focal areas of parakeratosis occasionally containing a few pyknotic neutrophils similar to those seen in the Munro microabscesses of psoriasis. The epidermis shows slight to moderate acanthosis with some elongation of the rete ridges, and slight intracellular edema and spongiosis. The dermis shows a mild chronic inflammatory infiltrate. Thus, the only major difference between psoriasis and seborrheic dermatitis is the presence of spongiosis in the latter.

Histogenesis. According to Pinkus and Mehregan, seborrheic dermatitis and psoriasis have a similar histogenesis, since in both diseases the papillary capillaries intermittently release neutrophils which then migrate through the epidermis and accumulate in the parakeratotic horny layer (see p. 140).

Stasis Dermatitis. Histologic examination shows either a subacute or a chronic dermatitis. Quite frequently, considerable amounts of hemosiderin are scattered through the dermis. Older lesions show numerous dilated capillaries embedded in a fibrotic dermis.

Histogenesis. Inadequate venous circulation in the legs is caused usually by thrombophlebitis or varicose veins and occasionally by congenital arteriovenous fistulae of the legs associated with a portwine nevus, the so-called Klippel-Trenaunay syndrome (Bluefarb and Adams). Any of these factors can cause venous and capillary stasis on the medial portions of the legs just above the ankles. The stasis leads to hypoxia and poor nutrition of the tissue and thus results in the dermatitis. Changes in the arterioles and venules consisting of intimal proliferation and medial hyperplasia are secondary; but arteriolar obstruction may be an important factor in the development of the ulcers in stasis dermatitis (Wiedmann).

Generalized Exfoliative Dermatitis or Generalized Erythroderma. The histologic picture shows either a subacute or a chronic dermatitis. If the dermatitis is subacute, one observes parakeratosis, marked intercellular and intracellular edema, acanthosis with elongation of the rete ridges, and migration of inflammatory cells through the epidermis, so-called exocytosis. The upper dermis shows edema and a considerable chronic inflammatory infiltrate (Fig. 7-4). If the edema in the upper stratum malpighii is pronounced, as seen especially in drug-induced generalized exfoliative dermatitis, marked oozing is apt to be present, in addi-tion to the exfoliation of the parakeratotic horny cells.

In the chronic type of generalized exfolia-tive dermatitis the histologic picture is that of a chronic dermatitis. Although the epi-dermis may have a psoriasiform appearance, the common presence of spongiosis and of eosinophils, and occasionally also of plasma cells, excludes psoriasis (Nicolis and Hel-wig). Each case of undetermined origin requires thorough histologic examination through multiple skin biopsies and a lymph node biopsy in order to rule out lymphoma. From 15 to 25 per cent of the cases of undetermined origin occur in association with lymphoma (Montgomery; Abrahams et al.; Nicolis and Helwig). Even if the his-tologic examination at first shows no evi-dence of lymphoma, it is advisable to per-form further biopsies at intervals (see below, Differential Diagnosis, and also p. 704).

Differential Diagnosis. Histologic differ-entiation of a vesicular or bullous contact dermatitis from erythema multiforme, espe-cially the mixed dermal-epidermal type, may be difficult on a histologic basis and may re-

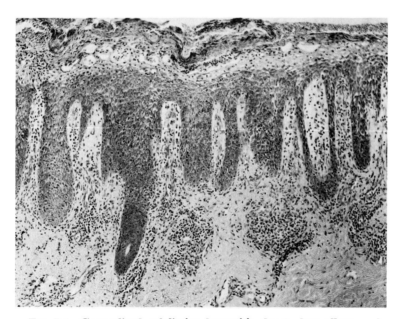

FIG. 7-4. **Generalized exfoliative dermatitis, due to drug allergy, sub-acute.** One observes parakeratosis, marked intercellular and intracellular edema, acanthosis with elongation of the rete ridges, and migration of inflammatory cells through the epidermis. The upper dermis shows edema and a considerable amount of the inflammatory infiltrate. (×100)

quire clinical information, since erythema multiforme may show invasion of the epidermis by mononuclear cells associated with spongiosis and formation of intraepidermal vesicles. However, in most cases of erythema multiforme with blisters there also are subepidermal vesicles or bullae. Furthermore, one often finds in instances of erythema multiforme with epidermal changes scattered necrotic keratinocytes as a characteristic feature (see p. 124). Differentiation of nummular dermatitis showing scattered and grouped papulo-vesicles from dermatitis herpetiformis may be difficult on a clinical basis. However, if early vesicles with their surrounding erythema are chosen for biopsy, dermatitis herpetiformis can be easily diagnosed through the presence of microabscesses at the tips of the papillae composed largely of neutrophils and containing occasionally also some eosinophils, and the presence of "nuclear dust" in the subpapillary dermis (see p. 119).

In regard to the diagnosis of chronic dermatitis,* it should be stressed that many diseases not belonging to the dermatitis-eczema group show either regularly or occasionally a histologic picture allowing no more specific a diagnosis than chronic dermatitis. Diseases that regularly show the nonspecific histologic picture of chronic dermatitis include pityriasis rosea, parapsoriasis en plaques, and pellagra. Many other diseases, especially psoriasis but also lichen planus, and pityriasis rubra pilaris, to name but a few, present a diagnostic histologic picture in clinically typical cases but may show a nonspecific histologic picture, that of a chronic dermatitis, in clinically not so typical cases. On the other hand, a chronic dermatitis may simulate the histologic picture of psoriasis through the presence of evenly elongated rete ridges. However, psoriasis, at least in typical cases, shows more pronounced parakeratosis, and, in addition, thinning of the suprapapillary epidermis, edema of the papillae with dilatation of the papillary capillaries, and, occa-

sionally, Munro microabscesses (see p. 138).

Early mycosis fungoides must always be kept in mind as a possible diagnosis when a section showing chronic dermatitis is examined, particularly if it shows a fairly marked dermal infiltrate. Often it is very difficult to establish or to rule out early mycosis fungoides in such instances. One should search for atypical mononuclear cells (so-called mycosis cells). Furthermore, a patchy infiltrate, mitotic figures, and Pautrier microabscesses are points in favor of mycosis fungoides. However, now and then a patchy infiltrate, some atypicality ("pleomorphism") in some of the mononuclear cells, and occasional mitotic figures are seen also in chronic dermatitis. This leaves Pautrier microabscesses as a most valuable differential diagnostic feature (see p. 698). Unfortunately, not all cases of mycosis fungoides show them even on "step sectioning." If the diagnosis is in doubt, it is advisable to request additional specimens for histologic examination.

DERMATOPATHIC LYMPHADENITIS

Any extensive itching dermatitis, but particularly generalized exfoliative dermatitis, whether due to lymphoma or not, may cause an asymptomatic enlargement of the subcutaneous lymph nodes, especially of the inguinal, axillary, and cervical lymph nodes. Dermatopathic lymphadenitis, also referred to as lipomelanotic reticulosis, being a reactive process, may occasionally occur in association with a pruritic cutaneous lymphoma; but as such it does not progress into lymphoma (Jarrett and Kellett). In some instances, however, a lymphoma may develop in a lymph node that previously was affected by dermatopathic lymphadenitis (Pautrier and Woringer) (see p. 701).

Histopathology. The capsule of the lymph node is well preserved. The lymph follicles may be increased in size and possess large germinal centers. The stroma of the lymph node shows areas of considerable proliferation of reticular cells or macrophages. These areas appear as pale patches because the reticular cells have a pale nucleus and abundant pale cytoplasm (Laipply). Although as a rule the architecture of the

---

* The term *chronic dermatitis* is used if there are both epidermal and nonspecific dermal changes; the term *chronic inflammation* is used if only dermal changes are present.

lymph node is well preserved, marked proliferation of the reticular cells may cause the architecture to appear hazy or even partially destroyed (Meessen). The reticular cells, being macrophages, show phagocytic activity and contain melanin and often also lipid material and hemosiderin. In addition, among the reticular cells as well as in the lymph follicles one finds a scattered infiltrate composed of eosinophils, neutrophils, plasma cells, and lymphocytes (Hurwitt).

Histogenesis. The melanin present in the lymph nodes, having been carried there from the skin, probably is responsible for the follicular hyperplasia, the proliferation of the reticular cells, and the inflammatory infiltrate. This is suggested by the work of Hohenadl and de Paola who, by injecting guinea pigs parenterally with melanin obtained from the choroid of cattle, produced the histologic picture of dermatopathic lymphadenitis. The lipid material in the lymph nodes gives a positive reaction for cholesterol and is doubly refractile (Pautrier and Woringer). Hohenadl and de Paola believe that the lipid accumulations in the cells are the result not of an increased storage but of a reduced breakdown of lipids.

Differential Diagnosis. The histologic changes in dermatopathic lymphadenitis differ from those seen in Hodgkin's disease, mycosis fungoides or follicular lymphoma by the preservation of the capsule, little or no destruction of the lymph node architecture, absence of Sternberg-Reed cells, and the presence of phagocytic activity in the reticular cells. On the other hand, the number of mitotic figures and the number and size of the lymph follicles are of little help in the differential diagnosis (Rappaport et al.).

MILIARIA

Miliaria occurs when sweating is associated with poral closure. There are two types: miliaria crystallina and miliaria rubra.

Miliaria crystallina occurs in sunburned areas and shows asymptomatic, small, superficial, clear, noninflammatory vesicles resembling dewdrops. The vesicles rapidly subside when sweating ceases or the horny layer overlying the vesicles exfoliates (Cage).

Miliaria rubra occurs following excessive sweating in parts of the skin covered by clothing. It may also occur following prolonged covering of the skin by occlusive polyethylene wraps. The lesions consist of pruritic small papulovesicles surrounded by erythema.

Histopathology. In *miliaria crystallina* one observes subcorneal vesicles. On serial sectioning the vesicles are found in direct communication with an underlying sweat duct (Shelley and Horvath).

In *miliaria rubra* spongiotic vesicles similar in appearance to those seen in dermatitis are found in the stratum malpighii. Serial sectioning will show these vesicles to be in continuity with a sweat duct. A chronic inflammatory infiltrate is seen around and within the vesicles as well as in the subjacent dermis (Sulzberger and Zimmerman; Loewenthal).

Histogenesis. In *miliaria crystallina* closure of the sweat pores in the stratum corneum is the result of mild damage to the epidermis induced by the preceding sunburn.

In *miliaria rubra* poral closure by hydration of the horny layer is the initial event blocking delivery of sweat (O'Brien; Papa and Kligman; Sulzberger and Harris). That poral closure is the primary event in miliaria rubra is shown by the fact that stripping off the stratum corneum with adhesive tape restores sweating (Papa and Kligman). The poral occlusion by hydration occurs without detectable anatomic plugging, since apparent obstructions blamed in the past for the poral occlusion, such as "keratin plugs" or "plugs caused by condensation of PAS-positive, diastase-resistant material" are found also in control sections (Sulzberger and Harris). The rapid restoration of sweating after tape stripping also has made it unlikely that intraepidermal rupture of the sweat duct takes place in miliaria rubra. It is likely, however, that poral closure leads to the escape of retained sweat from the intraepidermal sweat duct into the surrounding epidermis where the sweat acts as a primary irritant on account of its high concentration of sodium chloride and in this way causes periductal spongiosis and an inflammatory infiltration (Loewenthal).

ERYTHEMA TOXICUM NEONATORUM

This is a very common asymptomatic benign eruption of the newborn consisting of tiny macules, papules, and pustules. Occasionally, large areas of erythema are also

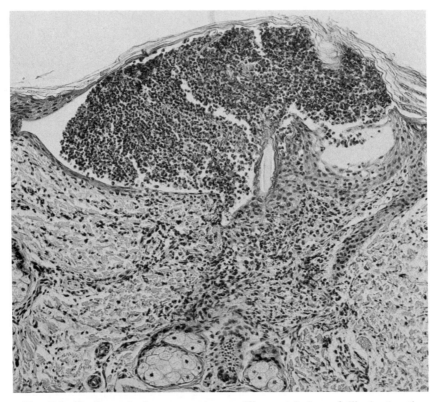

Fig. 7-5. **Erythema toxicum neonatorum.** The pustule has a follicular location and is filled with eosinophils. The outer root sheath beneath the pustule is infiltrated with eosinophils. (×100) (Dieter Lüders, M.D.)

present. The eruption clears spontaneously within a few days or weeks. The cause is unknown.

Histopathology. The macules and areas of erythema show only a few eosinophils in the upper dermis, largely in a perivascular location.

The papules show an accumulation of numerous eosinophils and some neutrophils among the cells of the outer root sheath of the hair from the entry of the sebaceous duct upward to the surface epidermis. In addition, eosinophils are present in the upper dermis.

The pustules form as a result of an upward migration of the eosinophils to the surface epidermis around the hair follicles (Lüders; Freeman et al.). Mature pustules usually have a subcorneal location (Fig. 7-5).

Differential Diagnosis. The subcorneal

pustules of staphylococcal pyoderma of the newborn (see p. 270) contain neutrophils rather than eosinophils and do not have a follicular distribution. Even though many eosinophils are present also in the vesicles of incontinentia pigmenti, the intraepidermal rather than subcorneal location of the vesicles and the presence of spongiosis in incontinentia pigmenti help in the differentiation.

PEMPHIGUS

There are two types of pemphigus, each of which has a variant: pemphigus vulgaris with pemphigus vegetans, and pemphigus foliaceus with pemphigus erythematosus. The bullae of pemphigus show acantholysis as a characteristic feature (see Table 7-1 and Glossary). In contrast, acantholysis is absent in the two types of pemphigoid: bul-

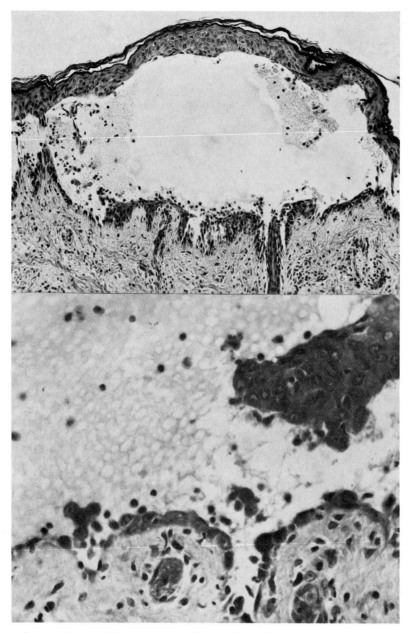

FIG. 7-6. **Pemphigus vulgaris.** (*Top*) The bulla lies in predominantly suprabasal position and leads at its periphery into suprabasal clefts. (×100) (*Bottom*) The floor of a bulla shows the basal layer adherent to the dermis. The cavity contains single acantholytic epidermal cells, as well as clusters. (×400)

lous pemphigoid and cicatricial pemphigoid (see pp. 115 and 119). On the other hand, acantholysis occurs not only in pemphigus but also in the following diseases: Darier's disease, familial benign pemphigus, transient acantholytic dermatosis, viral vesicles, and, occasionally, solar keratosis and squamous cell carcinoma.

PEMPHIGUS VULGARIS

Pemphigus vulgaris shows flaccid bullae. They break easily and leave denuded areas that tend to increase in size by progressive peripheral detachment of the epidermis. By the increase of lesions in size as well as in numbers large areas of the skin can become involved. Almost invariably, extensive oral lesions are present, and often oral lesions are the first manifestation of the disease. Prior to the availability of the corticosteroids the mortality in this disease was very high.

Histopathology. It is important that early bullae be selected for biopsy, preferably small ones that can be removed in their entirety with a skin punch. If there is reduced cohesion between the epidermal cells, as shown by a positive Nikolsky sign, it is advisable to use either a refrigerant spray before excising the blister with a punch or to excise it widely with a scalpel. If no recent blister is available, an old one may be moved into its neighboring skin by gentle vertical pressure with a finger (Asboe-

Hansen). Such a newly created cleavage will reveal the earliest histologic changes.

The earliest changes consist of intercellular edema and disappearance of the intercellular bridges in the lowermost epidermis. The resulting loss of coherence between the epidermal cells (acantholysis) leads to the formation first of clefts and then of bullae in predominantly suprabasal location (Fig. 7-6, *top*) (Civatte; Lever; Tappeiner and Pfleger). The basal cells, although separated from one another through the loss of intercellular bridges, remain attached to the dermis like a "row of tombstones" (Director). As a rule, there is little evidence of inflammation in pemphigus vulgaris during the early phase of blister formation. In rare instances, however, eosinophils invade the epidermis before acantholysis has become evident and this has been referred to as "eosinophilic spongiosis" by Emmerson and Wilson-Jones. The bullae contain single as well as clusters of epidermal cells that, because of the loss of coherence with their neighboring cells, have drifted into the bulla

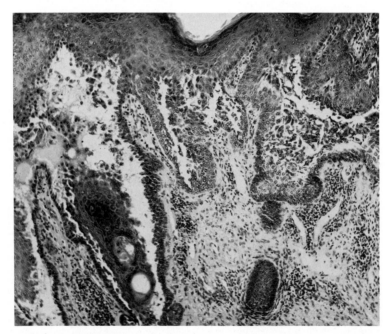

Fig. 7-7. **Pemphigus vulgaris.** There is an intra-epidermal, predominantly suprabasal bulla. The bulla cavity contains many acantholytic cells. In addition, there is irregular upward growth of papillae lined predominantly by a single layer of epidermal cells, so-called villi. (×200)

cavity. These acantholytic cells appear rounded, with a large hyperchromatic nucleus and homogeneous cytoplasm (Fig. 7-6, *bottom*). Frequently, one observes at the floor of the bulla, even in early bullae, irregular upward growth of papillae that are lined by a single row of basal cells, so-called villi, as well as downward proliferation of strands of epidermal cells into the spaces between the papillae (Fig. 7-7). Acantholysis may affect also the epithelium of the outer root sheath of the hair. As in the surface epidermis, clefts form predominantly right above the basal layer.

In older bullae, due to regeneration, the base of the bulla may consist of more than one layer of cells. Denuded areas usually show the basal cell layer still adherent to the dermis. During the stage of healing, irregular upward proliferation of villi and downward growth of epidermal strands may be present to a considerable degree. The histologic picture then approaches that of pemphigus vegetans.

The dermis beneath early bullae usually shows only slight inflammation, although a few eosinophils generally are present beneath and also within the bullae. In older lesions the number of inflammatory cells, including eosinophils and plasma cells, may be considerable.

In patients having only oral lesions specimens for biopsy are best taken, since intact blisters are rarely encountered, from the active border of a denuded area by means of a biopsy punch.

Cytologic examination, introduced by Tzanck, is useful for the rapid demonstration of acantholytic epidermal cells in the bullae of pemphigus vulgaris. For this purpose a smear is taken from the base of an early, freshly opened bulla and stained with Giemsa's or Papanicolaou's stain. Since, however, occasionally acantholytic epidermal cells are seen also in various nonacantholytic vesiculobullous or pustular diseases, cytologic examination represents merely a preliminary test that should not supplant the histologic examination (Graham et al.).

Histogenesis. On electron microscopic examination, the primary defect leading to acantholysis in pemphigus vulgaris was regarded by Wilgram et al., in 1961, to consist of damage to the tonofilaments; whereas in the opinion of Braun-Falco and Vogell the loss of the capability of epidermal cells to form desmosomal contacts was the primary event. When the work by Beutner et al. had established that in pemphigus antibodies are bound to the intercellular cement substance, re-examination of the early changes taking place in acantholysis led Hashimoto and Lever (1967) to the conclusion that dissolution of the intercellular cement substance was the primary event. This was particularly evident in oral lesions where only few desmosomes but largely intercellular cement substance provide for the coherence of the epithelial cells. Unlocking and dissolution of the desmosomes (E.M. Nos. 20 and 21) seemed to be a secondary event. Staining the intercellular cement with ruthenium red confirmed that acantholysis was, indeed, a result of dissolution of the intercellular cement substance. This substance underwent dissolution first in nondesmosomal areas and later in intradesmosomal areas.

Events taking place subsequent to the dissolution of the desmosomes are proliferation of microvilli in the intercellular spaces (E.M. Nos. 20 and 21), retraction of the tonofilaments to the perinuclear area (E.M. No. 20) and ultimately degeneration of the acantholytic cells. No dyskeratosis occurs, as a rule, because of this degeneration.

The reason why the cohesion of the basal cells with the dermis is not affected in pemphigus vulgaris (E.M. Nos. 20 and 21) has become evident by the failure of ruthenium red to penetrate into this area in normal skin, indicating that cement substance is absent there. Rather, the space between the basal cell plasma membrane with its half-desmosomes and the basal lamina is crossed by innumerable fine filaments, the anchoring filaments (Hashimoto and Lever, 1970).

Specific autoantibodies have been demonstrated to be present in the blood serum of patients with pemphigus vulgaris by means of *indirect* immunofluorescent testing (Beutner et al.). For indirect testing, first the patient's serum and then fluorescein-labeled antihuman gamma globulin are applied to sections of normal squamous epithelium, for instance, the mucosa of rabbit esophagus. The serum antibodies are found to be bound to the intercellular substance of the squamous epithelium, corresponding to the site at which blister formation takes place in pemphigus. The titer in the serum of patients with pemphigus vulgaris in general is proportional to the severity of the disease (Chorzelski et al., 1966; Sams and Jordon). Pemphigus antibodies are demonstrable also by *direct* immunofluorescent testing in sections of skin lesions from patients with pemphigus vulgaris. There they are found bound in vivo to the intercellular space of the epidermis. The fact that also complement is bound indicates that it is a true antigen-antibody reaction (Cormane and Chorzelski). The autoantibodies present in the serum and in the epidermis of patients with pemphigus vulgaris are of the IgG class (Grob and Inderbitzin).

In place of using fluorescein for labeling the antihuman gamma globulin, as required for immunofluorescent testing, peroxidase has been used as a label for *direct* immunologic testing of the skin of patients with pemphigus vulgaris, either by light microscopy (Fukuyama et al.) or by electron microscopy (Wolff and Schreiner). This method too has shown the pemphigus antibodies to be bound in vivo to the intercellular space of the epidermis.

Differential Diagnosis. In early bullae that are free of secondary changes caused by degeneration or regeneration of epidermal cells, the histologic picture of pemphigus vulgaris is highly diagnostic. There are only three conditions that may have the same his-

tologic appearance, namely pemphigus vegetans, familial benign pemphigus and transient acantholytic dermatosis. Since pemphigus vegetans merely is a variant of pemphigus vulgaris, quite naturally they resemble each other. However, the histologic resemblance to pemphigus vulgaris of the other two diseases is curious, since they have little in common clinically. (For differentiation of pemphigus vulgaris from familial benign pemphigus see p. 75; and from transient acantholytic dermatosis see p. 126.)

PEMPHIGUS VEGETANS

In the usual type of pemphigus vegetans, the so-called Neumann type, the disease begins and ends as pemphigus vulgaris. It differs from pemphigus vulgaris only by having many of the denuded areas heal, instead of with normal skin, with verrucous vegetations that in their early stage sometimes are studded with small pustules. A relatively benign variant of pemphigus vegetans

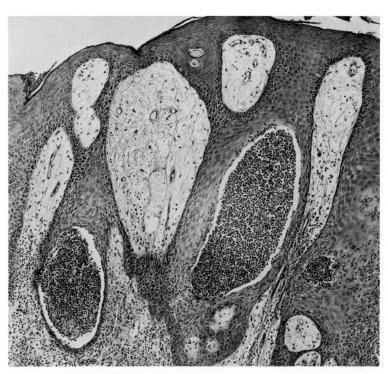

Fig. 7-8. **Pemphigus vegetans.** The section, obtained from a verrucous vegetation, shows considerable acanthosis and intraepidermal abscesses composed almost entirely of eosinophils. (×100).

is pyodermite végétante of Hallopeau: instead of bullae, pustules are the primary lesion. They are followed by the formation of gradually extending verrucous vegetations, especially in the intertriginous areas.

Histopathology. In the usual type of pemphigus vegetans, the so-called Neumann type, the early lesions, consisting of bullae and denuded areas, show essentially the same histologic picture as that seen in pemphigus vulgaris. However, the formation of villi and the downward proliferation of epithelial strands are much more pronounced than in pemphigus vulgaris. The verrucous vegetations that develop subsequently are characterized by considerable papillomatosis and acanthosis. Although acantholysis often is no longer apparent, not infrequently one observes intraepidermal abscesses composed almost entirely of eosinophils (Fig. 7-8). These abscesses, highly diagnostic of pemphigus vegetans, correspond to the bullae of earlier lesions (Lever). Old vegetations merely show considerable papillomatosis and hyperkeratosis with few or no eosinophils, so that the histologic picture is no longer diagnostic.

In pyodermite végétante of Hallopeau, the early lesions, consisting of pustules arising on normal skin, show acantholysis with formation of small clefts and cavities, many in suprabasal location. These cavities are filled with numerous eosinophils and degenerated, acantholytic epidermal cells (Röckl). A pronounced inflammatory infiltrate composed largely of eosinophils is present throughout the epidermis as well as in the upper dermis. The verrucous vegetations show the same histologic picture as those of the Neumann-type pemphigus vegetans, including the intraepidermal eosinophilic abscesses.

Histogenesis. Pemphigus vegetans is a variant of pemphigus vulgaris occurring in patients having an increased resistance to their disease. This increased resistance finds its expression in the presence of numerous eosinophils.

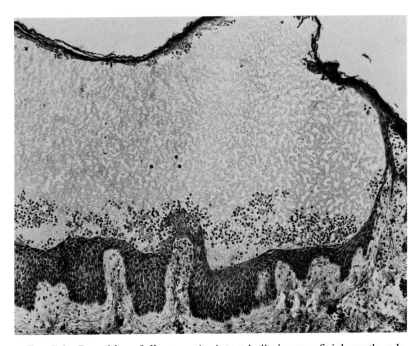

FIG. 7-9. **Pemphigus foliaceus.** An intact bulla in superficial, partly subcorneal position. Acantholysis is present at the base, as well as at the top, of the bulla. (×100)

PEMPHIGUS FOLIACEUS

Pemphigus foliaceus begins with flaccid bullae that usually arise on an erythematous base. Erythema, oozing and crusting are present from the beginning, not only around the bullae but also in other areas. The bullae break easily and, because of their superficial location, leave shallow erosions, rather than denuded areas, as in pemphigus vulgaris. Gradual extension of the lesions may lead to involvement of most of the body surface if not its entire surface. In the advanced stage bullae are few, and they may even be absent, so that the resemblance to generalized exfoliative dermatitis is great, except that pemphigus foliaceus has a positive Nikolsky sign. Also the presence of thick hyperkeratotic scales in some areas of erythema is common. In contrast with pemphigus vulgaris oral lesions occur very rarely. The prognosis of pemphigus foliaceus always has been better than that of pemphigus vulgaris, even prior to the availability of the corticosteroids.

In some instances pemphigus foliaceus presents a clinical picture suggestive of dermatitis herpetiformis, showing grouped papules, vesicles and bullae as well as erythematous patches with vesicles at their periphery (Floden and Gentele; Winkelmann and Roth; Barranco). Several of these patients responded well to the administration of sulfonamides or sulfones. The histologic picture, however, is that of pemphigus foliaceus.

"Fogo selvagem," a disease endemic in some parts of Brazil, is clinically and histologically indistinguishable from pemphigus foliaceus and can be regarded as identical with it (Furtado).

Histopathology. The earliest change in pemphigus foliaceus consists of areas of acantholysis in the upper epidermis, usually in the granular layer or right beneath it, leading to the formation of a cleft in a superficial, often a subcorneal location (Rook and Whimster; Lever).

This cleft may develop into a bulla in

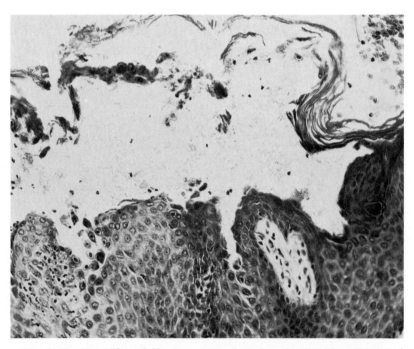

FIG. 7-10. **Pemphigus foliaceus.** An early lesion showing detachment of the horny and the granular layers without bulla formation. The epidermal cells at the base of the cleft show loss of intercellular bridges resulting in acantholysis. (×200)

FIG. 7-11. **Pemphigus foliaceus.**
This represents a late lesion showing considerable acanthosis and hyperkeratosis with cleft formation
and acantholysis in the granular
layer. The granular cells appear
shrunken and hyperchromatic; thus,
they resemble the grains of Darier's
disease. (×200)

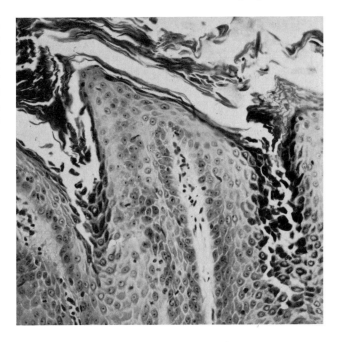

superficial, often subcorneal location, with acantholysis being present at the floor as well as at the roof of the bulla (Fig. 7-9). Usually, however, enlargement of the cleft leads to a detachment of the uppermost epidermis without formation of a bulla (Fig. 7-10). The cells bordering the cleft show absence of intercellular bridges and a tendency to break off into the space formed by the cleft. It should be emphasized that often the number of acantholytic cells bordering the bullae and clefts in pemphigus foliaceus is small, requiring a careful search for them. Occasionally, secondary clefts develop and result in detachment within the middle section of the epidermis. Detachment immediately above the basal layer, as seen typically in pemphigus vulgaris, occurs only very rarely and then over limited areas (Perry).

Older lesions show acanthosis, a mild degree of papillomatosis, and, in addition, hyperkeratosis and parakeratosis. The hyperkeratosis may be associated with keratotic plugging of the follicles. In areas of hyperkeratosis the granular layer is increased in thickness. A striking change frequently observed in older lesions of pemphigus foliaceus and diagnostic for this disease is the presence of dyskeratotic changes in the cells of the granular layer (Fig. 7-11). The granular cells show acantholysis, appear deeply basophilic and shrunken, and thus resemble the grains of Darier's disease.

The dermis shows a moderate number of inflammatory cells, among which eosinophils often are present.

Histogenesis. Electron microscopic examination reveals some early loss of intercellular cement substance in the lower epidermis associated with a decrease in the number of desmosomes and replacement by tortuous microvilli. However, acantholysis is most pronounced in the upper layers of the epidermis (E.M. No. 22) (Lever and Hashimoto). In the midepidermis many cells show perinuclear arrangement of the tonofilaments and homogenization of the perinuclear tonofilament bundles as evidence of dyskeratosis. In the granular cells the number of keratinosomes is greatly increased (Wilgram et al., 1964).

The autoantibodies encountered in pemphigus foliaceus are identical with those found in pemphigus vulgaris. They are IgG antibodies that are present in the blood serum and are bound in vivo with complement in the intercellular space of squamous epithelium.

Differential Diagnosis. The location of the bulla in pemphigus foliaceus is the same as in subcorneal pustular dermatosis and in impetigo. For their differentiation, see under subcorneal pustular dermatosis, p. 126.

PEMPHIGUS ERYTHEMATOSUS

Pemphigus erythematosus (Senear-Usher syndrome) represents either an abortive form or an initial stage of pemphigus foliaceus. In the former case the eruption remains localized; in the latter case it advances gradually into pemphigus foliaceus. Clinically, the lesions are the same as in pemphigus foliaceus. There is some clinical resemblance to lupus erythematosus and seborrheic dermatitis both in localization and in appearance. Thus, the facial lesions may show follicular hyperkeratosis, although atrophy as in lupus erythematosus does not occur.

Histopathology. The histopathologic picture is identical with that of pemphigus foliaceus (Percival; Perry and Brunsting). In older lesions follicular hyperkeratosis with acantholysis and dyskeratosis of the granular layer often is pronounced.

Histogenesis. Pemphigus erythematosus is identical with pemphigus foliaceus in its elec-

tron microscopic and immunologic manifestations. The opinion recently expressed by several authors that pemphigus erythematosus results from a "combination of pemphigus and lupus erythematosus" appears entirely unwarranted. The evidence cited by these authors consists of 9 cases of pemphigus erythematosus in which direct immunofluorescent testing revealed, in addition to the expected intercellular fluorescence, fluorescence at the dermal-epidermal junction, as seen in lupus erythematosus, but no other evidence of lupus erythematosus (Chorzelski et al., 1968; Bean and Lynch; Saikia and MacConnell). The fluorescence at the dermal-epidermal junction at best could be interpreted as evidence of the phenomenon that one autoimmune disease often is associated with laboratory evidence of another; but possibly, it was nonspecific, since fluorescence at the dermal-epidermal junction may be observed on exposed skin showing any kind of inflammation or dilatation of capillaries (Baart de la Faille and Baart de la Faille-Kuyper; Jablonska et al.).

Differential Diagnosis. Clinically the lesions of pemphigus erythematosus may resemble those of lupus erythematosus; but they differ sufficiently in their histologic appearance to make a differentiation possible. Even though both diseases may show

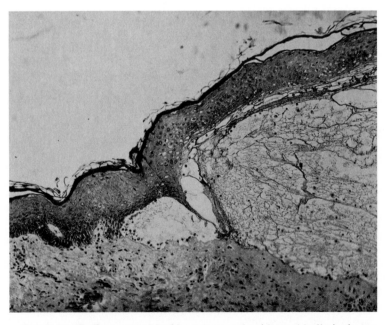

Fig. 7-12. **Bullous pemphigoid.** A large subepidermal bulla is shown. The bulla contains a net of fibrin but only few inflammatory cells. (×100)

follicular hyperkeratosis, acantholytic and dyskeratotic changes in the granular layer are seen only in pemphigus erythematosus, and hydropic degeneration and a patchy inflammatory infiltrate in the dermis occur only in lupus erythematosus. If bullae are present, they are located in the upper layers of the epidermis in pemphigus erythematosus; whereas in lupus erythematosus they have a subepidermal location, since they form secondary to the hydropic degeneration of the basal layer.

BULLOUS PEMPHIGOID

The disease is characterized by the presence of large, tense bullae over wide areas. Usually, the groins, the axillae and the flexor surfaces of the forearms show the largest number of bullae. When the bullae break, the resulting denuded areas in most cases do not materially increase in size as they do in pemphigus vulgaris; rather, they show a good tendency to heal. In addition to bullae, there also are areas of erythema with an irregular outline and central clearing. Bullae arise not only on noninflamed skin but also within the areas of erythema. Involvement of the oral mucosa usually is mild, and it may be absent. Bullous pemphigoid most commonly occurs in aged individuals but occasionally is seen in young adults and even in children (Fincher et al.; Jablonska et al.). Although in aged, debilitated people the disease may result in death, the prognosis in well-preserved individuals usually was good, even prior to the availability of corticosteroids, with the disease usually subsiding after having persisted for several months or years. Occasionally, there are recurrences.

Histopathology. The dermal changes in bullous pemphigoid differ, depending on whether the bulla selected for biopsy is located on normal-appearing or on erythematous skin, but the epidermal changes are the same in both, consisting of bullae arising through detachment of the epidermis from the dermis (Fig. 7-12) (Lever; Rook and Waddington; van der Meer). Early bullae are found fully beneath the epidermis; but

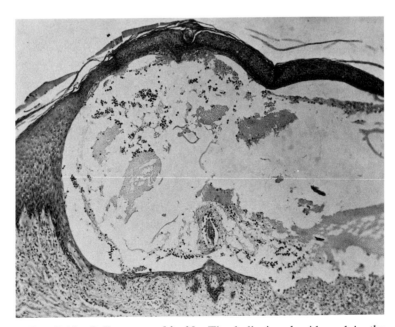

Fig. 7-13. **Bullous pemphigoid.** The bulla is subepidermal in the center but, on account of regeneration of the epidermis at the floor of the bulla, is intraepidermal at the periphery. In the area where the bulla is intraepidermal, more than the basal layer is adherent to the dermis, and there is no acantholysis. (×100)

after two days one can already observe regeneration of the epidermis at the floor of the bulla, beginning at the periphery and extending gradually over the entire floor (Fig. 7-13). This regeneration results in an intraepidermal location of the bulla. The epidermis at the roof of the bulla is intact at first, but in older bullae it may become necrotic and may then disintegrate with the exception of the horny layer. In this way, the bullae that form subepidermally may ultimately be subcorneal in location.

The dermal changes in noninflammatory bullae generally are slight. Beneath the bulla the dermis shows a rather sparse perivascular infiltrate consisting mainly of mononuclear cells with an admixture of a few eosinophils but hardly any neutrophils. In contrast to this sparse infiltrate beneath the bullae the bulla cavity contains often fairly numerous eosinophils and some neutrophils within a net of fibrin (Fig. 7-12). The peribullous area in some cases shows only a perivascular infiltrate, but in others shows, in addition, eosinophils intermingled with a few neutrophils in the upper dermis in close

approximation to the epidermis (Kresbach and Hartwagner; van der Meer).

The dermal changes in inflammatory bullae, on the other hand, consist of extensive perivascular accumulations of eosinophils intermingled with some mononuclear cells and neutrophils. Nuclear dust, due to the disintegration of eosinophils and neutrophils, is present (Fig. 7-14). This infiltrate extends throughout the upper dermis and at the periphery of the bulla it may form microabscesses at the tips of papillae (Fig. 7-15), similar to those seen in dermatitis herpetiformis (Jablonska and Chorzelski; Kresbach and Hartwagner; van der Meer).

Histogenesis. Several electron microscopic investigations have been carried out in bullous pemphigoid, but mainly on "noninflammatory bullae." Most authors, among them Braun-Falco and Rupec, Kobayasi, Wilgram, and Jakubowicz et al., found that blister formation occurred between the basal cells and basal lamina (E.M. No. 23). Kobayasi found this to be the case also in blisters that were induced by extending an existing blister by pressure with a finger into its neighboring skin. Schaumburg-

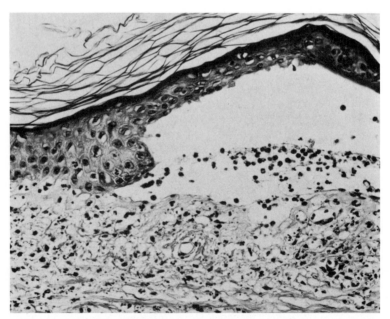

FIG. 7-14. **Bullous pemphigoid.** Bulla arising on erythematous skin. The dermis and the cavity of the bulla contain an inflammatory infiltrate containing many eosinophils. The dermis also shows nuclear dust, the result of disintegration of eosinophils and neutrophils. (×200)

FIG. 7-15. **Bullous pemphigoid.** An inflammatory bulla arising on erythematous skin shows at its periphery microabscesses at the tips of papillae that are similar to those seen in dermatitis herpetiformis. The predominant cell type, however, are eosinophils, in contrast with dermatitis herpetiformis, in which neutrophils usually predominate. (×100)

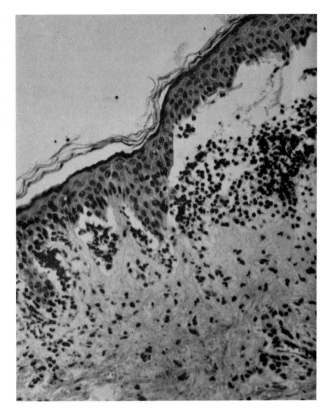

Lever et al., who investigated "inflammatory bullae," recognized three stages in the development of the blisters: (1) Edema is found in the dermis and epidermis together with a cellular infiltrate of eosinophils and histiocytes in the upper dermis; (2) the basal lamina develops discontinuities while eosinophils enter the epidermis and degranulate; and (3) in a fully developed blister the basal lamina is usually destroyed (E.M. No. 24), as it is in dermatitis herpetiformis. Also, as in dermatitis herpetiformis, precipitates of fibrin and amorphous protein are seen in the uppermost dermis.

Specific antibodies have been found in the blood serum of patients with bullous pemphigoid by indirect immunofluorescent testing. These serum antibodies are bound in vitro to the basement zone of normal skin or mucous membrane, so that in bullous pemphigoid, just as in pemphigus, the antibodies are bound at the site where blister formation takes place (Jordon et al., 1967). However, in contrast with pemphigus, no good correlation exists in bullous pemphigoid between the antibody titer in the serum and the severity of the disease (Christophers et al.; Sams and Jordon). Furthermore, in about 30 per cent of the patients with active lesions no circulating

antibodies can be demonstrated (Eng and Moncada). However, almost invariably, even in patients without circulating antibodies, antibodies at the dermal-epidermal junction can be demonstrated by direct immunofluorescent testing, using the patient's involved skin as substrate (Jordon et al., 1971; Burnham and Fine). The circulating antibodies, if present, always are of the IgG class. The in vivo subepidermally bound antibodies consist largely also of IgG, with an occasional admixture of IgA and/or IgM (Jordon et al., 1971; van der Meer; Welke et al.). In addition, complement is regularly present, indicating that the antibody binding represents an antigen-antibody reaction (Chorzelski and Cormane).

In the direct immunofluorescent test the in vivo bound immunoglobulins in bullous pemphigoid usually are arranged subepidermally in a linear fashion, as in lupus erythematosus. However, on electron microscopic examination, following labeling with peroxidase, the immunoglobulin deposits in bullous pemphigoid are located exclusively in the space between the basal cells and the basal lamina (Schaumburg-Lever et al.); whereas in lupus erythematosus the immunoglobulins are found mainly below the basal lamina (Ueki et al.).

Bullous pemphigoid, particularly on the basis of the immunologic studies, is recognized as a disease entity and no longer as a variant of dermatitis herpetiformis, as it has been in the past by some, especially in France (Degos). As a rule, dermatitis herpetiformis differs from bullous pemphigoid (a) by differences in its clinical appearance (absence of bullae and of oral lesions, grouping of lesions and their distribution on extensor surfaces); (b) by its excellent response to sulfapyridine or the sulfones; (c) by the prevalence of neutrophils in the lesions of dermatitis herpetiformis, in contrast to the prevalence of eosinophils in bullous pemphigoid; and (d) by different immunologic findings (in vivo subepidermal granular binding of IgA and absence of circulating antibodies in dermatitis herpetiformis, in contrast to the in vivo subepidermal linear binding of IgG and the usual presence of circulating antibodies in bullous pemphigoid). Still, in some instances a particular case may defy exact classification, as, for instance, a case reported by Honeyman et al. in which at first IgA was bound in vivo without circulating antibodies and four months later IgG was bound in vivo and circulating antibodies were present at a high titer.

A special situation exists in regard to chronic bullous eruptions in children. Besides bullous pemphigoid with in vivo bound IgG and usually also circulating antibodies (Fincher et al.; Jablonska et al.) there exists a disease referred to by Jordon et al. (1970) as *"bullous dermatosis of childhood"* in which all immunofluorescent tests are negative. It shares with bullous pemphigoid the predominance of bullae and self-limited duration, and with dermatitis herpetiformis the response to sulfapyridine and sulfones (Brehm et al.). In addition, clear-cut cases of papulovasicular dermatitis herpetiformis occur in rare instances in children, with in vivo deposits of IgA (Jablonska et al.).

Although the claim has been made repeatedly on the basis of one or a few individual cases that bullous pemphigoid may be a "dermadrome" of visceral malignancy, none of those who have had large series of cases have been able to confirm this (Lever; Rook and Waddington; Jordon et al., 1969).

Differential Diagnosis. Histologic differentiation of bullous pemphigoid from pemphigus vulgaris is not difficult because, even though in bullous pemphigoid the bullae as a result of regeneration may be located within the epidermis, they are never found above a "tombstone row" of basal cells (see p. 108), and acantholytic cells are not present in the bulla cavity. On the other hand, differentiation from other diseases associated with subepidermal bullae often is impossible. Bullae removed from areas without inflammation may not show any eosinophils and then are indistinguishable from bullae of epidermolysis bullosa or porphyria cutanea tarda, whereas bullae removed from areas of inflammation and showing an inflammatory infiltrate may be very difficult to differentiate from the bullae occurring in benign mucosal pemphigoid and dermatitis herpetiformis.

Differentiation of *benign mucosal pemphigoid* from bullous pemphigoid may be impossible in instances of benign mucosal pemphigoid showing a more or less extensive eruption of bullae, since such bullae may contain eosinophils both within their cavity and in the underlying dermis.

Differentiation of *dermatitis herpetiformis* from bullous pemphigoid lies in the degree rather than the type of changes, since in dermatitis herpetiformis (1) papillary microabscesses are present in greater number, extending over many neighboring papillae and resulting in a multilocular blister, which is rarely, if ever, seen in bullous pemphigoid; and (2) neutrophils predominate over eosinophils, especially in early lesions of dermatitis herpetiformis in contrast to bullous pemphigoid.

On the other hand, with few exceptions, differentiation of *erythema multiforme* from bullous pemphigoid is possible, since in erythema multiforme, in spite of the variability of the histologic picture from case to case, one finds that: (1) eosinophils and neutrophils, if present at all, are located largely perivascularly, rather near and within the dermal papillae; (2) if cells are seen near the dermal-epidermal junction, they are mononuclear cells, rather than eosinophils; and (3) epidermal changes often are prominent even in early lesions of erythema multiforme, which consist of exocytosis and spongiosis and intracellular edema in some, and of necrotic changes in others, whereby the necrosis may affect either individual keratinocytes or the entire epidermis.

BENIGN MUCOSAL PEMPHIGOID (CICATRICIAL PEMPHIGOID)

Bullae and denuded areas are present on the so-called orificial mucous membranes, particularly the oral mucosa, but occasionally also on the mucous membranes of the larynx, esophagus, nose, vulva and anus. Scarring occurs occasionally on these mucous membranes. The conjunctivae are frequently but not invariably inflamed without, however, showing blisters. Scarring to the point of near-blindness commonly results. Cutaneous lesions are present in about one third of the patients. They may be of two types: One type consists of a more or less extensive eruption of bullae that heal without scarring (Lever; Behlen and Mackay; Kleine-Natrop and Haustein). The other type consists of areas of erythema, mainly on the face and scalp, in which bullae erupt intermittently, ultimately followed by atrophic scarring.

Histopathology. The bullae on the skin and orificial mucous membranes form subepidermally. The dermal changes are not specific and thus not diagnostic. In cases with a more or less extensive eruption of bullae in which the bullae heal without scarring the bullae usually show only a slight to moderate perivascular infiltrate in which eosinophils may be present (Krafek and Streitmann; Kleine-Natrop and Haustein) or may be absent (Behlen and Mackay). The bullae in areas of scarring often show a considerable chronic inflammatory infiltrate and, in the later stages, fibrosis.

Histogenesis. Electron microscopic studies of oral lesions by Susi and Shklar seem to indicate that the initial changes take place in the basal lamina region with overproduction of basal lamina material. On the other hand, Caputo et al. found the basal lamina largely destroyed, in contrast with their findings in bullous pemphigoid in which the basal lamina was preserved at the floor of the blister. Their electron microscopic findings in cicatricial pemphigoid thus are similar to the electron microscopic findings in the "inflammatory bullae" of bullous pemphigoid described by Schaumburg-Lever et al. (see p. 117).

Immunofluorescent studies on patients with cicatricial pemphigoid have shown that, on direct immunofluorescent examination, the majority of patients have in vivo fixed immunoglobulins in the basement zone of involved skin or mucosa, mainly IgG with complement, but also occasionally IgA and rarely IgM (Holubar et al.; Griffith et al.; Kokoschka et al.; Dabelsteen et al.; Bean). In addition, circulating basement zone antibodies were observed on indirect testing by Dabelsteen et al. and by Bean. Dabelsteen et al. found in 7 of 8 patients in the serum basement zone antibodies, usually at a rather low titer, consisting of IgG and IgA in 6 patients and of IgA in 1. Bean, on testing with antihuman IgG, found in 3 of 12 patients IgG basement zone antibodies. Bean concluded that cicatricial pemphigoid and bullous pemphigoid are variants of the same basic disease process.

DERMATITIS HERPETIFORMIS

Dermatitis herpetiformis is a very chronic disease displaying in symmetrical distribution groups of papules and vesicles surrounded by erythema. In rare instances a few bullae are present. The extensor surfaces of the extremities, the shoulders, and the buttocks are affected predominantly. Lesions of the oral mucosa are absent (Tolman et al.). The eruption is well suppressed by sulfapyridine or the sulfones. As a rule, dermatitis herpetiformis occurs in adults and is very rarely seen in children (Ackerman and Tolman; Jablonska et al.).

"Bullous eruption of childhood" is regarded preferably as a separate disease rather than as a bullous variant of dermatitis herpetiformis (Jordon et al.) (see under Bullous Pemphigoid, p. 118).

Histopathology. The typical histologic features of dermatitis herpetiformis are best seen in erythematous, not yet blistering lesions and in the vicinity of early blisters. In these areas one observes at the tips of adjoining papillae accumulations of neutrophils and usually also of some eosinophils (Piérard). Early accumulations often consist entirely of neutrophils, whereas with increase in size to microabscesses they may have a significant admixture of eosinophils. As the microabscesses form, fibrin accumulates at the tips of the papillae, giving them a necrotic appearance. Subsequently, separations appear between the tips of adjoin-

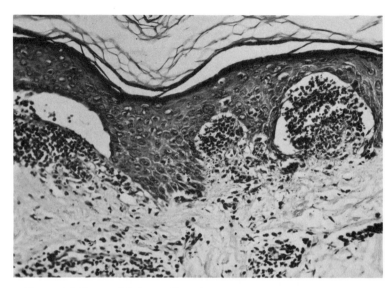

FIG. 7-16. **Dermatitis herpetiformis.** On the left side part of an early blister is seen. On the right two papillae show papillary microabscesses composed of neutrophils and an admixture of eosinophils. The accumulation of fibrin gives the papillae a necrotic appearance and results in separations between the tips of papillae and the epidermis, so that early blisters are multilocular (×200)

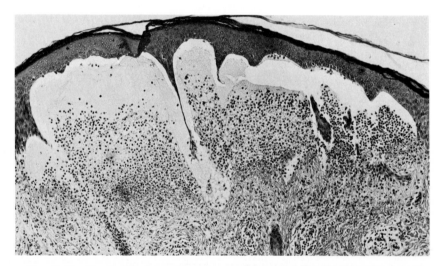

FIG. 7-17. **Dermatitis herpetiformis.** A fully developed blister no longer is multilocular. Some of the rete ridges that originally subdivided the blister can still be recognized. Most of the cells in the blister and around the dermal vessels are neutrophils. (×50)

ing papillae and the epidermis (Fig. 7-16) (van der Meer). At first, the interpapillary ridges of the epidermis remain attached to the dermis so that the blisters of dermatitis herpetiformis are multilocular when they are still too small to be clinically apparent. However, within one to two days the rete ridges lose their coherence with the dermis, and the blisters then become unilocular and clinically apparent (Fig. 7-17) (MacVicar et al.). Often at that time one may still see at the periphery of such unilocular blisters the characteristic papillary microabscesses. For this reason the inclusion of perivesicular skin in the biopsy is of considerable value.

The subpapillary dermis usually shows a moderately severe inflammatory infiltrate of neutrophils and eosinophils, many of which show disintegration of their nuclei to "nuclear dust." In addition, the underlying subpapillary vessels show a perivascular infiltrate composed of mononuclear cells as well as neutrophils and eosinophils (Kresbach and Hartwagner). As to be expected, a diagnostic histologic picture is not always seen in biopsies from patients with dermatitis herpetiformis. Thus, in a review of 105 biopsies by Connor et al., papillary microabscesses were present in only about one half, subepidermal vesicles in 61 per cent, and nuclear dust in the upper dermis in 77 per cent of the biopsies.

Histogenesis. The electron microscopic findings in dermatitis herpetiformis resemble changes seen during development of the "inflammatory bullae" in bullous pemphigoid (Schaumburg-Lever et al.). The only differences are the prevalence of neutrophils over eosinophils, especially in early lesions, and the earlier appearance and greater amount of fibrin present (E.M. No. 25), particularly in dermal papillae, where it often is attached to the dermal side of the basal lamina (E.M. No. 25, *inset*). In more advanced blisters the basal lamina has disappeared in many areas (Piérard and Kint; Jakubowicz et al.), just as has been noted in the "inflammatory bullae" of bullous pemphigoid (E.M. No. 25, *inset*).

Immunologic studies have revealed the absence of circulating antibodies, whereas direct immunofluorescent tests usually show deposits of IgA at the dermal-epidermal junction of uninvolved skin and in early erythematous areas. No IgA deposits are present within vesicles, where these deposits probably have been destroyed as the result of phagocytosis (van der Meer; Chorzelski et al.; Holubar et al.). In the great majority of cases the deposits of IgA are granular (van der Meer, 1969); but they may be continuous (Chorzelski et al.). The deposits of IgA are seen mainly at the tips of the dermal papillae. Occasionally the deposits are not limited to the subepidermal basement zone but are seen throughout the papillae (Chorzelski

et al.; van der Meer). Even though IgA, in association with complement, often is the only immunoglobulin present in dermatitis herpetiformis, some cases show also deposits of IgG, and rarely of IgM (van der Meer; Welke et al.). Since IgA deposits occur also in some cases of bullous pemphigoid in association with IgG (see p. 117), and furthermore in rare instances IgA deposits are absent in cases of dermatitis herpetiformis (Marks et al.), direct immunofluorescent testing does not represent an absolutely reliable method for the diagnosis of dermatitis herpetiformis.

The presence of early and extensive deposits of fibrin in the dermal papillae has been demonstrated by Mustakallio et al. by means of direct immunofluorescent testing, using a fluorescein-labeled antifibrinogen-containing serum. In the earliest lesions the fibrin is found as a crescentic deposition at the tips of papillae. Later the entire papilla is filled with globular fibrin deposits. According to Mustakallio et al., no crescentic or globular deposits of fibrin are found in bullous pemphigoid or erythema multiforme.

About two thirds of the patients with dermatitis herpetiformis have a mild, usually asymptomatic steatorrhea on the basis of a gluten sensitivity. A gluten-free diet improves the steatorrhea but not the dermatitis herpetiformis. Conversely, the sulfones do not improve the steatorrhea (Lyell). A jejunal biopsy shows atrophy of the villi. Since none of 10 patients with bullous pemphigoid showed jejunal changes on biopsy, Marks and Shuster regard the enteropathy as specific for dermatitis herpetiformis. Van der Meer (1972) has postulated that the relationship of the enteropathy to dermatitis herpetiformis may lie in the production of the IgA by the plasma cells of the "gut-associated" lymphoid tissue.

Differential Diagnosis. The presence of an early multilocular vesicle with a microabscess at the tip of each papilla can be regarded as diagnostic for dermatitis herpetiformis. However, microabscesses may be seen also in papillae adjoining the inflammatory bullae of bullous pemphigoid (Jablonska and Chorzelski; Kresbach and Hartwagner). It is, therefore, best to select for biopsy in patients suspected of having dermatitis herpetiformis, as Piérard has suggested, an erythematous area without clinically visible vesicles because, in the case of dermatitis herpetiformis, such an area is most apt to show a diagnostic multilocular vesicle, still too small to be clinically visible. The prevalence of neutrophils in the micro-abscesses certainly speaks in favor of a diagnosis of dermatitis herpetiformis; but a prevalence of eosinophils does not necessarily rule out dermatitis herpetiformis in favor of bullous pemphigoid.

ERYTHEMA MULTIFORME

Erythema multiforme is an acute, self-limited dermatosis showing in some patients a tendency to periodic recurrences. As the name implies, the lesions may be multiform. They include macules, papules, vesicles, and bullae. Quite commonly one observes so-called iris lesions, or target lesions, representing a macule or papule with a central vesicle. Not infrequently, some of the lesions are hemorrhagic. Erythema multiforme may be idiopathic, but it may occur also as a drug reaction. In addition, several infections can induce erythema multiforme, for instance with *Herpesvirus hominis,* or with *Mycoplasma pneumoniae,* a cause of primary atypical pneumonia (Cannell et al.).

There are two forms of severe erythema multiforme that start abruptly with high fever, prostration and a very extensive eruption. They are Stevens-Johnson disease, and the "subepidermal" type of Lyell's toxic epidermal necrolysis. Both have a high mortality, between 30 and 40 per cent, unless corticosteroids are given in large doses as soon as possible. Not infrequently they are caused by allergy to drugs.

In *Stevens-Johnson disease,* in addition to extensive inflammatory skin lesions, the mucous surfaces of the mouth and nose and the conjunctivae are severely involved.

In the "subepidermal" type of Lyell's *toxic epidermal necrolysis* the eruption begins with a widespread blotchy erythema. This soon is followed by large, flaccid bullae and detachment of the epidermis in large sheets, leaving the dermis exposed and giving the skin a scalded appearance. Involvement of the mucous membranes usually is less severe than in Stevens-Johnson disease. The "subepidermal" type usually occurs in adults and only rarely in small children.

It has become apparent in recent years that Lyell's toxic epidermal necrolysis includes two entirely different diseases (Lowney et al.; Lyell): (1) a "subcorneal" bacterial type, and (2) a "subepidermal" type. The "subcorneal" type does not affect mucous membranes and occurs predominantly in young children and is rarely fatal except during the first year of life. It is caused by coagulase-positive staphylococci of phage group 2, type 71 and is identical with Ritter's disease. (Further details, see p. 270.) The "subepidermal" type, described above, is regarded as a variant of severe erythema multiforme because of its acute course, its frequent occurrence as a drug allergy, its frequent association with Stevens-Johnson disease (according to Lyell, in 22 of 128 cases), and especially its histologic identity with the "epidermal type" of erythema multiforme (see below).

Histopathology. In a recent histologic description of erythema multiforme, Ackerman et al. described the "classical" type of erythema multiforme with target lesions. Both dermal and epidermal changes were present histologically. Ackerman et al. excluded cases with edematous or bullous lesions in which the changes are almost entirely dermal; and also excluded cases with predominantly epidermal necrotic changes. Review of many cases of erythema multiforme with multiple biopsies has revealed in some biopsies predominantly dermal changes, in others predominantly epidermal changes, and in still others both types of changes to a nearly equal degree. Thus, it seems best to distinguish histologically between three types of lesions in erythema multiforme: lesions of the dermal type, of the mixed dermal-epidermal type, and of the epidermal type (Orfanos et al.).

Dermal Type. Predominantly dermal changes are seen in the macular and erythematous lesions of erythema multiforme. One finds a fairly pronounced perivascular infiltrate of cells, largely mononuclear, but containing also admixtures of eosinophils and neutrophils. There may be pronounced edema of the papillary dermis. In cases in which the edema has led to the formation of a bulla, the epidermis together with part or all of the PAS-positive basement zone

FIG. 7-18. **Erythema multiforme, dermal type.** A fairly pronounced perivascular infiltrate composed largely of mononuclear cells is present. The upper dermis shows marked edema resulting in subepidermal blisters. (×100)

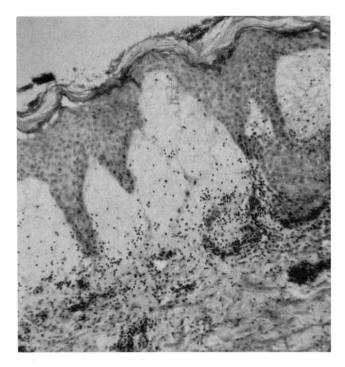

forms the top of the bulla, as described by MacVicar et al. (Fig. 7-18).

Mixed Dermal-Epidermal Type. This type, well described by Ackerman et al., is the most common type, and is seen in association with papular, plaquelike and target lesions. A mononuclear infiltrate is present around the superficial blood vessels and along the dermal-epidermal border, with the basal cells showing hydropic degeneration. The epidermis contains numerous scattered individually necrotic keratinocytes showing a strongly eosinophilic cytoplasm and pyknotic or absent nuclei. In some lesions the

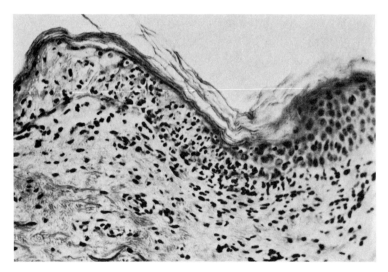

FIG. 7-19. **Erythema multiforme, epidermal type.** The epidermis shows on the left keratinocytes showing eosinophilic necrosis. (×200)

dermal mononuclear infiltrate extends into the epidermis; and mild spongiosis and intracellular edema may result in intraepidermal vesiculation. The hydropic degeneration of the basal cells in association with the focal necrosis of the epidermis may lead to the formation of subepidermal vesicles and bullae showing extensive necrosis of the overlying epidermis. Extravasated erythrocytes often are present in the upper dermis. Eosinophils, according to Ackerman et al., are uncommon and neutrophils and "nuclear dust" are absent, and there is no evidence of vasculitis.

Epidermal Type. Whereas the dermal changes in this type consist of only a mild mononuclear infiltrate around the superficial blood vessels, the epidermis in early lesions contains groups of keratinocytes showing eosinophilic necrosis (Fig. 7-19). The affected cells subsequently lose their nucleus and coalesce. In severely affected areas hydropic degeneration of the basal cells may result in subepidermal separation, and all keratinocytes appear necrotic, with only the horny layer remaining preserved. In other areas, however, there may be severe damage to the upper epidermal layers and less severe damage to the lower epidermal layers, resulting in intraepidermal cleavage (Orfanos et al.). These changes are identical with those occurring in toxic epidermal necrolysis, as described by Braun-Falco and by Tritsch. Tritsch points out in this connection that he observed the same histologic changes also in severe fixed drug eruptions.

Histogenesis. Electron microscopic examination of bullae of the dermal type have shown the basal lamina to be located on top of the blister and no significant alterations within the detached epidermis (Orfanos et al.). On the other hand, in blisters of the dermal-epidermal or epidermal type the basal lamina is destroyed in some instances; but, if present, it is located at the floor of the bulla. The basal cells show marked intracytoplasmic damage with a loss of organelles. Neutrophils and macrophages rich in lysosomes are seen in the lower epidermis phagocytizing the damaged keratinocytes (E.M. No. 26). In the midepidermis large, electron dense, dyskeratotic bodies may be located, corresponding to the cells with eosinophilic cytoplasm seen by light microscopy (Orfanos et al.; Prutkin and Fellner). In the necrotic epidermis of the epidermal type of erythema multiforme the damaged epidermal cells often contain few or no organelles (Orfanos et al.). The epidermal changes thus are the same as those described in the subepidermal type of Lyell's toxic epidermal necrolysis (Braun-Falco and Wolff).

Differential Diagnosis. For differentiation of erythema multiforme from bullous pemphigoid, see p. 118; and from herpes gestationis, see p. 125.

HERPES GESTATIONIS

Herpes gestationis is a rare eruption occurring during pregnancy and puerperium and showing vesicles and bullae associated with patchy erythema. Oral lesions may be present. Itching is severe. The clinical resemblance to bullous pemphigoid is often great. The cause is not known; but the fact that in women having had herpes gestationis oral contraceptives may bring on recurrences of the eruption suggests that herpes gestationis may be an "autoimmune progesterone" dermatosis (Lynch and Albrecht).

Histopathology. The bullae in herpes gestationis arise subepidermally. Areas of erythema may show in the epidermis considerable spongiosis as well as vacuolization of epidermal cells resulting in multiple intraepidermal microvesicles (Winer; Piérard et al.). The dermal infiltrate in some cases consists largely of mononuclear cells and some neutrophils with either no eosinophils (Winer) or only a few eosinophils (Piérard et al.); whereas in other cases eosinophils are present in large numbers and nuclear fragmentation ("nuclear dust") is prominent (Schaumburg-Lever et al.). Papillary microabscesses are absent.

Histogenesis. Electron microscopic examination of the epidermis at the periphery of bullae shows significant damage to epidermal cells, most pronounced in the basal cells but present also in the squamous cells, resulting in partial or complete necrosis of epidermal cells, with disappearance of all their organelles but partial preservation of the tonofilaments (Piérard et al.). The basal lamina is found at the floor of the bulla either fairly well preserved (E.M. No. 27) (Schaumburg-Lever et al.) or fragmented (Piérard et al.). Epidermal damage can be regarded as the main cause of bulla formation, just as in the epidermal type of erythema multiforme (Schaumburg-Lever et al.).

Immunofluorescent studies have revealed neither circulating antibodies nor in vivo bound immunoglobulins in the subepidermal basement zone. However, several authors have observed the presence of complement in the basement zone, either of C3 alone (Hentschel), or in association with C4 (Jablonska and Chorzelski), or with C5 (Provost and Tomasi).

Differential Diagnosis. It may be impossible to differentiate herpes gestationis from bullous pemphigoid if there are numerous eosinophils and nuclear dust; and from the dermal-epidermal type of erythema multiforme if there are a largely mononuclear infiltrate and epidermal spongiosis.

SUBCORNEAL PUSTULAR DERMATOSIS

This chronic disorder, first described by Sneddon and Wilkinson in 1956, shows pustules in annular and serpiginous arrangement, especially on the abdomen and in the axillary and inguinal folds. Oral lesions do not occur. The pustules are sterile. Like

dermatitis herpetiformis, the eruption responds well to sulfapyridine and the sulfones.

Histopathology. The pustules form directly beneath the stratum corneum (Fig. 7-20). The content of the pustules consists almost entirely of neutrophils, with only an occasional eosinophil. The stratum malpighii beneath the pustule contains a fairly small number of leukocytes and shows only in some areas rather mild intracellular edema and spongiosis. The underlying dermis, including the papillae, shows dilated capillaries and around them an infiltrate composed of neutrophils and a few eosinophils and mononuclear cells (Wolff).

In some instances, a few acantholytic cells are seen at the base of the pustule. They usually still show partial attachment to the epidermis at the base of the pustule but may lie free in the pustule among the neutrophils (Ellis). Since the pustules in subcorneal pustular dermatosis do not form on the basis of acantholysis, and acantholytic cells only appear later, one may regard their presence as being due to secondary acantholysis, caused probably by

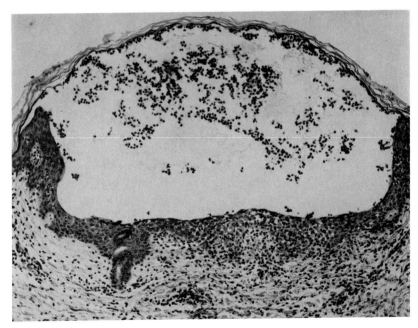

FIG. 7-20. **Subcorneal pustular dermatosis.** The pustule has formed beneath the horny layer. No acantholysis is present. (×100)

proteolytic enzymes present in the pustular content (Burns and Fine).

Histogenesis. Electron microscopic examination by Metz and Schröpl of the border of pustules have shown cytolytic degenerative changes in the upper epidermis, especially in the granular layer. The dissolution of the plasma membrane and of the cytoplasm of granular cells causes the formation of a subcorneal slit. The epidermal penetration of leukocytes and their subcorneal accumulation are regarded as events secondary to the cellular destruction in the stratum granulosum.

Differential Diagnosis. A histologic differentiation from impetigo usually is impossible, since as a rule bacteria cannot be demonstrated in the pustules of impetigo by staining methods.

A histologic differentiation from pemphigus foliaceus or pemphigus erythematosus also may be impossible, since one observes in both diseases subcorneal blisters with acantholysis that usually but not always is more pronounced in pemphigus foliaceus than in subcorneal pustular dermatosis. Thus, clinical information and a therapeutic test with sulfones may be necessary to arrive at a decision.

Although subcorneal pustules occur in both pustular psoriasis and subcorneal pustular dermatosis, spongiform pustules occur only in pustular psoriasis.

TRANSIENT ACANTHOLYTIC DERMATOSIS

In this condition, recently described by Grover and observed also by Wolff, pruritic, discrete, edematous papules and papulovesicles develop predominantly on the trunk. The eruption may be either localized or widespread and clears within a few weeks to months.

Histopathology. Suprabasal clefts and vesicles form on the basis of acantholysis. In some cases corps ronds and grains are present as seen in Darier's disease, while in others the predominance of acantholytic cells causes a resemblance to familial benign pemphigus.

Differential Diagnosis. The presence of either dyskeratotic changes or extensive acantholysis helps in the differentiation from pemphigus vulgaris; but a definitive differentiation probably requires clinical data.

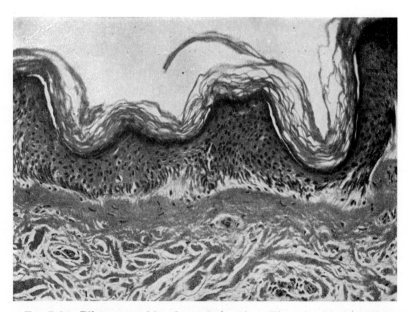

Fɪɢ. 7-21. **Blister caused by electrodesiccation.** The subepidermal blister shows as a diagnostic feature elongated, degenerated cytoplasmic processes protruding from the basal cells into the bulla cavity. Also the nuclei of the basal cells appear markedly stretched. (×200)

FRICTION BLISTERS

Friction blisters occur mainly on the soles as the result of prolonged walking, and on the palms and the palmar surfaces of the fingers as the result of repetitive actions required in certain occupations or sports.

Histopathology. In experimentally produced friction blisters intraepidermal cleavage and vesicles develop as the result of necrosis of keratinocytes in the stratum malpighii (Naylor). The cleavage lies always at the same level, with the roof of the blister being composed of the stratum corneum, the stratum granulosum and some amorphous cellular debris (Sulzberger et al.).

Of special interest is the histologic similarity of friction blisters to the blisters seen in the dominantly inherited epidermolysis bullosa of the hands and feet (see p. 70).

ELECTRIC BURNS

It is desirable that those working in dermatopathology be familiar with the effects of an electric current on the skin, such as is used during electrodesiccation or diathermy, because these modalities occasionally are used for the removal of tumors. The effects on small specimens are so severe that usually no other diagnosis than electric burn can be made.

Histopathology. The electrodesiccation or diathermy current causes a separation of the epidermis from the dermis. A diagnostic histologic feature is the fringe of elongated, degenerated cytoplasmic processes that protrudes from the lower end of the detached basal cells into the space separating the epidermis and the dermis (Fig. 7-21). The nuclei of the basal cells and often also of some of the higher lying epidermal cells appear stretched in the same direction as the fringe of cytoplasmic processes. In addition, the upper portion of the dermis shows homogenization due to coagulation necrosis (Winer and Levin).

BIBLIOGRAPHY

Dermatitis-Eczema and Dermatopathic Lymphadenitis

Abrahams, I., McCarthy, J. T., and Sanders, S. L.: 101 cases of exfoliative dermatitis. Arch. Derm., *87*:96, 1963.

Achten, G., and Delescluse, J.: Pathogenesis of allergic contact dermatitis. Arch. belges derm., *28*:47, 1973 (review).

Bandmann, H. J.: Beitrag zur Histopathologie allergischer epikutaner Testreaktionen. Hautarzt, *11*:258, 310, 355, and 393, 1960.

———: Monocyten bei experimentallem Kontaktekzem. Hautarzt, *18*:122, 1967.

Bluefarb, S. M., and Adams, L. A.: Arteriovenous malformation with angiodermatitis. Arch. Derm., *96*:176, 1967.

Braun-Falco, O., and Burg, G.: Celluläres Infiltrat und Capillaren bei Neurodermitis diffuse. Arch. Derm. Forsch., *249*:113, 1974.

Braun-Falco, O., and Petry, G.: Feinstruktur der Epidermis bei chronischem nummulärem Ekzem. Arch. klin. exp. Derm., *222*:219, 1965, and *224*:63, 1966.

Braun-Falco, O., and Wolff, H.H.: Zur Ultrastruktur der menschlichen Epidermis bei der allergischen Epicutantestreaktion. Arch. Derm. Forsch., *240*:23, 1971.

Calnan, C. D.: Eczema for me. Trans. St. John's Hosp. Derm. Soc., *54*:54, 1968.

Carr, R. D., Scarpelli, D. G., and Greider, M. H.: Allergic contact dermatitis. Light and electron microscopy. Dermatologica, *137*: 358, 1968.

Dvorak, H. F., Simpson, B. A., Bast, R. C., Jr., and Leskowitz S.: Cutaneous basophil hypersensitivity. J. Immunol., *107*:138, 1971.

Epstein, S.: Chlorpromazine photosensitivity. Arch. Derm., *98*:354, 1968.

Frichot, B. C., III, and Zelickson, A. S.: Steroids, lysosomes and dermatitis. Acta dermatoven., *52*:311, 1972.

Hall, J. B., Smith, J. G., Jr., and Burnett, S. C.: The lysosome in contact dermatitis: a histochemical study. J. Invest. Derm., *49*:590, 1967.

Hohenadl, L., and de Paola, D.: Über Gewebsreaktionen nach parenteraler Zufuhr von Melanin unter besonderer Berücksichtigung der lipomelanotischen Reticulose. Frankfurt. Z. Path., *69*:374, 1958.

Hurwitt, E.: Dermatopathic lymphadenitis. J. Invest. Derm., *5*:197, 1942.

Inderbitzin, T., Keel, A., and Blumental, G.: The identity of the permeability factor from lymph node cells (LNPF) with the permeability increasing factor (PIF). Int. Arch. Allergy, *29*:417, 1964.

Jarrett, A., and Kellett, H. S.: The association of generalized erythrodermia with superficial lymphadenopathy (lipomelanic reticulosis). Brit. J. Derm., *63*:343, 1951.

Kerl, H., Burg, G., and Braun-Falco, O.: Contact dermatitis in guinea pigs. Arch. Derm. Forsch., *249*:207, 1974.

Laipply, T. C.: Lipomelanotic reticular hyperplasia of lymph nodes. Arch. Intern. Med., *81*:19, 1948.

Macher, E.: Die Reaktion der regionären Lymphknoten beim tierexperimentellen allergischen Kontaktekzem. Hautarzt, *13*:126, 1962.

―――: Immunologische Mechanismen der Allergie. Z. Haut, *47*:307, 1972 (review).

Medenica, M., and Rostenberg, A.: A comparative light and electron microscopic study of primary irritant contact dermatitis and allergic contact dermatitis. J. Invest. Derm., *56*:259, 1971.

Meessen, H.: Zur Pathomorphologie des retikulären Gewebes unter besonderer Berücksichtigung der lipomelanotischen Retikulose. Hautarzt, *6*:1, 1955.

Metz, J.: Ultrastruktur der Spongiose beim allergischen Kontaktekzem. Dermatologica, *141*:315, 1970.

Miescher, G.: Abgrenzung des allergischen und toxischen Geschehens in morphologischer und funktioneller Sicht. Arch. klin. exp. Derm., *213*:297, 1961.

Montgomery, H.: Exfoliative dermatitis and malignant erythroderma. Arch. Derm. Syph., *27*:253, 1933.

Neumann, E., and Winter, V.: The character of cells with "altération cavitaire" (Leloir). Acta dermatoven., *45*:272, 1965.

Nicolis, G. D., and Helwig, E. B.: Exfoliative dermatitis. Arch. Derm., *108*:788, 1973.

Nordquist, B., and Rorsman, H.: Leukocytic migration in vitro as an indicator of allergy in eczematous contact dermatitis. Trans. St. John's Hosp. Derm. Soc., *53*:154, 1967.

Ogawa, M., Berger, P. A., McIntyre, O. R., et al.: IgE in atopic dermatitis. Arch. Derm., *103*:575, 1971.

Pautrier, L. M., and Woringer, F.: Mycosis fongoïdes généralisé, forme erythrodermique et tumorale: le ganglion mycosique. Bull. Soc. franç. derm. syph., *46*:498, 1939.

Pinkus, H., and Mehregan, A. H.: The primary histologic lesion of seborrheic dermatitis and psoriasis. J. Invest. Derm., *46*:109, 1966.

Prose, P. H., and Sedlis, E.: Morphologic and histochemical studies of atopic eczema in infants and children. J. Invest. Derm., *34*:149, 1960.

Prose, P. H., Sedlis, E., and Bigelow, M.: The demonstration of lysosomes in the diseased skin of infants with infantile eczema. J. Invest. Derm., *45*:448, 1965.

Rappaport, H., Winter, W. J., and Hicks, E. B.: Follicular lymphoma. Cancer, *9*:792, 1956.

Wiedmann, A.: Die arterielle Genese des Ulcus cruris "varicosum." Hautarzt, *5*:85, 1954.

Wolff, H. H., and Braun-Falco, O.: Zur Ultrastruktur dermaler Veränderungen bei der allergischen Epicutantestreaktion des Menschen. Arch. Derm. Forsch., *240*:219, 1971.

Miliaria

Cage, G. W.: Miliarias. *In* Fitzpatrick, T. B., et al. (eds.): General Practice. p. 383. New York, McGraw-Hill, 1971.

Loewenthal, L. J. A.: The pathogenesis of miliaria. Arch. Derm., *84*:2, 1961.

O'Brien, J. P.: The pathogenesis of miliaria. Arch. Derm., *86*:267, 1962.

Papa, C. M., and Kligman, A. M.: Mechanism of eccrine anidrosis. J. Invest. Derm., *47*:1, 1966.

Shelley, W. B., and Horvath, P. N.: Experimental miliaria in man. II. Production of sweat retention anhidrosis and miliaria crystallina by various kinds of injury. J. Invest. Derm., *14*:9, 1950.

Sulzberger, M. B., and Harris, D. R.: Miliaria and anhidrosis. III. Multiple small patches and the effects of different periods of occlusion. Arch. Derm., *105*:845, 1972.

Sulzberger, M. B., and Zimmerman, H. M.: Studies on prickly heat. J. Invest. Derm., *7*:61, 1946.

Erythema Toxicum Neonatorum

Freeman, R. G., Spiller, R., and Knox, J. M.: Histopathology of erythema toxicum neonatorum. Arch. Derm., *82*:586, 1960.

Lüders, D.: Histologic observations in erythema toxicum neonatorum. Pediatrics, *26*:219, 1960.

Pemphigus

Asboe-Hansen, G.: Blister-spread induced by finger pressure, a diagnostic sign of pemphigus. J. Invest. Derm., *34*:5, 1960.

Baart de la Faille, H., and Baart de la Faille-Kuyper, E. H.: Immunofluorescent studies of the skin in rosacea. Dermatologica, *139*:49, 1969.

Barranco, V. P.: Mixed bullous disease. Arch. Derm., *110*:221, 1974.

Bean, S. F., and Lynch, F. W.: Senear-Usher syndrome (Pemphigus erythematosus). Arch. Derm., *101*:642, 1970.

Beutner, E. H., Lever, W. F., Witebsky, E., et al.: Autoantibodies in pemphigus vulgaris. J.A.M.A., *192*:682, 1965.

Braun-Falco, O., and Vogell, W.: Elektronen-mikroskopische Untersuchungen zur Dynamik der Acantholyse bei Pemphigus vulgaris. Arch. klin. exp. Derm., *223*:338 and 533, 1965.

Chorzelski, T. P., von Weiss, J. F., and Lever, W. F.: Clinical significance of autoantibodies in pemphigus. Arch. Derm., *93*:570, 1966.

Chorzelski, T., Jablonska, S., and Blaszczyk, M.: Immunopathological investigation in the Senear-Usher syndrome (coexistence of pemphigus and lupus erythematosus). Brit. J. Derm., *80*:211, 1968.

Civatte, A.: Diagnostic histopathologique de la dermatite polymorphe douloureuse ou maladie de Duhring-Brocq. Ann. derm. syph., *3*:1, 1943.

Cormane, R. H., and Chorzelski, T. P.: "Bound" complement in the epidermis of patients with pemphigus vulgaris. Dermatologica, *134*:463, 1967.

Director, W.: Pemphigus vulgaris: a clinicopathologic study. Arch. Derm., *65*:155, 1952.

Emmerson, R. W., and Wilson-Jones, E.: Eosinophilic spongiosis in pemphigus. Arch. Derm., *97*:252, 1968.

Floden, C. H., and Gentele, H.: A case of clinically typical dermatitis herpetiformis (Morbus Duhring) presenting acantholysis. Acta dermatoven., *35*:128, 1955.

Fukuyama, K., Douglas, S. D., Tufanelli, D. L., and Epstein, W. L.: Immunohistochemical method of localization of antibodies in cutaneous disease. Am. J. Clin. Path., *54*:410, 1970.

Furtado, T. A.: Histopathology of pemphigus foliaceus. Arch. Derm., *80*:66, 1959.

Graham, J. H., Bingul, O., and Burgoon, C. B.: Cytodiagnosis of inflammatory dermatoses. Arch. Derm., *87*:118, 1963.

Grob, P. J., and Inderbitzin, T. M.: Serum immunoglobulins in pemphigus. J. Invest. Derm., *49*:282, 1967.

Hashimoto, K., and Lever, W. F.: An electron microscopic study of pemphigus vulgaris of the mouth with special reference to the intercellular cement. J. Invest. Derm., *48*:540, 1967.

————: An ultrastructural study of cell junctions in pemphigus vulgaris. Arch. Derm., *101*:287, 1970.

Jablonska, S., Chorzelski, T., and Maciejowska, E.: The scope and limitations of the immunofluorescence method in the diagnosis of lupus erythematosus. Brit. J. Derm., *83*:242, 1970.

Lever, W. F.: Pemphigus. Medicine, *32*:1, 1953.

————: Pemphigus and Pemphigoid. Springfield, Ill., Charles C Thomas, 1965.

Lever, W. F., and Hashimoto, K.: The etiology and treatment of pemphigus and pemphigoid. J. Invest. Derm., *53*:373, 1969.

Percival, G. H.: Diagnostic histologique du pemphigus foliacé et du syndrome de Senear-Usher. Arch. belg. derm. syph., *5*:278, 1949.

Perry, H. O.: Pemphigus foliaceus. Arch. Derm., *83*:52, 1961.

Perry, H. O., and Brunsting, L. A.: Pemphigus foliaceus. Arch. Derm., *91*:10, 1965.

Röckl, H.: Über die Pyodermite végétante von Hallopeau als benigne Form des Pemphigus vegetans von Neumann nebst einigen Bemerkungen zur Pyostomatitis vegetans von McCarthy. Arch. klin. exp. Derm., *218*:574, 1964.

Rook, A. J., and Whimster, I. W.: The histologic diagnosis of pemphigus. Brit. J. Derm., *62*: 443, 1950.

Saikia, N. K., and MacConnell, L. E. S.: Senear-Usher syndrome and internal malignancy. Brit. J. Derm., *87*:1, 1972.

Sams, W. M., Jr., and Jordon, R. E.: Correlation of pemphigus and pemphigoid antibody titers with activity of disease. Brit. J. Derm., *84*:7, 1971.

Tappeiner, J., and Pfleger, L.: Pemphigus vulgaris–Dermatitis herpetiformis. Arch. klin. exp. Derm., *214*:415, 1962.

Tzanck, A.: Le cytodiagnostic immediat en dermatologie. Ann. derm. syph., *8*:205, 1948.

Wilgram, G. F., Caulfield, J. B., and Lever, W. F.: An electron microscopic study of acantholysis in pemphigus vulgaris. J. Invest. Derm., *36*:373, 1961.

Wilgram, G. F., Caulfield, J. B., and Madgic, E. B.: An electron microscopic study of acantholysis and dyskeratosis in pemphigus foliaceus. J. Invest. Derm., *43*:287, 1964.

Winkelmann, R. K., and Roth, H. L.: Dermatitis herpetiformis with acantholysis or pemphigus with response to sulfonamides. Arch. Derm., *82*:385, 1960.

Wolff, K., and Schreiner, E.: Ultrastructural localization of pemphigus antibodies within the epidermis. Nature, *229*:59, 1971.

Bullous Pemphigoid

Braun-Falco, O., and Rupec, M.: Elektronen-mikroskopische Untersuchungen zur Dynamik der Blasenbildung bei bullösem Pemphigoid. Arch. klin. exp. Derm., *230*:1, 1967.

Brehm, K., Paul, E., and Schmitt, H.: Zur nosologischen Stellung der bullösen Variante der Dermatitis herpetiformis Duhring des Kindes. Hautarzt, *25*:379, 1974.

Burnham, T. K., and Fine, G.: Indirect cutaneous immunofluorescence. Arch. Derm., *105*: 52, 1972.

Chorzelski, T. P., and Cormane, R. H.: The presence of complement "bound" in vivo in the skin of patients with pemphigoid. Dermatologica, *137*:134, 1968.

Christophers, E., Braun-Falco, O., and Chorzelski, T.: Über das Verhalten von Autoantikörper bei bullösem Pemphigoid. Hautarzt, *18*:212, 1967.

Degos, R.: Bullous dermatoses. Proc. 11th Internat. Congr. Dermat., Acta dermatoven., *3*: 301, 1957.

Eng. A. M., and Moncada, B.: Bullous pemphigoid and dermatitis herpetiformis. Arch. Derm., *110*:51, 1974.

Fincher, D. F., Dupree, E., and Bean, S. F.: Bullous pemphigoid in childhood. Arch. Derm., *103*:88, 1971.

Honeyman, J. F., Honeyman, A., Lobitz, W. C., Jr., and Storrs, F. J.: The enigma of bullous pemphigoid and dermatitis herpetiformis. Arch. Derm., *106*:22, 1972.

Jablonska, S., and Chorzelski, T.: Kann das histologische Bild die Grundlage zur Differenzierung des Morbus Duhring mit dem Pemphigoid und Erythema multiforme darstellen? Derm. Wschr., *146*:590, 1963.

Jablonska, S., Chorzelski, T., Beutner, E. H., and Blaszczyk, M.: Juvenile dermatitis herpetiformis in the light of immunofluorescence studies. Brit. J. Derm., *85*:307, 1971.

Jakubowicz, K., Dabrowski, J., and Maciejewski, W.: Elektronenmikroskopische Untersuchungen bei bullösem Pemphigoid und Dermatitis herpetiformis Duhring. Arch. klin. exp. Derm., *238*:272, 1970.

Jordon, R. E., Beutner, E. H., Witebsky, E., et al.: Basement zone antibodies in bullous pemphigoid. J.A.M.A., *200*:751, 1967.

Jordon, R. E., Muller, S. A., Hale, W. L., and Beutner, E. H.: Bullous pemphigoid associated with systemic lupus erythematosus. Arch. Derm., *99*:17, 1969.

Jordon, R. E., Bean, S. F., Triftshauser, C. T., and Winkelmann, R. K.: Childhood bullous dermatitis herpetiformis. Arch. Derm., *101*: 629, 1970.

Jordon, R. E., Triftshauser, C. T., and Schroeter, A. L.: Direct immunofluorescent studies of pemphigus and bullous pemphigoid. Arch. Derm., *103*:486, 1971.

Kobayasi, T.: The dermo-epidermal junction in bullous pemphigoid. Dermatologica, *134*: 157, 1967.

Kresbach, H., and Hartwagner, A.: Zur Differentialdiagnose zwischen Dermatitis herpetiformis Duhring und bullösem Pemphigoid. Z. Haut, *43*:165, 1968.

Lever, W. F.: Pemphigus. Medicine, *32*:1, 1953.

———: Pemphigus and Pemphigoid. Springfield, Ill., Charles C Thomas, 1965.

Rook, A. J., and Waddington, E.: Pemphigus and pemphigoid. Brit. J. Derm., *65*:425, 1953.

Sams, W. S., Jr., and Jordon, R. E.: Correlation of pemphigoid and pemphigus antibody titers with activity of disease. Brit. J. Derm., *84*:7, 1971.

Schaumburg-Lever, G., Orfanos, C. E., and Lever, W. F.: Electron microscopic study of bullous pemphigoid. Arch. Derm., *106*:662, 1972.

Schaumburg-Lever, G., Rule, A., Schmidt-Ullrich, B., and Lever, W. F.: Ultrastructural localization of in vivo bound immunoglobulins in bullous pemphigoid. J. Invest. Derm., *64*: 47, 1975.

Ueki, H., Wolff, H. H., and Braun-Falco, O.: Cutaneous localization of human gamma-globulins in lupus erythematosus. Arch. Derm. Forsch., *248*:297, 1974.

van der Meer, J. B.: Dermatitis herpetiformis: a specific (immunopathological?) entity. University of Utrecht, 1972.

Welke, S., Jost, H., and Schwarz, J. A.: Immunologische Befunde bei Dermatitis herpetiformis und beim bullösen Pemphigoid. Z. Haut, *48*:943, 1973.

Wilgram, G. F.: Pemphigus and pemphigoid. *In* Zelickson, A. S. (ed.): Ultrastructure of Normal and Abnormal Skin. p. 335. Philadelphia, Lea and Febiger, 1967.

Benign Mucosal Pemphigoid

Bean, S. F.: Cicatricial pemphigoid. Arch. Derm., *110*:552, 1974.

Behlen, C. H., and Mackay, D. M.: Benign mucous membrane pemphigus with a generalized eruption. Arch. Derm., *92*:566, 1965.

Caputo, R., Bellone, A. G. and Crosti, C.: Pathogenesis of the blister in cicatricial pemphigoid and in bullous pemphigoid. Arch. Derm. Forsch., *247*:181, 1973.

Dabelsteen, E., Ullman, S., Thomsen, K., and Rygaard, J.: Demonstration of basement membrane autoantibodies in patients with benign mucous membrane pemphigoid. Acta dermatoven., *54*:189, 1974.

Griffith, M. R., Fukuyama, K., Tuffanelli, D., and Silverman, S., Jr.: Immunofluorescent studies in mucous membrane pemphigoid. Arch. Derm., *109*:195, 1974.

Holubar, K., Hönigsmann, H., and Wolff, K.: Cicatricial pemphigoid. Arch. Derm., *108*: 50, 1973.

Kleine-Natrop, H. E., and Haustein, U. F.: "Benignes Schleimhautpemphigoid" mit rascher Erblindung und generalisierten vernarbenden Hautveränderungen. Hautarzt, *19*:6, 1968.

Kokoschka, E. M., Kraft, D., Spängler, E., et al.: Narbenbildendes Pemphigoid. Hautarzt, *25*:227, 1974.

Krafek, A., and Streitmann, B.: Benignes Schleimhautpemphigoid mit generalisiertem Blasenschub auf der Haut. Derm. Wschr., *149*:297, 1964.

Lever, W. F.: Pemphigus conjunctivae with scarring of the skin. Arch. Derm. Syph., *46*:875, 1942, and *49*:113, 1944.

————: Pemphigus. Medicine, *32*:1, 1953.

Schaumburg-Lever, G., Orfanos, C. E., and Lever, W. F.: Electron microscopic study of bullous pemphigoid. Arch. Derm., *106*:662, 1972.

Susi, F. R., and Shklar, G.: Histochemistry and fine structure of oral lesions of mucous membrane pemphigoid. Arch. Derm., *104*:244, 1971.

Dermatitis Herpetiformis

Ackerman, A. B., and Tolman, M. D.: Papular dermatitis herpetiformis in childhood. Arch. Derm., *100*:286, 1969.

Chorzelski, T. P., Beutner, E. H., Jablonska, S., et al.: Immunofluorescence studies in the diagnosis of dermatitis herpetiformis and its differentiation from bullous pemphigoid. J. Invest. Derm., *56*:373, 1971.

Connor, B. L., Marks, R., and Wilson Jones, E.: Dermatitis herpetiformis. Trans. St. John's Hosp. Derm. Soc., *58*:191, 1972.

Holubar, K., Doralt, M., and Eggerth, G.: Immunofluorescence patterns in dermatitis herpetiformis. Brit. J. Derm., *85*:505, 1971.

Jablonska, S., and Chorzelski, T.: Kann das histologische Bild die Grundlage zur Differenzierung des Morbus Duhring mit dem Pemphigoid und Erythema multiforme darstellen? Derm. Wschr., *146*:590, 1963.

Jablonska, S., Chorzelski, T., Beutner, E. H., and Blaszczyk, R. M.: Juvenile dermatitis herpetiformis in the light of immunofluorescent studies. Brit. J. Derm., *85*:307, 1971.

Jakubowicz, K., Dabrowski, J., and Maciejewski, W.: Elektronenmikroskopische Untersuchungen bei bullösem Pemphigoid und Dermatitis herpetiformis Duhring. Arch. klin. exp. Derm., *238*:272, 1970.

Jordon, R. E., Bean, S. F., Triftshauser, C. T., and Winkelmann, R. K.: Childhood bullous dermatitis herpetiformis. Arch. Derm., *101*: 629, 1970.

Kresbach, H., and Hartwagner, A.: Zur Differentialdiagnose zwischen Dermatitis herpetiformis Duhring und bullösem Pemphigoid. Z. Haut, *43*:165, 1968.

MacVicar, D. N., Graham, J. H., and Burgoon, C. F., Jr.: Dermatitis herpetiformis, erythema multiforme and bullous pemphigoid: A comparative histopathological and histochemical study. J. Invest. Derm., *41*:289, 1963.

Marks, J., and Shuster, S.: Small-intestinal mucosa in pemphigoid and subcorneal pustular dermatosis. Arch. Derm., *100*:136, 1969.

Marks, J., Shuster, S., Young, S., et al.: The skin-gut relationship in dermatitis herpetiformis. Brit. J. Derm., *91* (suppl. 10):34, 1974.

Mustakallio, K. K., Blomquist, K., and Salo, O. P.: Papillary fibrin in dermatitis herpetiformis. Arch. belg. derm. syph., *26*:441, 1970.

Piérard, J.: De l'aspect histologique des plaques érythémateuses de la dermatite herpétiforme de Duhring. Ann. derm. syph., *90*:121, 1963.

Piérard, J., and Kint, A.: Dermatite herpétiforme et pemphigoide bulleuse. Ann. derm. syph., *95*:391, 1968.

Schaumburg-Lever, G., Orfanos, C. E., and Lever, W. F.: Electron microscopic study of bullous pemphigoid. Arch. Derm., *106*:662, 1972.

van der Meer, J. B.: Granular deposits of immunoglobulins in the skin of patients with dermatitis herpetiformis. An immunofluorescent study. Brit. J. Derm., *81*:493, 1969.

————: Dermatitis herpetiformis: a specific (immunopathological?) entity. University of Utrecht, 1972.

Welke, S., Jost, H., and Schwarz, J. A.: Immunologische Befunde bei Dermatitis herpetiformis und beim bullösen Pemphigoid. Z. Haut, *48*:943, 1973.

Erythema Multiforme

Ackerman, A. B., Penneys, N. S., and Clark, W. H.: Erythema multiforme exudativum: distinctive pathological process. Brit. J. Derm., *84*:554, 1971.

Braun-Falco, O.: Histopathologie des Lyell-Syndroms. In Braun-Falco, O., and Bandmann, H. J. (eds.): Das Lyell-Syndrom. pp. 61-80. Bern, Hans Huber, 1970.

Braun-Falco, O., and Wolff, H. H.: Zur Ultrastruktur der Epidermis beim Lyell-Syndrom. Arch. klin. exp. Derm., *236*:83, 1969.

Cannell, H., Churcher, G. M., and Milton-Thompson, G. J.: Steven-Johnson syndrome associated with Mycoplasma pneumoniae infection. Brit. J. Derm., *81*:196, 1969.

Lowney, E. D., Baublis, J. V., Kreye, G. M., et al.: The scalded skin syndrome in small children. Arch. Derm., *95*:359, 1967.

Lyell, A.: A review of toxic epidermal necrolysis in Britain. Brit. J. Derm., *79*:662, 1967.

MacVicar, D. N., Graham, J. H., and Burgoon, C. F., Jr.: Dermatitis herpetiformis, erythema multiforme, and bullous pemphigoid: a comparative histopathological and histochemical study. J. Invest. Derm., *41*:289, 1963.

Orfanos, C. E., Schaumburg-Lever, G., and Lever, W. F.: Dermal and epidermal types of erythema multiforme. Arch. Derm., *109*:682, 1974.

Prutkin, L., and Fellner, M. J.: Erythema multiforme bullosum. Acta dermatoven., *51*:429, 1971.

Tritsch, H.: Nekrolyse als histopathologisches Phänomen. Arch. klin. exp. Derm., *237*:295, 1970.

Herpes Gestationis

Hentschel, U.: Herpes gestationis (Milton), Derm. Monatsschr., *159*:904, 1973.

Jablonska, S., and Chorzelski, T.: Fortschritte auf dem Gebiet der Immunodermatologie. Zt. Haut, *49*:721, 1974.

Lynch, F. W., and Albrecht, R. J.: Hormonal factors in herpes gestationis. Arch. Derm., *93*:446, 1966.

Piérard, J., Thiery, M., and Kint, A.: Histologie et ultrastructure de l'herpes gestationis. Arch. belg. derm. syph., *25*:321, 1969.

Provost, T. T., and Tomasi, T. B.: Evidence for complement activation via the alternate pathway in skin diseases. J. Clin. Invest., *52*:1779, 1973.

Schaumburg-Lever, G., Saffold, O. E., Orfanos, C. E., and Lever, W. F.: Herpes gestationis. Histology and ultrastructure. Arch. Derm., *107*:888, 1973.

Winer, L. H.: Histologic observations in bullous Darier's disease, epidermolysis bullosa dystrophica and herpes gestationis. Proc. 11th Internat. Congr. Derm., Stockholm, 1957. Acta dermatoven., vol. 3, p. 362.

Subcorneal Pustular Dermatosis

Burns, R. E., and Fine, G.: Subcorneal pustular dermatosis. Arch. Derm., *80*:72, 1959.

Ellis, F. A.: Subcorneal pustular dermatosis. Arch. Derm., *78*:580, 1958.

Metz, J., and Schröpl, F.: Elektronenmikroskopische Untersuchungen bei subcornealer pustulöser Dermatose. Arch. klin. exp. Derm., *236*:190, 1970.

Wolff, K.: Ein Beitrag zur Nosologie der subcornealen pustulösen Dermatose (Sneddon-Wilkinson). Arch. klin. exp. Derm., *224*:248, 1966.

Transient Acantholytic Dermatosis

Grover, R. W.: Transient acantholytic dermatosis. Arch. Derm., *101*:426, 1970.

————: Transient acantholytic dermatosis. Arch. Derm., *104*:26, 1971.

Wolff, K.: Transient acantholytic dermatosis (Grover). Derm. Monatsschr., *158*:533, 1972.

Friction Blisters

Naylor, P. F. D.: Experimental friction blisters. Brit. J. Derm., *67*:327, 1955.

Sulzberger, M. B., Cortese, T. A., Jr., Fishman, L., and Wiley, H. S.: Studies on blisters produced by friction. J. Invest. Derm., *47*:456, 1966.

Electric Burns

Winer, L. H., and Levin, G. H.: Changes in the skin as a result of electric current. Arch. Derm., *78*:386, 1958.

8

Noninfectious Erythematous, Papular, and Squamous Diseases

URTICARIA

Urticaria is characterized by the presence of transient wheals having an erythematous, raised border and a blanched center. It is accompanied by itching. Large wheals in which the edema extends to the subcutaneous tissue are referred to as angioedema.

In *hereditary angioedema*, a rare form of dominantly inherited recurrent angioedema, the patient has a low serum level of an alpha-2 globulin that inhibits the esteratic activity of the activated first component of complement (Rosen and Austen). Itching is absent. Patients with this affliction may die from sudden laryngeal edema unless treated with epinephrine or tracheostomy.

Histopathology. An urticarial wheal shows edema of the dermis, whereas in lesions of angioedema the edema extends into the subcutaneous tissue (Beall). In a wheal the collagen bundles as well as the individual fibers are separated by edema. There is a polymorphous perivascular infiltrate composed of variously sized round cells, rather numerous neutrophils and a few eosinophils (Illig).

Histogenesis. Urticaria represents an anaphylactic reaction brought on by the release of histamine from mast cells. Certain complement factors, if activated, may cause a release of histamine from mast cells, as seen in hereditary angioedema (Lepow et al.).

ERYTHEMA ANNULARE CENTRIFUGUM

In this disorder one observes annular or serpiginous lesions with a red, raised, firm, wall-like border that in the course of weeks extends peripherally. Some lesions may be as large as 10 cm in diameter. The process may go on for years, with new lesions appearing successively. The preferred site of the eruption is the trunk.

Histopathology. A cellular infiltrate showing a fairly sharply demarcated perivascular "coat-sleeve-like" arrangement is present in the middle and lower portions of the dermis (Ellis and Friedman; Nordenskjöld and Wahlgren). The infiltrate consists of mononuclear cells.

Differential Diagnosis. The rather striking "coat-sleeve-like" perivascular arrangement of the infiltrate seen in erythema annulare centrifugum is encountered also in secondary syphilis. However, in secondary syphilis numerous plasma cells usually are present, and the intima and endothelial cells are swollen (see p. 301).

ERYTHEMA GYRATUM REPENS

This very rare but clinically highly characteristic dermatosis has been associated with a carcinoma in all reported cases. Clinically, there is a generalized mildly itching eruption consisting of parallel red bands with an annular and serpiginous arrangement resembling the grain of wood. The bands often show peripheral scaling. The clinical picture changes from day to day, since the bands of erythema move about 1 cm per day.

Histopathology. The histologic picture is nonspecific, merely showing a mild perivascular infiltrate of mononuclear cells (Gammel; Thomson and Stankler). In a case reported by Leavell et al. the epidermis showed spongiosis and the dermal infiltrate, in addition to mononuclear cells, contained eosinophils and melanophages.

ERYTHEMA DYSCHROMICUM PERSTANS

This extensive asymptomatic dermatosis begins with disseminated macules which by peripheral extension and coalescence form large patches with a polycyclic outline. At first the macules are erythematous but with increase in size they assume a blue-gray to ashy gray color. The disease progresses slowly and the discoloration persists. Most patients with this disorder are Latin-American.

Histopathology. In the early active stage many basal cells but also some squamous cells in the lower epidermis show vacuolization of their cytoplasm leading to liquefaction degeneration. The upper dermis shows a perivascular infiltrate of mononuclear cells and melanophages. Late lesions show as the only abnormality aggregates of melanophages (Knox et al.).

Histogenesis. Electron microscopic examination reveals within the affected keratinocytes, as ultrastructural counterpart of the liquefaction degeneration, many vacuoles delimited by a membrane. This is associated with widening of the intercellular spaces and retraction of desmosomes either to one cell or the other. Additional findings are discontinuities in the subepidermal basal lamina and presence in the dermis of melanophages containing aggregates of melanosomes enclosed by a lysosomal membrane (Soter et al.). It may be assumed that the liquefaction degeneration is the cause of the incontinence of pigment.

Differential Diagnosis. The histologic picture is not diagnostic. Similar inflammation and pigmentary incontinence may be seen in drug eruptions, especially in fixed drug erup-

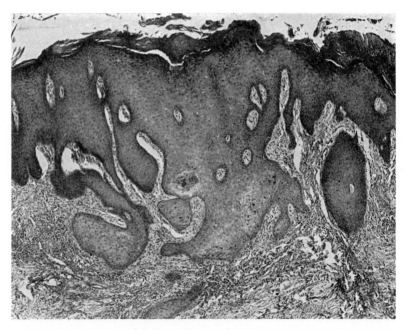

FIG. 8-1. **Prurigo nodularis.** There are hyperkeratosis and considerable acanthosis with irregular downward proliferation of the epidermis approaching pseudocarcinomatous hyperplasia. (×100)

tions (Knox et al.). The late lesions of erythema dyschromicum resemble those of the third stage of incontinentia pigmenti in showing melanophages in the upper dermis without evidence of inflammation.

PRURIGO SIMPLEX

Erythematous urticarial papules that are intensely pruritic are seen in symmetrical distribution, especially on the extensor surfaces of the extremities. In contrast with dermatitis herpetiformis, which prurigo simplex may resemble in its clinical appearance, there is no grouping of the lesions (Braun-Falco and von Eickstedt). In other cases, prurigo simplex greatly resembles arthropod bites (papular urticaria).

Histopathology. The histologic picture is nonspecific. Early papules show mild acanthosis, spongiosis with occasionally a small spongiotic vesicle, and parakeratosis. The upper dermis contains a mild, chronic inflammatory infiltrate in largely perivascular arrangement (Kocsard; Tritsch and Kantner). Excoriated papules show partial absence of the epidermis and, instead, are covered with a crust containing degenerated nuclei of inflammatory cells (Braun-Falco and von Eickstedt).

Differential Diagnosis. Dermatitis herpetiformis is easily excluded by the absence in prurigo simplex of microabscesses at the tips of papillae, and of neutrophils, eosinophils, and nuclear dust in the dermal infiltrate. The histologic picture of prurigo simplex resembles that of a subacute dermatitis, except that the papular lesion of prurigo simplex is much more limited in extent. A histologic differentiation from papular urticaria is not possible (Braun-Falco and von Eickstedt).

PRURIGO NODULARIS

There are discrete, raised, firm, hyperkeratotic lesions, usually from 2 to 10 mm in size but occasionally larger. They occur chiefly on the extensor surfaces of the extremities and are intensely pruritic.

Histopathology. One observes pronounced hyperkeratosis and acanthosis. There may be, in addition, papillomatosis and irregu-

lar downward proliferation of the epidermis (Fig. 8-1), approaching pseudocarcinomatous hyperplasia (see p. 482). The dermis shows a nonspecific inflammatory infiltrate with proliferation of fibroblasts. Even with routine stains a hyperplasia of cutaneous nerves may occasionally be observed; but this is more evident on silver impregnation: one often finds a considerable hyperplasia of nerve fibers and Schwann cells (Thies; Cowan, 1964, II). It seems likely that many cells having the appearance of fibroblasts in hematoxylin-eosin-stained sections in reality are Schwann cells (Cowan, 1964, I).

Histogenesis. Some authors have thought that the proliferation of neural elements was specific for prurigo nodularis (Thies). Cowan (1964, I), however, has described similar changes in lesions of lichen simplex chronicus. It thus seems likely that the neural proliferation is a secondary event. Prurigo nodularis may well represent, as suggested by Shaffer and Beerman, an exaggerated form of lichen simplex chronicus.

Differential Diagnosis. Multiple keratoacanthomas, which often show less of a central crater than the solitary keratoacanthoma, may be difficult to distinguish from prurigo nodularis, since both show marked epithelial hyperplasia (Ereaux and Schopflocher).

PSORIASIS

Psoriasis may be divided into psoriasis vulgaris in which pustules usually are absent, generalized pustular psoriasis, and localized pustular psoriasis. Generalized pustular psoriasis of von Zumbusch includes as variants generalized acrodermatitis continua of Hallopeau ("acral type of generalized pustular psoriasis") and impetigo herpetiformis ("exanthematous type of generalized pustular psoriasis"). There are three types of localized pustular psoriasis: (a) "psoriasis with pustules" (Schuppener), in which only one or several areas of psoriasis show pustules and the lesions may have an erythema-annulare-like configuration (Resneck and Cram), and the tendency to change into a generalized pustular psoriasis is not great; (b) localized acrodermatitis continua of Hallopeau, which occasionally changes into a generalized acrodermatitis continua; and (c) pustular psoriasis of the palms and soles, also called pustulosis palmaris et plantaris, which usually occurs without any other manifestation of psoriasis but occasionally is seen in association with psoriasis vulgaris. The relationship of Reiter's disease to psoriasis will be discussed in the description of Reiter's disease.

PSORIASIS VULGARIS

Psoriasis is a chronic disorder characterized by brownish-red papules and plaques. The lesions are sharply demarcated, dry, and usually covered with layers of fine silvery scales. As the scales are removed by gentle scraping, fine bleeding points usually are seen, the so-called Auspitz sign. The scalp, sacral region and extensor surfaces of the extremities are commonly involved, although in some patients the flexural and intertriginous areas are mainly affected. Involvement of the nails is common. In severe cases the disease may affect the entire skin and present itself as generalized erythrodermic psoriasis. Pustules generally are absent in psoriasis vulgaris, although occasionally pustular psoriasis of the palms and soles occurs with psoriasis vulgaris. Rarely, in psoriasis one or a few areas show pustules, referred to as "psoriasis with pustules." Also rarely, severe psoriasis vulgaris develops into generalized pustular psoriasis (see p. 141). Oral lesions do not occur in psoriasis vulgaris but may be seen in generalized pustular psoriasis.

Psoriatic arthritis characteristically involves the terminal interphalangeal joints; but, not infrequently, the large joints also are affected so that a clinical differentiation from rheumatoid arthritis often is impossible. However, the rheumatoid factor, determined by the latex fixation or the sheep red cell agglutination test, generally is absent.

Histopathology. The histologic picture of active psoriasis, as seen in the center of incipient papules and near the margin of advancing plaques (Soltani and Van Scott) is characterized by (1) regular elongation of the rete ridges with thickening in their lower portion, (2) elongation and edema of the papillae, (3) relative thinning of the suprapapillary portions of the stratum malpighii

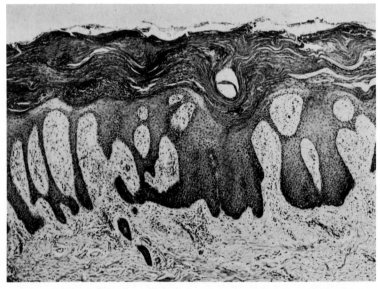

FIG. 8-2. **Psoriasis.** Low magnification. The rete ridges show regular elongation with thickening in their lower portion. The papillae are elongated and edematous. In addition, there is marked parakeratosis. (×50)

with occasional presence of a very small "spongiform pustule," (4) absence of granular cells, (5) parakeratosis, and (6) presence of Munro microabscesses (Fig. 8-2). Of all the listed features only the spongiform pustule is truly diagnostic of psoriasis, and in its absence the diagnosis of psoriasis rarely can be made with certainty on a histologic basis. In detail, the changes in active psoriasis are as follows:

The rete ridges show considerable elongation, and they extend downward to a uniform level. Often they are slender in their upper portion and thickened in their lower portion so that neighboring rete ridges often coalesce at their bases. There is as a rule neither intercellular nor intracellular edema in the rete ridges, in which even those cells that are located well above the basal layer show deep basophilia. Also, mitoses are not limited, as in normal skin, to the basal layer but are seen also in the two rows of cells above the basal layer (Van Scott and Ekel).

The papillae, in accordance with the elongation and basal thickening of the rete ridges, are elongated and club-shaped. They show edema, and the capillaries in the upper portion of the papillae are dilated. A mild to moderately severe inflammatory infiltrate is present in the upper dermis and the papillae. It consists of mononuclear cells, except in early lesions which, in addition, show neutrophils in the upper portion of the papillae (Pinkus and Mehregan). On histochemical examination, many of the mononuclear cells react like monocytes (Hundeiker).

The stratum malpighii overlying the papillae appears relatively thin on comparison with the markedly elongated rete ridges, and the cells may show intracellular edema. The epidermal cells located immediately beneath the parakeratotic stratum corneum may be intermingled with neutrophils (Fig. 8-3) (Gordon and Johnson). The histologic picture then is that of a small spongi-

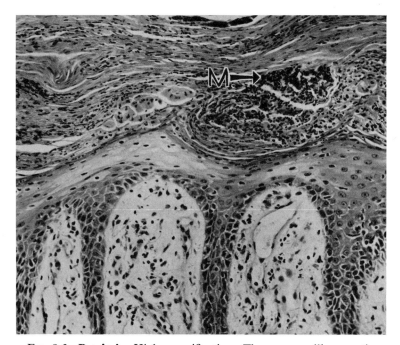

FIG. 8-3. **Psoriasis.** High magnification. The suprapapillary portions of the stratum malpighii are thinned and composed of cells showing intracellular edema. The epidermal cells located immediately beneath the parakeratotic stratum corneum are intermingled with neutrophils, suggestive of a spongiform pustule of Kogoj. A Munro abscess (M.) is located within the parakeratotic horny layer. (×200)

form pustule of Kogoj. Although it is only a micropustule it, nevertheless, is of the same type as the much larger macropustules seen in pustular psoriasis (see p. 142). Such a spongiform pustule, highly diagnostic for psoriasis and its variants, shows aggregates of neutrophils within the interstices of a spongelike network formed by degenerated and thinned epidermal cells (Rupec).

The stratum granulosum may be completely lacking in early, active lesions of psoriasis, but often areas without granular cells are seen intermingled with areas where they are present (Cox and Watson).

The horny layer in some instances consists entirely of parakeratotic cells and, since a direct relationship exists between the absence of keratohyaline granules and the presence of parakeratosis, there is concomitantly an absence of the stratum granulosum. However, not infrequently some orthokeratosis is present, with underlying granular cells.

The Munro microabscesses (Fig. 8-3) are located within parakeratotic areas of the horny layer. They consist of accumulations of pyknotic neutrophils that have migrated there from capillaries in the papillae through the suprapapillary epidermis. As a rule, Munro microabscesses are found easily in early lesions, whereas in older lesions they are few in number or absent (Burks and Montgomery).

An entirely typical histologic picture, as described above, is actually found in only a small percentage of biopsy specimens even if only clinically typical lesions of psoriasis are examined. Thus, Cox and Watson observed, in 33 of 107 lesions examined, that orthokeratosis was more extensive than parakeratosis. There were either vertical columns of orthokeratosis separating columns of parakeratosis or, less commonly, alternating horizontal layers of orthokeratosis and parakeratosis.

The bleeding points that may be produced by gentle scraping of the skin correspond to the tips of papillae. They are attributable to the following histologic changes: (1) parakeratosis, (2) intracellular edema of the

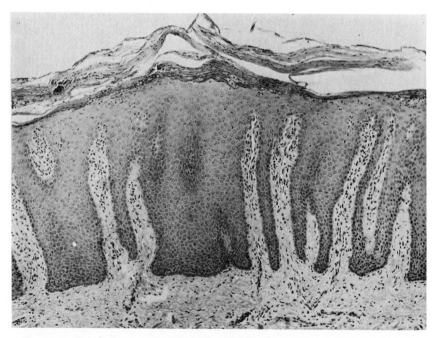

Fig. 8-4. **Psoriasis, erythrodermic types.** A diagnosis of psoriasis is possible if there are, as in this instance, small aggregates of neutrophils in the uppermost rete malpighii resulting in small spongiform pustules of Kogoj. (×50)

keratinocytes in the suprapapillary epidermis, and (3) dilatation of the capillaries in the upper portion of the papillae.

ERYTHRODERMIC PSORIASIS. The histologic picture in erythrodermic psoriasis in some instances shows enough of the characteristics of psoriasis to allow this diagnosis (Fig. 8-4). Frequently, however, the histologic appearance is indistinguishable from that of a chronic dermatitis (Abrahams et al.).

Histogenesis. In active lesions of psoriasis the rate of epidermal cell replication is greatly accelerated, as shown by the greatly increased number of mitotic figures and the greater number of premitotic cells labeled by tritiated thymidine (Weinstein and Van Scott). However, as yet it is not known by which means this excessive replication comes about. Rothberg et al. measured the transit time of cells from the basal layer to the skin surface by giving glycine-^{14}C systemically to human subjects and then measuring the specific activity of the glycine incorporated into the proteins of the horny layer. They found that, whereas the normal transit time to the skin surface is approximately 28 days, in very active lesions of psoriasis it was reduced to 3 to 4 days. Similarly, Weinstein and Van Scott, by injecting tritiated thymidine subepidermally into humans, found the transit time of cells through the stratum malpighii, i.e., from the basal cell layer to the uppermost row of the squamous cell layer, to be approximately 13 days in normal epidermis, but only 2 days in the epidermis of very active psoriatic lesions. An important question is whether the increase in epidermal replication is brought about solely by increased mitotic activity of the germinative epidermal cells or whether it is due also to a shortening of the reproductive cell cycle. Kinetic analyses by Weinstein and Frost based on autoradiographic studies using in vivo labeling of epidermal cells were interpreted by them as indicating a shortening of the reproductive cell cycle from 457 hours for normal germinative cells to 37.5 hours for psoriatic germinative cells. In addition, the duration of the various phases of the cell cycle seems to be altered in psoriatic epidermis. Goodwin et al., on correlating the number of mitotic figures with the number of cells labeled with tritiated thymidine in normal epidermis and in psoriatic epidermis, found a disproportionate increase in the number of mitotic figures in psoriatic epidermis: Whereas the number of cells in mitosis was increased more than

50 times, the increase in DNA synthesis was only 5-fold. Goodwin et al. believe that their findings can be explained by a shortening of the period of DNA synthesis (S-phase) in psoriatic epidermis from a normal of 16 hours to 8.5 hours, as found by Weinstein and Frost, and by a lengthening of the duration of mitotic division (M-phase) from 1½ hours in normal epidermis to about 4 hours in psoriatic epidermis, observed by Fisher and Wells.

The mitotic activity within different lesions of psoriasis can vary considerably. Cox and Watson, on correlating the degree of parakeratosis in the lowermost stratum corneum with the mitotic index of that area, found in psoriatic epidermis showing 91 to 100 per cent parakeratosis, on the average, 5 times as many mitotic figures as in psoriatic epidermis with only 0 to 20 per cent parakeratosis. Soltani and Van Scott found great variations of the mitotic activity even within individual lesions. On step sectioning lesions of psoriasis they found that initial "punctate" papules showed a mitotically very active parakeratotic center surrounded by a zone having a markedly thickened granular layer and only a slightly increased mitotic rate; and plaques with their greatest activity at their border showed parakeratosis and a high mitotic rate near the periphery and a thickened granular layer with a relatively low mitotic rate in the clinically less active center.

Electron microscopic studies indicate that psoriatic keratinocytes in the stratum malpighii are poorly developed and immature. In particular, tonofilaments are decreased in numbers and in diameter and lack their normal aggregation (Brody). The size and number of keratohyaline granules is greatly reduced and occasionally they are absent (Hashimoto and Lever). The horny cells also possess thin tonofilaments and often still contain organelles and a nucleus as parakeratotic cells. They often fail to form a marginal band and to lose their outer plasma membrane (Orfanos et al.). The intercellular spaces between all epidermal cells are widened because of a deficiency in the glycoprotein-rich cell surface coat so that intercellular adhesion is limited to the desmosomes (Mercer and Maibach; Orfanos et al.). On the other hand, the cell surface coat is thickened in the horny layer (Orfanos et al.).

The ultrastructure of the only diagnostic structure encountered in psoriasis, the spongiform pustule of Kogoj, has been described by Rupec. In the spongiform pustule, located in the upper portion of the suprapapillary epidermis, neutrophils lie intercellularly, rather than intracellularly, as had been assumed on the basis of light microscopic studies. It is a multilocular pustule in which the spongelike network is composed of degenerated and flattened keratinocytes. Close interactions between the infiltrating neutrophils and the keratinocytes can be observed, for instance, partial fusion of the two cell types and presence of neutrophilic granules within keratinocytes (Komura et al.).

The papillary capillaries show a wide lumen and a thin endothelium with areas of fenestration, as seen in the normal dermis (see p. 38). However, in psoriasis the gaps are wider and more numerous (Holzmann and Hoede; Braverman et al.). The migration of neutrophils through these gaps into the intercellular spaces of the epidermis has been described by Braverman et al.

The question whether the *primary lesion* of psoriasis resides in the epidermis or in the dermis is still undecided, although in recent years some evidence has been brought forth in favor of the epidermis being the primary site. The traditional view of the dermal origin of psoriasis still is maintained by Pinkus and Mehregan, who believe that the primary event in psoriasis is a periodic discharge of neutrophils from papillary capillaries and that the neutrophils then migrate into the epidermis to form first a spongiform pustule, which then by being carried to higher levels becomes a Munro microabscess. No reason is given by these authors for the periodic emission of neutrophils from the capillaries. It is, thus, of interest that Rupec in his electron microscopic description of the spongiform pustule regards a cytolysis of keratinocytes as the primary event in the formation of the spongiform pustule and the discharge of neutrophils from papillary capillaries as a response to the epidermal cell damage.

Among the adherents of a primary epidermal genesis of psoriasis is Braun-Falco, who on histochemical examination found that the earliest changes consisted of an increase in the activities of cytochrome oxidase, succinic dehydrogenase and phosphorylase within the epidermis. In addition, Christophers and Braun-Falco found that prolonged application of vitamin A acid to normal guinea pig skin accelerated the rate of epidermal replication to a level equal to that found in psoriasis but without causing a loss of keratohyaline granules and without inducing parakeratosis. Christophers and Braun-Falco therefore concluded that these two phenomena could not be the consequence of the rapid cell proliferation in psoriasis but resulted from a defect in cellular differentiation. The same conclusion was drawn by Fry and McMinn when they observed that topical treatment with a fluorinated corticosteroid caused the granular layer to reform before the rate of mitotic division had decreased. Fry has also pointed out that the rate of cellular proliferation in dominant congenital ichthyosiform erythroderma is equal to that of psoriasis and yet it has a well developed granular layer.

Two other theories have been advanced recently to explain the rapid rate of replication in the epidermis as a primary epidermal phenomenon. Vorhees et al. found a statistically significant decrease in adenosine $3',5'$-monophosphate, so-called cyclic AMP, in psoriatic epidermis and believe that this decrease could explain the accelerated cellular proliferation and the glycogen accumulation in psoriatic epidermis, since cyclic AMP regulates the glycogen metabolism and in cell cultures promotes differentiation and limits proliferation of cancer cells. Orfanos et al. believe that the rapid cellular proliferation in psoriatic epidermis may be explained by the phenomenon of loss of "contact inhibition of growth." Since electron microscopy has shown in psoriatic stratum malpighii a nearly complete absence of the glycoprotein-rich cell surface coat and as a result of its absence a decreased adhesiveness of the keratinocytes, it may be assumed that the psoriatic epidermis lacks the intercellular contact that is known to provide inhibition of uncontrolled cellular proliferation in tissue culture.

Differential Diagnosis. The only histologic feature that is highly diagnostic of psoriasis is the presence of spongiform micropustules of Kogoj. In their absence, occasionally the combined presence of all other features may permit a diagnosis of psoriasis, but usually these various features are not fully present in lesions of psoriasis with less than peak activity. Thus in many instances even a clinically typical lesion of psoriasis cannot be reliably differentiated from a chronic dermatitis; and in a clinically atypical lesion this differentiation almost invariably is impossible.

Even though Kogoj's spongiform pustule is highly diagnostic of the psoriasis group of diseases, including Reiter's disease, histologically typical spongiform pustules may occur in two other diseases: in candidiasis, particularly if clinically pustules are present (Degos et al.), and in geographic tongue, or superficial migratory glossitis (Dawson).

GENERALIZED PUSTULAR PSORIASIS (INCLUDING ACRODERMATITIS CONTINUA AND IMPETIGO HERPETIFORMIS)

Basically, generalized pustular psoriasis of von Zumbusch, acrodermatitis continua of Hallopeau, and impetigo herpetiformis represent the same disease process (Skog; Soltermann; Lapière; Baker and Ryan; Braverman et al.). There is considerable resemblance and overlapping in the clinical picture of these three diseases and they have the same histologic appearance. They differ mainly in the mode of onset and in the distribution of the lesions. Clinically, all three diseases show groups of shallow pustules on an erythematous base. All three may show oral pustules. Sudden exacerbations in association with chills and fever occur in all three diseases; and in the intervals between exacerbations all three diseases may show lesions having the clinical appearance of psoriasis.

Pustular psoriasis of von Zumbusch is generally diagnosed when the pustular eruption occurs in patients with pre-existing psoriasis either of the plaque type (Shelley and Kirschbaum) or of the erythrodermic type (Braverman et al.).

Acrodermatitis continua of Hallopeau is the term used if the pustular eruption either is limited to the distal portions of the fingers and toes, as in the localized type of acrodermatitis continua, or involves, in addition to the distal portions of the fingers and toes, extensive areas of the skin, as in the generalized type of acrodermatitis continua. Baker and Ryan refer to the generalized type of acrodermatitis continua simply as the "acral type of generalized pustular psoriasis." On the fingers and toes atrophy of the skin and permanent loss of the nails may occur.

Impetigo herpetiformis is diagnosed when the disease starts suddenly without any preceding lesions of psoriasis as an extensive

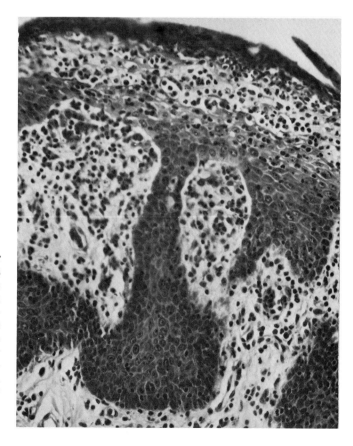

FIG. 8-5. **Generalized pustular psoriasis.** Early stage. There is acanthosis with elongation of the rete ridges. The upper stratum malpighii shows an early spongiform pustule formed through the migration of neutrophils from the papillary capillaries to the upper stratum malpighii where they aggregate within the interstices of a spongelike network formed by degenerated and thinned epidermal cells. (×300)

eruption of pustules on an erythematous base. This type, referred to as the "exanthematous type of generalized pustular psoriasis" by Baker and Ryan, may occur repeatedly during successive pregnancies (Katzenellenbogen and Feuerman) but may occur also without any known cause.

Histopathology. Whereas in ordinary psoriasis the spongiform pustule of Kogoj is a very small micropustule and is seen only in early, active lesions, it occurs as a macropustule in all three variants of pustular psoriasis and represents their characteristic histologic lesion. The spongiform pustule forms through migration of neutrophils from the papillary capillaries to the upper stratum malpighii where they aggregate within the interstices of a spongelike network formed by degenerated and thinned epidermal cells (Fig. 8-5) (Rupec). It may be pointed out that, prior to the electron microscopic study by Rupec, it had been assumed on the basis of light microscopy that in the spongiform pustule the neutrophils lie within edematous epidermal cells, rather than outside of thinned epidermal cells. With increase in the size of the pustule, the epidermal cells in the center of the pustule undergo complete cytolysis, so that a large single cavity forms. At the periphery of the pustule, however, the network of thinned epidermal cells persists for a much longer time (Fig. 8-6). As the neutrophils of the spongiform pustule move up into the horny layer, they become pyknotic and assume the appearance of a large Munro abscess (Shelley and Kirschbaum; Muller and Kitzmiller).

Aside from the presence of large spongiform pustules, the epidermal changes are very much like those seen in psoriasis, consisting of parakeratosis and elongation of the rete ridges. The upper dermis contains an infiltrate of mononuclear cells, and often neutrophils can be seen migrating from the capillaries in the papillae into the epidermis (Kingery et al.).

In the healing stage the lesions of all three diseases may present the same histologic appearance as ordinary psoriasis (Shelley and Kirschbaum).

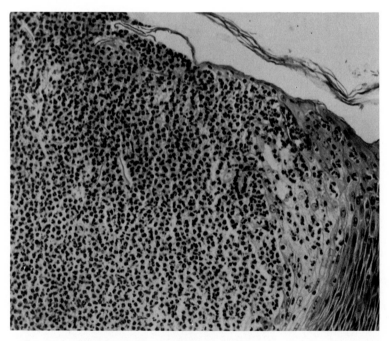

FIG. 8-6. **Acrodermatitis continua of Hallopeau.** A fully developed pustule is shown. The pustule is filled with neutrophils. At the periphery of the pustule, shown to the right, the epidermis has a spongiform appearance. (×200)

LOCALIZED PUSTULAR PSORIASIS (INCLUDING PUSTULAR PSORIASIS OF THE PALMS AND SOLES)

In two of the three types of localized pustular psoriasis, namely in "psoriasis with pustules" (see p. 135) (Schuppener) and in localized acrodermatitis continua of Hallopeau (see p. 135) the histologic picture is the same as that described for generalized pustular psoriasis.

The third type of localized pustular psoriasis, pustular psoriasis of the palms and soles, is a chronic, indolent disorder occurring on either the palms or the soles, or both. Crops of small deep-seated pustules are seen within areas of erythema and scaling. The acral portions of the fingers and toes, in contrast to acrodermatitis continua of Hallopeau, are spared.

Histopathology. A fully developed pustule is large, intraepidermal in location, unilocular and rounded at both sides (Fig. 8-7). It is elevated only slightly above the surface but, rather, extends into the underlying dermis. Many neutrophils are present within the cavity of the pustule. The epidermis surrounding the pustule shows slight acanthosis, and an inflammatory infiltrate can be seen beneath the pustule (Ashhurst).

Mature pustules thus do not show any resemblance to psoriasis. However, early pustules, especially if they still consist of several cavities, regularly show formations of typical, though small, spongiform pustules, most commonly at the junction of their lateral walls with the overlying epidermis (Piérard and Kint; Lever). This provides the histologic evidence for the relationship of the disease with psoriasis.

Histogenesis. Barber, in 1930, was the first to express the opinion that the pustular eruption of the palms and soles was a manifestation of psoriasis. This view was abandoned by many authors when Andrews maintained that focal infections caused the eruption which he renamed pustular bacterid. Other authors have preferred the descriptive and noncommittal term pustulosis palmaris et plantaris. The frequency with which on clinical examination different observers found lesions typical of psoriasis in association with pustular psoriasis of the palms and soles varies considerably. Thus, Everall found evidence of psoriasis in 19 per cent of his patients (13 of 70), Enfors and Molin in only 6 per cent (15 of 248), and Ashhurst in 2 per cent (1 of 43).

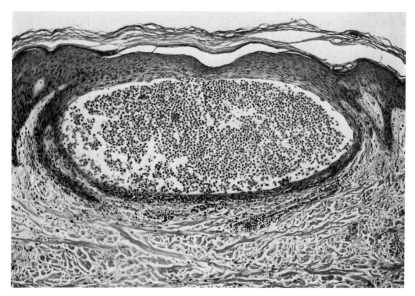

FIG. 8-7. **Localized pustular psoriasis: pustular psoriasis of the palms and soles.** A large intraepidermal unilocular pustule is present. On the right side and at the uppermost portion of the pustule spongiform pustule formation can still be recognized. (×100)

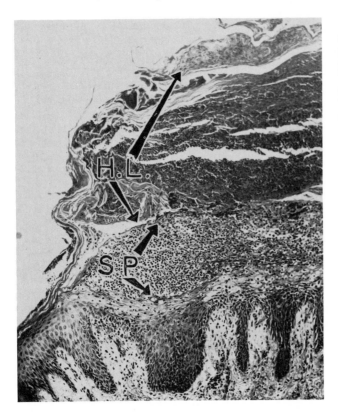

FIG. 8-8. **Reiter's disease.** Low magnification. There is a very thick parakeratotic horny layer (H.L.) permeated by numerous neutrophils. The upper stratum malpighii is the seat of a spongiform pustule (S.P.). The rete ridges are elongated, and the papillae show edema. (×100)

REITER'S DISEASE

In typical cases Reiter's disease consists of the triad of urethritis, arthritis, and conjunctivitis. Although, as a rule, the arthritis occurs in attacks and is followed by recovery, in some cases it progresses to cause permanent damage to the affected joints (Perry and Mayne; Khan and Hall). In about two thirds of the patients cutaneous lesions are present. They have a predilection for the glans penis, the palms and soles, and the subungual areas. On the glans penis the usual appearance is that of a brownish-red patch with central clearing referred to as balanitis circinata. On the palms and the soles early lesions consist of pustules. Gradually, the lesions on the palms and the soles become covered with thick horny crusts. Confluence of neighboring lesions leads to extensive horny excrescences. Occasionally, there are pustular or crusted, hyperkeratotic lesions elsewhere on the skin, which at first resemble pustular psoriasis but later may have the appearance of ordinary psoriasis (Perry and Mayne; Khan and Hall).

Histopathology. Early pustular lesions on the palms or soles show a spongiform macropustule in the upper epidermis (Fig. 8-8) (Weinberg et al.; Perry and Mayne). In addition, one observes parakeratosis and elongation of the rete ridges.

As the lesions age, the parakeratotic horny layer overlying the spongiform pustule thickens considerably (Figs. 8-8 and 8-9). The greatly thickened horny layer is the anatomic substrate for the horny excrescences seen clinically. The horny layer consists of parakeratotic cells intermingled with the pyknotic nuclei of neutrophils (Fig. 8-8).

In old lesions spongiform pustules are no longer seen, and the histologic picture usually is nonspecific, showing acanthosis and hyperkeratosis with only a few areas of parakeratosis; but occasionally, the histologic picture resembles psoriasis (Perry and Mayne).

Histogenesis. The cause of Reiter's disease is not known. An infectious nature of the disease has not been proved. The former designation of the hyperkeratotic palmar and plantar lesions as keratosis blennorrhagica, referring to gonorrhea, also was erroneous. A close relationship to psoriasis has been assumed for the cutaneous lesions because of their clinical resemblance to psoriasis and the presence of spongiform pustules (Perry and Mayne; Khan and Hall). Similarly, the arthritis of Reiter's disease resembles psoriatic arthritis clinically and also because of the absence of the rheumatoid factor in most cases (Wright and Reed; Khan and Hall).

Differential Diagnosis. The early spongiform macropustule seen in Reiter's disease is indistinguishable from the spongiform macropustule seen in pustular psoriasis. Slightly older lesions often can be identified as representing Reiter's disease in contradistinction to psoriasis by the presence of a greatly thickened horny layer.

PARAPSORIASIS

There are two types of parapsoriasis: parapsoriasis variegata and parapsoriasis en plaques. Both are very chronic and usually asymptomatic. They show a certain rela-

tionship with one another, since transitional forms exist between the two, such as the occasional development of poikiloderma-like changes in lesions of parapsoriasis en plaques (Fleischmajer et al.).

Clinically, one observes in *parapsoriasis variegata* an extensive eruption of brownish red, slightly raised, flattened, scaling papules in a netlike arrangement. Part of the reddish network gradually undergoes atrophy with telangiectases and mottled pigmentation, so that the eruption resembles poikiloderma atrophicans vasculare, from which it differs, however, by the netlike pattern. In some instances, fine petechiae are also seen (Musger).

Parapsoriasis en plaques is characterized by oval or elongated, slightly scaling patches located predominantly on the trunk. They possess little or no infiltration. Their color usually is red to brownish but in occasional instances is pale red to yellowish (Goldberg).

Histopathology. In *parapsoriasis variegata* the histologic picture at the beginning may be that of a nonspecific chronic dermatitis. However, as the disease progresses toward atrophy, the infiltrate appears in bandlike arrangement directly beneath a flattened and

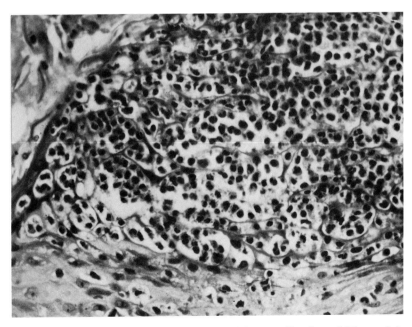

Fig. 8-9. **Reiter's disease, late stage.** High magnification of Figure 8-8. The spongiform nature of the pustule is very apparent. ($\times$400)

atrophic epidermis that may be invaded by the infiltrate (Walther). There also may be vacuolization of the cells of the basal layer, causing considerable resemblance to poikiloderma atrophicans vasculare (Grimmer). Small extravasations of red cells may be seen in the infiltrate (Musger).

In *parapsoriasis en plaques* the histologic picture is that of a chronic dermatitis (Goldberg; Fleischmajer et al.).

Relationship to Lymphoma. Some patients diagnosed as either parapsoriasis variegata or parapsoriasis en plaques have been found later to have lymphoma—usually mycosis fungoides, but occasionally also reticulum cell sarcoma (Kawada et al.). It is likely that in such cases the disease has been lymphoma from the beginning. The incidence of lymphoma varies in different reports. Thus, Keil and also Lapière have expressed the view that parapsoriasis en plaques is in most, if not in all cases, the precursor of mycosis fungoides. On the other hand, Samman reported that among 59 patients with parapsoriasis en plaques whom he had followed not one had shown progression to lymphoma. Both views represent extremes. The experience of most observers has been that in occasional instances the original diagnosis of parapsoriasis en plaques had to be changed to mycosis fungoides: in the series of Fleischmajer et al. in 6 of 13 patients; in Osmundsen's series in 3 of 21 patients; and in the series reported by Khan in 1 of 47 patients. The change in diagnosis was made after intervals varying from 2 to 30 years.

There seem to be no reliable clinical or histologic criteria for a decision whether or not a case of parapsoriasis ultimately will prove to be one of lymphoma, so that multiple biopsy studies over a prolonged period of time are required (Keil; Osmundsen).

PITYRIASIS ROSEA

Pityriasis rosea is a self-limited disorder lasting from 4 to 7 weeks. The lesions, found chiefly on the trunk, consist of round to oval salmon-colored patches following the lines of cleavage and showing peripherally attached, thin, cigarette-paper-like scales.

Histopathology. The histologic picture is that of a subacute or chronic dermatitis (see p. 98). The infiltrate in the upper dermis consists predominantly of small mononuclear cells, with a few neutrophils, eosino-

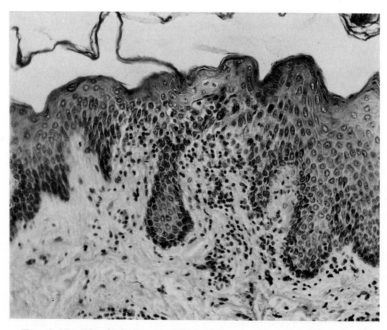

FIG. 8-10. **Pityriasis rosea.** The epidermis shows spongiosis and is invaded by an infiltrate of mononuclear cells. The upper dermis shows a chronic inflammatory infiltrate. (×200)

phils and histiocytes. In some of the lesions small mononuclear cells are seen migrating from the upper dermis into the epidermis. Spongiosis and intracellular edema occur at sites where the epidermis has been invaded by the cellular infiltrate (Fig. 8-10). Spongiotic vesicles are found in about half of the cases (Bunch and Tilley). In addition, mild acanthosis and focal parakeratosis are present.

GIANOTTI-CROSTI SYNDROME

In the Gianotti-Crosti syndrome, also referred to as acral papular eruption of childhood, one observes scattered erythematous papules symmetrically distributed over the extremities, the buttocks, and occasionally the face. The papules may appear hemorrhagic. The age of the patients varies from 9 months to 15 years, and the duration from 3 to 8 weeks.

Histopathology. The histologic appearance of the papules is nonspecific. A chronic inflammatory infiltrate is present in the upper dermis, extending into the papillae and occasionally also into the epidermis, causing spongiosis and parakeratosis. Small extravasations of erythrocytes may be observed in the upper dermis or the papillae (Winkelmann and Bourlond; Grimmer).

LICHEN PLANUS

Lichen planus is a subacute or a chronic dermatosis characterized by small, polygonal, violaceous papules that may coalesce into plaques. As a rule, itching is pronounced; but it may be slight or absent. The disease usually is limited to a few areas, the sites of predilection being the flexor surfaces of the forearms, the legs, the glans penis and the oral mucosa; but in some cases the eruption is very extensive.

Instead of consisting of the typical papules, the lesions of lichen planus may consist in part of vesicles and bullae (bullous lichen planus). In long-standing cases of lichen planus one may find considerable hyperplasia (hypertrophic lichen planus).

Occasionally, in early, extensive cases of lichen planus some lesions having the clinical and histologic appearance of lichen nitidus are present. (Concerning the rela-

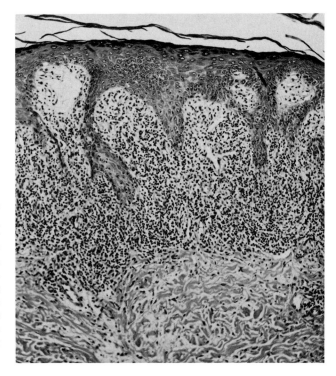

FIG. 8-11. **Lichen planus, early lesion.** There are hyperkeratosis, focal thickening of the granular layer, and acanthosis with irregular elongation of the rete ridges. The rete ridge in the center has a triangular saw-tooth configuration. The basal layer has been invaded by the inflammatory infiltrate and appears "wiped out." The infiltrate is band-like, and is sharply demarcated at its lower border. (×100)

tionship between lichen planus and lichen nitidus, see p. 153.)

The oral lesions of lichen planus are seen most commonly in the buccal region and usually consist of whitish papules often arranged in a reticular pattern. There also may be oral bullae, erosions and ulcers, occurring occasionally as the only manifestation of the disease (Shklar).

Lichen planopilaris (lichen planus follicularis) designates lichen planus with a follicular arrangement of some or all of the lesions. This type of lichen planus often affects the scalp. Loss of hair ensues in the involved areas, causing irregularly shaped patches of atrophic alopecia in the scalp resembling those seen in pseudopelade of Brocq and probably identical with it (Altman and Perry) (see p. 151). Other hairy areas, such as the axillae and the pubic region, may also be affected, but usually the alopecia in these areas is noncicatricial (Pagès et al.).

A rare, but rather characteristic form of lichen planus is the association of an atrophic, patchy alopecia of the scalp with bullae and painful ulcerations on the feet and toes resulting in permanent loss of the toenails. In addition, there may be cutaneous and oral lesions of lichen planus (Cram et al.; Male; Ebner).

Development of carcinoma is very rare in lesions of lichen planus of the skin (Kronenberg et al.); but it occurs occasionally in the lesions of the oral mucosa. The incidence of carcinoma of the oral mucosa according to Fulling is less than 1 per cent, and according to Jänner et al. is 4 per cent.

Histopathology. Typical papules of lichen planus show (1) hyperkeratosis, (2) hypergranulosis, (3) irregular acanthosis, (4) damage to the basal cell layer, and (5) a bandlike dermal infiltrate in close approximation to the epidermis (Fig. 8-11). This constellation of findings is sufficiently diagnostic so that in lichen planus, in contrast to psoriasis, for instance, a histologic diagnosis can usually be made—according to Ellis, in more than 90 per cent of the cases.

The horny layer is moderately thickened and, important for the diagnosis, contains few or no parakeratotic cells. Thus, parakeratotic cells were completely absent in 87 per cent of the specimens examined by Ellis.

The thickening of the stratum granulosum is irregular, showing so-called beading. The granular cells appear increased in size and contain coarser and more abundant keratohyaline granules than one observes normally.

The acanthosis in lichen planus affects the rete ridges as well as the stratum malpighii. The cells of the stratum malpighii appear eosinophilic because of advanced keratinization and, like the granular cells, are increased in size. The rete ridges show irregular lengthening, and some of the rete ridges are pointed at their lower end, giving them a saw-toothed appearance. Often the papillae between lengthened rete ridges are dome-shaped (Gougerot and Civatte).

The cells of the basal layer are visualized poorly in early lesions because of the close approximation of the dermal infiltrate to the basal layer, and its invasion between the basal cells. Where recognizable, the basal cells in early lesions show liquefaction degeneration. In fully developed lesions the lowest cell layer of the epidermis has the appearance of flattened squamous cells since, as a result of cytolysis, the basal cell layer has been "wiped out."

The infiltrate in the upper dermis is bandlike and quite sharply demarcated at its lower border. It "hugs" the epidermis, and in early lesions invades the epidermis so that the outline between epidermis and dermis becomes hazy ("moth-eaten"). The infiltrate is almost entirely mononuclear with only a few neutrophils being present. Histochemical staining reveals a preponderance of lymphocytes, but also a fairly large number of monocytes and macrophages, as shown by positive reactions for alphanaphtholacetate-esterase and acid phosphatase (Berger et al.). Mast cells are also present but no eosinophils or plasma cells. Occasionally, early small lesions of lichen planus have the histologic appearance of lichen nitidus (see p. 153).

In older lesions the cellular infiltrate decreases in density but the number of

FIG. 8-12. **Lichen planus, hyaline bodies.** Two hyaline bodies are present. The hyaline body on the right side lies just below the epidermis. The hyaline body on the left side lies in the lowermost epidermis and contains a narrow crescent of degenerating nuclear material. (×400)

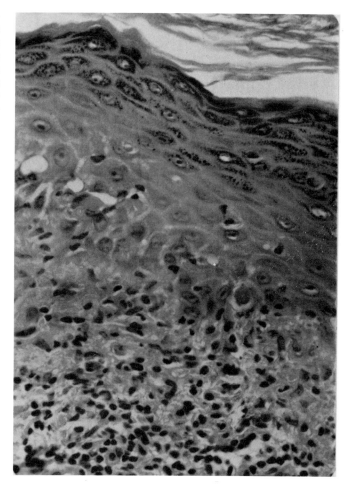

macrophages increases. Melanophages are present in the upper dermis, often in considerable number, since as a result of damage to the basal layer the basal cells are incapable of storing melanin ("incontinence of pigment"; see Glossary). Also, in some areas a basal cell layer has re-formed, and in such areas the dermal infiltrate no longer lies in close approximation to the epidermis. In the late stage some lesions may show considerable acanthosis, papillomatosis, and hyperkeratosis (*hypertrophic lichen planus*).

Quite frequently—according to Ellis, in 37 per cent of the cases—one observes hyaline or colloid bodies in the lower epidermis and within the infiltrate of the upper dermis. They average 10 μm in diameter and have a homogeneous, eosinophilic appearance (Fig. 8-12). They are PAS-positive and diastase-resistant because of their content of glycoproteins and are Feulgen-negative because they usually lack nuclear material. They represent degenerated basal cells and, even though they are found most commonly in lichen planus and lupus erythematosus, they may occur in any disease in which damage to the basal cells occur (Ebner and Gebhart).

Occasionally, small areas of separation are seen between the epidermis and the dermis. In some instances the separation increases to such extent that subepidermal

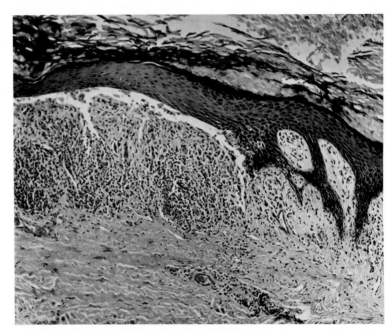

FIG. 8-13. **Lichen planus, bullous lesion.** Extensive separation of the epidermis from the dermis has taken place. (×100)

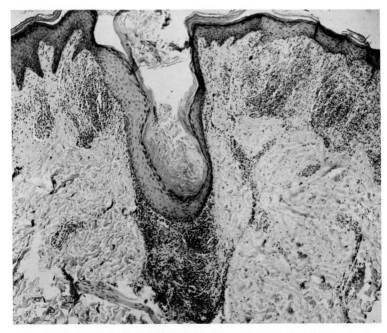

FIG. 8-14. **Lichen planopilaris.** There is a dilated hair follicle containing a keratotic plug. At the lower pole of the hair follicle is a dense chronic inflammatory infiltrate. In addition, there is a bandlike infiltrate beneath the epidermis. (×50)

bullae form (*bullous lichen planus*) (Fig. 8-13). These bullae form as a result of damage to the basal cells (Sarkany et al.). (See Classification of Blisters, see p. 96.)

The *oral lesions* of lichen planus differ in their histologic appearance from those of the skin as one would expect, since the oral mucosa normally shows parakeratosis without the presence of a granular layer (see p. 13). Thus, the lesions of the mouth show parakeratosis more commonly than hyperkeratosis, although alternate areas of both types of keratinization may be observed (Shklar). Also, rather than showing acanthosis, the epithelium often is thin. Ulcerations develop either consequent to the rupture of bullae or as a result of necrosis of the epithelium.

LICHEN PLANOPILARIS. Early lesions of lichen planopilaris, whether obtained from the glabrous skin or from hairy areas, show, in addition to a subepidermal infiltrate typical of lichen planus, a dense mononuclear infiltrate surrounding the hair follicle and the dermal hair papilla. Damage to the dermal hair papilla leads to obliteration of the hair. At first, the hair follicles are dilated and filled with a keratotic plug (Fig. 8-14) (Silver et al.). Later on, however, the hair follicles and sebaceous glands are no longer present, the epidermis is flattened, and the dermis shows fibrosis and a mild perivascular infiltrate (Altman and Perry). At this stage, both the clinical and histologic findings are indistinguishable from those of pseudopelade of Brocq (see p. 185).

Histogenesis. In lichen planus the primary damage seems to be in the basal cell layer where it manifests itself as liquefaction degeneration both by light microscopy and electron microscopy (Sarkany and Gaylarde). Secondary events, as seen by electron microscopy, are a dermal infiltrate that, on invading the epidermis, causes damage to the basal lamina, such as ruptures and splitting up (E.M. No. 28). The colloid or hyaline bodies, located either in the lowermost epidermis or the upper dermis (E.M. No. 28), can be seen to develop from damaged basal cells. They measure up to 10 μm in size and show a filamentous structure in which remnants of organelles can be seen occasionally (Ebner and Gebhart). In bullous lichen planus electron microscopic examination shows cytoly-

sis of the basal cell layer so that the roof of the blister is formed by the lower stratum spinosum (Ebner et al.).

Enzyme histochemical studies have revealed, as a result of severe damage to the basal cell layer, in the affected epidermis a marked reduction in respiratory enzyme activity, particularly in the activity of succinic dehydrogenase. Also the number of dopa-positive melanocytes is greatly decreased in areas of damage to the basal cell layer (Black and Wilson Jones).

Labeling of lichen planus lesions in vivo with tritiated thymidine, for the purpose of determining DNA synthesis, has shown in areas of severe basal cell damage little labeling in the basal layer. In other areas, however, labeled keratinocytes had migrated into the lichen planus lesions from the intact margins, replacing the eroded basal cell layer (Marks et al.). Similarly, tissue culture experiments have indicated that repopulation of the damaged basal cell layer occurs through migration of basal cells from nearby uninvolved areas rather than through mitotic activity at the site of damage (Presbury and Marks).

It is likely that the reduced mitotic activity in lichen planus, through a reduced rate of cellular proliferation, results in a prolonged retention of cells in the epidermis and thus in an increased degree of keratinization, as shown by a thickened horny layer, by hypergranulosis, and by eosinophilic staining of the keratinocytes in the stratum malpighii.

On direct immunofluorescent staining the lesions of lichen planus regularly reveal extensive deposits of fibrin in the upper part of the dermis, as well as finely granular aggregates of IgM along the basement zone. The colloid bodies show marked fluorescence for IgA, IgG and IgM as well as for complement and fibrin (Baart de la Faille-Kuyper and Baart de la Faille).

Differential Diagnosis. In the diagnosis of lichen planus on the glabrous skin it should be borne in mind that parakeratosis is not a feature of lichen planus and, if more than slight focal parakeratosis is present, a diagnosis of lichen planus should not be made on histologic grounds. Occasionally, difficulties arise in the differentiation of lichen planus from chronic discoid lupus erythematosus. The latter shows, however, hydropic degeneration of the basal cells during the entire course of the disease, rather than hydropic degeneration of the basal cells as a stage preceding their replacement by squamous cells. Chronic discoid lupus erythematosus, furthermore, shows a patchy rather than a bandlike infiltrate and, quite commonly, small areas of hemorrhage in the upper dermis. It may be difficult to differentiate long-standing hypertrophic lichen planus from lichen simplex chronicus, because in long-standing hypertrophic lichen planus the basal layer may show hardly any residual damage and the infiltrate may no longer be bandlike (Haber and Sarkany). Deeper sections still may show, however, in the case of lichen planus, areas of damage to the basal layer.

On the lips and in the mouth the differentiation of lichen planus from leukoplakia may cause difficulties, clinically as well as histologically. Both diseases may show hyperkeratosis and an inflammatory infiltrate close to the epidermis. Yet, thorough study of the epidermis reveals in leukoplakia some atypicality of the squamous cells. Furthermore, leukoplakia more than lichen planus is apt to show irregular proliferation of the rete ridges, and a conspicuous number of plasma cells. Lichen planopilaris of the scalp in its early phase must be differentiated from chronic discoid lupus erythematosus which also affects the hair follicles as well as the surface epidermis. Lupus erythematosus shows more prominent hydropic degeneration of the basal cells both in the epidermis and the hair follicles without their

replacement by squamous cells, and in addition it shows an interfollicular patchy infiltrate. In its late stage lichen planopilaris of the scalp, as already stated, may be indistinguishable from pseudopelade of Brocq.

Solitary lichenoid solar keratosis, a form of solar keratosis, may show a histologic picture indistinguishable from that of lichen planus, although in occasional cases some atypicality is present in the epidermis (see p. 470).

LICHEN NITIDUS

Lichen nitidus is characterized by asymptomatic, flat-topped, flesh-colored papules, 2 to 3 mm in size, that may occur in groups but do not coalesce. Their sites of predilection are the penis, arms and abdomen.

Histopathology. Each papule of lichen nitidus consists of a circumscribed infiltrate closely attached to the lower surface of the epidermis. Most of the cells within the infiltrate are mononuclear cells and histiocytes. Some of the latter may have the appearance of epithelioid cells (Fig. 8-15). A few multinucleated giant cells may be present. The dermal infiltrate often extends into the overlying epidermis to a slight degree.

The epidermis above the infiltrate is flattened and shows either hydropic degeneration or absence of the basal cell layer. In

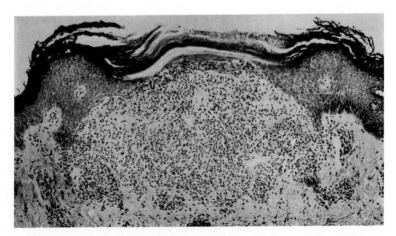

FIG. 8-15. **Lichen nitidus.** A circumscribed nest of cells lies in close approximation to the epidermis. The infiltrate consists of lymphoid and epithelioid cells. The epidermis above the infiltrate is flattened and has a parakeratotic horny layer. (×100)

the absence of the basal cell layer the overlying epidermis may become partially detached from the dermis (Ellis and Hill). The horny layer shows parakeratosis above the center of the infiltrate. At each lateral margin of the infiltrate, rete ridges tend to extend downward and seem to clutch the infiltrate in the manner of a claw clutching a ball.

Relationship Between Lichen Planus and Lichen Nitidus. The view that lichen nitidus represents a variant of lichen planus has been supported by several authors on the basis that both types of lesions are present simultaneously in some cases, clinically as well as histologically (Ellis and Hill; Gougerot and Civatte). Wilson and Bett reported 25 cases of extensive lichen planus, in which some of the lesions consisted of small miliary papules identical in their clinical appearance with those of lichen nitidus. On histologic examination some of the miliary papules resembled lichen planus, and others lichen nitidus, whereas a few showed features of both. It seems likely that very early small papules of lichen planus can resemble lichen nitidus histologically by having a flattened epidermis, but they differ in their subsequent evolution (Gougerot and Civatte). Therefore, they are different diseases. In particular, they differ in that in lichen nitidus the papule remains small and, besides epidermal flattening, develops parakeratosis, whereas in lichen planus the papule develops acanthosis and hyperkeratosis (Weiss and Cohen).

LICHEN STRIATUS

Lichen striatus is a fairly uncommon eruption that as a rule occurs in children. It manifests itself usually on one of the extremities as either a continuous or an interrupted band composed of small lichenoid papules. The eruption appears suddenly and usually involutes within a year. Itching is absent.

Histopathology. A fairly heavy chronic inflammatory infiltrate is seen around the subpapillary vessels and usually also around some of the deeper vessels. The infiltrate extends into some of the papillae (Pinkus). The epidermal changes are secondary and consist of intercellular and intracellular edema often associated with some exocytosis

and parakeratosis. In contrast to a dermatitis there usually is no acanthosis, and there even may be some atrophy. In about one half of the cases a few large, eosinophilic, dyskeratotic keratinocytes are seen in either the granular of the horny layer which, however, do not assume the proportions seen in the corps ronds of Darier's disease (Staricco).

PITYRIASIS RUBRA PILARIS

The primary lesions are pale red, hyperkeratotic papules, usually follicular in location. The papules gradually coalesce to form red, scaly plaques that in their clinical appearance resemble psoriasis. Ultimately, most of the body surface may be affected by a scaling erythroderma. Even at this late stage follicular keratotic papules usually can be detected, especially on the dorsa of the fingers.

Histopathology. The essential pathologic process is follicular hyperkeratosis. In addition, there is diffuse hyperkeratosis with focal parakeratosis. The epidermis shows acanthosis, usually of a slight degree. In the upper dermis a mild chronic inflammatory infiltrate is observed around the blood vessels (Brunsting and Sheard).

Differential Diagnosis. In spite of an occasional close clinical resemblance to psoriasis, pityriasis rubra pilaris does not resemble psoriasis histologically. For differentiation from phrynoderma (vitamin A deficiency) see page 412.

BIBLIOGRAPHY

Urticaria

Beall, G. N.: Urticaria. Medicine, *43*:131, 1964.

Illig, L.: Zur Pathogenese der cholinergischen Urticaria. Arch. klin. exp. Derm., *229*:231, 1967.

Lepow, I. H., Willms-Kretschmer, K., Patrick, R. A., and Rosen, F. S.: Gross and ultrastructural observations on lesions produced by intradermal injections of human C3a in man. Am. J. Path., *61*:13, 1970.

Rosen, F. S., and Austen, K. F.: The "neurotic edema" (hereditary angioedema). New Eng. J. Med., *280*:1356, 1969.

Erythema Annulare Centrifugum

Ellis, F., and Friedman, A. A.: Erythema annulare centrifugum (Darier's). Arch. Derm. Syph., *70*:496, 1954.

Nordenskjöld, A., and Wahlgren, F.: Erythema annulare centrifugum. Acta dermatoven., *35*: 281, 1955.

Erythema Gyratum Repens

Gammel, J. A.: Erythema gyratum repens. Arch. Derm. Syph., *66*:494, 1952.

Leavell, U. W., Winternitz, W. W., and Black, J. H.: Erythema gyratum repens and undifferentiated carcinoma. Arch. Derm., *95*:69, 1967.

Thomson, J., and Stankler, L.: Erythema gyratum perstans. Brit. J. Derm., *82*:406, 1970.

Erythema Dyschromicum Perstans

Knox, J. M., Dodge, B. G., and Freeman, R. G.: Erythema dyschromicum perstans. Arch. Derm., *97*:262, 1968.

Soter, N. A., Wand, C., and Freeman, R. G.: Ultrastructural pathology of erythema dyschromicum perstans. J. Invest. Derm., *52*: 155, 1969.

Prurigo Simplex

Braun-Falco, O., and von Eickstedt, U. M.: Beitrag zur Urticaria papulosa chronica. Hautarzt, *8*:534, 1957.

Kocsard, E.: The problem of prurigo. Austral. J. Derm., *6*:156, 1962.

Tritsch, H., and Kantner, M.: Neurohistologische Untersuchungen bei Prurigo simplex subacuta. Arch. klin. exp. Derm., *217*:355, 1963.

Prurigo Nodularis

Cowan, M. A.: Neurohistological changes in lichen simplex chronicus. Arch. Derm., *89*: 562, 1964, I.

———: Neurohistological changes in prurigo nodularis. Arch. Derm., *89*:754, 1964, II.

Ereaux, L. P., and Schopflocher, P.: Familial primary self-healing squamous epithelioma of skin. Arch. Derm., *91*:589, 1965.

Shaffer, B., and Beerman, H.: Lichen simplex chronicus and its variants. Arch. Derm. Syph., *64*:340, 1951.

Thies, W.: Neurohistologische Studie zur Differentialdiagnose des Prurigo nodularis Hyde und anderer Formen umschriebener Lichenifikation. Arch. klin. exp. Derm., *201*:539, 1955.

Psoriasis

Abrahams, J., McCarthy, J. T., and Sanders, S. L.: 101 cases of exfoliative dermatitis. Arch. Derm., *87*:96, 1963.

Andrews, G. C., and Machacek, G. F.: Pustular bacterids of the hands and feet. Arch. Derm. Syph., *32*:837, 1935.

Ashhurst, P. J. C.: Relapsing pustular eruptions of the hands and feet. Brit. J. Derm., *76*:169, 1964.

Baker, H., and Ryan, T. J.: Generalized pustular psoriasis. Brit. J. Derm., *80*:771, 1968.

Barber, H. W.: Acrodermatitis continua vel perstans (dermatitis repens) and psoriasis pustulosa. Brit. J. Derm., *42*:500, 1930.

Braun-Falco, O.: Zur Morphogenese der psoriatischen Hautreaktion. Arch. klin. exp. Derm., *216*:130, 1963.

Braverman, J. M., Cohen, I., and O'Keefe, E. O.: Metabolic and ultrastructural studies in a patient with pustular psoriasis (Von Zumbusch). Arch. Derm., *105*:189, 1972.

Brody, I.: The ultrastructure of the epidermis in psoriasis vulgaris as revealed by electron microscopy. J. Ultrastruct. Res., *6*:304, 1962.

Burks, J. W., and Montgomery, H.: Histopathologic study of psoriasis. Arch. Derm. Syph., *48*:479, 1943.

Christophers, E., and Braun-Falco, O.: Mechanism of parakeratosis. Brit. J. Derm., *82*: 268, 1970.

Cox, A. J., and Watson, W.: Histologic variations in lesions of psoriasis. Arch. Derm., *106*:503, 1972.

Dawson, T. A. Jr.: Microscopic appearance of geographic tongue. Brit. J. Derm., *81*:827, 1969.

Degos, R., Garnier, G., and Civatte, J.: Pustulose par *Candida albicans* avec lésions psoriasiformes rappelant le psoriasis pustuleux. Bull. Soc. franc, derm. syph., *69*:231, 1962.

Enfors, W., and Molin, L.: Pustulosis palmaris et plantaris. Acta dermatoven., *51*:289, 1971.

Everall, J.: Intractable pustular eruptions of the hands and feet. Brit. J. Derm., *69*:269, 1957.

Fisher, L. B., and Wells, G. C.: The mitotic rate and duration in lesions of psoriasis and ichthyosis. Brit. J. Derm., *80*:235, 1968.

Fry, L.: The nature of psoriasis. Brit. J. Derm., *80*:833, 1968.

Fry, L., and McMinn, R. M. H.: The action of chemotherapeutic agents on psoriatic epidermis. Brit. J. Derm., *80*:373, 1968.

Goodwin, P., Hamilton, S., and Fry, L.: A comparison between DNA synthesis and mitosis in uninvolved and involved psoriatic epidermis and normal epidermis. Brit. J. Derm., *89*:613, 1973.

Gordon, M., and Johnson, W. C.: Histopathology and histochemistry of psoriasis. Arch. Derm., *95*:402, 1967.

Hashimoto, K., and Lever, W. F.: Elektronen-mikroskopische Untersuchungen der Hautveränderungen bei Psoriasis. Derm. Wschr., *152*:713, 1966.

Holzmann, H., and Hoede, N.: Betrachtungen und Befunde zur multifaktoriellen Genese der Psoriasis vulgaris. Arch. klin. exp. Derm., *236*:15, 1969.

Hundeiker, M.: Monocyten im Infiltrat des Psoriasisherdes. Dermatologica, *140*:115, 1970.

Katzenellenbogen, I., and Feuerman, E. I.: Psoriasis pustulosa and impetigo herpetiformis single or dual entity? Acta dermatoven., *46*: 86, 1966.

Kingery, F. A. J., Chinn, H. D., and Saunders, T. S.: Generalized pustular psoriasis. Arch. Derm., *84*:912, 1961.

Komura, J., Takigawa, M., and Ofuji, S.: Epidermal cell–leukocyte interactions in spongiform pustules of Kogoj. Arch. Derm. Forsch., *249*:321, 1974.

Lapière, S.: A propos d'un cas d'impétigo herpétiforme. Arch. belg. derm. syph., *14*:146, 1958.

Lever, W. F.: *In* discussion to: Pay, D.: Pustular psoriasis. Arch. Derm., *99*:641, 1969.

Mercer, E. H., and Maibach, H. J.: Intercellular adhesion and surface coats of epidermal cells in psoriasis. J. Invest. Derm., *51*:213, 1968.

Muller, S. A., and Kitzmiller, K. W.: Generalized pustular psoriasis. Acta dermatoven., *42*: 504, 1962.

Orfanos, C. E., Schaumburg-Lever, G., Mahrle, G., and Lever, W. F.: Alterations of cell surfaces as a pathogenetic factor in psoriasis. Arch. Derm., *107*:38, 1973.

Piérard, J., and Kint, A.: Les "bactérides pustuleuses" d'Andrews. Arch. belg. derm. syph., *22*:83, 1966.

Pinkus, H., and Mehregan, A. H.: The primary histologic lesion of seborrheic dermatitis and psoriasis. J. Invest. Derm., *46*:109, 1966.

Resneck, J. S., and Cram, D. L.: Erythema annulare-like pustular psoriasis. Arch. Derm., *108*:687, 1973.

Rothberg, S., Crounse, R. G., and Lee, J. L.: Glycine-C^{14} incorporation into the proteins of normal stratum corneum and the abnormal stratum corneum of psoriasis. J. Invest. Derm., *37*:497, 1961.

Rupec, M.: Zur Ultrastruktur der spongiformen Pustel. Arch. klin. exp. Derm., *239*:30, 1970.

Schuppener, H. J.: Ausdrucksformen pustulöser Psoriasis. Derm. Wsch., *138*:841, 1958.

Shelley, W. B., and Kirschbaum, J. O.: Generalized pustular psoriasis. Arch. Derm., *84*:73, 1961.

Skog, E.: Familial acrodermatitis continua (Hallopeau)—psoriasis. Acta dermatoven., *38*: 345, 1958.

Soltani, K., and Van Scott, E. J.: Patterns and sequence of tissue changes in incipient and evolving lesions of psoriasis. Arch. Derm., *106*:484, 1972.

Soltermann, W.: Familiäre Psoriasis pustulosa unter dem Bilde der Impetigo herpetiformis. Dermatologica, *116*:313, 1958.

Van Scott, E. J., and Ekel, T. W.: Kinetics of hyperplasia in psoriasis. Arch. Derm., *88*: 373, 1963.

Vorhees, J. J., Duell, E. A., Bass, L. J., et al.: Decreased cyclic AMP in the epidermis of lesions of psoriasis. Arch. Derm., *105*:695, 1972.

Weinstein, G. D., and Frost, P.: Methotrexate for psoriasis. Arch. Derm., *103*:33, 1971.

Weinstein, G. D., and Van Scott, E. J.: Autoradiographic analysis of turnover times of normal and psoriatic epidermis. J. Invest. Derm., *45*:257, 1965.

Reiter's Disease

Khan, M. Y., and Hall, W. H.: Progression of Reiter's syndrome to psoriatic arthritis. Arch. Intern. Med., *116*:911, 1965.

Perry, H. O., and Mayne, J. G.: Psoriasis and Reiter's syndrome. Arch. Derm., *92*:129, 1965.

Weinberger, H. W., Ropes, M. W., Kulka, J. P., and Bauer, W.: Reiter's syndrome, clinical and pathologic observations. Medicine, *41*: 35, 1962.

Wright, V., and Reed, W. B.: The link between Reiter's syndrome and psoriatic arthritis. Ann. Rheum. Dis., *23*:12, 1964.

Parapsoriasis

Fleischmajer, R., Pascher, F., and Sims, C. F.: Parapsoriasis en plaques and mycosis fungoides. Dermatologica, *131*:149, 1965.

Goldberg, L.: Xantho-erythrodermia perstans (Crocker). Arch. Derm., *88*:901, 1963.

Grimmer, H.: Brocq'sche Krankheit. Z. Haut Geschlechtskr., *30*:xxxv, 1961.

Kawada, A., Takada, Y., Nishiwaki, S., et al.: A case of parapsoriasis en plaques of 18 years duration terminating with reticulum cell sarcoma. Dermatologica, *138*:19, 1969.

Keil, H.: Parapsoriasis en plaques disséminées and incipient mycosis fungoides. Arch. Derm. Syph., *37*:465, 1938; *38*:545, 1938.

Khan, M.: Parapsoriasis en plaques and myeosis fungoides. Z. Haut, *49*:547, 1974.

Lapière, S.: Evolution et pronostic du parapsoriasis en plaques. Ann. derm. syph., *9*: 609, 1949.

Musger, A.: Zur Frage der nosologischen Stellung der Parapsoriasis lichenoides Brocq. Hautarzt, *17*:280, 1966.

Osmundsen, P. E.: Parapsoriasis en plaques. Acta dermatoven., *48*:345, 1968.

Samman, P. D.: Survey of reticuloses and premycotic eruptions. Brit. J. Derm., *76*:1, 1964.

Walther, D.: Dermatitis lichenoides striata et reticularis partim hemorrhagica. Arch. Derm. Syph., *196*:110, 1953.

Pityriasis Rosea

Bunch, L. W., and Tilley, J. C.: Pityriasis rosea. Arch. Derm., *84*:79, 1961.

Gianotti-Crosti Syndrome

Grimmer, H.: Gianotti-Crosti Syndrom (Akrodermatitis papulosa eruptiva infantilis). Z. Haut Geschlechtskr., *42*:xlv, 1967.

Winkelmann, R. K., and Bourlond, A.: Infantile lichenoid acrodermatitis. Report of a case of Gianotti-Crosti syndrome. Arch. Derm., *92*:398, 1965.

Lichen Planus

Altman, J., and Perry, H. O.: The variations and course of lichen planus. Arch. Derm., *84*:179, 1961 (review).

Baart de la Faille-Kuyper, E. H., and Baart de la Faille, H.: An immunofluorescence study of lichen planus. Brit. J. Derm., *90*:365, 1974.

Berger, H., Hundeiker, M., and Engelhardt, A. W.: Über das Infiltrat im Lichen-ruber-Herd. Arch. klin. exp. Derm., *235*:394, 1969.

Black, M. M., and Wilson-Jones, E.: The role of the epidermis in the histopathogenesis of lichen planus. Arch. Derm., *105*:81, 1972.

Cram, D. L., Kierland, R. R., and Winkelmann, R. K.: Ulcerative lichen planus of the feet. Arch. Derm., *93*:692, 1966.

Ebner, H.: Lichen ruber planus mit Onychatrophic und narbiger Alopezie. Dermatologica, *147*:219, 1973.

Ebner, H., Erlach, E., and Gebhart, W.: Untersuchungen über die Blasenbildung beim Lichen ruber planus. Arch. Derm. Forsch., *247*:193, 1973.

Ebner, H., and Gebhart, W.: Beitrag zur Histochemie und Ultrastruktur der sogenannten hyalinen bzw. kolloiden Körperchen. Arch. Derm. Forsch., *242*:153, 1972.

Fulling, H. J.: Cancer development in oral lichen planus. Arch. Derm., *108*:667, 1973.

Gougerot, H., and Civatte, A.: Critères cliniques et histologiques des lichens plans cutanés et muqueux: délimitation. Ann. derm. syph., *80*:5, 1953.

Haber, H., and Sarkany, I.: Hypertrophic lichen planus and lichen simplex. Trans. St. John's Hosp. Derm. Soc., *41*:61, 1958.

Jänner, M., Muissus, E., and Rohde, B.: Lichen planus als fakultative Präkanzerose. Derm. Wschr., *153*:513, 1967.

Kronenberg, K., Fretzin, D., and Potter, B.: Malignant degeneration of lichen planus. Arch. Derm. *104*:304, 1971.

Male, O.: Über die ulzerös-atrophisierende Form des Lichen ruber planus. Z. Haut, *45*:1, 1970.

Marks, R., Black, M., and Wilson Jones, E.: Epidermal cell kinetics in lichen planus. Brit. J. Derm., *88*:37, 1973.

Pagès, F., Lapeyre, J., and Misson, R.: Syndrome de Lassueur-Graham-Little. Ann. Derm. Syph., *88*:272, 1961.

Presbury, D. G. C., and Marks, R. The epidermal disorder in lichen planus: an in vitro study. Brit. J. Derm., *90*:373, 1974.

Sarkany, I., Caron, G. A., and Jones, H. H.: Lichen planus pemphigoides. Trans. St. John's Hosp. Derm. Soc., *50*:50, 1964.

Sarkany, I., and Gaylarde, P. M.: Ultrastructural and light microscopic changes of the epidermo-dermal junction. Trans. St. John's Hosp. Derm. Soc., *57*:139, 1971.

Shklar, G.: Erosive and bullous oral lesions of lichen planus. Arch. Derm., *97*:411, 1968.

Silver, H., Chargin, L., and Sachs, P. M.: Follicular lichen planus (Lichen planopilaris). Arch. Derm. Syph., *67*:346, 1953.

Lichen Nitidus

Ellis, F. A., and Hill, W. F.: Is lichen nitidus a variety of lichen planus? Arch. Derm. Syph., *38*:568, 1938.

Gougerot, H., and Civatte, A.: Critères cliniques et histologiques des lichens plans cutanés et muqueux: délimitation. Ann. derm. syph., *80*:5, 1953.

Weiss, R. M., and Cohen, A. D.: Lichen nitidus of the palms and soles. Arch. Derm., *104*:538, 1971.

Wilson, H. T. H., and Bett, D. C. H.: Miliary lesions in lichen planus. Arch. Derm., *83*:920, 1961.

Lichen Striatus

Pinkus, H.: Lichen striatus and lichen planus. J. Invest. Derm., *11*:9, 1948.

Staricco, R. G.: Lichen striatus. Arch. Derm., *79*:311, 1959.

Pityriasis Rubra Pilaris

Brunsting, L. A., and Sheard, C.: Dark adaptation in pityriasis rubra pilaris. Arch. Derm. Syph., *43*:42, 1941.

9

Vascular Diseases

NONINFLAMMATORY PURPURAS

Purpura represents a hemorrhage into the skin. Lesions less than 3 mm in diameter are called petechiae. Larger lesions are called ecchymoses. Purpura occurs as the result of either noninflammatory or inflammatory changes within or around blood vessels.

Noninflammatory purpura occurs (a) on the basis of deficient collagen formation around capillaries: in *senile purpura* and in *scurvy*; (b) on the basis of sensitivity phenomena without vascular occlusion: in *idiopathic thrombocytopenic purpura* and in *autoerythrocyte sensitization*; and (c) on the basis of sensitivity phenomena with vascular occlusion: in *cryoglobulinemia,* in *coumarin necrosis,* in *thrombotic thrombocytopenic purpura,* and in *purpura fulminans.*

SENILE PURPURA

In senile purpura well defined ecchymoses are present on the dorsa of the forearms and hands of the elderly. Prolonged ingestion of corticosteroids is a predisposing factor.

Histopathology. The capillaries within the areas of extravasations appear fairly normal. However, the dermis in which the capillaries are located is altered. It shows solar elastosis (see p. 249) in its upper portion, and atrophy in its lower portion where the collagen is present largely as individual fibers rather than as bundles of fibers (Tattersall and Seville).

SCURVY

In scurvy, caused by a deficiency of ascorbic acid, the purpura usually consists of perifollicular petechiae, especially on the lower extremities. In addition, broken-off "corkscrew hairs" are seen in association with follicular hyperkeratosis. In long-standing scurvy, extensive ecchymoses may be present over the shins (Walker).

Histopathology. Extravasations of red cells are found predominantly in the vicinity of hair follicles without evidence of capillary changes or signs of inflammation. Extensive extravasations usually show deposits of hemosiderin both within and outside of macrophages (Walker). In many instances, intrafollicular keratotic plugs are seen.

Histogenesis. In scurvy there is both a decreased and an abnormal formation of collagen. On electron microscopic examination, the dermal fibroblasts appear shrunken and show a decreased amount of rough-surfaced endoplasmic reticulum (Hashimoto et al.). In the vicinity of the fibroblasts one observes increased amounts of extracellular filamentous or amorphous material. Much of this material fails to polymerize into collagen fibrils with normal periodicity (Ross and Benditt). The extravasation of red cells in scurvy is caused, however, not only by a decreased formation of perivascular collagen but also by discontinuities in the endothelial lining brought on by a vacuolar degeneration of endothelial cells (Hashimoto et al.).

IDIOPATHIC THROMBOCYTOPENIC PURPURA

In this disorder, petechiae and often also ecchymoses are present as the result of a greatly reduced platelet count. In addition, there may be hemorrhages from the nose, mouth or uterus.

Histopathology. Extravasations of red cells without evidence of inflammation are seen in the dermis.

Histogenesis. A humoral antiplatelet factor, which is an immunoglobulin and coats the platelets, causes an accelerated removal of such platelets in the spleen (Handin and Smith). The experimental reduction of platelets in the blood stream results, as electron microscopic examination has shown, in widened intercellular spaces in the endothelial lining of capillaries and defects in the capillary basal lamina. These two factors account for the extravasation of blood in thrombocytopenic purpura (Gore et al.).

AUTOERYTHROCYTE SENSITIZATION

Localized painful red swellings that develop into ecchymoses occur as recurrent attacks in women with a hysterical personality pattern.

Histopathology. Numerous extravasated red cells are present in the dermis and the subcutaneous fat. There is no evidence of vasculitis, but in a few instances a mild perivascular infiltrate of mononuclear cells has been found (Ratnoff and Agle). At a later stage, one finds in the dermis, in addition to decomposing red cells, hemosiderin, macrophages and fibroblasts (Waldorf and Lipkin).

Histogenesis. In a significant number of patients with autoerythrocyte sensitization the lesions are reproducible by the intradermal injection of the patient's blood (Ratnoff and Agle).

CRYOGLOBULINEMIA

Cryoglobulinemia occurs either as an idiopathic disease or in association with other diseases, particularly with macroglobulinemia and multiple myeloma but occasionally also with systemic lupus erythematosus and lymphoma. The cutaneous lesions consist of purpura and ulcers on the legs. Although in some cases only cutaneous vessels are affected, the vessels of the renal glomeruli, of the brain and of the lungs can also be involved, resulting in death (Ellis; McKenzie et al.).

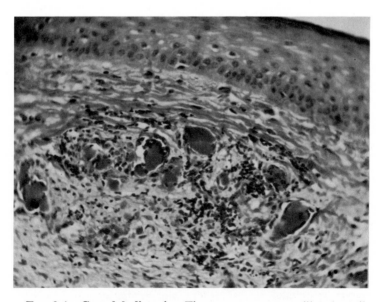

FIG. 9-1. **Cryoglobulinemia.** There are numerous dilated capillaries containing in their lumens an amorphous eosinophilic substance consisting largely of precipitated cryoglobulin. (×200)

Histopathology. Many dilated dermal capillaries of the legs contain in their lumen an amorphous eosinophilic substance consisting largely of precipitated cryoglobulin (Fig. 9-1). This intracapillary precipitate is visible in hematoxylin and eosin-stained sections (Ellis). However, it is best demonstrated by the PAS stain (Baughman and Sommer). Some capillaries are densely filled with erythrocytes, and extensive extravasations of red cells are present. The involved vessels may show swelling of their endothelial cells (Duperrat) or necrosis of their walls (McKenzie et. al.). Vascular changes similar to those in the dermis may be present in the subcutaneous tissue (McKenzie et al.). Although in early lesions an inflammatory infiltrate is absent, it may be present around the affected blood vessels in older lesions.

Histogenesis. The disease is caused by the presence in the serum of cryoglobulins which precipitate in the cold and redissolve on warming. These cryoprecipitates may contain either a single immunoglobulin (IgG, IgA or IgM) or a mixture of them and often contain also complement (Goldberg and Barnett). On precipitation they cause vascular damage. On direct immunofluorescence, the vessels of fresh lesions often show deposits of immunoglobulins of the same classes as those found in the cryoglobulin of the serum (Cream).

COUMARIN NECROSIS

In rare instances patients receiving coumarin therapy show between the third and tenth day of therapy one, and occasionally several, areas of petechiae and ecchymoses that rapidly culminate in necrosis. The extent of necrosis varies greatly. In the case of extensive necroses death may ensue (Koch-Weser).

Histopathology. One finds extensive occlusion of dermal veins and often also of subcutaneous veins with fibrin thrombi without signs of inflammation (Nalbandian et al.). This results in hemorrhagic infarcts and subsequent necrosis in the dermis and subcutaneous tissue. The petechiae correlate with ruptures of capillaries in the upper dermis, and coalescence of petechiae leads to ecchymoses.

Histogenesis. The necrosis most likely is caused by a toxic effect of coumarin on the vascular endothelium (Nalbandian et al.). Continued coumarin therapy does not aggravate the lesions.

THROMBOTIC THROMBOCYTOPENIC PURPURA

This rare syndrome has a rapid onset and a fulminating fatal course. Death possibly may be prevented by the early administration of heparin. The syndrome is the result of disseminated intravascular coagulation and develops on the basis of widespread vascular damage, as it may occur in the course of systemic lupus erythematosus, glomerulonephritis, or systemic infections such as meningococcemia (Umlas and Kaiser).

Thrombotic thrombocytopenic purpura has the following five major manifestations: (1) "microangiopathic" hemolytic anemia often associated with jaundice, (2) thrombocytopenic purpura, (3) central nervous system symptoms, (4) severe renal impairment, and (5) fever. The disseminated intravascular coagulation represents a consumption coagulopathy with depletion of platelets, fibrinogen, prothrombin, and other factors (Umlas and Kaiser). The extensive thrombosis of small blood vessels causes small hemorrhages in many organs of the body, including occasionally the skin (Luttgens; Haim et al.). In particular, melena, hematuria and hemoptysis may occur.

Cutaneous manifestations, aside from jaundice, consist of petechiae and ecchymoses due to the thrombocytopenia. There may be, in addition, areas of hemorrhagic necrosis that may be covered by large bullae (Luttgens; Haim et al.).

Histopathology. The cutaneous lesions and at times even areas free of lesions show occlusion of capillaries by an amorphous eosinophilic PAS-positive material containing fibrin and platelets (Haim et al.). There is no significant perivascular inflammation. The presence of fibrin in the thrombi can be proved by a positive reaction with fluorescein-labeled rabbit antihuman fibrin antibodies (Craig and Gitlin). In addition, the skin may show more or less extensive extravasations of red cells.

In the absence of diagnostic findings in the skin it may be possible to establish the diagnosis of thrombotic thrombocytopenic purpura by demonstrating the presence of thrombi in the small blood vessels either through random biopsy of a lymph node (Ruffolo et al.), through aspiration of bone marrow (Ruffolo et al.), or through a biopsy of the gingiva, a highly vascular tissue (Goldenfarb and Finch).

Autopsy reveals the widespread presence of thrombi in the small blood vessels of many organs, especially the kidneys, adrenals, spleen, pancreas, myocardium, and brain (Ruffolo et al.).

PURPURA FULMINANS

Purpura fulminans is characterized by the sudden occurrence of large areas of ecchymoses that undergo necrosis, mainly on the lower extremities. Large bullae may overlie the ecchymoses. Purpura fulminans occurs most commonly in children recovering from an infection, such as scarlet fever or varicella; but it may occur without a preceding illness (Cram and Soley) and even in adults (Case Records of the Massachusetts General Hospital). The lesions progress rapidly with severe systemic toxicity. The disease usually is fatal within a few days, although the administration of heparin may prove life-saving.

Histopathology. In the dermis the blood vessels in the vicinity of the areas of necrosis are occluded by platelet-fibrin thrombi. No inflammation surrounds the blood vessels, but the presence of a large amount of hemorrhage in the dermis indicates the loss of vascular integrity (Case Records of Massachusetts General Hospital). The epidermis and portions of the dermis often show necrosis. At sites of bullae the epidermis is detached from the dermis.

In addition to the skin, the subcutaneous fat and occasionally also some of the internal organs show thrombosis of small vessels and hemorrhagic necrosis (Chambers et al.).

Histogenesis. Purpura fulminans, like thrombotic thrombocytopenic purpura, results from a consumption coagulopathy. Depletion of platelets, fibrinogen, prothrombin, and various coagulation factors is caused by disseminated intravascular coagulation (Cram and Soley). Probably in cases following an infectious disease a bacterial endotoxin by virtue of its antigenicity has sensitized the vascular endothelium (Case Records of the Massachusetts General Hospital).

INFLAMMATORY PURPURAS (VASCULITIS)

The following types of purpura are caused by inflammatory changes in the walls of blood vessels, i.e., a vasculitis: (1) allergic vasculitis, a neutrophilic type of vasculitis; (2) pityriasis lichenoides et varioliformis of Mucha-Habermann, and (3) purpura pigmentosa chronica, both representing lymphoid types of vasculitis; (4) purpura associated with periarteritis nodosa, allergic granulomatosis, and Wegener's granulomatosis. These four types of inflammatory purpura will be discussed in this chapter. Two other types will be discussed elsewhere, namely: (5) bacterial purpura, usually caused by meningococci (see p. 275); and (6) purpura due to drug allergy (see p. 239).

ALLERGIC VASCULITIS (ANAPHYLACTOID PURPURA)

This disorder, in which purpuric lesions usually are present, is characterized histologically by damage to the small cutaneous vessels and an infiltrate of neutrophils showing fragmentation of nuclei (karyorrhexis or leukocytoclasis). It can be divided into an acute type, the Henoch-Schönlein type, which frequently is associated with systemic manifestations, and a chronic type, the Gougerot-Ruiter type, in which systemic manifestations usually are absent (Winkelmann and Ditto). Intermediate cases, between these two types, occur.

In the acute Henoch-Schönlein type, petechiae and often also ecchymoses are present. One observes frequently also erythema and in some cases vesicles, bullae and ulcers. Fever and malaise are present. Systemic manifestations are frequent and may consist of arthralgia (Schönlein's purpura), crises of abdominal pain with melena (Henoch's purpura), hematuria due to either focal or diffuse glomerulitis, and dyspnea, due to pulmonary infiltrates (McCoombs). In severe cases, referred to by Zeek as hypersensitivity angiitis and characterized by marked pulmonary and renal involvement, death occurs within a few days or weeks, usually with renal failure as the cause of death. As a rule, Henoch-Schönlein purpura lasts about 4 weeks, but recurrences develop in about 40 per cent of the cases (Allen et al.). Even though the renal lesions often are reversible, death from either acute or chronic renal failure occurs in some of the patients (Ansell).

In the chronic Gougerot-Ruiter type, the eruption is often polymorphous. Petechiae are present in most but not in all patients and are limited largely to the legs, with only occasional occurrence on the thighs and arms. Other cutaneous manifestations are macules, papules, nodules, blisters, and ulcers. The eruption often shows remissions and exacerbations (Ruiter, 1957).

The so-called *purpura hyperglobulinemica of Waldenström,* in which petechiae on the legs of many years duration are associated with a polyclonal hypergammaglobulinemia, is regarded by some authors as a disease entity, possibly as an autoimmune disease because of its occasional association with Sjögren's syndrome or lupus erythematosus (Kyle et al.). It seems, however, more likely that this disorder represents a chronic allergic vasculitis of the Gougerot-Ruiter type in which the amounts of serum gamma globulin have increased gradually, as it is known to occur (Wang et al.). In favor of the latter view are also that in both diseases there is a neutrophilic vasculitis with fragmentation of nuclei (Goltz and Good; Holubar et al.) and, further, that there are cases on record in which after many years duration the purpura cleared and the values for gamma globulin reverted to normal (Shapiro et al.).

Histopathology. The histologic changes in allergic vasculitis of the skin are the same in the acute and the chronic type, except that

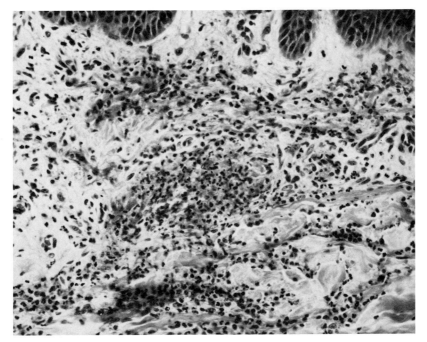

FIG. 9-2. **Allergic vasculitis (anaphylactoid purpura).** The capillaries show swelling of the endothelial cells and deposition of fibrinoid material around them. A rather severe inflammatory infiltrate is present, especially around the capillaries. It is composed largely of neutrophils, many of which show fragmentation of their nuclei (karyorrhexis). No extravasation of erythrocytes is present, probably as a result of occlusion of the capillaries. (×200)

extravasation of red cells is less pronounced in the chronic type and may even be absent. The two outstanding features in allergic vasculitis are vascular changes and a cellular infiltrate containing many neutrophils.

The vascular changes are limited to the small blood vessels in the dermis, except in the relatively rare cases of the chronic type having nodular lesions (see below). The dermal vessels show swelling of their endothelial cells and deposits of strongly eosinophilic strands of fibrin within and around their walls. The perivascular deposits of fibrin cause splitting up of the perivascular collagen into argyrophilic fibers (Ruiter, 1962). In sections stained with hematoxylin and eosin the deposits of fibrin and the marked edema combine to give the perivascular collagen a smudgy appearance that has been referred to as fibrinoid degeneration. Actual necrosis of the perivascular collagen, however, is seen only rarely in conjunction with ulcerative lesions (Winkelmann and Ditto). If the vascular changes are severe, swelling of the endothelial cells may result in occlusion of the lumen.

The cellular infiltrate is present predominantly around the dermal blood vessels, but often also within the vascular walls so that the outline of the blood vessels may appear indistinct (Fig. 9-2). The infiltrate consists mainly of neutrophils and varying numbers of eosinophils, with only a few mononuclear cells. A characteristic feature is the presence of many scattered nuclear fragments, often referred to as nuclear dust, resulting from the disintegration of neutrophils (karyorrhexis or leukocytoclasis). In addition to its perivascular location, the infiltrate is found scattered through the upper dermis in association with fibrin deposits between and within collagen bundles. Extensive extravasations of erythrocytes are present as a rule; but the extravasations may be slight or absent in chronic cases of allergic vasculitis. Vesicles, if present, usually form subepidermally (Ruiter and Hadders). Often, the detached epidermis is necrotic. The ulcers seen in occasional cases are the result of vascular necrosis and subsequent cutaneous infarction (Winkelmann and Ditto).

Lesions of prolonged duration may show, in addition to extravasated red cells, deposits of hemosiderin as the result of decomposition of red cells. The walls of capillaries may show hyaline thickening. In cases of long duration the infiltrate usually is less pronounced, but it continues to consist mainly of neutrophils and to contain nuclear dust.

The nodular lesions occasionally seen in cases of chronic allergic vasculitis and referred to as *nodular dermal allergid* of Gougerot (Gougerot and Duperrat; Laymon) show extension of the involvement to the small arteries and veins present at the dermal-subcutaneous border. These vessels show, similar to the dermal vessels, an infiltrate composed largely of neutrophils and deposits of fibrin within and around their walls. In contrast to periarteritis nodosa, the walls show no areas of necrosis.

Visceral Lesions. In the rapidly fatal cases of hypersensitivity angiitis a widespread vasculitis of small blood vessels is found in many organs (Zeek). Otherwise the only organ that is frequently affected is the kidney, with involvement in about 40 per cent of the cases with the acute Henoch-Schönlein type of allergic vasculitis. There may be either a focal or a diffuse glomerulitis characterized by occlusion of lobules of glomeruli by fibrinoid material (Ansell). Occasionally, the small intestine shows focal areas of vasculitis during crises of abdominal pain (Ansell).

Allergic vasculitis of the skin may occur as part of allergic granulomatosis (see p. 171) and of Wegener's granulomatosis (see p. 172). On the other hand, its association with periarteritis nodosa is rather rare (Winkelmann and Ditto).

Histogenesis. Electron microscopic studies by Ruiter and Molenaar as well as by Perrot et al. have shown in allergic vasculitis as main findings: (1) marked swelling of the endothelial cells; (2) extravasation of corpuscular elements through spaces between endothelial cells and breaks in the basal lamina; (3) marked sponge-like thickening of the pericapillary basal lamina resulting from an increased production of basal lamina material by pericapillary fibroblasts and from infiltration of the basal lamina by diffusing plasma molecules; and (4) thick coating of the pericapillary basal lamina and collagen fibrils with filamentous fibrin.

Direct immunofluorescent studies have revealed in most, but not in all cases of allergic vasculitis vascular deposits of IgG and complement, and in some instances also deposits of IgM (Schroeter et al.). It is likely that these deposits have a pathogenetic significance, especially in view of the similarity of allergic vasculitis with the Arthus phenomenon. The Arthus phenomenon occurs in sensitized animals at the site of a subcutaneous injection of the specific antigen. Histologically, it resembles a neutrophilic vasculitis with leukocytoclasis and, immunologically, it shows as the primary event the vascular deposition of antigen-antibody complexes, followed by complement-dependent leukocytic infiltration (Cochrane). Occasionally, the histologic picture of a leukocytoclastic vasculitis is seen also in other diseases associated with deposits of immunoglobulins and complement: for instance, in dermatitis herpetiformis, lupus erythematosus, and cryoglobulinemia (Cormane; Nir et al.).

PITYRIASIS LICHENOIDES ET VARIOLIFORMIS (MUCHA-HABERMANN)

This disorder occurs in two forms that differ in severity. Transitions between the two forms occur (Nasemann et al.; Marks et al.). Both are chronic and asymptomatic and show on histologic examination a lymphoid type of vasculitis.

The milder form, called pityriasis lichenoides chronica, is characterized by recurrent crops of brownish-red papules, mainly on the trunk, that are covered with a scale and show a very slow evolution.

The more severe form, called pityriasis lichenoides et varioliformis acuta, consists of a fairly extensive eruption, mainly on the trunk, characterized by papules that may become vesicular before developing into papulonecrotic, occasionally hemorrhagic lesions. Within a few weeks individual lesions heal without leaving a scar. Although the indi-

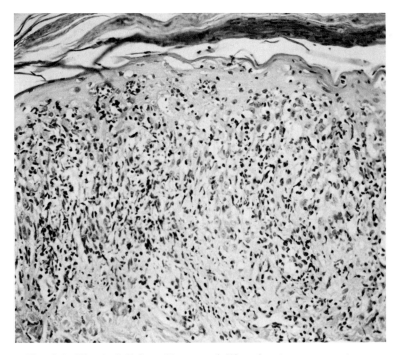

FIG. 9-3. **Pityriasis lichenoides et varioliformis.** A pronounced mononuclear infiltrate is present in the dermis and is seen invading the epidermis. The epidermis appears degenerated. It contains several small vesicles and also small accumulations of red cells. (×200)

vidual lesions follow an acute course, the disorder, because of the continuous development of new lesions, is chronic and extends over several months or even many years. In a few reported instances, pityriasis lichenoides et varioliformis acuta has shown, in addition to hemorrhagic papules, numerous scattered ulcers 2 to 5 cm in diameter, and a high temperature extending over several months (Degos et al.; Burke et al.).

Lymphomatoid papulosis represents a variant of pityriasis lichenoides et varioliformis acuta in which the histologic appearance of the infiltrate suggests lymphoma (see below). Clinically, such cases may show, in addition to papules, some ulcers, but there is no fever and the course is protracted. The malignant histologic appearance thus is in contrast with the benign clinical course. Still, in 2 of the approximately 30 cases reported so far, death from reticulum cell lymphoma has occurred, after 7 and 18 years, respectively (Kawada et al.; Black and Wilson Jones).

Histopathology. In the mild lichenoid type one observes a perivascular infiltrate composed largely of mononuclear cells. The infiltrate does not invade the walls of the vessels and extravasations of red cells thus do not occur (Szymanski). The infiltrate extends into the papillae and into the epidermis, where one observes spongiosis and a thickened, parakeratotic horny layer. Occasionally, there are degenerative changes in the epidermis with swelling and degeneration of some of the malpighian cells so that the histologic picture approaches that of the more severe form, pityriasis lichenoides et varioliformis acuta (Piérard and Van Steenbergen).

In the more severe lichenoid and varioliform type, one observes vascular changes consisting of a pronounced mononuclear infiltrate around capillaries, with the capillaries showing endothelial swelling and permeation of their walls by the infiltrate. This results in usually only mild, focal extravasations of erthrocytes, representing a lymphoid vasculitis (Piérard and Van Steenbergen; Szymanski). Not only lymphoid cells but also, as a fairly characteristic feature of the disease, a few erythrocytes often are seen "trapped" within the epidermis (Fig. 9-3). Pronounced intercellular and intracellular edema may oc-

cur in the epidermis, leading to a reticular degeneration and necrosis of the epidermis (Nasemann et al.). Finally, disintegration of the epidermis may occur and result in an erosion or even ulceration.

In general, pityriasis lichenoides et varioliformis acuta differs from allergic vasculitis by the absence of neutrophils, of so-called nuclear dust and of fibrinoid deposits around the capillaries. In some cases, however, especially those with ulcers, these features are present to some extent (Burke et al.; Muller and Schulze).

In LYMPHOMATOID PAPULOSIS one observes within the cellular infiltrate of pityriasis lichenoides et varioliformis acuta varying numbers of large, atypical cells with a hyperchromatic, irregularly shaped nucleus resembling mycosis fungoides cells (Black and Wilson Jones). They may be so large and atypical that they resemble the cells of metastatic carcinoma or malignant melanoma (Macaulay). In other instances multinucleated cells resembling Sternberg-Reed giant cells are present (Valentino and Helwig; Schimpf and Pons). In such cases the presence of vasculitis, the diapedesis of red cells into the dermis and the epidermis, and also clinical data aid in arriving at the right diagnosis.

Histogenesis. Direct immunofluorescent studies have revealed the absence of immunoglobulins and complement within and around the capillaries, suggesting that pityriasis lichenoides et varioliformis is not an "immune complex disorder." Enzyme histochemical and electron microscopic data suggest that the inflammatory infiltrate is composed largely of histocytes rather than lymphocytes, since many cells in the infiltrate are rich in hydrolytic enzyme activity and, on electron microscopy, their cytoplasm is rich in organelles including lysosomes. The vascular damage, especially of the endothelium, is rather mild on electron microscopic examination (Black and Marks).

PURPURA PIGMENTOSA CHRONICA (MAJOCCHI-SCHAMBERG)

Four diseases comprise this group, namely, purpura annularis telangiectodes of Majocchi, progressive pigmentary dermatosis of Schamberg, pigmented purpuric lichenoid dermatitis of Gougerot and Blum, and ecze-

FIG. 9-4. **Purpura pigmentosa chronica (Majocchi-Schamberg).** The capillaries of a papilla show swelling of their endothelial cells and are surrounded by extravasated erythrocytes and a lymphoid infiltrate. (×400)

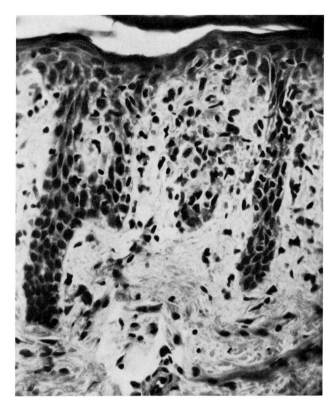

matidlike purpura of Doucas and Kapetanakis. They are closely related to one another so that often they cannot be differentiated on clinical or histologic grounds. Therefore, their separation into different entities is not warranted (Randall et al.; Pfleger). The term *purpura pigmentosa chronica* appears suitable for this disease.

Clinically, the primary lesion consists of purpuric puncta appearing in groups and extending slowly so that patches of various sizes form. Gradually, telangiectatic puncta may appear as the result of capillary dilatation, and pigmentation as the result of hemosiderin deposits. In some cases telangiectasia predominates (Majocchi's disease), and in others pigmentation (Schamberg's disease). Not infrequently, clinical signs of inflammation are present, such as erythema, papules, and scaling (Gougerot-Blum disease), or papules, scaling, and lichenification (eczematidlike purpura). Often, the disorder is limited to the lower extremities, but it may be extensive. Mild pruritus may be present, but there are no systemic symptoms.

Histopathology. The basic process is a lymphoid type of vasculitis, limited to the upper dermis. In early lesions the capillaries of the upper dermis, including those located in the papillae, show swelling of their endothelial cells. Small amounts of extravasated red cells usually are found in the vicinity of the capillaries (Fig. 9-4). A cellular infiltrate, consisting largely of lymphocytes together with some histiocytes and occasionally a few neutrophils, is present in the upper dermis, especially in the vicinity of the capillaries (Randall et al.; Doucas and Kapetanakis). The infiltrate may invade the epidermis and provoke mild spongiosis of the stratum malpighii and patchy parakeratosis (Mosto and Casala).

In older lesions the capillaries often show dilatation of their lumen and proliferation of their endothelium. Extravasated red cells may no longer be present, but frequently one finds hemosiderin, though in varying amounts. The inflammatory infiltrate is less pronounced than in the early stage.

Histogenesis. On electron microscopic examination, damage to the capillaries is rather mild and the cellular infiltrate consists largely of monocytes and histiocytes, rather than of lymphocytes (Berger and Hagedorn). The composition of the infiltrate thus is similar to that in Mucha-Habermann disease (see above). The presence of fairly numerous monocytes and histiocytes as well as the occasional presence of spongiosis, as seen also in contact dermatitis, suggests that purpura pigmentosa chronica represents a delayed hypersensitivity reaction (Illig and Kalkoff).

Differential Diagnosis. Purpura pigmentosa chronica may resemble stasis dermatitis because inflammation, dilatation of capillaries, extravasation of erythrocytes, and deposits of hemosiderin occur in both. However, the process extends much deeper into the dermis in stasis dermatitis, and in addition fibrosis of the dermis and fibrous thickening of the walls of medium-sized vessels in the lower dermis commonly are present (see p. 102). Anaphylactoid purpura differs from purpura pigmentosa chronica by the pre-dominance of neutrophils in the infiltrate, the presence of nuclear dust in the infiltrate, and the deposits of fibrinoid material within and around the walls of dermal vessels.

GRANULOMA FACIALE

This disorder, also called granuloma faciale eosinophilicum, consists occasionally of one but usually of several asymptomatic, soft, brownish-red, slowly enlarging patches nearly always limited to the face. Except for dilatation of the follicular openings, the surface of the skin appears normal.

Histopathology. A dense polymorphous infiltrate is found (Fig. 9-5). Although located mainly in the upper half of the dermis, it extends in some areas into the lower dermis and occasionally even into the subcutaneous tissue. Quite characteristically, the infiltrate does not invade the epidermis or the pilosebaceous appendages but is separated from them by a narrow "grenz" zone of normal collagen (Lever; Pfleger and Tappeiner).

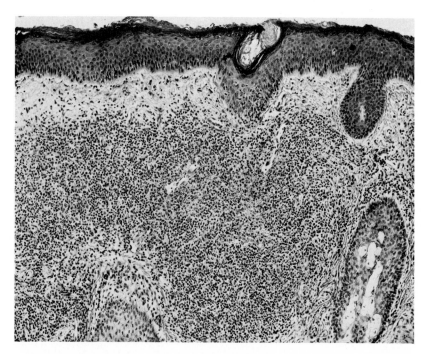

FIG. 9-5. **Granuloma faciale.** A dense infiltrate containing many eosinophils is present in the dermis. The infiltrate does not invade the epidermis or the sebaceous gland shown on the right but is separated from them by a zone of normal collagen. (×100)

Fig. 9-6. **Granuloma faciale.** Two types of cells, eosinophils and histiocytes, predominate in the inflammatory infiltrate. Some nuclei in the infiltrate are fragmented. The capillary shown is dilated and shows strongly eosinophilic fibrinoid material within and around its wall. (×400)

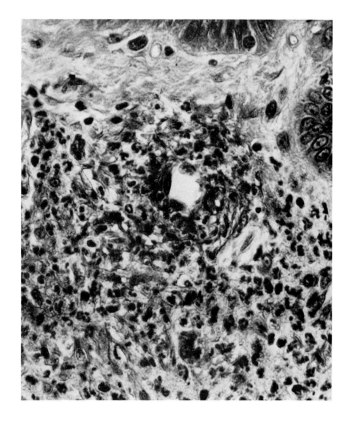

The pilosebaceous appendages are well preserved.

The polymorphous infiltrate consists, in large part, of neutrophils and eosinophils; but mononuclear cells, i.e., lymphocytes and histiocytes, as well as plasma cells and mast cells are also present. Frequently, the nuclei of some of the eosinophils and neutrophils are fragmented, thus forming nuclear dust, especially in the vicinity of the capillaries (Pinkus; Johnson et al.). There is evidence of vasculitis, since many capillaries are dilated and show strongly eosinophilic fibrinoid material within and around their walls (Fig. 9-6). A few extravasated red cells are often seen. In many cases deposits of hemosiderin are present in the upper dermis as the result of extravasation of red cells (Pedace and Perry). The presence of foam cells has been noted in a few instances (Lever; McCarthy).

Areas of fibrosis are present in some lesions; but their presence does not necessarily relate to the age of the lesion, and it does not indicate a tendency of the lesion to regress, which it seldom does.

Histogenesis. Direct immunofluorescent studies have shown IgG, IgM, IgA, and complement in the subepidermal basement zone as a thick band and around the capillaries of the upper dermis in a reticulated pattern (Schroeter et al.). The fact that three immunoglobulins are found in two different locations suggests that the reaction is nonspecific, in contrast to the reaction in allergic vasculitis (see p. 163).

Differential Diagnosis. The arrangement and the composition of the infiltrate in granuloma faciale result in a diagnostic histologic picture. Granuloma faciale shares with erythema elevatum diutinum the presence of a dense inflammatory infiltrate containing numerous neutrophils and of vasculitis. However, erythema elevatum diutinum differs from granuloma faciale by the nearly complete absence of eosinophils and by the lack of a "grenz" zone of normal collagen beneath the epidermis.

ERYTHEMA ELEVATUM DIUTINUM

This rare disorder shows persistent, brownish-red to purple papules, nodules, and plaques located in symmetrical distribution on the extensor surfaces of the extremities, on the elbows and knees, and on the dorsa of the hands and feet. At first the lesions are soft, but later they become hard as the result of fibrosis. Some patients show during the early phase of their disease bullae on normal appearing skin, and, even later on, bullae may be seen on some of the plaques (Vollum).

Extracellular cholesterosis, originally described by Urbach et al. as a lipoidosis, is now regarded as erythema elevatum diutinum with secondary lipid deposits (Herzberg; Laymon).

Histopathology. In its early stage erythema elevatum diutinum shows a dense, predominantly perivascular infiltrate composed largely of neutrophils intermingled with some mononuclear cells, and occasionally also with some eosinophils and plasma cells (Haber). Some of the neutrophils show fragmentation of their nuclei, so-called nuclear dust (Nordenskjöld and Wahlgren; Cream et al.). There is widespread vasculitis characterized by swelling of the endothelial cells and deposits of strongly eosinophilic fibrinoid material within and around the vessel walls (Mraz and Newcomer). Occasionally, one also sees a few extravasated erythrocytes (Herzberg). The bullae that are present in some patients arise subepidermally (Vollum).

In the late fibrous stage the cellular infiltrate is less pronounced, but even then neutrophils predominate (Mraz and Newcomer). The capillaries still may show deposits of fibrinoid material or show merely fibrous thickening.

The lipid material which may be present in lesions of the late fibrous stage has been deposited as a secondary event in damaged tissue. It is doubly refractile and, therefore, probably consists largely of cholesterol esters. It may be located entirely extracellularly (Urbach; Mraz and Newcomer), or both extracellularly and intracellularly (Herzberg), or entirely intracellularly (Kalkoff).

Histogenesis. Direct immunofluorescent studies have revealed perivascular deposits of IgG, IgA, IgM, complement, fibrin, transferrin and alpha-2-macroglobulin (Cream et al.). Since substances were found that, like transferrin and alpha-2-macroglobulin, are not involved in immune reactions, it is apparent that the deposits are not specific but have leaked out because of damage to the vessels.

ACUTE FEBRILE NEUTROPHILIC DERMATOSIS (SWEET)

This disorder, first described by Sweet in 1964, shows tender, raised, dark-red plaques, that usually are from 0.5 to 2.0 cm in diameter, but may be larger. They are found mainly on the face and extremities, and only rarely on the trunk. The eruption is associated with fever and leukocytosis. The eruption may last from one to eight months. There may be recurrences. Most patients are women. In about one third of the patients vesicles or pustules are seen on some of the plaques (Goldman and Moschella).

Histopathology. There is a dense perivascular infiltrate composed largely of neutrophils, many of which show leukocytoclasis (Sweet). In addition, there are some mononuclear cells, such as lymphocytes and histiocytes, and rarely a few eosinophils (Crow et al.). Although the capillaries may show endothelial swelling, there is no evidence of a true vasculitis, such as deposits of fibrinoid material around the capillaries or extravasation of red cells (Goldman and Moschella). The dermal papillae show edema which in some instances results in subepidermal blisters (Evans and Evans).

Differential Diagnosis. The prevalence of neutrophils with "nuclear dust" and presence of subepidermal blisters are found also in erythema elevatum diutinum; but acute febrile neutrophilic dermatosis lacks the perivascular fibrin deposits.

PERIARTERITIS NODOSA

Periarteritis nodosa represents a disease of largely the medium-sized muscular-type arteries. The most commonly affected arteries are those of the gastrointestinal tract, kidney, heart and muscles. The central nervous system is rarely affected, and the lungs almost never (Zeek, 1952). Also, the skin is only rarely involved in systemic periarteritis nodosa.

FIG. 9-7. **Periarteritis nodosa.** Low magnification. An artery (A) at the cutaneous-subcutaneous border shows the granulation stage of periarteritis nodosa. Above the artery is an ulcer that probably was caused by the occlusion of the artery. (×50)

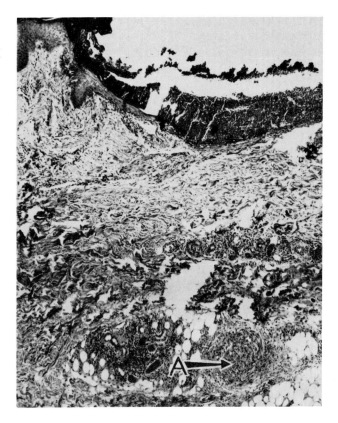

The clinical symptoms depend on the sites involved. The most common clinical manifestations are fever, weakness, abdominal pain, hypertension due to renal involvement, cardiac insufficiency, and polyneuritis with polymyositis (Arkin). Periarteritis nodosa follows an intermittent course. While nearly always fatal without treatment, early intensive corticosteroid therapy results in survival of nearly half the patients (Frohnert and Sheps). Renal insufficiency is the most common cause of death (Alarcón-Segovia and Brown).

Among the cutaneous manifestations of systemic periarteritis nodosa one observes only in rare instances the "classical" tender cutaneous-subcutaneous nodules. Such nodules, if present, may be associated with either a localized or an extensive livedo reticularis, characterized by a mottled or reticulated purplish erythema, and with ulcerations at the site of thrombosed arteries. More commonly than nodules one observes in systemic periarteritis nodosa widespread erythema, purpura and ulcerations caused by

a necrotizing vasculitis in the dermis (Borrie). In the absence of cutaneous lesions the diagnosis of periarteritis nodosa can best be established by renal biopsy (Patalano and Sommers).

Benign Cutaneous Periarteritis Nodosa. Periarteritis nodosa can occur as a benign disease limited to the skin (Fisher and Orkin; Diaz-Perez and Winkelmann). It may be associated with peripheral neuropathy (Borrie) or with Crohn's disease (Verbov and Stansfeld). In this variant cutaneous or subcutaneous nodules appear in crops, mainly on the lower extremities. In addition, focal livedo reticularis and cutaneous ulcerations are often present. After many years' duration the disease gradually subsides. Since nodules are regularly present in the benign cutaneous form and are only rarely encountered in the systemic form, they are suggestive of a good prognosis (Borrie).

Histopathology. The name *periarteritis* is misleading, for the lesions actually represent a panarteritis (Fig. 9-7). The term *nodosa* is based on the fact that the arteritis is focal and thus can cause nodose swellings (Zeek, 1952).

On a histologic basis the changes taking place in the arteries may be divided into four stages (Arkin):

In the first—the degenerative stage—foci of necrosis form, usually first in the media or the adventitia, but soon they extend also to the intima (Zeek, 1953). At the site of the necrosis a small aneurysm may form with perivascular hemorrhage when it ruptures (Zeek, 1952).

In the second—the inflammatory stage— the necrotic area within the artery is densely infiltrated with inflammatory cells, mainly neutrophils but also eosinophils and mononuclear cells (Fig. 9-8). The infiltrate extends to the perivascular tissue. The lumen of affected arteries may become thrombosed.

In the third—the granulation stage—the necrotic part of the vascular wall is replaced by granulation tissue, and the intima shows proliferation leading to partial or even complete occlusion of the lumen.

In the fourth—the fibrotic stage—the destroyed vascular wall is replaced by scar tissue. The lumen may show reduction in size, obliteration, or recanalization.

In the skin of patients with systemic periarteritis nodosa the small and medium-sized arteries at the dermal-subcutaneous border and in the subcutaneous tissue may be affected. A subcutaneous hemorrhage may occur when a small aneurysm of an affected artery ruptures. The subcutaneous nodules form as the result of reparative tissue proliferation around a necrotic artery (Alarcón-Segovia and Brown). Cutaneous ulcers result from the occlusion of an artery (Fig. 9-7). In patients with systemic periarteritis nodosa showing areas of erythema or purpura, widespread necrotizing vasculitis of the dermal capillaries is found characterized by thrombus formation and necrosis of the capillary walls with or without an inflammatory infiltrate (Ketron and Bernstein; Borrie).

The BENIGN CUTANEOUS FORM OF PERIARTERITIS NODOSA shows in the dermal-subcutaneous nodules the same histologic picture as that seen in the dermal-subcutaneous nodules of the malignant systemic form, i.e., involvement of the small and medium-

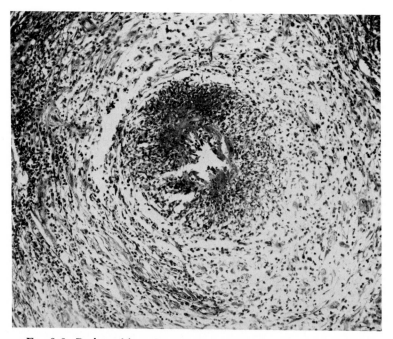

FIG. 9-8. **Periarteritis nodosa.** High magnification. An artery located in the lower dermis shows partial necrosis of its wall and invasion by inflammatory cells. (×200)

sized arteries at the dermal-subcutaneous border and in the subcutaneous fat (Miescher; Fisher and Orkin; Borrie; Diaz-Perez and Winkelmann).

Differential Diagnosis. The nodular lesions of periarteritis nodosa show a fairly diagnostic histologic picture, namely, necrosis in the small to medium-sized muscular-type arteries. The subcutaneous nodules of nodular dermal allergid show a fibrinoid vasculitis but not necrosis of vascular walls (see p. 162). In allergic granulomatosis the cutaneous or subcutaneous nodules, in addition to showing necrosis of the walls of arteries, show granulomatous lesions in the walls of arteries as well as extravascularly (see below).

ALLERGIC GRANULOMATOSIS

The separation of allergic granulomatosis from periarteritis nodosa by Churg and Strauss in 1951 has been generally accepted because, even though allergic granulomatosis shows necrotizing lesions of the medium-sized and small muscular-type arteries in nearly the same distribution as that seen in periarteritis nodosa, it differs from periarteritis nodosa by (1) respiratory symptoms, usually asthma, preceding the terminal illness by several years; (2) the presence of pulmonary infiltrations during the terminal illness in contrast to the usual absence of pulmonary lesions in periarteritis nodosa; (3) pronounced eosinophilia both in the circulating blood and in the lesions; and (4) the presence of granulomatous lesions in the walls of arteries as well as extravascularly. Cutaneous manifestations are frequent in allergic granulomatosis. They consist of cutaneous and subcutaneous nodules and of purpuric papular lesions.

After the prodromal phase of asthma has passed, the terminal illness lasts as in periarteritis nodosa from a few months to several years. Common causes of death are cardiac or renal failure and cerebral hemorrhage (Churg and Strauss). As in periarteritis nodosa, the administration of large doses of corticosteroids has improved the prognosis also of allergic granulomatosis (Varriale et al.).

Histopathology. The lesions of the small and medium-sized muscular-type arteries are the same as in periarteritis nodosa except that (1) the arteries in the lungs are also involved, (2) the walls of arteries show granulomas, and (3) similar granulomas are present in great numbers, independent of arteries (Churg and Strauss; Rose and Spencer; Varriale et al.).

The granulomas possess a central core consisting of two elements, namely, collagen imbued with fibrinoid material and degenerated cells, largely eosinophils. Around this core lie numerous epithelioid cells and multinucleated giant cells, often in a radial arrangement. Some neutrophils and lymphoid cells are present throughout the granulomas. Not infrequently, a small necrotic vessel is seen near the center of the granulomas (Churg and Strauss; Zeek, 1953).

The cutaneous and subcutaneous nodules are composed of numerous granulomas showing marked fibrinoid alteration in their center. Because of their typical appearance the histologic examination of such nodules is often very helpful in establishing the diagnosis of allergic granulomatosis (Churg and Strauss). Purpuric lesions in the skin result from the presence of a severe allergic vasculitis in dermal vessels, characterized by inflammatory infiltration and deposits of fibrinoid material (Varriale et al.).

WEGENER'S GRANULOMATOSIS

Wegener's granulomatosis, like allergic granulomatosis, represents a variant of periarteritis nodosa with sufficiently distinctive clinical and histologic findings to deserve separate consideration. It is characterized by the following triad: (1) necrotizing granulomatous lesions mainly in the upper and lower respiratory tract, such as the nose, nasal sinuses, nasopharynx, glottis, trachea, bronchi, and lungs, but often also in other viscera; (2) generalized focal necrotizing vasculitis, involving small arteries and veins, present almost always in the lungs and, more or less widely disseminated, at other sites; and (3) focal necrotizing glomerulitis, often associated with interstitial necrotizing vasculitis and granulomas in the extraglomerular tissue. The most common cause of death is uremia (Godman and Churg; Friend).

The disease begins in two thirds of the patients with upper respiratory tract symptoms, while in one third the lungs are the first organ involved (Eisner and Harper). Because of the renal involvement the prognosis is extremely grave in Wegener's granulomatosis. However, there exists a "limited" form of Wegener's granulomatosis in which in spite of the presence of massive pulmonary and extrapulmonary lesions, including cutaneous lesions, renal lesions do not develop and thus the patients stay alive (Carrington and Liebow; Cassan et al.).

Cutaneous lesions are present in the early stage of the disease in about one fourth of the patients, and at the height of the disease, in about one half of the patients (Reed et al.). Oral lesions occur in nearly all patients. The cutaneous lesions, aside from edema of the nose and crusting of the nostrils, may consist of papulonecrotic lesions (Reed et al.), nodules with central ulceration (Knoth et al.), ulcers (Godman and Churg), and, especially in the later stage of the disease, petechial or ecchymotic lesions (Budzilovich and (Wilens). Subcutaneous nodules are only rarely encountered (Fauci and Wolff). Oral lesions, in analogy with the lesions of the respiratory tract, consist of ulcers, especially on the palate, buccal mucosa, and gums (Reed et al.).

Histopathology. Of the two types of lesions, necrotizing granulomas and necrotizing vasculitis, the granulomas are characterized by variously sized, often confluent areas of necrosis surrounded by a polymorphous infiltrate containing neutrophils, lymphoid cells and plasma cells but only rarely a few eosinophils. Epithelioid cells are few or absent. Multinucleated giant cells, however, are common (Godman and Churg). The necrotizing vasculitis involving small arteries and veins is characterized by fibrinous deposits and a polymorphous inflammatory infiltrate. Whereas in some areas both type of lesions are seen, in others only one type of lesion is present (Fauci and Wolff).

The cutaneous papules usually show only a necrotizing vasculitis with thrombosis of the lumen. The thrombosis explains the frequent presence of central ulceration (Reed et al.; Fauci and Wolff). Occasionally, however, necrotizing granulomas are also present (Kraus et al.). The purpuric lesions generally show a necrotizing vasculitis with thrombosis and subsequent extravasation of erythrocytes (Budzilovich and Wilens). The cutaneous ulcers and the cutaneous and subcutaneous nodules show necrotizing granulomas either with or without necrotizing vasculitis (Knoth et al.; Kraus et al.; Fauci and Wolff). Intimal proliferation and thrombosis may obliterate the lumen of vessels to such a degree that staining of the elastic laminae may be necessary for their recognition (Knoth et al.).

Differential Diagnosis. Wegener's granulomatosis differs in its cutaneous manifestations from periarteritis nodosa by showing (1) involvement of small arteries and veins, rather than predominantly of medium-sized arteries, and (2) necrotizing granulomatous formations. The latter differ from the granulomas seen in allergic granulomatosis by the sparsity of eosinophils and by the lack of radial arrangement of the epithelioid and giant cells around the areas of necrosis.

LETHAL MIDLINE GRANULOMA OF THE FACE

The disease begins insidiously with edema of the nose and congestion of the nasal passages. This is followed by perforation of the nasal septum and ulcerations of the hard palate. Ultimately, there is extensive mutilating destruction in the center of the face, leading almost invariably to death, usually within 12 to 18 months after onset of the disease.

Histopathology. During the patient's life biopsies show, as a rule, a nonspecific, chronic inflammatory infiltrate. Still, in some instances atypical cells with hyperchromatic nuclei are seen which are suggestive of lymphoma (Resnick and Skerrett); and occasionally, the extensive examination carried out at autopsy has shown evidence of disseminated lymphoma (Walton; Kassel et al.).

In most instances, however, autopsy has not revealed evidence of systemic involvement, as one would expect if lymphoma regularly were the underlying cause of lethal midline granuloma of the face. Therefore, Walton divided the disease into classical, nonlymphomatous cases and cases with lymphoma. Kassel et al., however, concluded that, besides cases that were instances of typical lymphoma, also the so-called classical cases of lethal midline granuloma of the face represented a peculiar type of lymphoma that was not recognizable as such in the beginning. Kassel et al. have therefore suggested the term *midline malignant reticulosis* for the classical cases of lethal midline granuloma of the face. Kassel et al. have stated that, in regard to the difficulty of recognizing the process as being lymphoma in the beginning, the situation was akin to that in mycosis fungoides which in its early stage also shows only inflammation. These authors, furthermore, pointed out that it had been not only their experience but also the impression gained by Spear and Walker and by Resnick and Skerrett that on autopsy the cellular infiltrate resembled that seen in mycosis fungoides by showing cells analogous to the "mycosis cell" characterized by a large, irregular and hyperchromatic nucleus.

The view that all cases of lethal midline granuloma of the face are lymphoma, either overt lymphoma or "polymorphic reticulosis," has been expressed also by Eichel and Mabery who believe that both types might be cured by aggressive radiation in the early stage.

Differential Diagnosis. Even though in the early stage the clinical differentiation from Wegener's granulomatosis may be difficult, it is now generally agreed that lethal midline granuloma of the face is not a localized form of Wegener's granulomatosis. The main point of differentiation is that lethal midline granuloma of the face, on histologic examination, shows no evidence of arteritis.

TEMPORAL GIANT CELL ARTERITIS

Temporal arteritis may be unilateral or bilateral and may be associated with an involvement of other cranial arteries, including cerebral and retinal arteries. It occurs in the elderly and is characterized clinically by unilateral or bilateral pain of the forehead, erythema and edema of the skin overlying the involved arteries, and occasionally ulcerations of the scalp that may be linear or extensive. The involved temporal artery and its branches may be palpable. Because of the rather frequent involvement of the retinal artery sudden visual impairment in either one or both eyes is common. Usually the arteritis resolves, unless death occurs on the basis of involvement of cerebral arteries.

Histopathology. On biopsy of an obstructed temporal or other cranial artery one finds a panarteritis that is unevenly distributed (Hitch). The primary event is a degeneration of the internal elastic lamina, resulting in a digestion of the degenerated portions of the internal elastic lamina by macrophages that evolve into multinucleated giant cells (Luger and Wuketich). In addition, there is an infiltrate of mononuclear cells and plasma cells between the intima and media, and thickening of the intima by fibrinoid degeneration and fibrosis so that the lumen of the artery is reduced and even obliterated in some areas (Kinmont and McCallum).

Biopsy of a cutaneous ulceration may show at the base of the ulcer a few arteries showing proliferative changes and stenosis of the lumen similar to but less conspicuous than those usually found in the temporal artery (Barefoot and Lund).

Differential Diagnosis. In contrast to periarteritis nodosa there is no frank necrosis of the arterial wall. The presence of giant cells is of diagnostic importance. For the demonstration of the damage to the internal elastic lamina an elastic tissue stain is necessary.

MALIGNANT ATROPHIC PAPULOSIS (DEGOS)

This rare but characteristic disease begins with crops of asymptomatic, slightly raised, yellowish-red papules that gradually develop an atrophic porcelain-white center. Similar lesions may occur also on the bulbar conjuctiva and the oral mucosa. In the majority of cases systemic manifestations develop, from a few weeks to several years after the onset of the cutaneous lesions. Usually, the systemic disease consists of recurrent attacks of abdominal pain and ends in death from intestinal perforations. Less commonly, death occurs from cerebral infarctions (Winkelmann et al.). However, as pointed out by Black and Wilson Jones in 1971, of the 45 patients reported up to that time 11 had had

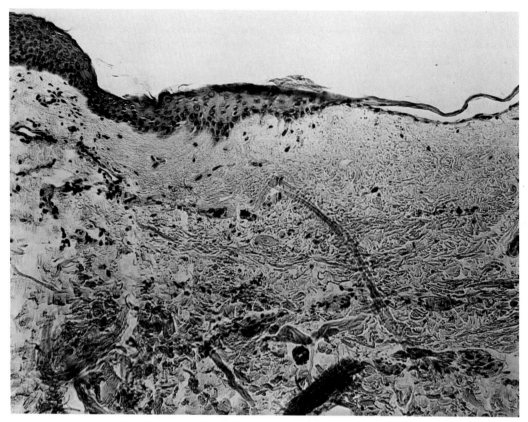

FIG. 9-9. **Malignant atrophic papulosis (Degos).** The margin of a lesion is shown. Within the lesion, consisting of an ischemic infarct, the stratum malpighii is markedly atrophic and the collagen shows hyaline degeneration with nearly complete absence of fibroblasts. (×140) (Ruben Nomland, M.D., and Jack M. Layton, M.D.)

only cutaneous lesions, with the longest period of follow-up being 14 years.

Histopathology. The essential finding in the skin is an ischemic infarct that is wedge-shaped, with the broad base located at the epidermis. It results from intimal proliferation in an arteriole located either in the lowermost dermis (Degos; Schuermann and Hornstein; Strole et al.) or in the subcutaneous fat (Kociolek et al.). The intimal proliferation may occlude the artery directly or cause occlusion by means of a thrombus.

In an early lesion the area of ischemic infarction shows swelling of the dermal collagen and an accumulation of mucin both around and within the collagen bundles (Mauss et al.; Black and Wilson Jones; Feuerman et al.). In a late lesion one finds marked atrophy of the stratum malpighii associated with slight hyperkeratosis (Fig. 9-9). Within the infarct the collagen shows hyaline degeneration with nearly complete absence of fibroblasts, and the capillaries appear indistinct because of degeneration of their walls. In such late lesions mucin can no longer be demonstrated within the necrobiotic area but only at its margins where there is a moderately dense perivascular round-cell infiltrate (Black and Wilson Jones).

The mucin present first within the necrobiotic area and later at its periphery contains acid mucopolysaccharides. Consequently it stains with alcian blue but not with PAS and shows metachromasia with toluidine blue (Mauss et al.). It should be pointed out that the affected arteriole below the area of infarction often is not seen on routine sectioning but is found only on step sectioning.

On autopsy vascular lesions are seen most commonly in the small intestine (Degos; Nomland and Layton; Strole et al.). In some instances vascular lesions are found also in the brain, the kidneys (Strole et al.), and the myocardium (Nomland and Layton); and in rare instances the brain is the only site of internal involvement (Winkelmann et al.). If lesions are present, inspection of the small intestine during autopsy reveals scattered white patches representing subserosal ischemic infarcts, analogous to those seen on the skin. In addition, areas of ulceration and perforation are found. On histologic examination, the arteries at the sites of the subserosal infarcts are occluded either by subendothelial fibrosis (Strole et al.) or by thrombosis (Degos; Nomland and Layton). In patients dying from cerebral involvement the brain shows focal infarctions associated with thrombosis of many of the small arteries and veins of that area (Winkelmann et al.).

SEGMENTAL HYALINIZING VASCULITIS (LIVEDO RETICULARIS WITH ULCERATION, ATROPHIE BLANCHE)

In this condition one observes on the lower portions of the legs, particularly on the ankles and on the dorsa of the feet, purpuric macules and recurrent, painful ulcers healing with hypopigmented atrophic areas that often are surrounded by hyperpigmentation. The disease often runs a protracted course.

Livedo reticularis, a netlike bluish discoloration of the skin of the legs may be present (Barker et al.; Feldaker et al.) or may be absent (Bard and Winkelmann). The ulcerations may be seasonal, occurring in winter (Barker et al.) or in summer (Feldaker et al.), or they may occur at irregular intervals (Gray et al.; Bard and Winkelmann; Issroff and Whiting). The healing of the ulcers with hypopigmented atrophic areas is responsible for the name atrophie blanche, first proposed by Milian in 1929. It should be noted, however, that occasionally the lesions of atrophie blanche form without preceding ulceration (Nelson; Schuppener); or ulcers follow, rather than precede, the development of the atrophic areas (Nelson). Since the essential lesion consists of a segmental hyaline intimal thickening of the dermal vessels, the term segmental hyalinizing vasculitis proposed by Bard and Winkelmann and used also by Piérard and Geerts appears preferable to the other designations.

Histopathology. Numerous capillaries of the dermis show focal endothelial proliferation and thickening of their wall caused by the deposition of eosinophilic hyaline basement membrane material that is PAS-positive and diastase-resistant. This is followed by occlusion of the lumen by a thrombus composed of loose fibrinoid material (Gray et al.; Bard and Winkelmann). Subsequently, there may be recanalization. The dermis in early lesions is apt to show hemorrhage and necrosis, and in older lesions hemosiderin deposits and fibrosis. The affected vessels are surrounded by a mild to moderate inflammatory infiltrate consisting largely of lymphoid cells and histiocytes (Gray et al.).

Histogenesis. The essential change consists of thickening of the walls of dermal capillaries brought on by the deposition of basement membrane material and resulting in ischemic infarction (Feldaker et al.; Gray et al.; Piérard and Geerts). The perivascular inflammation is a secondary phenomenon. Thus, a vasculitis in the true sense does not exist, as the designation segmental hyalinizing vasculitis chosen by Bard and Winkelmann might suggest. Rather, it seems to be a process characterized by degenerative changes in the capillary walls (Gray et al.).

Differential Diagnosis. A histologic differentiation from stasis dermatitis usually is possible, since stasis dermatitis shows only slight thickening of the capillary walls.

BIBLIOGRAPHY

Noninflammatory Purpuras

Baughman, R. D., and Sommer, R. G.: Cryoglobulinemia presenting as "factitial ulceration." Arch. Derm., *94*:725, 1966.
Case Records of the Massachusetts General Hospital, Case 29-1969: Purpura fulminans. New Eng. J. Med., *281*:153, 1969.
Chambers, W. N., Holyoke, J. B., and Wilson, R. F.: Purpura fulminans. New Eng. J. Med., *247*:933, 1952.
Craig, J. M., and Gitlin, D.: The nature of the hyaline thrombi in thrombotic thrombocytopenic purpura. Am. J. Path., *33*:251, 1957.

Cram, D. L., and Soley, R. L.: Purpura fulminans. Brit. J. Derm., *80*:323, 1968.

Cream, J. J.: Immunofluorescent studies of the skin in cryoglobulinaemic vasculitis. Brit. J. Derm., *84*:48, 1971.

Duperrat, B.: Manifestations cutanées de la cryoglobulinémie. Arch. belg. derm. syph., *13*: 310, 1957.

Ellis, F. A.: The cutaneous manifestations of cryoglobulinemia. Arch. Derm., *89*:690, 1964.

Goldberg, L. S., and Barnett, E. V.: Essential cryoglobulinemia. Arch. Int. Med., *125*:145, 1970.

Goldenfarb, P. B., and Finch, S. C.: Thrombotic thrombocytopenic purpura. JAMA, *226*:644, 1973.

Gore, J., Takada, M., and Austin, J.: Ultrastructural basis of experimental thrombocytopenic purpura. Arch. Path., *90*:197, 1970.

Haim, S., Tatarski, I., Zeltzer, M., and Amikam, S.: Disseminated intravascular coagulation presenting with cutaneous symptoms. Dermatologica, *141*:239, 1970.

Handin, R., and Smith, A. L.: Immunoidiopathic or immunogenic thrombocytopenic purpura. New Eng. J. Med., *286*:720, 1970.

Hashimoto, K., Kitabchi, A. E., Duckworth, W. C., and Robinson, N.: Ultrastructure of scorbutic human skin. Acta dermatoven., *50*:9, 1970.

Koch-Weser, J.: Coumarin necrosis. Ann. Int. Med., *68*:1365, 1968.

Luttgens, W. F.: Thrombotic thrombocytopenic purpura with extensive hemorrhagic gangrene of the skin and subcutaneous tissue. Ann. Intern. Med., *46*:1207, 1957.

McKenzie, A. W., Earle, J. H. O., Lockey, E., and Mitchell-Heggs, G. B.: Essential cryoglobulinaemia. Brit. J. Derm., *73*:22, 1961.

Nalbandian, R. M., Mader, J. J., Barrett, J. L., *et al.*: Petechiae, ecchymoses, and necrosis of skin induced by coumarin congeners. J.A.M.A., *192*:603, 1965.

Ratnoff, O. D., and Agle, D.: Psychogenic purpura: a re-evaluation of the syndrome of autoerythrocyte sensitization. Medicine, *47*:475, 1968.

Ross, R., and Benditt, E. P.: Wound healing and collagen formation. IV. Distortion of ribosomal patterns of fibroblasts in scurvy. J. Cell Biol., *22*:365, 1964.

Ruffolo, E. H., Pease, G. L., and Cooper, T.: Thrombotic thrombocytopenic purpura. Arch. Intern. Med., *110*:78, 1962.

Tattersall, R. N., and Seville, R.: Senile purpura. Quart. J. Med., *19*:151, 1950.

Umlas, J., and Kaiser, J.: Thrombohemolytic thrombocytopenic purpura (TTP). A disease or a syndrome? Am. J. Med., *49*:723, 1970.

Waldorf, D. S., and Lipkin, G.: Sensitization to erythrocytes. J.A.M.A., *203*:597, 1968.

Walker, A.: Chronic scurvy. Brit. J. Derm., *80*: 625, 1968.

Inflammatory Purpuras

Allen, D. M., Diamond, L. K., and Howell, D. A.: Anaphylactoid purpura in children (Schönlein-Henoch syndrome). Am. J. Dis. Child., *99*:833, 1960.

Ansell, B. M.: Henoch-Schönlein purpura with particular reference to the prognosis of the renal lesion. Brit. J. Derm., *82*:211, 1970.

Berger, H., and Hagedorn, M.: Elektronenmikroskopische Befunde bei der Purpura pigmentosa progressiva. Arch. Derm. Forsch., *247*:245, 1973.

Black, M. M., and Marks, R.: The inflammatory reaction in pityriasis lichenoides. Brit. J. Derm., *87*:533, 1972.

Black, M. M., and Wilson Jones, E.: "Lymphomatoid" pityriasis lichenoides: a variant with histologic features simulating a lymphoma. Brit. J. Derm., *86*:329, 1972.

Burke, D. P., Adams, R. M., and Arundell, F. D.: Febrile ulceronecrotic Mucha Habermann's disease. Arch. Derm., *100*:200, 1969.

Cochrane, G. G.: Mediators of the Arthus and related reactions. Progr. Allergy, *11*:1, 1967.

Cormane, R. H.: Neutrophilen-vermittelte Immunreaktionen. Hautarzt, *25*:254, 1974.

Degos, R., Duperrat, B., and Daniel, F.: Le parapsoriasis ulcéronécrotique hyperthermique. Ann. derm. syph., *93*:481, 1966.

Doucas, C., and Kapetanakis, J.: Eczematidlike purpura. Dermatologica, *106*:86, 1953.

Goltz, R. W., and Good, R. A.: Benign hyperglobulinemic purpura. Arch. Derm., *83*:26, 1961.

Gougerot, H., and Duperrat, B.: The nodular dermal allergides of Gougerot. Brit. J. Derm., *66*:283, 1954.

Holubar, K., Lechner, K., and Pfleger, L.: Zur Pathogenese der Purpura hyperglobulinaemica. Hautarzt, *15*:112, 1964.

Illig, L., and Kalkoff, K. W.: Zum Formenkreis der Purpura pigmentosa progressiva. Hautarzt, *21*:497, 1970.

Kawada, A., Anekoji, K., and Miyamoto, M., *et al.*: Unusual manifestation of malignant reticulosis of the skin: cutaneous lesion simulating parapsoriasis guttata. Dermatologica, *138*:369, 1969.

Kyle, R. A., Gleich, G. J., Bayrd, E. D., and Vaughan, J. H.: Benign hypergammaglobulinemic purpura of Waldenström. Medicine, *50*:113, 1971.

Laymon, C. W.: The nodular dermal allergid. Arch. Derm., *82*:163, 1960.

Macaulay, W. L.: Lymphomatoid papulosis. Arch. Derm., *97*:23, 1968.

Marks, R., Black, M., and Wilson Jones, E.: Pityriasis lichenoides. Brit. J. Derm., *86*: 215, 1972.

McCombs, R. P.: Systemic "allergic" vasculitis. J.A.M.A., *194*:1059, 1965.

Mosto, S. J., and Casala, A. M.: Disseminated pruriginous angiodermatitis (itching purpura). Arch. Derm., *91*:351, 1965.

Muller, S. A., and Schulze, T. W., Jr.: Mucha-Habermann disease mistaken for reticulum cell sarcoma. Arch. Derm., *103*:423, 1971.

Nasemann, T., Markowski, R., and Jakubowicz, K.: Zur histologischen Differentialdiagnose der Pityriasis lichenoides et varioliformis acuta Mucha-Habermann. Hautarzt, *17*:395, 1966.

Nir, M. A., Pick, A. I., Schreibman, S., and Feuerman, E. J.: Mixed IgG-IgM cryoglobulinemia with follicular pustular purpura. Arch. Derm., *109*:539, 1974.

Perrot, H., Leung, T. K., Leung, J., *et al.*: Etude ultrastructurale des lesions vasculaires dermiques du trisyndrome de Gougerot (vasculite leucocytoclasique). Arch. derm. Forsch., *241*:44, 1971.

Pfleger, L.: Zur Pathogenese unklarer Purpuraformen. Arch. Derm. Syph., *197*:187, 1954.

Piérard, J., and Van Steenbergen, E. P.: A propos du parapsoriasis varioliforme et de son histologie. Ann. derm. syph., *84*:630, 1957.

Randall, S. J., Kierland, R. R., and Montgomery, H.: Pigmented purpuric eruptions. Arch. Derm. Syph., *64*:177, 1951.

Ruiter, M.: Über die sogenannte Arteriolitis (Vasculitis) allergica cutis. Hautarzt, *8*: 293, 1957.

————: Vascular fibrinoid in cutaneous "allergic" arteriolitis. J. Invest. Derm., *38*:85, 1962.

Ruiter, M., and Hadders, H. N.: Predominantly cutaneous form of necrotizing angiitis. J. Path. Bact., *77*:71, 1959.

Ruiter, M., and Molenaar, I.: Ultrastructural changes in arteriolitis (vasculitis) allergica cutis superficialis. Brit. J. Derm., *83*:14, 1970.

Schimpf, A., and Pons, F.: Zum Krankheitsbild des Pseudolymphoma cutis ("lymphomatoid papulosis" Macaulay). Z. Haut, *48*:913, 1973.

Schroeter, A. L., Copeman, P. W. M., Jordon, R. E., *et al.*: Immunofluorescence of cutaneous vasculitis associated with systemic disease. Arch. Derm., *104*:254, 1971.

Shapiro, C. M., Texidor, T. A., Robbins, K. C., and Rabiner, S. F.: Clinical remission of purpura hyperglobulinemica. Arch. Int. Med., *124*:81, 1969.

Szymanski, F. J.: Pityriasis lichenoides et varioliformis acuta. Arch. Derm., *79*:7, 1959.

Valentino, L. A., and Helwig, E. B.: Lymphomatoid papulosis. Arch. Path., *96*:409, 1973.

Wang, P., Hofmann, N., and Hornstein, O. P.: CAF-elektrophoretische und immunelektrophoretische Untersuchungen bei Patienten mit Vasculitis allergica Ruiter. Arch. Derm. Forsch., *246*:222, 1973.

Winkelmann, R. K., and Ditto, W. B.: Cutaneous and visceral syndromes of necrotizing or "allergic" angiitis. Medicine, *43*:59, 1964.

Zeek, P. M.: Periarteritis nodosa and other forms of necrotizing angiitis. New Eng. J. Med., *248*:764, 1953.

Granuloma Faciale

Johnson, W. C., Higdon, R. S., and Helwig, E. B.: Granuloma faciale. Arch. Derm., *79*: 42, 1959.

Lever, W. F.: Eosinophilic granuloma of the skin: its relation to erythema elevatum diutinum and eosinophilic granuloma of the bone. Arch. Derm. Syph., *55*:194, 1947.

McCarthy, P. L.: Granuloma faciale. Arch. Derm., *77*:458, 1958.

Pedace, F. J., and Perry, H. O.: Granuloma faciale. Arch. Derm., *94*:387, 1966.

Pfleger, L., and Tappeiner, S.: Über das eosinophile Granulom des Gesichtes. Arch. f. Derm. u. Syph., *193*:1, 1951.

Pinkus, H.: Granuloma faciale. Dermatologica, *105*:85, 1952

Schroeter, A. L., Copeman, P. W. M., Jordon, R. E., *et al.*: Immunofluorescence of cutaneous vasculitis associated with systemic disease. Arch. Derm., *104*:254, 1971.

Erythema Elevatum Diutinum

Cream, J. J., Levine, G. M., and Calnan, D. D.: Erythema elevatum diutinum. Brit. J. Derm., *84*:393, 1971.

Haber, H.: Erythema elevatum diutinum. Brit. J. Derm., *67*:121, 1955.

Herzberg, J. J.: Die extracelluläre Cholesterinose (Kerl-Urbach), eine Variante des Erythema elevatum diutinum. Arch. klin. exp. Derm., *205*:447, 1958.

Kalkoff, K. W.: Zur Behandlung des Erythema elevatum diutinum mit 3-sulfanilamido-6-methoxypyridazin (Lederkyn). Derm. Wschr., *142*:788, 1960.

Laymon, C. W.: Erythema elevatum diutinum. Arch. Derm., *85*:22, 1962.

Mraz, J. P., and Newcomer, V. D.: Erythema elevatum diutinum. Arch. Derm., *96*:235, 1967.

Nordenskjöld, A., and Wahgren, F.: Erythema elevatum diutinum. Acta dermatoven., *40*:317, 1960.

Urbach, E., Epstein, E., and Lorenz, K.: Extrazelluläre Cholesterinose. Arch. f. Derm. u. Syph., *166*:243, 1932.

Vollum, D. I.: Erythema elevatum diutinum—vesicular lesions and sulphone response. Brit. J. Derm., *80*:178, 1968.

Acute Febrile Neutrophilic Dermatosis (Sweet)

Crow, K. D., Kerdel-Vegas, F., and Rook, A.: Acute febrile neutrophilic dermatosis. Sweet's syndrome. Dermatologica, *139*:123, 1969.

Evans, S., and Evans, C. C.: Acute febrile neutrophilic dermatosis. Two cases. Dermatologica, *143*:153, 1971.

Goldman, G. C., and Moschella, S. L.: Acute febrile neutrophilic dermatosis (Sweet's syndrome). Arch. Derm., *103*:654, 1971.

Sweet, R. D.: An acute febrile dermatosis. Brit. J. Derm., *76*:349, 1964.

Periarteritis Nodosa, Allergic Granulomatosis, Wegener's Granulomatosis

Alarcón-Segovia, D., and Brown, A. L.: Classification and etiologic aspects of necrotizing angiitides. Proc. Mayo Clin., *39*:205, 1964.

Arkin, A.: A clinical and pathological study of periarteritis nodosa. Am. J. Path., *6*:401, 1930.

Borrie, P.: Cutaneous polyarteritis nodosa. Brit. J. Derm., *87*:87, 1972.

Budzilovich, G. N., and Wilens, S. L.: Fulminating Wegener's granulomatosis. Arch. Path., *70*:653, 1960.

Carrington, C. B., and Liebow, A. A.: Limited forms of angiitis and granulomatosis of Wegener's type. Am. J. Med., *41*:497, 1966.

Cassan, S. M., Coles, D. T., and Harrison, E. G., Jr.: The concept of limited forms of Wegener's granulomatosis. Am. J. Med., *49*:366, 1970.

Churg, J., and Strauss, L.: Allergic granulomatosis, allergic angiitis, and periarteritis nodosa. Am. J. Path., *27*:277, 1951.

Diaz-Perez, J. L., and Winkelmann, R. K.: Cutaneous periarteritis nodosa. Arch. Derm., *110*:407, 1974.

Eisner, B., and Harper, F. B.: Disseminated Wegener's granulomatosis with breast involvement. Arch. Path., *87*:545, 1969.

Fauci, A. S., and Wolff, S. M.: Wegener's granulomatosis: studies in eighteen patients and a review of the literature. Medicine, *52*:535, 1973.

Fisher, I., and Orkin, M.: Cutaneous form of periarteritis nodosa. Arch. Derm., *89*:180, 1964.

Friend, D. S.: Wegener's granulomatosis. Arch. Intern. Med., *111*:703, 1963.

Frohnert, P. P., and Sheps, S. G.: Long-term follow-up study of periarteritis nodosa. Am. J. Med., *43*:8, 1967.

Godman, G. C., and Churg, J.: Wegener's granulomatosis. Arch. Path., *58*:533, 1954.

Ketron, L. W., and Bernstein, J. C.: Cutaneous manifestations of periarteritis nodosa. Arch. Derm. Syph., *40*:929, 1939.

Knoth, W., Beneke, G., and Kuntz, E.: Zur Kenntnis der Wegenerschen Granulomatose. Hautarzt, *16*:289, 1965.

Kraus, Z., Vortel, V., Fingerland, A., *et al.*: Unusual cutaneous manifestations in Wegener's granulomatosis. Acta dermatoven., *45*:288, 1965.

Miescher, G.: Über kutane Formen der Periarteritis nodosa. Dermatologica, *92*:225, 1946.

Patalano, V. J., and Sommers, S. C.: Biopsy diagnosis of periarteritis nodosa. Arch. Path., *72*:1, 1961.

Reed, W. B., Jensen, A. K., Konwaler, B. E., and Hunter, D.: The cutaneous manifestations in Wegener's granulomatosis. Acta dermatoven., *43*:250, 1963.

Rose, G. A., and Spencer, H.: Polyarteritis nodosa. Quart. J. Med., *50*:43, 1957.

Ruiter, M.: The so-called cutaneous type of periarteritis nodosa. Brit. J. Derm., *70*:102, 1958.

Varriale, P., Minogue, W. F., and Alfenito, J. C.: Allergic granulomatosis. Arch. Intern. Med., *113*:235, 1964.

Verbov, J., and Stansfeld, A. G.: Cutaneous polyarteritis nodosa and Crohn's disease. Trans. St. John's Hosp. Derm. Soc., *58*:261, 1972.

Zeek, P. M.: Periarteritis nodosa: a critical review. Am. J. Clin. Path., *22*:777, 1952.

————: Periarteritis nodosa and other forms of necrotizing angiitis. New Eng. J. Med., *248*:764, 1953.

Lethal Midline Granuloma of the Face

Eichel, B. S., and Mabery, T. E.: The enigma of the lethal midline granuloma. Laryngoscope, *78*:1367, 1968.

Kassel, S. H., Echevarria, R. E., and Guzzo, F. P.: Midline malignant reticulosis (so-called lethal midline granuloma). Cancer, *23*:920, 1969.

Resnick, N., and Skerrett, P. V.: Lethal midline granuloma of the face. Arch. Intern. Med., *103*:116, 1959.

Spear G. S., and Walker, W. G.: Lethal midline granuloma (granuloma gangrenescens) at autopsy. Bull. Johns Hopkins Hosp., *99*:313, 1956.

Walton, E.: Reticulo-endothelial sarcoma arising in the nose and palate (granuloma gangrenescens). Am. J. Clin. Path., *13*:279, 1960.

Temporal Giant Cell Arteritis

Barefoot, S. W., and Lund, H. Z.: Temporal (giant cell) arteritis associated with ulcerations of scalp. Arch. Derm., *93*:79, 1966.

Hitch, J. M.: Dermatologic manifestations of giant-cell (temporal, cranial) arteritis. Arch. Derm., *101*:409, 1970.

Kinmont, P. D. C., and McCallum, D. I.: Skin manifestations of giant-cell arteritis. Brit. J. Derm., *76*:299, 1964.

Luger, A., and Wuketich, S.: Kopfschwartennekrose bei temporaler Riesenzellarteriitis. Derm. Wschr., *153*:89, 1967.

Malignant Atrophic Papulosis

Black, M. M., and Wilson Jones, E.: Malignant atrophic papulosis (Degos syndrome). Brit. J. Derm., *85*:290, 1971.

Degos, R.: Malignant atrophic papulosis: a fatal cutaneo-intestinal syndrome. Brit. J. Derm., *66*:304, 1954.

Feuerman, E. J., Dollberg, L., and Salvador, O.: Malignant atrophic papulosis with mucin in the dermis. Arch. Path., *90*:310, 1970.

Kociolek, M., Winiarski, J., and Gina, J.: Papulosis atrophicans maligna Degos. Derm. Monatsschr., *155*:55, 1969.

Mauss, J., Reichenberger, M., and Zambal, S.: Papulosis atrophicans maligna (Degos). Hautarzt, *20*:389, 1969.

Nomland, R., and Layton, J. M.: Malignant papulosis with atrophy (Degos). Fatal cutaneointestinal syndrome. Arch. Derm., *81*:181, 1960.

Schuermann, H., and Hornstein, O.: Papulosis atrophicans maligna. Hautarzt, *13*:531, 1962.

Strole, W. E., Jr., Clark, W. H., Jr., and Isselbacher, K. J.: Progressive arterial occlusive disease (Köhlmeyer-Degos). New Eng. J. Med., *276*:195, 1967.

Winkelmann, R. K., Howard, F. M., Perry, H. O., and Miller, R. H.: Malignant papulosis of skin and cerebrum. Arch. Derm., *87*:54, 1963.

Segmental Hyalinizing Vasculitis

Bard, I. W., and Winkelmann, R. K.: Livedo vasculitis. Arch. Derm., *96*:489, 1967.

Barker, N. W., Hines, E. A., Jr., and Craig, W. M.: Livedo reticularis: a peripheral arteriolar disease. Am. Heart J., *21*:592, 1941.

Feldaker, M., Hines, E. A., Jr., and Kierland, R. R.: Livedo reticularis with summer ulcerations. Arch. Derm., *72*:31, 1955.

Gray, H. R., Graham, J. H., Johnson, W., and Burgoon, C. F., Jr.: Atrophie blanche: Periodic painful ulcers of the lower extremities. Arch. Derm., *93*:187, 1966.

Issroff, S. W., and Whiting, D. A.: Low molecular weight dextran in the treatment of livedo reticularis with ulceration. Brit. J. Derm., *85*(suppl. 7):26, 1971.

Milian, G.: Les atrophies cutanées syphilitiques. Bull. Soc. franç. derm. syph., *36*:865, 1929.

Nelson, L. M.: Atrophie blanche en plaque. Arch. Derm., *72*:242, 1955.

Piérard, J., and Geerts, M. L.: Vascularite hyalisante segmentaire (Livedo vasculitis). Arch. belg. derm. syph., *27*:103, 1971.

Schuppener, H. J.: Zur Kenntnis der Atrophia alba (atrophie blanche Milian). Arch. klin. exp. Derm., *204*:500, 1957.

10

Inflammatory Diseases of the Epidermal Appendages and of Cartilage

ACNE VULGARIS

Acne vulgaris occurs predominantly during adolescence and in early adult life. It affects mainly the face, the upper back, and the upper chest. Clinically, two types of lesions occur. One is the comedo located either in an open follicle as a "blackhead" or in a closed follicle as a "whitehead." The second type of lesion is inflammatory and begins either as a follicular papule that may evolve into a pustule, or as a nodule that may evolve into a cyst. Inflammatory lesions only rarely develop at sites of comedones, but usually arise in normal-appearing follicles.

Histopathology. A comedo contains keratinized cells, sebum and some microorganisms; but in routinely fixed sections one sees only keratinized cells, since fixation has removed the lipid material. The black color at the tip of open comedones is due to melanin (see below).

The follicular papules of acne are characterized by a predominantly lymphocytic perifollicular infiltrate. On careful searching one may find small areas of beginning disintegration of the follicular wall (Strauss and Kligman).

Pustules in intrafollicular location and containing predominantly neutrophils usually form after the follicular wall has ruptured. Only rarely is the pustule caused by a bacterial, impetiginous folliculitis (Strauss and Kligman).

Nodules occur at the sites of ruptured follicles where sebum, free fatty acids, bacteria and keratinized cells have escaped from the follicle into the dermis. The perifollicular infiltrate may develop into a cyst containing numerous neutrophils and, in addition, mononuclear cells, plasma cells, and foreign body giant cells. Frequently, keratin particles are seen near giant cells.

During healing the inflammatory infiltrate is replaced by fibrosis. Also, epidermis from the remaining follicular wall may grow around and encapsulate part of the inflammatory mass (Strauss and Kligman).

Histogenesis. The most important factor in the development of the acne lesion seems to be the erosion and subsequent disruption of the follicular wall. Since it is generally agreed that the fatty acids are the only component of the follicular content capable of producing a sufficiently severe irritation to bring about an erosion and disruption of the follicular wall, the following hypothesis regarding the pathogenesis of acne is favored by many (Van Scott and McCardle; Strauss and Pochi, 1965; Freinkel):

At puberty, under the influence of androgens, the sebaceous glands develop, the follicular walls hypertrophy, and some of the enlarged follicular walls mechanically block the flow of sebum from the follicle. Bacteria flourish in this nutrient-rich environment, and *Corynebacterium acnes* is especially favored by the relative anaerobiasis within the follicle. The lipolytic enzymes elaborated by *C. acnes* act on the sebum triglycerides to produce the fatty acids which are capable of eroding and disrupting the follicular wall and thus allow the follicular content to enter the dermis.

The theory attributing a key role to the lipase elaborated by *C. acnes* in causing follicular ruptures is supported by the fact that tetracycline exerts a pronounced bacteriostatic effect on *C. acnes;* and suppression of *C. acnes* and of its lipolytic action would seem to explain the beneficial effect of tetracycline on acne vulgaris (Freinkel et al.; Puhvel and Reisner).

Even though sebaceous secretion is usually increased in acne and the sebaceous secretion is androgen-stimulated, there is, according to Strauss and Pochi (1969), no evidence of overproduction of androgens in patients with acne vulgaris, with the rare exceptions when acne is secondary to the presence of an ovarian tumor or secondary to Cushing's syndrome. However, the recent finding by Sansone and Reisner that skin with acne converts testosterone to dihydrotestosterone at a rate 2 to 20 times greater than normal skin is significant because it indicates that, even though acne vulgaris is not a systemic hormonal disorder, it may be caused by a hormonal disturbance in its target organ, the sebaceous gland.

The difference in melanin content between open and closed comedones is due to the fact that the melanocytes normally present in the upper portion of the infundibulum produce very little melanin in closed comedones; whereas in open comedones numerous, large, enzymatically active melanocytes are present (Kaidbey and Kligman).

ACNE ROSACEA

Acne rosacea affects mainly the center of the face, but occasionally also the sides of the face. Three types of acne rosacea occur: the erythematous telangiectatic type, the glandular hyperplastic type, and the papular type. These three types may occur together. The erythematous telangiectatic type often shows, besides erythema and telangiectasia, follicular pustules and occasionally cystic nodules. The glandular hyperplastic type causes an enlargement of the

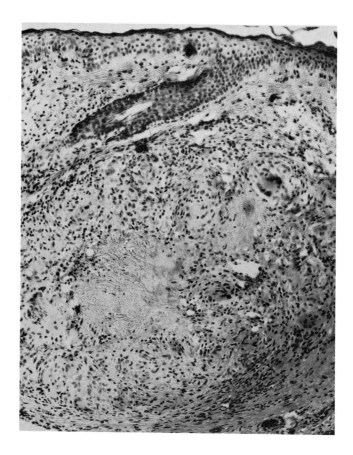

FIG. 10-1. **Acne rosacea, papular type.** A tubercle showing central necrosis and at its periphery an inflammatory infiltrate is present. Formerly a lesion of this type was diagnosed as *lupus miliaris disseminatus faciei.* (×100)

nose called rhinophyma. The papular type shows numerous moderately firm, slightly raised papules 1 to 3 mm in diameter, usually associated with erythema. Formerly, some cases of papular acne rosacea were mistakenly diagnosed as either rosacealike tuberculid or lupus miliaris disseminatus faciei because of the presence of granulomatous "tuberculoid" formations on histologic examination (see below, under Histogenesis).

Histopathology. In the erythematous telangiectatic type of acne rosacea a nonspecific inflammatory infiltrate is present in the dermis, often arranged around dilated capillaries (Marks and Harcourt-Webster). As in acne vulgaris, the pustules consist of intrafollicular accumulations of neutrophils, and the cystic nodules are made up of intradermal accumulations of neutrophils, mononuclear cells, plasma cells and foreign body giant cells.

In the glandular hyperplastic type of acne rosacea the sebaceous glands are increased in size and number. The sebaceous ducts are dilated and filled with keratinous material. In addition, the capillaries are dilated and a chronic inflammatory infiltrate is present in the upper dermis (Marks and Harcourt-Webster).

In the papular type of acne rosacea the papules may show merely a nonspecific chronic inflammatory infiltrate. Frequently, however, small groups of epithelioid cells are found scattered in the round-cell infiltrate, and occasionally the papules contain quite typical tubercles composed of epithelioid cells and a few giant cells surrounded by a round-cell infiltrate. A tuberculoid infiltrate was found in 10 per cent of their cases of acne rosacea by Laymon and Schoch; in 11 per cent by Marks and Harcourt-Webster, and in 21 per cent by van Ketel. Necrosis in the tubercles may be absent or present (Fig. 10-1). In some cases one may find islands of epithelioid cells with only a slight admixture of lymphoid cells, as seen in sarcoidosis; and occasionally such "naked" tubercles predominate in the infiltrate (Fig. 10-2) (Laymon).

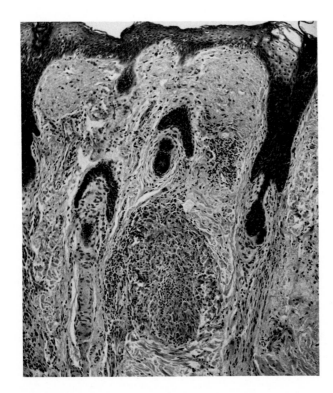

Fig. 10-2. **Acne rosacea, papular type.** An epithelioid cell tubercle showing no necrosis and only a very slight inflammatory infiltrate at its periphery is present, resembling sarcoidosis. Formerly a lesion of this type was diagnosed as *rosacealike tuberculid.* (×100)

Histogenesis. The realization that granulomatous, "tuberculoid" formations can be present in lesions of papular acne rosacea and that their presence does not indicate the existence of tuberculosis or of a tuberculid has come only very slowly; and even nowadays some authors continue the tradition of featuring rosacealike, or micropapular, tuberculid and lupus miliaris disseminatus faciei as tuberculids.

According to this traditional view, micropapular tuberculid shows a tuberculoid granuloma with little or no central caseation; whereas in lupus miliaris disseminatus faciei the tuberculoid granuloma shows a large focus of central caseation.

The impossibility of separating micropapular tuberculid and lupus miliaris disseminatus faciei either on a clinical or a histologic basis is evident in a recent article by Scott and Calnan describing 12 cases, of which 4 showed caseation in the center of the granuloma and 8 showed noncaseating granulomas. The authors found no proof of a tuberculous genesis and used as diagnostic designation the term *acne agminata*. They hesitate to identify acne agminata with the papular type of acne rosacea because erythema and telangiectasia regarded by them as prerequisites for a diagnosis of acne rosacea were absent. In contrast to the view expressed by Scott and Calnan, many other authors have regarded micropapular tuberculid as identical with rosacealike tuberculid and both conditions as representing acne rosacea (Laymon and Schoch; Michelson; van Ketel; Mullanax and Kierland). Even a special term, *lupoid rosacea* was introduced by Laymon.

Some authors, such as Flegel, and Pinkus and Mehregan, even though they no longer regard lupus miliaris disseminatus faciei as a tuberculid, still regard it as an entity. On the other hand, Strauss regards it as related to acne rosacea, since a follow-up study revealed that in 7 of his 13 patients the eruption of lupus miliaris disseminatus faciei was followed by acne rosacea either of the papular ("lupoid") type or of the erythematous type.

The presence of tuberculoid structures with or without central caseation in acne rosacea usually is explained as a foreign-body reaction against keratinized cells of disintegrating hair structures. However, Grosshans et al. regard the granulomatous formations as a delayed hypersensitivity reaction to the mite *Demodex* folliculorum since they frequently found particles of *Demodex* folliculorum in the granulomas of acne rosacea on serial sections.

Differential Diagnosis. The tuberculoid granulomas may be suggestive of lupus vulgaris in the presence of central caseation and of sarcoidosis in its absence. As a matter of fact, a differentiation of acne rosacea from lupus vulgaris or sarcoidosis may be impossible on histologic grounds. It is a good rule never to make a diagnosis of tuberculosis or sarcoidosis on biopsy specimens obtained from the face without adequate supporting evidence.

DISSEMINATE INFUNDIBULO-FOLLICULITIS

This eruption, first described by Hitch and Lund in 1968, consists of firm, closely set, skin-colored, follicular papules having the appearance of exaggerated cutis anserina. The trunk and proximal portions of the extremities are the areas of predilection. The eruption usually is recurrent but may be persistent (Wolf and Tolmach).

Histopathology. The histologic findings, although not specific, are characteristic. There is spongiosis of the uppermost portion of the hair follicle, the so-called infundibulum. The adjoining dermis shows a fairly mild inflammatory infiltrate. Exocytosis of inflammatory cells from the dermis into the spongiotic areas is usually seen (Hitch and Lund, 1968 and 1972).

TRICHORRHEXIS INVAGINATA (NETHERTON)

In this nearly always recessively inherited condition occurring almost exclusively in the female, the scalp hair is short, sparse and brittle. Trichorrhexis invaginata usually is found in association with ichthyosis linearis circumflexa, characterized by migratory polycyclic lesions of erythema (Hurwitz et al.) (see p. 62). In a few instances, however, as in Netherton's original case, trichorrhexis invaginata has been found to be associated with the recessive type of congenital ichthyosiform erythroderma (see p. 61).

Histopathology. Trichorrhexis invaginata or bamboo hair, on histologic examination of a scalp biopsy or on microscopic examination of a plucked hair, shows invagination of the distal portion of the hair shaft (as "ball") into its proximal portion (as "cup") (Altman and Stroud).

Histogenesis. The invagination of the hair results from a transient defect in the keratinization of both hair shaft and inner root sheath in the keratogenous zone of the hair so that the inner root sheath no longer can act as a splint and the distal portion of the hair is wedged into its proximal portion (Julius and Keeran).

TRICHOSTASIS SPINULOSA

Clinically one observes slightly raised follicular spines resembling comedones in the center of the face of older persons (Braun-Falco and Vakilzadeh). The same condition may occur occasionally on the trunk and limbs and may affect also younger persons (Sarkany and Gaylarde).

Histopathology. Each affected hair follicle contains in its infundibular portion numerous hairs, usually between 6 and 20 hairs, enveloped in a keratinous sheath (Sarkany and Gaylarde).

Histogenesis. The retained hairs are telogen or club hairs of the vellus type that all have been produced successively by the same hair matrix and have not been shed because of an abnormal angulation between the infraseboglandular and the supraseboglandular portions of the hair follicle (Braun-Falco and Vakilzadeh).

ALOPECIA AREATA

Alopecia areata is characterized by complete or nearly complete absence of hair in one or several circumscribed areas. There is no visible evidence of inflammation. The scalp is the most common site of lesions. In most cases there is complete regrowth of hair. In occasional instances the entire scalp is involved (alopecia totalis) as well as other hair-bearing portions of the skin (alopecia universalis). In such cases the loss of hair usually is permanent.

Histopathology. In the vicinity of expanding patches of alopecia areata where hair usually can be pulled out easily one finds a significant increase in the percentage of telogen or club hairs. Thus, Van Scott found in biopsies obtained from patches of alopecia areata an increase in the percentage of telogen hairs from an average of 26 per cent to 42 per cent. The "telogenization" and subsequent shedding of hair is followed by the appearance of early anagen hairs that seem

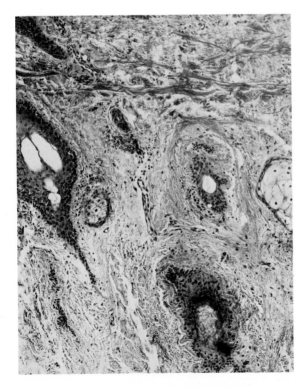

Fig. 10-3. **Alopecia areata, scalp.** In the center are two small hair structures, each surrounded by a thick sheath of connective tissue representing the fibrous root sheath; they are early anagen hair. The hair structure on the left with an epithelial column extending downward from it into a fibrous root sheath represents a telogen hair. (×50)

to be restrained from proceeding beyond this stage. The entire hair appears diminutive, including its papilla. The bulb of such early anagen hairs is located, on the average, only 2 mm below the skin surface, rather than 3.5 mm, as is the bulb of normal anagen hair (Van Scott). A thick, homogenized connective tissue stalk representing the fibrous root sheath extends from each early anagen hair downward to the original depth of the hair bulb (Fig. 10-3). An inner root sheath is present in each of the early anagen hair structures, but the hair itself is thin, short and incompletely keratinized. The sebaceous glands, however, are not altered in their size or appearance.

A chronic inflammatory infiltrate composed of mononuclear cells is found around the bulbs of the early anagen hairs. This infiltrate is present even in cases of many years' duration (Goos). It often extends into the hair bulb and external root sheath of the early anagen hairs, and may extend also into the connective tissue stalk beneath each early anagen hair. The infiltrate is seen extending to the surface epidermis only in early, rapidly advancing cases where it then may cause spongiosis of the lower portion of the surface epidermis (Goos). The inflammatory infiltrate around the early anagen hair bulbs appears loosely arranged, surrounding them like a "swarm of bees" (Kalkoff and Macher).

Histogenesis. On the basis of the good response of alopecia areata to corticosteroids it appears likely that the inflammatory infiltrate represents the primary event and that secondarily, through an enzymatic disturbance, it causes telogenization, shedding of the telogen hair and arrest of growth in the early anagen stage of the hair (Braun-Falco and Zaun). The early anagen hairs, although arrested in their growth, show an intensive alkaline phosphatase activity in their papillae (Kopf and Orentreich).

Differential Diagnosis. For differentiation from trichotillomania, see below.

TRICHOTILLOMANIA

Although the temporary hair loss resulting from compulsive hair pulling does not result in well demarcated patches of alopecia as they are usually seen in alopecia areata,

differentiation between the two conditions on clinical grounds can be almost impossible, since occasionally also alopecia areata may show a "moth-eaten" type of thinning of the hair.

Histopathology. The most striking histologic finding in trichotillomania is the presence of many hairs in the catagen stage characterized by the transformation of the follicular epithelium in the lower portion of the follicles into a cord of undifferentiated basaloid cells. The hair shaft in such follicles may appear soft and wrinkled (Mehregan).

No perifollicular inflammatory infiltrate is present; but, as the result of the trauma of extracting hair, small areas of hemorrhage may be found within and around involuting hair follicles. The follicular infundibulum may contain no hair but may be dilated through the presence of a keratin plug (Muller and Winkelmann).

Differential Diagnosis. A histologic differentiation of alopecia areata from trichotillomania is usually possible, since alopecia areata, in contrast to trichotillomania, shows numerous early anagen hairs and a loosely arranged perifollicular inflammatory infiltrate.

ALOPECIA CICATRISATA (PSEUDOPELADE BROCQ)

In alopecia cicatrisata, also referred to as pseudopelade of Brocq, one finds scattered through the scalp irregularly defined and confluent patches of alopecia that in the early stage may show mild perifollicular erythema but in the late stage show smooth atrophy without any signs of inflammation. Characteristically, a few solitary hairs often persist for a long time within the patches of atrophy.

Histopathology. In the early stage one finds a moderately severe, predominantly perifollicular infiltrate composed of mononuclear cells. The infiltrate is present around the upper and middle thirds of the hair follicles but spares the lower third (Miescher and Lenggenhager). It invades the walls of the follicles and the sebaceous glands. A mild inflammatory infiltrate occasionally is seen also around the subpapillary vessels (Laymon). Slight follicular hyperkeratosis may be present (Miescher and Lenggen-hager). Gradually, the infiltrate destroys the hair follicles and the sebaceous glands.

In the late stage there is extensive fibrosis of the dermis with only traces of an inflammatory infiltrate. The follicles and the sebaceous glands are absent, but the arrectores pilorum and sweat glands often are still preserved, at least in part.

Histogenesis. Several authors (Spier and Keilig; Gay Prieto; Waldorf; Cram et al.) believe that alopecia cicatrisata represents lichen planopilaris of the scalp. They point out that (1) in occasional cases of alopecia cicatrisata lesions of lichen planopilaris are found outside the scalp; (2) the histologic appearance of the perifollicular infiltrate in the scalp is very similar in both diseases; and (3) in some cases of alopecia cicatrisata histologic examination reveals, in addition to the perifollicular infiltrate, the presence of extrafollicular, subepidermal infiltrates having the same histologic appearance as lichen planus. Altman and Perry assume that there are two forms of lichen planopilaris: an acute form having distinct follicular spinous lesions, and a chronic form showing only slight follicular keratosis but ending in atrophy, and that the latter form is identical with alopecia cicatrisata.

Other authors, however (Laymon; Miescher and Lenggenhager; Keining and Rathjens; Ronchese), maintain that alopecia cicatrisata differs clinically and histologically from lichen planopilaris and therefore should be maintained as a disease entity.

Degos et al., and Juon have denied the existence of alopecia cicatrisata as an autonomous disease on the basis that it represents the atrophic final stage of several scarring diseases, including not only lichen planopilaris but also chronic discoid lupus erythematosus, circumscribed scleroderma and folliculitis decalvans. All these diseases, according to Degos et al., and Juon, may end in a "pseudopeladic state." It can be maintained, however, that circumscribed scleroderma and folliculitis decalvans in their active phase are quite distinct from alopecia cicatrisata. This then leaves lichen planus and discoid lupus erythematosus as the two diseases that may be indistinguishable from alopecia cicatrisata throughout their course, clinically as well as histologically. The possibility exists that all cases of alopecia cicatrisata represent either lichen planus or lupus erythematosus and that alopecia cicatrisata does not exist as an independent disease (Male).

Differential Diagnosis. In typical cases of discoid lupus erythematosus, in contrast to alopecia cicatrisata, the inflammatory infiltrate not only is located around hair follicles and sebaceous glands but also is distributed in a patchy fashion throughout the dermis. In addition, the basal layer of the epidermis, and often also the basal layer of the outer root sheath, shows liquefaction degeneration. Also, there is more pronounced hyperkeratosis not limited to the follicles.

Circumscribed scleroderma is characterized by thickening and homogenization of the collagen bundles extending into the subcutaneous tissue. Flattening of the surface epidermis occurs only in the late stage.

Folliculitis decalvans, which represents a folliculitis of the scalp, shows in its early stage intrafollicular pustules. Often, the perifollicular infiltrate contains a good number of plasma cells, which are absent in alopecia cicatrisata (Miescher and Lenggenhager).

ALOPECIA MUCINOSA

Alopecia mucinosa, first described by Pinkus in 1957, shows two types of lesions: grouped follicular papules and red, raised, boggy, occasionally nodular plaques. The lesions are devoid of hair, but except in the scalp this is not a conspicuous feature. An idiopathic, benign form and a "malignant" form associated from the very beginning with lymphoma are recognized.

The benign form is either localized to the head and neck or disseminated with lesions occurring also on the trunk and limbs. Usually, the lesions resolve spontaneously within 2 months to 2 years, but occasionally they persist for many years (Emmerson).

The malignant form consists of disseminated plaques having the clinical appearance of mycosis fungoides rather than of alopecia mucinosa. The histologic finding of alopecia mucinosa in these cases is a secondary phenomenon. No case of transformation of a benign case of alopecia mucinosa into mycosis fungoides is known (Braun-Falco, 1957; Kim and Winkelmann).

Histopathology. The histologic picture is characterized by a reticular degeneration of the epithelial cells in sebaceous glands and outer root sheaths, leading to a disruption of

FIG. 10-4. **Alopecia mucinosa.** The sebaceous gland on the left shows a "reticular" degeneration of its cells associated with the presence of mucin. (×40) (Armed Forces Institute of Pathology, No. 57-13780)

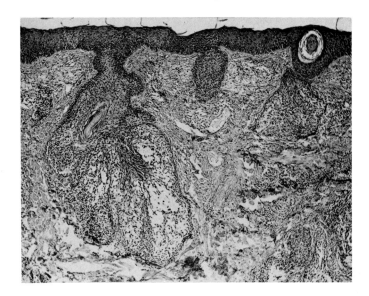

FIG. 10-5. **Alopecia mucinosa.** The cells of the outer root sheath have undergone degeneration with accumulation of mucin, whereas the sebaceous lobule in the center shows as yet no degeneration. (×100)

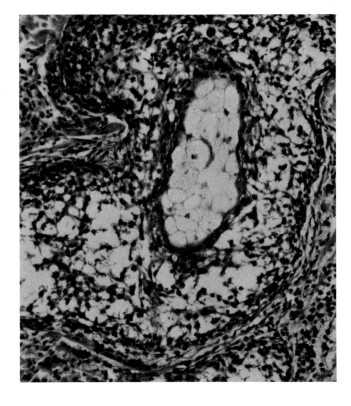

these cells and the formation of cystic spaces (Fig. 10-4) (Johnson et al.). This usually is followed by the accumulation of mucin within the hair follicles and sebaceous glands (Fig. 10-5). Occasionally, however, no mucin is found, probably because it was removed during fixation on account of its solubility in water (Braun-Falco, 1970). The mucin consists of acid mucopolysaccharides that stain metachromatically with Giemsa's stain and stain with alcian blue. The mucin is only partially removed by hyaluronidase, indicating the presence of hyaluronic acid and of sulfated acid mucopolysaccharides (Johnson et al.). The mucin does not stain with PAS except when small amounts of glycogen from the damaged root sheath cells are present in it (Emmerson).

The inflammatory infiltrate in the benign form of alopecia mucinosa is variable in its intensity, but often it is pronounced, especially in boggy nodular plaques. The infiltrate, no matter how dense, consists of benign inflammatory cells, largely mononuclear cells, with an admixture of eosinophils (Emmerson). In some instances, PAS-positive, diastase-resistant material representing neutral mucopolysaccharides is found in the dermis (Okun and Kay).

In patients having mycosis fungoides in association with their alopecia mucinosa the dermal infiltrate is that of mycosis fungoides,

and Pautrier microabscesses may be present in the epidermis and in the upper part of hair follicles (see p. 700).

Histogenesis. The presence of mucin can be explained on the basis of mucophanerosis secondary to cell damage (Braun-Falco, 1957). Autoradiography using ^{35}S-sulfate shows no increased rate of synthesis of sulfated acid mucopolysaccharides, according to Langner et al., thus confirming Braun-Falco's hypothesis.

FOX-FORDYCE DISEASE

This disease occurs almost exclusively in women. It is characterized by the presence of discrete, firm, follicular, pruritic papules in areas where apocrine glands are found, namely, in the axillae, the areolae, and the pubic and perineal regions.

Histopathology. Fox-Fordyce disease, as established by Shelley and Levy, represents an "apocrine miliaria." The primary event

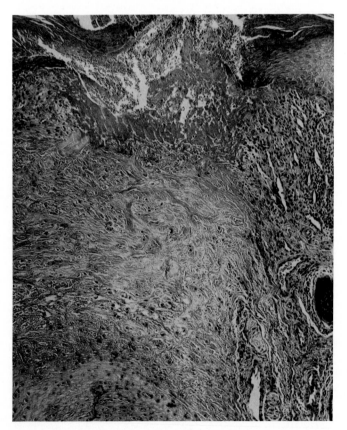

Fig. 10-6. **Chondrodermatitis nodularis helicis.** The epidermis shows an ulcer in the center. The collagen beneath the ulcer shows degeneration with loss of nuclei. On the right one sees richly vascularized granulation tissue. At the bottom the thickened perichondrium is seen. (×50)

is the formation of a keratotic plug in the uppermost portion of the hair follicle, the infundibulum. This keratotic plug obstructs the ostium of the apocrine duct as it emerges from the follicular wall. A spongiotic vesicle is seen located within the follicular wall where the apocrine duct may have ruptured. The formation of this "apocrine sweat retention vesicle" is followed by acanthosis of the infundibulum and by an inflammatory infiltrate occupying the dermis outside the infundibulum and extending to the vesicle within the follicular wall. Since the vesicle within the follicular wall is small, usually it can be found only when step sections are studied (Mevorah et al.; Macmillan and Vickers).

CHONDRODERMATITIS NODULARIS HELICIS

In this condition one nodule and rarely several nodules are found usually on the apex of the helix of the ear. Occasionally, a nodule may be located, instead, on the antihelix. The nodules are very tender, are hyperkeratotic or crusted, and usually measure less than 1 cm in diameter. Those of long duration often show ulceration.

Histopathology. The epidermis may show a large keratotic, partly parakeratotic plug causing an invagination of the epidermis. In some cases there is instead a central erosion or ulceration covered with a crust. The dermis in the center of the lesion shows degenerated collagen devoid of nuclei (Fig. 10-6). At the periphery of the lesion there is richly vascularized granulation tissue composed of lymphocytes, plasma cells, histiocytes, and fibroblasts (Newcomer et al.; Shuman and Helwig). Within the vascularized granulation tissue structures resembling those seen in glomus tumors may be seen occasionally. However, since the cells having the appearance of glomus cells lack the rich supply of nerves seen in glomus tumors, one may regard the structures resembling glomus tumors as reactive, hyperplastic changes in arteriovenous anastomoses that normally are present in the ear (Haber).

The perichondrium is thickened and shows cellular infiltration. Frequently, but not always, changes in the cartilage are present. When present, they may vary from merely a diminution in the number of nuclei to focal degeneration.

Histogenesis. Originally it had been assumed that the primary event was degeneration of the cartilage. However, recent authors (Newcomer et al.; Gropper; Shuman and Helwig) have pointed out that degenerative changes in the aural cartilage similar to those that may be seen in chondrodermatitis nodularis helicis are commonly found in old age and, furthermore, that changes in the aural cartilage may be absent in chondrodermatitis nodularis helicis. It is now assumed that in chondrodermatitis nodularis helicis the initial damage occurs in the dermis, and that probably the basically poor blood supply of the ear in conjunction with repeated minor traumas is responsible for the lesion. It is possible that the presence of structures resembling glomus tumors accounts for the great tenderness of the lesion.

RELAPSING POLYCHONDRITIS

In this disease one observes, in association with fever, malaise and arthralgia, intermittent attacks of painful erythema and edema of the ears. Ultimately, the ears become soft and flabby because of degeneration of the cartilage. There also is degeneration of the cartilage of the nose, larynx, trachea and bronchi, of the costochondral junctions, and of the cartilage of the peripheral joints (Dolan et al.). There may be dilatation of the aortic ring with aneurysmal dilatation of the aorta (Hainer and Hamilton). Death may result from tracheal and bronchial obstruction (Verity et al.).

Histopathology. Histologically, there is chondrolysis associated with chondritis and perichondritis. The overlying dermis of the ear usually appears normal (Thurston and Curtis). The involvement of the cartilage is characterized by loss of basophilia caused by the release of the basophilic acid mucopolysaccharides from their attachment to proteins. This is accompanied by pyknosis of the chondrocytes. An elastic tissue stain shows clumping and destruction of the cartilaginous elastic fibers (Feinerman et al.). An inflammatory infiltrate consisting largely of monocytes and macrophages permeates the cartilage, with lymphocytes and plasma cells at the periphery of the infiltrate (Hundeiker et al.).

Histogenesis. Proteolysis of the chondroitin-sulfate–protein complex with release of acid mucopolysaccharides appears to be the primary factor in the chondrolysis (Feinerman et al.). Lysosomal enzymes released by the monocytes of the infiltrate play a role in the proteolysis (Hundeiker et al.). It can be assumed that the chondrolysis takes place on the basis of an immune mechanism since indirect immunofluorescent testing has revealed the presence of anti-cartilage antibodies in the serum of patients with relapsing polychondritis (Rogers et al.).

BIBLIOGRAPHY

Acne Vulgaris

Freinkel, R. K.: Pathogenesis of acne vulgaris. New Eng. J. Med., *280*:1161, 1969.

Freinkel, R. K., Strauss, J. S., Yip, S. Y., and Pochi, P. E.: Effect of tetracycline on the composition of sebum in acne vulgaris. New Eng. J. Med., *273*:850, 1965.

Kaidbey, K. H., and Kligman, A. M.: Pigmentation in comedones. Arch. Derm., *109*:60, 1974.

Puhvel, S. M., and Reisner, R. M.: Effect of antibiotics on the lipases of *Corynebacterium acnes* in vitro. Arch. Derm., *106*:45, 1972.

Sansone, G., and Reisner, R. M.: Differential rates of conversion of testosterone to dihydrotestosterone in acne and in normal human skin—a possible pathogenic factor in acne. J. Invest. Derm., *56*:366, 1971.

Strauss, J. S., and Kligman, A. M.: The pathologic dynamics of acne vulgaris. Arch. Derm., *82*:779, 1960.

Strauss, J. S., and Pochi, P. E.: Intracutaneous injection of sebum and comedones. Arch. Derm., *92*:443, 1965.

———: Recent advances in androgen metabolism and their relation to the skin. Arch. Derm., *100*:621, 1969.

Van Scott, E. J., and McCardle, R. C.: Keratinization of the duct of the sebaceous gland and growth cycle of the hair follicle in the histogenesis of acne in human skin. J. Invest. Derm., *27*:405, 1956.

Acne Rosacea

Flegel, H.: Zur Spezifität einiger tuberkuloidgranulomatöser Hautaffektionen. Arch. klin. exp. Derm., *205*:112, 1957.

Grosshans, E. M., Kremer, M., and Maleville, J.: Demodex folliculorum und die Histogenese der granulomatösen Rosacea. Hautarzt, *25*: 166, 1974.

Laymon, C. W.: Lupoid rosacea. A.M.A. Arch. Derm.. *63*:409, 1951.

Laymon, C. W., and Schoch, E. P., Jr.: Micropapular tuberculid and rosacea. Arch. Derm. Syph., *58*:286, 1948.

Marks, R., and Harcourt-Webster, J. N.: Histopathology of rosacea. Arch. Derm., *100*: 623, 1969.

Michelson, H. E.: Does the rosacea-like tuberculid exist? Arch. Derm., *78*:681, 1958.

Mullanax, M. G., and Kierland, R. R.: Granulomatous rosacea. Arch. Derm., *101*:206, 1970.

Pinkus, H., and Mehregan, A. H.: A Guide to Dermatohistopathology. p. 229. New York, Appleton-Century-Crofts, 1969.

Scott, K. W., and Calnan, C. D.: Acne agminata. Trans. St. John's Hosp. Derm. Soc., *53*:60, 1967.

Strauss, H.: Katamnestische Untersuchungen von Fällen mit Tuberkulid. Arch. f. Derm. u. Syph. *198*:417, 1954.

van Ketel, W. G.: Rosacea-like tuberculid of Lewandowsky. Dermatologica, *116*:201, 1958.

Disseminate Infundibulofolliculitis

Hitch, J. M., and Lund, H. Z.: Disseminate and recurrent infundibulo-folliculitis. Arch. Derm., *97*:432, 1968.

———: Disseminate and recurrent infundibulofolliculitis. Arch. Derm., *105*:580, 1972.

Wolf, M., and Tolmach, J.: Disseminate and recurrent infundibulo-folliculitis. Arch. Derm., *103*:552, 1971.

Trichorrhexis Invaginata

Altman, J., and Stroud, J.: Netherton's syndrome and ichthyosis linearis circumflexa. Psoriasiform ichthyosis. Arch. Derm., *100*:550, 1969.

Hurwitz, S., Kirsch, N., and McGuire, I.: Reevaluation of ichthyosis and hair shaft abnormalities. Arch. Derm., *103*:266, 1971.

Julius, C. E., and Keeran, M.: Netherton's syndrome in a male. Arch. Derm., *104*:422, 1971.

Netherton, E. W.: A unique case of trichorrhexis nodosa: "bamboo hairs." Arch. Derm., *78*:483, 1958.

Trichostasis Spinulosa

Braun-Falco, O., and Vakilzadeh, F.: Trichostasis spinulosa. Hautarzt, *18*:501, 1967.

Sarkany, J., and Gaylarde, P. M.: Trichostasis spinulosa and its management. Brit. J. Derm., *84*:311, 1971.

Alopecia Areata

Braun-Falco, O., and Zaun, H.: Über die Beteiligung des gesamten Capillitiums bei Alopecia areata. Hautarzt, *13*:342, 1962.

Eckert, J., Church, R. E., and Ebling, F. J.: The pathogenesis of alopecia areata. Brit. J. Derm., *80*:203, 1968.

Goos, M.: Zur Histopathologie der Alopecia areata. Arch. derm. Forsch., *240*:160, 1971.

Kalkoff, K. W., and Macher, E.: Über das Nachwachsen der Haare bei der Alopecia areata und maligna nach intracutaner Hydrocortisoninjektion. Hautarzt, *9*:441, 1958.

Kopf, A. W., and Orentreich, N.: Alkaline phosphatase in alopecia areata. Arch. Derm., *76*:288, 1957.

Van Scott, E. J.: Morphologic changes in pilosebaceous units and anagen hairs in alopecia areate. J. Invest. Derm., *31*:35, 1958.

Trichotillomania

Mehregan, A. H.: Trichotillomania. Arch. Derm., *102*:129, 1970.

Muller, S. A., and Winkelmann, R. K.: Trichotillomania. Arch. Derm., *105*:535, 1972.

Alopecia Cicatrisata

Altman, J., and Perry, H. O.: The variations and course of lichen planus. Arch. Derm., *84*:179, 1961.

Cram, D. L., Kierland, R. R., and Winkelmann, R. K.: Ulcerative lichen planus of the feet. Arch. Derm., *93*:692, 1966.

Degos, R., Rabut, R., Duperrat, B., and Leclerq, R.: L'état pseudo-peladique. Réflexions à propos de cent cas d'alopécies cicatricielles en aires, d'apparence primitive du type pseudopelade. Ann. derm. syph., *81*:5, 1954.

Gay Prieto, J.: Pseudopelade of Brocq: Its relationship to some forms of cicatricial alopecias and to lichen planus. J. Invest. Derm., *24*:323, 1955.

Juon, M.: Le problème des états pseudopeladiques ou pseudopeladoides dans le cadre des alopécies cicatricielles. Dermatologica, *133*:66, 1966.

Keining, E., and Rathjens, B.: Versuch einer Abgrenzung des Graham Little-Syndroms. Derm. Wschr., *132*:1016, 1955.

Laymon, C. W.: The cicatricial alopecias. J. Invest. Derm., *89*:99, 1947.

Male, O.: Über die ulzerös-atrophisierende Form des Lichen ruber planus. Z. Haut, *45*:17, 1970.

Miescher, G., and Lenggenhager, R.: Über Pseudopelade Brocq. Dermatologica, *94*:122, 1947.

Ronchese, F.: Pseudopelade. Arch. Derm., *82*:336, 1960.

Spier, H. W., and Keilig, W.: Lichen ruber follicularis decalvans (Graham Little-Syndrom) und seine Beziehungen zur Pseudopelade Brocq. Hautarzt, *4*:457, 1953.

Waldorf, D. S.: Lichen planopilaris. Arch. Derm., *93*:684, 1966.

Alopecia Mucinosa

Braun-Falco, O.: Mucophanerosis intrafollicularis et seboglandularis. Derm. Wschr., *136*:1289, 1957.

———: In the discussion of Zambal, Z.: Ablagerungen in der Haut bei Alopecia mucinosa. Arch. klin. exp. Derm., *237*:115, 1970.

Emmerson, R. W.: Follicular mucinosis. Brit. J. Derm., *81*:395, 1969.

Johnson, W. C., Higdon, R. S., and Helwig, E. B.: Alopecia mucinosa. Arch. Derm., *79*:395, 1959.

Kim, R., and Winkelmann, R. K.: Follicular mucinosis (alopecia mucinosa). Arch. Derm., *85*:490, 1962.

Langner, A., Jablonska, S., and Darzynkiewicz, Z.: Studies on the origin of the mucin in mucinosis follicularis. Acta dermatoven., *49*:76, 1969.

Okun, M. R., and Kay, F.: Follicular mucinosis (alopecia mucinosa). Arch. Derm., *89*:809, 1964.

Pinkus, H.: Alopecia mucinosa. Arch. Derm., *76*:419, 1957.

Fox-Fordyce Disease

Macmillan, D. C., and Vickers, H. R.: Fox-Fordyce disease. Brit. J. Derm., *84*:181, 1971.

Mevorah, B., Duboff, G. S., and Wass, R. W.: Fox-Fordyce disease in prepubescent girls. Dermatologica, *136*:43, 1968.

Shelley, W. B., and Levy, E. J.: Apocrine sweat retention in man. II. Fox-Fordyce disease (apocrine miliaria). Arch. Derm., *73*:38, 1956.

Chondrodermatitis Nodularis Helicis

Gropper, H.: Chondrodermatitis chronica nodularis helicis in Verbindung mit Studien am Ohrmuschelknorpel. Derm. Wschr., *130*:979, 1954.

Haber, H.: Chondrodermatitis nodularis chronica helicis. Hautarzt, *11*:122, 1960.

Newcomer, V. D., Steffen, C. G., Sternberg, T. H., and Liechtenstein, L.: Chondrodermatitis nodularis chronica helicis. Arch. Derm., *68*:241, 1953.

Shuman, R., and Helwig, E. B.: Chondrodermatitis helicis. Am. J. Clin. Path., *24*:126, 1954.

Relapsing Polychondritis

Dolan, D. L., Lemmon, G. B., Jr., and Teitelbaum, S. L.: Relapsing polychondritis. Am. J. Med., *41*:285, 1966.

Feinerman, L. K., Johnson, W. C., Weiner, J., and Graham, J. H.: Relapsing polychondritis. Dermatologica, *140*:369, 1970.

Hainer, J. W., and Hamilton, G. W.: Aortic abnormalities in relapsing polychondritis. New Eng. J. Med., *280*:1166, 1969.

Hundeiker, M., Brehm, K., and Go, M.: Infiltrat und Knorpelzerstörung bei Polychondritis. Z. Haut, *45*:437, 1970.

Rogers, P. H., Boden, G., and Tourtellotte, C. D.: Relapsing polychondritis with insulin resistance and antibodies to cartilage. Am. J. Med., *55*:243, 1973.

Thurston, C. S., and Curtis, A. C.: Relapsing polychondritis. Arch. Derm., *93*:664, 1966.

Verity, M. A., Larson, W. M., and Madden, S. C.: Relapsing polychondritis. Am. J. Path., *42*:251, 1963.

11

Inflammatory Diseases Due to Physical Agents and Foreign Substances

POLYMORPHOUS LIGHT ERUPTION

Allergy to sunlight may produce in exposed areas the following types of eruption: (1) a papular type; (2) a papulovesicular type; (3) an eczematous type; (4) a plaque type; and (5) a diffuse erythematous type. Not infrequently, several of these five types of eruption are present together.

In the papular type, scattered edematous papules are present. In the papulovesicular type, the papules are associated with vesicles. In the eczematous type, one observes diffuse erythema with edema, scaling and crusting, as in contact dermatitis. Lesions of the plaque type are red, slightly edematous, and indurated. They show a close clinical resemblance to the early lesions of chronic discoid lupus erythematosus as well as to those of Jessner's lymphocytic infiltration of the skin. The lesions of the diffuse erythematous type have the clinical appearance of lupus erythematosus except for the strict limitation to sun-exposed areas.

Polymorphous light eruption may be acute or chronic. In the acute type, the action spectrum of the eruption is confined to sunburn radiation in the range from 290 to 320 nm (Fisher et al.). The eruption starts within a few hours to one day after sun exposure and involutes spontaneously within one to two weeks if no additional exposure to sunlight occurs. In the chronic type the action spectrum is found not only in the sunburn range but also in the long ultraviolet (320-400 nm) and visible (above 400 nm) ranges

(Frain-Bell et al.). Also nonexposed areas may be involved in the chronic type and the eruption may persist through the winter. In most instances, polymorphous light eruption responds well to treatment with antimalarial drugs of the 4-aminoquinoline group, such as chloroquine.

Histopathology. In the papular, the papulovesicular, the eczematous, and the diffuse erythematous types of eruption, the histologic picture is nonspecific (Everett et al.).

In the plaque type the histologic picture shows a patchy infiltrate of lymphoid cells resembling that seen in early lesions of lupus erythematosus, except that the infiltrate is more apt to be arranged around blood vessels than around the pilosebaceous structures, and liquefaction degeneration of the cells of the basal layer is absent (Fig. 11-1) (Wright and Winer). Yet, a differentiation is not always possible since in early lesions of discoid lupus erythematosus hydropic degeneration of the basal layer may be absent (see p. 424). In addition, the plaque type of polymorphous light eruption must be differentiated from Jessner's lymphocytic infiltration, lymphoma, and pseudolymphoma of Spiegler-Fendt. For this differentiation see p. 426.

Histogenesis. Phototesting with wave lengths shorter than 320 nm is valuable in establishing the existence of light sensitivity, but it does not rule out lupus erythematosus, since approximately one third of patients with lupus erythematosus give positive phototests with short ultraviolet rays (Fisher et al.). However, im-

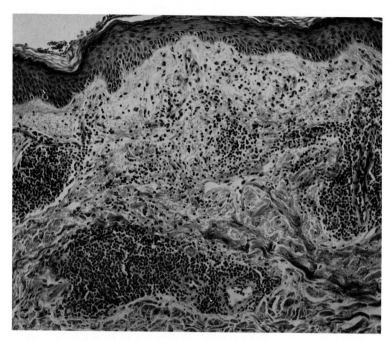

FIG. 11-1. **Polymorphous light eruption, plaque type.** A patchy infiltrate of lymphoid cells is present in the dermis, as in discoid lupus erythematosus. However, there is no hydropic degeneration of the basal cells. (×100)

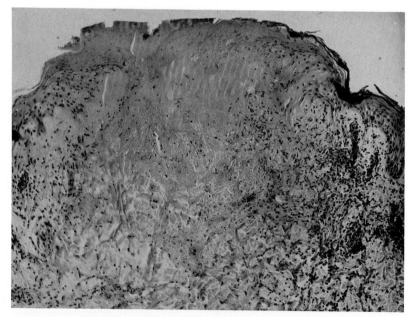

FIG. 11-2. **Hydroa vacciniforme.** There is necrosis of the epidermis and of the subjacent dermis at the site of the blister. The area of necrosis is walled off by a chronic inflammatory infiltrate. (×100)

munofluorescent testing usually permits a distinction, since, on direct testing, deposits of IgG and complement are found in lesions of lupus erythematosus but not in those of polymorphous light eruption (Lester et al.; Chorzelski et al.). On the other hand, antinuclear antibodies, although commonly present in the serum of patients with systemic lupus erythematosus (see p. 431), are rarely found at a significant titer in the serum of patients with either discoid lupus erythematosus or polymorphous light eruption (Peterson and Fusaro). It should be mentioned, however, that Burnham et al., using tumor imprints as substrate, found antinuclear antibodies in the serum of 31 per cent of the patients with polymorphous light eruption, as compared with 46 per cent of the patients with chronic discoid lupus erythematosus.

Differential Diagnosis. Before accepting polymorphous light eruption as diagnosis it is necessary not only to exclude lupus erythematosus and the other above-mentioned diseases but also porphyria of the papular and papulovesicular types. For the latter differentiation see p. 398.

HYDROA VACCINIFORME

Hydroa vacciniforme is a recurring vesicular or papulovasicular eruption on light-exposed cutaneous surfaces that heals with scars. It usually starts in early childhood. A nonscarring variant eruption is referred to as hydroa aestivale. Both types of hydroa respond well to treatment with drugs of the 4-aminoquinoline group.

Histopathology. In hydroa vacciniforme, one finds at the site of the blister necrosis of the epidermis and of the subjacent dermis (Fig. 11-2). The area of necrosis in the dermis appears homogeneous and eosinophilic. A cellular infiltrate surrounds the area of necrosis (McGrae and Perry).

Histogenesis. McGrae and Perry, as well as Musger, have recently stressed that hydroa vacciniforme represents a disease entity that should not be regarded as a variant of polymorphous light eruption because of its onset in early childhood and healing with scarring. Its close relationship with polymorphous light eruption, however, is attested by (1) the existence of a nonscarring variant referred to as hydroa aestivale, (2) the existence of a polymorphous light eruption showing papulovesicles in association with other types of light-sensitivity erup-

tions, and (3) the same good response to drugs of the 4-aminoquinoline group as seen in polymorphous light eruption. It is, of course, important in every case of hydroa vacciniforme to rule out the existence of erythropoietic protoporphyria (see p. 397).

ACTINIC RETICULOID

In this persistent light eruption, encountered largely in elderly males, photosensitivity extends from the sunburn ultraviolet range (290 to 320 nm) to visible light (above 400 nm). The patients at first show erythema, papules and lichenified plaques only in exposed areas, but gradually the eruption spreads to cover most of the skin surface as a generalized erythroderma. The skin of the face may show sufficient thickening to result in deep furrows (Ive et al.). The eruption clears only slowly when the patient is confined to a darkened room illuminated by incandescent bulbs rather than by fluorescent lighting (Brown et al.).

Histopathology. The infiltrate in the dermis is dense and extends not only throughout the dermis but also into the subcutaneous fat. The cells of the infiltrate are largely lymphoid cells and histiocytes, with an admixture of eosinophils and plasma cells. However, the similarity to lymphoma, especially mycosis fungoides, is often great not only on account of the extent of the infiltrate but also because of the presence of hyperchromatic nuclei resembling mycosis cells and their invasion into the epidermis where they may form aggregates resembling Pautrier microabscesses.

In spite of its clinical and histologic resemblance to lymphoma, actinic reticuloid is benign and reversible. In one patient, however, a reticulum cell lymphoma developed after the actinic reticuloid had existed for 9 years (Jensen and Sneddon). The authors leave the question open whether this was a chance occurrence of two unrelated diseases or whether the actinic reticuloid transformed into a lymphoma.

Histogenesis. Phototesting has established that patients with actinic reticuloid have particularly reduced threshold for erythema on exposure to longwave ultraviolet radiation and to visible light (Brown et al.). The existence of a photocontact

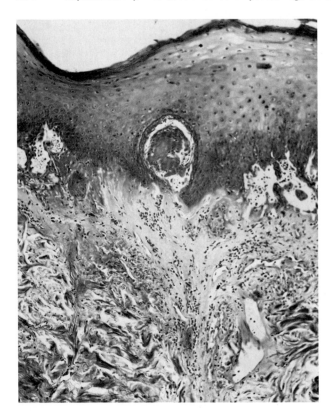

FIG. 11-3. **Late radiodermatitis.** The epidermis shows acanthosis and downward growth around a telangiectatic blood vessel. Many irregularly dilated lymphatics are located directly beneath the epidermis. The collagen shows degeneration. (×100)

dermatitis in such patients must be excluded by photopatch tests, for instance with tetrachlorsalicylanilide (Ive et al.). Degos et al. were able to passively transfer the photoallergy of a patient with actinic reticuloid to two normal persons by the Prausnitz-Küstner technique.

RADIATION DERMATITIS

An early (acute) stage and a late (chronic) stage of radiation dermatitis are recognized Early radiation dermatitis develops after large doses of x-radiation or radium. Erythema develops within about a week. This may heal with desquamation and pigmentation. If the dose was high enough, painful blisters may develop at the site of erythema. In that case, healing usually takes place with atrophy, telangiectasia and irregular hyperpigmentation. Subsequent to very large doses ulceration will occur, generally within 2 months. Such an ulcer may heal ultimately with severe atrophic scarring, or it may not heal.

Late (chronic) radiation dermatitis occurs from a few months to many years after the administration of fractional doses of x-rays or radium. The skin shows atrophy, telangiectasia and irregular hyperpigmentation. Ulceration may be seen within the areas of atrophy, as well as foci of hyperkeratosis. Squamous cell carcinomas or basal cell epitheliomas may develop. The former tend to arise in areas of severe radiation damage, and the latter in areas where the radiation damage is rather mild (Lazar and Cullen).

Histopathology of Early Radiation Dermatitis. There is both intracellular and intercellular edema of the epidermis with pyknosis of the nuclei. The cells of the hair follicles, sebaceous glands and sweat glands also show degenerative changes. An inflammatory infiltrate is seen throughout the dermis and it may permeate the epidermis. Some of the blood vessels are dilated, whereas others, especially the larger ones in the deeper portions of the dermis, show edema of their walls, endothelial proliferation, and even thrombosis (Epstein). The collagen bundles show edema. In severe cases the epidermis undergoes necrosis and detaches itself from the dermis; and in the presence

FIG. 11-4. **Late radiodermatitis.** The walls of the vessels (V.) show fibrotic thickening. A large vessel (L.V.) at the junction of dermis and subcutis shows thrombosis. The collagenous bundles of the dermis appear sclerotic. (×50)

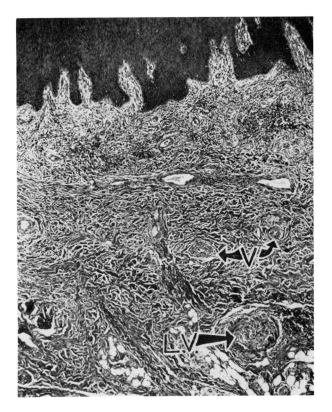

of ulceration not only the epidermis but also the upper dermis have become necrotic. The area of necrosis then is surrounded by neutrophils.

Histopathology of Late Radiation Dermatitis. The epidermis is irregular, showing atrophy in some areas and variable hyperplasia in others. Hyperkeratosis is common. The cells of the stratum malpighii show degenerative changes, such as edema and homogenization. In addition, they may show a disorderly arrangement and individual cell keratinization. The nuclei may show atypicality. The epidermal changes thus are similar to those seen in solar keratosis. The epidermis also may show irregular downward growth and even may grow around telangiectatic vessels, which thus may become nearly enclosed in the epidermis (Fig. 11-3).

In the dermis the collagen bundles are swollen and often show hyalinization. They may stain irregularly and appear palely eosinophilic in some areas and deeply eosinophilic in others. In response to the degeneration of collagen there is formation of new collagen throughout the dermis. Striking and rather typical changes may be observed on the blood vessels. Those located in the deeper portions of the dermis often show fibrous thickening of their walls so that the lumen may be nearly or entirely occluded (Fig. 11-4). Some of the vessels show thrombosis and recanalization. The vessels of the upper dermis may show telangiectasia. Also, there may be lymphedema in the subepidermal region. Hair structures and sebaceous glands are absent, but the sweat glands usually are preserved at least in part, except in areas of severe injury.

In severe cases of late radiation dermatitis ulceration occurs. The deep-lying large blood vessels in the region of such ulcers often show complete occlusion.

The squamous cell carcinomas arising in late radiation dermatitis often show a high degree of malignancy, with a tendency to metastasize. Frequently, they are of the spindle cell type (Sims and Kirsch) (see p. 478). Basal cell epitheliomas tend to be less invasive and destructive (Anderson and Anderson; Totten et al.). The occurrence of a fibrosarcoma is rare. A few quite convincing cases have been reported (Blom-Ides; Maggiora et al.); but in most instances the diagnosis of spindle-celled squamous cell carcinoma cannot be ruled out conclusively because this differentiation may be nearly impossible (see p. 584).

Differential Diagnosis. The epidermal changes of late radiation dermatitis may be similar to those of either an atrophic or a hyperplastic solar keratosis. However, the dermal changes differ. In solar keratosis there is basophilic degeneration of the collagen limited to the upper dermis, whereas in late radiation dermatitis degenerative changes of the collagen extend deep into the dermis.

CALCANEAL PETECHIAE (BLACK HEEL)

An asymptomatic pigmented macular lesion is found on one or both heels, immediately above the hyperkeratotic border of the foot. The margin is ill defined and speckled. The lesion is traumatic in origin and due to any sport leading to slamming the foot against a shoe, such as basketball, tennis, or football. The importance of the lesion lies in its resemblance to a malignant melanoma.

Histopathology. Extravasated erythrocytes are found in the papillae (Crissey and Peachey). In addition, rounded collections of amorphous, yellow-brown material are seen in the stratum corneum, representing lysed red blood cells (Vakilzadeh and Happle). The amorphous material does not stain blue with Perl's stain, as hemosiderin would do. However, positive peroxidase and benzidine reactions prove that the material is derived from hemoglobin (Kirton and Price).

SCABIES

Scabies, caused by the itch mite *Acarus scabiei,* presents burrows as its characteristic lesion. The burrows, produced by the female mite, occur mainly on the palms, the palmar and lateral aspects of the fingers, the web spaces between the fingers, the flexor surfaces of the wrists, the nipples of women, and the genitals of men. They appear as fine, tortuous blackish threads a few millimeters long. Often a vesicle is visible near the blind end of the burrow. In addition to the burrows, scabies presents a papular pruritic eruption that usually is most pronounced on the abdomen, the lower portions of the buttocks, and the anterior axillary folds. In some patient itching nodules persist for several months after successful treatment.

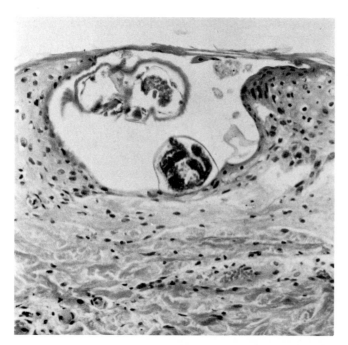

Fig. 11-5. **Scabies.** A female mite is located within a subcorneal burrow. (×400)

In especially susceptible individuals, such as mongoloids who experience only slight itching (Haydon and Caplan) and patients with leukemia who apparently have a lowered resistance to infection with scabies (Logan et al.), the clinical picture of so-called Norwegian scabies may result. Such patients show widespread erythroderma with crusting and scaling but no obvious burrows.

Histopathology. Histologic examination reveals the burrow in almost its entire length to be located within the horny layer. Only the extreme, blind end of the burrow either is in contact with or extends into the stratum malpighii. The female mite is situated at the blind end of the burrow (Fig. 11-5). Its head is located within the stratum malpighii (Heilesen). Intracellular and intercellular edema is present in the stratum malpighii near the mouth parts of the mite to such an extent that often vesicle formation results. Thus, the mite takes its food in fluid form. The dermis beneath the burrow shows a chronic inflammatory infiltrate composed predominantly of lymphoid cells.

The persistent scabetic nodules may show an inflammatory infiltrate containing lymphoid cells and numerous eosinophils (Konstantinov and Stanoeva). In some instances, however, the nodules show, similar to persistent arthropod bites or stings (see p. 201), a histologic picture resembling lymphoma (Thomson et al.).

Whereas it often is very difficult to locate the mite in histologic sections of ordinary scabies, Norwegian scabies shows the horny layer riddled with innumerable mites, so that nearly every section shows several parasites (Fig. 11-6) (Burks et al.; Haydon and Caplan).

SUBCUTANEOUS DIROFILARIASIS

Infection with the filarial worm *Dirofilaria conjunctivae* may be contracted in southern Florida. Mosquitoes are the vector. Clinically, a tender subcutaneous nodule is seen.

Histopathology. The subcutaneous nodule shows a central abscess within which one

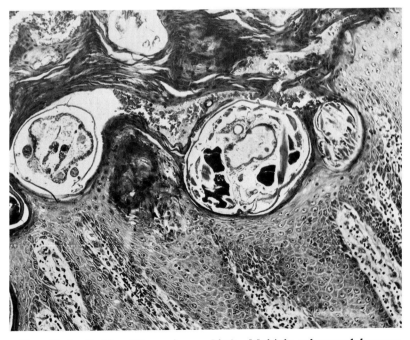

Fig. 11-6. **Scabies (Norwegian scabies).** Multiple subcorneal burrows containing female mites are present. There are also hyperkeratosis, acanthosis, and a marked dermal cellular infiltrate. (×200) (Robert N. Buchanan, Jr., M.D.)

sees transverse and diagonal sections of a usually dead filarial worm. Transverse sections measure 250 to 300 μm in diameter. The worm characteristically possesses a thick laminated cuticle showing longitudinal ridges (Fisher et al.). Surrounding the abscess are fibroblasts, epithelioid cells, and a few giant cells. Peripherally, there is a diffuse, nonspecific inflammatory reaction.

ONCHOCERCIASIS

Onchocerciasis occurs in Central America, Venezuela and tropical Africa. It is transmitted by black flies. Through their proboscis the infective larvae of *Onchocerca* enter the human skin. They mature to the adult stage in the subcutaneous tissue. The adult worms become clinically apparent as asymptomatic subcutaneous nodules, called onchocercomas, of which there usually are only a few, ranging in size from 0.5 to 2.0 cm. The adult worms do not cause any harm; however, their progeny, consisting of millions of microfilaria, live in the dermis and the aqueous humor of the eyes where they provoke inflammatory changes after several years. Clinically, onchocercal dermatitis is characterized by itching, edema, thickening, wrinkling and spotty depigmentation of the skin. In the eyes, iritis may result in blindness. The microfilaria in the anterior chamber of the eyes can be visualized by slit lamp examination.

Histopathology. The onchocercomas show at their periphery a chronic inflammatory infiltrate with areas of fibrosis. Their center consists of dense fibrous tissue containing transverse and diagonal sections of adult worms, measuring from 100 to 500 μm in their transverse diameter (Fig. 11-7). Some of them may be alive at the time of biopsy. Dead worms are surrounded by an inflammatory reaction containing foreign-body giant cells. Microfilariae, hatched by female worms, are seen within lymphatic vessels of the onchocercomas, through which they are disseminated in the skin. They measure from 5 to 9 μm in diameter and from 150 to 360 μm in length (Piers and Fasal).

In onchocercal dermatitis the skin every-

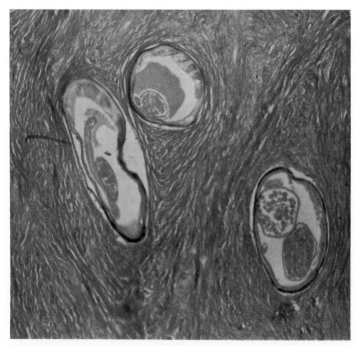

FIG. 11-7. **Onchocerciasis.** Within a dense fibrous tissue located in the subcutis transverse and diagonal sections of the adult filaria *Onchocera* are seen. ($\times$50)

where contains numerous microfilaria within the dermis. They are seen in greatest number close to the epidermis. In early infections histologic changes in the dermis are minimal, but in the course of years chronic inflammatory cells accumulate around the vessels, and ultimately fibrosis of the dermis and flattening of the epidermis result (Connor et al.).

Histogenesis. The slow development of the cutaneous and also of the ocular changes suggests that microfilariae, as they gradually disintegrate, act as a source of foreign protein and that the dermatitis and iritis are the result of a delayed hypersensitivity (Connor et al.).

ARTHROPOD BITES AND STINGS

Mosquito bites evoke an early toxic response which is urticarial and a later allergic response characterized by papules (Bandmann and Bosse).

Stings of bees, wasps or hornets may produce three types of reaction: an acute necrotic response, a subacute inflammatory response, or a chronic lymphoid response (Horen). The bites of ticks may result in persistent papular or nodular lesions with or without ulceration that cause a diagnostic problem clinically as well as histologically.

Hypersensitivity to insect bites, especially from fleas, mosquitoes or bedbugs, may result in papular urticaria (see below).

Histopathology. Mosquito bites show mainly neutrophils during the early toxic response, and a mononuclear infiltrate of lymphoid cells and plasma cells during the later allergic response. Eosinophils are few or absent (Bandmann and Bosse).

The acute necrotic response and the subacute inflammatory response to stings of bees, wasps or hornets have a nonspecific histologic appearance. On the other hand, the lymphoid response to these stings or to the bites of ticks is at least suggestive in its histologic appearance. In situations where the diagnosis is missed clinically, the histologic examination then can be of value.

In the chronic lymphoid reaction, the dermis presents a dense inflammatory infiltrate that may even extend into the subcutaneous fat. It consists of lymphoid cells and histiocytes with an admixture of eosinophils and plasma cells. Some of the histiocytes may show hyperchromatic nuclei. Also multinucleated histiocytic cells may occur (Allen). Frequently, one finds large lymphoid follicles with germinal centers (Winer and Strakosch; Allen; Tobias). Occasionally, in the case of tick bites, parts of the tick are found in the dermis.

Differential Diagnosis. At first glance the dense infiltrate, and the presence of hyperchromatic nuclei and of eosinophils may suggest mycosis fungoides; or the multinucleated histiocytic cells, if present, may suggest Hodgkin's disease because of their resemblance to Sternberg-Reed cells. However, the presence of lymphoid follicles, like those in Spiegler-Fendt pseudolymphoma, point toward a benign, reactive process such as arthropod bites or stings.

PAPULAR URTICARIA

This eruption, also known as lichen urticatus, is the result of hypersensitivity to bites from certain insects, especially mosquitoes, fleas and bedbugs. One observes edematous papules and papulovesicles which because of severe itching usually are excoriated. The eruption is more commonly found in children than in adults, and, if caused by mosquitoes, is limited to the summer months. The lesions of papular urticaria are clinically and histologically indistinguishable from those of prurigo simplex (see p. 135).

Histopathology. The stratum malpighii shows intercellular and intracellular edema and occasionally a spongiotic vesicle. A chronic inflammatory infiltrate is present around the vessels of the upper dermis (Shaffer et al.).

FOREIGN-BODY REACTIONS

Some foreign substances, when injected or when implanted accidentally into the skin, produce a foreign-body reaction. Others produce, but only in persons who are sensitized to the foreign substance, an allergic granulomatous reaction (see p. 204). In addition, certain substances formed within the body may produce a foreign-body reaction when deposited in the dermis or in the subcutaneous tissue. Such endogenous foreign-

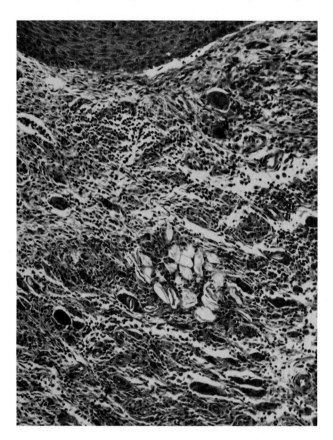

FIG. 11-8. **Foreign-body granuloma caused by a silk suture.** The silk suture is located in the center of the field. Around it there is a severe inflammatory infiltrate containing numerous foreign-body giant cells. (×200)

body reactions are produced, for instance, by urates in gout, and by keratinous material in calcifying epithelioma of Malherbe, in ruptured epidermal and pilar cysts, and in acne vulgaris.

Histopathology. A foreign-body reaction typically shows macrophages and foreign-body giant cells around the foreign material. In addition, lymphoid cells and plasma cells are present in most types of foreign-body reactions. Frequently, some of the foreign material is seen near macrophages and foreign-body giant cells, a finding that, of course, is of great diagnostic value. Substances producing foreign-body reactions are, for instance, silk or nylon sutures (Fig. 11-8), paraffin, silica, surgical glove starch powder, and human hair.

An *allergic* granulomatous reaction to a foreign body typically shows a tuberculoid pattern consisting of epithelioid cells with or without giant cells, and with or without caseation necrosis. Phagocytosis of the for-

eign substance is slight or absent. Substances producing an allergic granulomatous reaction are, for instance, zirconium, beryllium, and certain dyes used in tattoos.

PARAFFINOMA

Foreign-body reactions following injections of oily substances—for instance, mineral oil (paraffin), cottonseed oil, sesame oil, or camphor oil—occur as irregular plaque-like indurations of the skin and subcutaneous tissue. Ulceration may develop. The interval between the time of injection and the development of induration or ulceration may be many years (Rupec et al.).

Histopathology. Paraffinomas have a "Swiss cheese" appearance because of the presence of numerous ovoid or round cavities of varying size (Fig. 11-9). These cavities represent spaces occupied by the oily substance (Conrad et al.). The spaces between the cavities are taken up in part by

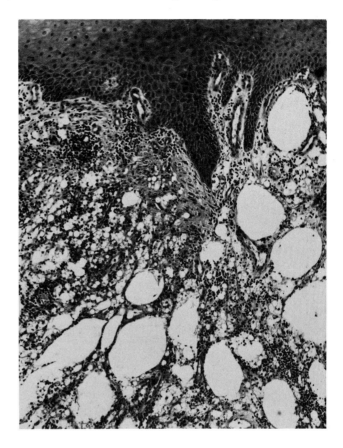

FIG. 11-9. **Lipid granuloma caused by mineral oil (paraffinoma).** The many large and small ovoid or round cavities that give the section a "Swiss cheese" appearance represent spaces filled with mineral oil (paraffin). (×200)

fibrotic connective tissue and in part by a cellular infiltrate of macrophages, histiocytes, and lymphoid cells. Some of the macrophages have the appearance of foam cells. Variable numbers of multinucleated foreign-body giant cells are present.

In frozen sections of paraffinoma the foreign material stains orange with Sudan, though less so than neutral fat. If the foreign substance consists of paraffin or other mineral oils, rather than vegetable oils, the osmic acid stain, the bromine-silver stain, and the phospholipid reaction of Baker are negative (Rupec et al.). As Best et al. and Newcomer et al. have shown with osmic acid, and Urbach et al. with bromine-silver, these stains are of particular value in differentiating spontaneous lipogranulomas, such as the lipogranulomatosis subcutanea of Rothmann and Makai, from reactions to injections of mineral oil, such as paraffin. Since osmic acid and bromine-silver stain only substances containing unsaturated carbon linkages, they stain animal and vegetable lipids but not mineral oil.

SILICA GRANULOMA

Silica granulomas result from the contamination of wounds with particles of soil or glass, which contain silicon dioxide (silica). Such wounds heal at first, and then, many months or years later, indurated nodules develop in the skin or the subcutaneous tissue. A similar reaction may result from the introduction of talcum powder (magnesium silicate) into open wounds (Macher; Tye et al.).

Histopathology. The usual histologic picture shows a diffuse inflammatory infiltrate containing numerous macrophages and multinucleated giant cells without organization into a tuberculoid granuloma (Epstein; Epstein et al., 1963; Tye et al.). In some cases, however, the inflammatory reaction is slight, and numerous epithelioid cell tubercles containing multinucleated giant cells are present

(Sommerville and Milne; Arzt). In either case the diagnosis of silica granuloma is greatly facilitated by the presence within the infiltrate of colorless crystalline particles, varying in size from being barely visible to 100 μm in length; they represent silica crystals. When examined with polarized light, these particles are doubly refractile (Epstein). Furthermore, spectrographic analysis (Arzt) or x-ray diffraction studies (Tye et al.) will reveal the presence of silicon.

Histogenesis. According to Shelley and Hurley (1960) and Epstein et al. (1963), the long interval that usually elapses between the injury and the appearance of the silica granuloma is caused by the very slow conversion of the large particles of silica introduced into the tissue to colloidal silica. These authors showed by means of intradermal injections of silica particles of various size that only silica in colloidal form having a particle size between 1 and 100 nm produces a reaction, whereas larger particles, like those present in suspensions of silica, or small particles, like those present in true molecular solutions of silica, cause no reaction. Inasmuch as injections of colloidal silica regularly produce a reaction, and since the reaction consists primarily of macrophages phagocytizing the colloidal silica, it seems likely that the development of silica granulomas represents a foreign-body reaction rather than an allergic phenomenon. It is possible, however, that in cases characterized by epithelioid cell tubercles developing many years after the injury, as described by Sommerville and Milne and by Arzt, the epithelioid cell reaction is the result of an allergic sensitization to silica.

STARCH GRANULOMA

Starch granulomas result from the accidental contamination of wounds with surgical glove powder. Such powder consists of cornstarch that has been treated with epichlorhydrin so that the powder can be autoclaved. As the result of this treatment the powder acts as a foreign body.

Histopathology. A foreign-body reaction with multinucleated giant cells is present. Scattered through the infiltrate one observes ill defined ovoid basophilic structures measuring 10 to 20 μm in diameter. They react with PAS and methenamine silver and, on examination in polarized light, are birefringent, showing a Maltese cross configuration (Leonard).

INTERDIGITAL PILONIDAL SINUS

In barbers the implantation of human hair in the interdigital web spaces may cause small, asymptomatic or slightly tender openings (Joseph and Gifford).

Histopathology. Histologic examination reveals a sinus tract lined by epidermis and containing one or several hairs, thus resembling a hair follicle. Either the sinus tract encases the hair completely or, if the hair extends deeper than the sinus tract, one finds at the lower end of the hair a foreign-body giant cell reaction intermingled with inflammatory cells (Joseph and Gifford; Goebel and Rupec).

ZIRCONIUM GRANULOMA

Deodorant sticks containing zirconium lactate and creams containing zirconium oxide may cause in the areas to which they are applied a persistent eruption composed of soft reddish-brown papules.

Histopathology. Histologic examination shows large aggregates of epithelioid cells forming tubercles without caseation. A few giant cells and a moderate lymphoid cell infiltrate are present (LoPresti and Hambrick). Thus, the histologic picture is indistinguishable from that of sarcoidosis. Because of the small size of the zirconium particles, they cannot be detected on examination with polarized light (Williams and Skipworth). Their presence, however, can be proved by spectrographic analysis (Baler).

Histogenesis. Zirconium granulomas develop on the basis of an allergic sensitization to zirconium, since (1) they occur only in individuals sensitized to zirconium (Shelley and Hurley, 1958); (2) they consist of epithelioid cell granulomas; and (3) autoradiographic analysis of experimentally induced lesions in sensitized individuals reveals no zirconium within the epithelioid cells, as is typical of granulomas that have formed on the basis of a delayed hypersensitivity reaction (Epstein et al., 1962).

SYSTEMIC BERYLLIOSIS

Beryllium granulomas of the skin may form in two different ways (Grier et al.). They may arise as a manifestation of systemic berylliosis, in which case particles of beryllium, after their inhalation and after they have produced pulmonary berylliosis, reach the skin through the blood circulation. On the other hand, purely local beryllium granulomas may develop following a laceration through which beryllium enters the skin directly. For discussion of local beryllium granuloma, see below.

The cutaneous granulomas of systemic berylliosis usually consist of only a few papular lesions over which the skin remains intact. In the four instances observed by Stoeckle et al. among 535 patients with systemic berylliosis, the cutaneous lesions cleared even though the pulmonary lesions progressed and caused death due to respiratory failure in 36 per cent of the patients.

Histopathology. The cutaneous granulomas of systemic berylliosis are indistinguishable from sarcoidosis, since they show very slight or no caseation (Stoeckle et al.).

The lungs of patients with systemic berylliosis show one of two histologic patterns: either a widely disseminated cellular infiltration with little tendency to form granulomas; or, in the less common pattern, well formed granulomas indistinguishable from those of sarcoidosis (Stoeckle et al.).

Histogenesis. Systemic berylliosis develops on the basis of a delayed hypersensitivity reaction. This has been shown by means of in vitro testing: The lymphocytes of patients with systemic berylliosis, when exposed to beryllium oxide in vitro, (1) undergo blastogenic transformation (Hanifin et al.); and (2) produce MIF (macrophage migration inhibitory factor). This factor present in the cell-free supernatant of the incubated lymphocytes inhibits the migration of normal guinea pig peritoneal exudate cells out of capillary tubes (Henderson et al.).

LOCAL BERYLLIUM GRANULOMA

Local beryllium granulomas were observed some years ago from cuts with fluorescent light tubes, which were coated at that time with a mixture containing zinc-beryllium silicate (Neave et al.).

The cutaneous granulomas following laceration show as their first sign incomplete healing of the laceration, followed by swelling, induration and tenderness, and, finally, central ulceration.

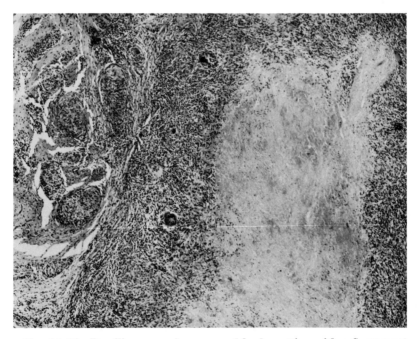

FIG. 11-10. **Beryllium granuloma caused by laceration with a fluorescent light bulb.** There is a large area of caseation necrosis surrounded by a tuberculoid granulomatous infiltrate. (×100)

Histopathology. The cutaneous granulomas following laceration, in contrast to the cutaneous granulomas of systemic berylliosis, show pronounced caseation necrosis. The necrosis may affect the entire center of the lesion (Fig. 11-10) (Neave et al.). Often a collar of lymphoid cells surrounds some of the epithelioid cell islands, giving them the appearance of true tubercles. Most likely the lymphoid cells are monocytes from which the epithelioid cells develop (Hanifin et al.). Schaumann bodies like those in sarcoidosis are present occasionally (Grier et al.). The epidermis shows acanthosis and may show ulceration. No particles of beryllium are seen in histologic sections, but its presence has been demonstrated by spectrographic analysis (Dutra).

TATTOO GRANULOMA

Allergic reactions to tattoos have been observed most commonly to cinnabar, a red dye containing mercuric sulfide, but occasionally also to chrome green, a tervalent chrome compound, and to cobalt blue. The reactions can be of two types, either an allergic dermatitis or an allergic granulomatous reaction.

Histopathology. Ordinarily, tattoos show diffusely scattered granules of dye that seem to be located not only within macrophages but also extracellularly in the dermis without any inflammatory reaction (Rostenberg et al.).

In cases of an allergic dermatitis, such as may occur against mercuric sulfide (Madden) or against chrome green (Rostenberg et al.), a pronounced inflammatory infiltrate is present in the dermis composed largely of lymphoid cells but also containing histiocytes, eosinophils and a few plasma cells. The tattoo granules are found predominantly in macrophages. The epidermis shows acanthosis and spongiosis.

In cases of an allergic granulomatous reaction, as has been observed against mercuric sulfide (Sulzberger and Tolmach), chrome green (Loewenthal), or cobalt blue (Björnberg), the reaction may consist entirely of epithelioid cell granulomas resembling sarcoidosis. There may be, in addition, a "nonsarcoidal" foreign-body reaction showing lymphoid cells, macrophages, and foreign-body giant cells. In epithelioid cell granulomas the tattoo granules are located extracellularly (Sulzberger and Tolmach); and in foreign-body granulomas both extracellularly and within macrophages and foreign-body giant cells (Loewenthal).

Histogenesis. Electron microscopic examination of tattoo marks without an allergic reaction shows most tattoo granules to be intracellular in location, largely within macrophages where they often lie within membrane-bound lysosomes. In addition, some tattoo granules are found free in the dermis (Abel et al.).

BIBLIOGRAPHY

Polymorphous Light Eruption

Brown, S., Lane, P. R., and Magnus, I. A.: Skin photosensitivity from fluorescent lighting. Brit. J. Derm., *81*:420, 1969.

Burnham, T. K., Neblett, T. R., Fine, G., and Bank, P.: The immunofluorescent tumor imprint technique. Arch. Derm., *99*:611, 1969.

Chorzelski, T., Jablonska, S., and Blaszczyk, M.: Immunopathologic investigations in lupus erythematosus. J. Invest. Derm., *52*:333, 1969.

Degos, R., Civatte, J., Akhound-Zadeh, H., *et al.*: Actino-réticulose. Photo-allergie avec infiltrat hématodermique. Ann. derm. syph., *97*:121, 1970.

Everett, M. A., Crockett, W., Lamb, J. H., and Minor, D.: Light-sensitive eruptions in American Indians. Arch. Derm., *83*:243, 1961.

Fisher, D. A., Epstein, J. H., Kay, D. N., and Tuffanelli, D. L.: Polymorphous light eruption and lupus erythematosus. Arch. Derm., *101*:458, 1970.

Frain-Bell, W., Mackenzie, L. A., and Witham, E.: Chronic polymorphous light eruption. Brit. J. Derm., *81*:885, 1969.

Ive, F. A., Magnus, I. A., Warin, R. P., and Wilson Jones, E.: "Actinic reticuloid;" a chronic dermatosis associated with severe photosensitivity and the histologic resemblance to lymphoma. Brit. J. Derm., *81*:469, 1969.

Jensen, N. E., and Sneddon, I. B.: Actinic reticuloid with lymphoma. Brit. J. Derm., *82*:287, 1970.

Lester, R. S., Burnham, T. K., Fine, G., and Murray, K.: Immunologic concepts of light reactions in lupus erythematosus and polymorphous light eruptions. Arch. Derm., *96*:1, 1967.

McGrae, J. D., and Perry, H. O.: Hydroa vacciniforme. Arch. Derm., *87*:618, 1963.

Musger, A.: Zur nosologischen Stellung der als Hydroa vacciniforme bezeichneten Hautveränderungen. Z. Haut, *46*:1, 1971.

Peterson, W. C., Jr., and Fusaro, R. M.: Antinuclear factor in light sensitivity and lupus erythematosus. Arch. Derm., *87*:563, 1963.

Wright, E. T., and Winer, L. H.: Histopathology of allergic solar dermatitis. J. Invest. Derm., *34*:103, 1960.

Radiation Dermatitis

Anderson, N. P., and Anderson, H. E.: Development of basal cell epithelioma as a consequence of radiodermatitis. Arch. Derm. Syph., *63*:586, 1951.

Blom-Ides, C.: Sarcoma in Röntgenoderma. Acta dermatoven., *30*:47, 1950.

Epstein, E.: Radiodermatitis. Springfield, Ill., Charles C Thomas, 1962.

Lazar, P., and Cullen, S. I.: Basal cell epithelioma and chronic radiodermatitis. Arch. Derm., *88*:172, 1963.

Maggiora, A., Bujard, E., and Jadassohn, W.: Beitrag zur Frage des Röntgensarkoms. Derm. Wschr., *147*:209, 1963.

Sims, C. F., and Kirsch, N.: Spindle-cell epidermoid epithelioma simulating sarcoma in chronic radiodermatitis. Arch. Derm. Syph., *57*:63, 1948.

Totten, R. S., Antypas, P. G., Dupertuis, S. M., *et al.*: Pre-existing roentgen-ray dermatitis in patients with skin cancer. Cancer, *10*:1024, 1957.

Calcaneal Petechiae (Black Heel)

Crissey, J. T., and Peachey, J. C.: Calcaneal petechiae. Arch. Derm., *83*:501, 1961.

Kirton, V., and Price, M. W.: "Black Heel." Trans. St. John's Hosp. Derm. Soc., *51*:80, 1965.

Vakilzadeh, F., and Happle, R.: Die Tennisferse (Black Heel). Z. Haut, *49*:285, 1974.

Scabies

Burks, J. W., Jung, R., and George, W. M.: Norwegian scabies. A.M.A. Arch. Derm., *74*:131, 1956.

Haydon, J. R., Jr., and Caplan, R. M.: Epidemic scabies. Arch. Derm., *103*:168, 1971.

Heilesen, B.: Studies on *Acarus scabiei* and scabies. Acta dermatoven., *16* (Suppl. XIV), 1946.

Konstantinov, D., and Stanoeva, L.: Persistent scabious nodules. Dermatologica, *147*:321, 1973.

Logan, J. C. P., Grant, P. W., and Keczkes, K.: Norwegian scabies and lymphatic leukaemia. Brit. J. Derm., *79*:303, 1967.

Thomson, J., Cochrane, T., Cochran, R., and McQueen, A.: Histology simulating reticulosis in persistent nodular scabies. Brit. J. Derm., *90*:421, 1974.

Subcutaneous Dirofilariasis

Fisher, B. K., Homayouni, M., and Orihel, T. C.: Subcutaneous infection with Dirofilaria. Arch. Derm., *89*:837, 1964.

Onchocerciasis

Connor, D. H., Williams, P. H., Helwig, E. B., and Winslow, D. J.: Dermal changes in onchocerciasis. Arch. Path., *87*:193, 1969.

Piers, F., and Fasal, P.: Onchocerciasis. *In* Simons, R.D.G.Ph. (ed.): Handbook of Tropical Dermatology. vol. 2, p. 950. Amsterdam, Elsevier Press, 1953.

Arthropod Bites and Stings

Allen, A. C.: Persistent "insect bites" (dermal eosinophilic granulomas) simulating lymphoblastomas, histiocytoses, and squamous cell carcinomas. Am. J. Path., *24*:367, 1948.

Bandmann, H. J., and Bosse, K.: Histologie des Mückenstiches (Aedes aegypti). Arch. klin. exp. Derm., *231*:59, 1967.

Horen, W. P.: Insect and scorpion sting. J.A.M.A., *221*:894, 1972.

Shaffer, B., Jacobsen, C., and Beerman, H.: Histopathologic correlation of lesions of papular urticaria and positive skin test reactions to insect antigens. Arch. Derm., *70*:437, 1954.

Tobias, N.: Tickbite granuloma. J. Invest. Derm., *12*:255, 1949.

Winer, L. H., and Strakosch, E. A.: Tickbites— *Dermacentor variabilis* (Say). J. Invest. Derm., *4*:249, 1941.

Foreign-Body Reactions

Abel, E. A., Silberberg, I., and Queen, D.: Studies of chronic inflammation in a red tattoo by electron microscopy and histochemistry. Acta dermatoven., *52*:453, 1972.

Arzt, L.: Foreign body granulomas and Boeck's sarcoid. J. Invest. Derm., *24*:155, 1955.

Baler, G. R.: Granulomas from topical zirconium in poison ivy dermatitis. Arch. Derm., *91*:145, 1965.

Best, E. W., Mason, H. L., DeWeerd, J. W., and Dahlin, D. C.: Sclerosing lipogranuloma of the male genitalia produced by mineral oil. Proc. Mayo Clin., *28*:623, 1953.

Björnberg, A.: Allergic reaction to cobalt in light blue tattoo markings. Acta dermatoven., *41*:259, 1961.

Conrad, A. H., Conrad, A. H., Jr., and Weiss, R. S.: Sesame oil tumors. J.A.M.A., *121*:237, 1943.

Dutra, F. R.: Beryllium granulomas of the skin. Arch. Derm. Syph., *60*:1140, 1949.

Epstein, E.: Silica granuloma of the skin. A.M.A. Arch. Derm., *71*:24, 1955.

Epstein, W. L., Skahen, J. R., and Krasnobrod, H.: Granulomatous hypersensitivity to zirconium: Localization of allergen in tissue and its role in formation of epithelioid cells. J. Invest. Derm., *38*:223, 1962.

————: The organized epithelioid cell granuloma: differentiation of allergic (zirconium) from colloidal (silica) types. Am. J. Path., *43*:391, 1963.

Goebel, M., and Rupec, M.: Interdigitaler pilonidaler Sinus. Derm. Wschr., *153*:341, 1967.

Grier, R. S., Nash, P., and Freiman, D. J.: Skin lesions in persons exposed to beryllium compounds. J. Industr. Hyg. Toxicol., *30*:228, 1948.

Hanifin, J. M., Epstein, W. L., and Cline, M. J.: In vitro studies of granulomatous hypersensitivity to beryllium. J. Invest. Derm., *55*:284, 1970.

Henderson, W. R., Fukuyama, K., Epstein, W. L., and Spitler, L. E.: In vitro demonstration of delayed hypersensitivity in patients with berylliosis. J. Invest. Derm., *58*:5, 1972.

Joseph, H. L., and Gifford, H.: Barber's interdigital pilonidal sinus. Arch. Derm., *70*:616, 1954.

Leonard, D. D.: Starch granulomas. Arch. Derm., *107*:101, 1973.

Loewenthal, L. J. A.: Reactions in green tattoos. A.M.A. Arch. Derm., *82*:237, 1960.

LoPresti, P. J., and Hambrick, G. W.: Zirconium granuloma following treatment of Rhus dermatitis. Arch. Derm., *92*:188, 1965.

Macher, E.: Die Bedeutung des Talkumgranuloms in der Dermatologie. Hautarzt, *4*:529, 1954.

Madden, J. F.: Reactions in tattoos. Arch. Derm. Syph., *40*:256, 1939.

Neave, H. J., Frank, S. B., and Tolmach, J.: Cutaneous granulomas following laceration by fluorescent light bulbs. Arch. Derm. Syph., *61*:401, 1950.

Newcomer, V. D., Graham, J. H., Schaffert, R. R., and Kaplan, L.: Sclerosing lipogranuloma resulting from exogenous lipids. Arch. Derm., *73*:361, 1956.

Rostenberg, A., Jr., Brown, R. A., and Caro, M. R.: Discussion of tattoo reactions with report of a case showing a reaction to a green color. Arch. Derm. Syph., *62*:540, 1950.

Rupec, M., Treeck, W., and Braun-Falco, O.: Zum Paraffingranulom. Derm. Wschr., *151*:129, 1965.

Shelley, W. B., and Hurley, H. J.: The allergic origin of zirconium deodorant granulomas. Brit. J. Derm., *70*:75, 1958.

————: The pathogenesis of silica granulomas in man: a non-allergic colloidal phenomenon. J. Invest. Derm., *34*:107, 1960.

Sommerville, J., and Milne, J. A.: Pseudotuberculoma silicoticum. Brit. J. Derm., *62*:105, 1950.

Stoeckle, J. D., Hardy, H. L., and Weber, A. L.: Chronic beryllium disease. Am. J. Med., *46*:545, 1967.

Sulzberger, M. B., and Tolmach, J. A.: Allergische Aufflammungs-Reaktionen in roten Tätowierungen. Hautarzt, *10*:110, 1959.

Tye, M. J., Hashimoto, K., and Fox, F.: Talc granulomas of the skin. J.A.M.A., *198*:1370, 1966.

Urbach, F., Wine, S. S., Johnson, W. C., and Davies, R. E.: Generalized paraffinoma (sclerosing lipogranuloma). Arch. Derm., *103*:277, 1971.

Williams, R. M., and Skipworth, G. B.: Zirconium granulomas of the glabrous skin following treatment of Rhus dermatitis. Arch. Derm., 80:273, 1959.

12

Noninfectious Granulomas

SARCOIDOSIS

Sarcoidosis is a systemic granulomatous disease of undetermined etiology. One distinguishes between a subacute, transient type of sarcoidosis and a chronic, persistent type.

In subacute, transient sarcoidosis one encounters erythema nodosum in association with hilar adenopathy, fever and often also migrating polyarthritis and acute iritis. The disease subsides within a few months without sequelae. Cutaneous manifestations, other than erythema nodosum, do not occur (Putkonen; James et al.). Occasionally, there is enlargement of some of the subcutaneous lymph nodes, such as the submental or cervical lymph nodes (Wood et al.).

In chronic, persistent sarcoidosis cutaneous lesions are encountered in about one fourth of the patients. The most common type of cutaneous lesion consists of brownish-red or purplish papules and plaques. By central clearing, annual or circinate lesions may result. Next in frequency is the so-called lupus pernio, consisting of purplish papules and plaques on the nose, cheeks and ears. A rather rare form of sarcoidosis is the lichenoid form in which small papular lesions are either widespread (Thal), limited to a few areas (Brunner and Robin), or arranged in well demarcated patches (Thal; Nozaki).

Rather rare manifestations of sarcoidosis are the erythrodermic type of sarcoidosis characterized by extensive, sharply demarcated, brownish-red, slightly scaling patches with little or no palpable infiltration (Lever

and Freiman). Subcutaneous nodules of sarcoidosis also are rare and may occur either in association with cutaneous lesions or in their absence (Marten and Warner).

Histopathology. The lesions of erythema nodosum occurring in subacute, transient sarcoidosis have the same histologic appearance as "idiopathic" erythema nodosum (Wood et al.).

The cutaneous lesions of chronic, persistent sarcoidosis are characterized, just as are the lesions in other organs, by the presence of circumscribed granulomas of epithelioid cells, so-called epithelioid cell tubercles.

The papules, plaques and lupus-perniotype lesions show variously sized aggregates of epithelioid cells scattered irregularly through the dermis, with occasional extension into the subcutaneous tissue (Barrie and Bogoch). In the erythrodermic form the infiltrate shows rather small granulomas of epithelioid cells in the upper dermis (Lever and Freiman; Wigley and Musso; Nagai and Kato). In the subcutaneous nodules the epithelioid cell tubercles lie in the subcutaneous fat (Grimmer).

In typical lesions of sarcoidosis of the skin the well demarcated islands of epithelioid cells contain only few giant cells or none at all (Fig. 12-1). A slight to moderate admixture of lymphoid cells is present, particularly at the margins of the epithelioid cell granulomas (Fig. 12-2). As histochemical stains have shown, these lymphoid cells are monocytes from which the epithelioid cells develop

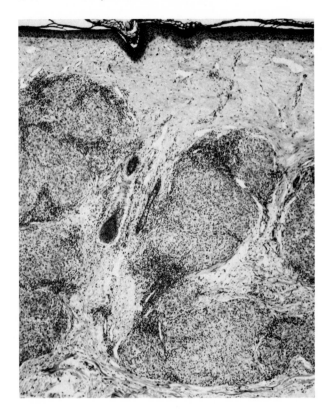

FIG. 12-1. **Sarcoidosis.** Low magnification. There are large islands of epithelioid cells with only a slight admixture of lymphocytes. (×50)

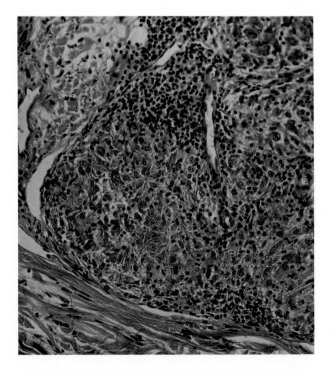

FIG. 12-2. **Sarcoidosis.** High magnification of Figure 12-1. The island of epithelioid cells is sharply demarcated. A "sprinkling" of lymphoid cells is present at the margin of the island. Histochemical stains have shown the presence of lysosomal enzymes in the lymphoid cells which thus are monocytes, and not lymphocytes. (×200)

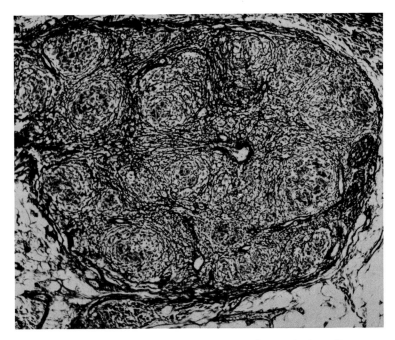

FIG. 12-3. **Sarcoidosis.** Foot's reticulum stain. Reticulum fibers surround and permeate the epithelioid cell granulomas composing this lesion. At the margin of the lesion one can observe the aggregation of reticulum fibers into collagen fibers. (×100)

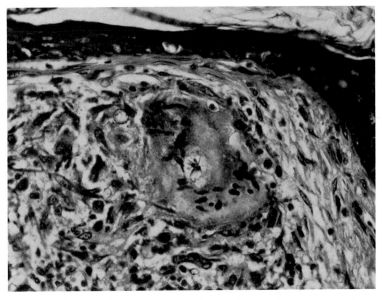

FIG. 12-4. **Sarcoidosis.** A large giant cell contains an asteroid inclusion body. (×400)

(Mustakallio and Niemi; Hundeiker). Not infrequently, a slight degree of necrosis, having the appearance of coagulation necrosis, is found in the center of some of the granulomas. The slight necrosis is characterized by granular eosinophilic degeneration of the cytoplasm of the epithelioid cells with coalescence of the cytoplasm of neighboring cells (Barrie and Bogoch). If a reticulum stain is employed, one sees a network of reticulum fibers surrounding and permeating the epithelioid cell granulomas (Fig. 12-3). In older lesions one can observe within the epithelioid cell granulomas not only reticulum fibers but also some collagen fibers resistant to silver impregnation (Barrie and Bogoch). Also in older lesions a moderate number of giant cells may be found. They are apt to be quite large and irregular in shape. Occasionally, they contain Schaumann bodies or asteroid bodies. Schaumann bodies are round or oval, laminated, and calcified, especially at their periphery. They stain dark blue because of the presence of calcium. Asteroid bodies (Fig. 12-4) stain best with phosphotungstic acid–hematoxylin which stains the center brownish-red and the spikes blue (Lever and Freiman). The significance of the Schaumann and the asteroid bodies is not known. Neither is specific for sarcoidosis, since they have been observed in other granulomas, such as tuberculosis, leprosy, and berylliosis. If the granulomas of sarcoidosis involute, fibrosis extends from the periphery toward the center, with gradual disappearance of the epithelioid cells (Barrie and Bogoch).

Systemic Lesions. In the chronic, persistent type of sarcoidosis, a diagnosis of sarcoidosis should not be made on the basis of its clinical and radiologic manifestations alone, because it may resemble, among other diseases, tuberculosis and lymphoma. Since material for a Kveim test (see below) often is not available, a biopsy is essential for the diagnosis. In the acute, transient type of sarcoidosis, on the other hand, the symptom complex is unique, so that a biopsy may not be required.

In the chronic, persistent type of sarcoidosis the disease often is widespread even in the absence of symptoms. In patients with skin lesions, such lesions are the obvious site for biopsy. If there are no palpable lymph nodes or other lesions present near the surface, a random biopsy of a lung will result in positive findings in nearly 100 per cent of the cases—even in patients without positive x-ray findings—and biopsy of the liver in 80 per cent (Israel and Sones). Also, a random gastrocnemius muscle biopsy often shows sarcoidosis (Israel and Sones). In doubtful cases mediastinoscopy under general anesthesia and biopsy of a mediastinal lymph node may be advisable (Israel).

Among organs producing clinical manifestations in the chronic, persistent type of sarcoidosis, the lungs are the most common organ to do so—in about 50 per cent of the cases, according to James et al. The lesions may be either nodular or disseminated with extensive parenchymal fibrosis of the lungs. In the latter type of involvement cavities form not infrequently and aspergillosis with pulmonary hemorrhage may ensue (Israel and Ostrow).

In about 25 per cent of the patients ocular manifestations occur, consisting most commonly of a chronic iridocyclitis. Splenomegaly exists in about 17 per cent. In about 12 per cent osseous granulomas are present, causing swelling of one or several phalanges of the fingers and toes and appearing as cysts in roentgenograms; and 8 per cent of the patients have involvement of salivary glands, usually of the parotid gland (James et al.). In about 5 per cent one encounters paresis of a cranial nerve, most commonly of the facial nerve (James et al.). Asymptomatic enlargement of the hilar lymph nodes is present in 70 per cent, of peripheral lymph nodes in 30 per cent, and of the liver in 20 per cent (James et al.; Maycock et al.).

Sarcoidosis, although usually a benign disease, may lead to death. In the large series of patients reviewed by Maycock et al. and by James et al., 6.2 per cent and 5 per cent of the patients, respectively, died as a result of sarcoidosis. The most common cause of death from sarcoidosis is insufficiency of the right side of the heart resulting from massive involvement of the lungs with parenchymal fibrosis. Rather rare is death from pulmonary hemorrhage (see above) or from tuberculosis superimposed on sarcoidosis of the lungs. Another possible fatal complication is renal insufficiency resulting from hypercalcemia and hypercalciuria (Longcope and Freiman) or from sarcoidal glomerulonephritis (McCoy and Fisher). In very rare instances only, death results from massive involvement of the myocardium (Pascoe), or of the liver (Mistilis et al.). A rare fatal complication also is hypopituitarism from involvement of either the pituitary gland or the hypothalamus (Selenkow et al.).

Histogenesis. In sarcoidosis a particular state of host reactivity exists characterized by a depression of delayed hypersensitivity reactions. Thus, there is: (1) depression of the phytohemagglutinin-stimulated transformation of lymphocytes into blast cells in vitro, measured by the percentage of lymphocytes that, as indication of DNA-synthesis, are labeled with tritiated thymidine (Langner et al.); (2) a weakened response to skin tests with tuberculin and other antigens, such as are used in testing for mumps, pertussis, trichophytosis and candidiasis (Sones and Israel); (3) failure to reject homografts (Elton and Andrew); and (4) failure of potent allergens, e.g., dinitrochlorobenzene and paradinitrodiphenylaniline, to induce contact sensitivity (Epstein and Maycock). In contrast to the depression in delayed or cellular hypersensitivity, the immediate or humoral hypersensitivity is unimpaired.

The Kveim test, which consists of the intradermal injection of a heat-sterilized suspension of sarcoidal tissue, preferably spleen or lymph nodes, is a useful test; but, unfortunately, material for this test often is unavailable. The test is positive in 80 to 90 per cent of the patients with sarcoidosis (James et al.). For the evaluation of this test, a histologic examination of the test site 6 to 8 weeks after the injection is required. This shows, in the case of a positive reaction, well-defined epithelioid cell granulomas, as in sarcoidosis (Rupec et al.). If the histologic examination is carried out sooner than the 6 weeks that are necessary for the development of the epithelioid-cell granuloma, the prevalence of pregranulomatous monocytes and the presence of necrosis may interfere with the evaluation of the test (Steigleder et al.; Rupec et al.). It is not known whether the Kveim test represents an isomorphic effect or, as Danbolt assumes, a specific hypersensitivity to a cellular protein present in human sarcoidal tissue.

Electron microscopic examination of sarcoidal granulomas has shown that the round cells present at the periphery of the granulomas that were formerly regarded as lymphocytes, possess lysosomes in which acid phosphatase and other lysosomal enzymes are present (see p. 55). Thus, they are blood monocytes from which the epithelioid cells develop. The epithelioid cells fail to show any evidence of bacterial fragments, unlike the macrophages seen in granulomas caused by mycobacteria, although they contain both electron-light and electron-dense lysosomes (E.M. No. 29), some autophagic vacuoles, and complex, laminated residual bodies (Azar and Lunardelli). The giant cells form through the coalescence of epithelioid cells with partly fused plasma membranes (see p. 55 for details). The Schaumann bodies seem to form from laminated residual bodies of lysosomes. The asteroid bodies consist of collagen showing the typical 64 to 70 nm periodicity. It seems most likely that the collagen got trapped between epithelioid cells during the stage of giant cell formation (Azar and Lunardelli).

Differential Diagnosis. The histologic differentiation of lesions of sarcoidosis from lupus vulgaris may be very difficult, and occasionally it is impossible. There is no absolute histologic criterion by which the two diseases can be differentiated with certainty. As a rule, the infiltrate in sarcoidosis tends to lie scattered throughout the dermis, whereas in lupus vulgaris the infiltrate is located close to the epidermis. Furthermore, sarcoidosis usually shows only few lymphoid cells at the periphery of the granulomas, giving them the appearance of "naked epithelioid cell tubercles," whereas lupus vulgaris often shows a marked inflammatory reaction around and between the granulomas. Also, the granulomas of sarcoidosis usually show much less central necrosis than the granulomas of lupus vulgaris (Civatte). The epidermis in sarcoidosis is either normal or atrophic, whereas in lupus vulgaris, in addition to atrophy, there may be areas of ulceration, acanthosis, and pseudocarcinomatous hyperplasia. Aside from the Kveim test, the only laboratory procedures by which the two diseases can be differentiated with certainty are culture and guinea-pig inoculation, which are usually positive for tubercle bacilli in lupus vulgaris and always negative in sarcoidosis.

The foreign-body granulomas occurring in systemic berylliosis and in response to the local application of zirconium (occasionally incorporated into deodorant sticks and into creams) are indistinguishable from the granulomas seen in sarcoidosis. Clinical data are necessary for their differentiation (Epstein and Allen).

Tuberculoid leprosy also may be difficult to distinguish from sarcoidosis, since only 7 per cent of the cases with tuberculoid leprosy show acid-fast bacilli, and then only a few, so that they may easily be overlooked (Azulay). The most likely place to find bacilli is within degenerated dermal nerves. As a rule, the epithelioid cell granulomas of tuberculoid leprosy form around dermal nerves that are undergoing necrosis. Thus, the epithelioid cell granulomas of tuberculoid leprosy, like those of sarcoidosis, often show central necrosis. Since, however, the granulomas of tuberculoid leprosy, in contrast with those of sarcoidosis, follow nerves they often appear elongated (Wiersema and Binford).

CHEILITIS GRANULOMATOSA (MIESCHER-MELKERSSON-ROSENTHAL)

This disorder is characterized by fluctuating or recurrent chronic swelling, usually of one lip but occasionally of both lips. Associated with this there may be recurrent facial pareses and a lingua plicata (Hornstein). Occasionally, one observes, either in addition to or sometimes in place of swelling of the lips, swelling of the forehead, the chin, the cheeks, the eyelids, or the tongue (Wagner and Oberste-Lehn). In rare instances enlargement of cervical or submental lymph nodes is present (Hornstein; Klaus and Brunsting).

Histopathology. In the skin one observes focal accumulations of either a tuberculoid or a lymphoid-plasma-cellular infiltrate. Usually, both types of infiltrate are seen, and occasionally there are also small "naked" epithelioid cell granulomas, as in sarcoidosis (Miescher; Hornstein; Laymon). Lymph nodes, if involved, show the same histologic features as the skin, including the occasional presence of epithelioid cell granulomas (Hering and Scheid).

Histogenesis. The cause of the disorder is unknown. A relationship to sarcoidosis which had been originally assumed by some authors (Hering and Scheid), does not exist. The granulomas may represent a foreign-body reaction arising in response to degenerative changes in the tissue, especially the subcutaneous fat (Laymon).

CHEILITIS GLANDULARIS

This condition is characterized by swelling of the lower lip and occasionally also of the upper lip. When the lip is squeezed, droplets of a mucoid fluid emerge from the mucosa of the lip and from the vermilion border. In about 20 per cent of the cases, squamous cell carcinoma of the vermilion border develops (Michalowski).

Histopathology. Heterotopic salivary glands are present deep in the vermilion border and in the neighboring mucosa of one or both lips. Thus, numerous salivary gland lobules are seen where normally they are absent or present in only small number (Ruelens-van Haeverbeek). An infiltrate of lymphoid cells, histiocytes and plasma cells surrounds the acini of the salivary glands. Their ducts are dilated and contain eosinophilic material (Schweich).

Although some authors assume that the squamous cell carcinomas developing in cheilitis glandularis arise in the glandular ducts (Schweich; Ruelens-van Haeverbeek), Michalowski regards them as being of solar origin. He reasons that heterotopia of the salivary glands causes protrusion of the lower lip and thus increases its exposure to the rays of the sun.

GRANULOMA ANNULARE

The lesions consist of small, firm, asymptomatic nodules that are flesh-colored or pale red and often are grouped in a ringlike or circinate fashion. There usually are several lesions; but there may be just one or there may be many. The lesions are found most commonly on the hands and feet. Though chronic, the lesions subside after a number of years. Unusual variants of granuloma annulare include a generalized form consisting of hundreds of papules which are either discrete or confluent but only rarely show an annular arrangement (Dicken et al.; Haim et al.). Other rare forms are perforating granuloma annulare with umbilicated lesions occurring either in a localized (Owens and Freeman) or a generalized distribution (Izumi); and subcutaneous granuloma annulare in which subcutaneous nodules occur, especially in children, either alone or in association with intradermal lesions (Draheim et al.; Rubin and Lynch; Kerl). These subcutaneous nodules have the same clinical appearance as rheumatoid nodules (see p. 222).

A certain correlation between generalized papular granuloma annulare and diabetes mellitus has been observed by several authors (Romaine et al.; Haim et al.).

Histopathology. The histologic picture of granuloma annulare is characterized by focal degeneration of collagen and by reactive inflammation and fibrosis. The epidermis appears normal except in the rare instances of perforating granuloma annulare. The degeneration of collagen consists either of one to a few large foci of complete collagen degeneration or of numerous small foci of incomplete collagen degeneration. Most commonly, one observes only small foci of incomplete collagen degeneration; less com-

monly, large foci of complete as well as small foci of incomplete collagen degeneration; and rarely, only one large focus of complete collagen degeneration.

Foci of complete degeneration consist of large, sharply demarcated areas of collagen degeneration surrounded by histiocytes in palisading or radial arrangement and an infiltrate containing lymphoid cells and fibroblasts (Fig. 12-5). Within the area of complete collagen degeneration the collagen appears pale and homogeneous and contains only a few pyknotic nuclei.

Foci of incomplete degeneration consist of usually small, ill defined areas in which some of the collagen bundles appear normal while others are found in various stages of degeneration, ranging from a slight decrease in the degree of eosinophilic staining to disappearance and replacement by basophilic mucinous material. In addition, an infiltrate of lymphoid cells, histiocytes and fibroblasts is seen, often in a single-row alignment, in the spaces between the partially degenerated and partially normal collagen bundles. Also new collagen is being laid down. In areas thus affected the collagen bundles present an

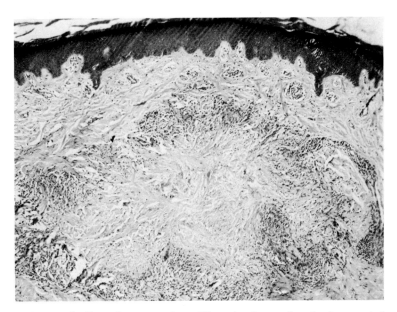

FIG. 12-5. **Granuloma annulare.** There is a large, sharply demarcated focus of complete collagen degeneration containing only very few nuclei. It is surrounded by an infiltrate composed largely of histiocytes in palisading arrangement. (×50)

irregular, disorderly arrangement (Fig. 12-6). The mucinous material, consisting of fine threads and granules (see Plate 1, facing p. 74), shows a metachromatic staining reaction with Giemsa's stain or toluidine blue (Gray et al.).

Occasionally, a few isolated, "naked" giant cells with irregularly arranged nuclei are present (Gray et al.). Also, in rare instances there are a few aggregates of histiocytes that resemble epithelioid cells to such an extent that the aggregates have the appearance of tuberculoid granulomas (Laymon and Fisher; Gray et al.). Not infrequently, small deposits of lipid material are encountered extracellularly in areas of collagen degeneration (Gray et al.; Wood and Beerman).

In the rare cases of perforating granuloma annulare foci of complete collagen degeneration surrounded by palisading histiocytes are located directly beneath the epidermis. Part of the degenerated collagen is being released through a "transepidermal elimination canal" (Owens and Freeman; Duncan et al.; Izumi). In other instances of perforating granuloma annulare, however, there merely is a central ulcer rather than true transepidermal elimination (Delaney et al.).

The subcutaneous nodules of granuloma annulare show multiple large foci of complete collagen degeneration with peripheral palisading of histiocytes. The foci of degeneration usually show, instead of homogeneous pale staining as in cutaneous granuloma annulare, strongly eosinophilic staining. This represents fibrinoid degeneration resulting from fibrinous exudation (Kerl). Peripheral to the foci of degeneration there is a chronic inflammatory infiltrate (Draheim et al.; Rubin and Lynch).

Differential Diagnosis. The type of granuloma annulare with small areas of incomplete collagen degeneration may show such inconspicuous changes that they can be overlooked. However, the presence of single

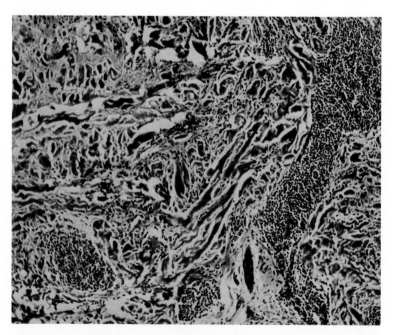

FIG. 12-6. **Granuloma annulare.** In the left upper quadrant is an ill defined area of incomplete degeneration of collagen. Some of the collagen bundles are in various stages of degeneration; others appear normal. Note the disorderly arrangement of the collagen bundles. Peripheral to the area of collagen degeneration a marked perivascular inflammatory infiltrate is present. (×100)

rows of fibroblasts between collagen bundles and some disorder in the arrangement of the collagen bundles should raise one's suspicion and set off a search for foci of collagen degeneration.

The type of granuloma annulare showing multiple, fairly conspicuous areas of incomplete collagen degeneration may greatly resemble necrobiosis lipoidica, in which a similar pattern of collagen degeneration may be present (see below). As a matter of fact, all the histologic and histochemical features seen in necrobiosis lipoidica may occur at times in granuloma annulare (Ellis and Kirby-Smith; Wood and Beerman). However, necrobiosis lipoidica differs from granuloma annulare as a rule by (1) the presence of a larger number of giant cells, (2) more pronounced vascular changes, (3) more extensive hyalinization of collagen, (4) more extensive deposits of lipids, and (5) smaller amounts or absence of mucin.

The type of granuloma annulare showing one or several large areas of complete collagen degeneration in the dermis presents a similar histologic picture as that seen in subcutaneous rheumatoid nodules except that in the latter the areas of degeneration are located in the subcutaneous layer, usually are larger, and show eosinophilic fibrinoid degeneration.

A differentiation of subcutaneous granuloma annulare from rheumatoid nodule is not possible on clinical or histologic grounds. Thus, in the absence of any rheumatoid disease, it is best to regard such nodules as subcutaneous granuloma annulare (Kerl) (see p. 222).

In spite of the histologic differences usually present in these three diseases, the fact stands out that granuloma annulare, necrobiosis lipoidica, and rheumatoid nodule have a common histologic pattern based on a focal degeneration of collagen. This suggests a similar pathogenesis for them (Wood and Beerman).

NECROBIOSIS LIPOIDICA

Clinically, one observes usually on the shins one or several sharply but irregularly demarcated patches. They appear yellowish in the center and violaceous at the periphery. The center of the lesions gradually becomes atrophic and shows telangiectases, and it may break down to form an ulcer. In addition to the shins, lesions may be present elsewhere on the legs. In about 15 per cent of the cases lesions are present also in areas other than the legs, especially on the thighs, hands, fingers, forearms, face and scalp (Muller and Winkelmann, 1966, I). In rare instances lesions are present in areas exclusive of the legs, particularly on the face and scalp (Dowling and Wilson Jones). Lesions located in areas other than the legs often are raised and firm and have a nodular or annular appearance so that clinically the lesions resemble granuloma annulare (Ellis; Balabanow et al.).

About three quarters of the patients with necrobiosis lipoidica are female; and approximately two thirds have clinical diabetes mellitus (Muller and Winkelmann, 1966, I).

Histopathology. On histologic examination the epidermis may be normal, but often it is atrophic and may be absent, owing to ulceration of the lesion. Two types of reaction may be observed in the dermis, namely a necrobiotic and a granulomatous type of reaction. Cases with the latter type of reaction at one time were referred to as granulomatosis disciformis (Miescher and Leder). However, combinations of the two types of reaction and transitions between them occur so frequently that now they are regarded as variants of the same process and not as two different processes. Also, at one time the necrobiotic type of reaction was regarded as typical for the diabetic type of necrobiosis lipoidica, and the granulomatous type of reaction as typical for the nondiabetic type. Although this is so to some extent, there are too many exceptions, so that the histologic appearance cannot be correlated with the presence or absence of diabetes in any specific case (Gray et al.; Muller and Winkelmann, 1966, II). It is of interest that a large proportion of lesions of necrobiosis lipoidica located in areas other than the legs show a predominantly granulomatous reaction.

In the *necrobiotic* type of reaction, poorly defined areas of necrobiosis of collagen are seen throughout the dermis, but especially

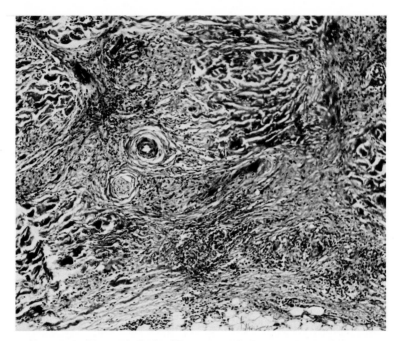

FIG. 12-7. **Necrobiosis lipoidica, necrobiotic type of reaction.** Much of the collagen appears degenerated. An inflammatory infiltrate is scattered through the areas of degeneration. A vessel in the center shows intimal thickening. (×100)

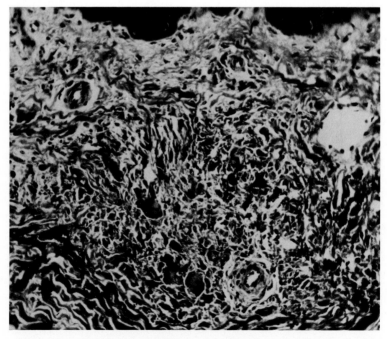

FIG. 12-8. **Necrobiosis lipoidica, necrobiotic type of reaction.** Several foreign-body giant cells are located within an area of collagen degeneration. Two fibrotic vessels are present. (×200)

in the lower portions (Fig. 12-7). The collagen bundles in these areas appear split up and amorphous and are intermingled with basophilic, mucinous material. Frequently, young collagen fibers are seen near the areas of collagen degeneration. Because of the continuous process of degeneration and regeneration the collagen fibers and bundles extend in various directions, resulting in considerable disorder of the collagen. In some areas the collagen bundles appear thickened, hyalinized, and in close approximation to one another.

At the margin of the areas of necrobiosis, as well as scattered through the dermis and often extending into the subcutaneous fat, one finds a cellular infiltrate composed of lymphoid cells, histiocytes, fibroblasts and occasional groups of epithelioid cells. Scattered foreign-body giant cells frequently are present and are of considerable diagnostic value (Gray et al.) (Fig. 12-8). In some cases histiocytes and epithelioid cells lie in fairly well circumscribed groups intermingled with a few giant cells, giving the infiltrate a granulomatous appearance (Laymon and Fisher). Cases with conspicuous granuloma formation are intermediate between the necrobiotic and the granulomatous type of necrobiosis lipoidica (see below).

The blood vessels, particularly in the middle and lower dermis, often exhibit thickening of their walls with proliferation of their endothelial cells. The process may lead to partial and, occasionally, even to complete occlusion of the lumen. Vascular changes of this type are seen particularly near areas in which the collagen bundles appear thickened and hyalinized. Whereas the vascular changes often are conspicuous in lesions of the lower legs, they are mild or absent elsewhere (Wilson Jones).

Staining for lipids with scarlet red frequently, but not always, reveals numerous granules of lipid extracellularly in areas of collagen degeneration. Occasionally, a few foam cells are also noted (Nicholas). The fact that occasionally the lesions contain no

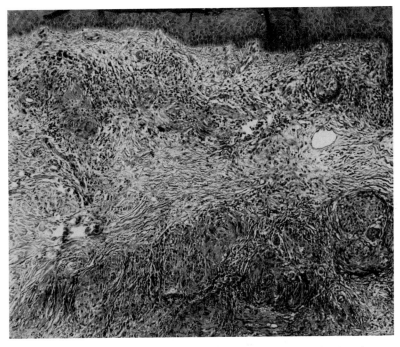

FIG. 12-9. **Necrobiosis lipoidica, granulomatous type.** The dermis contains scattered granulomas composed of histiocytes, epithelioid cells, and giant cells. There is fibrosis but only slight focal necrobiosis of the collagen. (×100)

lipids (Leifer) indicates that the presence of lipids is purely a secondary phenomenon, a "lipid phanerosis" secondary to collagen degeneration (Gertler). The extracellular lipid deposits on staining with scarlet red stain a rusty brown in contrast with the neutral fat in the subcutaneous layer and the fat in the sebaceous glands, which stain orange red. The lipid deposits probably consist of neutral fat, phospholipids, and small amounts of free cholesterol (Hildebrand et al.). Cholesterol esters cannot be present in significant amounts, since the granules only rarely show double refraction (Laymon and Fisher; Mehregan and Pinkus).

In the *granulomatous* type of reaction, the dermis contains scattered granulomatous foci composed of histiocytes, epithelioid cells, and giant cells (Fig. 12-9). One observes extensive fibrosis and hyalinization of the collagen, but areas of necrobiosis and deposits of lipids are not conspicuous and occasionally are even absent (Miescher and Leder; Muller and Winkelmann, 1966, I). Also, vascular changes usually are mild. In some lesions of necrobiosis lipoidica, especially those located on the face and scalp, numerous multinucleated giant cells are present (Fig. 12-10) (Dowling and Wilson Jones). Asteroid bodies may be present in some of these giant cells (Tappeiner).

Histogenesis. Some authors have expressed their belief that the necrobiosis of collagen is due to vascular changes, and that in cases in which diabetes exists, the diabetes is the cause of the vascular changes (Hildebrand et al.; Knoth and Füller). However, it is quite likely that the vascular changes are merely a part of the process of necrobiosis, hyalinization, and fibrosis of collagen. This would explain not only why vascular changes are occasionally absent but also why, when they are present, they are much more pronounced on the legs, where normally the vascular walls contain a good deal of collagen, than in other areas, where the vascular walls have less collagen (Wilson Jones). Many authors, such as Wood and Beerman, and Muller and Winkelmann (1966, I), regard focal degeneration of collagen as the primary event in necrobiosis lipoidica. Wood and Beerman have pointed out that since focal degeneration of the collagen is the primary event also in granuloma annulare and in rheumatoid nodules, these three diseases have a similar pathogenesis.

About two thirds of the patients with necrobiosis lipoidica have clinical diabetes mellitus. Occasionally, diabetes develops several years after the appearance of the cutaneous lesions

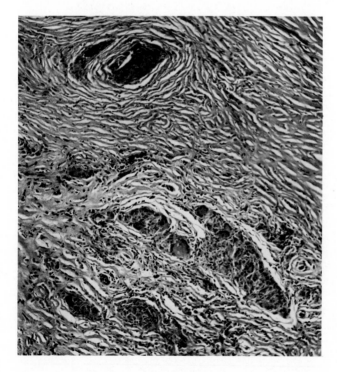

FIG. 12-10. **Necrobiosis lipoidica, granulomatous type.** Islands containing epithelioid cells and giant cells are closely surrounded by hyalinized bundles of collagen. (×200).

(Muller and Winkelmann, 1966, I); and nearly one half of the patients with "nondiabetic" necrobiosis lipoidica show an abnormal cortisone glucose tolerance test, e.g., 13 of the 32 patients tested by Komisaruk, by Mobacken et al., and by Muller and Winkelmann (1966, I). Nevertheless, this leaves a significant number of patients with necrobiosis lipoidica without evidence of diabetes. For instance, cases have been reported in which the cutaneous lesions had been present for 10 to 20 years without the development of diabetes (Smith). Only long-range follow-up studies will prove or disprove the postulate by Muller and Winkelmann (1966, I) that diabetes mellitus will occur in all nondiabetic patients having necrobiosis lipoidica who attain sufficient age. Diabetes seems to be particularly rare in patients in whom the lesions are present in areas exclusive of the legs. Thus, Wilson Jones found diabetes in only 1 of 21 patients with lesions confined to the face and scalp.

Differential Diagnosis. As already pointed out, differentiation from granuloma annulare may be difficult (see p. 217). This difficulty is rarely encountered in lesions of necrobiosis lipoidica located on the legs because in that location hyalinization of the collagen and thickening of the vessel walls usually are pronounced, and as a rule more giant cells and more lipid are present than are seen in granuloma annulare. However, lesions of necrobiosis lipoidica in locations other than the legs may be indistinguishable from granuloma annulare in their histologic features (Ellis; Wood and Berman; Gray et al.).

Occasionally, the granulomatous type of necrobiosis lipoidica shows well defined granulomas containing epithelioid cells and giant cells so that the histologic picture resembles that of sarcoidosis (Mehregan and Pinkus; Muller and Winkelmann, 1966, II; Dowling and Wilson Jones). However, the hyalinization of the collagen and often also the presence of foci of necrobiosis and of extracellular lipids aid in the differential diagnosis (Mehregan and Pinkus).

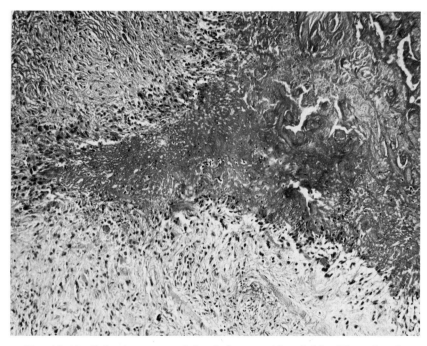

FIG. 12-11. **Subcutaneous nodule of rheumatoid arthritis.** There is a large central zone of fibrinoid degeneration surrounded by histiocytes in palisade arrangement. (×100)

RHEUMATOID NODULES

Subcutaneous rheumatoid nodules occur most commonly in rheumatoid arthritis and rheumatic fever. Recently, their occurrence in systemic lupus erythematosus has been described (Hahn et al.; Dubois et al.). The nodules develop near bony structures, often in the vicinity of a joint. They may or may not be attached to the overlying skin. Their size usually varies from a few millimeters to 2 cm; but they may be larger (Bennett et al.).

Subcutaneous nodules that are indistinguishable both clinically and histologically from rheumatoid nodules but are not accompanied by a rheumatoid disease occur occasionally in children (Beatty; Lowney and Simons) and rarely in adults (Kerl). Since subsequently none of these patients had a rheumatoid disease, but intradermal lesions of granuloma annulare appeared in several of them, it is best to regard such "pseudorheumatoid" nodules as subcutaneous granuloma annulare (see p. 217).

Histopathology. A rheumatoid nodule shows several sharply demarcated foci of fibrinoid collagen degeneration surrounded by histiocytes in palisade arrangement. In the intermediary stroma of the nodule one observes a chronic inflammatory infiltrate with some proliferation of blood vessels and fibrosis (Fig. 12-11) (Watt and Baumann). Although inflammatory changes prevail in the nodules of rheumatic fever, and proliferative changes predominate in the nodules of rheumatoid fever, nevertheless this difference is based on the age of the lesion, so that young nodules of rheumatoid fever have an appearance similar to those of rheumatic fever (Bennett et al.).

BIBLIOGRAPHY

Sarcoidosis

Azar, H. A., and Lunardelli, C.: Collagen nature of asteroid bodies of giant cells in sarcoidosis. Am. J. Path., *57*:81, 1969.

Azulay, R. D.: Histopathology of skin lesions in leprosy. Internat. J. Leprosy, *39*:244, 1971.

Barrie, H. J., and Bogoch, A.: The natural history of the sarcoid granuloma. Am. J. Path., *29*:451, 1953.

Brunner, M. J., and Robin, M.: Lichen-scrofulosorum-like lesions associated with sarcoidosis. Arch. Derm. Syph., *60*:1212, 1949.

Civatte, J.: Sarcoidose et infiltrats tuberculoides. Ann. derm. syph., *90*:5, 1963.

Danbolt, N.: Kveim's reaction and its significance in sarcoidosis research. Acta dermatoven., *42*:354, 1962.

Elton, R. F., and Andrew, J. H.: Homograft survival in sarcoidosis. Arch. Derm., *94*:403, 1966.

Epstein, W. L., and Allen, J. R.: Granulomatous hypersensitivity after use of zirconium-containing poison oak lotion. J.A.M.A., *190*:940, 1964.

Epstein, W. L., and Maycock, R. L.: Induction of allergic contact dermatitis in patients with sarcoidosis. Proc. Soc. Exp. Biol. Med., *96*: 786, 1957.

Grimmer, H.: Morbus Besnier-Boeck-Schaumann (Sarkoidose). Z. Haut Geschlechtskr., *39*:xv, 1965.

Hundeiker, M.: Zur Abstammung der Zellen des Sarkoidosegranuloms. Hautarzt, *20*:164, 1969.

Israel, H. L.: The diagnosis of sarcoidosis. Ann. Int. Med., *68*:1323, 1968.

Israel, H. L., and Ostrow, A.: Sarcoidosis and aspergillosis. Am. J. Med., *47*:243, 1967.

Israel, H. L., and Sones, M.: Selection of biopsy procedures for sarcoidosis diagnosis. Arch. Intern. Med., *113*:255, 1964.

James, D. G., Siltzbach, L. E., Sharma, O. P., and Carstairs, L. S.: A tale of two cities. A comparison of sarcoidosis in London and New York. Arch. Int. Med., *123*:187, 1969.

Langner, A., Moskalewska, K., and Proniewska, M.: Studies on the mechanism of lymphocyte transformation inhibition in sarcoidosis. Brit. J. Derm., *81*:829, 1969.

Lever, W. F., and Freiman, D. G.: Sarcoidosis: a report of a case with erythrodermic lesions, subcutaneous nodes and asteroid inclusion bodies in giant cells. Arch. Derm. Syph., *57*: 639, 1948.

Marten, R. H., and Warner, J.: Subcutaneous nodular sarcoid. Trans. St. John's Hosp. Derm. Soc., *53*:160, 1967.

Maycock, R. L., Bertrand, P., Morrison, C. E., and Scott, J. H.: Manifestations of sarcoidosis. Am. J. Med., *35*:67, 1963.

McCoy, R. C., and Fisher, C. C.: Glomerulonephritis associated with sarcoidosis. Am. J. Path., *68*:339, 1972.

Mistilis, S. P., Green, J. R., and Schiff, L.: Hepatic sarcoidosis with portal hypertension. Am. J. Med., *36*:470, 1964.

Mustakallio, K. K., and Niemi, M.: Histochemie der Lysosomenzyme des Sarkoidosegranuloms. Derm. Wschr., *152*:1454, 1966.

Nagai, R., and Kato, Y.: Erythrodermisches Sarkoid. Hautarzt, *13*:550, 1962.

Nozaki, T.: Sarcoidosis with lichenoid type eruption. Jap. J. Derm., *82*:47, 1972.

Pascoe, H. R.: Myocardial sarcoidosis. Arch. Path., *77*:299, 1964.

Putkonen, T.: Symptomenkomplex der beginnenden Sarkoidose. Derm. Wschr., *152*:1455, 1966.

Rupec, M., Korb, G., and Behrend, H.: Feingewebliche Untersuchungen zur Entwicklung des positiven Kveim-Tests. Arch. klin. exp. Derm., *237*:811, 1970.

Selenkow, H. A., Tyler, H. R., Matson, D. D., and Nelson, D. H.: Hypopituitarism due to hypothalamic sarcoidosis. Am. J. Med. Sci., *238*:456, 1959.

Sones, M., and Israel, H. L.: Altered immunologic reactions in sarcoidosis. Ann. Int. Med., *40*:260, 1954.

Steigleder, G. K., Silva, A., Jr., and Nelson, C. T.: Histopathology of the Kveim test. Arch. Derm., *84*:828, 1961.

Thal, M.: Zur Klinik der lichenoiden Form des Boeck'schen Sarcoids. Dermatologica, *111*:87, 1955.

Wiersema, J. P., and Binford, C. H.: The identification of leprosy among epithelioid cell granulomas of the skin. Internat. J. Leprosy, *40*:10, 1972.

Wigley, J. E. M., and Musso, L. A.: A case of sarcoidosis with erythrodermic lesions. Brit. J. Derm., *63*:398, 1951.

Wood, B. T., Behlen, C. H., II, and Weary, P. E.: The association of sarcoidosis, erythema nodosum and arthritis. Arch. Derm., *94*:406, 1966.

Cheilitis Granulomatosa

Hering, H., and Scheid, P.: Kritische Bemerkungen zum Melkersson-Rosenthal-Syndrom als Teilbild des Morbus Besnier-Boeck-Schaumann. Arch. f. Derm. u. Syph., *197*:344, 1954.

Hornstein, O.: Über die Pathogenese des sogenannten Melkersson-Rosenthal Syndroms (einschliesslich der "Cheilitis granulomatosa" Miescher). Arch. klin. exp. Derm., *212*:570, 1961.

Klaus, S. N., and Brunsting, L. A.: Melkersson's syndrome (persistent swelling of the face, recurrent facial paralysis and lingua plicata): report of a case. Proc. Mayo Clin., *34*:365, 1959.

Laymon, C. W.: Cheilitis granulomatosa and Melkersson-Rosenthal syndrome. Arch. Derm., *83*:112, 1963.

Miescher, G.: Über essentielle granulomatöse Makrocheilie (Cheilitis granulomatosa). Dermatologica, *91*:57, 1945.

Wagner, G., and Oberste-Lehn, H.: Zur Kenntnis der Symptomatologie der Granulomatosis idiopathica. Z. Haut Geschlechtskr., *32*:166, 1963.

Cheilitis Glandularis

Michalowski, R.: Cheilitis glandularis, heterotopic salivary glands and squamous cell carcinoma of the lips. Brit. J. Derm., *74*:445, 1962.

Ruelens-van Haeverbeek, A.: A propos de la cheilite glandulaire de Puente. Arch. belg. derm. syph., *25*:147, 1969.

Schweich, L.: Cheilitis glandularis simplex (Puente and Acevedo). Arch. Derm., *89*:301, 1964.

Granuloma Annulare

Delaney, T. J., Gold, S. C., and Leppard, B.: Disseminated perforating granuloma annulare. Brit. J. Derm., *89*:523, 1973.

Dicken, C. H., Carrington, S. G., and Winkelmann, R. K.: Generalized granuloma annulare. Arch. Derm., *99*:556, 1969.

Draheim, J. H., Johnson, L. C., and Helwig, E. B.: A clinico-pathological analysis of "rheumatoid" nodules occurring in 54 children. Am. J. Path., *35*:678, 1959.

Duncan, W. C., Smith, J. D., and Knox, J. M.: Generalized perforating granuloma annulare. Arch. Derm., *108*:570, 1973.

Ellis, F. A., and Kirby-Smith, H.: Necrobiosis lipoidica and granuloma annulare. Arch. Derm. Syph., *45*:40, 1942.

Gray, H. R., Graham, J. H., and Johnson, W. C.: Necrobiosis lipoidica: a histopathological and histochemical study. J. Invest. Derm., *44*:369, 1965.

Haim, S., Friedman-Birnbaum, R., and Shafrir, A.: Generalized granuloma annulare: Relationship to diabetes mellitus as revealed in 8 cases. Brit. J. Derm., *83*:302, 1970.

Izumi, A. K.: Generalized perforating granuloma annulare. Arch. Derm., *108*:708, 1973.

Kerl, H.: Knotige rheumatische Hautmanifestationen und ihre Differentialdiagnose. Z. Haut, *47*:193, 1972.

Laymon, C. W., and Fisher, I.: Necrobiosis lipoidica (diabeticorum?). A histologic study and comparison with granuloma annulare. Arch. Derm. Syph., *59*:150, 1949.

Owens, D. W., and Freeman, R. G.: Perforating granuloma annulare. Arch. Derm., *103*:64, 1971.

Romaine, R., Rudner, E. J., and Altman, J.: Papular granuloma annulare and diabetes mellitus. Arch. Derm., *98*:152, 1968.

Rubin, M., and Lynch, F. W.: Subcutaneous granuloma annulare. Arch. Derm., *93*:416, 1966.

Wood, M. G., and Beerman, H.: Necrobiosis lipoidica, granuloma annulare, and rheumatoid nodule. J. Invest. Derm., *34*:139, 1960.

Necrobiosis Lipoidica

Balabanow, K., Durmischew, A., and Karajachev, G.: Ein Fall von Nekrobiosis lipoidica diabeticorum mit ungewöhnlicher Lokalisation. Z. Haut, *47*:217, 1972.

Dowling, G. B., and Wilson Jones, E.: Atypical (annular) necrobiosis lipoidica of the face and scalp. Dermatologica, *135*:11, 1967.

Ellis, F. A.: Necrobiosis lipoidica. A form of granuloma annulare. Arch. Derm. Syph., *43*: 822, 1941.

Gertler, W.: Die nosologische Stellung der Granulomatosis (tuberculoides) pseudosklerodermiformis symmetrica chronica (Gottron). Derm. Wschr., *141*:241, 1960.

Gray, H. R., Graham, J. H., and Johnson, W. C.: Necrobiosis lipoidica: a histopathological and histochemical study. J. Invest. Derm., *44*: 369, 1965.

Hildebrand, A. G., Montgomery, H., and Rynearson, E. H.: Necrobiosis lipoidica diabeticorum. Arch. Intern. Med., *66*:851, 1940.

Knoth, W., and Füller, H.: Zur Patho- und Histogenese der Nekrobiosis lipoidica "diabeticorum." Arch. f. Derm. u. Syph., *199*: 109, 1955.

Komisaruk, E.: Cortisone glucose tolerance test in necrobiosis lipoidica. Arch. Derm., *90*: 208, 1964.

Laymon, C. W., and Fisher, I.: Necrobiosis lipoidica (diabeticorum?). Arch. Derm. Syph., *59*:150, 1949.

Leifer, W.: Necrobiosis lipoidica diabeticorum in a nondiabetic person. Arch. Derm. Syph., *44*:717, 1941.

Mehregan, A. H., and Pinkus, H.: Necrobiosis lipoidica with sarcoid reaction. Arch. Derm., *83*:143, 1961.

Miescher, G., and Leder, M.: Granulomatosis disciformis chronica et progressiva. Dermatologica, *97*:25, 1948.

Mobacken, H., Gisslen, H., and Johannisson, G.: Granuloma annulare. Acta dermatoven., *50*: 440, 1970.

Muller, S. A., and Winkelmann, R. K.: Necrobiosis lipoidica diabeticorum. Arch. Derm., *93*:272, 1966, I.

————: Necrobiosis lipoidica diabeticorum. Arch. Derm., *94*:1, 1966, II.

Nicholas, L.: Necrobiosis lipoidica diabeticorum with xanthoma cells. Arch. Derm. Syph., *48*: 606, 1943.

Smith, J. G., Jr.: Necrobiosis lipoidica. Arch. Derm., *74*:280, 1956.

Tappeiner, S.: Zur Klinik und Histologie der Granulomatosis disciformis chronica et progressiva (Miescher) (Atypisches Sarkoid). Arch. f. Derm. u. Syph., *194*:341, 1952.

Wilson Jones, E.: Necrobiosis lipoidica presenting on the face and scalp. Trans. St. John's Hosp. Derm. Soc., *57*:202, 1971.

Wood, M. G., and Beerman, H.: Necrobiosis lipoidica, granuloma annulare, and rheumatoid nodule. J. Invest. Derm., *34*:139, 1960.

Rheumatoid Nodules

Beatty, E. C.: Rheumatic-like nodules occurring in nonrheumatic children. Arch. Path., *68*: 154, 1959.

Bennett, G. A., Zeller, J. W., and Bauer, W.: Subcutaneous nodules of rheumatoid arthritis and rheumatic fever. Arch. Path., *30*:70, 1940.

Dubois, E. L., Friou, G. J., and Chandor, S.: Rheumatoid nodules and rheumatoid granulomas in systemic lupus erythematosis. J.A.M.A., *220*:515, 1972.

Hahn, B. H., Yardley, J. H., and Stevens, M. D.: Rheumatoid "nodules" in systemic lupus erythematosus. Ann. Int. Med., *72*:49, 1970.

Kerl, H.: Knotige rheumatische Hautmanifestationen und ihre Differentialdiagnose. Z. Haut, *47*:103, 1972.

Lowney, E. D., and Simons, H. M.: "Rheumatoid" nodules of the skin. Arch. Derm., *88*: 853, 1963.

Watt, T. L., and Baumann, R. R.: Pseudoxanthomatous rheumatoid nodules. Arch. Derm., *95*:156, 1967.

13

Inflammatory Diseases of the Subcutaneous Fat

CLASSIFICATION OF PANNICULITIS

No generally agreed on classification of panniculitis exists. While certain forms of panniculitis are regarded by some as an entity and by others as merely a variant, there exist several well established forms of panniculitis, with either a characteristic histologic picture or an established etiology. Some of them will be discussed in this chapter, among them subcutaneous nodular fat necrosis in pancreatitis, cold panniculitis, sclerema neonatorum, and subcutaneous fat necrosis of the newborn, and some are discussed in other chapters, including subcutaneous sarcoidosis (see p. 209), subcutaneous granuloma annulare (see p. 217), and lupus erythematosus panniculitis (see p. 434).

The problem of classification concerns the remainder of nodose lesions, as they occur predominantly on the legs. These nodose lesions, with the exception of acute erythema nodosum, are chronic and show variations of their histologic picture on the basis of duration so that different histologic interpretations could be made during different stages (Pierini et al.). In most instances of panniculitis an early stage of nonspecific inflammation with varying degrees of vascular changes is followed by a stage characterized by phagocytosis of fat and by a more or less pronounced granulomatous reaction, and ultimately by fibrosis. Since different areas of the same lesion may show different stages, a punch biopsy often is insufficient for the adequate evaluation of a process, which would require excision of an entire node or at least a large part of it. Often, therefore, when merely a small specimen is submitted, only a diagnosis of panniculitis without further classification can be rendered. But even with adequate histologic material it may be difficult to assign every case to a recognized entity, and only adequate follow-up will make a diagnosis possible.

A simplified classification of panniculitis recognizes an acute and a chronic form of erythema nodosum and includes under the latter, in accordance with Fine and Meltzer, subacute nodular migratory panniculitis, as described by Vilanova and Piñol, and by Perry and Winkelmann. Furthermore, erythema induratum is an entity, since, in addition to a tuberculoid infiltrate and vascular lesions, it usually shows in its later stage areas of necrosis, in contrast to erythema nodosum. Nodular vasculitis, as described by Montgomery et al., can be classified as a variant of erythema induratum. Additional entities with a characteristic histologic picture are superficial migratory thrombophlebitis and Weber-Christian disease. It appears doubtful, however, that adiponecrosis subcutanea of Rothmann and Makai qualifies as an entity, since most, if not all, cases described as such can be assigned either to the chronic form of erythema nodosum, or to erythema induratum, or to Weber-Christian disease.

ERYTHEMA NODOSUM

An acute form and a chronic form of erythema nodosum exist that differ in their clinical manifestations but not in their histologic characteristics.

In the *acute form of erythema nodosum,* the lesions consist of tender, red or livid red nodes raised slightly above the level of the skin. They vary from 1 to 5 cm in diameter and usually are confined to the anterior surface of the legs, although they may occur elsewhere. Without breaking down, they involute generally within a few weeks, although, as the result of the intermittent appearance of new lesions, the disease may extend over several months.

In the *chronic form of erythema nodosum* one or several red, subcutaneous nodules are found on the legs. Tenderness is slight or absent. The nodules through peripheral extension change into plaques. Older plaques often show central clearing. The duration of the disease may be from a few months to a few years.

Histopathology. The histologic changes are present mainly in the subcutaneous tissue. The dermis merely shows a moderate amount of a perivascular, chronic inflammatory infiltrate.

In early lesions of *acute erythema nodosum,* the subcutaneous tissue shows scattered accumulations of lymphoid cells and of varying numbers of neutrophils both in the fibrous septa between fat lobules and between individual fat cells. A few histiocytes and occasionally, eosinophils are present; but plasma cells are absent. As a rule, the infiltrate appears massive in only a few areas. Elsewhere it consists of numerous small, scattered, irregularly outlined aggregates wedged in among the fat cells, giving the fat lobules a "lacelike" appearance. Abscess formation or necrosis of the fatty tissue does not occur. The fibrous septa of the subcutaneous tissue show edema and swelling of the collagenous fibers (Bäfverstedt, 1968).

The small blood vessels within the fibrous septa often show marked involvement; and occasionally also the medium-sized veins show alterations (Fig. 13-1). Thus, many

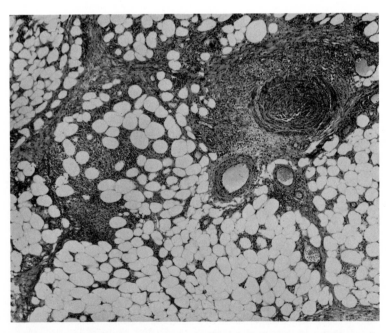

FIG. 13-1. **Erythema nodosum.** A chronic inflammatory infiltrate is scattered among the fat cells, giving the fat lobules a lacelike appearance. A medium-sized vein shows invasion of its wall by an inflammatory infiltrate and intimal proliferation. (×50)

authors believe that a vasculitis represents the primary and predominant lesion (Winer; Vilanova and Piñol). In some cases, however, the blood vessels are only slightly affected (Miescher; Perry and Winkelmann) or show no involvement (Löfgren and Wahlgren; Röckl). In cases with vascular changes one observes invasion of the vascular walls by the inflammatory infiltrate and intimal proliferation. Complete occlusion or thrombosis, however, do not occur. Extravasation of red cells into the tissue of the septa is a rather common finding (Perry and Winkelmann).

In older lesions of acute erythema nodosum neutrophils usually are absent. Lymphoid cells and histiocytes predominate, and giant cells are present, often in significant numbers. In some instances one finds small nodules in which histiocytes are lying in either a radial or a palisadelike arrangement around a small central fissure (Fig. 13-2) (Miescher). The giant cells usually show an irregular arrangement of their nuclei. They may lie alone or in association with a few histiocytes. Formations suggestive of tuberculoid granulomas, however, are encountered very rarely.

In *chronic erythema nodosum,* the findings are the same as in older lesions of acute erythema nodosum. The most striking finding as a rule is the presence of histiocytes and giant cells. Thickening of capillary walls with proliferation of endothelial cells in the fibrous septa has been stressed as an important feature by some (Vilanova and Piñol; Fine and Meltzer); but it may be slight or absent (Bäfverstedt, 1954; 1968; Perry and Winkelmann).

Histogenesis. Although the cause of erythema nodosum cannot always be established, in many instances the acute form of erythema nodosum occurs as a reaction against an infectious or allergic antigen. The greater number of cases of erythema nodosum of the acute type occur after an attack of streptococcal tonsillitis, and either beta-hemolytic streptococci can be cultured from the throat or the patient has an elevated anti-streptolysin-O titer (Favour and Sosman). In addition, primary infections with coccidioidomycosis or with histoplasmosis can elicit an attack of erythema nodosum (Medeiros et al.).

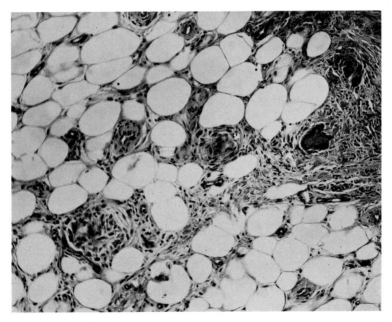

Fɪɢ. 13-2. **Erythema nodosum.** An older lesion shows two small nodules composed of histiocytes and, to the right, several giant cells of the foreign-body type. (×200)

Also, erythema nodosum may be part of the symptom complex of subacute, transient sarcoidosis which consists, in addition to lesions of the acute form of erythema nodosum, of hilar adenopathy, fever, arthralgia and often also acute iritis (see p. 209). Furthermore, erythema nodosum may occur in association with regional enteritis (see p. 273), and Behçet's disease (see p. 274). Allergy to some drugs, such as sulfathiazole (Miescher), gold sodium thiomalate (Stone et al.), and the contraceptive drugs, occasionally may cause erythema nodosum.

Differential Diagnosis. For differentiation from erythema induratum, see page 231. In cases of erythema nodosum showing severe vascular involvement, periarteritis nodosa must be excluded. In the latter disease, however, medium-sized arteries rather than veins and small-caliber dermal blood vessels are affected, and there is necrosis of the walls of involved vessels. Superficial migratory thrombophlebitis shows a large vein in the center of the lesion.

SUPERFICIAL MIGRATORY THROMBOPHLEBITIS

Multiple, tender, often cordlike nodules are present, usually on the legs but occasionally on the arms instead. In some instances the nodules slowly migrate along the course of a vein. The nodules may arise in crops. Ulceration does not occur.

Histopathology. A large vein at the border between the dermis and the subcutaneous tissue that is well endowed with thick muscular and elastic layers shows an inflammatory infiltrate permeating all layers of its wall. A thrombus usually occludes the entire lumen (Fig. 13-3) (Röckl). The inflammatory infiltrate extends only a short distance into the tissue surrounding the vein (Montgomery et al.). In early lesions the infiltrate shows a fairly large number of neutrophils, whereas later it is composed mainly of lymphocytes, histiocytes, and a few giant cells (Ruiter). When recanalization of the lumen takes place, intravasal and intra-

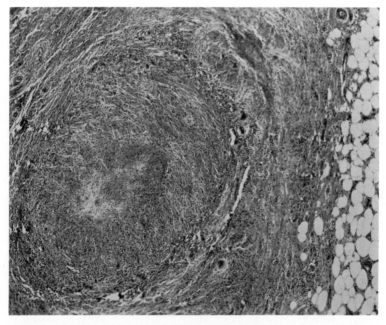

FIG. 13-3. **Superficial migratory thrombophlebitis.** A large vein shows an inflammatory infiltrate permeating all layers of its wall. The infiltrate contains several giant cells. The lumen of the vein is occluded by a thrombus. (×50)

FIG. 13-4. **Erythema in-
duratum.** Low magnification.
The infiltrate is limited to the
subcutaneous fat, where it is
located between the fat cells,
replacing them in part. (×25)

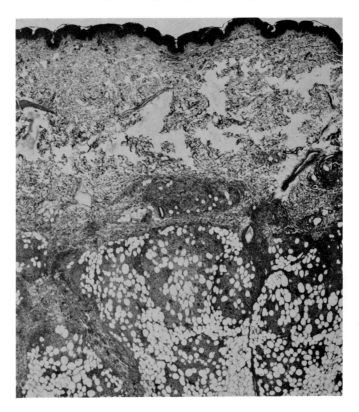

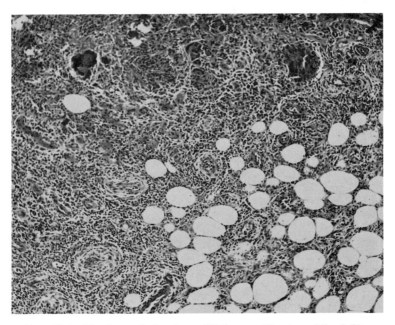

FIG. 13-5. **Erythema induratum.** High magnification. The infiltrate
in the area shown is tuberculoid in appearance, being composed largely
of epithelioid cells and giant cells. Many of the small vessels show
proliferation of their walls. (×200)

mural granulomas with giant cells are often seen (Röckl).

ERYTHEMA INDURATUM

The lesions in erythema induratum consist of chronic, painless but somewhat tender, deep-seated subcutaneous infiltrations on the legs, especially the calves. Gradually, the infiltrations extend to the surface, forming bluish-red plaques that often ulcerate before healing with an atrophic scar. Recurrences are common and often are precipitated by the onset of cold weather. Women are much more commonly affected than men.

Histopathology. In early lesions the histologic changes are limited to the subcutaneous tissue (Fig. 13-4), but in lesions that are farther advanced the infiltrate extends into the dermis. The histologic picture is characterized by (1) a granulomatous, tuberculoid infiltrate, (2) vascular changes, and (3) areas of caseation necrosis.

The infiltrate may be largely nonspecific, although usually it shows at least in some areas a granulomatous, tuberculoid structure, provided that the lesion is at least a few weeks old and an adequate specimen has been taken for biopsy. Sometimes it is necessary to cut deeper into the block of tissue to find areas with a granulomatous, tuberculoid structure. In such areas one finds epithelioid and giant cells, occasionally in tubercle arrangement (Fig. 13-5). In areas of nonspecific infiltration lymphoid and plasma cells predominate. Both the tuberculoid and nonspecific infiltrates extend between the fat cells, largely replacing them.

Vascular changes are extensive and usually severe. Arteries and veins of small and medium size show invasion of their walls by a dense inflammatory infiltrate, leading to endothelial swelling and to edema of the vessel wall (Montgomery et al.; Eberhartinger; Schneider and Undeutsch). Thrombosis and occlusion of the lumen result (Fig. 13-6). The occlusion may result in caseation necrosis.

Caseation necrosis is a fairly late development and therefore is lacking in about one half of the cases in which a biopsy is carried out (Andersen; Förström and Hannuksela). In lesions in which ulceration has taken place caseation necrosis usually is ex-

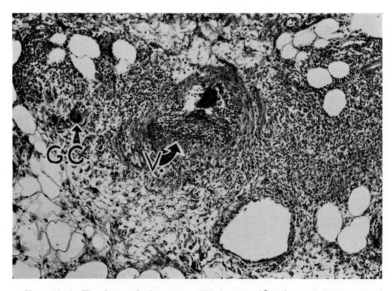

FIG. 13-6. **Erythema induratum.** High magnification. A large vessel (V.) in the subcutaneous fat is invaded by inflammatory cells and thrombosed. At the right of the vessel, the inflammatory infiltrate is nonspecific; at the left, epithelioid cells and a Langhans type of giant cell (G.C.) are located. (×200)

tensive. In areas of caseation necrosis the fat cells may still be partially preserved, while the invading infiltrate between the fat cells has been transformed into an amorphous, finely granular, eosinophilic material in which some pyknotic nuclei are present.

Cases showing evidence of vasculitis but only minor tuberculoid changes and absence of caseation necrosis have been called *nodular vasculitis* and have been regarded as a "nontuberculous" type of erythema induratum by Montgomery et al., and by others. However, abandonment of the tuberculous etiology for erythema induratum (see below) has made this subdivision unnecessary. In reality, nodular vasculitis merely represents either an early or a mild manifestation of erythema induratum (Pierini et al.).

Histogenesis. Because of the presence of a tuberculoid infiltrate and, often also, of caseation necrosis, erythema induratum has been regarded by many authors up to the present time as a form of tuberculosis, or at least as a tuberculid, for instance by Andersen, and by Förström and Hannuksela. Three factors speak against a tuberculous etiology: (1) Inoculation of tissue from lesions into guinea pigs (Telford) and culturing of such tissue (Eberhartinger) have given no evidence for tuberculosis; (2) active tuberculosis occurs with no greater frequency in patients with erythema induratum than in the general population (Eberhartinger); and (3) erythema induratum does not respond to antituberculous treatment but responds to the administration of corticosteroids (Eberhartinger; Van der Lugt).

Several authors in recent years have expressed their belief that in erythema induratum the primary event is a vasculitis of subcutaneous arteries and veins (Eberhartinger; Schneider and Undeutsch). According to Schneider and Undeutsch, any fat necrosis following vascular damage can develop a tuberculoid appearance.

Differential Diagnosis. Histologic differentiation of erythema induratum from erythema nodosum rarely causes difficulties, even though vascular changes and giant cells may occur also in erythema nodosum. First, the infiltrate in erythema nodosum is much less massive than in erythema induratum and usually consists only of small scattered aggregates; second, caseation is regularly absent in erythema nodosum, whereas in erythema induratum one often finds at least a few areas

of caseation necrosis; third, even though giant cells and histiocytes occur in erythema nodosum, tuberculoid structures are very rarely encountered; and fourth, in erythema nodosum the vasculitis, if present at all, is much less pronounced than in erythema induratum.

Lesions of erythema induratum showing a pronounced tuberculoid infiltrate, extensive caseation, and ulceration may resemble scrofuloderma. However, scrofuloderma shows no significant vascular changes, and usually tubercle bacilli can be found on staining with Ziehl-Neelsen's stain.

For differentiation from gummatous syphilis, see page 304.

RELAPSING FEBRILE NODULAR NONSUPPURATIVE PANNICULITIS (WEBER-CHRISTIAN DISEASE)

This disease is characterized by the appearance of crops of tender nodules and plaques in the subcutaneous fat, usually in association with mild fever. The lower extremities are predominantly involved, but lesions can occur also on the trunk, the upper extremities, and rarely also on the face (Pambor et al.). As the lesions involute, they may leave a depression in the skin. The overlying skin as a rule shows no involvement other than mild erythema. In occasional instances the nodules liquefy, the overlying skin breaks down, and an oily liquid is discharged (liquefying panniculitis).

Histopathology. The subcutaneous lesions of Weber-Christian disease pass through three stages. The first two stages occur while there is induration clinically. During the third stage depression of the skin may develop. The first stage is found only rarely on histologic examination because it is of short duration. It is probable that it does not always occur. Most sections show a combination of the changes of the second and the third stages. In some cases, however, a biopsy has shown only a nonspecific picture of inflammatory cells, without the presence of a significant number of foam cells on whose presence the diagnosis depends (Pinals).

In the first (acute inflammatory) stage one observes degeneration of fat cells accom-

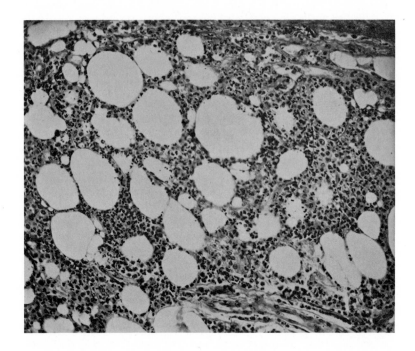

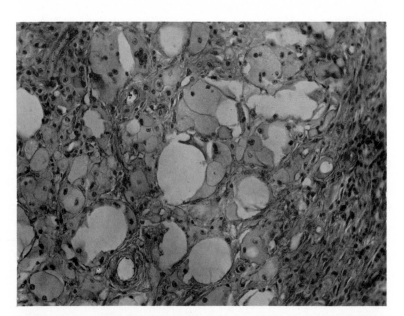

FIG. 13-7. **Relapsing febrile nodular nonsuppurative panniculitis.** (*Top*) First stage. An acute inflammatory infiltrate composed predominantly of neutrophils is seen between the fat cells. (×100) (*Bottom*) Second and third stages. The left side and the center of the field show the second stage: foam cells (macrophages) invading and digesting the fat cells. The right side shows the third stage: replacement by fibrotic connective tissue. (×100)

panied by an inflammatory infiltrate composed of neutrophils, lymphocytes, and histiocytes. Neutrophils may predominate (Fig. 13-7, *top*) (Ungar; Lever). Abscess formation does not occur.

In the second (macrophagic) stage the infiltrate consists predominantly of histiocytes. A few lymphocytes and plasma cells are also present. Many histiocytes in the vicinity of fat cells have the appearance of foam cells (macrophages) as the result of digesting fat from degenerated fat cells. Many foam cells are quite large, and some of them are multinucleated. In some areas numerous macrophages with foamy cytoplasm replace the fat cells completely (Fig. 13-7, *bottom*). A few foreign-body type giant cells without foamy cytoplasm may also be present (Kooij).

In the third (fibrotic) stage fibroblasts intermingled with lymphocytes and some plasma cells gradually replace the foam cells. Collagen is laid down, with resulting fibrosis.

The epidermis and dermis show no involvement in Weber-Christian disease. In some cases the larger subcutaneous vessels show mild changes, such as endothelial proliferation, as well as edema and thickening of their walls (Cummins and Lever; Steinberg).

In cases of liquefying panniculitis (Shaffer; Binkley; Hoyos et al.), the second (macrophagic) stage is followed by liquefaction of the foam cell infiltrate instead of by fibrosis. One finds an amorphous matrix in which foam cells, as well as lymphocytes and neutrophils, are situated.

Systemic Lesions. In the approximately 12 autopsies on record three types of lesions have been described: first, involvement of the mesenteric, omental, and retroperitoneal fat (Milner and Mitchinson); second, involvement of the fatty bone marrow, resulting in hypoplastic anemia (Spain and Folsy; Ungar; Steinberg); and third, involvement of the intravisceral adipose tissue in liver and spleen, causing focal necroses and subsequent invasion of these organs by fat-digesting macrophages, resulting in hepatomegaly and splenomegaly (Mostofi and Engleman; Schoen et al.; Arnold and Bainborough).

Among the nonfatal extracutaneous manifestations painful osteolytic lesions have been repeatedly described. On histologic exami-

nation the bone lesions have shown fat necrosis, chronic inflammation, fat-laden macrophages, and multinucleated giant cells (Pinals).

Differential Diagnosis. The histologic appearance of Weber-Christian disease is diagnostic during the second stage because in no other condition is there such preponderance of foam cells in the subcutaneous fat. The subcutaneous nodular fat necrosis occurring either in pancreatitis or with pancreatic carcinoma may resemble Weber-Christian disease clinically by showing, in addition to subcutaneous lesions, also involvement of visceral fat, of bone marrow, and of bones, but histologically it shows more pronounced necrosis of the fat cells, with the presence of "ghostlike" cells having thick "shadowy" walls and no nuclei.

LIPOGRANULOMATOSIS SUBCUTANEA OF ROTHMANN AND MAKAI

On the basis of present evidence it is very doubtful that lipogranulomatosis subcutanea of Rothmann and Makai exists as an entity, because there is too much divergence among the cases described under this diagnosis.

Some cases of lipogranulomatosis of Rothmann and Makai are identical with Weber-Christian disease as, for instance, the case described by Pambor et al. This patient, in the authors' opinion, at first had lipogranulomatosis of Rothmann and Makai "without fever or malaise and with the lesions developing gradually rather than in crops;" but this later changed into Weber-Christian disease with a fatal outcome.

Other cases, like the one described by Laymon and Peterson concerning a child who had tender "bumps" developing over a period of three months and showing absence of fat necrosis on histologic examination, differed in no way from erythema nodosum. And the three middle-aged women described by Röckl and Thies who had recurring, ulcerated nodules showing on histologic examination necrosis and granulomas probably had erythema induratum.

SUBCUTANEOUS NODULAR FAT NECROSIS IN PANCREATITIS

Subcutaneous nodules on the basis of fat necrosis may occur in patients with either pancreatitis or pancreatic cancer. The pretibial region is the most common site of the nodules; but they may occur also on the thighs, the buttock, and elsewhere. In some instances, the nodules discharge a turbid, oily material through fistular ducts (de Graciansky). There may be, in addition, polyarthritis caused by periarticular fat necrosis, and extensive intraperitoneal fat necrosis (Mullin et al.).

Histopathology. Foci of fat necrosis are observed in the subcutaneous tissue. They consist of "ghostlike" fat cells having thick "shadowy" walls and no nuclei (Szymanski and Bluefarb). Basophilic calcium granules are often seen within the areas of fat necrosis. A polymorphous infiltrate consisting of neutrophils, lymphoid cells, histiocytes, foam cells, and foreign-body giant cells surrounds the foci of fat necrosis (Mullin et al.). There may be areas of hemorrhage, in addition (Schrier et al.).

Histogenesis. The subcutaneous fat necrosis often carries considerable diagnostic significance since, in the case of pancreatic carcinoma, the tumor may still be asymptomatic at the time the necrosis takes place. The subcutaneous fat necrosis is due to the action of lipase on the neutral fat. Since the lipase is carried to the subcutaneous fat by way of the lymphatics, the serum levels of pancreatic enzymes, such as lipase and amylase, may be normal at the time of their determination, even though previously they were elevated (Schrier et al.; de Graciansky).

Differential Diagnosis. Although the presence of pretibial nodules may suggest erythema nodosum clinically, this diagnosis is easily ruled out histologically because erythema nodosum does not show fat necrosis. For differentiation from Weber-Christian disease, see p. 223.

COLD PANNICULITIS

Infants and, occasionally, also older children and adults may develop red, indurated and tender plaques or nodules at sites exposed to cold weather, especially on the face but also the legs (Rotman). In some instances, similar nodules have been seen on one or both cheeks of infants who had held a popsicle in their mouth (Duncan et al.). The plaques or nodules appear from 1 to 3 days after exposure and subside spontaneously within 2 weeks.

Histopathology. At the onset of the reaction to cold an infiltrate of lymphoid and histiocytic cells is observed around the blood vessels at the dermal-subdermal junction. At the height of the reaction on the third day some of the fat cells in the subcutaneous tissue have ruptured and coalesced into cystic structures (Duncan et al.). A rather marked inflammatory infiltrate is present around the cystic structures and between the fat cells. In addition to the lymphoid and histiocytic cells, a few neutrophils and eosinophils may be present (Solomon and Beerman).

Histogenesis. The lesions of cold panniculitis can be reproduced in the patients by holding an ice cube to their skin (Duncan et al.). Applying an ice cube to the skin for 50 seconds produces nodules in all newborn infants, in 40 per cent of infants 6 months old, and occasionally in 9-month-old infants (Epstein and Oren). It is known that the fatty acids of the subcutaneous fat are more highly saturated in the newborn than in the adult and that therefore the fat solidifies more readily at a lowered temperature than in the adult (see also under sclerema neonatorum). As shown by Adams et al., in pigs fed varying types of fat, cold panniculitis could be produced only in those who had been fed saturated fatty acids and thus had a high fatty acid saturation of their fat.

SCLEREMA NEONATORUM

Sclerema neonatorum is characterized by a diffuse, rapidly spreading hardening of the entire subcutaneous fat of infants during the first few days of life. The entire skin has a waxlike appearance and feels cold, tight and indurated. With few exceptions, death occurs within a few days. On autopsy the subcutaneous tissue appears greatly thickened, hardened and lardlike.

Histopathology. The subcutaneous tissue owes its thickening to an increase in size of the fat cells and to the presence of wide intersecting fibrous bands (Kellum et al.). Many of the fat cells are filled with rosettes of fine needlelike clefts. In frozen sections these clefts are found to be occupied by crystals. The crystals fail to stain with fat stains. They are doubly refractile in the polarizing microscope (Horsfield and Yardley). In most instances, no evidence of fat necrosis or inflammation is present (Kellum et al.). Still, in some cases one can see fat necrosis and an inflammatory reaction with giant cells (Zeek and Madden; Flory), but they are much less extensive and pronounced than in subcutaneous fat necrosis of the newborn.

In most cases of sclerema the changes in the fatty tissue were found to be limited to the subcutaneous fat when an autopsy was performed (Kellum et al.). In two cases of sclerema, however, autopsy revealed in the visceral fat lesions that were histologically identical with those observed in the subcutaneous fat. In one of these cases (Zeek and Madden) the lesions were widely distributed, while in the other case (Flory) they were limited to a few areas, namely the perirenal and retroperitoneal fat.

Histogenesis. The subcutaneous fat of the normal newborn, in comparison to adult subcutaneous fat, has greater amounts of saturated fatty acids, lower amounts of unsaturated fatty acids, a higher melting point, and a lower solidification point. The alterations in the subcutaneous fatty acids of infants with sclerema neona-torum represent an exaggeration of the normal newborn pattern. Thus, the increased ratio of saturated to unsaturated fatty acids in the subcutaneous triglycerides could be responsible for the physical changes of the subcutaneous fat in sclerema neonatorum (Kellum et al.). The increased ratio of saturated to unsaturated fatty acids probably is due to the fact that the enzyme systems involved in the desaturation of palmitic acid and stearic acid develop more slowly in newborn with sclerema than in the normal newborn (Horsfield and Yardley). The doubly refractile crystals in the fat cells consist of triglycerides, as Horsfield and Yardley have shown by means of x-ray diffraction.

SUBCUTANEOUS FAT NECROSIS OF THE NEWBORN

Subcutaneous fat necrosis of the newborn does not represent a localized form of sclerema neonatorum, as has been assumed by some authors in the past, but differs from it clinically as well as histologically, and in its prognosis.

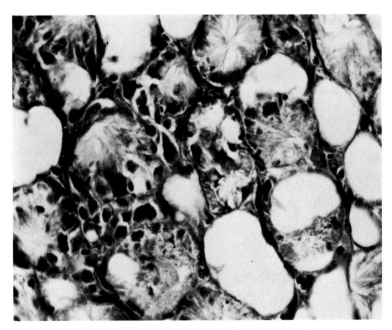

Fig. 13-8. **Subcutaneous fat necrosis of the newborn.** Several fat cells contain needle-shaped clefts in a radial arrangement. These clefts are indicative of fat crystals. The fat crystals themselves are not visible because lipids have been extracted by the processing of the tissue. An inflammatory infiltrate containing many foreign-body giant cells is present between the fat cells. (×400)

Subcutaneous fat necrosis of the newborn occurs shortly after birth as nodules and plaques in the subcutis. They disappear spontaneously after a few weeks or months. The general health is not affected. The cause is not known. It is not likely that trauma plays a role in the development of the lesions.

Histopathology. Histologic examination shows in the subcutaneous tissue areas of fat necrosis infiltrated by inflammatory cells and foreign-body giant cells. Many of the remaining fat cells, as well as the giant cells, contain needle-shaped clefts which in the fat cells often lie in radial arrangement (Fig. 13-8). In frozen sections the clefts are seen to contain doubly refractile crystals. Calcium deposits are scattered through the necrotic fat (Noojin et al.). In some instances extensive areas of calcification are present which may require several years to involute (Wesener).

Differential Diagnosis. Even though needle-shaped clefts are found in the fat cells of both diseases, sclerema neonatorum differs from subcutaneous fat necrosis of the newborn by (1) showing either little or no fat necrosis, inflammation, or giant cell infiltration, (2) the absence of calcium deposits, and (3) the presence of wide fibrous bands in the subcutaneous tissue (Kellum et al.).

HEREDITARY EDEMA OF THE LEGS (MILROY'S DISEASE)

Congenital lymphedema, which is dominantly inherited, is characterized by indolent, persistent swelling of the lower extremities. In patients several years old or older the lymphedema is associated with only slight pitting edema on pressure.

Histopathology. In congenital lymphedema the collagen bundles of the dermis appear homogenized and widened (Tappeiner). The subcutaneous fat is permeated by thick strands of collagen, and pools of lymph fluid are seen in spaces devoid of endothelial lining (Rosenberg).

Histogenesis. Lymphangiograms have shown the lymphatic vessels to be hypoplastic. It is possible that the primary disturbance is a retardation in the absorption of albumin by the lymphatics from the tissue (Calnan).

PROGRESSIVE LIPODYSTROPHY

Progressive lipodystrophy shows progressive disappearance of the subcutaneous fat in certain areas of the body. Most cases are of the cephalothoracic type, involving the face, the neck, the upper extremities, and the upper trunk. In other cases the atrophy of the fat extends from the crest of the ilium downward. In lipo-atrophic diabetes there is generalized rather than localized loss of fat.

Histopathology. The involved regions show complete absence of the subcutaneous fat. The dermis lies directly on the fascia or muscle (Taylor and Honeycutt).

BIBLIOGRAPHY

Classification of Panniculitis

Fine, R. M., and Meltzer, H. D.: Chronic erythema nodosum. Arch. Derm., *100*:33, 1969.

Montgomery, H., O'Leary, P. A., and Barker, N. W.: Nodular vascular diseases of the legs. J.A.M.A., *128*:335, 1945.

Perry, H. O., and Winkelmann, R. K.: Subacute nodular migratory panniculitis. Arch. Derm., *89*:170, 1964.

Pierini, L. E., Abulafia, J., and Wainfeld, S.: Idiopathic lipogranulomatous hypodermitis. Arch. Derm., *98*:290, 1968.

Vilanova, X., and Piñol, J. A.: Subacute nodular migratory panniculitis. Brit. J. Derm., *71*:45, 1959.

Erythema Nodosum

Bäfverstedt, B.: Erythema nodosum migrans. Acta dermatoven., *34*:181, 1954.

———: Erythema nodosum migrans. Acta dermatoven., *48*:381, 1968.

Favour, C. B., and Sosman, M. C.: Erythema nodosum. Arch. Intern. Med., *80*:435, 1947.

Fine, R. M., and Meltzer, H. D.: Chronic erythema nodosum. Arch. Derm., *100*:33, 1969.

Löfgren, S., and Wahlgren, F.: On the histopathology of erythema nodosum. Acta dermatoven., *29*:1, 1949.

Medeiros, A. A., Marty, S. D., Tosh, F. E., and Chin, T. D. Y.: Erythema nodosum and erythema multiforme as clinical manifestations of histoplasmosis in a community outbreak. New Eng. J. Med., *274*:415, 1966.

Miescher, G.: Zur Histologie des Erythema nodosum. Acta dermatoven., *27*:447, 1947.

Perry, H. O., and Winkelmann, R. K.: Subacute nodular migratory panniculitis. Arch. Derm., *89*:170, 1964.

Röckl, H.: Die Bedeutung der Histopathologie für die Diagnostik knotiger Unterschenkel-Dermatosen. Hautarzt, *19*:540, 1968.

Stone, R. L., Claflin, A., and Penneys, N. S.: Erythema nodosum following gold sodium thiomalate therapy. Arch. Derm., *107*:602, 1973.

Vilanova, X., and Piñol, J. A.: Subacute nodular migratory panniculitis. Brit. J. Derm., *71*:45, 1959.

Winer, L. H.: Histopathology of nodose lesions of the extremities. Arch. Derm. Syph., *63*: 347, 1951.

Superficial Migratory Thrombophlebitis

Montgomery, H., O'Leary, P. A., and Barker, N. W.: Nodular vascular diseases of the legs. J.A.M.A., *128*:335, 1945.

Röckl, H.: Die Bedeutung der Histopathologie für die Diagnostik knotiger Unterschenkel-Dermatosen. Hautarzt, *19*:540, 1968.

Ruiter, M.: Über die sogenannte Thrombophlebitis migrans. Arch. f. Derm. u. Syph., *197*: 22, 1953.

Erythema Induratum

Andersen, S. la C.: Erythema induratum (Bazin) treated with isoniazid. Acta dermatoven., *50*: 65, 1970.

Eberhartinger, C.: Das Problem des Erythema induratum Bazin. Arch. klin. exp. Derm., *217*:196, 1963.

Förström, L., and Hannuksela, M.: Antituberculous treatment of erythema induratum Bazin. Acta dermatoven., *50*:143, 1970.

Montgomery, H., O'Leary, P. A., and Barker, N. W.: Nodular vascular diseases of the legs. J.A.M.A., *128*:335, 1945.

Pierini, L. E., Abulafia, J., and Wainfeld, S.: Idiopathic lipogranulomatous hypodermitis. Arch. Derm., *98*:290, 1968.

Schneider, W., and Undeutsch, W.: Vasculitiden des subcutanen Fettgewebes. Arch. klin. exp. Derm., *221*:600, 1965.

Telford, E. D.: Lesions of the skin and subcutaneous tissue in diseases of the peripheral circulation. Arch. Derm. Syph., *36*:952, 1937.

Van der Lugt, L.: Some remarks about tuberculosis of the skin and tuberculids. Dermatologica, *131*:266, 1965.

Nonsuppurative Panniculitis (Weber-Christian disease)

Andsersen, S. la C.: Eryhtema induratum (Bazin) treated with isoniazid. Acta dermatoven., *50*:65, 1970.

Binkley, J. S.: Relapsing febrile nodular nonsuppurative panniculitis. J.A.M.A., *113*:113, 1939.

Cummins, L. J., and Lever, W. F.: Relapsing febrile nodular nonsuppurative panniculitis (Weber-Christian disease). Arch. Derm. Syph., *38*:415, 1938.

Hoyos, N., Shaffer, B., and Beerman, H.: Liquefying nodular panniculitis. Arch. Derm., *94*: 436, 1966.

Kooij, R.: Weber-Christian disease, a form of spontaneous panniculitis. Dermatologica, *101*: 332, 1950.

Laymon, C. W., and Peterson, W. C., Jr.: Lipogranulomatosis subcutanea (Rothmann-Makai). Arch. Derm., *90*:288, 1964.

Lever, W. F.: Nodular nonsuppurative panniculitis (Weber-Christian disease). Arch. Derm. Syph., *59*:31, 1949.

Milner, R. D. G., and Mitchinson, M. J.: Weber-Christian disease. J. Clin. Path., *18*:150, 1965.

Mostofi, F. K., and Engleman, E.: Fatal relapsing febrile nonsuppurative panniculitis. Arch. Path., *43*:417, 1947.

Pambor, M., Kemnitz, P., and Theuring, F.: Panniculitis nodularis febrilis "non-suppurativa" (Morbus Pfeifer-Weber-Christian) mit foudroyant-letalem Verlauf nach langjährigem afebrilem Bestehen. Derm. Monatsschr., *155*: 330, 1969.

Pinals, R. S.: Nodular panniculitis associated with an inflammatory bone lesion. Arch. Derm., *101*:359, 1970.

Röckl, H., and Thies, W.: Herdförmige chronisch rezidivierende Krankheitszustände des subcutanen Fettgewebes. Zur Histopathogenese der Lipogranulomatosis. Hautarzt, *8*: 58, 1957.

Schoen, K., Reingold, I. M., and Meister, L.: Relapsing nodular nonsuppurative panniculitis with lung involvement. Ann. Intern. Med., *49*:687, 1958.

Shaffer, B.: Liquefying nodular panniculitis. Arch. Derm. Syph., *38*:535, 1938.

Spain, D. M., and Foley, J. M.: Nonsuppurative panniculitis (Weber-Christian's disease). Am. J. Path., *20*:783, 1944.

Steinberg, B.: Systemic nodular panniculitis. Am. J. Path., *29*:1059, 1953 (discussion of systemic lesions).

Ungar, H.: Relapsing febrile nodular inflammation of adipose tissue (Weber-Christian syndrome): report of a case with autopsy. J. Path. Bact., *58*:175, 1946.

Subcutaneous Nodular Fat Necrosis in Pancreatitis

de Graciansky, P.: Weber-Christian syndrome of pancreatic origin. Brit. J. Derm., *79*:278, 1967.

Mullin, G. T., Caperton, E. M., Jr., Crespin, S. R., and Williams, R. C., Jr.: Arthritis and skin lesions resembling erythema nodosum in pancreatic disease. Ann. Int. Med., *68*:75, 1968.

Schrier, R. W., Melmon, K. L., and Fenster, L. F.: Subcutaneous nodular fat necrosis in pancreatitis. Arch. Intern. Med., *116*:832, 1965.

Szymanski, F. J., and Bluefarb, S. M.: Nodular fat necrosis and pancreatic disease. Arch. Derm., *83*:224, 1961.

Cold Panniculitis

Adams, J. E., Foster, J. H., Faulk, W. H., *et al.*: Experimental production of subcutaneous fat necrosis by general hypothermia: relation to the chemical composition of the fat. Surg. Forum, *5*:556, 1954.

Duncan, W. C., Freeman, R. G., and Heaton, C. L.: Cold panniculitis. Arch. Derm., *94*:722, 1966.

Epstein, E. H., Jr., and Oren, M. E.: Popsicle panniculitis. New Eng. J. Med., *282*:966, 1970.

Rotman, H.: Cold panniculitis in children. Arch. Derm., *94*:720, 1966.

Solomon, L. M., and Beerman, H.: Cold panniculitis. Arch. Derm., *88*:897, 1963.

Sclerema Neonatorum

Flory, C. M.: Fat necrosis of the newborn. Arch. Path., *45*:278, 1948.

Horsfield, G. I., and Yardley, H. J.: Sclerema neonatorum. J. Invest. Derm., *44*:326, 1965.

Kellum, R. E., Ray, T. L., and Brown, G. R.: Sclerema neonatorum. Arch. Derm., *97*:372, 1968.

Zeek, P., and Madden, E. M.: Sclerema adiposum neonatorum of both internal and external adipose tissue. Arch. Path., *41*:166, 1946.

Subcutaneous Fat Necrosis of the Newborn

Kellum, R. E., Ray, T. L., and Brown, G. R.: Sclerema neonatorum. Arch. Derm., *97*:372, 1968.

Noojin, R. O., Pace, B. F., and Davis, H. G.: Subcutaneous fat necrosis of the newborn: certain etiologic considerations. J. Invest. Derm., *12*:331, 1949.

Wesener, G.: Zur Klinik und Therapie der Adiponecrosis subcutanea neonatorum. Arch. klin. exp. Derm., *206*:531, 1957.

Hereditary Edema of the Legs

Calnan, J.: Lymphedema. The case for doubt. Brit. J. Plast. Surg., *21*:32, 1968.

Rosenberg, W. A.: Hereditary edema of the legs (Milroy's disease). Arch. Derm. Syph., *42*:1113, 1940.

Tappeiner, J.: Störungen der Lymphzirkulation als diagnostisches Problem des Dermatologen. Hautarzt, *20*:412, 1969.

Progressive Lipodystrophy

Taylor, W. B., and Honeycutt, W. M.: Progressive lipodystrophy and lipoatrophic diabetes. Arch. Derm., *84*:31, 1961.

14

Eruptions Due to Drugs

Allergic reactions to drugs may cause various eruptions identical in their clinical appearance with cutaneous diseases occurring also as idiopathic entities. For instance, drugs may cause urticaria, erythema multiforme, erythema nodosum, dermatitis, including generalized exfoliative dermatitis, folliculitis, and purpura due to either allergic vasculitis or thrombocytopenia. The histologic picture is the same in these diseases whether they are due to a drug or occur in their idiopathic form.

Several histologic changes more or less specific for drug eruptions will be discussed.

FIXED DRUG ERUPTION

Fixed drug eruptions are circumscribed lesions that recur persistently at the same site with each administration of the allergenic drug. The most common type of fixed drug eruption consists of one or several slightly elevated, erythematous patches that may become bullous and on healing leave pigmented areas. Fixed drug eruptions occur most commonly after the ingestion of either phenolphthalein or one of the barbiturates or phenylbutazone.

Histopathology. The histologic changes observed in fixed drug eruption suggest that it is a variant of erythema multiforme. Just as in erythema multiforme, the reaction may be predominantly dermal or epidermal, or it may take place in both the dermis and the epidermis. The latter type reaction is the most common.

The frequent presence of hydropic degeneration of the basal cell layer leads to "pigmentary incontinence," characterized by the presence of large amounts of melanin within macrophages in the upper dermis (Tarnowski). In addition, scattered individually necrotic keratinocytes with eosinophilic cytoplasm and pyknotic nucleus are frequently seen (Furuya et al.). Bullae form by detachment of the epidermis from the dermis (Stritzler and Kopf). Not infrequently, the epidermis shows extensive colliquation necrosis, even in areas where it has not yet become detached. The appearance of the epidermis then is similar to that seen in so-called toxic epidermal necrolysis (see p. 124) (Tritsch et al.).

BULLAE AND SWEAT GLAND NECROSIS IN DRUG-INDUCED COMA

Patients who are in a coma due to an accident or illness, or after a suicidal dose of a narcotic drug may show within a few hours areas of erythema at sites of trauma or pressure. Subsequently, usually within 24 hours, vesicles and bullae develop in the areas of erythema. The incidence of bullae depends on the severity of the coma and thus is highest in patients who subsequently die. In addition to narcotic drugs, carbon monoxide poisoning also can produce the lesions (Leavell et al.). The most common locations of bullae are the hands, wrists, scapulae, sacrum, knees, legs, ankles or heels.

Histopathology. The epidermis shows extensive necrosis. Where it is necrotic throughout the bullae arise subepidermally, but in areas of early necrosis showing eosinophilia of the cytoplasm and decreased staining of the nuclei small intraepidermal vesicles may be seen (Mandy and Ackerman). Where the epidermis is necrotic in its upper layers but not in its lower layers even large bullae can form within the epidermis (Achten et al.).

The secretory cells of the sweat glands show necrosis characterized by eosinophilic homogenization of their cytoplasm and by pyknosis or disappearance of their nuclei (Achten et al.). The sweat ducts usually appear less severely damaged but often also show pale staining or necrosis similar to the secretory cells (Brehmer-Andersson and Pedersen). It is of interest that the sweat gland necrosis is limited to areas where there are skin lesions. In patients who survive the necrotic sweat gland epithelium is replaced by normal appearing epithelial cells within about two weeks (Mandy and Ackerman).

The dermis beneath the bullae contains a sparse polymorphous infiltrate composed of neutrophils, eosinophils, lymphoid cells and histiocytes. In addition, some extravasated erythrocytes are often present (Mandy and Ackerman).

Histogenesis. The necrosis of the epidermis and sweat glands as well as the blister formation are the result of both generalized and local hypoxia (Achten et al.). Coma, whether the result of an accident, an illness or a drug, causes generalized hypoxia by depressing blood circulation and respiration. Carbon monoxide may act, in addition, by its binding to hemoglobin. Trauma, especially pressure, causes local hypoxia by decreasing local blood flow (Mandy and Ackerman).

DRUG-INDUCED PHOTOSENSITIVITY

One distinguishes photoallergic from phototoxic drug eruptions. Photoallergic drug eruptions, in contrast to phototoxic drug eruptions, represent a cell-mediated, delayed immunologic response.

PHOTOALLERGIC DRUG ERUPTION

In photoallergy, light is required for the allergic reaction to occur. The role of light consists of altering either the hapten itself or the avidity with which the hapten combines with the carrier protein to form a complete photoantigen (Harber and Baer). Among the photoallergenic drugs are: the sulfonamides; the thiazides, such as chlorothiazide (Diuril, a diuretic and antihypertensive agent) and tolbutamide (Orinase, an oral antidiabetic agent), both of which are aromatic sulfonamides; griseofulvin; and the phenothiazines, such as chlorpromazine, a psychosedative. A photoallergic drug eruption causes a photocontact dermatitis in all light-exposed areas. Like any allergic contact dermatitis, it causes itching (Hägermark et al.).

Histopathology. The histologic appearance of a photocontact dermatitis is that of an allergic contact dermatitis and as such shows epidermal spongiosis and microvesiculation, a perivascular lymphoid-cell infiltrate and exocytosis (Willis and Kligman) (see p. 100).

PHOTOTOXIC DRUG ERUPTION

If given in sufficiently large doses, certain internally administered drugs, in association with exposure to sunlight, may produce a phototoxic dermatitis, which represents an intensified sunburn and as such does not cause any itching (Hägermark et al.). Among the drugs known to elicit a phototoxic response are, in the first place, all drugs capable of producing a photoallergic reaction, provided that they are given in sufficiently high concentrations (Harber and Baer). Other commonly prescribed phototoxic drugs are certain tetracyclines, such as demeclocycline hydrochloride (Declomycin) and doxycycline (Vibramycin) (Frost et al.), and the psoralens.

Histopathology. A phototoxic drug eruption does not have a diagnostic histologic appearance. There merely is a nonspecific dermal inflammatory infiltrate.

CHLORPROMAZINE PIGMENTATION

Chlorpromazine, when given in high doses for several years as a tranquilizer to psychiatric patients, may produce in exposed areas of the skin a slate-gray discoloration resembling the discoloration seen in argyria. The exposed parts of the bulbar conjunctive also may show darkening (Hays et al.).

Histopathology. The amount of melanin in the basal layer of the epidermis may be normal (Hays et al.; Zelickson) or increased (Hashimoto et al.). Considerable accumulations of pigment are found throughout the dermis within macrophages, especially in the vicinity of the capillaries. The pigment has the staining properties of melanin in that it stains black with the Fontana-Masson silver stain and is decolorized by hydrogen peroxide (Hays et al.).

In patients on prolonged medication with chlorpromazine who have died of unrelated causes, autopsy may reveal in many internal organs melaninlike material that stains black with the Fontana-Masson silver stain and can be decolorized by hydrogen peroxide. This material is found throughout the entire reticuloendothelial system and to a lesser degree in the parenchymal cells of the liver, kidneys and endocrine glands, in myocardial fibers, and in cerebral neurons (Greiner and Nicolson).

Histogenesis. Electron microscopic examination has confirmed the presence of many melanosome complexes within the lysosomes of dermal macrophages. In addition, one observes round or bizarrely shaped bodies, measuring 0.2 to 3 μm in diameter and possessing such great electron-density that no internal structure is recognizable (Zelickson; Hashimoto et al.). These bodies are located in macrophages, endothelial cells, pericytes, Schwann cells, and fibroblasts, usually within lysosomes. At times both the electron-dense bodies and melanosome complexes are found within the same lysosome. Zelickson has interpreted the electron-dense bodies as a drug metabolite of chlorpromazine, and Hashimoto as a lipoprotein complex that is conjugated with chlorpromazine or its metabolites. It has become apparent, however, that histochemically the dense bodies react like melanin (Greiner and Nicolson), and Blois has furthermore shown that chlorpromazine binds to melanin with a high degree of selectivity, whereby chlorpromazine acts as electron donor and melanin as the acceptor. Thus, it can be assumed that the electron-dense bodies represent complexes of melanin with chlorpromazine. It is apparent that, in contrast to melanin, the chlorpromazine-melanin complexes are not metabolized by the human body. Since the chlor-

promazine-melanin complexes are found also within neutrophils and monocytes of the circulating blood, it can be assumed that these complexes are carried from the dermis via the circulating blood to the various internal organs (Satanove). It is likely that, in addition to an inability of the body to metabolize the melanin-chlorpromazine complexes, there is an overproduction of melanin. Hashimoto assumes that chlorpromazine, analogous to the silver particles in argyria (see p. 244), stimulates the epidermal melanocytes to an increased production of melanin. Other authors have cited evidence that chlorpromazine stimulates the secretion of MSH (melanin-stimulating hormone) by the pituitary gland (Scott and Nading).

DRUG-INDUCED LUPUS ERYTHEMATOSUS

Several drugs may induce a syndrome identical with systemic lupus erythematosus. The drugs that do this most commonly are procainamide, which is used against cardiac arrhythmia, hydralazine, an antihypertensive drug, and diphenylhydantoin (Dilantin), an anticonvulsive drug. It is likely that the development of a systemic-lupus-erythematosuslike syndrome under medication with these drugs represents an uncovering of a latent systemic lupus erythematosus, rather than an allergic reaction (Alarcon-Segovia et al.).

Drug-induced systemic lupus erythematosus is clinically, pathologically and serologically indistinguishable from spontaneously arising systemic lupus erythematosus. However, cutaneous and renal manifestations are rarer in drug-induced than in spontaneous systemic lupus erythematosus, and pleuropulmonary manifestations are somewhat more common (Dubois). The LE-cell phenomenon and antinuclear antibodies are always present (Weiss and Swift). Usually, but not always, when the medication is discontinued, the clinical and laboratory manifestations subside (Dubois).

Histopathology. The histologic picture of the cutaneous lesions is the same as that in systemic lupus erythematosus (see p. 428).

Histogenesis. A considerable difference exists between naturally arising and drug-induced systemic lupus erythematosus on direct immunofluorescent testing. Whereas 14 of 26 patients with naturally arising systemic lupus erythematosus showed fluorescence at the epidermal-dermal border of normal-appearing skin, only 1 of 16 patients with procaine-induced systemic lupus erythematosus showed fluorescence (Grossman et al.).

BROMODERMA

Prolonged ingestion of bromides may cause the formation of raised verrucous plaques, which are called bromoderma. They occur usually on the lower extremities.

Histopathology. One observes papillomatosis and considerable downward proliferation of the epidermis, often to such a degree as to produce the picture of pseudocarcinomatous hyperplasia. Islands of epidermis may be found deep in the dermis. Frequently, intraepidermal abscesses are present in the surface epidermis as well as in the downward proliferations of the epidermis (Fig. 14-1). The intraepidermal abscesses are densely filled with neutrophils, eosinophils, histiocytes, and desquamated squamous cells, most of which appear necrotic although some resemble acantholytic cells (Schirren and Wehrmann).

The dermis shows an extensive infiltrate that may reach into the subcutaneous layer. It is composed of a great variety of cells, including lymphoid cells, plasma cells, and histiocytes. Usually, neutrophils are numerous, and abscesses may be found scattered through the infiltrate. The number of eosinophils is variable, but in most cases they are quite numerous (Leibl). The blood vessels are increased in number and dilated, and they show proliferation of their endothelium (Teller). Often, areas of necrosis and of hemorrhage are present within the dermis.

Differential Diagnosis. The histologic picture of bromoderma is suggestive but not diagnostic. Intraepidermal abscesses also occur in blastomycosis and pemphigus vegetans. Blastomycosis is easily differentiated by its numerous giant cells and the presence of yeast cells within them. On the other hand, differentiation from pemphigus vegetans may cause difficulties, especially since acantholytic cells may be seen occasionally in the intraepidermal abscesses of bromoderma. Generally, pemphigus vegetans has a less extensive dermal infiltrate and con-

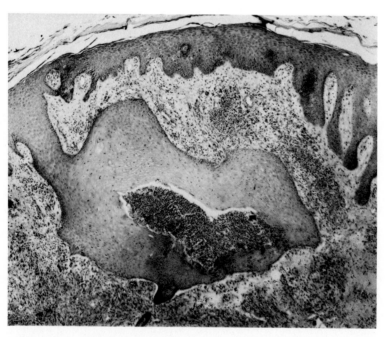

Fig. 14-1. **Bromoderma.** There is downward proliferation of the epidermis. A large intraepidermal abscess is shown. The dermis contains a dense inflammatory infiltrate. (×50)

tains a larger proportion of eosinophils in both the intraepidermal abscesses and the dermal infiltrate. For differentiation from iododerma, see below.

IODODERMA

Iododerma is characterized clinically by raised vegetating lesions that resemble those of bromoderma. However, as a rule there is less verrucous proliferation, and there is a greater tendency to ulceration. The face is commonly affected (Rosenberg et al.).

Histopathology. Iododerma differs from bromoderma by showing less epithelial proliferation. Frequently, the invasion of the epidermis by the inflammatory infiltrate destroys the epidermis, resulting in ulceration. At the margin of such ulcers one often finds intraepidermal abscesses and pseudocarcinomatous hyperplasia (Gehrels). The dermal infiltrate may resemble that seen in bromoderma (Jones et al.). In some cases it is composed to a large extent of neutrophils (Rosenberg et al.), while in other cases

mononuclear cells predominate, some of which may show mitotic figures and hyperchromatic nuclei, so that distinction from lesions of mycosis fungoides in the tumor stage may be difficult (Hollander and Fetterman). However, the presence of vascular proliferation with endothelial swelling, of neutrophilic abscesses, and of hemorrhages in the dermis aids in the differentiation (Jones et al.).

Histogenesis. In a case of iododerma described by Rosenberg et al. the patient's lymphocytes in culture underwent blastogenic transformation when they were exposed to ^{131}I-labeled serum albumin, but they failed to do so on exposure to potassium iodide. Since (1) iodine caused transformation of the patient's lymphocytes only when it was present as a hapten with serum albumin, (2) no circulating antibodies could be demonstrated in the patient's serum, and (3) the lymphocyte transformation test is correlated to delayed rather than immediate hypersensitivity, Rosenberg et al. concluded that the iododerma in their patient had formed on the basis of delayed hypersensitivity.

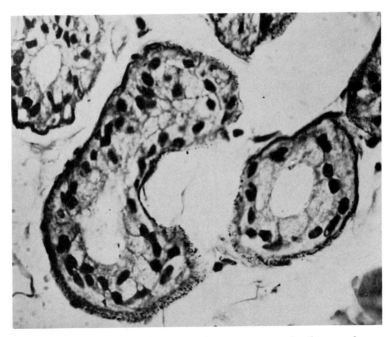

FIG. 14-2. **Argyria.** Silver granules are present in the membrana propria of the sweat glands. In some places the granules are so dense that they form a solid black band. (×400)

ARGYRIA

This condition, caused by prolonged ingestion of silver salts or their application to the mucous membranes of the upper respiratory tract, is characterized by a slate-gray discoloration of the skin, especially in the exposed areas, and often also of the oral mucosa and conjunctivae.

Histopathology. Silver is found in the dermis extracellularly as fine, small, round, brownish-black granules that appear fairly uniform in size. In contrast, silver is never seen in the epidermis or its appendages. The silver granules measure less than 1 μm in diameter and lie singly as well as in groups. Although visible in routine stains, the silver granules stand out much more clearly when sections are examined with a darkfield microscope. The silver granules then appear as brilliantly refractile white particles against a dark background. Many more granules can be seen by this method than with direct illumination.

The silver granules are present in greatest number in the hyaline basement zone, or membrana propria, surrounding the sweat glands (Fig. 14-2). In addition, silver granules are seen in high concentration in the connective tissue sheaths around the hair follicles and sebaceous glands, around as well as in the walls of capillaries, in the arrectores pilorum, and in the nerves (Hill and Montgomery). Silver granules are also found in the dermal papillae and scattered diffusely through the dermis. Elastic tissue stains reveal a predilection of the granules of silver for elastic fibers. The location of silver in elastic fibers explains the presence of fingerlike chains of granules projecting into the dermal papillae (Hill and Montgomery). The silver granules also show an affinity to areas of solar elastosis (Schröpl et al.).

In addition to silver, which is equally distributed throughout the exposed and the unexposed skin, one finds an increase in the amounts of melanin, particularly in the exposed skin. Increased amounts of melanin are present in some cases only in the epidermis (Mehta et al.) whereas in other cases melanin is found also within melanophages scattered through the upper dermis (Hill and Montgomery).

Deposits of silver are found also in internal organs, particularly in the connective tissue of the liver and spleen. Analogous to the marked involvement of the hyaline basement zone around the sweat glands, the hyaline basement zone around the seminiferous tubules of the testes is particularly rich in silver granules (Prose).

Histogenesis. On electron microscopy the silver granules lie almost entirely extracellularly within the dermis. The silver granules consist of aggregates of microgranules, in which the microgranules vary from 3 to 70 nm in diameter (Prose) and average 40 nm (Hönigsmann et al.). The silver granules are round, ovoid or irregularly shaped and, in contrast to their rather uniform size on light microscopy, vary considerably in size on electron microscopy, measuring from 13 to 1,000 nm in diameter according to Prose, and up to 300 nm according to Mehta et al.

The silver granules are located predominantly in the basal lamina surrounding the sweat glands, and in the basal lamina around endothelial cells, nerve fibers and smooth muscle cells (Hönigsmann et al.). Localization in the subepidermal basal lamina surrounding hair follicles and sebaceous glands is less pronounced (Mehta et al.). In the elastic fibers the silver granules are located exclusively among the protofilaments of the skeleton fibrils and not in the amorphous substance, the elastin (Hönigsmann et al.). Only occasionally some silver granules are found within lysosomes of fibroblasts (Mehta et al.) or macrophages (Hönigsmann et al.).

The increase in the amount of melanin in the basal cell layer and in the upper dermis can be explained by the fact that the presence of silver in the skin stimulates melanocytic activity. Silver is assumed to act either through the increasing of oxidative processes (Robert and Zürcher) or by reacting with epidermal sulfhydryl groups thus reducing the inhibition that sulfhydryl groups normally exert on the enzyme system governing melanin synthesis (Buckley). It is well known that melanocytic activity is stimulated not only by deposits of silver in the skin but also by deposits of other heavy metals—for instance, iron in hemochromatosis (see p. 411), and mercury in mercury pigmentation (see below).

The question arises whether the slate-gray pigmentation of argyria is caused solely by the deposits of silver, or by the increase in the amount of melanin, or by both the silver and the melanin. The fact that the pigmentation is more pronounced in sun-exposed areas probably cannot be explained solely by an increased deposit of silver granules in areas of solar elastosis, as suggested by Schröpl et al. On the other hand, the marked degree of pigmentation and the slate-gray hue, which results from the Tyndall effect of deeply deposited pigment, make it appear unlikely that the pigmentation is caused solely by the increase in melanin, which is moderate, as a rule, and is limited to the epidermis and uppermost dermis. It thus appears most likely that both the deposits of silver and the increase in melanin contribute to the pigmentation (Czitober et al.).

Differential Diagnosis. Histologic differentiation of argyria from other kinds of pigmentation rarely causes any difficulty because of the uniform size and characteristic distribution of the silver granules. The easiest procedure proving that the granules contain silver is to place sections into a solution consisting of 1 per cent of potassium ferricyanide in 20 per cent sodium thiosulfate, which will result in removal of the silver (Pearse). If a positive identification of the silver deposits in histologic sections is desired, this can be accomplished by means of neutron-activation analysis (Czitober et al.).

MERCURY PIGMENTATION

Regular application of a mercury-containing cream to the face and neck over many years may produce a slate-gray pigmentation of the skin in the areas to which the cream has been applied. Generally, the pigmentation is most pronounced on the eyelids, in the nasolabial folds and the folds of the neck (Lamar and Bliss).

Histopathology. Irregular brownish black granules are found in the upper dermis, located partially free in the dermis and partially within macrophages (Lüders et al.). Darkfield examination of sections reveals the granules to be brilliantly refractile (Burge and Winkelmann). On staining with silver nitrate the amount of melanin in the basal layer of the epidermis may be within normal limits (Lüders et al.) or may be increased (Burge and Winkelmann).

Histogenesis. By electron microscopy, the mercury particles measure approximately 14 nm in diameter and are aggregated into irregular granules up to 340 nm in size. Many granules are associated with elastic fibers, while others are situated free among the collagen fibers and in macrophages either within lysosomes or free in the cytoplasm (Burge and Winkelmann).

Since clinically the pigmentation is most pronounced in skin folds that are protected from the sun, and histologically there may be no increase in the amount of melanin, it can be concluded that most of the pigmentation is caused by the presence of mercury rather than of melanin.

Differential Diagnosis. Mercury pigmentation differs from a tattoo by the more superficial location of the granules and by refractility of the granules on darkfield examination. A positive identification of the granules as mercury granules can be made by submitting unstained sections to neutron-activation analysis (Burge and Winkelmann).

ARSENICAL KERATOSIS AND CARCINOMA

Inorganic arsenic was a frequently used oral medication for a number of dermatoses until in the 1930's evidence accumulated that, besides its long known tendency to form arsenical keratoses on the palms and soles, inorganic arsenic quite frequently caused carcinoma of the skin (Montgomery). In the 1950's it had become apparent that inorganic arsenic could cause visceral carcinoma, especially of the bronchi and of the genitourinary system (Sommers and McManus). The most common form in which inorganic arsenic had been administered was Fowler's solution, containing 1 per cent of potassium arsenite.

Arsenical keratoses of the palms and soles are verrucous pale papules without surrounding inflammation. They occurred quite frequently. Thus, Fierz, in a follow-up study of 262 patients who had received Fowler's solution from 6 to 26 years prior to his study, found arsenical keratoses of the palms and soles in 40.4 per cent of the patients. In one of them a metastasizing carcinoma had developed on the left palm. The minimal latent period had been 2½ years, and the average latent period 6 years.

Cutaneous carcinomas following arsenic ingestion are often multiple and usually are located on the trunk. They consist of erythematous, scaling, occasionally crusted patches that slowly increase in size. In Fierz's series 8 per cent of the patients had cutaneous carcinoma. Since the average latency had been 14 years, many more of his patients could be expected to develop a cutaneous carcinoma in the future.

Visceral carcinoma had been the cause of death in 4 of Fierz's 11 patients who had died. Three had died of bronchial carcinoma, and one of carcinoma of the liver. That several more of Fierz's patients were due to die from arsenic-induced visceral carcinoma could be concluded from the observation of Sommers and McManus that the latent period for arsenic-induced visceral carcinoma varied from 13 to 50 years, with an average of 24 years.

Since Bowen's disease is the usual cutaneous carcinoma produced by arsenic, the relationship between Bowen's disease and visceral carcinoma, first pointed out by Graham and Helwig in 1959, is of interest. If one takes only those cases of Bowen's disease in which the lesions are in nonexposed areas, and thus are not caused by sun exposure, there is an association with internal carcinoma in about one third of the cases (Peterka et al.). It is likely that in such cases arsenic is the common denominator, causing both Bowen's disease and internal carcinoma. According to Graham and Helwig, the lesions of Bowen's disease appear, on the average, 8.5 years sooner than the internal carcinoma.

Histopathology. In early *arsenical keratoses* of the palms and soles there may be hyperkeratosis and acanthosis without evidence of atypicality. However, on cutting deeper into the tissue block, atypicality may become apparent. In well developed arsenical keratoses the findings are those of a squamous cell carcinoma in situ and are analogous to Bowen's disease or a solar keratosis. One observes disorder in the arrangement of the squamous cells and nuclear atypicalities, such as hyperchromasia, clumping or dyskeratosis (Hundeiker and Petres). Atrophy of the epidermis and basophilic degeneration of the upper dermis, as seen in some solar keratoses, are absent in arsenical keratoses. Evidence of development into an invasive squamous cell carci-

noma may be seen in some arsenical keratoses.

Concerning the type of *cutaneous carcinoma* following arsenic ingestion, at one time it was thought that most of these were superficial basal cell epitheliomas (Fierz; Ehlers); but, as had been pointed out in 1941 by Montgomery and Waisman and was emphasized again lately by Hundeiker and Petres, nearly all, if not all, arsenical carcinomas of the skin are squamous cell carcinomas, usually located in situ, analogous to Bowen's disease. Often they show invasion into the dermis, especially in larger lesions when step sectioning is carried out. Vacuolization of the epidermal cells, originally thought by Montgomery and Waisman to be typical of arsenical cutaneous carcinoma, is only occasionally seen and can occur also in Bowen's disease and squamous cell carcinoma not caused by arsenic. Rather, one finds the usual cellular changes of Bowen's disease: disorder in the arrangement of the cells and hyperchromasia, clumping and dyskeratosis of the nuclei (see p. 473).

Histogenesis. In vitro experiments concerning the effects of inorganic arsenic on human epidermal cells have shown that arsenic depresses premitotic DNA replication. Incubation with inorganic arsenic and subsequent exposure of the cell cultures to ultraviolet light, causes interruption of the enzymatic "dark repair mechanism" in the epidermal cells. Arsenic seems to block, among other enzymes, predominantly DNA polymerase through attaching itself to sulfhydryl groups. These effects of arsenic on DNA synthesis may explain its carcinogenic effect (Jung and Trachsel).

BIBLIOGRAPHY

Fixed Drug Eruption

Furuya, T., Sekido, N., and Ishihara, F.: Beitrag zum fixen Arzneimittelexanthem. Arch. klin. exp. Derm., *225*:375, 1966.

Stritzler, C., and Kopf, A. W.: Fixed drug eruption caused by 8-chlorotheophylline in Dramamine with clinical and histologic studies. J. Invest. Derm., *34*:319, 1960.

Tarnowski, W. M.: Fixed drug eruption due to tetracyclines. Acta dermatoven., *50*:117, 1970.

Tritsch, H., Orfanos, C., and Lückerath, J.: Nekrolytische Arznei-Exantheme. Hautarzt, *19*:24, 1968.

Bullae and Sweat Gland Necrosis in Drug-Induced Coma

Achten, G., Ledoux-Corbusier, M., and Thys, J. P.: Intoxication à l'oxyde de carbone et lésions cutanées. Ann. derm. syph., *98*:421, 1971.

Brehmer-Andersson, E., and Pedersen, N. B.: Sweat gland necrosis and bullous skin changes in acute drug intoxication. Acta dermatoven., *49*:157, 1969.

Leavell, U. W., Farley, C. H., and McIntire, J. S.: Cutaneous changes in a patient with carbon monoxide poisoning. Arch. Derm., *99*:429, 1969.

Mandy, S., and Ackerman, A. B.: Characteristic traumatic skin lesions in drug-induced coma. J.A.M.A., *213*:253, 1970.

Drug-Induced Photosensitivity

Blois, M. S., Jr.: On chlorpromazine binding in vivo. J. Invest. Derm., *45*:475, 1965.

Frost, P., Weinstein, G. P., and Gomez, E. C.: Phototoxic potential of minocycline and doxocycline. Arch. Derm., *105*:681, 1972.

Greiner, A. C., and Nicolson, G. A.: Pigmentary deposit in viscera associated with prolonged chlorpromazine therapy. Canad. M.A.J., *91*:627, 1964.

Hägermark, O., Wennersten, G., and Almeyda, J.: Cutaneous side effects of phenothiazines. Brit. J. Derm., *84*:605, 1971.

Harber, L. C., and Baer, R. L.: Pathogenic mechanisms of drug-induced photosensitivity. J. Invest. Derm., *58*:327, 1972.

Hashimoto, K., Wiener, W., Albert, J., and Nelson, R. G.: An electron microscopic study of chlorpromazine pigmentation. J. Invest. Derm., *47*:296, 1966.

Hays, G. B., Lyle, C. B., Jr., and Wheeler, C. E., Jr.: Slate-gray color in patients receiving chlorpromazine. Arch. Derm., *90*:471, 1964.

Satanove, A.: Pigmentation due to phenothiazines in high and prolonged doses. J.A.M.A., *191*:263, 1965.

Scott, G. T., and Nading, L. K.: Relative effectiveness of phenothiazine tranquilizing drugs causing release of MSH. Proc. Soc. Exp. Biol. Med., *106*:88, 1961.

Willis, I., and Kligman, A. M.: The mechanism of photoallergic contact dermatitis. J. Invest. Derm., *51*:378, 1968.

Zelickson, A. S.: Skin pigmentation and chlorpromazine. J.A.M.A., *194*:670, 1965.

Drug-Induced Lupus Erythematosus

Alarcon-Segovia, D., Wakin, K. G., Worthington, J. W., and Ward, L. E.: Clinical and experimental studies on the hydralazine syndrome and its relationship to systemic lupus erythematosus. Medicine, *46*:1, 1967.

Dubois, E. L.: Procainamide induction of a systemic lupus erythematosus-like syndrome. Medicine, *48*:217, 1969,

Grossman, J., Callerame, M. L., and Condemi, J. J.: Skin immunofluorescence studies on lupus erythematosus and other antinuclear-antibody-positive diseases. Ann. Intern. Med., *80*:496, 1974.

Weiss, R. S., and Swift, S.: The significance of a positive L. E. phenomenon. Arch. Derm., *72*:103, 1955.

Bromoderma

Leibl, K.: Bromoderma tuberosum. Derm. Wschr., *137*:681, 1958.

Schirren, C., and Wehrmann, R.: Experimentelle Untersuchungen zur Ausscheidung von Brom bei Bromoderma tuberosum. Arch. klin. exp. Derm., *217*:50, 1963.

Teller, H.: Bromoderma und Jododerma tuberosum. Derm. Wschr., *143*:273, 1961.

Iododerma

Gehrels, P. E.: Zum Krankheitsbild des Jododerma tuberosum. Z. Haut Geschlechtskr., *30*:246, 1961.

Hollander, L., and Fetterman, G. H.: Fatal iododerma. Arch. Derm. Syph., *34*:228, 1936.

Jones, L. E., Pariser, H., and Murray, P. F.: Recurrent iododerma. Arch. Derm., *78*:353, 1958.

Rosenberg, F. R., Einbinder, J., Walzer, R. A., and Nelson, C. T.: Vegetating iododerma. Arch. Derm., *105*:900, 1972.

Argyria

Buckley, W. R.: Localized argyria. Arch Derm., *88*:531, 1963.

Czitober, H., Frischauf, H., and Leodolter, I.: Quantitative Untersuchungen bei universeller Argyrose mittels Neutronenaktivierungsanalyse. Virchows Arch., Abt. A, *350*:44, 1970.

Hill, W. R., and Montgomery, H.: Argyria. Arch. Derm. Syph., *44*:588, 1941.

Hönigsmann, H., Konrad, K., and Wolff, K.: Argyrose (Histologie und Ultrastruktur). Hautarzt, *24*:24, 1973.

Mehta, A. C., Dawson-Butterworth, K., and Woodhouse, M. A.: Argyria. Electron microscopic study of a case. Brit. J. Derm., *78*:175, 1966.

Pearse, A. G. E.: Histochemistry, Theoretical and Applied. ed. 3, p. 1151. Edinburgh, Churchill Livingstone, 1972.

Prose, P. H.: An electron microscopic study of human generalized argyria. Am. J. Path., *42*:293, 1963.

Robert, P., and Zürcher, H.: Pigmentstudien. I. Über den Einfluss von Schwermetallverbindungen, Hämin, Vitaminen, mikrobiellen Toxinen, Hormonen und weiteren Stoffen auf die Dopamelaninbildung in vitro und die Pigmentbildung in vivo. Dermatologica, *100*:217, 1950.

Schröpl, F., Oehlschlaegel, G., and Drabner, J.: Schwermetallnachweis in der Haut bei Argyrose mittels Neutronenaktivierungsanalyse. Arch. klin. exp. Derm., *231*:398, 1968.

Mercury Pigmentation

Burge, K. M., and Winkelmann, R. K.: Mercury pigmentation. An electron microscopic study. Arch. Derm., *102*:51, 1960.

Lamar, L. M., and Bliss, B. O.: Localized pigmentation of the skin due to topical mercury. Arch. Derm., *93*:450, 1966.

Lüders, G., Fischer, H., and Hensel, U.: Hydrargyrosis cutis mit allgemeinen Vergiftungserscheinungen nach langdauernder Anwendung quecksilberhaltiger Kosmetica. Hautarzt, *19*:61, 1968.

Arsenical Keratosis and Carcinoma

Ehlers, G.: Klinische und histologische Untersuchungen zur Frage arzneimittelbedingter Arsen-Tumoren. Z. Haut, *43*:763, 1968.

Fierz, U.: Katamnestische Untersuchungen über die Nebenwirkungen der Therapie mit anorganischem Arsen bei Hautkrankheiten. Dermatologica, *131*:41, 1965.

Graham, J. H., and Helwig, E. B.: Bowen's disease and its relationship to systemic cancer. Arch. Derm., *80*:133, 1959.

Hundeiker, M., and Petres, J.: Morphogenese und Formenreichtum der arseninduzierten Präkanzerosen. Arch. klin. exp. Derm., *231*:355, 1968.

Jung, E. G., and Trachsel, B.: Molekularbiologische Untersuchungen zur Arsencarcinogenese. Arch. klin. exp. Derm., *237*:819, 1970.

Montgomery, H.: Arsenic as an etiologic agent in certain types of epithelioma. Arch. Derm. Syph., *32*:218, 1935.

Montgomery, H., and Waisman, M.: Epithelioma attributable to arsenic. J. Invest. Derm., *4*:365, 1941.

Peterka, E. S., Lynch, F. W., and Goltz, R. W.: An association between Bowen's disease and internal cancer. Arch. Derm., *84*:623, 1961.

Sommers, S. C., and McManus, R. G.: Multiple arsenical cancers of skin and internal organs. Cancer, *6*:347, 1953.

15

Degenerative Diseases

SOLAR (ACTINIC) DEGENERATION

Senile changes in areas of the skin not regularly exposed to sunlight manifest themselves clinically only in thinning of the skin and a decrease in the amount of subcutaneous fat. On the other hand, in the exposed skin of older persons there often are pronounced changes, especially in individuals with a fair complexion. These changes are, however, the result of chronic sun exposure, rather than of age. In exposed areas, especially on the face, the skin shows wrinkling and furrowing as well as thinning. In addition, there may be an irregular distribution of pigment. In the nuchal region, the skin, after many years of exposure to the sun, may appear thickened and furrowed. The term *cutis rhomboidalis nuchae* is used for this.

Histopathology. In skin not regularly exposed to sunlight the only histologic change of old age consists of a diminution in the number and the diameter of the elastic fibers (Mitchell).

In skin exposed to the sun, especially in individuals with a fair complexion, hyperplasia of the elastic tissue is usually evident on histologic examination by age 30, even though clinically the skin may appear normal. No white person past 40 was found by Kligman to have normal elastic tissue in the skin of the face. The elastic fibers may appear not only increased in number and thicker but also curled and tangled.

In patients with clinically evident solar degeneration of the exposed skin, staining with hematoxylin and eosin reveals in the upper dermis basophilic degeneration of the collagen separated from a somewhat atrophic epidermis by a narrow band of normal collagen. In the areas of basophilic degeneration the bundles of eosinophilic collagen have been replaced by amorphous granular material (Plate 2, facing p. 250).

With elastic tissue stains, the areas of basophilic degeneration stain like elastic tissue and, therefore, are referred to as consisting of elastotic material (Fig. 15-1). The elastotic material usually consists of aggregates of thick, interwoven bands in the upper dermis; but in areas of severe solar degeneration the elastotic material may have an amorphous rather than a fibrous appearance and may extend into the lower portions of the dermis, rather than being confined to upper dermis (Mitchell).

On staining with silver nitrate, the distribution of melanin in the basal cell layer may appear irregular, in that areas of hyperpigmentation alternate with areas of hypopigmentation (Mitchell).

Histogenesis. Electron microscopic examination of areas of solar degeneration has shown them to be composed of: (1) elastic fibers that contain in their amorphous matrix only very few normal skeleton fibrils but numerous irregularly thickened, electron-dense skeleton fibrils which in longitudinal sectioned elastic fibers have the appearance of "tiger stripes" (Ledoux-Corbusier and Achten) (E.M. No. 30); (2) a decreased number of collagen fibrils, with those present showing a diminished electron density, a diminished contrast in cross striation, and a splitting up into microfibrils at their ends; and (3) extensive amorphous material containing microfibrils (E.M. No. 30).

Various views have been expressed in the interpretation of these findings, although it is generally agreed that there is both a decrease in amount and also degeneration of collagen fibrils. In regard to the elastic fibers most authors believe that the electron-dense inclusions represent degenerated skeleton fibrils (Mitchell; Ebner; Ledoux-Corbusier and Achten), although Braun-Falco regards the inclusions as enclosed disintegrated collagen fibrils. But there is disagreement concerning the nature of the extensive amorphous material containing microfibrils. The traditional view is that this material including the microfibrils forms as a result of degeneration, either of collagen (Niebauer and Stockinger; Mitchell; Kretzberg and Klingmüller), or of elastic tissue (Banfield and Brindley), or of both (Rasheed et al.). In contrast to the traditional view that solar degeneration is purely a degenerative process, several authors (Ebner; Braun-Falco; Berger) have stressed the presence within the elastotic material of actively secreting fibroblasts with a well developed, dilated rough endoplasmic reticulum. It appears likely that, as the result of the chronic solar damage, the fibroblasts are no longer capable of secreting the type of microfibrils that can be synthesized into collagen and elastin, but secrete abnormal microfibrils and amorphous material.

The elastotic material that histochemically stains like elastic tissue and by electron microscopy consists largely of amorphous material containing microfibrils, on the basis of its chemical, physical and enzymatic reactions resembles elastic tissue more than collagenous tissue. Thus, (1) amino acid analyses indicate that the elastotic material, like elastic tissue, has a much lower hydroxyproline content than does collagen (Felsher); (2) the elastotic material shows the same brilliant autofluorescence as do normal elastic fibers on examination with the fluorescence microscope (Niebauer and Stockinger); and (3) both the elastotic material and elastic tissue are susceptible to elastase digestion (Findlay).

In the elastotic material the amount of acid mucopolysaccharides is increased, as shown by staining with alcian blue. A considerable proportion of the acid mucopolysaccharides is sulfated, since incubation with hyaluronidase removes only from 50 to 75 per cent of the acid mucopolysaccharides. The basophilia of elastotic material, however, is not affected by the incubation with hyaluronidase, so that it can be concluded that the basophilia is not caused by the presence of acid mucopolysaccharides (Sams and Smith).

The irregular distribution of pigmentation seen in some patients with solar degeneration is caused largely by an impairment of pigment transfer from melanocytes to keratinocytes, according to electron microscopic studies by Olson et al. They found some keratinocytes containing many melanosomes and others containing few or no melanosomes. The latter were surrounded by dendrites laden with melanosomes.

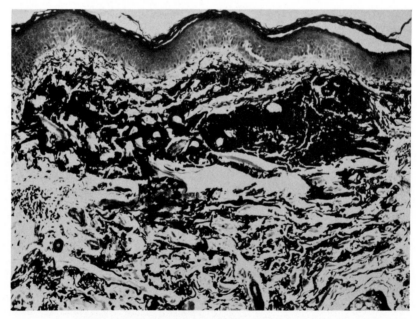

FIG. 15-1. **Solar (actinic) degeneration.** Elastic tissue stain. In the upper dermis, separated from the epidermis by a narrow band of normal collagen, there are aggregates of thick, interwoven bands of elastotic material staining like elastic tissue. (×100)

PLATE 2

Solar degeneration. Basophilic degeneration is present in the upper dermis. There the collagen bundles have been replaced by amorphous material staining faintly basophilic on staining with hematoxylin and eosin. (×100).

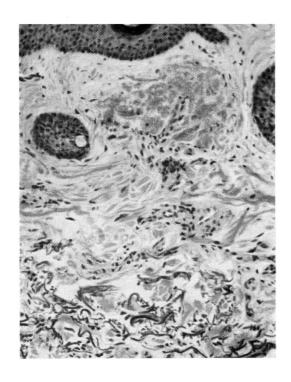

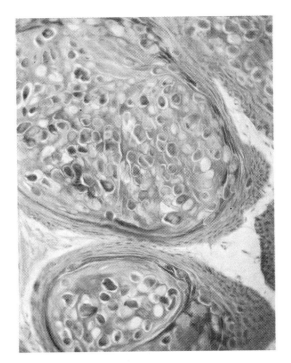

Molluscum contagiosum. In the horny layer numerous large basophilic molluscum bodies lie enmeshed in a network of eosinophilic horny fibers. (×350)

Differential Diagnosis. For differentiation of solar elastosis from pseudoxanthoma elasticum, see page 78.

NODULAR ELASTOSIS WITH CYSTS AND COMEDONES (FAVRE AND RACOUCHOT)

Some patients with pronounced solar degeneration of the facial skin show, especially lateral to the eyes, multiple comedones as well as yellowish nodules, which measure up to 4 mm in diameter and contain a central comedo.

Histopathology. In addition to pronounced solar elastosis, one observes in the dermis dilated pilosebaceous openings and large round cysts that are lined by a flattened epidermis and represent greatly extended hair follicles (Favre and Racouchot; Helm). Both the dilated pilosebaceous openings and the cysts are filled with layered horny material and a lipoid substance similar to sebum. The sebaceous glands are atrophic.

KYRLE'S DISEASE

Kyrle's disease together with three unrelated diseases form the group of perforating lesions with transepidermal elimination (Table 15-1). The other three diseases are perforating folliculitis, elastosis perforans serpiginosa, and reactive perforating collagenosis. The latter two diseases have so typical a histologic picture that they are easily diagnosed. On the other hand, Kyrle's disease and perforating folliculitis may be difficult to differentiate histologically, except in sections showing the area of perforation. In addition, they also show some histologic resemblance.

Kyrle's disease is a rare disorder. Thus, in 1968, Carter and Constantine, besides their own five cases, accepted only 12 of the 45 cases reported in the literature up to that

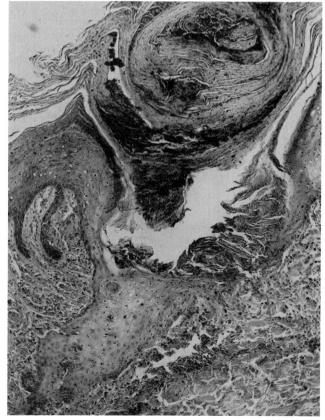

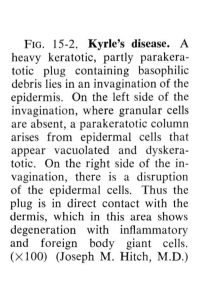

FIG. 15-2. **Kyrle's disease.** A heavy keratotic, partly parakeratotic plug containing basophilic debris lies in an invagination of the epidermis. On the left side of the invagination, where granular cells are absent, a parakeratotic column arises from epidermal cells that appear vacuolated and dyskeratotic. On the right side of the invagination, there is a disruption of the epidermal cells. Thus the plug is in direct contact with the dermis, which in this area shows degeneration with inflammatory and foreign body giant cells. (×100) (Joseph M. Hitch, M.D.)

time as valid examples of Kyrle's disease. It is perhaps significant that, in turn, Pinkus and Mehregan have expressed their belief that the five cases described by Carter and Constantine were instances of perforating folliculitis, a rather common disease, rather than of Kyrle's disease.

Kyrle's disease, which Kyrle in 1916 named hyperkeratosis follicularis et parafollicularis in cutem penetrans, is characterized by a more or less extensive eruption of hyperkeratotic papules, 2 to 8 mm in size, containing a central, cone-shaped plug that can be removed with the aid of a curette. The papules may be follicular or extrafollicular in location and may coalesce into verrucous plaques. The extensor surfaces of the extremities are the most common sites of involvement.

Histopathology. A heavy keratotic, partly parakeratotic plug occupies an invagination of the epidermis. It is possible that some of the plugs occupy hair follicles, but often the invaginations merely resemble hair follicles. Basophilic debris that does not stain like elastic tissue is present within most plugs (Fig. 15-2) (Thyresson; Constantine and Carter). The parakeratosis within each plug extends down to the epidermis of the invagination, usually at its deepest point (Tappeiner et al.) but occasionally at more than one point (Constantine and Carter). The epidermal invagination shows a well developed granular layer, except at the point or points at which the parakeratotic cells of the plug are in contact with the epidermis of the invagination. At sites of absence of the granular layer one observes within the epidermal invagination in early lesions a focus of vacuolated dyskeratotic cells extending to the basal cell layer, and at a later stage a focus where epidermal cells are absent and the keratotic plug has perforated into the dermis through the area of disruption of epidermal cells. Wherever the keratotic plug is in direct contact with the dermis, one observes a rather pronounced granulomatous reaction composed of inflammatory and foreign body giant cells (Thyresson; Prakken; de Graciansky et al.). The epidermal cells bordering the site of perforation proliferate and surround the granulomatous focus in the dermis. Subsequently, the granulomatous material is moved upward by the continuing epidermal cell proliferation

around it and ultimately forms the basophilic debris within the keratotic plug (Constantine and Carter; Aram et al.). Although the granulomatous focus in the dermis may show a mild degree of collagen degeneration, there is neither an increase in the amount nor signs of degeneration of the elastic tissue (Abele and Dobson).

It should be pointed out that perforation of the keratotic plug is a stage that is not always reached. Thus, absence of perforation does not rule out Kyrle's disease. In cases without perforation no basophilic debris is found in the keratotic plug; nevertheless, parakeratotic cells are present in the plug, and at least at one site of the epidermal invagination there are dyskeratotic cells, although it may require serial sections to find this site (Constantine and Carter).

Histogenesis. Constantine and Carter as well as Tappeiner et al. have come to the conclusion that the presence of dyskeratotic cells at one site, and occasionally at more than one site, of the epidermal invagination causes a speeding up of keratinization and results in the formation of parakeratotic cells in the horn plug. Because of overrapid keratinization, the parakeratotic column gradually extends deeper into the abnormal epidermis, resulting ultimately in the perforation of the parakeratotic column into the dermis. Perforation thus is not the cause of Kyrle's disease, as Kyrle had thought, but represents the consequence or final event of the abnormally speeded up keratinization. Tappeiner et al. have pointed out the similarity of the parakeratotic column in Kyrle's disease to that seen in porokeratosis Mibelli. In both conditions a parakeratotic column forms as the result of rapid and faulty keratinization of dyskeratotic cells; but, whereas in Kyrle's disease the dyskeratotic cells are used up and disruption of the epithelium occurs, the clone of dyskeratotic cells can maintain itself in porokeratosis Mibelli by extending peripherally.

Differential Diagnosis. For differentiation from perforating folliculitis, see below and Table 15-1; from elastosis perforans serpiginosa, see page 255 and Table 15-1.

PERFORATING FOLLICULITIS

Perforating folliculitis, first described by Mehregan and Coskey in 1968, is a fairly common disorder, in contrast to the rarity of Kyrle's disease which it resembles. As in Kyrle's disease, one observes erythematous

TABLE 15-1. Group of Four Diseases Forming Perforations of Epidermis With Subsequent Transepidermal Elimination

	Primary Defect	Type of Epidermal Disruption	Eliminated Material
Kyrle's disease	Focus of dyskeratotic, rapidly proliferating cells in epidermis	Rapid proliferation causes parakeratotic column in epidermal invagination and ultimate exhaustion of supply of cells in dyskeratotic focus, resulting in disruption.	Elimination of granulomatous focus as basophilic debris into epidermal invagination
Perforating folliculitis	Hyperkeratotic plug in hair follicle containing a curled-up hair	Hair causes perforation.	Elimination of basophilic debris and eosinophilic elastic fibers into the hair follicle
Elastosis perforans serpiginosa	Formation of numerous coarse elastic fibers in dermal papillae	Formation of narrow winding channels through acanthotic epidermis	Elimination of basophilic debris and eosinophilic elastic fibers into narrow channels
Reactive perforating collagenosis	Trauma causes subepidermal focus of necrobiotic basophilic collagen.	Overlying epidermis develops areas of disruption.	Elimination of necrobiotic basophilic collagen bundles into cup-shaped epidermal depression

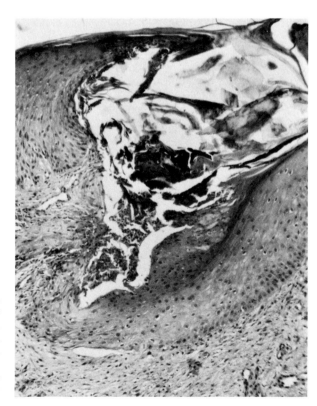

FIG. 15-3. **Perforating folliculitis.** A greatly dilated hair follicle contains keratotic material intermingled with basophilic debris. On the left side, a perforation of the follicular epithelium is seen within the infundibular region. Degenerated dermal material is eliminated through this perforation. (×50)

papules, 2 to 8 mm in diameter with a central keratinous plug that can be removed. In contrast to Kyrle's disease, the papules always are follicular, show no tendency to coalesce, and are limited in their distribution to the arms, thighs and buttocks.

Histopathology. Within a dilated hair follicule one finds orthokeratotic and parakeratotic material that is intermingled with basophilic debris composed of degenerated collagen and inflammatory cells, and with brightly eosinophilic degenerated elastic fibers. In addition, a curled-up hair is often (but not always) present. One or several small areas of perforation of the follicular epithelium are seen within the infundibular region, some distance above the level of the sebaceous glands (Fig. 15-3). At the sites of perforation the dermis shows a focal inflammatory infiltrate containing degenerated collagen and, as a characteristic feature, degenerated elastic fibers that have lost their orceinophilic staining property and stain brightly eosinophilic (Mehregan and Coskey; Streitmann). This focus of inflammation and degeneration then is surrounded by proliferating follicular epithelium and is thus moved upward into the follicular cavity and ultimately eliminated through the follicular opening to the surface. Staining for elastic tissue shows no increase in the number of elastic fibers in the dermis.

Histogenesis. According to Mehregan and Coskey, the perforations in perforating folliculitis are caused by a hair. They found that a portion of a curled-up hair is usually present in close approximation to the areas of disruption, and occasionally a hair shaft is found within the area of perforation or even in the dermis surrounded by a foreign body granuloma. On the other hand, Streitmann, who found no hair, believes that the primary event is an eosinophilic degeneration of elastic fibers near the area of perforation, and that subsequently the degenerated elastic fibers evoke an inflammatory reaction, break through the follicular epithelium into the follicular cavity and are eliminated.

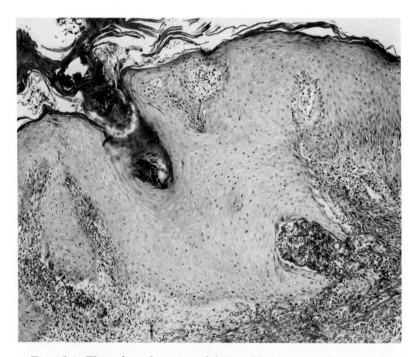

FIG. 15-4. **Elastosis perforans serpiginosa.** The upper and lower portions of a narrow channel winding through the epidermis are shown. The upper portion of the channel contains basophilic necrotic material with a small keratotic plug on top. The lower portion of the channel contains, in addition to basophilic necrotic material, degenerated elastic fibers. (×100)

Differential Diagnosis. In Kyrle's disease the keratinous plug may be extrafollicular in location, the perforation may be present deep in the invagination at the bottom of the keratinous plug, and, above all, no eosinophilic degeneration of elastic fibers is found. For differential diagnosis from elastosis perforans serpiginosa see below.

ELASTOSIS PERFORANS SERPIGINOSA

In this fairly rare disorder one observes hyperkeratotic papules with small central areas of scaling, 1 to 5 mm in diameter, that are grouped or arranged in an annular or circinate fashion. The lesions usually are confined to one area, most commonly the nape of the neck, the face, or the upper extremities; in rare instances the lesions are widely disseminated (Rasmussen; Pedro and Garcia). Occasionally, the disease is associated with mongoloid idiocy or with other connective tissue disorders, such as Ehlers-Danlos disease, pseudoxanthoma elasticum, or Marfan's syndrome (Rasmussen).

Histopathology. The basic change in elastosis perforans serpiginosa is a focal increase in both the amount and the size of the elastic fibers in the uppermost dermis and particularly in the dermal papillae. The elastic fibers in the papillae are recognizable even in section routinely stained with hematoxylin and eosin as amorphous material filling the papillae (Fig. 15-4). Thus, the diagnosis of elastosis perforans serpiginosa usually can be suspected from hematoxylin and eosin stained sections, although differentiation from the other three diseases with transepidermal elimination may be difficult, since they too contain amorphous material in close approximation to the epidermis. However, on staining with Verhoeff's stain for elastic tissue the great increase in the amount and the size of the elastic fibers in the uppermost dermis and particularly in the dermal papillae becomes apparent and makes differentiation from any other disease easy, since it is

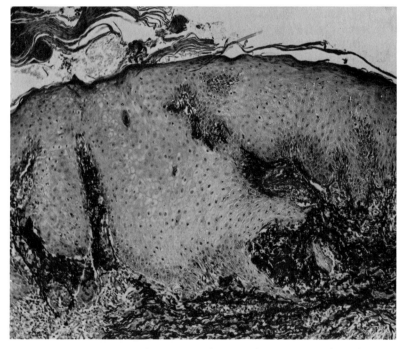

FIG. 15-5. **Elastosis perforans serpiginosa.** Elastic tissue stain. The great increase in both the amount and the size of the elastic fibers in the uppermost dermis and particularly in the dermal papillae is pathognomonic for elastosis perforans serpiginosa. (×100)

pathognomonic for elastosis perforans serpiginosa (Fig. 15-5).

Staining with hematoxylin and eosin shows the presence of an inflammatory infiltrate in the dermal papillae and the areas of downward proliferation of the epidermis which partially engulf the aggregates of elastic fibers and the associated inflammatory infiltrate. The acanthotic epidermis contains narrow, irregularly winding channels that lead, as serial sections show, from the dermis either to a pilosebaceous follicle or, more commonly, to the surface of the epidermis. These eliminating channels, in their lower portion, show many thick elastic fibers that stain brightly eosinophilic with hematoxylin and eosin and no longer stain with elastic tissue stains (Mehregan). In addition, the channels contain basophilic necrotic material consisting of degenerated epidermal cells and of the pyknotic nuclei of inflammatory cells (Whyte and Winkelmann). The upper portion of the channel often contains a plug containing keratin as well as basophilic necrotic material and eosinophilic elastic fibers.

Histogenesis. That the orceinophilic material present in the uppermost dermis and the dermal papillae actually is elastic tissue has been established through digestion of this material by elastase (Marshall and Lurie) and by electron microscopic studies (Cohen and Hashimoto). The elastic fibers in the uppermost dermis, on electron microscopy, appear much longer and thicker and show branching. In addition, there are many young, very small elastic fibers that are surrounded by numerous microfibrils (Meves and Vogel). The primary event apparently is an increase in elastic tissue formation and the appearance of abnormal, coarse elastic fibers. The altered composition of these fibers leads to their elimination through the epidermis in association with epidermal proliferation (Hitch and Lund). Although the invaginated epidermis surrounding the plugs may suggest pilosebaceous follicles, and although the winding channels through which the altered elastic tissue is extruded may suggest intraepidermal sweat ducts, it seems that, as a rule, the extrusion occurs without any relationship to these structures (Whyte and Winkelmann).

Differential Diagnosis. Both Kyrle's disease and perforating folliculitis share with elastosis perforans serpiginosa the presence of a central keratotic plug and of a perforation through which degenerated material is being eliminated. Perforating folliculitis, in addition, shows, like elastosis perforans serpiginosa, the elimination of degenerated eosinophilic elastic fibers. However, neither of the two shows the great increase in elastic tissue seen in elastosis perforans serpiginosa in the uppermost dermis and particularly in the dermal papillae on staining with elastic tissue stains.

REACTIVE PERFORATING COLLAGENOSIS

This rare dermatosis may be recessively inherited and thus has been reported to occur in siblings (J. Weiner; A. L. Weiner). The lesions usually begin to appear in infancy or childhood and consist of papules, 5 to 10 mm in diameter, which become umbilicated with a removable keratotic plug and involute within 6 to 8 weeks. However, new lesions continue to appear, frequently as a result of minor trauma. The lesions are often haphazardly distributed and usually are discrete, but they may be linear at sites of trauma. As a rule, the trauma is mild, but in one patient many lesions formed within lacerations caused by broken glass (Woringer and Laugier).

Histopathology. Early, nonumbilicated lesions show in their center a widened dermal papilla containing necrobiotic, deeply basophilic collagen. The suprapapillary epidermis is very thin, and in the center of the papilla it may consist only of the stratum corneum (Mehregan et al.). At this early stage, no inflammatory infiltrate is present.

Older, umbilicated lesions, in which the basophilic collagen has been largely eliminated through perforations in the thin suprapapillary epidermis, have a cup-shaped central area of depression filled by a large plug containing parakeratotic keratin, basophilic collagen and numerous pyknotic nuclei of inflammatory cells. The epidermis, which at this stage is located beneath the plug, is markedly atrophic and in several areas shows interruptions by thin, basophilic bundles of collagen extending in a vertical direction, indicating that they are being extruded from the underlying dermis (Bovenmyer). The upper dermis shows an inflammatory infiltrate. Elastic tissue stains show no increase in the number of elastic fibers in the dermis and also no elastic fibers in the keratotic plug or in the areas of disruption in the epidermis. At the periphery of the cup-shaped depression the epidermis may show hyperplasia (Woringer and Laugier).

Histogenesis. In response to a minor injury the collagen within a circumscribed area of the upper dermis undergoes necrobiosis and becomes basophilic. The overlying epidermis, in becoming atrophic, develops areas of disruption through which degenerated basophilic collagen bundles and inflammatory cells are being extruded (Mehregan et al.).

HYPERKERATOSIS LENTICULARIS PERSTANS (FLEGEL)

This rare dermatosis, first described in 1958 by Flegel, consists of asymptomatic hyperkeratotic papules, from 1 to 5 mm in size, located predominantly on the dorsa of the feet and on the lower legs. Removal of the adherent, thick, horny scale causes slight bleeding. Larger papules often have, in addition to the central horny scale, a peripherally attached collarette of fine scaling. The disorder starts in later life and persists indefinitely. Its occurrence in three generations, observed by Bean (1972), suggests that hyperkeratosis lenticularis perstans is transmitted by an autosomal dominant gene.

Histopathology. In some instances, the histologic picture is nonspecific, showing hyperkeratosis with occasional areas of parakeratosis, irregular acanthosis intermingled with areas of flattening of the stratum malpighii, and vascular dilation with a moderate amount of perivascular round cell infiltration (Bean, 1969). It seems, however, that if the specimen is obtained from a well developed, markedly hyperkeratotic lesion, a fairly characteristic histologic picture may be seen, even though it is not diagnostic. As described by Flegel, and in subsequent cases by Kocsard et al., by Raffle and Rogers, and by Krinitz and Schäfer, a greatly thickened horny layer overlies a flattened malpighian layer. At the margins of the lesion the malpighian layer forms a papillomatous elevation resembling a church spire. The der-

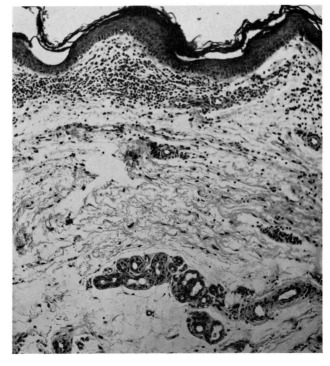

FIG. 15-6. **Acrodermatitis chronica atrophicans.** There is atrophy of the stratum malpighii. A band-like infiltrate is separated from the epidermis by a narrow zone of normal collagen. The dermis shows interstitial edema and atrophy of the collagen bundles. Because of this atrophy, the thickness of the dermis is markedly decreased, and the sweat glands lie unusually close to the epidermis. (×100)

mal infiltrate is composed largely of lymphoid cells and is located as a narrow band close to the epidermis, with a rather sharp demarcation at its lower border.

ACRODERMATITIS CHRONICA ATROPHICANS

This disorder occurs on the extremities, usually over their extensor surfaces. There is an initial inflammatory stage that is followed by an atrophic stage. The affected areas of the skin in the initial stage appear reddish and slightly edematous, but gradually they become atrophic and then present a bluish-red or brownish, atrophic, wrinkled appearance. Because of the decrease in the amount of subcutaneous fat at the sites of atrophy, the subcutaneous veins are clearly visible. In some cases areas of fibrous thickening develop within the atrophic skin, either as indurated bands, especially in the ulnar or tibial region; or as nodules, especially near joints; or as plaques, especially on the dorsa of the feet.

Histopathology. In the initial inflammatory stage the histologic picture is nonspecific, consisting of a largely perivascular chronic inflammatory infiltrate. In the early atrophic stage, however, the histologic findings are diagnostic. One observes atrophy of the epidermis, with absence of the rete ridges. Directly beneath the epidermis there is a narrow zone of connective tissue separating a bandlike chronic inflammatory infiltrate from the epidermis. In addition, one finds scattered areas of inflammatory infiltration throughout the dermis, especially around the blood vessels, and also in the subcutaneous fat. The infiltrate is composed predominantly of lymphoid cells, but it also contains histiocytes. The entire dermis shows interstitial edema separating the bundles of collagen into fibers. In addition, there is a marked decrease in the amount of collagen. Ultimately, the dermis measures only one half or a quarter of its normal thickness (Fig. 15-6). There is a gradual loss of elastic tissue until finally it is completely absent (Korting et al.).

The hairs and sebaceous glands undergo atrophy early in the disease and usually are entirely absent in the atrophic stage. However, as a rule the sweat glands are preserved. Because of the thinness of the dermis, they lie unusually close to the epidermis (Montgomery and Sullivan). The subcutaneous tissue also undergoes atrophy, with decrease in the number and size of the fat cells.

After several years' duration an atrophic stage is reached in which the findings are no longer diagnostic, since one sees merely an atrophic epidermis and atrophy of the dermis and of the subcutaneous fat without an inflammatory infiltrate.

The areas of fibrous thickening of the skin show coarse, hyalinized collagen bundles beneath an atrophic epidermis and dermis (Hardmeier).

Differential Diagnosis. In the late atrophic stage of acrodermatitis chronica atrophicans the atrophy of the collagen and loss of elastic tissue cause resemblance to the findings in early striae distensae (see p. 264). The histologic changes in the areas of fibrous thickening may be indistinguishable from those of scleroderma (Grimmer).

PRETIBIAL PIGMENTED PATCHES IN DIABETES

Circumscribed, round to oval, pigmented, often slightly depressed macules, from 2 to 10 mm in diameter, are found on the shins in about 17 per cent of adults with diabetes, but also in about 3 per cent of adults without diabetes (Bauer et al.). The role of trauma in the development of these lesions is difficult to evaluate. Most patients give no specific history of trauma. On the other hand, the pretibial area is particularly exposed to frequent minor traumas (Kerl).

Histopathology. The findings are not diagnostic. The upper dermis shows a mild perivascular infiltrate of lymphoid and histiocytic cells, an increase in the number of capillaries, fibroblastic proliferation, and small amounts of hemosiderin (Fisher and Danowski; Kerl). The capillaries often show thickening of their walls, with increased deposits of a PAS-positive, diastase-resistant material in a fibrillary pattern representing neutral mucopolysaccharides of the basement membrane.

Histogenesis. On electron microscopy the fibrillar PAS-positive, diastase-resistant material corresponds to an increase in the thickness and in the number of layers of the pericapillary basal lamina (Auböck). Although this is a characteristic finding in diabetic microangiopathy, it is not specific for it, and in the skin it can be the result of capillary proliferation.

Differential Diagnosis. Since proliferation of capillaries with thickening of their walls, deposits of hemosiderin, and fibrosis may occur in any mild dermal inflammation, the diagnosis of pretibial pigmented patches and their association with diabetes has to be based on clinical rather than on histologic considerations. The pretibial pigmented patches differ from necrobiosis lipoidica by showing neither necrobiosis nor giant cells.

BULLOSIS DIABETICORUM

In rare instances patients with diabetes may show recurrent eruptions of spontaneously arising bullae on their hands and feet. The bullae can attain a fairly large size and are slow in healing. The coexistence of bullosis diabeticorum with pretibial pigmented patches has been observed (Kurwa et al.; Kerl and Kresbach).

Histopathology. In some instances the bullae are unilocular and show a subepidermal location (Kurwa et al.; Kerl). In other instances, they were reported as unilocular with intraepidermal location (Allen and Hadden). Conceivably, they could have arisen subepidermally. However, in cases reported by Cantwell and Martz and by Kerl and Kresbach the bullae were multilocular with intraepidermal location, making a subepidermal formation unlikely. In addition, Kerl and Kresbach found the surrounding epidermis to be necrotic, as seen also in toxic epidermal necrolysis (see p. 124).

Histogenesis. The mechanism for the development of the bullae is not known. The absence of diabetic neuropathy in several of the reported cases indicates that this is not the cause (Cantwell and Martz). Kerl and Kresbach believe that the bullae arise as the result of trophic damage to the epidermis.

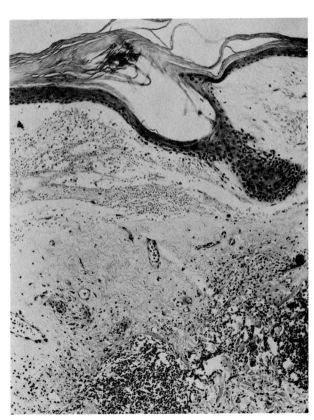

FIG. 15-7. **Lichen sclerosus et atrophicus.** There are hyperkeratosis with follicular plugging, atrophy of the stratum malpighii, marked lymphedema of the upper dermis and an inflammatory infiltrate in the mid-dermis. The edema in the subepidermal dermis is so marked that a bulla has resulted. (×100)

LICHEN SCLEROSUS ET ATROPHICUS

This disorder is characterized by the presence of flat-topped white macules that may coalesce to form white patches usually showing only slight induration. Fine, comedolike follicular plugs often are seen on the surface of the macules.

Lichen sclerosus et atrophicus is much more common in women than in men. In both men and women the genitals are the most frequent site of involvement. In women, involvement of the genitals is known as kraurosis vulvae (see p. 261); and in men, as balanitis xerotica obliterans (see p. 264). Frequently only the genital region is involved, but there may be extragenital lesions, either together with the genital involvement or alone.

Extragenital lesions of lichen sclerosus et atrophicus usually are limited in extent and are found most commonly as sharply outlined patches on the trunk and neck. Occasionally, however, lichen sclerosus et atrophicus occurs as an extensive eruption (Gottschalk and Cooper).

A patch of lichen sclerosus et atrophicus, whether solitary or part of an extensive eruption, may become bullous in its center. Older patches of lichen sclerosus et atrophicus often feel indurated, but they still can be distinguished from morphea by their distinctive epidermal changes both clinically and histologically (Steigleder and Raab). However, in occasional instances of extensive involvement, lesions of lichen sclerosus et atrophicus and of morphea coexist in the same patient (Bergfeld and Lesowitz; Wallace).

Histopathology. In lichen sclerosus et atrophicus one observes (1) hyperkeratosis with keratotic plugging, (2) atrophy of the stratum malpighii with hydropic degeneration of basal cells, (3) pronounced edema and homogenization of the collagen in the upper dermis, and (4) an inflammatory infiltrate in the middermis (Fig. 15-7).

The hyperkeratosis is so marked that often the horny layer is thicker than the atrophic stratum malpighii. The stratum malpighii may be reduced to a few layers of flattened cells. The cells of the basal layer show hydropic degeneration. The rete ridges often are completely absent, although they may persist in a few areas and even show some irregular downward proliferation. In such proliferations hydropic degeneration of the basal cells usually is pronounced.

Beneath the epidermis there is a broad zone of pronounced lymphedema. Within this zone the collagenous fibers are swollen and homogeneous and contain only a few nuclei. They stain poorly with eosin and other connective tissue stains. The blood and lymph vessels are dilated, and there may be areas of hemorrhage. Elastic fibers are sparse, and in older lesions they are absent within the area of lymphedema (Steigleder and Raab). In areas of severe lymphedema clinically visible bullae may form; they are found in subepidermal location (Gottschalk and Cooper). In addition, shrinkage within the area of lymphedema may occur during the process of dehydration of the specimen, resulting in the formation of pseudobullae, which are located intradermally (Piper).

An inflammatory infiltrate is present in the dermis except in lesions of long duration. The younger the lesion, the more superficial is the location of the infiltrate. In very early lesions and at the periphery of somewhat older lesions the infiltrate may be found in the uppermost dermis, in direct apposition to the basal layer (Miller). Soon, however, a narrow zone of edema and homogenization of the collagen displaces the inflammatory infiltrate farther down so that in well developed lesions the infiltrate is found in the middermis. The infiltrate can be patchy, but often it is bandlike. It consists largely of lymphoid cells intermingled with some histiocytes. In older lesions in which the infiltrate is slight or absent, the collagen bundles in the lower dermis may appear swollen, homogeneous, and hyperchromatic, as in scleroderma (Fig. 15-8).

Histogenesis. Electron microscopic studies suggest that the primary changes consist of a degeneration of collagen fibrils which often lack cross striation and at times have the appearance of empty tubes (Mann and Cowan). In many fibroblasts the cisternae of the endoplasmic reticulum are dilated and empty, indicative of a reduced collagen synthesis (Klug and Sönnichsen). In some areas, however, new collagen

FIG. 15-8. **Lichen sclerosus et atrophicus.** In this older lesion only a very slight inflammatory infiltrate is seen. There are, however, hydropic degeneration of the basal cells and lymphedema of the upper dermis. The collagen bundles in the lower dermis appear swollen, homogeneous, and hyperchromatic, as in scleroderma. (×50)

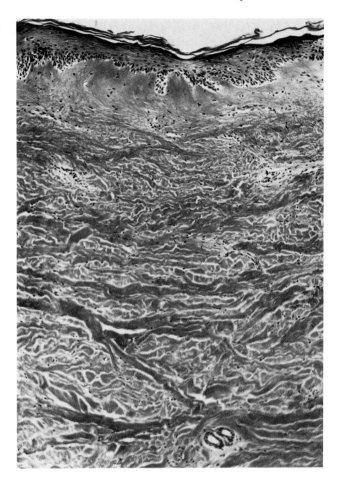

fibrils are seen in irregular arrangement and showing a variable but generally reduced diameter (Forssman et al.). Considerable edema often separates the basal cells from one another (Klug and Sönnichsen). Thus, the hydropic degeneration of the basal cells observed by light microscopy in reality is an intercellular edema. In addition, however, the basal cells themselves show degenerative changes (Mann and Cowan). There is nearly complete absence of melanosomes within the keratinocytes which, according to Mann and Cowan, is the result of a degeneration and disappearance of the melanocytes, whereas Klug and Sönnichsen attribute it to an inhibition of the transfer of melanosomes from the melanocytes to keratinocytes.

Differential Diagnosis. Very early lesions may resemble lichen planus because of the apposition of the inflammatory infiltrate to the basal layer. However, the basal cells are not replaced by flattened squamous cells, as in lichen planus, but appear hydropic; and

usually in lichen sclerosus et atrophicus a subepidermal zone of edema has already begun to form in some areas. Older lesions of lichen sclerosus et atrophicus with thickening and hyperchromasia of the collagen bundles in the lower dermis and only a slight inflammatory infiltrate may resemble morphea. Nevertheless, in morphea the epidermis, although it may be thin, shows neither hydropic degeneration of the basal cells nor follicular plugging, and the upper dermis shows no zone of edema (Steigleder and Raab).

KRAUROSIS VULVAE

Lichen sclerosus et atrophicus of the vulva, often referred to as kraurosis vulvae, is characterized by sharply demarcated whitish lesions that involve most of the vulva, including the labia majora and minora, and often extend to the perineum, the perianal region, and the inguinal folds. Atrophy of the labia and narrowing of the vaginal orifice ensue. In contrast with lichen sclerosus et atrophicus of the skin, which rarely itches, pruritus in the vulvar region often is severe. In most instances, when lichen sclerosus et atrophicus involves the vulvar, perianal and inguinal regions it is limited to these areas, but occasionally lesions of lichen sclerosus et atrophicus are encountered elsewhere on the skin. Lichen sclerosus et atrophicus of the vulva may occur in prepubertal children. Whereas in adults the lesions usually progress, in children there often is improvement with time (Clark and Muller).

Although lichen sclerosus et atrophicus of the skin never undergoes malignant degeneration, lichen sclerosus et atrophicus of the vulva can progress to leukoplakia and squamous cell carcinoma. In the experience of several authors, the development of carcinoma is a rare event. Some have stated that they have never observed it (McAdams and Kistner; Oberfield); while Barker and Gross, Höfs, and Grimmer have reported the development of vulvar carcinoma only once among 42, 23 and 57 patients, respectively. On the other hand, Wallace has reported 12 instances of carcinoma in 290 patients; Suurmond, 9 instances in 55 patients; and Balus, 18 instances in 75 patients.

Histopathology. Lichen sclerosus et atrophicus of the vulva (kraurosis vulvae) shows the same histologic picture as it does on the skin, with the exception that lesions on the mucous membranes show no keratotic plugs (Fig. 15-9) (Barker and Gross). Irregular downward proliferations of the epithelium in which the basal cells show considerable hydropic degeneration are seen more often and more extensively than on the skin (Fig. 15-10). They should not be confused with the early atypical proliferations of leukoplakia, which do not contain basal cells with hydropic degeneration (Fig. 15-11).

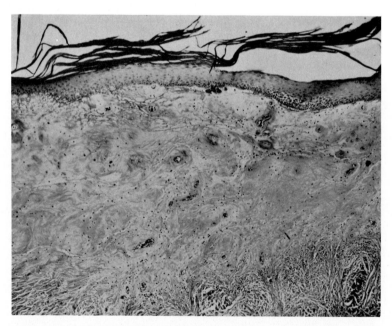

FIG. 15-9. **Kraurosis vulvae (lichen sclerosus et atrophicus).** There are hyperkeratosis, atrophy of the stratum malpighii, and marked lymphedema of the upper dermis with homogenization of the collagen. (×100)

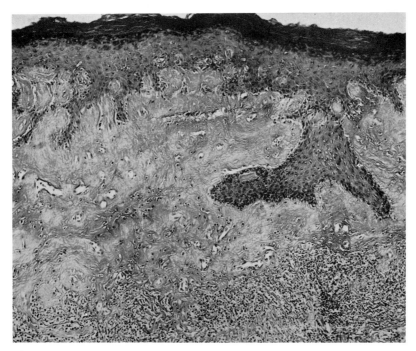

FIG. 15-10. **Kraurosis vulvae (lichen sclerosus et atrophicus).** There are edema of the upper dermis and a bandlike inflammatory infiltrate beneath the edematous zone. In addition, there is irregular downward proliferation of the rete ridges with hydropic degeneration of the basal cells. The latter feature is typical of lichen sclerosus et atrophicus and rules out leukoplakia. (×100)

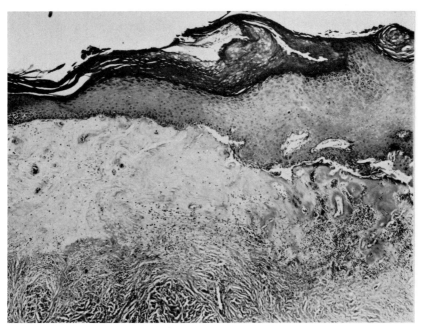

FIG. 15-11. **Kraurosis vulvae (Lichen sclerosus et atrophicus).** On the right side leukoplakia has developed characterized by irregular thickening of the epidermis and disorderly arrangement of the cells. (×100)

BALANITIS XEROTICA OBLITERANS

Balanitis xerotica obliterans, the term applied to lichen sclerosus et atrophicus of the glans penis and prepuce, shows white, atrophic, slightly edematous areas that may lead to phimosis. In rare instances carcinoma supervenes (Roederer; Tritsch; Wallace).

Histopathology. The histologic picture is that of lichen sclerosus et atrophicus. Because of the absence of follicles in the area of involvement, no keratotic plugging occurs (Laymon).

STRIAE DISTENSAE

Striae distensae occur most commonly on the abdomen, the buttocks, the thighs, and in the inguinal region. They consist of bands of thin wrinkled skin which are reddish at first, then purple, and finally white.

Histopathology. The epidermis is thin and flattened. There is a decrease in the thickness of the dermis. The collagen fibers lie separated from one another rather than united into collagen bundles (Epstein et al.). Elastic fibers are absent in the center of the lesion, whereas at the periphery they appear curled and clumped (Chernosky and Knox).

In older striae, as a result of regeneration, one observes in the upper dermis many rather straight collagen bundles arranged parallel to the skin surface and intermingled with numerous fairly straight and thin elastic fibers. Beneath this area, absence of elastic fibers persists (Pinkus et al.).

Histogenesis. Striae distensae occur in conditions associated with an increased production of glucocorticoids by the adrenal glands. Among these are (1) pregnancy, (2) obesity, (3) adolescence, and, especially, (4) Cushing's disease (Hauser; Epstein et al.). In obesity the increased adrenocortical activity is a consequence of the obesity, and the production of glucocorticoids returns to normal on reducing the body weight (Simkin and Arce). Also, the occurrence of striae in nonobese adolescents noted in 35 per cent of the girls and in 15 per cent of the boys examined by Sisson, is associated with an increased 17-ketosteroid excretion. Striae may form also on prolonged medication with corticosteroids; and occasionally they form following the prolonged local application of corticosteroid creams to the skin under occlusive dressings (Chernosky and Knox), and to the inguinal region even without occlusion (Epstein et al.). The action of the glucocorticoids consists of a suppression of fibroblastic activity (Hauser). Overextension of the skin is of significance only so far as the localization and direction of the striae is concerned.

MACULAR ATROPHY (ANETODERMA)

Macular atrophy, or anetoderma, is characterized by atrophic oval patches located mainly on the upper trunk. The skin of the patches is thin and bluish white, and bulges slightly. The lesions may give the palpating finger the same sensation as does a hernial orifice. Two types of macular atrophy are generally distinguished: the Jadassohn type, in which intially the atrophic lesions appear red and, on histologic examination, show an inflammatory infiltrate, and the Schweninger and Buzzi type, which clinically and histologically is noninflammatory from the beginning. However, not every case can be clearly assigned to one or the other of these two types, as pointed out by Deluzenne, since some clinically noninflammatory cases show in early lesions evidence of an inflammatory infiltrate when examined histologically.

Histopathology. In most cases reported as the Jadassohn type and in some cases reported as the Schweninger and Buzzi type the early lesions show a moderately pronounced perivascular infiltrate of lymphoid-histiocytic cells (Feldman). In two recently reported cases, however, the early inflammatory lesions showed a perivascular infiltrate in which neutrophils or eosinophils predominated and "nuclear dust" was present, resulting in a histologic picture of vasculitis (Neumann and Vacátko; Cramer). Even during the early inflammatory stage the elastic tissue is already greatly decreased or even absent within the lesions.

In noninflammatory cases of the Schweninger and Buzzi type the only abnormality usually is the absence of elastic tissue, so that the sections show no abnormality when stained with hematoxylin and eosin (Varadi and Saqueton). In some cases, however, the collagen bundles appear swollen and homogenized (Duperrat; Korting et al.).

ACROOSTEOLYSIS

The term acroosteolysis refers to lytic changes on the distal phalanges. Three types are recognized: (1) familial; (2) idiopathic, nonfamilial; and (3) occupational, associated with vinyl chloride polymerization.

The *familial type* affects mainly the phalanges of the feet and is associated with recurrent ulcers on the soles (Meyerson and Meier).

The *idiopathic type* affects mainly the distal phalanges of the fingers, causing shortening of the fingers. This may be associated with Raynaud's phenomenon. In one case, reported by Meyerson and Meier, numerous yellowish papules, 2 to 4 mm in size, were present, mainly on the arms.

Occupational acroosteolysis, like the idiopathic type, causes shortening of the fingers due to osteolysis. This often is associated with Raynaud's phenomenon and progressive thickening of the skin of the hands and forearms simulating scleroderma. There may be erythema of the hands, and the thickening may consist of papules and plaques (Markowitz et al.).

Histopathology. The histologic changes in the papules of idiopathic and occupational acroosteolysis consists of thickening of the collagen bundles. Staining for elastic tissue shows disorganization of the elastic fibers which in some areas are thin and fragmented and in others are condensed into thick bundles (Meyerson and Meier; Markowitz et al.).

ULERYTHEMA OF EYEBROWS AND CHEEKS

Ulerythema of the eyebrows, referred to as *ulerythema ophryogenes,* starts in childhood with redness and thinning of the hairs in the lateral portions of the eyebrows and ends with atrophy of the skin and hair loss in these areas (Davenport).

Ulerythema of the cheeks, referred to as *folliculitis ulerythematosa reticulata,* also starts in childhood. Starting with perifollicular erythema it ends with perifollicular atrophy on the cheeks. As the result of numerous follicular pits the atrophy on the cheeks has a honeycombed appearance (MacKee and Cipollaro).

Histopathology. The histologic findings are not diagnostic. In both conditions one observes hair follicles filled with horny material. There is perifollicular inflammation and dermal fibrosis with absence of the sebaceous glands.

BIBLIOGRAPHY

Solar (Actinic) Degeneration

Banfield, W. G., and Brindlay, D. C.: Preliminary observations on senile elastosis using the electron microscope. J. Invest. Derm., *41*:9, 1963.

Berger, H.: Elektronenmikroskopische Befunde zur Bindegewebsneubildung bei aktinischer Elastose. Derm. Monatsschr., *155*:251, 1969.

Braun-Falco, O.: Die Morphogenese der senil-aktinischen Elastose. Arch. klin. exp. Derm., *235*:138, 1969.

Ebner, H.: Über die Entstehung des elastotischen Materials. Z. Haut, *44*:889, 1969.

Favre, M., and Racouchot, J.: L'élastéidose cutanée nodulaire à kystes et à comédons. Ann. derm. syph., *78*:681, 1951.

Felsher, Z.: Observations on senile elastosis. J. Invest. Derm. *37*:163, 1961.

Findlay, G. H.: On elastase and the elastic dystrophies of the skin, Brit. J. Derm., *66*:16, 1954.

Helm, F.: Nodular cutaneous elastosis with cysts and comedones (Favre-Racouchot syndrome). Arch. Derm., *84*:666, 1961.

Kligman, A. M.: Early destructive effect of sunlight on human skin. J.A.M.A., *210*:2377, 1969.

Kretzberg, R., and Klingmüller, G.: Senile elastosis. Z. Haut, *43*:(105), 1968.

Ledoux-Corbusier, M., and Achten, G.: Elastosis in chronic radiodermatitis. An ultrastructural study. Brit. J. Derm., *91*:287, 1974.

Mitchell, R. E.: Chronic solar dermatosis: a light and electron microscopic study of the dermis. J. Invest. Derm., *48*:203, 1967.

Niebauer, G., and Stockinger, L.: Über die senile Elastose. Arch. klin. exp. Derm., *221*:122, 1965.

Olson, R. L., Nordquist, J., and Everett, M. A.: The role of epidermal lysomes in melanin physiology. Brit. J. Derm., *83*:189, 1970.

Rasheed, A., El-Hefnawi, H., Nagy, G., and Wiskemann, A.: Elektronenmikroskopische Untersuchungen bei Xeroderma pigmentosum. Arch. klin. exp. Derm., *234*:321, 1969.

Sams, W. M., Jr., and Smith, J. G., Jr.: The histochemistry of chronically sun-damaged skin. J. Invest. Derm., *37*:447, 1961.

Kyrle's Disease

Abele, D. C., and Dobson, R. L.: Hyperkeratosis penetrans (Kyrle's disease). Arch. Derm., 83:277, 1961.

Aram, H., Szymanski, F. J., and Bailey, W. E.: Kyrle's disease. Arch. Derm., 100:453, 1969.

Carter, V. H., and Constantine, V. S.: Kyrle's disease. I. Clinical findings in five cases and review of literature. Arch. Derm., 97:624, 1968.

Constantine, V. S., and Carter, V. H.: Kyrle's disease. II. Histopathologic findings in five cases and review of the literature. Arch. Derm., 97:633, 1968.

de Graciansky, P., Boulle, S., Boulle, M., and Dalion, J.: La maladie de Kyrle. Ann. derm. syph., 82:8, 1955.

Kyrle, J.: Hyperkeratosis follicularis et parafollicularis in cutem penetrans. Arch f. Derm. u. Syph., 123:466, 1916.

Pinkus, H., and Mehregan, A. H.: A Guide to Dermatohistopathology. p. 343. New York, Appleton-Century-Crofts, 1969.

Prakken, J. R.: Kyrle's disease. Acta dermatoven., 34:360, 1954.

Tappeiner, J., Wolff, K., and Schreiner, E.: Morbus Kyrle. Hautarzt, 20:296, 1969.

Thyresson, N.: Hyperkeratosis follicularis et parafollicularis in cutem penetrans. Acta dermatoven., 31:287, 1951.

Perforating Folliculitis

Mehregan, A. H., and Coskey, R. J.: Perforating folliculitis. Arch. Derm., 97:394, 1968.

Streitmann, B.: Ein Beitrag zu den das Follikelepithel durchbrechenden Prozessen. Z. Haut, 45:195, 1970.

Elastosis Perforans Serpiginosa

Cohen, A. S., and Hashimoto, K.: Electron microscopic observations on the lesions of elastosis perforans serpiginosa. J. Invest. Derm., 35:15, 1960.

Hitch, J. M., and Lund, H. Z.: Elastosis perforans serpiginosa. Arch. Derm., 79:407, 1959.

Marshall, J., and Lurie, H. I.: Keratosis follicularis serpiginosa (Lutz). Dermatologica, 113:13, 1956.

Mehregan, A. H.: Elastosis perforans serpiginosa. Arch. Derm., 97:381, 1968. (Review)

Meves, C., and Vogel, C.: Elektronenmikroskopische Untersuchungen an einem Fall von Elastosis perforans serpiginosa. Dermatologica, 143:210, 1973.

Pedro, S. D., and Garcia, R. L.: Disseminate elastosis perforans serpiginosa. Arch. Derm., 109:84, 1974.

Rasmussen, J. E.: Disseminated elastosis perforans serpiginosa in four mongoloids. Brit. J. Derm., 86:9, 1972.

Whyte, H. J., and Winkelmann, R. K.: Elastosis perforans (perforating elastosis). J. Invest. Derm., 35:113, 1960.

Reactive Perforating Collagenosis

Bovenmyer, D. A.: Reactive perforating collagenosis. Arch. Derm., 102:313, 1970.

Laugier, P., and Woringer, F.: Réflexions au sujet d'un collagénome perforant verruciforme. Ann. derm. syph., 90:29, 1936.

Mehregan, A. H., Schwartz, O. D., and Livingood, C. S.: Reactive perforating collagenosis. Arch. Derm., 96:277, 1967.

Weiner, A. L.: Reactive perforating collagenosis. Arch. Derm., 102:540, 1970.

Weiner, J.: Kyrle's disease: Hyperkeratosis follicularis et parafollicularis in cutem penetrans in siblings. Arch. Derm., 95:329, 1967.

Woringer, F., and Laugier, P.: Collagenoma perforans verruciforme. Derm. Wchschr., 147:63, 1963.

Hyperkeratosis Lenticularis Perstans (Flegel)

Bean, S. F.: Hyperkeratosis lenticularis perstans. Arch. Derm., 99:705, 1969.

————: The genetics of hyperkeratosis lenticularis perstans. Arch. Derm., 106:72, 1972.

Flegel, H.: Hyperkeratosis lenticularis perstans. Hautarzt, 9:362, 1958.

Kocsard, E., Bear, C. L., and Constance, T. J.: Hyperkeratosis lenticularis perstans (Flegel). Dermatologica, 136:35, 1968.

Krinitz, K., and Schäfer, I.: Hyperkeratosis lenticularis perstans. Derm. Monatsschr., 157:438, 1971.

Raffle, E. J., and Rogers, J.: Hyperkeratosis lenticularis perstans. Arch. Derm., 100:423, 1969.

Acrodermatitis Chronica Atrophicans

Grimmer, H.: Akrodermatitis chronica atrophicans. Z. Haut Geschlechtskr., 36:XVII, 1964.

Hardmeier, T.: Zur Histopathologic der fibroiden Knoten bei Akrodermatitis chronica atrophicans. Arch. klin. exp. Derm., 232:373, 1968.

Korting, G. W., Hoede, N., and Holzmann, H.: Zur Frage des Elastikaverhaltens bei einigen sklerosierenden und atrophisierenden Hautkrankheiten. Hautarzt, 20:351, 1969.

Montgomery, H., and Sullivan, R. R.: Acrodermatitis atrophicans chronica. Arch. Derm. Syph., 51:32, 1945.

Pretibial Pigmented Patches in Diabetes

Auböck, L.: Elektronenmikroskopische Untersuchungen der prätibialen Pigmentflecke. Z. Haut, *46*:624, 1971.

Bauer, M. F., Levan, N. E., Frankel, A., and Bach, J.: Pigmented pretibial patches. Arch. Derm., *93*:282, 1966.

Fisher, E. R., and Danowski, T. S.: Histologic, histochemical, and electron microscopic features of the skin spots of diabetes mellitus. Am. J. Clin. Path., *50*:547, 1968.

Kerl, H.: Zur Frage der prätibialen Pigmentflecke bei Diabetes mellitus (Diabetische Dermopathie). Z. Haut, *46*:619, 1971.

Bullosis Diabeticorum

Allen, G. E., and Hadden, D. R.: Bullous lesions of the skin in diabetes (bullosis diabeticorum). Brit. J. Derm., *82*:216, 1970.

Cantwell, A. R., Jr., and Martz, W.: Idiopathic bullae in diabetics. Bullosis diabeticorum. Arch. Derm., *96*:42, 1967.

Kerl, H.: Bullosis diabeticorum. Derm. Monatsschr., *158*:148, 1972.

Kerl, H., and Kresbach, H.: Zu einigen Aspekten der "Bullosis diabeticorum." Hautarzt, *25*:60, 1974.

Kurwa, A., Roberts, P., and Whitehead, R.: Concurrence of bullous and atrophic skin lesions in diabetes mellitus. Arch. Derm., *103*:670, 1971.

Lichen Sclerosus et Atrophicus

Balus, L.: Lichen sclerosus et atrophicus der Vulvagegend als präcanceröser Zustand. Hautarzt, *22*:199, 1971.

Barker, L. P., and Gross, P.: Lichen sclerosus et atrophicus of the female genitalia. Arch. Derm., *85*:362, 1962.

Bergfeld, W. F., and Lesowitz, S. A.: Lichen sclerosus et atrophicus. Arch. Derm., *101*:247, 1970.

Clark, J. A., and Muller, S. A.: Lichen sclerosus et atrophicus in children. Arch. Derm., *95*:476, 1967.

Forssmann, W. G., Holzmann, H., and Cabré, J.: Elektronenmikroskopische Untersuchungen der Haut beim Lichen sclerosus et atrophicus. Arch. klin. exp. Derm., *220*:584, 1964.

Gottschalk, H. R., and Cooper, Z. K.: Lichen sclerosus et atrophicus with bullous lesions and extensive involvement. Arch. Derm. Syph., *55*:433, 1947.

Grimmer, H.: Lichen sclerosus et atrophicus (Kraurosis) vulvae. Z. Haut, *42*:(113), 1967.

Höfs, W.: Lichen sklerosus et atrophicus, Kraurosis vulvae und Balanitis xerotica obliterans. Derm. Wschr., *149*:217, 1964.

Klug, H., and Sönnichsen, N.: Elektronenoptische Untersuchungen bei Lichen sklerosus et atrophicus. Derm. Mschr., *158*:641, 1972.

Laymon, C. M.: Lichen sclerosus et atrophicus and related disorders. Arch. Derm. Syph., *64*:620, 1961.

Mann, P. R., and Cowan, M. A.: Ultrastructural changes in four cases of lichen sclerosus et atrophicus. Brit. J. Derm., *89*:223, 1973.

McAdams, A. J., Jr., and Kistner, R. W.: The relationship of chronic vulvar disease, leukoplakia, and carcinoma in situ to carcinoma of the vulva. Cancer, *11*:740, 1958.

Miller, R. F.: Lichen sclerosus et atrophicus with oral involvement. Arch. Derm., *76*:43, 1957.

Oberfield, R. A.: Lichen sclerosus et atrophicus and kraurosis vulvae. Are they the same disease? Arch. Derm., *83*:806, 1961.

Piper, H. G.: Lichen sklerosus et atrophicus partim bullosus. Derm. Wschr., *143*:137, 1961.

Roederer, J.: Un cas d'épithelioma sur balanitis xerotica obliterans post-operationem. Bull. Soc. franç. derm. syph., *60*:327, 1953.

Steigleder, G. K., and Raab, W. P.: Lichen sclerosus et atrophicus. Arch. Derm., *84*:219, 1961.

Suurmond, D.: Lichen sclerosus et atrophicus of the vulva. Arch. Derm., *90*:143, 1964.

Tritsch, H.: Adenoides Plattenepithel-Carcinom bei Lichen sclerosus et atrophicus. Arch. klin. exp. Derm., *232*:187, 1968.

Wallace, H. J.: Lichen sclerosus et atrophicus. Trans. St. John's Hosp. Derm. Soc., *57*:9, 1971.

Striae Distensae

Chernosky, M. E., and Knox, J. M.: Atrophic striae after occlusive corticosteroid therapy. Arch. Derm., *90*:15, 1964.

Epstein, N. W., Epstein, W. L., and Epstein, J. H.: Atrophic striae in patients with inguinal intertrigo. Arch. Derm., *87*:450, 1963.

Hauser, W.: Zur Frage der Entstehung der Striae cutis atrophicae. Derm. Wschr., *138*:1291, 1958.

Pinkus, H., Keech, M. K., and Mehregan, A. H.: Histopathology of striae distensae with special reference to striae and wound healing in the Marfan syndrome. J. Invest. Derm., *46*:283, 1966.

Simkin, B., and Arce, R.: Steroid excretion in obese patients with colored abdominal striae. New Eng. J. Med., *266*:1031, 1962.

Sisson, W. R.: Colored striae in adolescent children. J. Pediat., *45*:520, 1954.

Macular Atrophy (Anetoderma)

Cramer, H. J.: Zur Histopathogenese der Dermatitis atrophicans maculosa. Derm. Wschr., *147*:230, 1963.

Deluzenne, R.: Les anétodermies maculeuses. Ann. derm. syph., *83*:618, 1956.

Duperrat, B.: Anétodermie type Schweninger-Buzzi. Bull. Soc. franç. derm. syph., *61*:11, 1954.

Feldman, S.: Macular atrophy (Schweninger and Buzzi type). Arch. Derm. Syph., *38*:117, 1938.

Korting, G. W., Cabré, J., and Holzmann, H.: Zur Kenntnis der Kollagenveränderungen bei der Anetodermie vom Typus Schweninger-Buzzi. Arch. klin. exp. Derm., *218*:274, 1964.

Neumann, E., and Vacátko, S.: Kutane Form der Arteriitis als Vorläufer einer Atrophia maculosa. Derm. Wschr., *140*:1008, 1959.

Varadi, D. P., and Saqueton, A. C.: Perifollicular elastolysis. Brit. J. Derm., *83*:143, 1970.

Acroosteolysis

Markowitz, S. S., McDonald, C. J., Fethiere, W., and Kerzner, M. S: Occupational acroosteolysis. Arch. Derm., *106*:219, 1972.

Meyerson, L. B., and Meier, G. C.: Cutaneous lesions in acroosteolysis. Arch. Derm., *106*:224, 1972.

Ulerythema of Eyebrows and Cheeks

Davenport, D. D.: Ulerythema ophryogenes. Arch. Derm., *89*:74, 1964.

MacKee, G. M., and Cipollaro, A. C.: Folliculitis ulerythematosa reticulata. Arch. Derm., *57*:281, 1948.

16

Bacterial Diseases

IMPETIGO

Impetigo is caused by group A beta-hemolytic streptococci, except in newborn babies, infants and young children in whom it is usually caused by coagulase-positive staphylococci largely belonging to phage group 2, type 71 (Wannamaker). Although staphylococci can often be grown from streptococcal impetigo they are secondary invaders (Dajani et al.). Bullae represent the primary lesion of streptococcal impetigo, but the bullae soon rupture so that heavy yellowish crusts represent the clinical picture usually seen in streptococcal impetigo. On the other hand, in staphylococcal bullous impetigo occurring almost exclusively in newborn babies, in infants, and in young children the bullae can persist for several days (see below).

Streptococcal impetigo, if caused by group A streptococci with an M antigen, especially M-type 49, may result in an acute glomerulonephritis about 3 weeks after onset of the impetigo (Kaplan et al.). As a rule, the nephritis following impetigo has a favorable long-term prognosis.

Histopathology. In both the streptococcal and the staphylococcal varieties of impetigo the bulla arises directly beneath the horny layer (see Classification of Bullae, p. 96). The bulla contains numerous neutrophils (Fig. 16-1). Occasionally, a few acantholytic cells can be observed at the floor of the bulla as the result of the proteolytic action of the neutrophils (Steigleder).

The stratum malpighii underlying the bulla shows spongiosis, and neutrophils can be seen migrating through it. The upper dermis contains a moderately severe inflammatory infiltrate of neutrophils and lymphoid cells.

At a later stage, when the bulla has ruptured, the horny layer is absent, and a crust composed of serous exudate and the nuclear debris of neutrophils may be seen covering the stratum malpighii.

Differential Diagnosis. A histologic differentiation from subcorneal pustular dermatosis is impossible (Ellis). The presence of a few acantholytic cells may lead to confusion with pemphigus foliaceus; but aside from the fact that the number of acantholytic cells is small, impetigo differs from pemphigus foliaceus by the presence of numerous neutrophils in the bulla cavity.

BULLOUS IMPETIGO, RITTER'S DISEASE

In newborn babies, in infants and rarely also in young children, impetigo is caused by coagulase-positive staphylococci of phage group 2, type 71. It may show bullae that can persist for several days without rupturing. In severe infections a clinical picture develops that has been known as Ritter's disease for nearly a hundred years and consists of generalized erythema followed within a few hours by detachment of the upper epidermis in large sheets. It is unfortunate that

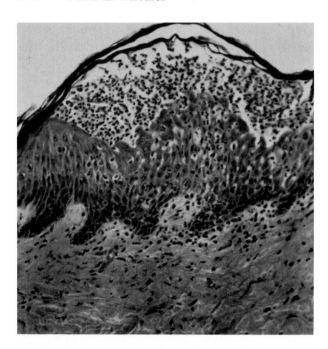

FIG. 16-1. **Impetigo.** A subcorneal pustule containing numerous neutrophils is present. The underlying stratum malpighii shows spongiosis, and neutrophils are seen migrating through it. (×200)

terms like "scalded skin syndrome," "toxic epidermal necrolysis," and "Lyell's disease" have become attached to severe staphylococcal impetigo as well as to severe erythema multiforme (see p. 124). These two diseases, even though they have some clinical resemblance, differ from one another in their etiology, histology, course, and treatment (Lowney et al.; Lyell).

Ritter's disease in infants runs an acute course and, even without antibiotic treatment, rarely is fatal, except in newborn babies. It must be kept in mind that the disease is transmissible and can cause nursery epidemics (Melish and Glasgow). In recent years a few instances of Ritter's disease, or staphylococcal scalded skin syndrome, have been reported also in adults either with chronic renal failure and deficiency in cell-mediated immunity (Levine and Norden; Reid et al.) or with severe septicemia due to a phage group 2 Staphylococcus (Rothenberg et al.).

Histopathology. In bullous staphylococcal impetigo the histologic picture is identical with that described above for impetigo. In Ritter's disease, in which one observes clinically detachment of the upper epidermis in large sheets, there is a zone of cleavage in the upper portion of the epidermis, usually close to the stratum corneum. The detaching or detached upper portion of the epidermis consists of degenerated cells showing eosinophilic necrosis, whereas the lower portion of the epidermis consists of basophilic viable cells (Koblenzer).

Histogenesis. Coagulase-positive staphylococci of phage group 2, type 71 isolated from patients with Ritter's disease, grown in culture, and injected subcutaneously or intraperitoneally into newborn mice, have reproduced the disease both clinically and histologically. Clinically, the mice show bullae and a positive Nikolsky sign followed by spontaneous detachment of the upper layers of the epidermis. Histologically, the mice show intraepidermal cleavage largely at the level of the stratum granulosum. The intraepidermal bullae of the mice proved to be sterile; but staphylococci could be recovered from the sites into which they had been injected. This suggests that the epidermal lesion in Ritter's disease is caused by a soluble toxin produced by the staphylococci (Melish and Glasgow; Dick and Baird).

Differential Diagnosis. Both Ritter's disease and severe erythema multiforme, when of the toxic epidermal necrolysis or Lyell type, show extensive epidermal detachment and thus resemble each other clinically, a situation that has resulted in both diseases being referred to as Lyell's disease. However, histologically the two diseases can be easily differentiated because in severe erythema multiforme the entire, or nearly the entire epidermis detaches itself, whereas in Ritter's disease only the uppermost portion of the epidermis becomes detached (see p. 124).

ECTHYMA

Ecthyma is essentially ulcerated impetigo. It occurs chiefly below the knees but occasionally also on the arms. It is streptococcal in origin, since skin cultures are always positive for group A beta-hemolytic streptococci. In addition, coagulase-positive staphylococci as secondary invaders can frequently be cultured from the lesions (Kelly et al.).

Histopathology. A nonspecific ulcer is seen, with numerous neutrophils being present both in the dermis and in the serous exudate at the floor of the ulcer.

ERYSIPELAS

Erysipelas is an acute superficial cellulitis of the skin caused by streptococci. It is characterized by the presence of a well demarcated, slightly indurated, dusky red area having an advancing, palpable border. In certain individuals erysipelas has a tendency to recur periodically in the same area.

Histopathology. The dermis shows marked edema and dilatation of the lymphatics and capillaries. There is a diffuse infiltrate composed chiefly of neutrophils. The infiltrate extends throughout the dermis and, occasionally, into the subcutaneous fat. It shows a loose arrangement around the dilated blood and lymph vessels. If sections are stained with Giemsa's or Gram's stain, streptococci may be found distributed in the tissue.

In cases of recurring erysipelas the lymph vessels of the dermis and subcutaneous tissue show fibrotic thickening of their walls with partial or complete occlusion of the lumen (Tappeiner and Pfleger).

ACUTE SUPERFICIAL FOLLICULITIS (IMPETIGO BOCKHART)

Impetigo Bockhart, caused by staphylococci, is characterized by an eruption of small pustules, many of which are pierced by a hair.

Histopathology. Impetigo Bockhart presents a subcorneal pustule situated in the opening of a hair follicle. The upper portion of the hair follicle is surrounded by a considerable inflammatory infiltrate composed predominantly of neutrophils.

ACUTE DEEP FOLLICULITIS (FURUNCLE)

A furuncle, caused by staphylococci, consists of a tender, red perifollicular swelling terminating in suppuration and necrosis.

Histopathology. A furuncle presents a perifollicular abscess composed mainly of neutrophils. The hair with its follicular wall and sebaceous gland is destroyed in the process.

CHRONIC SUPERFICIAL FOLLICULITIS (ACNE VARIOLIFORMIS; ACNE NECROTICA MILIARIS)

Acne varioliformis is characterized by the presence of small indolent follicular papules and pustules along the frontal hairline. The lesions undergo central necrosis and usually heal with small pitted scars.

Acne necrotica miliaris of the scalp is a diminutive variety of acne varioliformis. Because of the superficial location of the necrosis, no hair loss ensues.

Histopathology. The histologic changes in both acne varioliformis and in acne necrotica miliaris consist of an intrafollicular subcorneal pustule and an acute perifollicular infiltrate. A superficial perifollicular abscess may form, leaving a small area of necrosis. In the case of acne varioliformis but not in the case of acne necrotica miliaris, the area of necrosis often is sufficiently large to result in healing with fibrosis and scar formation (Montgomery).

CHRONIC DEEP FOLLICULITIS (FOLLICULITIS BARBAE; FOLLICULITIS DECALVANS; FOLLICULITIS KELOIDALIS NUCHAE)

Folliculitis barbae is a deep-seated infection of the bearded region in men. There are follicular papules and pustules followed by erythema, crusting, and boggy infiltration of the skin. Abscesses may or may not be present. Scarring and permanent hair loss usually ensue.

Folliculitis decalvans occurs predominantly in men and shows throughout the scalp crops of follicular papules, pustules, and abscesses healing with atrophy and permanent hair loss.

Folliculitis keloidalis nuchae represents a chronic folliculitis on the nape of the neck of men. It causes hypertrophic scarring. In early cases one observes follicular papules, pustules, and, occasionally, abscesses. The lesions are replaced gradually by fibrous nodules.

Histopathology. In all three forms of chronic deep folliculitis one observes in early lesions a perifollicular infiltrate composed largely of neutrophils but also containing lymphoid cells, histiocytes, and plasma cells. The infiltrate develops into a perifollicular abscess. Older lesions show chronic granulation tissue containing numerous plasma cells, as well as lymphoid cells and fibroblasts (Meinhof and Braun-Falco). Often, numerous foreign body giant cells are present around remnants of hair follicles. Particles of keratin may be located near the giant cells (Moyer and Williams). As healing takes place, fibrosis is seen. If there is hypertrophic scar formation, as in folliculitis keloidalis nuchae, numerous thick bundles of sclerotic collagen are present.

FOLLICULAR OCCLUSION TRIAD (HIDRADENITIS SUPPURATIVA; ACNE CONGLOBATA; PERIFOLLICULITIS CAPITIS ABSCEDENS ET SUFFODIENS)

The three diseases included into the follicular occlusion triad have a similar pathogenesis and similar histopathologic findings. Occasionally two of the three diseases, and rarely all three diseases, are encountered in the same patient (Pillsbury et al.). All three diseases represent a chronic, recurrent, deep-seated folliculitis resulting in abscesses and cysts. Healing takes place with the formation of sinus tracts and with considerable scarring.

In *hidradenitis suppurativa,* the chronic suppurative and scarring process affects the axillary and anogenital regions. Early lesions consist of red, tender nodules that become fluctuant and finally discharge pus. The development of deep-seated abscesses leads to the discharge of pus through sinus tracts. Severe scarring results (Brunsting).

Acne conglobata, an entity different from acne vulgaris, occurs mainly on the back, buttocks and chest and rarely on the face or the extremities. In addition to comedones, fluctuant nodules discharging pus or a mucoid material occur, together with deep-seated abscesses discharging through sinus tracts (Strauss).

In *perifolliculitis capitis abscedens et suffodiens,* nodules and abscesses, as described for acne conglobata, occur in the scalp (Moschella).

Histopathology. Early lesions in all three diseases show a perifolliculitis with an extensive infiltrate composed of neutrophils, lymphoid cells and histiocytes. Abscess formation results and leads to destruction of the cutaneous appendages. In response to this destruction granulation tissue infiltrates the area, containing, in addition to lymphoid and plasma cells, foreign body giant cells near the remnants of hair follicles. As the abscesses extend deeper into the subcutaneous tissue, draining sinus tracts develop that are lined with epidermis. In areas of healing extensive fibrosis may be seen.

Histogenesis. Hidradenitis suppurativa traditionally is regarded as an infection of apocrine glands (Shaughnessy et al.). This deduction is based on the occurrence of the disease in apocrine-gland-bearing areas. However, the histologic resemblance of hidradenitis suppurativa to the other two diseases and the occasional occurrence with them make a purely apocrine genesis for hidradenitis suppurativa unlikely, since the other two diseases occur in areas generally free of apocrine glands. It even appears doubtful that the diseases comprising the follicular occlusion triad are caused primarily by bacterial infection. The beneficial effect of the internal administration of corticosteroids suggests that the three diseases represent antigen-antibody reactions resulting in tissue breakdown.

PYODERMA GANGRENOSUM

The lesions of pyoderma gangrenosum, of which there may be one or several, begin as a fluctuant nodule in the skin that ulcerates. The ulcer enlarges peripherally. The skin at the edge of the ulcer is purplish red and undermined. In about 40 per cent of the cases, pyoderma gangrenosum is associated with ulcerative colitis (Perry and Brunsting; Sluis). In rare instances, it is associated with Crohn's disease, also called regional enteritis (Stathers et al.), or with a chronic rheumatoidlike polyarthritis (Lazarus et al.).

Histopathology. The histologic appearance is not diagnostic. In the region of the ulcer the epidermis is absent. The upper dermis shows necrosis and is permeated by an acute inflammatory infiltrate. Farther down, the infiltrate is chronic inflammatory in nature, consisting of lymphoid cells, plasma cells, histiocytes, and fibroblasts. Frequently a few foreign body giant cells are present (Stathers et al.). The number of blood vessels is increased, but aside from minimal endothelial proliferation they appear normal (Perry and Brunsting; Kresbach; de Bast et al.). The cellular infiltrate may extend deep into the subcutaneous tissue. Fibrosis occurs in areas of healing. The epidermis at the edge of an ulcer may show considerable hyperplasia.

Histogenesis. In a significant number of patients with pyoderma gangrenosum, but by no means in all of them, immunoelectrophoresis has revealed the presence of a monoclonal gammopathy. Several patients were found to have an abnormal IgA component (Sluis; Schröpl), whereas others had an IgG gammopathy (Imhof et al.) or an IgM gammopathy (Cream). In several other patients abnormalities of the delayed hypersensitivity response were present: There was anergy inasmuch as the patients could not be actively sensitized by various antigens, such as dinitrochlorobenzene, tuberculin or mumps antigen. Also the patients' lymphocytes failed to produce macrophage migration inhibition factor (MIF) in vitro in response to

tuberculin or streptokinase-streptodornase. On the other hand, their lymphocytes showed an adequate blastogenic response in vitro to phytohemagglutinin; and no abnormalities in their humoral immunity were detected (Lazarus et al.). The good response of patients with pyoderma gangrenosum to the systemic administration of corticosteroids suggests that antigen-antibody reactions play a role in the pathogenesis of pyoderma gangrenosum and may be responsible for the tissue breakdown leading to the formation of the ulcers. In any case, there is no evidence that microorganisms play a role in the causation of pyoderma gangrenosum.

CROHN'S DISEASE (REGIONAL ENTERITIS)

Regional enteritis, a disease of unknown etiology, is characterized by sharply demarcated areas of inflammation that may occur anywhere in the gastrointestinal tract from the stomach to the anus. Nearly half of the patients with regional enteritis have perianal lesions. They may consist of ulcers, fissures, and sinus tracts arising from perianal abscesses (Korting). The perianal lesions are indolent, bleed easily and heal with scarring. The lesions occasionally extend to the gluteal fold. The perianal lesions usually occur in association with intestinal lesions, but they may precede them (McCallum and Kinmont).

In addition to the specific perianal lesions, regional enteritis in rare instances is associated with pyoderma gangrenosum (see above) or with erythema nodosum.

Histopathology. The perianal lesions show the same aspect as the intestinal lesions. Frequently, noncaseating granulomas with giant cells are present. The presence of a conspicuous number of giant cells aids in the differentiation from sarcoidosis or tuberculosis (Korting).

APHTHOSIS; BEHÇET'S SYNDROME

Aphthae commonly occur in the mouth as recurrent ulcers. Usually, they are small, but occasionally they may consist of fairly large, irregularly shaped ulcers measuring more than 1 cm in diameter.

Behçet's syndrome consists of an association of the oral aphthae with recurrent ulcers on the external genitals and with uveitis, forming the so-called triple syndrome. However, the uveitis is frequently absent. Instead, there may be additional manifestations.

Among the cutaneous manifestations occasionally seen in Behçet's syndrome are numerous small pustules, painful nodose lesions on the legs resembling erythema nodosum, and recurrent attacks of thrombophlebitis of the superficial veins of the legs, often manifesting itself as superficial migratory thrombophlebitis (see p. 228) (Forman; Schneider). Systemic manifestations include pneumonitis, gastrointestinal ulcerations, and recurrent attacks of central nervous system lesions, including meningoencephalitis, cranial nerve palsies, and cerebellar and spinal cord lesions (Sigel and Larson). In patients with central nervous system lesions the prognosis is guarded, with a mortality exceeding 30 per cent (Pallis and Fudge).

Histopathology. The aphthae show as earliest lesion an invasion of the oral epithelium by lymphocytes and monocytes (Lehner, 1969). After the destruction of the epithelium a nonspecific ulcer ensues showing necrotic material and neutrophils near its surface and lymphoctes and monocytes farther down (Lehner, 1969). Although in some aphthae vascular changes, such as obliterating endarteritis, have been described (Curth; O'Duffy et al.), vascular involvement has been found to be mild or absent in most cases (Ship et al.; Lehner, 1969). Even in the same patient severe vasculitis can be present in some lesions and absent in others (Nethercott and Lester). Also, evidence of vasculitis has been observed in late lesions in contrast with early lesions (Civatte and Belaich). The same variability that exists in regard to the presence of vascular lesions in the aphthae is encountered also in the description of the central nervous system lesions. Whereas some authors found no vascular disease in the central nervous system of patients who had died of neurologic complications (Pallis and Fudge), other authors have stressed the presence at autopsy of perivascular infiltration and thrombosis of small vessels (Schottland et al.).

Histogenesis. An attempt has been made by some authors to prove that in patients with simple aphthae or with aphthae of Behçet's disease the aphthae form on the basis of an autoimmune response. Thus, Lehner (1967) found that fetal oral mucosa stimulated in vitro the transformation of lymphocytes obtained from such patients; and that cell-bound antibodies, as measured by the lymphocyte transformation test, were present in increased amounts during exacerbations, and were absent or decreased during remissions (Lehner, 1968). It further has been demonstrated that the peripheral lymphocytes of patients with aphthosis exert a cytotoxic effect in vitro on normal oral epithelial cells, reducing their survival time to a much greater degree than the lymphocytes of patients with other types of oral lesions (Rogers et al.). Saito et al. have expressed agreement with the concept that delayed hypersensitivity plays a role in the formation of aphthae, since they observed by electron microscopy that in the very early stage the epithelium overlying aphthae was being invaded by macrophages, exactly as in contact dermatitis. In contrast to this view, O'Duffy et al., who have expressed the view that aphthae form as a result of a vasculitis, have stated that the presence of cellular antibodies could be a secondary event and their presence thus did not necessarily prove the existence of an autoimmune process.

ACUTE SEPTICEMIA

Three types of acute fulminating septicemia have cutaneous manifestations that are diagnostically significant. They comprise those caused by meningococci, staphylococci, and pseudomonas.

ACUTE MENINGOCOCCEMIA

In fulminating septicemic infections with *Neisseria meningitidis,* extensive purpura is seen. Death may occur within 12 to 24 hours. On autopsy, extensive hemorrhage is found in many internal organs, especially the lungs, brain, kidneys and adrenals. In the past, vascular collapse and death had been attributed to massive bilateral hemorrhage into the adrenal glands and was known as the Waterhouse-Friderichsen syndrome. However, it has been known for some time that this syndrome could occur in the absence of significant damage to the adrenals (Ferguson and Chapman). It is now recognized that the generalized hemorrhagic diathesis is caused by the consumptive depletion of plasma clotting factors and the resulting disseminated intravascular coagulation (Winkelstein et al.). The disseminated intravascular coagulation, in addition to causing widespread hemorrhage, also interferes with the microcirculation and function of vital organs and thus leads to death. Disseminated intravascular coagulation, which occurs not only in acute septicemias but also in thrombotic thrombocytopenic purpura (see p. 159) and purpura fulminans (see p. 160), is often amenable to therapy with anticoagulants such as heparin. The existence of disseminated intravascular coagulation is easily established by a number of coagulation tests, such as platelet count, prothrombin time, and activated partial thromboplastin time.

Other septicemias that occasionally may cause rapid death through disseminated intravascular coagulation are those caused by hemolytic streptococci and *Diplococcus pneumoniae.*

Histopathology. The cutaneous petechiae and ecchymoses in acute meningococcemia show in many of the dermal vessels thrombi composed of fibrin and platelets. The walls of such vessels generally show considerable damage, even necrosis (Hill and Kinney). Large and small areas of hemorrhage are present in the tissue.

In addition, a severe vasculitis is found in the dermis, with presence of many neutrophils, as well as nuclear dust. It is likely that the endotoxin of meningococci causes the vasculitis as a Shwartzman phenomenon (Shapiro et al.). Many meningococci can be demonstrated in and around vessels as gram-negative diplococci located not only in the cytoplasm of endothelial cells and neutrophils but also extracellularly (Hill and Kinney; Shapiro et al.).

ACUTE STAPHYLOCOCCAL SEPTICEMIA

Acute staphylococcal septicemia resembles acute meningococcemia in the appearance of the skin lesions, except that the purpuric lesions often are associated with pustules. Puncture of the pustules and staining of smears with Gram's stain reveal the presence of gram-positive cocci (Plaut). The purpura in acute staphylococcal septicemia, like that of acute meningococcemia,

is caused largely by disseminated intravascular coagulation but also by vasculitis.

PSEUDOMONAS SEPTICEMIA

The classical and diagnostic cutaneous lesion of *Pseudomonas aeruginosa* septicemia is referred to as *ecthyma gangrenosum.* Pseudomonas septicemia usually occurs in debilitated, moribund, leukemic or severely burned patients, particularly after they have received treatment with multiple antibiotics. The cutaneous lesions may be single but usually are multiple. They consist of punched-out ulcers, about 1 cm in diameter, that may be preceded by purulent or hemorrhagic bullae (Hall et al.). In Tzanck-smears prepared from the base of the lesions gram-negative rods can be identified, confirming the diagnosis. Because of the rapid fatality of pseudomonas septicemia early institution of intravenous treatment with gentamicin sulfate is indicated.

Histopathology. Pseudomonas bacilli invade the walls first of deep subcutaneous veins and later of superficial vessels at sites where ulcers form. The superficial vessels become thrombosed as their walls undergo necrosis. Inflammatory cells are absent (Dorff et al.).

CHRONIC SEPTICEMIA

Meningococcemia and gonococcemia can occur as a chronic intermittent, benign eruption.

CHRONIC MENINGOCOCCEMIA

In individuals with partial immunity to *Neisseria meningitidis,* an infection with this organism produces chronic meningococcemia. This is characterized by recurrent attacks of fever, each lasting about 12 hours, associated with migratory joint pains and a papular and petechial eruption. Positive blood cultures are obtained during the febrile attacks.

Histopathology. The cutaneous lesions of chronic meningococcemia, in contrast to those of acute meningococcemia, show no bacteria and no vascular thrombosis or necrosis. Instead, one observes a perivascular infiltrate composed largely of lymphoid cells and only a few neutrophils (Ognibene and Ditto; Nielsen). In petechial areas one may find, in addition to a limited area of perivascular hemorrhage, a fairly high percentage of neutrophils and also fibrinoid material in the walls of the vessels so that the histologic picture resembles that of an allergic vasculitis (Nielsen). Meningococci cannot be demonstrated, not even through direct immunofluorescent testing (Ognibene and Ditto).

CHRONIC GONOCOCCEMIA

As in chronic meningococcemia, patients with chronic gonococcemia have intermittent attacks of fever and polyarthralgia. Also, the cutaneous lesions are similar, except that the lesions have predominantly an acral distribution and, in addition to papules and petechiae, there often are vesicopustules with a hemorrhagic halo and rarely hemorrhagic bullae. Blood cultures are positive for *Neisseria gonorrhoeae* only during attacks of fever.

Histopathology. The capillaries in the upper dermis and middermis are surrounded by an infiltrate of neutrophils, a variable admixture of mononuclear cells, and red cells. There often is nuclear dust, as in allergic vasculitis. Fibrinoid material may be seen in the walls of some vessels and fibrin thrombi in some lumina (Shapiro et al.). Pustular lesions show a predominance of neutrophils within both the pustule and the dermis (Björnberg). Bullae are subepidermal in location (Ackerman).

Bacteria almost never can be found by staining methods in tissue sections, and even cultures are only rarely positive for *N. gonorrhoeae* (Holmes et al.). However, after application, either to fresh or to deparaffinized sections, of fluorescein isothiocyanate-labeled rabbit antigonococcus globulin that has been mixed with lissamine rhodamine B-labeled normal rabbit globulin, gonococci can be seen by fluorescence microscopy to be located around capillaries, proving that the skin lesions are caused by gonococci. The reason why the fluorescent antibody technic is successful in demonstrating gonococci lies

in the fact that it is not dependent on living organisms, as are bacterial staining methods (Kahn and Danielsson).

TUBERCULOSIS

When a normal, not previously infected guinea pig is inoculated intradermally with an adequate dose of *Mycobacterium tuberculosis,* a hard nodule develops at the site of the inoculation after 8 to 12 days. The nodule soon ulcerates. The regional lymph nodes become enlarged and ultimately may drain pus. This represents the primary or Ghon complex. Histologic examination of the primary ulcer 10 to 14 days after inoculation reveals an acute inflammatory infiltrate with many neutrophils and many tubercle bacilli. Areas of tissue necrosis are present. During the third and fourth week after inoculation the histologic picture gradually changes. First mononuclear cells and then epithelioid cells appear and replace the neutrophils. During the fourth week after inoculation distinct tubercles or tuberculoid structures appear both at the site of the inoculation and in the regional lymph nodes. Simultaneously with the formation of tuberculoid structures the number of tubercle bacilli decreases rapidly (Sulzberger).

A typical tubercle consists of an accumulation of epithelioid cells surrounded by a wall of mononuclear cells. Usually, a few giant cells are present among the epithelioid cells. The epithelioid cells in the center of the tubercle may show various degrees of necrosis. If such typical tubercles are present, one speaks of a tuberculous infiltrate. In tuberculosis, however, one frequently does not find typical tubercles but only irregular accumulations of epithelioid cells within an inflammatory infiltrate, with or without necrosis and with or without giant cells. In that case one speaks of a tuberculoid infiltrate.

The presence of a tuberculous or a tuberculoid infiltrate does not necessarily mean tuberculosis. Such infiltrate may be seen in various other conditions: (1) It can be produced by several other infectious diseases, especially syphilis, leprosy and several deep fungus infections. The Jadassohn-Lewandowsky law states that wherever microorganisms are being subdued by immunologic reactions, tubercles or tuberculoid structures have a tendency to appear (Sulzberger). (2) It can occur in instances of hypersensitivity to foreign substances, such as zirconium, beryllium, and certain dyes used in tattoos (see p. 204). (3) Some foreign-body reactions not associated with hypersensitivity show a tuberculoid structure, for instance, silk or nylon sutures, paraffin, silica, surgical glove starch powder, and human hair (see p. 203). Disintegrating hair structures are held responsible also for the presence of tubercles or tuberculoid structures in the papular type of acne rosacea, formerly referred to erroneously as lupus miliaris disseminatus faciei and rosacealike tuberculoid (see p. 182).

The establishment of a diagnosis of tuberculosis requires proof of the presence of tubercle bacilli. Their demonstration in the histologic sections of some forms of cutaneous tuberculosis, particularly in lupus vulgaris, very rarely is possible with acid-fast staining; and, even though fluorescent staining for mycobacteria with auramine or rhodamine is superior to acid-fast staining (Wilner et al.), it is apt to give negative results in lupus vulgaris (Steigleder). Both guinea pig inoculation and bacterial cultures should be carried out. Cultures on special media will grow within 3 to 4 weeks, whereas guinea pig inoculations require from 6 to 7 weeks for a positive result (Slany). Cultures are required also for isolating the atypical mycobacteria some of which cause lesions that both clinically and histologically resemble those caused by *Mycobacterium tuberculosis* (Weed and Macy) (see p. 283).

Tuberculosis of the skin may be divided into primary and reinfection tuberculosis. The diagnosis of the various types of cutaneous tuberculosis is dependent on a correlation of a number of factors, such as the presence or absence of bacteria in the histologic sections, the amount of necrosis, the amount of inflammatory infiltrate, the depth of the tuberculous or tuberculoid infiltrate, and the type of epidermal response.

Areas of necrosis, on histologic examination, show a loss of their cellular outline. One observes eosinophilic granular material in which, unless the necrosis is advanced, some nuclei still are present. However, most of the nuclei show pyknosis (shrinkage) or karyorrhexis (fragmentation). The amount of necrosis, often referred to as caseation necrosis, usually is proportional to the number of bacteria present (see under Histogenesis).

Histogenesis. Prior to the results obtained by histochemical studies, the mononuclear cells present at the periphery of epithelioid cell granulomas, as seen in tuberculosis and sarcoidosis, had been thought to be lymphocytes. It has since become generally recognized that the high content of lysosomal enzymes in most of these cells clearly establishes them as monocytes. As such they are derived from the bone marrow and are carried to the sites of the granulomas through the blood stream (see p. 54). Within the granulomas, the monocytes develop into macrophages. Macrophages, in turn, give rise to both epithelioid cells and giant cells.

Electron microscopic studies have shown that tubercle bacilli are phagocytized by macrophages through the formation of membrane-lined phagosomes. Through interaction with primary lysosomes containing hydrolytic enzymes, such as acid phosphatase, the phagosomes develop into digestive vacuoles or secondary lysosomes (Dumont and Sheldon). Whether the disease progresses or is contained depends on whether the macrophages, before disintegrating, are able to kill all or nearly all tubercle bacilli within them, or whether they disintegrate first and thus release many viable bacilli. In the latter case, however, the bacilli are phagocytized by a new series of macrophages. With each new series of macrophages their bactericidal ability may increase (Shima et al.). Disintegrating macrophages form areas of necrosis ("caseation"). On the other hand, macrophages capable of digesting the bacilli within them, in the process of digesting them assume the appearance of epithelioid cells. In addition, since in many infections more macrophages enter the area than are needed to engulf the organisms present, macrophages that never have ingested bacilli can develop into epithelioid cells (Papadimitriou and Spector).

Multinucleated giant cells usually form by fusion of nonproliferating, i.e., tritiated-thymidine negative, macrophages or epithelioid cells. As macrophages mature into epithelioid cells and lose their ability to divide they show a greater tendency to fuse into multinucleated giant cells (Carter and Roberts).

Delayed Hypersensitivity. Infection with tubercle bacilli in previously noninfected individuals results in a delayed hypersensitivity reaction that is elicited by proteins present in the bacilli. In nonsensitized individuals an infection with tubercle bacilli at first attracts neutrophils, but as soon as thymus-derived lymphocytes have become specifically sensitized to *M. tuberculosis* they will by means of their lymphokines attract monocytes and stimulate them to develop into macrophages. Macrophages are much more capable of digesting and destroying tubercle bacilli than are neutrophils. The antibodies in sensitized individuals are carried by T-lymphocytes, as is typical of delayed hypersensitivity reactions, and are not freely circulating in the blood serum as are the immunoglobulins.

When, for the purpose of testing, the antigen is applied to the skin as PPD tuberculin, in which tuberculoproteins are present as "purified protein derivative," it causes in sensitized individuals at first an influx of relatively few antibody-carrying lymphocytes, resulting in an antigen-antibody reaction. This reaction leads not only to tissue destruction but also, through the lymphokines of the specifically sensitized T-lymphocytes, to the accumulation of monocytes which, by developing into macrophages, remove the local damage produced by the antigen-antibody reaction. The predominantly perivascular accumulation of monocytes produces the positive tuberculin reaction within 24 to 48 hours after its injection. Thus, the response to tuberculin is similar to the response to patch tests observed in contact dermatitis, which also is a delayed hypersensitivity reaction (see p. 100).

PRIMARY TUBERCULOSIS

Primary infection with tuberculosis occurs only very rarely on the skin. In the great majority of cases it presents itself in the lung as the so-called Ghon complex or primary complex. This consists of a small necrotic lesion at the periphery of one lung associated with a necrotic lesion in the hilar lymph nodes. The Ghon complex in the lung does not become chronic. It either heals or extends rapidly. Extension may be limited to the lungs or may be generalized through hematogenous dissemination. In the latter case miliary tuberculosis develops.

Tuberculous Chancre

Primary infection of the skin with tuberculosis has always been a rare event. In the past, when tuberculosis was common, it was reported mainly in children (O'Leary and Harrison); whereas nowadays it is reported mainly in adults, for instance as the result of mouth-to-mouth artificial respiration (Heil-man and Muschenheim), of inoculation during an autopsy (Minkowitz et al.), or of sexual contact (de Bast et al.). Usually, the cutaneous lesion consists of an asymptomatic crust-covered ulcer, referred to as tuberculous chancre. The regional lymph nodes are enlarged, and may suppurate and produce draining sinuses.

Histopathology. The histologic development of the lesion is very much like that observed in experimental cutaneous inoculation of the guinea pig (see p. 276) (O'Leary and Harrison). During the early stage of the disease the histologic picture is that of an acute neutrophilic reaction with areas of necrosis resulting in ulceration. Numerous tubercle bacilli are present, particularly in the areas of necrosis. After 2 weeks monocytes and macrophages predominate, but necrosis within the infiltrate remains a prominent feature. Three to 6 weeks after onset, epithelioid cells and giant cells begin to appear. As the proportion of epithelioid cells and giant cells gradually increases, the number of tubercle bacilli decreases until their number is so greatly reduced that it may be impossible to demonstrate them in histologic sections, and the only proof of their presence is through animal inoculations and positive cultures. Simultaneous with the decrease in the number of tubercle bacilli in the lesion, the tuberculin test with PPD, previously negative, becomes positive (see above under Histogenesis).

Generalized Miliary Tuberculosis of the Skin

The cutaneous lesions consist of papules and pustules, 3 to 5 mm in diameter, on erythematous bases.

Histopathology. The center of the lesions consists of neutrophils, cellular debris and numerous tubercle bacilli. This is surrounded by a zone of macrophages (Schermer et al.).

REINFECTION TUBERCULOSIS

The immunity acquired by the primary infection almost always protects, at least for several years. After such a latent period reinfection may occur. Reinfection tuberculosis often is limited to one organ, so that, in cases in which the skin is affected, no active tuberculosis may be found elsewhere.

FIG. 16-2. **Lupus vulgaris.** Low magnification. There are several tubercles. The large tubercle in the center shows slight caseation necrosis. (×100)

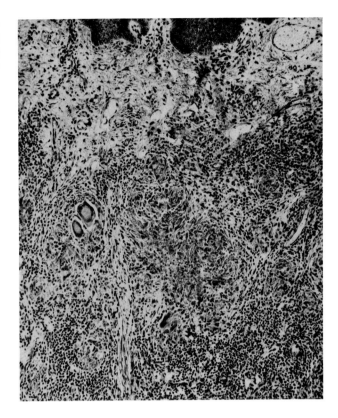

Nevertheless, from 10 to 20 per cent of the patients with lupus vulgaris have either pulmonary tuberculosis or tuberculosis of the bones or joints (Horwitz).

In reinfection tuberculosis one may find, depending on the degree of resistance of the patient, a slight amount of necrosis, as in lupus vulgaris, a moderate amount of necrosis, as in tuberculosis verrucosa cutis, or a considerable amount of necrosis, as in scrofuloderma and tuberculosis cutis orificialis. The regional lymph nodes are not involved.

Lupus Vulgaris

In lupus vulgaris the lesions are found most commonly on the face. They consist of well demarcated reddish-brown patches containing deep-seated nodules, each about 1 mm in size. If the blood is pressed out of the skin with a glass slide (diascopy), these nodules stand out clearly as yellowish-brown macules. Because of their yellowish-brown color the nodules are referred to as apple-jelly nodules. In the course of time the affected areas become atrophic, with contrac-

tion of the tissue. It is a characteristic feature of lupus vulgaris that new lesions may appear in areas of atrophy. Superficial ulceration or verrucous thickening of the skin occurs occasionally. Squamous cell carcinoma develops at the margin of ulcers in rare instances.

Histopathology. Tubercles or tuberculoid structures composed of epithelioid cells and giant cells are present. Caseation necrosis within the tubercles is slight and may be absent (Fig. 16-2). Although usually the giant cells are of the Langhans type with peripheral arrangement of the nuclei, some can be of the foreign-body type, with irregular arrangement of the nuclei (Fig. 16-3). In addition, there is an infiltrate of mononuclear cells. In the vicinity of the tubercles or tuberculoid structures the mononuclear cells, on staining for lysosomal enzymes, show positive staining, indicating that they are monocytes, whereas farther away they do not stain and thus can be interpreted as lymphocytes (Shima et al.) (see also under Histogenesis, p. 277).

The extent and density of the mononuclear infiltrate are variable. In some instances, especially in cases showing ulceration, the inflammatory infiltrate dominates the histologic picture, so that one has to search for occasional tuberculoid structures; in other cases the inflammatory infiltrate is slight.

Both the tubercles or tuberculoid structures and the mononuclear infiltrate usually are most pronounced in the upper dermis, but in some areas they may extend into the subcutaneous layer. They cause destruction of the cutaneous appendages. In areas of healing, extensive fibrosis may be present.

Secondary changes in the epidermis are common. The epidermis may undergo atrophy and subsequently destruction causing ulceration; or it may become hyperplastic, showing acanthosis, hyperkeratosis, and papillomatosis. At the margin of ulcers, pseudocarcinomatous hyperplasia and in rare instances squamous cell carcinoma may be found.

Tubercle bacilli are present in such small numbers that their presence very rarely can be demonstrated by staining methods. Even cultures and guinea pig inoculations are not always successful. Thus, among 31 cases of lupus vulgaris, van der Lugt had 7 in whom both cultures and guinea pig inoculations gave negative results.

Differential Diagnosis. For differentiation from sarcoidosis, see page 213; for differentiation from atypical mycobacterial diseases, see page 283.

Tuberculosis Verrucosa Cutis

Tuberculosis verrucosa cutis and its variant verruca necrogenica represent virulent infections of the skin in patients with a rather high degree of immunity. In tuberculosis verrucosa cutis one observes usually a single lesion presenting as a verrucous plaque with inflammatory border, showing gradual peripheral extension. The verrucous surface shows fissures from which pus often can be expressed. Verruca necrogenica differs from tuberculosis verrucosa cutis only in the mode by which it is contracted, namely from handling cadavers, and by its small size.

Histopathology. The histologic picture

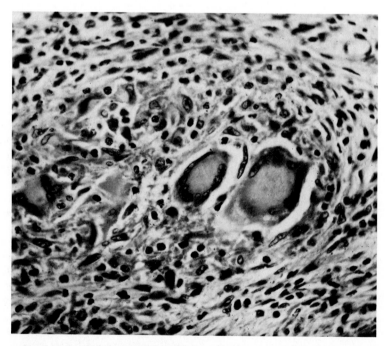

FIG. 16-3. **Lupus vulgaris.** High magnification of Figure 16-2. A tubercle contains several giant cells of the Langhans type with peripheral arrangement of the nuclei. (×400)

shows hyperkeratosis, papillomatosis and acanthosis. Beneath the epidermis one observes an acute inflammatory infiltrate. Abscess formation may be seen in the upper dermis or within downward extensions of the epidermis. In the middermis tuberculoid structures with a moderate amount of necrosis are usually present. Tubercle bacilli are more numerous than in lupus vulgaris and occasionally can be demonstrated histologically (Montgomery).

Scrofuloderma

Scrofuloderma, also called tuberculosis colliquativa cutis, represents a direct extension to the skin of an underlying tuberculous infection present most commonly in a lymph node or a bone. The lesion first manifests itself as a bluish-red painless swelling that breaks open and then forms an ulcer with irregular, undermined bluish borders.

Histopathology. The center of the lesion usually shows nonspecific changes, such as abscess formation or ulceration. In the deeper portions and at the periphery of the lesion, however, one usually sees, if the biopsy specimen is adequate, tuberculoid structures with a considerable amount of necrosis together with a pronounced inflammatory reaction (Fig. 16-4) (Montgomery). Usually, the number of tubercle bacilli is sufficient to enable one to find them in the histologic sections.

Differential Diagnosis. For differentiation from erythema induratum, see page 231; from gummatous syphilis, see page 304.

Tuberculosis Cutis Orificialis

The lesions are shallow ulcers with a granulating base, occurring near the mucosal orifices of patients with advanced internal tuberculosis. Most patients have a low degree of immunity, and some show anergy to *M. tuberculosis,* as found in miliary tuberculosis. The condition is very rare nowadays.

Histopathology. The histologic picture may show merely an ulcer surrounded by a nonspecific inflammatory infiltrate. Yet in most instances tuberculoid formations with pronounced necrosis are found deep in the

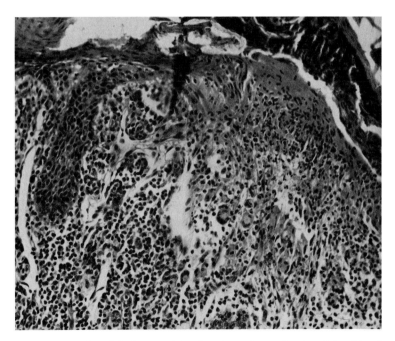

FIG. 16-4. **Scrofuloderma.** Margin of an ulcer. On the right side of the photograph one observes necrosis of epidermis and dermis. In the center are tuberculoid structures. On the left the infiltrate is composed of lymphocytes and plasma cells. (×200)

dermis. Tubercle bacilli are easily demonstrated in the sections even when the histologic appearance is nonspecific.

TUBERCULIDS

The tuberculids, a term first proposed by Darier in 1896, comprise, according to most present-day dermatologic texts, the following four dermatoses: erythema induratum, the papulonecrotic tuberculid, lichen scrofulosorum, and lupus miliaris disseminatus faciei. However, there is no convincing argument in favor of a tuberculous genesis of any of these four diseases (Flegel).

Histogenesis. At present the generally accepted view is that tuberculids are caused by the hematogenous dissemination of tubercle bacilli from a focus, often extrapulmonary in location, into the skin, where they are rapidly destroyed. The fact that in most instances no active focus of tuberculosis can be found has led to two hypotheses. According to one hypothesis the skin is "hyperergic" (Spier and Röckl); and according to the other hypothesis, the skin has a "decreased immunologic resistance" (Miescher). The existence of a "hyperergic" reactivity of the skin in the absence of a clinically active focus of tuberculosis is not in accord with immunologic concepts; these hold that if the skin is in a state of "hyperergic" reaction, the focus from which the dissemination is taking place also should be in a "hyperergic" state and thus should show an acute necrotizing inflammation that would be clinically noticeable (Flegel). The other theory, postulating that a clinically obscure focus could cause the development of tuberculous lesions in the skin because the skin had a "decreased immunologic resistance" against tubercle bacilli, also fails to satisfy immunologic concepts; these hold that a decrease in the resistance of the skin against tubercle bacilli should be accompanied by a decrease of resistance against tubercle bacilli in the primary focus also, resulting in an activation of the tuberculosis in the focus also. It thus becomes evident that the concept of the existence of tuberculids is incompatible with immunologic facts. It is a relic of the times when a tuberculoid histology was tantamount to tuberculosis. If any further evidence were needed to disprove the existence of the tuberculids, the lack of response of the tuberculids to antituberculous therapy may be cited, as has been reported, for instance, by Chantraine and van der Lugt.

Of the four types of so-called tuberculids, lupus miliaris disseminatus faciei and erythema induratum have already been discussed. Lupus miliaris disseminatus faciei (see p. 182) is regarded as a manifestation of the papular type of acne rosacea; and erythema induratum is thought to represent a vasculitis of subcutaneous arteries and veins with subsequent fat necrosis and tuberculoid reaction. The other two types of tuberculids, the papulonecrotic tuberculid and lichen scrofulosorum, do not represent disease entities, since they can be identified with other diseases.

PAPULONECROTIC TUBERCULID. This condition is described clinically as showing indolent papules appearing in crops and undergoing central necrosis. The histologic findings are said to show a small area of necrosis involving the upper dermis and the overlying epidermis. The area of necrosis is surrounded by an infiltrate largely nonspecific in type but usually containing tuberculoid structures at its periphery. Vascular changes are regularly present and consist of the invasion of the walls of vessels by an inflammatory infiltrate and the thickening of these walls.

The extent of the vascular changes makes it very likely that the so-called papulonecrotic tuberculid basically represents a form of vasculitis (Krüger). Cases described as papulonecrotic tuberculid can be classified largely as pityriasis lichenoides et varioliformis of Mucha and Habermann (see p. 163).

LICHEN SCROFULOSORUM. This condition is said to occur mainly in children. The lesions, present chiefly on the trunk, consist of indolent papules, 1 to 2 mm in size. Their color varies from that of normal skin to a pale red. The histologic picture, according to Montgomery, shows epithelioid cell tubercles without caseation. It thus is indistinguishable from sarcoidosis.

On the basis of the clinical and histologic data it can be assumed that most patients described as having lichen scrofulosorum had sarcoidosis with lichenoid or micropapular lesions. Cases of lichenoid or micropapular sarcoidosis having the clinical appearance of lichen scrofulosorum have been described in recent years, for instance, by

Brunner and Robin, by Ockuly and Montgomery, by Thal, and by Kanaar. The only two cases reported in recent years with the diagnosis of lichen scrofulosorum were those described by Schuhmachers. They can be regarded as instances of generalized papular granuloma annulare.

INFECTIONS WITH ATYPICAL MYCOBACTERIA

Among the so-called atypical mycobacterial infections of the skin those caused by *Mycobacterium marinum* are by far the most common. Infections with this organism, formerly also referred to as *M. balnei,* can take place through minor abrasions incurred while bathing in swimming pools (Philpott et al.) or in ocean water (Zeligman; Jolly and Seabury) or while cleaning home aquariums (Adams et al.).

Clinically, most of the lesions caused by *M. marinum* are solitary and consist of indolent, dusky red, hyperkeratotic, papillomatous papules, nodules or plaques. Superficial ulceration is seen occasionally. The fingers, knees, elbows and feet are most commonly affected. In some instances the infection consists of a primary verrucous nodule at the periphery of an extremity and of ascending multiple subcutaneous nodules, as seen in sporotrichosis (Dickey; Adams et al.). The period of incubation usually is 3 weeks. Although spontaneous healing usually takes place within a few months, in some patients the cutaneous infection may persist for years (Zeligman).

In contrast to the infection with *M. marinum,* infections with other atypical mycobacteria are extremely rare. Only one instance of cutaneous infection with group I *M. kansasii* has been reported (Maberry et al.), and only very few with group II scotochromogens (Knox et al.; Cott et al.) and with group IV mycobacteria (Brock et al.). The clinical appearance of infections with these organisms is similar to infections with *M. marinum,* but the infection does not always occur through exposure in water.

Histopathology. Early lesions not more than 2 or 3 months old show a nonspecific inflammatory infiltrate composed of neutrophils, monocytes and macrophages. In lesions about 4 months old a few multinucleated giant cells and a few small epithelioid cell granulomas usually are present; and in lesions 6 months old or older, typical tubercles or tuberculoid structures may be seen (Mansson et al.). Areas of necrosis are only occasionally present in the center of the granulomas. The epidermis often shows papillomatosis and hyperkeratosis, and there may be central ulceration.

Acid-fast organisms usually can be identified in histologic sections of early lesions that show a nonspecific inflammatory infiltrate (Adams et al.). On the other hand, tuberculoid granulomas generally show no acid-fast organisms, unless areas of central necrosis are present (Scholz-Jordan et al.).

In histologic sections the atypical mycobacteria appear slightly larger than *M. tuberculosis* and show transverse striation (Philpott et al.). If acid-fast bacilli cannot be detected in histologic sections, in most instances they still can be identified by culture or by animal inoculation, except in healing lesions.

Histogenesis. All atypical mycobacteria show good growth in culture media at a temperature of 30° C., whereas *M. tuberculosis* requires 37° C. for optimal growth. None of the atypical mycobacteria are pathogenic to guinea pigs as is *M. tuberculosis;* but most of them can multiply in mice; *M. marinum,* however, is pathogenic to mice only if inoculated into their foot pads (Cott et al.).

Differential Diagnosis. The granulomatous reaction produced by the atypical mycobacteria is very similar to that seen in tuberculosis verrucosa cutis or lupus vulgaris so that cultures and animal inoculations are necessary for their differentiation.

BURULI ULCERATION

This infection, caused by an atypical mycobacterium, *M. ulcerans,* is common in some parts of central Africa and consists of a solitary large ulcer in an exposed area of the skin.

Histopathology. At the base of the ulcer one observes extensive areas of necrosis characterized by a "ghost outline" of tissue structure (Connor and Lunn). Acid-fast organisms are found in large quantities in the necrotic tissue without any associated inflammatory reaction.

Histogenesis. It is assumed that the widespread destruction of tissue in the absence of inflammation is caused by a toxic substance elaborated by *M. ulcerans*. Like other atypical mycobacteria, *M. ulcerans* shows optimal cultural growth at 30° C. It is pathogenic to mice when inoculated into their foot pads (Cott et al.).

LEPROSY

Leprosy, caused by *Mycobacterium leprae*, affects predominantly the skin and peripheral nerves. Aside from the initial manifestation of leprosy referred to as the indeterminate form, leprosy can be divided into five clinical forms forming a spectrum. The form of disease arising in the individual patient depends on the degree of his resistance. On the one end of the spectrum is tuberculoid leprosy (TT) with a very high degree of immunity and only one or very few asymmetrically arranged lesions showing but rarely a few bacilli. This is followed by the borderline-tuberculoid form (BT), the true borderline form (BB), the borderline-lepromatous form (BL), and lepromatous leprosy (LL). The number of lesions and the number of bacilli within the lesions increase with diminishing immunity. Thus, lepromatous leprosy shows widespread lesions with very many bacilli. Only tuberculoid leprosy with its very high degree of resistance represents a stable form, all the other forms being unstable. The disease may move spontaneously from BT to BL and ultimately develop into lepromatous leprosy; whereas under treatment with diaminodiphenylsulfone the disease may move in the opposite direction as far as BT (Pettit).

Clinical Appearance. In *indeterminate leprosy,* which may occur in the beginning of the disease, either a single hypochromic or erythematous macule or several such macules are present. Frequently, the lesions are hypoesthetic (Kwittken and Peck). Indeterminate leprosy may heal spontaneously or under treatment, or it may go on to any of the other forms of leprosy (Azulay).

Tuberculoid leprosy often shows only a single cutaneous lesion and at most very few asymmetrically arranged lesions. They are large, well defined macules characterized by hypoesthesia, hypopigmentation, hair loss, and impairment of sweating. The superficial nerves in the vicinity of the lesion may be palpable.

Lepromatous leprosy, representing the completely anergic type, initially has cutaneous and mucosal lesions, with neural changes occurring later. There usually are numerous symmetrically arranged lesions which, although macular at first, develop into nodules and diffuse infiltrates. Involvement of the eyebrows and forehead often results in a leonine facies. The lesions themselves are not hypoesthetic, although through involvement of the large peripheral nerves disturbances of sensation develop, as well as trophic disturbances and nerve paralyses.

Borderline leprosy exhibits clinical features of both tuberculoid and lepromatous leprosy, often with prevalence of either one or the other, so that the patient has either borderline tuberculoid, true borderline, or borderline lepromatous leprosy. Often at the beginning, borderline leprosy resembles tuberculoid leprosy. clinically, but the large macules are symmetrically distributed, more numerous, and less sharply demarcated than in tuberculoid leprosy (Kwittken and Peck).

Reactional leprosy may show one of two types of reaction: erythema nodosum leprosum, and Lucio's phenomenon. Erythema nodosum leprosum is seen most commonly in lepromatous leprosy and rarely in borderline lepromatous leprosy. It occurs during treatment as a reaction against the large number of damaged lepra bacilli. Clinically, the reaction has greater resemblance to erythema multiforme than to erythema nodosum, showing tender, red plaques as well as areas of erythema and occasionally also purpura and vesicles, but only rarely ulceration. The reaction is accompanied by high fever, malaise and arthralgia (Kramarsky et al.).

The Lucio phenomenon occurs in patients with lepromatous leprosy showing diffuse infiltration of the skin. Numerous erythematous, infiltrated, tender plaques appear in crops, ulcerate and heal with atrophic scarring. Fever and malaise are present (Donner and Shively).

Histopathology. INDETERMINATE LEPROSY shows a scattered nonspecific chronic inflam-

FIG. 16-5. **Tuberculoid leprosy.** The infiltrate shows epithelioid cell granulomas showing a slight admixture of monocytes, particularly at their margins. Thus, the histologic picture resembles that of sarcoidosis. (×100)

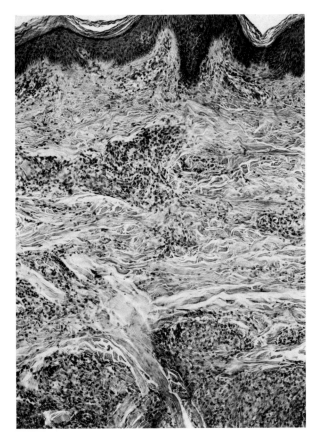

matory infiltrate in the dermis. In the cutaneous nerves occasionally isolated bacilli are found on acid-fast staining (Kwittken and Peck). In cases developing toward lepromatous leprosy, fairly numerous lepra bacilli and occasional foamy macrophages may be present; and in those developing toward tuberculoid leprosy a few epithelioid cell granulomas may be found (Case Records of the Massachusetts General Hospital, Case 21-1970).

TUBERCULOID LEPROSY shows epithelioid cell granulomas that often are indistinguishable from those seen in sarcoidosis (Wiersema and Binford). The presence of a tuberculoid infiltrate and the scarcity or absence of bacilli are, in accord with the Jadassohn-Lewandowsky law (see p. 276), the result of a very good tissue immunity against the lepra bacillus. A mild mononuclear cell infiltrate is present and occasionally giant cells, as in sarcoidosis (Fig. 16-5). Since the epithelioid cell granulomas of tuberculoid leprosy form around dermal nerves that are undergoing necrosis, the granulomas of tuberculoid leprosy, like those of sarcoidosis, often show central necrosis. In contrast with lepromatous leprosy, the infiltrate in tuberculoid leprosy, if present in the upper dermis, does not necessarily remain separated from the epidermis by a free grenz zone but may press against and even invade the epidermis (Fields). Lepra bacilli usually are absent in quiescent lesions; but they may be found in small numbers if the specimen for biopsy is taken from the active margin of an extending lesion (Wiersema and Binford).

Differentiation of tuberculoid leprosy from sarcoidosis can be very difficult (see p. 214). The following features aid in the differentiation: (1) Occasionally in tuberculoid leprosy, if the biopsy specimen has been taken from the active margin of the lesion, bacilli may be found in the necrotic center of some of the granulomas on staining with the Fite

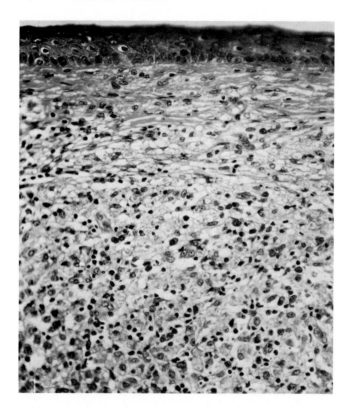

FIG. 16-6. **Lepromatous leprosy.** The infiltrate is separated from the flattened epidermis by a narrow zone of normal collagen. Macrophages with abundant foamy cytoplasm, so-called lepra cells, predominate. (×200)

stain; (2) in sections impregnated with silver, remnants of nerve tissue may be found in the necrotic center of some of the granulomas of tuberculoid leprosy; and (3) since the granulomas of tuberculoid leprosy, in contrast to those of sarcoidosis, follow nerves, they often appear elongated (Wiersema and Binford).

LEPROMATOUS LEPROSY shows, as a rule, an extensive cellular infiltrate that almost invariably is separated from the flattened epidermis by a narrow grenz zone of normal collagen. The infiltrate causes the destruction of the cutaneous appendages. It extends into the subcutaneous fat. Macrophages with abundant foamy or vacuolated cytoplasm, so-called lepra cells or Virchow cells, predominate (Fig. 16-6). They resemble xanthoma cells. On staining with fat stains they are shown to contain lipid, largely neutral fat and phospholipids rather than cholesterol. Because of the absence of cholesterol the lipid is, in contrast with the lipid in xanthomata, not doubly refractile. Using the Fite stain, innumerable acid-fast, red-staining bacilli are seen, measuring about 0.5 by 5 μm in size. They are found particularly within the lepra cells, where they often lie in bundles, like packs of cigars, or, if degenerated, in large clumps called globi (Fig. 16-7). In contrast with tuberculoid leprosy, the nerves in the skin, even though they may show considerable numbers of lepra bacilli, remain well preserved for a long time, and thus there is much less anesthesia in the cutaneous lesions of lepromatous leprosy than in those of tuberculoid leprosy (Wiersema and Binford).

The large peripheral nerves in lepromatous leprosy contain large numbers of lepra bacilli, as many as are seen in the cutaneous infiltrate, with a minimal amount of inflammation. The Schwann sheaths are invaded, resulting in their destruction and subsequent fibrosis. Demyelinization ultimately is followed by axonal degeneration (Job and Desikan).

Autopsy reveals even in clinically quiescent cases bacilli in many organs, especially in the liver and the lymph nodes, including the visceral lymph nodes, as well as in the spleen, the adrenals, and the testes (Desikan). The presence of bacillary depositions in the viscera explains the tendency to relapse.

BORDERLINE LEPROSY shows a wide range of histologic changes, depending on whether a case is one of borderline tuberculoid, true borderline, or borderline lepromatous. Generally, the cutaneous lesions show features of both tuberculoid and lepromatous leprosy so that aggregates of foamy macrophages and of epithelioid cells may occur side by side. Usually, acid-fast bacilli can be found with ease within the macrophages (Kwittken and Peck).

REACTIONAL LEPROSY. In erythema nodosum leprosum, which actually is a misnomer, histologic examination reveals the presence of a neutrophilic vasculitis characterized by swelling of the endothelial cells, fibrinoid deposits within and around the vascular walls and a perivascular infiltrate of neutrophils and macrophages. Many bacilli are present in the macrophages, the vessel walls and the vessel lumina (Kramarsky et al.; Wemambu et al.).

The Lucio phenomenon with its tendency to ulcerations shows a much more severe neutrophilic vasculitis than is seen in erythema nodosum leprosum characterized by degeneration of the endothelial cells, and extensive permeation of even larger vessels with fibrin, neutrophils and eosinophils (Kramarsky et al.). As in erythema nodosum leprosum, acid-fast organisms are present in great numbers even within vascular lumina.

Histogenesis. Concerning their *immunologic reactivity,* patients with lepromatous leprosy, in contrast with those having tuberculoid or borderline leprosy, are deficient in their cell-mediated immunologic reactions. On the other hand, their humoral antibody production is unimpaired (Turk and Waters). Thus, their lymph nodes contain numerous plasma cells, and their serum levels for IgG and IgA are elevated (Sheagren et al.). As evidence of their deficient cell-mediated immunologic reactivity patients with lepromatous leprosy are anergic to intradermal testing with lepromin, tuberculin and other allergens which elicit delayed-type skin responses (Bullock). Furthermore, dinitrochlorobenzene sensitizes only 50 per cent of patients with leproma-

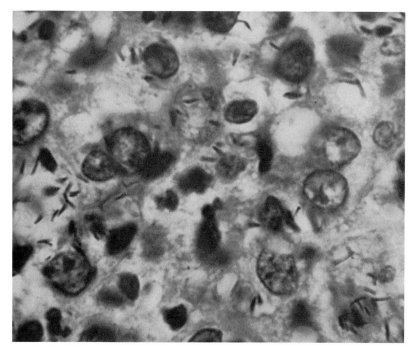

FIG. 16-7. **Lepromatous leprosy.** Fite stain. Numerous acid-fast lepra bacilli are present. They are found particularly within the lepra cells, where they tend to lie in bundles. (×800)

tous leprosy, whereas 95 per cent of a normal population will become sensitized (Waldorf et al.). Also, in vitro transformation of lymphocytes into lymphoblasts after stimulation with phytohemagglutinin usually does not occur; and after stimulation with lepromin the lymphocytes of patients with lepromatous leprosy produce little or no macrophage migration inhibiting factor (MIF) (Katz et al.).

The *lepromin skin test,* consisting of the intradermal injection of a preparation containing killed lepra bacilli, serves as a measure of tissue resistance against leprosy. It is regarded as positive if after 3 weeks a papule, 5 mm or more in diameter, has formed at the site of injection. The test is always negative in lepromatous leprosy, and usually is also negative in borderline leprosy. It is always positive in tuberculoid leprosy, while in indeterminate leprosy it may be positive or negative (Moschella).

Mycobacterium leprae so far has not been grown on any culture media. However, like *M. marinum, M. leprae* can multiply if injected into the footpads of mice (Shepard). Abundant growth with formation of granulomas will take place when *M. leprae* is inoculated into thymectomized and irradiated mice (Rees et al.). However, the armadillo has recently been found to be by nature much more susceptible to *M. leprae* than the mouse, since lepromatous leprosy develops in one third of the animals after the intravenous or intradermal inoculation of *M. leprae* (Kirchheimer and Storrs). On electron microscopy, each mycobacterium shows the electron-dense cytoplasm to be lined by a trilaminal plasma membrane. Outside of this one finds the bacterial cell wall surrounded by a radiolucent area, the waxy coating typical of mycobacteria (Kramarsky et al.).

Bacterial Phagocytosis. Lepra bacilli are found in the skin, particularly in macrophages and Schwann cells. In *tuberculoid leprosy,* the Schwann cells of the cutaneous nerves contain the lepra bacilli including their waxy coat. During the cell-mediated immune response against *M. leprae,* macrophages digest both the bacilli and the Schwann cells that contain them. After the digestion, only macrophages with the appearance of epithelioid cells remain. The epithelioid cells in tuberculoid leprosy are free of mycobacteria and contain no lipid. On electron microscopy, the epithelioid cells show a strongly positive reaction for acid phosphatase within numerous, well preserved primary lysosomes (Job).

In *lepromatous leprosy,* on the other hand, it is evident that the macrophages are incapable of digesting the lepra bacilli adequately. Light microscopy shows that although the macrophages at first cause some damage to the bacilli, nevertheless, the bacilli multiply to such an extent that they are present as globi in huge numbers. Electron microscopic examination reveals that initially the bacilli are engulfed by phagocytic vacuoles into which primary lysosomes discharge their contents, causing partial lysis of the mycobacteria (Kramarsky et al.). However, the multiplication of the mycobacteria is so rapid that the phagocytic vacuoles suffer damage as they become filled with lipid derived from the waxy coat of the mycobacteria (Imaeda). Thus, the foamy appearance of the macrophages evident by light microscopy is revealed by elecron microscopy to be due to the presence of greatly enlarged, lipid-laden phagocytic vacuoles (Job). These lipid-laden vacuoles no longer are accessible to lysosomal enzymes which are found in considerable concentration in the cytoplasm of the macrophages but outside of the phagocytic vacuoles (Job).

In *borderline leprosy* bacterial growth activity and the cellular response are balanced so that the mycobacteria do not multiply uninhibitedly, as they do in lepromatous leprosy. On electron microscopy, many cells are intermediate between macrophages and epithelioid cells and the phagolysosomes within them contain rather well preserved mycobacteria and no free lipid material (Imaeda).

The two variants of *reactional leprosy* can be explained by the rapid death of many mycobacteria and a resulting reaction between mycobacterial antigen and circulating antibody occurring in association with the fixation of complement (Turk and Waters). Analogous to the Arthus phenomenon, the two types of leprosy reactions are due to the deposition of immune complexes. On fluorescence microscopy granular deposits of immunoglobulins and complement are seen around blood vessels in areas of neutrophilic infiltration (Wemambu et al.).

Differential Diagnosis. The resemblance, and the consequent need to differentiate between lepromatous leprosy and xanthoma, and between tuberculoid leprosy and sarcoidosis require re-emphasis, even though the differences have already been stressed in the histologic description.

ANTHRAX

Anthrax, caused by *Bacillus anthracis,* is enzootic in many countries. In the United States, anthrax occurs occasionally among workers in tanneries and wool-scouring mills through the handling of infected hides, wool, or hair imported from Asia (Matz and Brugsch). The lesion starts as a papule, enlarges, ulcerates, and then becomes covered with a black eschar. Marked erythema and edema surround the lesion. Characteristically, pain is slight or absent. Often there is regional lymphadenopathy with slight tenderness.

Histopathology. At the site of the ulcer the epidermis is destroyed and the ulcerated surface is covered with necrotic tissue. There is marked edema of the dermis. Numerous erythrocytes and neutrophils are present throughout the dermis and the subcutaneous tissue. The blood vessels are dilated, and their walls show diffuse degenerative changes.

Anthrax bacilli are present in large numbers and can be recognized in sections stained with routine stains, but they are visualized best in sections stained with Gram's stain. The anthrax bacillus is a large rod-shaped, square-ended, gram-positive bacillus, 6 to 10 μm long and 1 to 2 μm thick. In the tissue it is usually surrounded by a well defined capsule. Anthrax bacilli are found particularly in the necrotic tissue at the surface of the ulcer; but the dermis also contains numerous bacilli, whereas the subcutaneous tissue usually contains only a few. It is worth noting that phagocytosis of the bacilli by either neutrophils or histiocytes is absent (Lebowich et al.).

TULAREMIA

Tularemia, an infectious disease caused by *Francisella tularensis,* can be acquired by man through direct contact with rodents, or it can be transmitted from rodents to man by biting insects, such as mosquitoes, deerflies (Klock et al.), or ticks (Young et al.). It occurs in four types: (1) ulceroglandular, the most common type, (2) oculoglandular, (3) pulmonary, and (4) typhoidal. Specific cutaneous lesions occur only in the ulceroglandular type.

In the ulceroglandular type, one or several ulcers occur as primary lesions at the site of infection, usually on the hands. Tender subcutaneous nodes may form along the lymph vessels draining the primary lesion or lesions. Nodes may also occur at the site of the regional lymph nodes.

Histopathology. The primary ulcer shows at its base a nonspecific inflammatory infiltrate containing several granulomas with central necrosis so that each granuloma shows three zones: (1) a central zone of necrosis, consisting of finely granular eosinophilic material, nuclear fragments, and a few erythrocytes; (2) an intermediate zone composed of epithelioid cells with a few multinucleated giant cells and lymphoid cells; and (3) an outer zone consisting largely of lymphoid cells but containing also some histiocytes, plasma cells, and extravasated erythrocytes (Schuermann and Reich). Older lesions may show epithelioid cell tubercles that have no central necrosis and are surrounded by only a slight inflammatory reaction and thus may have an appearance resembling that of sarcoidosis.

The tender nodes along lymph vessels show in the subcutaneous tissue a histologic picture similar to that seen in the primary ulcer of tularemia, namely, multiple granulomas in which three zones can be recognized (Lawless). The central zones of necrosis in the granulomas may attain much greater size than in the primary ulcer (Reich).

F. tularensis, although present, does not stain in tissue sections. It can be demonstrated, however, in the exudate from cutaneous lesions or in tissue sections by the direct fluorescent-antibody technic with fluorescein-conjugated antiserum (Young et al.).

Differential Diagnosis. The histologic picture differs clearly from that of tuberculosis whenever the arrangement in three zones is present. Differentiation from sporotrichosis (see p. 325) and lymphogranuloma venereum (see p. 356), however, may be impossible.

CHANCROID

Chancroid, or "soft chancre," caused by *Hemophilus ducreyi,* is a venereal disease causing one or several ulcers, chiefly in the genital region. The ulcers possess little if any induration and often have an undermined border. Regional lymphadenitis is common and, unless treated, often results in an inguinal abscess, called bubo.

Histopathology. The histologic changes observed beneath the ulcer are sufficiently distinct to permit a diagnosis of chancroid in many instances (Heyman et al.). The lesion consists of three vertically arranged zones (Sheldon and Heyman) and shows characteristic vascular changes (Pund et al.). The surface zone at the floor of the ulcer is rather narrow and consists of neutrophils, fibrin, erythrocytes, and necrotic tissue. The next zone is fairly wide and contains many newly formed blood vessels showing marked proliferation of their endothelial cells (Sheldon and Heyman). As the result of the endothelial proliferation within the vessels, their lumina are often occluded, resulting in thrombosis. In addition, there are degenerative changes in the walls of the vessels. The deep zone is composed of a dense infiltrate of plasma cells and lymphoid cells.

Demonstration of Ducrey bacilli in tissue sections by staining with Giemsa's stain, Gram's stain or polychrome methylene blue is only rarely possible. They are most apt to be found between the cells of the surface zone (Sheldon and Heyman). In smears, Ducrey bacilli usually can be fairly easily seen as gram-negative rods, 1 to 2 μm long and 0.5 μm wide, arranged in pairs or short chains (Borchardt and Hoke).

GRANULOMA INGUINALE

Granuloma inguinale, also called donovanosis, is a venereal disease caused by *Calymmatobacterium granulomatis,* which is found in the lesions as intracytoplasmic inclusion bodies, called Donovan bodies. *Calymmatobacterium granulomatis* is a gram-negative bacterium that grows only in a medium containing yolk of fertilized chicken eggs (Goldberg et al.).

Granuloma inguinale occurs in the genital or perianal region either as a single lesion or as several lesions. The lesions consist of ulcers filled with exuberant granulation tissue that bleeds easily. The border is elevated and often has a serpiginous outline. Due to the fact that the lesions spread by peripheral extension they may attain a large size. Years later the lesions heal with a thick, fibrous contracted scar. In occasional instances squamous cell carcinoma supervenes (Beerman and Sonck; Davis).

Histopathology. The epidermis is absent in the center of the lesion, while at the border it shows acanthosis, which may reach the proportions of pseudocarcinomatous hyperplasia (Beerman and Sonck). A dense infiltrate is present in the dermis composed predominantly of histiocytes and plasma cells.

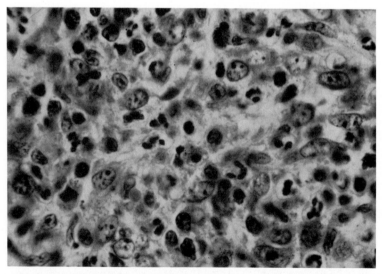

FIG. 16-8. **Granuloma inguinale.** The dense infiltrate is composed predominantly of histiocytes and plasma cells. There is a diffuse sprinkling of neutrophils. Several of the histiocytes contain within their cytoplasm aggregates of Donovan bodies. (×400)

Scattered throughout this infiltrate one finds small abscesses composed of neutrophils. The number of lymphoid cells is conspicuously small.

Intracytoplasmic inclusion bodies, the Donovan bodies, are present within a variable number of histiocytes. The parasitized histiocytes, or macrophages, possess abundant cytoplasm and may measure 20 μm or more in diameter. Their cytoplasm has a multicystic appearance. Within the cystic compartments of the cytoplasm one sees groups of small, ovoid bodies measuring 1 to 2 μm in diameter (Fig. 16-8). In the cross sections of large histiocytes several dozen such bodies may be observed.

The Donovan bodies are difficult to recognize in sections stained with hematoxylin and eosin. In sections stained with Giemsa's stain they may be seen as bipolar, encapsulated bodies. They are better visualized when a silver stain is used. The Donovan bodies then appear black and have the shape of a closed safety pin because of their elongated ovoid contour and intense bipolar staining reaction (Torpin et al.). The capsule surrounding the Donovan bodies does not show up in silver stains. By far the best method for visualizing the Donovan bodies in tissue sections is to cut sections one-half

micron thick from blocks processed for electron microscopy and to stain these sections with toluidine blue. The Donovan bodies then appear as dark, ovoid structures located within vacuolar compartments of macrophages. The number of Donovan bodies within each vacuole varies greatly, from 1 to 20 (Dodson et al.). Each Donovan body is surrounded by a wide, clear or finely granular capsule (Davis).

Since the diagnosis of granuloma inguinale rests on the demonstration of the Donovan bodies, it may be pointed out that often it is easier to find them in smears made from crushed, fresh biopsy material and stained with Wright-Giemsa stain than in routinely fixed tissue sections.

Histogenesis. Electron microscopic examination of Donovan bodies has confirmed the presence of a homogeneous electron-lucid capsule surrounding the bacteria within histiocytes. The bacterial cell wall inside the capsule appears corrugated. The trilaminar plasma membrane is located medial to the cell wall. The corrugated appearance of the cell wall and the fact that division takes place by invagination of both the cell wall and plasma membrane are features typical of gram-negative bacteria (Davis and Collins). The vacuoles in which the Donovan bodies are located are lined by a trilaminar limit-

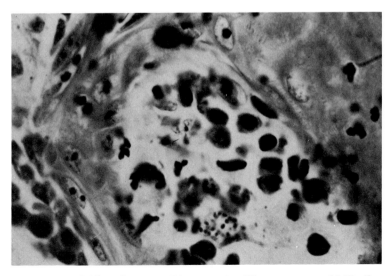

FIG. 16-9. **Rhinoscleroma.** Giemsa stain. There are several Mikulicz cells, the cytoplasm of which is pale, foamy, and vacuolated. One Mikulicz cell contains in its cytoplasm many Frisch bacilli, which appear here as small, round, deeply staining bodies. (×900)

ing membrane (Dodson et al.). This suggests that the vacuoles represent phagolysosomes.

Differential Diagnosis. The parasitism of histiocytes is strikingly similar to that observed in rhinoscleroma, histoplasmosis, and leishmaniasis. However, the small size of the Donovan bodies and the presence of small abscesses in the infiltrate usually make differentiation from these diseases possible (see Table 19-1, p. 335).

A difficult problem may be posed by the marked epidermal proliferation present occasionally in granuloma inguinale (Beerman and Sonck). Several biopsies may be necessary to decide whether it represents merely pseudocarcinomatous hyperplasia (see p. 482) or squamous cell carcinoma.

RHINOSCLEROMA

Rhinoscleroma is a chronic infectious but only mildly contagious disease in which the nose, the pharynx, the larynx, the trachea, and occasionally also the skin of the upper lip are infiltrated with hard granulomatous masses. The disorder always begins in the nose.

Histopathology. The cellular infiltrate is very rich in plasma cells and contains two striking structures: the Mikulicz cell and Russell bodies. Because of their presence the histologic picture of rhinoscleroma is diagnostic (Convit et al.).

The Mikulicz cell is a large histiocyte measuring up to 100 μm in diameter. It has a pale, foamy, vacuolated cytoplasm and an eccentric nucleus. One finds within the cytoplasm of the Mikulicz cells many bacilli, called *Klebsiella rhinoscleromatis* or Frisch bacilli (Fig. 16-9). They can be seen even in sections stained with hematoxylin and eosin but are better visualized with Giemsa's stain or a silver stain. They are short, gram-negative rods, measuring 1 to 2 μm in length, and are surrounded by PAS-positive material (Fisher and Dimling; Hoffmann et al.). Although it is likely, it has not been proved that rhinoscleroma is caused by this organism, since so far the disease has not been reproduced by cultures of Frisch bacilli.

The Russell bodies are round to ovoid formations, measuring from 20 to 40 μm in diameter. Thus they are twice as large as a normal plasma cell. They have a homogeneous, bright red, light-refractile cytoplasm and no nucleus (Fig. 16-10). They form within plasma cells as a result of cellular degeneration and finally are expelled (see p. 53).

In older lesions marked fibrosis is present (Kline and Brody). The mucosal epithelium overlying the cellular infiltrate often shows

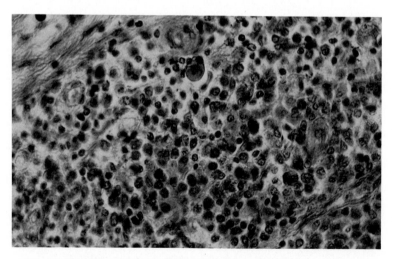

FIG. 16-10. **Rhinoscleroma.** The infiltrate contains many plasma cells and one Russell body. The Russell body is larger than the cells in the infiltrate. It has a homogeneous, brilliant red, light refractile cytoplasm. (×400)

hyperplasia which may be so pronounced as to give rise to a mistaken diagnosis of squamous cell carcinoma (Fisher and Dimling).

Histogenesis. Electron microscopy reveals numerous vacuoles of varying size within the Mikulicz cells. Some vacuoles contain one or a few bacteria, each of them surrounded by a wide, electron-lucid, finely granular, mucinous capsule. However, many vacuoles merely contain electron-lucid, finely granular material similar to the capsular mucopolysaccharide of the bacteria (Cain and Kraus; Hoffmann et al.). Since the vacuoles are lined by a limiting membrane, they can be regarded as phagolysosomes (Hoffmann et al.).

Differential Diagnosis. Parasitized histiocytes are observed also in granuloma inguinale, histoplasmosis, and leishmaniasis. For their differentiation, see Oriental Leishmaniasis (p. 334 and Table 19-1, p. 335). Rhinoscleroma differs from the other three diseases by the abundance of plasma cells and the presence of Russell bodies; therefore, the Russell bodies are of considerable diagnostic value. However, they are not specific for rhinoscleroma because they may occur in other diseases when an infiltrate rich in plasma cells is present—for instance, in syphilis, lupus vulgaris, squamous cell carcinoma, and mycosis fungoides.

BIBLIOGRAPHY

Impetigo

Dajani, A. S., Ferrieri, P., and Wanamaker, L.: Endemic superficial pyoderma in children. Arch. Derm., *108*:517, 1973.

Dick, H. M., and Baird, E.: An animal model for staphylococcal toxic epidermal necrolysis. Brit. J. Derm., *86*(suppl. 8):28, 1972.

Ellis, F. A.: Subcorneal pustular dermatosis. Arch. Derm., *78*:580, 1958.

Kaplan, E. L., Anthony, B. F., Chapman, S. S., and Wannamaker, L. W.: Epidemic acute glomerulonephritis associated with type 49 streptococcal pyoderma. Am. J. Med., *48*:9, 1970.

Kelly, C., Taplin, D., and Allen, A. M.: Streptococcal ecthyma. Arch. Derm., *103*:306, 1971.

Koblenzer, P. J.: Acute epidermal necrolysis (Ritter von Rittershain-Lyell). Arch. Derm., *95*:608, 1967.

Levine, J., and Nooden, C. W.: Staphylococcal scalded-skin syndrome in an adult. New Eng. J. Med., *287*:1339, 1972.

Lowney, E. D., Baublis, J. V., Kreye, G. M., *et al.*: The scalded skin syndrome in small children. Arch. Derm., *95*:359, 1967.

Lyell, A.: A review of toxic epidermal necrolysis in Britain. Brit. J. Derm., *79*:662, 1967.

Melish, M. E., and Glasgow, L. A.: The staphylococcal scalded-skin syndrome. New Eng. J. Med., *282*:1114, 1970.

Reid, L. H., Weston, W. L., and Humbert, J. R.: Staphylococcal scalded skin syndrome. Arch. Derm., *109*:239, 1974.

Ritter von Rittershain, G.: Die exfoliative Dermatitis jüngerer Säuglinge. Centralzeit. Kinderheilk., *2*:3, 1878.

Rothenberg, R., Renna, F. S., Drew, T. M., and Feingold, D. S.: Staphylococcal scalded skin syndrome in an adult. Arch. Derm., *108*:408, 1973.

Steigleder, G. K.: Zur Differentialdiagnose des Pemphigus vulgaris aus dem Blasengrundausstrich. Arch. klin. exp. Derm., *202*:1, 1955.

Wannamaker, L. W.: Differences between streptococcal infections of the throat and of the skin. New Eng. J. Med., *282*:23 and 78, 1970.

Erysipelas

Tappeiner, J., and Pfleger, L.: Zur Histopathologie cutaner Lymphgefässe beim chronisch-rezidivierenden Erysipel der unteren Extremitäten. Hautarzt, *15*:218, 1964.

Chronic Superficial Folliculitis

Montgomery, H.: Acne necrotica miliaris of the scalp. Arch. Derm. Syph., *36*:40, 1937.

Chronic Deep Folliculitis

Meinhof, W., and Braun-Falco, O.: Über die Folliculitis sycosiformis atrophicans barbae Hoffmann (Sycosis lupoides Milton-Brocq, Ulerythema sycosiforme Unna). Derm. Wschr., *152*:153, 1966.

Moyer, D. G., and Williams, R. M.: Perifolliculitis capitis abscedens et suffodiens. Arch. Derm., *85*:378, 1962.

Follicular Occlusion Triad

Brunsting, H. A.: Hidradenitis suppurativa; abscess of the apocrine sweat glands. Arch. Derm. Syph., *39*:108, 1939.

Moschella, S. L., Klein, M. H., and Miller, R. J.: Perifolliculitis capitis abscedens et suffodiens. Arch. Derm., *96*:195, 1967.

Pillsbury, D. M., Shelley, W. B., and Kligman, A. M.: Dermatology. p. 481. Philadelphia, W. B. Saunders, 1956.

Shaughnessy, D. M., Greminger, R. R., Margolis, I. B., and Davis, W. C.: Hidradenitis suppurativa. J.A.M.A., *222*:320, 1972.

Strauss, J. S.: Acne conglobata. *In* Fitzpatrick, T. B., *et al.* (eds.): Dermatology in General Practice. p. 368. New York, McGraw-Hill, 1971.

Pyoderma Gangrenosum

Cream, J. J.: Pyoderma gangrenosum with a monoclonal IgM red cell agglomerating factor. Brit. J. Derm., *84*:223, 1971.

de Bast, C., Achten, G., and Moriame, G.: Pyoderma gangrenosum. Arch. belg. derm. syph., *25*:111, 1969.

Imhof, J. W., Schutter, G. J. N. V., Hart, H. C., and Zegers, B. J. M.: Monoclonal gammopathy (IgG) and chronic ulcerative dermatitis (phagedenic pyoderma). Acta med. scand., *186*:289, 1969.

Kresbach, H.: Ein Beitrag zum Problem der sogenannten Pyodermia ulcerosa. Arch. klin. exp. Derm., *208*:128, 1959.

Lazarus, G. S., Goldsmith, L. A., Rocklin, R. E., *et al.*: Pyoderma gangrenosum, altered delayed hypersensitivity, and polyarthritis. Arch. Derm., *105*:46, 1972.

Perry, H. O., and Brunsting, L. A.: Pyoderma gangrenosum. Arch. Derm., *75*:380, 1957.

Schröpl, F.: Dermatitis ulcerosa (pyoderma gangrenosum) mit IgA-Paraproteinamia. Arch. klin. exp. Derm., *228*:430, 1967.

Sluis, I.v.d.: Two cases of pyoderma (ecthyma) gangraenosum associated with the presence of an abnormal serum protein (IgA-paraprotein). Dermatologica, *132*:409, 1966.

Stathers, G. M., Abbott, L. G., and McGuinness, A. E.: Pyoderma gangrenosum in association with regional enteritis. Arch. Derm., *95*:375, 1967.

Crohn's Disease

Korting, G. W.: Zur perianalen Erscheinungsweise der Crohnschen Krankheit. Hautarzt, *19*:553, 1968.

McCallum, D. I., and Kinmont, P. D. C.: Dermatological manifestations of Crohn's disease. Brit. J. Derm., *80*:1, 1968.

Aphthosis; Behçet's Syndrome

Civatte, J., and Belaich, S.: Histopathologic picture of aphthae in Behçet's syndrome. Brit. J. Derm., *91* (suppl. 10):27, 1974.

Curth, H. O.: L'aphthose. Ann. derm. syph., *83*:130, 1956.

Forman, L.: Behçet's disease. Brit. J. Derm., *63*:417, 1951.

Lehner, T.: Stimulation of lymphocyte transformation by tissue homogenates in recurrent oral ulceration. Immunology, *13*:159, 1967.

———: Autoimmunity in oral diseases, with special reference to recurrent oral ulceration. Proc. Roy. Soc. Med., *61*:515, 1968.

———: Pathology of recurrent oral ulceration and oral ulceration in Behçet's syndrome. J. Path., *97*:481, 1969.

Nethercott, J., and Lester, R. S.: Azathioprine therapy in incomplete Behçet syndrome. Arch. Derm., *110*:432, 1974.

O'Duffy, J. D., Carney, J. A., and Deodhar, S.: Behçet's disease. Ann. Int. Med., *75*:561, 1971.

Pallis, C. A., and Fudge, B. J.: Neurological complications of Behçet's syndrome. Arch. Neurol., *75*:1, 1956.

Rogers, R. S., III, Sams, W. M., Jr., and Shorter, R. G.: Lymphocytotoxicity in recurrent aphthous stomatitis. Arch. Derm., *109*:361, 1974.

Saito, T., Honma, T., Sato, T., and Fujioka, Y.: Auto-immune mechanisms as a probable aetiology of Behçet's syndrome; an electron microscopic study of the oral mucosa. Virchows Arch. (Abt. A, Path. Anat.), *353*:261, 1971.

Schneider, W.: Zur Frage der arteriellen Beteiligung beim Morbus Behçet (Aphthosis Touraine). Z. Haut Geschlechtskr., *39*:185, 1965.

Schottland, D. L., Wolf, S. M., White, H. M., and Durbin, H. V.: Neurologic aspects of Behçet's disease. Am. J. Med., *34*:544, 1963.

Ship, I. I., Merritt, A. D., and Stanley, H. R.: Recurrent aphthous ulcers. Am. J. Med., *32*: 32, 1962.

Sigel, N., and Larson, R.: Behçet's syndrome. Arch. Intern. Med., *115*:203, 1965.

Acute Septicemia

Dorff, G. I., Geimer, N. F., Rosenthal, D. R., and Rytel, M. W.: Pseudomonas septicemia. Illustrated evolution of its skin lesion. Arch. Int. Med., *128*:591, 1971.

Ferguson, J. H., and Chapman, O. D.: Fulminating meningococcic infections and the so-called Waterhouse-Friderichsen syndrome. Am. J. Path., *24*:763, 1948.

Hall, J. H., Callaway, J. L., Tindall, J. P., and Smith, J. G., Jr.: *Pseudomonas aeruginosa* in dermatology. Arch. Derm., *97*:312, 1968.

Hill, W. R., and Kinney, T. D.: The cutaneous lesions in acute meningococcemia. J.A.M.A., *134*:513, 1947.

Plaut, M. E.: Staphylococcal septicemia and pustular purpura. Arch. Derm., *99*:82, 1969.

Shapiro, L., Teisch, J. A., and Brownstein, M. H.: Dermatohistopathology of chronic gonococcal sepsis. Arch. Derm., *107*:403, 1973.

Winkelstein, A., Songster, C. L., Caras, T. S., *et al.*: Fulminant meningococcemia and disseminated intravascular coagulation. Arch. Int. Med., *124*:55, 1969.

Chronic Septicemia

Ackerman, A. B.: Hemorrhagic bullae in gonococcemia. New Eng. J. Med., *282*:793, 1970.

Björnberg, A.: Benign gonococcal sepsis. Acta dermatoven., *50*:313, 1970.

Holmes, K. K., Counts, G. W., and Beaty, H. N.: Disseminated gonococcal infection. Ann. Int. Med., *74*:979, 1971.

Kahn, G., and Danielsson, D.: Septic gonococcal dermatitis. Arch. Derm., *99*:421, 1969.

Nielsen, L. T.: Chronic meningococcemia. Arch. Derm., *102*:97, 1970.

Ognibene, A. J., and Ditto, M. R.: Chronic meningococcemia. Arch. Int. Med., *114*:29, 1964.

Shapiro, L., Teisch, J. A., and Brownstein, M. H.: Dermatohistopathology of chronic gonococcal sepsis. Arch. Derm., *107*:403, 1973.

Tuberculosis

Carter, R. L., and Roberts, J. D. B.: Macrophages and multinucleate giant cells in nitrosoquinoline-induced granulomata in rats: an autoradiographic study. J. Path., 105:285, 1971.

de Bast, C., Moriame, G., and Ledoux-Corbusier, M.: Chancre tuberculeux d'inoculation. Arch. belg. derm. syph., *27*:323, 1971.

Dumont, A., and Sheldon, H.: Changes in the fine structure of macrophages in experimentally produced tuberculous granulomas in hamsters. Lab. Invest., *14*:2034, 1965.

Heilman, K. M., and Muschenheim, C.: Primary cutaneous tuberculosis resulting from mouth-to-mouth respiration. New Eng. J. Med., *273*:1035, 1965.

Horwitz, O.: Lupus vulgaris cutis in Denmark 1895-1954. Its relation to the epidemiology of other forms of tuberculosis. Acta tuberc. scand., *suppl. 49*:1, 1960.

Minkowitz, S., Brandt, L. J., Rapp, Y., and Radlauer, C. B.: "Prosector's wart" (cutaneous tuberculosis) in a medical student. Am. J. Clin. Path., *51*:261, 1969.

Montgomery, H.: Histopathology of the various types of cutaneous tuberculosis. Arch. Derm. Syph., *35*:698, 1937.

Papadimitriou, J. M., and Spector, W. G.: The origin, properties and fate of epithelioid cells. J. Path., *105*:187, 1971.

O'Leary, P. A., and Harrison, M. W.: Inoculation tuberculosis. Arch. Derm. Syph., *44*:371, 1941.

Schermer, D. R., Simpson, C. G., Haserick, J. R., and Van Ordstrand, H. S.: Tuberculosis cutis miliaris acuta generalisata. Arch. Derm., *99*:64, 1969.

Shima, K., Dannenberg, A. M., Jr., Ando, M., *et al.*: Macrophage accumulation, division, maturation and digestive and microbicidal capacities in tuberculous lesions. Am. J. Path., *67*:159, 1972.

Slany, E.: Moderne Behandlung der Hauttuberkulosen. Hautarzt, *25*:218, 1974.

Steigleder, G. K.: Diagnostische Möglichkeiten der Dermatohistopathologie. Hautarzt, *19*:447, 1968.

Sulzberger, M. B.: Dermatologic Allergy. p. 211. Springfield, Ill., Charles C Thomas, 1940.

van der Lugt, L.: Some remarks about tuberculosis of the skin and tuberculids. Dermatologica, *131*:266, 1965.

Weed, L. A., and Macy, N. E.: Tuberculosis— Problem in diagnosis and eradication. Am. J. Clin. Path., *53*:136, 1970.

Wilner, G., Nassar, S. A., Siket, A., and Azar, H. A.: Fluorescent staining for mycobacteria in sarcoid and tuberculous granulomas. Am. J. Clin. Path., *51*:584, 1969.

Tuberculids

Brunner, M. J., and Robin, M.: Lichen-scrofulosorum-like lesions associated with sarcoidosis. Arch. Derm. Syph., *60*:1212, 1949.

Chantraine, R.: Un traitement efficace des tuberculides papulonécrotiques rebelles. Arch. belg. derm. syph., *14*:369, 1958.

Flegel, H.: Die Stellung des Tuberkulids im Rahmen der Tuberkulose. Derm. Wschr., *145*:609, 1962.

Kanaar, P.: Micropapular sarcoidosis in two brothers. Dermatologica, *138*:347, 1969.

Krüger, H.: Das Trisymptom von Gougerot im Rahmen der allergischen Vasculitis. Arch. klin. exp. Derm., *213*:496, 1961.

Miescher, G.: Mikrobenstreuung und Infektionsimmunität. Hautarzt, *2*:347, 1951.

Montgomery, H.: Histopathology of the various types of cutaneous tuberculosis. Arch. Derm. Syph., *35*:698, 1937.

Ockuly, O. E., and Montgomery, H.: Lichenoid tuberculosis. J. Invest. Derm., *14*:415, 1950.

Schuhmachers, R.: 2 Fälle eines lichenoiden Tuberkulids (= Lichen scrophulosorum). Hautarzt, *18*:81, 1967.

Spier, H. W., and Röckl, H.: Differentialdiagnose und Therapie entzündlicher knotiger Dermatosen, insbesondere der unteren Extremitäten. Fortschr. prakt. Derm. Venerol., *3*:98, 1960.

Thal, M.: Zur Klinik der lichenoiden Form des Boeck'schen Sarkoids. Dermatologica, *111*: 87, 1955.

van der Lugt, L.: Some remarks about tuberculosis of the skin and tuberculids. Dermatologica, *131*:266, 1965.

Infections with Atypical Mycobacteria

Adams, R. M., Remington, J. S., Steinberg, J., and Seibert, J. S.: Tropical fish aquariums. A source of *Mycobacterium marinum* infections resembling sporotrichosis. J.A.M.A., *211*:457, 1970.

Brock, J. M., Kennedy, C. B., and Clark, W. H., Jr.: Cutaneous infection with atypical mycobacterium. Arch. Derm., *82*:918, 1960.

Cott, R. E., Carter, D. M., and Sall, T.: Cutaneous disease caused by atypical mycobacteria. Arch. Derm., *95*:259, 1967.

Dickey, R. F.: Sporotrichoid mycobacteriosis caused by *M. marinum (balnei)*. Arch. Derm., *98*:385, 1968.

Jolly, H. W., Jr., and Seabury, J. H.: Infections with *Mycobacterium marinum*. Arch. Derm., *106*:32, 1972.

Knox, J. M., Gever, S. G., Freeman, R. G., and Whitcomb, F.: Atypical acid-fast organism infection of the skin. Arch. Derm., *84*:386, 1961.

Maberry, J. D., Mullins, J. F., and Stone, O. J.: Cutaneous infection due to *Mycobacterium kansasii*. J.A.M.A., *194*:1135, 1965.

Mansson, T., Brehmer-Andersson, E., Wittbeck, B., and Grabb, R.: Aquarium-borne infection with *Mycobacterium marinum*. Acta dermatoven., *50*:119, 1970.

Philpott, J. A., Jr., Woodburns, A. R., Philpott, O. S., et al.: Swimming pool granuloma. Arch. Derm., *88*:158, 1963.

Scholz-Jordan, D., Fasske, E., and Schröder, K. H.: Chronische Infektion durch Mycobakterium marinum aus einem Aquarium. Z. Haut, *49*:9, 1974.

Zeligman, I.: *Mycobacterium marinum* granuloma. Arch. Derm., *106*:26, 1972.

Buruli Ulceration

Connor, D. H., and Lunn, H. F.: Buruli ulceration. Arch. Path., *81*:183, 1966.

Cott, R. E., Carter, D. M., and Sall, T.: Cutaneous disease caused by atypical mycobacteria. Arch. Derm., *95*:259, 1967.

Leprosy

Azulay, R. D.: Histopathology of skin lesions in leprosy. Internat. J. Leprosy, *39*:244, 1971. (Review)

Bullock, W. E.: Studies of immune mechanisms in leprosy. New Eng. J. Med., *278*:298, 1968.

Case Records of the Massachusetts General Hospital, Case 21-1970. Indeterminate leprosy. New Eng. J. Med., *282*:1144, 1970.

Desikan, K. V., and Job, C. K.: A review of postmortem findings in 37 cases of leprosy. Internat. J. Leprosy, *36*:32, 1968.

Donner, R. S., and Shively, J. A.: The "Lucio phenomenon" in diffuse leprosy. Ann. Int. Med., *67*:831, 1967.

Fields, J. P.: Leprosy. Arch. Derm., *100*:650, 1969.

Imaeda, T.: Electron microscopy of leprosy lesions. Derm. Internat., *7*:116, 1968.

Job, C. K.: *Mycobacterium leprae* in nerve lesions of lepromatous leprosy. Arch. Path., *89*:195, 1970.

Job, C. K., and Desikan, K. V.: Pathologic changes and their distribution in peripheral nerves in lepromatous leprosy. Internat. J. Leprosy, *36*:257, 1968.

Katz, S. I., De Betz, B. H., and Zaias, N.: Production of macrophage inhibitory factor by patients with leprosy. Arch. Derm., *103*:358, 1971.

Kirchheimer, W. F., and Storrs, R. C.: Lepromatoid leprosy in the armadillo. Internat. J. Leprosy, *39*:693, 1971.

Kramarsky, B., Edmondson, H. A., Peters, R. L., and Reynolds, T. B.: Lepromatous leprosy in reaction. Arch. Path., *85*:516, 1968.

Kwittken, J., and Peck, S. M.: Borderline leprosy. Arch. Derm., *95*:50, 1967.

Moschella, S. L.: A current review of leprosy. Cutis, *10*:27, 1972. (Review)

Pettit, J. H. S.: Recent advances in leprosy. Austral. J. Derm., *9*:285, 1968.

Rees, R. J. W., Waters, M. F. R., Weddell, A. G. M., and Palmer, E.: Experimental lepromatous leprosy. Nature, *215*:599, 1967.

Sheagren, J. N., Block, J. B., Trautman, J. R., and Wolff, S. M.: Immunological reactivity in patients with leprosy. Ann. Int. Med., *70*:295, 1969.

Shepard, C. C.: The experimental disease that follows the injection of human leprosy bacilli into foot-pads of mice. J. Exp. Med., *112*: 445, 1960.

Turk, J. L., and Waters, M. F. R.: Cell-mediated immunity in patients with leprosy. Lancet, *2*:243, 1969.

Waldorf, D. S., Sheagren, J. N., Trautman, J. R., et al.: Impaired delayed hypersensitivity in patients with lepromatous leprosy. Lancet, *2*:773, 1966.

Wemambu, S. N. C., Turk, J. L., Waters, M. F. R., and Rees, R. J. W.: Erythema nodosum leprosum; a clinical manifestation of the Arthus phenomenon. Lancet, *2*:933, 1969.

Wiersema, J. P., and Binford, C. H.: The identification of leprosy among epithelioid cell granulomas of the skin. Internat. J. Leprosy, *40*: 10, 1972.

Anthrax

Lebowich, R. J., McKillip, B. G., and Conboy, J. R.: Cutaneous anthrax. Am. J. Clin. Path., *13*:505, 1943.

Matz, M. H., and Brugsch, H. G.: Anthrax in Massachusetts, 1943 to 1962. J.A.M.A., *188*: 635, 1964.

Tularemia

Klock, L. E., Olsen, P. F., and Fukushima, T.: Tularemia epidemic associated with deerfly. J.A.M.A., *226*:149, 1973.

Lawless, T. K.: Tularemia. Arch. Derm. Syph., *44*:147, 1941. (Review)

Reich, H.: Zur Kenntnis der Tularämie hautnaher (regionaler) Lymphknoten. Arch. f. Derm. u. Syph., *192*:175, 1950.

Schuermann, H., and Reich, H.: Zur Klinik und Histologie des cutan lokalisierten tularämischen Primäraffekts. Arch. f. Derm. u. Syph., *190*:579, 1950.

Young, L. S., Bicknell, D. S., Archer, B. G., *et al.*: Tularemia epidemic: Vermont, 1968. New Eng. J. Med., *280*:1253, 1969.

Chancroid

Borchardt, K. A., and Hoke, A. W.: Simplified laboratory technique for diagnosis of chancroid. Arch. Derm., *102*:188, 1970.

Heyman, A., Beeson, P. B., and Sheldon, W. A.: Diagnosis of chancroid. J.A.M.A., *129*:935, 1945.

Pund, E. R., Greenblatt, R. B., and Huie, G. B.: The role of biopsy in diagnosis of venereal disease. Am. J. Syph., *22*:495, 1938.

Sheldon, W. H., and Heyman, A.: Studies on chancroid. Am. J. Path., *22*:415, 1946.

Granuloma Inguinale

Beerman, H., and Sonck, C. E.: The epithelial changes in granuloma inguinale. Am. J. Syph., *36*:501, 1952.

Davis, C. M.: Granuloma inguinale. J.A.M.A., *211*:632, 1970.

Davis, C. M., and Collins, C.: Granuloma inguinale: an ultrastructural study of *Calymmatobacterium granulomatis*. J. Invest. Derm., *53*:315, 1969.

Dodson, R. F., Fritz, G. S., Hubler, W. R., Jr., et al.: Donovanosis: a morphologic study. J. Invest. Derm., *62*:611, 1974.

Goldberg, J., Weaver, R. H., and Packer, H.: Studies on granuloma inguinale. I. Bacteriologic behavior of Donovania *granulomatis*. Am. J. Syph., *37*:60, 1953.

Torpin, R., Greenblatt, R. B., and Pund, E. R.: Granuloma inguinale (venereum) in the female. Am. J. Surg., *44*:551, 1939.

Rhinoscleroma

Cain, H., and Kraus, B.: Feinstrukturelle Befunde und Probleme bei langjähriger Skleromerkrankung. Virchows Arch. (Abt. A, Path. Anat.), *357*:345, 1972.

Convit, J., Kerdel-Vegas, F., and Gordon, B.: Rhinoscleroma. Arch. Derm., *84*:55, 1961.

Fisher, E. R., and Dimling, C.: Rhinoscleroma. Arch. Path., *78*:501, 1964.

Hoffmann, E., Loose, L. D., and Harkin, J. C.: The Mikulicz cell in rhinoscleroma. Am. J. Path., *73*:47, 1973.

Kline, P. R., and Brody, E. R.: Scleroma. Arch. Derm. Syph., *59*:606, 1949.

17

Treponemal Diseases

SYPHILIS

Acquired syphilis occurs on the skin in two stages: early and late. The early stage comprises primary and secondary syphilis; the late stage, tertiary syphilis. During the early stage the causative organism, *Treponema pallidum (Spirochaeta pallida),* often can be demonstrated in the cutaneous lesions by dark-field examination of tissue fluid or by silver staining or fluorescent antibody staining of tissue sections (see p. 276). During the late stage no spirochetes can be demonstrated in the cutaneous lesions.

Primary syphilis is characterized by the syphilitic, or hard, chancre, which usually is a single lesion but may be multiple. The typical, or hunterian, chancre is represented by a brownish-red, indurated round papule or plaque with an eroded surface, usually measuring from 1 to 2 cm in diameter. Occasionally, the chancre shows ulceration. The regional lymph nodes are enlarged.

Secondary syphilis is characterized by a more or less generalized eruption composed usually of macules or papules brownish red in color. In the anogenital region the papules may become large, verrucous, and moist; then they are called condylomata lata. (They must be differentiated from condylomata acuminata, a variety of verruca; see p. 352.) In some instances the cutaneous eruption, due to the presence of scaling, resembles psoriasis (psoriasiform syphilis). Occasionally, pustules develop, either primarily as follicular papulopustules, or secondarily on

plaques where the pustules are followed by crusting. Ulcerating lesions in secondary syphilis are very rare and occur only in severe cases, so-called lues maligna. The ulcers may be covered by thick crusts. On the palms and the soles discrete, hyperkeratotic, centrally pitted papules may be present (syphilis cornée).

Occasionally, a benign, self-limited hepatitis occurs during secondary syphilis with tenderness and enlargement of the liver and in some cases also jaundice. In rare instances an acute nephrosis occurs in secondary syphilis characterized by massive edema, albuminuria, and elevated triglycerides and cholesterol, but with normal renal function.

Tertiary syphilis often shows only a single lesion, but occasionally there are several lesions. A superficial nodular type and a deep gummatous type occur. Lesions of the nodular type show a smooth, atrophic center and an active serpiginous border composed of nodules that may be superficially ulcerated. Lesions of the gummatous type begin as a soft cutaneous or subcutaneous swelling, which breaks down to form one or several ulcers having a punched-out appearance. In rare instances juxta-articular nodes occur. They are painless, slowly growing, subcutaneous, fibrous nodules, often symmetrically situated in the vicinity of joints. The elbows and the knees are the sites of predilection.

Histopathology. The fundamental pathologic changes in syphilis are (1) swelling and proliferation of endothelial cells, and

(2) a predominantly perivascular infiltrate composed of lymphoid cells and many plasma cells. In tertiary syphilis usually one finds, in addition, a granulomatous infiltrate of epithelioid and giant cells, often with necrosis in the center of the granulomas.

PRIMARY SYPHILIS. In the typical primary lesion the epidermis shows acanthosis at the margin of the lesion. Toward the center the epidermis gradually becomes thinner and appears edematous and permeated by inflammatory cells. In the center the epidermis

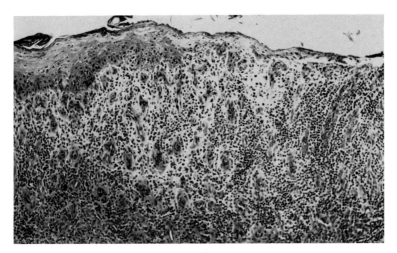

FIG. 17-1. **Primary syphilis.** Low magnification. The margin of an erosion is shown. The epidermis gradually becomes thinner as it approaches the erosion. (×100)

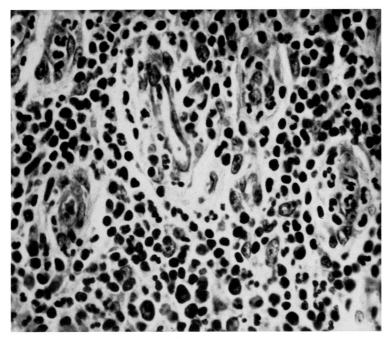

FIG. 17-2. **Primary syphilis.** High magnification of Figure 17-1. The capillaries show proliferation of their endothelial cells. Many plasma cells are present in the dense infiltrate. (×400)

may be absent (Fig. 17-1). An infiltrate composed of lymphoid cells and many plasma cells is present in the dermis. It is compact in the center, while at the margin it consists of individual perivascular islands. The capillaries show considerable proliferation of their endothelial cells (Fig. 17-2). Their walls may be invaded by the cellular infiltrate.

On staining with a silver stain, such as Levaditi's stain or the Warthin-Starry stain, spirochetes usually can be found in the dermis around the walls of capillaries. The number of spirochetes in the epidermis is small, in contrast with yaws and pinta (Ferris and Turner). In using staining methods with silver, it must be remembered that these methods also stain reticulum fibers. Thus, it often is difficult to differentiate between spirochetes and reticulum fibers. For this reason, fluorescent antibody staining methods are being used not only on smears but also on tissue sections. However, frozen sections, rather than formalin-fixed sections, are required (Yobs et al.).

Histologic examination of swollen regional lymph nodes in primary syphilis most commonly reveals a chronic inflammatory infiltrate containing many plasma cells. In addition, there is endothelial proliferation and follicular hyperplasia. Spirochetes are numerous and nearly always can be identified with the Warthin-Starry stain. In some instances noncaseating granulomas resembling those of sarcoidosis can be found (Hartsock et al.).

Histogenesis. Electron microscopic examination of lesions of early syphilis has revealed the presence of *T. pallidum* mainly in the perivascular areas of the dermis, and to a lesser extent in the intercellular spaces of the epidermis (Hasegawa). In the dermis, some spirochetes are found within phagolysosomes of endothelial cells, macrophages, neutrophils and plasma cells (Azar et al.). Similarly, some spirochetes have been demonstrated also within epidermal cells (Metz and Metz). *T. pallidum* shows at both ends 3 or 4 basal nodules. From each of the 6 to 8 nodules a long fibril extends to the other end of the cytoplasmic body. These fibrils, about 10 nm thick, are located between the plasma membrane and the outer cell wall. Being contractile, they are responsible for the contractile and spiral motions of the spirochete (Klingmüller et al.).

SECONDARY SYPHILIS. In secondary syphilis the number of spirochetes seen in sec-

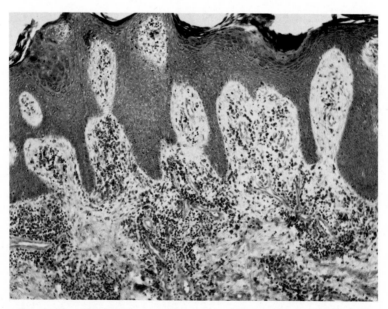

FIG. 17-3. **Secondary syphilis.** Low magnification. The vessels throughout the dermis show endothelial proliferation. The cellular infiltrate is located around the vessels in coat-sleevelike arrangement. (×100)

Fig. 17-4. **Secondary syphilis.** High magnification of Figure 17-3. The perivascular infiltrate contains many plasma cells. (×200)

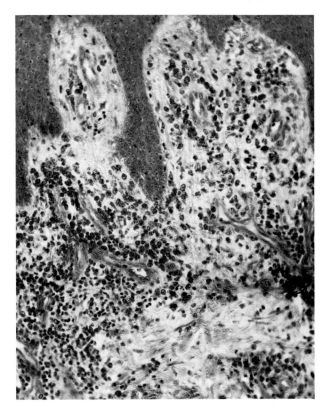

tions stained with a silver stain varies with the type of lesion. In the macular lesions of early secondary syphilis, spirochetes cannot be found as a rule. In papular lesions and, especially, in condylomata lata they are almost always present in sufficient numbers to be found in the dermis.

The *macular lesions* of early secondary syphilis usually do not present a diagnostic histologic picture. The superficial capillaries show swelling of their endothelium and are surrounded by a slight infiltrate of lymphoid cells and plasma cells. However, the number of plasma cells is not sufficiently large to be of diagnostic value.

Papular lesions as a rule have a fairly diagnostic appearance. Not only the superficial but also the deeper vessels of the dermis are involved. They show marked endothelial swelling and proliferation and are surrounded by a pronounced infiltrate (Fig. 17-3.) This perivascular coat-sleeve-like arrangement stands out very clearly in the lower dermis. In the upper dermis, in addi-

tion to the perivascular infiltrate, there may be a diffuse scattering of cells. Usually, a significantly high number of plasma cells is present in the infiltrate (Fig. 17-4). Not infrequently, small discrete epithelioid cell granulomas, some of them with giant cells, are present in the infiltrate even in early secondary syphilis (Kahn and Gordon).

In the differential diagnosis erythema annulare centrifugum may have to be considered in the presence of a pronounced infiltrate in perivascular arrangement; and sarcoidosis in the presence of epithelioid-cell granulomas. However, the vascular changes and presence of plasma cells aid in arriving at a diagnosis of syphilis.

Condylomata lata show the same changes in the dermis as the papular lesions. In addition, the epidermis shows considerable acanthosis, with broadening and elongation of the rete ridges, intracellular and intercellular edema of the epidermal cells, and migration of neutrophils through the epidermis.

Psoriasiform secondary syphilis may show

epidermal changes similar to those of psoriasis, but the dermal infiltrate is that of secondary syphilis and not of psoriasis.

Follicular papulopustular secondary syphilis, in addition to a perivascular coat-sleeve infiltrate containing many plasma cells, often shows small granulomas consisting of epithelioid and giant cells in the perifollicular region (Mikhail and Chapel).

Ulcerating lesions, which may occur in the very rare lues maligna, in addition to pronounced endothelial swelling and proliferation, may show accumulation of fibrinoid material within many vessels. This causes partial to complete occlusion of the lumen and may result in infarction necrosis of the upper dermis and epidermis (Fisher et al.). It is possible, however, that defective cell-mediated immunity plays an important role in the pathogenesis (Petrozzi et al.).

Syphilis cornée shows a central keratotic, in part parakeratotic, plug invaginating the epidermis (Kerdel-Vegas et al.). The dermis shows the usual changes of secondary syphilis.

In addition to finding small sarcoidlike granulomas in papular and follicular lesions of early secondary syphilis, one may find in lesions of late secondary syphilis extensive aggregates of epithelioid cells and giant cells intermingled with many lymphoid and plasma cells, as seen typically in tertiary syphilis (Lantis et al.). Conversely, lesions of early tertiary syphilis may show vascular changes and many plasma cells without any epithelioid and giant cell reaction. Thus, it is not always possible on the basis of histologic examination to assign cutaneous lesions of syphilis to either secondary or tertiary syphilis.

The *hepatitis* that may occur in secondary syphilis, on biopsy of the liver, shows a pericholangitis consisting of an infiltration of the portal tracts by round cells and neutrophils and scattered foci of necrosis in the parenchyma (Sobel and Wolf).

The *nephrosis* of secondary syphilis shows mild proliferative changes in the glomeruli (Bhorade et al.). It represents an immune-complex disease, since, on immunofluorescent microscopy, deposits of IgG and complement are seen as granular deposits along the glomerular basement membrane (Braunstein et al.; Bhorade et al.).

TERTIARY SYPHILIS. In tertiary syphilis one observes an infiltrate composed of lymphoid cells, plasma cells, histiocytes, fibroblasts, and granulomas containing epithelioid and giant cells. Usually, but not always, the number of plasma cells is prominent. The

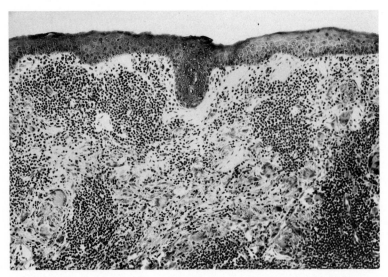

FIG. 17-5. **Nodular tertiary syphilis.** Several islands of epithelioid and multinucleated giant cells are present. They are surrounded by an infiltrate containing a large proportion of plasma cells. (×100)

infiltrate is massive in the center but tends to have a perivascular arrangement at the periphery. Vascular changes are prominent. The vessels may show thickening of their walls, permeation of their walls with plasma cells and lymphoid cells, and proliferation of their endothelial cells, causing narrowing of the lumina. Caseation necrosis is frequent. It is likely that the caseation necrosis is not due to the vascular changes, because often the vascular changes are as severe in areas without caseation as in those with caseation. Rather, the caseation is part of the immune phenomenon occurring in tertiary syphilis. The granulomas of tertiary syphilis basically are a reaction of cellular immunity, but their occurrence is due to a renewed activity of *T. pallidum,* resulting from a decrease in circulating humoral antibodies against *T. pallidum* (Wigfield). In the healing stage lesions of tertiary syphilis show numerous fibroblasts. The process ends in fibrosis. Tertiary syphilis occurs in the skin in two forms: nodular and gummatous.

In *nodular tertiary syphilis* the granulomatous process is limited to the dermis. As a rule, the number of epithelioid and multinucleated giant cells is small. Occasionally, however, these cells are fairly numerous in the center of the lesion (Fig. 17-5). Caseation necrosis is usually not extensive, and it may be absent. If it is extensive, ulceration results.

In *gummatous tertiary syphilis* the granulomatous process is more extensive than in the nodular form and involves the subcutaneous tissue in addition to the dermis. Epithelioid and giant cells are numerous, and massive caseation necrosis occurs in the center of the lesion (Fig. 17-6). The epithelioid and giant cells are located mainly in the vicinity of the areas of caseation. Because of the deep extension of the process, not only the vessels of the dermis, as in nodular tertiary syphilis, but also the large vessels of the subcutaneous layer are markedly involved (Holtzmann and Hassenpflug).

Differentiation of nodular tertiary syphilis

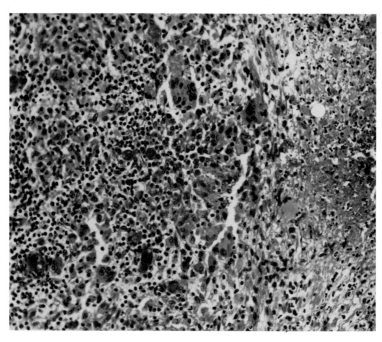

FIG. 17-6. **Gummatous tertiary syphilis.** On the left side of the field the infiltrate consists of lymphoid cells and plasma cells. In the center, numerous epithelioid and multinucleated giant cells are present. On the right side is seen part of the large area of caseation necrosis that forms the center of the gumma. (×200)

from lupus vulgaris may be impossible if caseation is slight or absent, since many plasma cells can also occur in lupus vulgaris. The gummatous type of tertiary syphilis greatly resembles scrofuloderma and erythema induratum. Scrofuloderma differs by not showing vascular changes; but erythema induratum, in which obliterative vascular changes similar to those of gummatous tertiary syphilis may be found, often cannot be excluded without clinical data.

In *juxta-articular nodes* the histologic picture varies with the age of the lesion. Early lesions are fairly cellular and present, embedded in a dense fibrous tissue, granulomatous areas composed of epithelioid cells, lymphocytes, and plasma cells, with an occasional multinucleated giant cell (Tuta and Coombs). Older lesions show an increasing amount of fibrosis and hyalinization. In the late stage the node is composed entirely of hyalinized collagen with little or no cellular infiltrate (Freeman). The center may contain amorphous material and occasionally also cholesterol clefts (Kalz and Newton).

SYPHILIS OF INTERNAL ORGANS. Without going into details about the histologic appearance of the lesions of syphilis in the internal organs, it may be pointed out that late syphilis may cause two types of reactions in the internal organs: gumma and diffuse interstitial inflammation. The latter reaction is more common.

The gummata in internal organs show the same histologic changes as those observed in the skin.

Diffuse interstitial syphilitic inflammation manifests itself as accumulations of lymphoid and plasma cells around the small blood vessels. As a result of the long-continued inflammation, there is gradual degeneration of the parenchymatous structures and their replacement by fibrous tissue. This type of reaction produces, for instance, syphilitic hepatic cirrhosis. Syphilis of the aorta is also of the diffuse type. It affects predominantly the thoracic portion of the aorta, in which one observes (1) fragmentation and loss of the elastic tissue of the media, (2) an inflammatory infiltrate with a predominance of plasma cells around the blood vessels, including the vasa vasorum, and (3) formation of fibrous scar tissue (Sohn and Levine).

General paresis shows perivascular accumulations of lymphoid cells and plasma cells in the meninges and in the cortex of the brain. In addition, there is etxensive degeneration of the cortex. In contrast with general paresis, tabes does not show inflammatory changes. The essential lesion is degeneration of the posterior columns of the spinal cord.

YAWS (FRAMBESIA TROPICA)

Yaws is caused by *Treponema pertenue,* which is morphologically indistinguishable from *Treponema pallidum.* Yaws is endemic in humid regions in the tropical belt around the globe. It is not a venereal disease but is transmitted by direct contact between children, usually with the hands (Guthe). Three stages are recognized. They may, however, overlap.

The *primary lesion* starts in childhood as a papule which often enlarges and becomes papillomatous and crusted.

Secondary yaws develops subsequently and consists of crops of infectious, relapsing skin lesions consisting of frambesiform (raspberrylike) papillomata, resembling the primary lesion. Healing takes place with atrophic scarring (Lanigan-O'Keeffe et al.).

Late or tertiary yaws develops in adolescence or in later life. It has two principal cutaneous manifestations: hyperkeratotic lesions confined to the palms and soles, and ulcerating lesions. The ulcerating lesions, comparable with gummas, develop from preexisting lesions, either from the primary lesion or from the secondary lesions. Ulcerations at the mucocutaneous borders of the mouth and of the nose may progress to considerable destruction in the mouth and the upper respiratory tract; these destructive lesions are referred to as rhinopharyngitis mutilans, or gangosa. In addition, the bones may show extensive destructive lesions. However, the central nervous system and the cardiovascular system show no clinical involvement.

Histopathology. The PRIMARY LESION shows considerable acanthosis and papillomatosis. There is pronounced edema of the epidermis, and numerous neutrophils are seen migrating into the epidermis, leading to the formation of intraepidermal microabscesses. The dermis shows a dense infiltrate composed predominantly of plasma cells but containing also neutrophils, lymphoid cells, histiocytes, fibroblasts, and a few eosinophils. In contrast with syphilis, the blood vessels show little or no endothelial proliferation (Williams; Hasselmann, 1957).

The SECONDARY LESIONS show the same histologic appearance as the primary lesion. Although the secondary lesions of yaws resemble condylomata lata in their epidermal changes, they differ from condylomata lata by a diffuse rather than a perivascular arrangement of the infiltrate and by the absence of vascular changes.

In LATE YAWS the ulcerative lesions greatly resemble those seen in late syphilis in their histologic appearance (Williams). Even then, however, vascular changes are slight or absent (Hasselmann, 1957). The hyperkeratotic lesions on the palms and soles have a nonspecific histologic appearance, showing considerable acanthosis, hyperkeratosis, and parakeratosis, with only a slight inflammatory infiltrate in the dermis (Hasselmann, 1952).

The causative organism, *T. pertenue,* can be demonstrated in the lesions during the first two stages of the disease when on silver impregnation large numbers of organisms can be seen between the epidermal cells. Thus an important biologic difference exists between *T. pertenue,* which is almost entirely epidermotropic, and *T. pallidum,* which is largely mesodermotropic (Hasselmann, 1952).

PINTA

Pinta, like yaws, is caused by a treponema that is morphologically indistinguishable from *T. pallidum.* It is called *Treponema carateum.* Pinta is endemic in Central America. It is not a venereal disease but is transmitted by personal contact. Three stages exist.

The *primary lesion* starts as a red papule, which by peripheral extension grows into an oval or a rounded patch 10 cm in diameter or larger. Often small papules surround the extending primary lesion and gradually merge with it. The lesion shows scaling but no oozing.

In the *secondary stage* disseminated lesions appear. These are called pintids. They, too, show peripheral enlargement and may coalesce. Often they are covered with scales and thus may resemble psoriasis. At first the lesions are red, but later they assume a purple or a slate color, depending on the amount of melanin present in them.

The *tertiary stage* is characterized by the presence of dyschromic lesions that consist of alternating areas of hyperpigmentation and depigmentation resembling vitiligo.

Pinta is a benign but, especially in the tertiary stage, a disfiguring disease. No lesions of the bones, the central nervous system, or the cardiovascular system occur.

Histopathology. The PRIMARY LESION shows mild acanthosis. There is edema of the epidermis with migration of lymphoid cells into the epidermis. The basal layer shows liquefaction degeneration and loss of melanin. The upper dermis contains abundant melanophages. Thus even in this early stage the pigment mechanism is greatly disturbed. In addition to the melanophages, the upper dermis contains a fairly heavy cellular infiltrate composed of plasma cells, lymphoid cells, and occasional histiocytes and neutrophils (Pardo-Castello and Ferrer). Swelling of the endothelium of the dermal blood vessels is either mild or absent (Hasselmann). On silver impregnation the causative organism, *T. carateum,* can be demonstrated in great numbers between the cells of the epidermis.

In the SECONDARY STAGE the lesions show essentially the same histologic changes as the primary lesion, including the presence of many treponemata.

In the TERTIARY STAGE the hyperpigmented areas show atrophy of the epidermis with absence of melanin in the basal layer. The upper dermis, however, contains accumulations of melanophages intermingled with a moderate number of lymphoid cells. Treponemata still are present in considerable number among the cells of the epidermis. The depigmented lesions show atrophy of the epidermis, complete absence of melanin, even in the dermis, no inflammatory infiltrate, and no treponemata. They represent the final stage of the disease. However, some early depigmented lesions still may show a mild inflammatory infiltrate in the dermis and treponemata in the epidermis (Pardo-Castello and Ferrer).

Histogenesis. Electron microscopic examination has revealed in the depigmented areas of tertiary or late pinta the absence of basal epidermal melanocytes (Rodriguez et al.). Langerhans cells, on the other hand, are present; and some of them contain a few melanosomes enclosed within lysosomes.

BIBLIOGRAPHY

Syphilis

Azar, H. H., Pham, T. D., and Kurban, A. K.: An electron microscopic study of a syphilitic chancre. Arch. Path., *90*:143, 1970.

Bhorade, M. S., Carag, H. B., Lee, H. J., et al.: Nephropathy of secondary syphilis. J.A.M.A., *216*:1159, 1971.

Braunstein, G. D., Lewis, E. J., Galvanek, E. G., et al.: The nephrotic syndrome associated with secondary syphilis. Am. J. Med., *48*: 643, 1970.

Ferris, H. W., and Turner, T. B.: Comparative histology of yaws and syphilis in Jamaica. Arch. Path., *24*:703, 1937.

Fisher, D. A., Chang, L. W., and Tuffanelli, D. L.: Lues maligna. Arch. Derm., *99*:70, 1969.

Freeman, H. E.: Juxta-articular nodules. Arch. Derm. Syph., *43*:206, 1941.

Hartsock, R. J., Halling, L. W., and King, F. M.: Luetic lymphadenitis. Am. J. Clin. Path., *53*:304, 1970.

Hasegawa, T.: Electron microscopic observations on the lesions of condyloma latum. Brit. J. Derm., *81*:367, 1969.

Holtzmann, H., and Hassenpflug, K.: Tertiär-syphilitische Lymphknotenbeteiligung vom granulierenden Typ bei einem Kranken mit plattenartigen Gummen der Haut. Arch. klin. exp. Derm., *215*:230, 1962.

Kahn, L. B., and Gordon, W.: Sarcoid-like granulomas in secondary syphilis. Arch. Path., *92*:334, 1971.

Kalz, F., and Newton, B. L.: Syphilitic juxta-articular nodules. Arch. Derm. Syph., *48*:626, 1943.

Kerdel-Vegas, F., Kopf, A. W., and Tolmach, J. A.: Keratoderma punctatum syphiliticum: report of a case. Brit. J. Derm., *66*:449, 1954.

Klingmüller, G., Ishibashi, Y., and Radke, K.: Der elektronenmikroskopische Aufbau des Treponema pallidum. Arch. klin. exp. Derm., *233*:197, 1968.

Lantis, L. R., Petrozzi, J. W., and Hurley, H. J.: Sarcoid granuloma in secondary syphilis. Arch. Derm., *99*:748, 1969.

Metz, J., and Metz, G.: Electronenmikroskopischer Nachweis von *Treponema pallidum* in Hauteffloreszenzen der unbehandelten Lues I und II. Arch. Derm. Forsch., *243*:241, 1972.

Mikhail, G. R., and Chapel, T. A.: Follicular papulopustular syphilid. Arch. Derm., *100*: 471, 1969.

Petrozzi, J. W., Lockshin, N. A., and Berger, B. J.: Malignant syphilis. Arch. Derm., *109*: 387, 1974.

Sobel, H. J., and Wolf, E. H.: Liver involvement in early syphilis. Arch. Path., *93*:565, 1972.

Sohn, D., and Levine, S.: Luetic aneurysms of the aortic valve, sinus of Valsalva, and aorta. Am. J. Clin. Path., *46*:99, 1966.

Tuta, J. A., and Coombs, R. A.: Symmetric syphilitic granulomas of the elbow. Arch. Derm. Syph., *46*:375, 1942.

Wigfield, A. S.: Immunological phenomena in syphilis. Brit. J. Vener. Dis., *41*:275, 1965.

Yobs, A. R., Brown, L., and Hunter, E. F.: Fluorescent antibody technique in early syphilis. Arch. Path., *77*:220, 1964.

Yaws

Guthe, T.: Clinical, serological and epidemiological features of framboesia tropica (yaws) and its control in rural communities. Acta dermatoven., *49*:343, 1969.

Hasselmann, C. M.: Experimental evidence and clinical studies as basis for nomenclature in frambesia tropica (yaws). Arch. Derm., *66*: 107, 1952.

————: Comparative studies on the histopathology of syphilis, yaws and pinta. Brit. J. Vener. Dis., *33*:5, 1957.

Lanigan-O'Keeffe, F. M., Holmes, J. G., and Hill, D.: Infections and active yaws in a midland city. Brit. J. Derm., *79*:325, 1967.

Williams, H. U.: Pathology of yaws. Arch. Path., *20*:596, 1935.

Pinta

Hasselmann, C. M.: Studien über die Histopathologie von Pinta, Frambösie und Syphilis. Arch. klin. exp. Derm., *201*:1, 1955.

————: Comparative studies on the histopathology of syphilis, yaws and pinta. Brit. J. Vener. Dis., *33*:5, 1957.

Pardo-Castello, V., and Ferrer, I.: Pinta. Arch. Derm. Syph., *45*:843, 1942.

Rodriguez, H. A., Albores-Saavedra, J., Lozano, M. M., et al.: Langerhans' cells in late pinta. Arch. Path., *91*:302, 1971.

18

Fungal Diseases

TINEA (DERMATOPHYTOSIS)

Among the dermatophytes causing superficial infections two—*Trichophyton rubrum* and *Pityrosporum orbiculare*—are by far the most common. Still, the following fungi should be listed as potential causes of superficial fungus infections:

Microsporum audouini, M. canis
Trichophyton mentagrophytes, T. rubrum, T. schoenleinii, T. tonsurans, T. verrucosum, T. violaceum
Epidermophyton floccosum
Pityrosporum orbiculare

Clinically, eight regional types of fungal infections can be recognized: tinea capitis, tinea barbae, tinea corporis, tinea cruris, tinea of the hands and feet, onychomycosis, favus, and tinea versicolor.

Tinea capitis presently is caused in the United States mainly by *Trichophyton tonsurans* (Zaslow and Derbes). Formerly—up to about 1960—*Microsporum audouini* and *Microsporum canis* were the fungi most commonly causing tinea capitis. *Trichophyton violaceum* has been the cause in only exceptional cases. In contrast with the two types of *Microsporum* that show fluorescence in Wood's light and cause scalp infections in children only, the two types of *Trichophyton* do not fluoresce in Wood's light and occasionally affect the scalp of adults. In all four types of tinea capitis the affected hairs tend to break off either at the level of the scalp or slightly above it. Whereas *M. audouini*

and *T. violaceum* usually produce only a slight inflammatory reaction, *M. canis* and *T. tonsurans* may result in pronounced inflammation of the affected areas of the scalp, so-called kerion celsi. In addition, *T. tonsurans* often shows follicular pustules.

Tinea barbae, rare in the United States, may be caused by *Trichophyton mentagrophytes* or by *Trichophyton verrucosum (faviforme)*. Infection of the bearded region with *T. verrucosum* is referred to also as cattle ringworm, since usually it is contracted from cattle. Both *T. mentagrophytes* and *T. verrucosum* cause a kerionlike soft, nodular inflammatory infiltration in the bearded region of men (Birt and Wilt). *T. verrucosum* infections may also affect the scalp.

Tinea corporis may be caused by *Microsporum canis* or by *Trichophyton mentagrophytes, T. rubrum,* and *T. verrucosum (faviforme)*, with *T. rubrum* being by far the most common cause in the United States. If caused by *M. canis*, tinea corporis manifests itself as several annular lesions with a raised papulovesicular border and central clearing. If caused by *T. mentagrophytes*, one finds one or at the most a few annular lesions showing little or no central clearing. If caused by *T. rubrum*, there are large patches showing central clearing and a polycyclic scaling border which may be quite narrow and "threadlike." Occasionally, *T. rubrum* causes an asymptomatic perifolliculitis in circumscribed areas. It is seen most commonly on the legs in association with an infection of the soles by *T. rubrum* (Cremer; Wilson et al.); but it may occur in other areas (Mikhail). If caused by *T. verrucosum,* tinea corporis manifests itself as grouped follicular pustules, referred to as agminate folliculitis (Birt and Wilt).

Tinea cruris, usually caused by *Trichophyton rubrum* and occasionally by *T. mentagrophytes* or *Epidermophyton floccosum,* produces sharply demarcated areas, often with a raised border, on the upper and inner surfaces of the thighs opposite the scrotum. From there the eruption can extend to the scrotum and to the perineal and perianal regions.

Tinea of the feet and hands is caused usually by *Trichophyton rubrum* and occasionally by *T. mentagrophytes.* In cases of infection with *T. rubrum* the soles and sometimes also the palms show diffuse erythema and superficial scaling; and in cases of infection with *T. mentagrophytes* the lesions consist of maceration between the toes and an erythematous, vesicular eruption on the soles and palms.

Onychomycosis, caused usually by *Trichophyton rubrum,* shows disintegration of the nail substance.

Favus, rare in this country, is caused by *Trichophyton schoenleinii.* It affects mainly the scalp, where it produces inflammation with formation of perifollicular hyperkeratotic crusts, called scutula. Destruction of the hair ensues. Healing takes place with scarring.

Tinea versicolor, caused by *Pityrosporum orbiculare,* generally affects the upper trunk, where one finds areas of brownish discoloration. The surface of the discolored areas on gentle scraping shows fine branny scaling.

Histopathology. For the demonstration of fungi in histologic sections, two stains can be used: the periodic acid-Schiff (PAS) reaction (see p. 48), staining fungi deeply red, and the methenamine silver nitrate method, staining fungi black. The reason for the positive staining of fungi with the PAS reaction is the presence of cellulose and chitin in their cell walls, two substances that are rich in polysaccharides (Kligman et al.). The PAS reaction of fungi, being caused by polysaccharides, is diastase-resistant, in contrast to the PAS reaction of glycogen. Whenever the

PAS reaction is being used for the demonstration of fungi it is advisable to clear the tissue sections of glycogen by exposing them to diastase prior to the PAS reaction, since glycogen granules may resemble fungal spores (Fetter).

In histologic sections fungi may present two structures: hyphae (or mycelia) and spores. Hyphae are threadlike structures that may be septate or nonseptate; they grow by extending and branching. Spores appear as round or ovoid bodies; they grow by budding.

TINEA OF THE GLABROUS SKIN. In tinea of the glabrous skin, which includes tinea corporis, tinea cruris, and tinea of the feet and hands, fungi occur only in the horny layer of the epidermis, and they never invade hair follicles, with two exceptions—*Trichophyton rubrum* and *T. verrucosum* (see below). In histologic sections stained with the PAS reaction or with methenamine silver nitrate the number of fungi present in the horny layer is small. In infection with *Microsporon* or *Trichophyton* only hyphae are seen, and in infections with *Epidermophyton floccosum* chains of spores are present.

In the absence of demonstrable fungi, no diagnostic picture is presented by fungal infections of the glabrous skin. Depending on the degree of reaction of the skin to the presence of fungi, one sees the histologic picture of an acute, a subacute, or a chronic dermatitis (see p. 98). If blisters are present, as they may be in tinea of the feet or hands due to *Trichophyton mentagrophytes,* they present the histologic picture of intraepidermal "spongiotic" vesicles like those seen in dermatitis.

Two fungal infections of the glabrous skin occasionally are associated with an invasion of hair follicles and a subsequent perifolliculitis, namely, infections with *Trichophyton rubrum* and with *T. verrucosum.*

The *nodular perifolliculitis* caused by *Trichophyton rubrum* shows on staining with the PAS reaction or with methenamine silver nitrate numerous mycelia and spores not only within hair follicles but also in the inflammatory infiltrate of the dermis. The spores present in the dermis may form short chains and may be larger than those present in the hair follicles, especially when located within multinucleated giant cells, up to 6 μm in size (Mikhail). The fungal elements reach the dermis through a break in the follicular wall. The dermal infiltrate shows, besides central necrosis and occasionally also suppuration, lymphoid cells, histiocytes, epithelioid cells and scattered multinucleated giant cells (Wilson et al.).

In the *agminate folliculitis* caused by *Trichophyton verrucosum (faviforme)* one finds, on staining with the PAS reaction, mycelia and spores within hair follicles (Birt and Wilt). The dermis around the hair follicles, however, contains no fungi. Depending on the severity and also on the stage of the inflammatory reaction, one observes in the dermis predominantly either an acute or a chronic inflammatory infiltrate around the hair follicles.

TINEA VERSICOLOR. In contrast to other fungal infections of the glabrous skin, the horny layer in lesions of tinea versicolor contains abundant amounts of fungal elements. *Pityrosporum orbiculare* is present as both hyphae and spores (Fig. 18-1). This combination of hyphae and spores is often referred to as "spaghetti and meat balls."

Histogenesis. The causative fungus of tinea versicolor is *Pityrosporum orbiculare* which occurs on the skin of the trunk in more than 90 per cent of normal subjects as a yeastlike organism consisting only of spores (Roberts). In addition, a few short rods resembling hyphae are seen in 8 per cent of normal subjects. In patients with tinea versicolor, *Pityrosporum orbiculare* becomes dimorphous by forming, in addition to spores, numerous septate hyphae and then becomes pathogenic (McGinley et al.). The reason for this dimorphous transformation may lie in the extracellular accumulation of glycogen in the epidermis that is seen by electron microscopy only in patients with tinea versicolor (Keddie). The thick-walled hyphae of *Pityrosporum orbiculare* are from 1 to 3 μm thick and thus are much thicker than normal horny cells which measure only about 0.3 μm in diameter. Nevertheless, the hyphae are frequently seen not only between horny cells but also inside them (Keddie). In cultures, *P. orbiculare* forms only spores.

TINEA CAPITIS AND TINEA BARBAE. In tinea capitis and tinea barbae, fungi are usually demonstrable in the hair follicles, with the exception of infections due to *Trichophyton tonsurans* or *T. verrucosum (faviforme)*

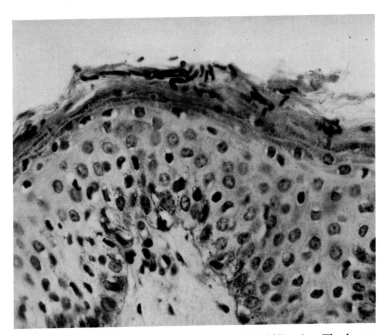

FIG. 18-1. **Tinea versicolor.** Periodic acid-Schiff stain. The horny layer contains hyphae and spores. ($\times$400)

where fungi may no longer be found (see below). The fungi in tinea capitis and in tinea barbae, if still present in the hair follicles, generally are found both within and around the hair. The fungi descend in the hair to a line about 30 μm distal to the zone of keratinization (Graham et al.). The dermis, which contains no fungi, shows a perifollicular infiltrate of varying intensity, depending on the degree of reaction of the patient. The infiltrate is most pronounced in patients with kerion celsi. In addition to a chronic inflammatory infiltrate, multinucleated giant cells may be present in the vicinity of disrupted or degenerated hair follicles (Graham et al.).

Tinea capitis due to *Trichophyton tonsurans* and tinea capitis or barbae due to *T. verrucosum (faviforme)* often show clinically a pronounced kerion celsi reaction and follicular pustules. Histologically, they show a marked inflammatory reaction consisting largely of neutrophils within the hair follicles and a chronic inflammatory infiltrate surrounding the hair follicles. Not infrequently in cases with a severe inflammatory reaction fungi can no longer be demonstrated either by microscopic examination or by culture (Birt and Wilt; Zaslow and Derbes). However, direct immunofluorescent studies with fluorescein-labeled antihuman gamma globulin have shown in such cases reactivity, indicating the presence of antibody within the hair follicles, both inside and around hairs (Zaslow and Derbes).

Favus. Mainly hyphae and only a few spores of *Trichophyton schoenleinii* are present in the stratum corneum of the epidermis, around and within hairs (Fig. 18-2), and in the scutula. The scutula consist of keratinized as well as parakeratotic cells, exudate, and inflammatory cells intermingled with hyphae and spores that are well preserved at the periphery but appear degenerated and granular in the center of the scutula. The dermis shows in active areas a pronounced inflammatory infiltrate containing multinucleated giant cells and many plasma cells in association with degenerating hair follicles. In older areas there is fibrosis with absence of pilosebaceous structures (Graham et al.).

Histogenesis. The formation of kerion celsi in the scalp or the bearded region in response to certain fungi, especially *Microsporon canis,*

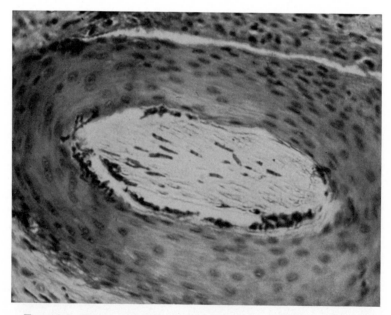

Fig. 18-2. **Favus.** Periodic acid-Schiff stain. The cross section of a hair follicle is shown. The fungus *Trichophyton schoenleinii* is present, largely as hyphae, within and around the hair. ($\times$400)

Trichophyton tonsurans, and *T. verrucosum (faviforme)* can be regarded as an immunologic reaction. In favor of this view are: (1) the tendency to self-healing of lesions of the kerion celsi type; (2) the occasional absence of fungi in markedly reactive lesions caused by *Trichophyton verrucosum (faviforme)* (Birt and Wilt) or by *T. tonsurans* (Zaslow and Derbes); and (3) the presence of antibodies within hair follicles infected with *T. tonsurans* (Zaslow and Derbes).

ERYTHRASMA

Erythrasma is caused by *Corynebacterium minutissimum,* a diphtheroid bacterium rather than a fungus, as had been formerly thought (Sarkany et al.).

Erythrasma shows well demarcated, reddish-brown, slightly scaling patches in intertriginous areas, especially in the groins, or in the axillae, or between the toes. The affected areas show a coral red fluorescence in Wood's light.

Histopathology. The causative organism is present in the horny layer in small amounts as rods and filaments. They are PAS-positive, diastase-resistant.

CANDIDIASIS

Candida albicans is a dimorphous fungus, exhibiting on the skin both yeast and filamentous growth. It exists in a commensal relationship with man. The spectrum of infection may be divided into three groups (Maize and Lynch):

(1) Acute mucocutaneous candidiasis, caused by environmental changes that act either locally, like heat and sweating, or systemically, like antibiotic or corticosteroid therapy. It results in a localized and self-limited infection of intertriginous areas, either alone or in association with oral, vulvar or paronychial lesions.

(2) Acute systemic candidiasis, in which host resistance is depressed. Thus, in patients with advanced lymphoproliferative disorders, especially Hodgkin's disease and leukemia, and debilitated patients under treatment with corticosteroids or immunosuppressive drugs, visceral organs may become involved, usually with fatal outcome. The skin is spared in most instances. Three types of

involvement are recognized, namely, candida meningitis; candida endocarditis occurring usually after cardiac surgery; and disseminated candidiasis affecting most commonly the kidneys but often also the lungs, the brain, the liver, as well as other organs (Bendel and Race; Louria et al.). In the rare instances in which skin lesions are present they consist of papules, pustules and ulcers (Hamada et al.; Balandran et al.).

(3) Chronic mucocutaneous candidiasis, in which defects of cell-mediated immunity lead to widely disseminated cutaneous lesions. Oral, vulvar and paronychial lesions are also often present, but systemic lesions do not occur (Kirkpatrick et al.). Of the three types of chronic mucocutaneous candidiasis, one type (a) is characterized by the congenital absence of the thymus and has lethal immunologic deficiencies as, for instance, the DiGeorge's syndrome associated with hypoparathyroidism, and the "Swiss type" of immunologic deficiency in which there is hypoplasia not only of the thymus but of all lymphoid tissue, resulting in both defective cell-mediated immunity and hypogammaglobulinemia. Death usually occurs before the age of two, not from candidiasis but from viral pneumonia. The second type (b) is associated with nonlethal immunologic deficiencies, and multiple endocrinopathies exist (Montes et al.). While the candidiasis starts in early childhood and often is associated with "candidal granulomas" the endocrine deficiencies, such as hypoparathyroidism, hypothyroidism, hypoadrenalism or diabetes, develop several years later. The third, or adult, type (c) occurs either in patients with benign thymoma (Schoch) or with malignant disease, especially Hodgkin's disease, or in patients receiving prolonged treatment with corticosteroids or immunosuppressive drugs.

Candidal granuloma of the face and scalp, occurring in children as a manifestation of chronic mucocutaneous candidiasis usually in association with endocrinopathies, manifests itself as numerous hyperkeratotic crusted lesions.

Histopathology. *Superficial candidiasis* of the skin has as primary lesion a subcorneal pustule resembling that of impetigo (Maibach and Kligman). In some instances the pus-

TABLE 18-1. Histologic Appearance of the Tissue and the Fungi in Fungal Diseases

Disease	Histologic Appearance of Tissue	Average Size of Spores (Micrometers)	Appearance of Fungus in Dermis
Candidiasis	When invasive: nonspecific chronic inflammatory infiltrate.	4	Hyphae and a few spores.
North American blastomycosis	Epithelial hyperplasia; giant cells and inflammatory infiltrate with formation of small abscesses.	10	Thick-walled spores in giant cells and tissue. Budding forms.
Paracoccidioido-mycosis	Like North American blastomycosis.	30	Spores with multiple budding resembling a marine pilot's wheel.
Chromoblasto-mycosis	Like North American blastomycosis.	10	Thick-walled dark-brown spores, often in clusters. Some cells possess cross walls.
Coccidioido-mycosis	Verrucous nodules: like blastomycosis, except that caseation may occur. Subcutaneous abscesses; central necrosis surrounded by a granulomatous infiltrate.	40	Thick-walled spores with granular cytoplasm. The larger spores contain endospores.
Cryptococcosis	Gelatinous reaction shows many spores; granulomatous reaction shows fewer spores.	7	Spores with wide gelatinous capsule.
Histoplasmosis	Chronic inflammatory infiltrate with foci of necrosis.	3	Numerous spores surrounded by a clear halo lie in the cytoplasm of large histiocytes.
Sporotrichosis	Primary lesion: nonspecific inflammatory infiltrate. Subcutaneous nodules: three zones—suppurative, tuberculoid, and round cell.	5	Usually, spores can be seen only if diastase is used prior to PAS. Occasionally asteroid forms of spores are present.
Actinomycosis	Nonspecific inflammatory infiltrate with abscess formation.	150	Large irregularly lobulated granules with radiating, branching filaments.

tules have a spongiform appearance so that they are indistinguishable from the spongiform pustules of Kogoj seen in pustular psoriasis (Degos et al.; see p. 142). The fungal organisms are present, usually in small amounts only, in the stratum corneum. They consist of hyphae and ovoid spores, some of the latter in the budding stage. The hyphae, which are septate and show branching, measure from 2 to 4 μm in diameter; and the size of the ovoid spores varies from 3 to 5 μm (Table 18-1) (Louria et al.).

Candidal granuloma shows pronounced papillomatosis and hyperkeratosis and a dense infiltrate in the dermis composed of lymphoid cells, neutrophils, plasma cells, and multinucleated giant cells. The infiltrate may extend into the subcutis (Hauser and Rothman). *Candida albicans* usually is present only in the stratum corneum (Hauser and

Rothman; Degos et al.; Kugelman et al.). In rare instances, however, fungal elements are found also within hairs (Hellier et al.) or in the dermis (Papazian and Koch; Ezold and Schönborn).

Acute systemic candidiasis shows in the rarely encountered cutaneous lesions areas of necrosis with spores and hyphae of *Candida albicans* present in the surrounding cellular infiltrate (Hamada et al.; Balandran et al.). In the internal organs there are widespread tangled masses of spores and hyphae, often with only a slight inflammatory reaction (Bendel and Race).

Histogenesis. Of interest is the close relationship existing between chronic mucocutaneous candidiasis and deficient cell-mediated immunity; whereas no such relationship exists to humoral immunity. As evidence of inadequate cell-mediated immunity one finds in patients with chronic mucocutaneous candidiasis: (1) cutaneous anergy on intradermal testing with various antigens, such as *Candida albicans* antigen, PPD tuberculin, etc.; (2) failure to become sensitized through repeated patch tests with dinitrochlorobenzene; (3) poor response of the patient's lymphocytes to in vitro stimulation with either *C. albicans* antigen or phytohemagglutinin, with little or no increase in tritiated thymidine uptake by the lymphocytes; and (4) failure of the lymphocytes to produce macrophage migration inhibitory factor (MIF) when the lymphocytes are incubated with *C. albicans* antigen (Kirkpatrick et al.).

GRANULOMA GLUTEALE INFANTUM

Granuloma gluteale infantum, recently described by Tappeiner and Pfleger, is regarded by some as a manifestation of cutaneous candidiasis (Delacrétaz et al.). Since, however, several observers have failed to find *Candida albicans,* it seems that granuloma gluteale infantum is primarily caused by the prolonged use of corticosteroid creams in infants with diaper dermatitis and that the candidal infection present in some infants is a secondary event (Altmeyer; Uyeda et al.).

Clinically, granuloma gluteale infantum shows asymptomatic, round to oval, smooth, raised nodules, brownish in color, of firm consistency, from 1 to 3 cm in diameter, symmetrically distributed over the buttocks and the inguinal region of infants (Tappeiner and Pfleger).

Histopathology. A dense polymorphous inflammatory infiltrate is seen throughout the dermis composed of various types of mononuclear cells as well as neutrophils and eosinophils (Tappeiner and Pfleger). In some of the cases staining with the PAS reaction or cultures reveal the presence of *Candida albicans* (Uyeda et al.). In addition, fungal elements were observed in the dermis by Delacrétaz et al.

ACRODERMATITIS ENTEROPATHICA

This recessively inherited disorder starts as a rule in infancy and is characterized by (1) a cutaneous eruption on the extremities and in the periorificial areas, (2) diarrhea, and (3) diffuse partial alopecia. The cutaneous lesions consist of areas of erythema associated with vesicles and pustules as well as with scaling and crusting. Paronychia and stomatitis are common. In many patients, but not in all, *Candida albicans* can be cultured from some of the lesions. This is, however, a secondary phenomenon. The cause is a zinc deficiency, and oral therapy with zinc sulfate results in complete healing (Michaelsson).

Histopathology. The blisters in several cases have shown suprabasal separation with acantholytic cells present in the blister cavity (Piper; Rodin and Goldman). In addition to suprabasal clefts, similar clefts may be seen in the midsection of the epidermis or in subcorneal location (Juljulian and Kurban). Thus, distinction from pemphigus may be difficult on a histologic basis.

Autopsy has revealed in one case absence of the thymus and of the germinal centers in the spleen and lymph nodes. However, since the serum immunoglobulins were normal, it is possible that the atrophy of the lymphoid tissue was due to stress (Rodin and Goldman).

ASPERGILLOSIS

Cutaneous aspergillosis usually occurs in patients whose host defenses have been altered either by severe primary disease such as leukemia or by immunosuppressive therapy. In most instances, cutaneous lesions occur as part of a fatal systemic aspergillosis. They may consist of subcutaneous abscesses

(Cawley; Young et al.), intradermal cellulitis (Young et al.), or pustules (Allan and Anderson). In primary cutaneous aspergillosis one to several nodules (Boelaert et al.) or even many nodules (Cahill et al.) may be found.

Histopathology. The skin lesions show intradermal or subcutaneous dissemination of aspergillus hyphae in great amounts. The hyphae are best demonstrated by the methenamine silver stain (Young et al.). The hyphae are septate and show branching at an acute angle (Cahill et al.; Boelaert et al.). They may show terminal bulbous dilatation. Spores are absent. There may be abscesses (Young et al.) or areas of necrosis (Cahill et al.; Boelaert et al.) with a granulomatous response consisting largely of multinucleated giant cells at their periphery (Cawley).

MUCORMYCOSIS

Mucormycosis represents a rare fungal infection occurring in debilitated persons, especially in those with diabetes, leukemia, or extensive burns. The most common sites are the nasal sinuses with rapid spread to the orbit and brain, the lungs, and the intestinal tract; but infection of the palate (Taylor et al.) and of the skin have also been reported. The infection is caused by one of the fungi of the genera *Rhizopus* and *Mucor.*

The clinical findings consist in the case of infection of the nasal sinuses of asymptomatic periorbital edema and ophthalmoplegia; in the case of infection of the palate, of severe tissue necrosis; and in the case of the skin, of indurated nodules (Meyer et al.) or burned areas showing extensive dry, black necrosis (Rabin et al.).

Histopathology. Within areas of nonspecific necrosis or granulation tissue, one observes very large, long, branching nonseptate hyphae (Fig. 18-3) (Taylor et al.). Numerous entangled hyphae may be present as thrombi within dermal blood vessels (Meyer et al.). The hyphae are easily located because of their large size, up to 30 μm in width (Rabin et al.). They stain well with the PAS reaction. No spores are seen.

NORTH AMERICAN BLASTOMYCOSIS

North American blastomycosis, caused by *Blastomyces dermatitidis,* occurs in three forms: primary cutaneous inoculation blasto-

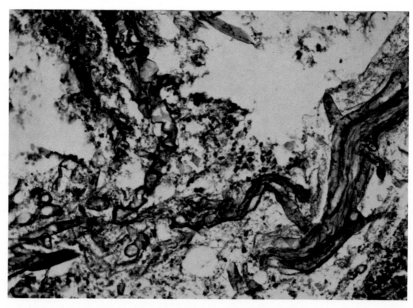

FIG. 18-3. **Mucormycosis.** PAS-stain. Very large, long, nonseptate hyphae are seen within an area of necrotic tissue. The ring-shaped structures represent cross sections of hyphae. (×200)

TABLE 18-2. Some Clinical Data Concerning the "Deep" Fungal Infections

Disease	Occurrence of Primary Cutaneous Inoculation	Existence of a Benign Systemic Form With Only Cutaneous Lesions	May Go On to Generalized Systemic Disease	Lymphoma or Medication With Corticosteroids May Activate the Disease
North American blastomycosis	very rare	very rare	no	
Paracoccidioidomycosis	no	no		
Chromoblastomycosis	no	very common	no	
Coccidioidomycosis	very rare	very rare	no	
Cryptococcosis	no	rare	yes	yes
Histoplasmosis	very rare	very rare	no	yes
Sporotrichosis	very common	rare	yes	yes

mycosis, pulmonary blastomycosis, and systemic blastomycosis (Harrell and Curtis).

Primary cutaneous inoculation blastomycosis is very rare and seems to occur only as a laboratory or autopsy-room infection (Table 18-2). It starts at the site of injury on a hand or wrist as an indurated ulcerated solitary lesion, which has been called chancriform. It is followed by lymphangitis and lymphadenitis of the affected arm. Small nodules may be present along the involved lymph vessel. Spontaneous healing takes place within a few weeks or months (Wilson et al.).

Pulmonary blastomycosis, the usual route of acquiring the infection, may be asymptomatic or produce mild to moderately severe, acute pulmonary signs, such as fever, chest pain, cough, and hemoptysis. In rare instances, acute pulmonary blastomycosis is accompanied by erythema nodosum (Smith et al.). The pulmonary lesions either resolve or progress into chronic pulmonary blastomycosis with cavity formation.

In systemic blastomycosis the lungs are the primary site of infection. Granulomatous and suppurative lesions may occur in many different organs, but most commonly they are found, aside from the lungs, in the skin,

the bones and the central nervous system. The mortality rate of systemic blastomycosis, which prior to the advent of amphotericin B was in excess of 80 per cent, has decreased to about 10 per cent (Witorsch and Utz). It has long been recognized, however, that there is a benign systemic form of blastomycosis in which cutaneous lesions are the only clinical manifestation (Wilson et al.; Macauley; Klapman et al.). It may be pointed out that the same phenomenon of a benign systemic form with only cutaneous lesions occurs, though rarely, in most other deep mycoses subsequent to pulmonary infection, for instance in coccidioidomycosis, cryptococcosis, histoplasmosis, and sporotrichosis, and occurs commonly in chromoblastomycosis (Table 18-2) (Procknow and Loosli).

The cutaneous lesions occurring in systemic blastomycosis may be solitary or may be numerous. They occur in two types: either as verrucous lesions, the more common type, or as ulcerative lesions (Witorsch and Utz). Verrucous lesions show central healing with scarring and a slowly advancing, raised, verrucous border that is beset by a large number of pustules or small crusted abscesses. Ulcerative lesions begin as pustules and develop into ulcers with a granulating base. In addition, subcutaneous abscesses may occur which usually develop as an extension of bone lesions. In the benign systemic form of blastomycosis with only cutaneous lesions, the lesions usually are of the verrucous type. There often are only one or two lesions, with the face being the most common site of involvement (Klapman et al.).

Histopathology. In primary cutaneous inoculation blastomycosis, the primary lesion shows a nonspecific inflammatory infiltrate without epithelioid or giant cells. Numerous organisms, many in a budding state, are present. The nodules that may be found along the lymphatic vessel show an identical histologic picture. The regional lymph nodes, however, already show a granulomatous reaction with numerous giant cells; and the organisms are located predominantly in the giant cells (Wilson et al.).

The verrucous lesions seen in systemic blastomycosis show acanthosis, papillomatosis, and considerable downward prolif-

eration of the epidermis. Intraepidermal abscesses often are present. Occasionally, multinucleated giant cells are completely enclosed by the proliferating epidermis (Fig. 18-4). The dermis is permeated by a polymorphous infiltrate. Neutrophils usually are present in large numbers and form small abscesses in the dermis. Multinucleated giant cells are scattered throughout the dermis. Usually they lie alone and not within groups of epithelioid cells. Occasionally, however, one observes tuberculoid formations but without evidence of caseation necrosis (Moore). In the ulcerative lesions the dermal changes are the same as in the verrucous lesions, but the epidermis is absent.

The spores of *Blastomyces dermatitidis* are fairly numerous in histologic sections. Often, they are found lying free in the tissue, particularly in the abscesses. However, they occur in their largest number within the giant cells. One or several spores may lie within a giant cell (Fig. 18-5). When in this location, the spores are easily spotted,

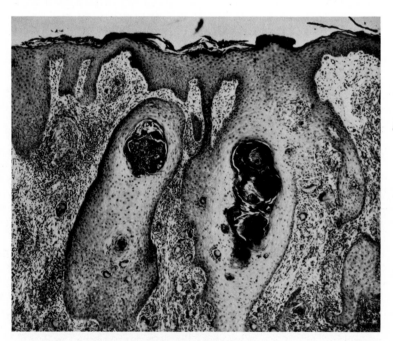

FIG. 18-4. **North American blastomycosis.** Low magnification. There is marked epidermal hyperplasia. Many multinucleated giant cells are present in the dermis and are also enclosed in the downward proliferations of the epidermis. (×50)

even in sections stained with routine stains. Being unstained, the spores resemble small round holes punched out of the cytoplasm of the giant cells. On high magnification the spores are seen to have a thick wall, which gives them a double-contoured appearance. They measure 8 to 15 μm in diameter, and on the average, 10 μm. Occasionally, budding forms are seen in sections. As in most fungal infections, many more spores are visualized in sections stained with the PAS reaction or with methenamine silver than in routinely stained sections.

Of great value is the demonstration of the spores of *Blastomyces dermatitidis* in tissue sections by direct immunofluorescence (Rezai and Haberman; Kaplan and Kraft). The required antiserum is prepared in rabbits with pure cultures of fungi and is conjugated with fluorescein isothiocyanate. The antiserum can be applied to fresh as well as to formalin-fixed tissue sections. Digestion of sections in a 1 per cent trypsin solution for one hour at 37°C., prior to applying the conjugate, enhances the staining reaction. Previous staining with hematoxylin and eosin does not interfere with the procedure.

Corresponding antisera are valuable also for the demonstration of the spores of *Coc-cidioides immitis, Cryptococcus neoformans, Histoplasma capsulatum,* and *Sporotrichum schenckii.*

The histologic appearance of the visceral lesions in North American blastomycosis is analogous to that of the cutaneous lesions. The number of neutrophils often is great, and numerous abscesses may be present (Littman et al.).

Differential Diagnosis. The verrucous lesions of systemic blastomycosis must be differentiated from tuberculosis verrucosa cutis, chromoblastomycosis, and cryptococcosis. Tuberculosis verrucosa cutis shows no spores in the tissue. In addition, the number of neutrophils is smaller, and areas of caseation necrosis usually are present. The distinctive features of chromoblastomycosis and cryptococcosis are discussed under those headings (see below).

PARACOCCIDIOIDOMYCOSIS

Paracoccidioidomycosis, also called South American blastomycosis, is a chronic granulomatous disease caused by *Paracoccidioides brasiliensis.* It is almost invariably fatal in its usual systemic form, unless amphotericin B and sulfonamides are used in treatment

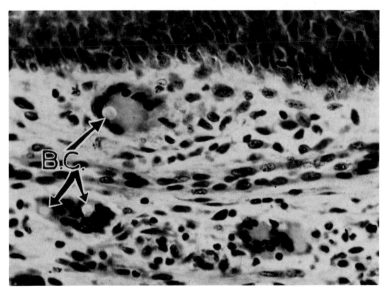

FIG. 18-5. **North American blastomycosis.** High magnification of Figure 18-4. Three blastomyces cells (B.C.), or spores, are shown lying in the cytoplasm of giant cells. ($\times$400)

(Wilson). The disease occurs exclusively in South and Central America, mainly in Brazil.

P. brasiliensis gains entrance into the human body through inhalation. The lungs are the site of the primary infection which may be asymptomatic and then can be recognized only through a positive paracoccidioidin skin test (Londero and Ramos). The primary pulmonary infection may be followed by active pulmonary lesions. From the lungs hematogenous dissemination to other viscera and to the skin can take place.

In systemic paracoccidioidomycosis the lungs are always involved, producing a clinical picture that greatly resembles chronic pulmonary tuberculosis (Salfelder et al.).

In about one half of the patients with systemic paracoccidioidomycosis granulomatous, ulcerated lesions are encountered in the mouth, nose, larynx, or pharynx. The oral lesions may extend to the neighboring skin (Londero and Ramos). Rarely, there are multiple, widely scattered cutaneous lesions as the result of hematogenous dissemination. They may be papular, pustular, nodular, papillomatous or ulcerated (Furtado).

In addition, intestinal lesions may occur, leading to perforation. Adrenal insufficiency due to destruction of the adrenal glands, uncommon in other systemic mycoses except histoplasmosis, is seen occasionally (Murray et al.). Involvement of other organs occurs, but usually is asymptomatic.

Histopathology. Examination of cutaneous or mucosal lesions reveals in some areas a granulomatous infiltrate showing epithelioid and giant cells in association with an acute inflammatory infiltrate and abscess formation (Götz). The fungus spores may lie within giant cells or may lie free in the infiltrate, especially in the abscesses. They are best demonstrated with the PAS reaction or with methenamine silver.

Many of the fungus spores present in the tissue show only single buds or no buds at all; and, in order to detect the diagnostic multiple budding, often many sections will have to be searched (Salfelder et al.). In spores with multiple budding peripheral buds are distributed over the whole surface of the ball-shaped fungus cell. Because of the protrusion of the peripheral buds, the yeast cells in cross sections have the appearance of a "steering wheel" or "marine pilot's wheel." While nonbudding or singly budding spores measure from 5 to 20 μm in diameter, spores with multiple budding may measure up to 60 μm in size.

Occasionally, histologic examination does not reveal spores with multiple budding. The resemblance to North American blastomycosis then is such that cultural studies are necessary for differentiation (Perry et al.).

CHROMOBLASTOMYCOSIS

Chromoblastomycosis may occur in the skin either as a cutaneous or as a subcutaneous infection (Derbes and Friedman). In both types the disease usually remains localized and is benign. Both types formerly were thought to result from the contamination of minor wounds by the fungus present in the soil or in vegetation. In recent years, however, evidence has been accumulating that chromoblastomycosis may be acquired through the inhalation of the spores and that the lesions are produced by hematogenous dissemination (Caplan). This would explain why in occasional cases there are numerous widely disseminated cutaneous lesions (Azulay and Serruya), or widely separated cutaneous lesions (Ariewitsch; Caplan), or osseous lesions (Ariewitsch). Caplan also observed in the chest x-ray film of a patient with chromoblastomycosis multiple areas of calcification in the absence of tuberculin reactivity.

The cutaneous type of chromoblastomycosis is caused by one of four closely related fungi that appear alike in the tissue: *Phialophora verrucosa, Cladosporium carrionii, Fonsecaea pedrosi,* and *Fonsecaea compacta.* The lesions are located usually on the lower extremities and consist of verrucous nodules and plaques. While some of the lesions heal with scarring, new ones may appear in the vicinity as the result of spreading of the fungus through the superficial lymphatic vessels (Derbes and Friedman).

The subcutaneous type of chromoblastomycosis is caused by *Cladosporium gougerotii* (formerly called *Sporotrichum gougerotii).* It consists of a solitary, asymptomatic subcutaneous abscess located most commonly on the hands, forearms, and ankles (Young and Ulrich; Kempson and Sternberg).

Cerebral chromoblastomycosis is caused by a fungus different from those causing cutaneous chromoblastomycosis and is not associated with lesions of the skin. This fungus, called *Cladosporium trichoides,* in contrast to the organisms causing cutaneous chromoblastomycosis, shows not only spores but also mycelia (Symmers; Watson).

Histopathology. The cutaneous type of chromoblastomycosis resembles North American blastomycosis in its histologic appearance. There is considerable hyperplasia of the epidermis. The dermis shows extensive infiltration with a polymorphous granulation tissue containing many multinucleated giant cells and small abscesses composed of neutrophils. Tuberculoid formations may be present, but caseation necrosis is absent, as it is in North American blastomycosis (Moore et al.; French and Russell). In some cases there are numerous aggregates of epithelioid cells, each aggregate having a small abscess in its center (Nödl).

In the subcutaneous type of chromoblasto-mycosis the abscess is lined by a fibrous wall that on its inner side shows a granulomatous reaction composed of histiocytes, epithelioid cells, and usually also giant cells. The center of the abscess consists of necrotic debris and numerous neutrophils (Kempson and Sternberg).

The causative organisms in both the cutaneous and subcutaneous type are found within giant cells as well as free in the tissue, especially in the abscesses. They appear as conspicuous dark-brown, thick-walled, ovoid or spherical spores, varying in size from 6 to 12 μm (French and Russell). They lie either singly or in chains or clusters (Fig. 18-6). Reproduction is by intracellular wall formation and splitting, not by budding. In some of the spores cross walls can be seen.

COCCIDIOIDOMYCOSIS

Coccidioidomycosis is caused by *Coccidioides immitis.* It is endemic in the southwestern United States, especially in the San Joaquin Valley in California, and in northern Mexico. Like blastomycosis it occurs in three forms: primary cutaneous inocula-

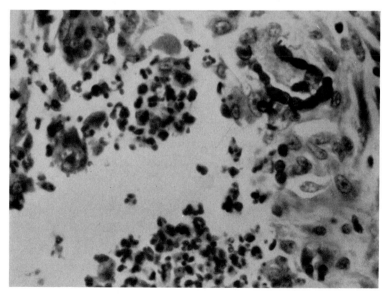

FIG. 18-6. **Chromoblastomycosis.** Periodic acid-Schiff stain. Epithelioid cells and multinucleated giant cells form the wall of an abscess. Two chains of fungal spores are located in the right upper corner. In addition, three fungal spores lie in the right center. ($\times$400)

tion coccidioidomycosis, pulmonary coccidioidomycosis, and systemic coccidioidomycosis (Harrell and Honeycutt).

Primary cutaneous inoculation coccidioidomycosis is very rare. In a few instances it occurred, like primary cutaneous inoculation blastomycosis, as a laboratory or an autopsy-room infection (Wilson et al.; Tremble and Doucette; Overholt and Hornick); but in addition, it has occurred, in contrast with primary cutaneous inoculation blastomycosis, also as a naturally occurring infection through injuries by thorns or splinters (Levan and Huntington; Winn). A tender ulcerated nodule forms at the site of inoculation which may enlarge into a granulomatous, ulcerated plaque. This is followed, as in the case of accidental inoculation with *Blastomyces dermatitidis,* by regional lymphangitis and lymphadenitis. Healing usually takes place within a few months; but in one patient meningitis developed, requiring prolonged intrathecal treatment with amphotericin B (Winn).

Pulmonary coccidioidomycosis, the usual route of infection, is very common in endemic areas; and, on the basis of positive skin tests with coccidioidin, it has been estimated that there are 10 million persons in the United States who have been infected with coccidioidomycosis (Wilson). The infection may be asymptomatic; but in about 40 per cent of those infected, symptoms of an acute respiratory infection develop which usually subside without sequelae. Development of erythema nodosum is not uncommon. In some instances the pulmonary lesions progress into chronic pulmonary disease with cavity formation before finally healing. Cutaneous lesions do not occur.

Systemic coccidioidomycosis follows the primary pulmonary infection in only about 1 of each 1,000 cases. Prior to the availability of amphotericin B, it had a mortality rate of about 50 per cent (Wilson). Many organs, especially the meninges, the lungs, the bones, and the lymph nodes, may be involved. Cutaneous lesions occur in 15 to 20 per cent of the cases (Levan and Huntington). They consist either of verrucous nodules and plaques or of subcutaneous abscesses, which may break through the skin. In rare instances the only clinical manifestation of systemic coccidioidomycosis consists of one or a few cutaneous nodules or plaques, and the prognosis is good (Table 18-2) (Levan and Kwong).

Histopathology. In primary cutaneous inoculation coccidioidomycosis one observes a dense inflammatory infiltrate of neutrophils, eosinophils, lymphoid cells, and plasma cells with an occasional giant cell. Small abscesses may be present (Tremble and Doucette). Spores are present, and in some cases hyphae also (Levan and Huntington). The regional lymph nodes show a well developed granulomatous reaction consisting of epithelioid and giant cells, and spores are found within and outside the giant cells.

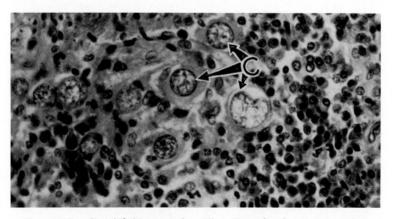

Fig. 18-7. **Coccidioidomycosis.** The *Coccidioides* spores (C) are large—larger than those of other fungi—and show considerable variation in size. Their cytoplasm is granular. (×400)

The nodose skin lesions occurring in primary pulmonary coccidioidomycosis have the same histologic appearance as those in idiopathic erythema nodosum (Winer).

The verrucous nodules and plaques of the skin in systemic coccidioidomycosis resemble blastomycosis in their histologic aspects. However, there is less tendency to abscess formation, and caseation necrosis may occur (Moore). The causative organisms are found as spores free in the tissue as well as within multinucleated giant cells. As a rule, they are present in large numbers.

The subcutaneous abscesses of systemic coccidioidomycosis resemble scrofuloderma in their histologic appearance. Surrounding a central area of necrosis one observes a granulomatous infiltrate that is tuberculoid in type and composed of lymphoid cells, plasma cells, epithelioid cells, and some giant cells. Numerous spores are present extracellularly as well as intracellularly in giant cells (Moore).

The spores of *Coccidioides immitis* vary greatly in size, from 10 to 80 μm (Fig. 18-7). Their average size is about 40 μm. Thus, *Coccidioides* is much larger than either *Blastomyces, Cryptococcus,* or *Phialophora.* The spores are spherical and thick-walled and have a granular cytoplasm. Multiplication takes place by the formation of endospores, which may be seen lying inside the larger spores (Fig. 18-8). The endospores are released into the tissue by rupture of the wall of the spore. Endospores may measure up to 10 μm in diameter.

CRYPTOCOCCOSIS

Cryptococcosis, though quite rare, occurs throughout the world. The causative fungus, *Cryptococcus neoformans,* is found in avian excreta and in the soil. The respiratory tract is the only known portal of entry into the body. The resulting pulmonary cryptococcosis may be symptomatic or asymptomatic. In the latter case the fact that an infection with cryptococcosis has taken place can be established, as in the case of histoplasmosis, only by testing, the most reliable test being the indirect immunofluorescent technique for the presence of circulating antibodies in the patient (Warr et al.).

In patients with active disease cryptococcosis often manifests itself as a widespread systemic disease with predominant involvement of the brain and meninges, and presence of the fungus in the spinal fluid. This form is invariably fatal unless amphotericin B is being administered. Cutaneous lesions are found in 10 to 15 per cent of the cases of systemic cryptococcosis. In rare instances lesions of the oral mucosa also occur (Cawley et al.).

In some instances, systemic cryptococcosis after the primary pulmonary infection, rather than being widespread, may show only one or a few lesions without central nervous system involvement, for instance, in the skin, the lymph nodes, the bones or the eyes (Littman and Walter). In cases in which only cutaneous lesions are present, the disease usually takes a benign course, ending with

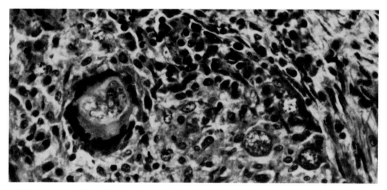

FIG. 18-8. **Coccidioidomycosis.** A large *Coccidioides* spore lies within a giant cell. The *Coccidioides* spore contains numerous endospores. ($\times$400)

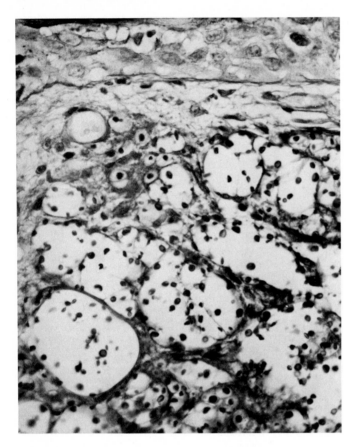

FIG. 18-9. **Cryptococcosis.** A large mass of spores is located directly beneath the epidermis. Each spore is surrounded by a wide gelatinous capsule. (×400) (S. William Becker, M.D.)

healing of the lesions, even without treatment (Gandy; Brier et al.; Rook and Woods). In some instances, however, systemic cryptococcosis with lesions initially limited to the skin is followed by a wide dissemination of the disease, with fatal ending (Table 18-2) (Sarosi et al.).

The cutaneous lesions vary in appearance and may consist of papules, nodules, infiltrated plaques, ulcers, or subcutaneous abscesses (Moore). Ulcers are the most common lesion and they may show a raised, papillomatous border (Hübschmann).

The dissemination of cryptococcosis in the presence of lymphoma, such as Hodgkin's disease (Gendel et al.; Noble and Fajardo) and leukemia (Cawley et al.), has been repeatedly observed as a result of the depressed immune response. For the same reason, the prolonged administration of corticosteroids may be followed by cryptococcosis (Table 18-2) (Ruiter and Ensink; Sarosi et al.; Collins et al.).

Histopathology. Two types of histologic reactions to infection with *Cryptococcus neoformans* may occur in the skin: gelatinous and granulomatous. Both types may be seen in the same skin lesion (Moore). In patients with only cutaneous lesions the reaction is apt to be granulomatous as indication of an effective host response (Noble and Fajardo). Gelatinous lesions show numerous organisms in aggregates and only very little tissue reaction (Fig. 18-9). Granulomatous lesions, on the other hand, show a pronounced tissue reaction consisting of histiocytes, giant cells, lymphoid cells, and fibroblasts; and areas of necrosis may be seen. The organisms are present in much smaller number than in the gelatinous lesions. They are found mainly within giant cells and histiocytes, but they are encountered also free in the tissue.

Cryptococcus neoformans, a spherical to ovoid spore measuring from 4 to 12 μm in diameter, multiplies, as does *Blastomyces dermatitidis,* by budding. Usually it is surrounded by a wide gelatinous capsule. In sections stained with hematoxylin and eosin or with the PAS reaction the capsule does not stain; but it stains metachromatically purple with methylene blue (Linell et al.), blue with alcian blue (Ruiter and Ensink), and red with mucicarmine (Littman and Walter) because of the presence of acid mucopolysaccharides. When the alcian blue stain and the PAS reaction are combined, the yeast cell stains red and the surrounding capsule blue. Generally, yeast cells located within a granulomatous infiltrate, and especially those that have been phagocytized, show only a narrow capsule, and some of them may show no capsule at all.

Histogenesis. The characteristic mucinous capsule of *Cryptococcus neoformans,* on electron microscopy, is seen to consist of a fine, radially arranged fibrillar material, with the fibrils being long and intertwined and having a beaded appearance (Collins et al.).

HISTOPLASMOSIS

Histoplasmosis is caused by the fungus *Histoplasma capsulatum.* This fungus exists in the soil of endemic areas and usually enters the body by inhalation, although in very rare instances it enters by primary cutaneous inoculation. On the basis of positive histoplasmin tests it has been estimated that 30 million persons in the United States have undergone pulmonary infection with *Histoplasma capsulatum,* most of whom live in the central eastern states, where in some areas 80 per cent of the population react positively (Rubin et al.).

The primary pulmonary infection is entirely asymptomatic in approximately 70 per cent of the cases; while in 30 per cent of the infected persons the primary infection produces acute pulmonary histoplasmosis, a disease resembling influenza. Usually, the process heals; it may, however, progress into chronic pulmonary histoplasmosis with cavities, resembling tuberculosis and having a mortality of about 30 per cent, unless it is treated with amphotericin B (Yates). Systemic histoplasmosis occurs in only 1 to 2 of every 10,000 persons infected with histoplasmosis. It is a severe systemic disease

which formerly was almost invariably fatal, but, if adequately treated with amphotericin B, has a mortality of only 7 per cent (Reddy et al.).

Thus histoplasmosis, like blastomycosis and coccidioidomycosis, occurs in three forms: primary cutaneous inoculation histoplasmosis, pulmonary histoplasmosis, and systemic histoplasmosis.

Primary cutaneous inoculation histoplasmosis, a very rare event, is benign and self-limited in duration. It has been reported as an accidental autopsy-room infection (Tosh et al.) and as a penile lesion (Curtis and Grekin). The cutaneous lesion consists of an ulcer and is associated with regional lymphadenopathy.

Systemic histoplasmosis presents a variable clinical picture. Virtually any organ in the body may be involved. Often, the lymph nodes are markedly enlarged. Pulmonary and adrenal involvement may be a prominent feature. Even though amphotericin B has greatly improved the chances of survival it does not, as a rule, prevent the development of adrenal insufficiency in patients having adrenal lesions, so that adrenal insufficiency presently is the commonest cause of death in systemic histoplasmosis (Sarosi et al.).

Cutaneous and especially mucosal lesions occur in about one half of the patients with systemic histoplasmosis (Miller et al.). Most commonly, one encounters indurated plaques that undergo ulceration. In some cases, the skin shows purpuric lesions that may undergo ulceration, or crusted lesions (Miller et al.). Also in some instances a generalized pruritic erythroderma occurs (Samovitz and Dillon; Cramer). This usually is associated with cutaneous or oral ulcers, a feature that is highly suggestive of generalized cutaneous histoplasmosis.

In rare instances, systemic histoplasmosis, instead of disseminating widely, causes only localized lesions either in the oral cavity (Curtis and Grekin; Nejedly and Baker) or in an area of the skin (Symmers) and ultimately heals (Table 18-2).

The simultaneous occurrence of systemic histoplasmosis and lymphoma has been repeatedly described (Ende et al.; Curtis and Grekin). As in other deep mycoses, such as cryptococcosis or sporotrichosis, the depressed immune response induced by lymphoma may cause activation of histoplasmosis.

Histopathology. Histologic examination of a lesion of primary cutaneous inoculation histoplasmosis shows essentially the same findings as the cutaneous and mucosal lesions of localized or widely disseminated systemic histoplasmosis. One finds superficial ulceration and foci of necrosis in a chronic inflammatory infiltrate. A few giant cells may be present (Miller et al.; Nejedly and Baker). The diagnostic feature in all forms of histoplasmosis is the presence of macrophages with abundant cytoplasm that is engorged with numerous spores (Baum et al.; Dumont and Piché).

Histoplasma capsulatum, in sections stained with hematoxylin and eosin, appears as round or oval bodies surrounded by a clear space that is suggestive of a capsule. Including this clear space, the spores measure from 2 to 4 μm in diameter. However, on staining with the PAS reaction or with methenamine silver, *Histoplasma capsulatum* shows no capsule. Instead, the inner portion of the clear space stains more intensely than the center of the spore and thus is shown to represent the cell wall of the fungus, while the outer part of the clear space forms a halo separating the cell wall of the fungus from the cytoplasm of the macrophage. In the past, this halo has been interpreted as an artifact produced by shrinkage of the cytoplasm of the macrophage away from the rigid fungus cell wall (Kligman and Baldridge; Binford). Electron microscopy, however, has shown that the spores of *H. capsulatum* within the cytoplasm of macrophages are enclosed individually in vacuoles, most of which have the aspect of phagosomes, since they are lined by a continuous trilaminar membrane. It is the area between the fungus cell wall and the trilaminar membrane of phagosomes that appears as halo on light microscopy. On electron microscopy, this area is partly filled with granular or cytoplasmic material (Dumont and Piché). *H. capsulatum* is a dimorphous fungus that in culture at temperatures below 35°C grows as a mycelial fungus elaborating large spores (8 to 16 μm) and small spores

(2 to 5 μm). When inhaled only the small spores multiply by budding within macrophages (Rippon).

Differential Diagnosis. The histologic appearance of histoplasmosis, characterized by the presence of parasitized macrophages within a chronic inflammatory infiltrate, is much like that of rhinoscleroma, granuloma inguinale, and cutaneous leishmaniasis. For their differential diagnosis, see Table 19-1, page 335. It may be pointed out, in addition, that only in histoplasmosis the causative organism is stained by the usual fungal stains, such as the PAS reaction and methenamine silver.

SPOROTRICHOSIS

Sporotrichosis, caused by *Sporotrichum schenckii,* occurs in four forms: (1) primary cutaneous inoculation sporotrichosis; (2) asymptomatic pulmonary sporotrichosis; (3) unifocal systemic sporotrichosis; and (4) multifocal systemic sporotrichosis. Primary cutaneous inoculation sporotrichosis is by far the most common of clinically apparent forms. However, the use of the sporotrichin skin test has revealed that in certain areas, such as Louisiana and Arizona, up to 10 per cent of the population have had an asymptomatic pulmonary infection with sporotrichosis (Lynch et al.). Development of either unifocal or multifocal systemic sporotrichosis from an asymptomatic pulmonary infection, although rare, occurs particularly in patients with a depressed immune response as for instance in patients with lymphoma or those receiving corticosteroids for a prolonged period of time (Lynch et al.).

Primary cutaneous inoculation sporotrichosis starts with a painless papule, located most commonly on a hand or arm. It may grow into an ulcer with an elevated border or into a verrucous plaque (Lurie). Subsequently, a chain of asymptomatic nodules appears along the lymph vessel draining the area. These lymphatic nodules may undergo suppuration with subsequent ulceration. Systemic sporotrichosis very rarely develops from primary cutaneous inoculation sporotrichosis, with only one proven instance, reported by Seabury and Dascomb.

Unifocal systemic sporotrichosis subsequent to asymptomatic pulmonary infection may affect the lungs, a single joint or symmetrical joints, the genitourinary tract, and, rarely, the brain (Wilson et al.). Chronic pulmonary sporotrichosis greatly resembles pulmonary tuberculosis (Baum et al.).

Multifocal systemic sporotrichosis nearly always shows widely scattered cutaneous lesions. They start as nodules or as subcutaneous abscesses (Stroud) and undergo ulceration. While some patients have only cutaneous lesions (Krause), others show either from the beginning or in the later course of the disease lytic bone lesions and chronic arthritis (Stroud). Such patients can be improved or cured with potassium iodide given alone or in combination with amphotericin B (Cawley; Parker et al.). Some patients with involvement of many visceral organs or of the brain have died (Collins; Geraci et al.).

Histopathology. Primary lesions of sporotrichosis that are only a few weeks old and are ulcerated usually show a nonspecific inflammatory infiltrate composed of neutrophils, lymphoid cells, plasma cells, and histiocytes (Fetter). If the primary lesion is older and possesses an elevated border or appears verrucous, small intraepidermal abscesses are found in the hyperplastic epidermis; and the dermis, similar to blastomycosis, shows scattered through an inflammatory infiltrate not only giant cells and small granulomas but also small abscesses (Fetter; Lurie; Itani).

The lymphatic nodules of primary cutaneous inoculation sporotrichosis as well as the cutaneous nodules of multifocal systemic sporotrichosis, at first show scattered granulomas within an inflammatory infiltrate. At a later stage, through coalescence, the nodules may show the characteristic arrangement of the infiltrate in three zones: a central "suppurative" zone composed of neutrophils, surrounded by a "tuberculoid" zone and peripheral to it a "round cell" zone of lymphoid cells and plasma cells (Lurie; Stroud).

Usually, it is not possible to recognize the causative organisms of *Sporotrichum schenckii* in sections stained with the PAS reaction. The reason is that, because of their small size and varying shape, the spores cannot be distinguished from glycogen granules that often are present in large numbers and also are PAS-positive. It is, therefore, advisable to clear the tissue sections of glycogen, as Fetter has suggested, by exposing them to a 1:1,000 solution of malt diastase at 37° C. for 1 hour prior to staining them with the PAS reaction. The spores

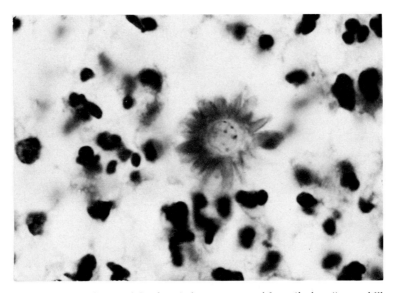

FIG. 18-10. **Sporotrichosis.** A large spore with radiating "asteroid" elongations is shown. (×1350) (Hermann Pinkus, M.D.)

then appear as small, budding, round to oval bodies 4 to 6 μm in diameter that stain more strongly at their periphery than at their center (Fetter and Tindall). In some cases small cigar-shaped bodies 4 to 8 μm in length are also present (Stroud). Asteroid bodies have been observed only rarely in cases of sporotrichosis occurring in the United States (Moore and Ackerman; Pinkus and Grekin). On the other hand, they are found regularly in cases of sporotrichosis occurring in South Africa (Lurie). They show radiating eosinophilic elongations arranged around a central spore (Fig. 18-10). In only a very few cases can clumps of branching, nonseptate hyphae be demonstrated with the PAS reaction (Maberry et al.; Stroud).

Differential Diagnosis. Without finding the fungus in sections a diagnosis of sporotrichosis can only be suspected. The subcutaneous abscesses of tularemia and of systemic coccidioidomycosis may have the same histologic appearance as the cutaneous and subcutaneous nodules and abscesses of sporotrichosis.

ACTINOMYCOSIS

Actinomycosis is caused by *Actinomyces israelii,* an anaerobic or microaerophilic, gram-positive bacterium, formerly thought to be a fungus. *A. israelii* frequently is found as a saprophyte in tonsillar crypts or carious teeth. Actinomycosis usually occurs at three sites: the cervicofacial area, the lungs, and the intestinal tract. Very rarely, *A. israelii,* is one of the organisms causing mycetoma (see p. 327).

Cervicofacial actinomycosis produces an area of "wooden" hardness of the skin over one mandible with multiple draining sinuses discharging purulent material that often contains the characteristic yellowish "sulfur granules."

Pulmonary actinomycosis produces areas of infiltration of the lungs with or without abscess formation. The infection may extend to the thoracic wall, which becomes indurated and shows multiple draining sinuses, often containing "sulfur granules."

Intestinal actinomycosis affects primarily a portion of the intestinal tract, especially the appendix, the cecum, or the rectum, from which multiple draining sinuses extend either to the abdominal wall or to the perineum (Fry et al.). "Sulfur granules" are often present in the discharge.

In rare instances, hematogenous dissemination may lead to intermittently draining, subcutaneous abscesses in widely separated areas (Graybill and Silverman).

Histopathology. Histologic examination

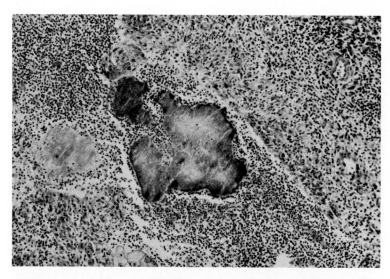

FIG. 18-11. **Actinomycosis.** A large basophilic and lobulated "sulfur granule" of *Actinomyces israelii* is present, measuring several hundred micrometers in diameter. (×100)

of the indurated skin shows extensive granulation tissue containing abscesses that may enlarge into sinuses. The granulation tissue is nonspecific in appearance. In the early phase of the disease the tissue surrounding the abscesses is composed of lymphoid cells, plasma cells, histiocytes, and fibroblasts, while in the late phase fibroblasts may predominate. Thus, the diagnosis can be established only by finding the "sulfur granules." They occur almost exclusively in abscesses or sinuses. Therefore, in selecting a site for biopsy an area containing purulent material should be chosen.

The "sulfur granules" of *Actinomyces israelii* may measure several hundred micrometers in diameter and thus are large enough to be visible macroscopically. In histologic sections the "sulfur granules" appear irregularly lobulated (Fig. 18-11). On staining with hematoxylin and eosin, they appear homogeneous in the center and show clubbing at the periphery (McQuown). On staining with the Gram stain, the center of the granules is seen to consist of basophilic, gram-positive, branching filaments, about 1 μm in diameter. The filaments thus are thinner than the hyphae of the fungi causing maduromycosis (see below) whose diameter varies from 2 to 5 μm (Zaias et al.).

NOCARDIOSIS

Nocardiosis is caused by *Nocardia asteroides,* an aerobic, gram-positive, acid-fast bacterium. Nocardiosis represents a primary infection of the lungs or of the brain, with a tendency to hematogenous dissemination. Very rarely, *N. asteroides* is one of the organisms causing mycetoma, a purely cutaneous infection (see below).

Pulmonary nocardiosis causes abscesses and occasionally draining sinuses of the chest wall, resembling those of pulmonary actinomycosis. In contrast to pulmonary actinomycosis, pulmonary nocardiosis shows no "sulfur granules" in the discharge of the draining sinuses (Robboy and Vickery). Pulmonary nocardiosis, however, shows a much greater tendency to hematogenous dissemination than does pulmonary actinomycosis. It disseminates especially to the brain but also to the subcutaneous tissue and to

many internal organs and then results in death (Welsh et al.).

Histopathology. In the subcutaneous tissue, as well as in other organs, one finds abscesses composed of neutrophils and surrounded by fibroblastic proliferation (Welsh et al.).

The organisms of *Nocardia asteroides* present in the areas of suppuration do not stain with hematoxylin and eosin. Being gram-positive, however, they appear in sections stained with a Gram stain as basophilic, branching filaments, approximately 1 μm in diameter. These filaments, rather than aggregating into sulfur granules, like *Actinomyces israeli,* have a tendency to break up into short segments like *Mycobacterium tuberculosis*. The possibility of confusion with *M. tuberculosis* is increased by the fact that *N. asteroides* nearly always is acid-fast, although not as strongly as *M. tuberculosis*. However, branching of the filaments, as seen in nocardiosis, is not seen in tuberculosis (Peabody and Seabury).

MYCETOMA AND MADUROMYCOSIS

Mycetoma and maduromycosis look clinically alike. Both represent an indolent infection characterized by draining sinuses occurring most frequently on a foot.

Mycetoma is caused by a group of filamentous bacteria, among which *Nocardia brasiliensis* and *Streptomyces madurae* are the most common. In rare instances, *Nocardia asteroides,* commonly the cause of nocardiosis, and *Actinomyces israelii,* commonly the cause of actinomycosis, produce a mycetoma on the hands or feet (Vasarinsh).

Maduromycosis is caused by a group of true fungi with thick, septate hyphae, including *Allescheria boydii, Madurella grisea* and *Madurella mycetomi* (Montes et al.).

Differentiation between mycetoma and maduromycosis is important because of the different responses to treatment. On the one hand, the filamentous bacteria producing mycetoma often respond to treatment with sulfonamides or sulfones (or to treatment with penicillin in cases of infection with the bacterium *Actinomyces israelii*). On the other hand, the fungi causing maduromycosis usually are resistant to all forms of drug therapy.

Although much more common in tropical regions, both mycetoma and maduromycosis are seen occasionally in the United States (Zaias et al.). Both show, usually on a foot but occasionally on a hand, subcutaneous nodules that eventuate in abscesses and draining sinuses. Gradually, the muscles and tendons are damaged, and osteomyelitis develops. Granules are discharged from the draining sinuses. These granules are black in cases of maduromycosis caused by *Madurella grisea* and *M. mycetomi* (Butz and Ajello; Heyd et al.); whereas the grains are colorless in mycetoma and in maduromycosis caused by *Allescheria boydii*.

Mycetoma as well as maduromycosis are local infections without tendency to systemic spreading. This is of particular importance when comparing *Nocardia brasiliensis,* one of the causes of mycetoma, with *Nocardia asteroides,* the cause of nocardiosis, since nocardiosis often ends in fatal systemic dissemination. There is, however, on record the case of one patient in whom *Nocardia brasiliensis* caused a fatal systemic infection; but this patient had multiple myeloma as basic disease (Mahvi).

Histopathology. The histologic picture in mycetoma and maduromycosis is essentially the same as that described for actinomycosis (Khandari et al.; Zaias et al.). The granules are found within abscesses. A Gram stain is of considerable value in distinguishing between mycetoma and maduromycosis, since the delicate, branching filaments within the grains of bacterial mycetoma are gram-positive, whereas the broad, septate hyphae of the fungi causing maduromycosis are not stained with Gram's stain (Zaias et al.). Fungal stains are of no value in distinguishing between mycetoma and maduromycosis, since both the filaments of mycetoma and the hyphae of maduromycosis stain with the PAS reaction and with methenamine silver.

BIBLIOGRAPHY

Tinea and Erythrasma

Birt, A. R., and Wilt, J. C.: Mycology, bacteriology, and histopathology of suppurative ringworm. Arch. Derm., 69:441, 1954.

Cremer, G.: A special granulomatous form of mycosis on the lower legs caused by *Trichophyton rubrum Castellani.* Dermatologica, 107:28, 1953.

Fetter, B. F.: Human cutaneous sporotrichosis due to *Sporotrichum schenckii;* technique for demonstration of organisms in tissue. Arch. Path., 71:416, 1961.

Graham, J. H., Johnson, W. C., Burgoon, C. F., and Helwig, E. B.: Tinea capitis. Arch. Derm., 89:528, 1964.

Keddie, F. M.: A novel cellular reaction caused by tinea versicolor: extracellular glycogen deposits. J. Invest. Derm., 53:363, 1969.

Kligman, A. M., Mescon, H., and DeLamater, E. D.: The Hotchkiss-McManus stain for the histopathologic diagnosis of fungus diseases. Am. J. Clin. Path., 21:86, 1951.

McGinley, K. J., Lantis, L. R., and Marples, R. R.: Microbiology of tinea versicolor. Arch. Derm., 102:168, 1970.

Mikhail, G. R.: Trichophyton rubrum granuloma. Internat. J. Derm., 9:41, 1970.

Roberts, S. O. B.: *Pityrosporum orbiculare*: incidence and distribution on clinically normal skin. Brit. J. Derm., 81:264, 1969.

Sarkany, I., Taplin, D., and Blank, H.: Incidence and bacteriology of erythrasma. Arch. Derm. 85:578, 1962.

Wilson, J. W., Plunkett, O. A., and Gregersen, A.: Nodular granulomatous perifolliculitis of the legs caused by *Trichophyton rubrum.* Arch. Derm., 69:258, 1954.

Zaslow, L., and Derbes, V. J.: The immunologic nature of kerion celsi formation. Dermat. Internat., 8:1, 1971.

Candidiasis

Altmeyer, P.: Die Bedeutung fluorierter Glucocorticoide in der Aetiopathogenese des Granuloma glutaeale infantum (Tappeiner und Pfleger). Z. Haut, 48:621, 1973.

Balandran, L., Rothschild, H., Pugh, N., and Seabury, J.: A cutaneous manifestation of systemic candidiasis. Ann. Int. Med., 78:400, 1973.

Bendel, W. L., Jr., and Race, G. J.: Acute disseminated candidiasis in aplastic anemia. Arch. Intern. Med., 108:916, 1961.

Degos, R., Garnier, G., and Civatte, J.: Pustulose par Candida albicans avec lésions psoriasiformes rappelant le psoriasis pustuleux. Bull. Soc. franç. derm. syph., 59:231, 1962.

Delacrétaz, J., Grigoriu, D., de Crousaz, H., *et al.*: Candidose nodulaire de la région inguinogénitale et de fesses (granuloma glutaeale infantum). Dermatologica, 144:144, 1972.

Ezold, M., and Schönborn, C.: Über ein Granuloma candidamyceticum des Erwachsenen, behandelt mit Amphotericin B. Z. Haut Geschlechtskr., *37*:379, 1964.

Hamada, T., Miyamoto, T., and Nagahama, M.: An autopsy case of candidiasis cutis profunda generalisata. Jap. J. Derm., Series B, *77*:39, 1967.

Hauser, F. V., and Rothman, S.: Monilial granuloma. Arch. Derm. Syph., *61*:297, 1950.

Hellier, F. F., LaTouche, C. G., and Rowell, N. R.: Monilial granuloma treated by amphotericin B in an achondroplastic with bronchiectasis. Brit. J. Derm., *75*:375, 1963.

Juljulian, H. H., and Kurban, A. K.: Acantholysis, a feature of acrodermatitis enteropathica. Arch. Derm., *103*:105, 1971.

Kirkpatrick, C. H., Rich, R. R., and Bennett, J. E.: Chronic mucocutaneous candidiasis: model-building in cellular immunity. Ann. Int. Med., *74*:955, 1971.

Kugelman, T. P., Cripps, D. J., and Harrell, E. R., Jr.: Candida granuloma with epidermophytosis. Arch. Derm., *88*:150, 1963.

Louria, D. B., Stiff, D. P., and Bennett, B.: Disseminated moniliasis in the adult. Medicine, *41*:307, 1962.

Maibach, H. I., and Kligman, A. M.: The biology of experimental human cutaneous moniliasis (*Candida albicans*). Arch. Derm., *85*:233, 1962.

Maize, J. C., and Lynch, P. J.: Chronic mucocutaneous candidiasis of the adult. Arch. Derm., *105*:96, 1972.

Michaelsson, G.: Zinc therapy in acrodermatitis enteropathica. Acta dermatoven., *54*:377, 1974.

Montes, L. F., Bradford, L. G., Lauderdale, R. O., and Taylor, C. D.: Prolonged oral treatment of chronic mucocutaneous candidiasis with amphotericin B. Arch. Derm., *104*:45, 1971.

Papazian, C. E., and Koch, R.: Monilial granuloma with hypothyroidism. New Eng. J. Med., *262*:16, 1960.

Piper, E. L.: Acrodermatitis enteropathica in an adult. Arch. Derm., *76*:221, 1957.

Rodin, A. E., and Goldman, A. S.: Autopsy findings in acrodermatitis enteropathica. Am. J. Clin. Path., *51*:315, 1969.

Schoch, E. P., Jr.: Thymic conversion of *Candida albicans* from commensalism to pathogenism. Arch. Derm., *103*:311, 1971.

Tappeiner, J., and Pfleger, L.: Granuloma glutaeale infantum. Hautarzt, *22*:383, 1971.

Uyeda, K., Nakayasu, K., and Takaishi, Y.: Kaposi sarcoma-like granuloma on diaper dermatitis. Arch. Derm., *107*:605, 1973.

Aspergillosis

Allan, G. W., and Anderson, D. H.: Generalized aspergillosis in an infant 18 days of age. Pediatrics, *26*:432, 1960.

Boelaert, J., Deschilder, J., de Vos, A., and Coninx, S.: Aspergillose cutanée dans un cas de transplantation rénale. Arch. belg. derm. syph., *26*:561, 1970.

Cahill, K. M., El Mofty, A. M., and Kawaguchi, T. P.: Primary cutaneous aspergillosis. Arch. Derm., *96*:545, 1967.

Cawley, E. P.: Aspergillosis and the aspergilli. Arch. Int. Med., *80*:423, 1947.

Young, R. C., Bennett, J. E., Vogel, C. L., *et al.*: Aspergillosis. Medicine, *49*:147, 1970.

Mucormycosis

Meyer, R. D., Kaplan, M. H., Ang, M., and Armstrong, D.: Cutaneous lesions in disseminated mucormycosis. J.A.M.A., *225*:737, 1973..

Rabin, E. R., Lundberg, G. D., and Mitchell, E. T.: Mucormycosis in severely burned patients. New Eng. J. Med., *264*:1286, 1961.

Taylor, R., Shklar, G., Budson, R., and Hackett, R.: Mucormycosis of the oral mucosa. Arch. Derm., *89*:419, 1964.

North American Blastomycosis

Harrell, E. R., and Curtis, A. C.: North American blastomycosis. Am. J. Med., *27*:750, 1959 (review).

Kaplan, W., and Kraft, D. E.: Demonstration of pathogenic fungi in formalin-fixed tissues by immunofluorescence. Am. J. Clin. Path., *52*:420, 1969.

Klapman, M. H., Superfon, N. P., and Solomon, L. M.: North American blastomycosis. Arch. Derm., *101*:653, 1970.

Littman, M. L., Wicker, E. H., and Warren, A. S.: Systemic North American blastomycosis. Am. J. Path., *24*:339, 1948.

Macaulay, W. L.: Is cutaneous blastomycosis a systemic disease? Arch. Derm., *73*:560, 1956.

Moore, M.: Mycotic granulomata and cutaneous tuberculosis: a comparison of the histopathologic response. J. Invest. Derm., *6*:149, 1945.

Procknow, J. J., and Loosli, C. G.: Treatment of the deep mycoses. Arch. Intern. Med., *101*:765, 1958.

Rezai, H. R., and Haberman, S.: The use of immunofluorescence for identification of yeast-like fungi in human infections. Am. J. Clin. Path., *46*:433, 1966.

Smith, J. G., Jr., Harris, J. S., Conant, N. F., and Smith, D. T.: An epidemic of North American blastomycosis. J.A.M.A., *158*:641, 1955.

Wilson, J. W., Cawley, E. P., Weidman, F. D., and Gilmer, W. S.: Primary cutaneous North American blastomycosis. Arch. Derm., *71*:39, 1955.

Witorsch, P., and Utz, J. P.: North American blastomycosis: a study of 40 patients. Medicine, *47*:169, 1968.

Paracoccidioidomycosis

Furtado, T. A.: Mechanism of infection in South American blastomycosis. Derm. tropica, *2*:27, 1963.

Götz, H.: Klinische und experimentelle Studien über das Granuloma paracoccidioides. Arch. f. Derm. u. Syph., *198*:507, 1954.

Londero, A. T., and Ramos, C. D.: Paracoccidioidomycosis. Am. J. Med., *52*:771, 1972.

Murray, H. W., Littman, M. L., and Roberts, R. B.: Disseminated paracoccidioidomycosis (South American blastomycosis). Am. J. Med., *56*:209, 1974.

Perry, H. O., Weed, L. A., and Kierland, R. R.: South American blastomycosis. Arch. Derm. Syph., *70*:477, 1954.

Salfelder, K., Doehnert, G., and Doehnert, H. R.: Paracoccidioidomycosis. Anatomic study with complete autopsies. Virchows Arch. (Abt. A, Path. Anat.), *348*:51, 1969.

Wilson, J. W.: Therapy of systemic fungus infections in 1961. Arch. Int. Med., *108*:292, 1961.

Chromoblastomycosis

Ariewitsch, A. M.: Über die Metastasierung der Chromomykose-Infektion. Derm. Wschr., *153*:685, 1967.

Azulay, R. D., and Serruya, J.: Hematogenous dissemination in chromoblastomycosis. Arch. Derm., *95*:57, 1967.

Caplan, R. M.: Epidermoid carcinoma arising in extensive chromoblastomycosis. Arch. Derm., *97*:38, 1968.

Derbes, V. J., and Friedman, L.: Chromoblastomycosis. Derm. tropica, *3*:201, 1964.

French, A. J., and Russell, S. R.: Chromoblastomycosis. Arch. Derm. Syph., *67*:129, 1953.

Kempson, R. L., and Sternberg, W. H.: Chronic subcutaneous abscess caused by pigmented fungi, a lesion distinguishable from cutaneous chromoblastomycosis. Am. J. Clin. Path., *39*:598, 1963.

Moore, M., Cooper, Z. K., and Weiss, R. S.: Chromomycosis (chromoblastomycosis). J.A.M.A., *122*:1237, 1943.

Nödl, F.: Zur Histologie der Chromomykose. Z. Haut Geschlechtskr., *35*:305, 1963.

Symmers, W. S. C.: A case of chromoblastomycosis (cladosporiosis) occurring in Britain as a complication of polyarteritis treated with cortisone. Brain, *83*:37, 1960.

Watson, K. C.: Cerebral chromoblastomycosis. J. Path. Bact., *84*:233, 1962.

Young, J. M., and Ulrich, E.: Sporotrichosis produced by *Sporotrichum gougeroti*. Arch. Derm., *67*:44, 1953.

Coccidioidomycosis

Harrell, E. R., and Honeycutt, W. M.: Coccidioidomycosis, a traveling fungus disease. Arch. Derm., *87*:188, 1963.

Levan, N. E., and Huntington, R. W., Jr.: Primary cutaneous coccidioidomycosis in agricultural workers. Arch. Derm., *92*:215, 1965.

Levan, N. E., and Kwong, M. Q.: Coccidioidomycosis: persistent pulmonary lesion, solitary "disseminated" lesion of face. Arch. Derm., *87*:511, 1963.

Moore, M.: Mycotic granulomata and cutaneous tuberculosis: a comparison of the histopathologic response. J. Invest. Derm., *6*:149, 1945.

Overholt, E. L., and Hornick, R. B.: Primary cutaneous coccidioidomycosis. Arch. Intern. Med., *114*:149, 1964.

Tremble, J. R., and Doucette, J.: Primary cutaneous coccidioidomycosis. Arch. Derm., *74*:405, 1956.

Wilson, J. W.: Factors which may increase severity of coccidioidomycosis. Lab. Invest., *11*:1146, 1962.

Wilson, J. W., Smith, C. E., and Plunkett, O. A.: Primary cutaneous coccidioidomycosis—the criteria for diagnosis and a report of a case. Calif. Med., *79*:233, 1955.

Winer, L. H.: Histopathology of the nodose lesion of acute coccidioidomycosis. Arch. Derm. Syph., *61*:1010, 1950.

Winn, W. A.: Primary cutaneous coccidioidomycosis. Arch. Derm., *92*:221, 1965.

Cryptococcosis

Brier, R. L., Mopper, C., and Stone, J.: Cutaneous cryptococcosis. Arch. Derm., *75*:262, 1957.

Cawley, E. P., Grekin, R. H., and Curtis, A. C.: Torulosis. J. Invest. Derm., *14*:327, 1950.

Collins, D. N., Oppenheim, J. A., and Edwards, M. R.: Cryptococcosis associated with systemic lupus erythematosus. Arch. Path., *91*:78, 1971.

Gandy, W. M.: Primary cutaneous cryptococcosis. Arch. Derm. Syph., *62*:97, 1950.

Hübschmann, K., Trapl, J., and Fragner, P.: Zum Problem der Diagnostik und Pathogenese der Kryptokokkose. Hautarzt, *10*:534, 1959.

Linell, F., Magnusson, B., and Norden, A.: Cryptococcosis. Acta dermatoven., *33*:103, 1953.

Littman, M. L., and Walter, J. E.: Cryptococcosis: Current status. Am. J. Med., *45*:922, 1968 (review).

Moore, M.: Cryptococcosis with cutaneous manifestations. J. Invest. Derm., *28*:159, 1957.

Noble, R. C., and Fajardo, L. F.: Primary cutaneous cryptococcosis. Am. J. Clin. Path., *57*:13, 1972.

Rook, A., and Woods, B.: Cutaneous cryptococcosis. Brit. J. Derm., *74*:43, 1962.

Ruiter, M., and Ensink, G. J.: Acute primary cutaneous cryptococcosis. Dermatologica, *128*:185, 1964.

Sarosi, G. A., Silberfarb, P. M., and Tosh, F. E.: Cutaneous cryptococcosis, a sentinel of disseminated disease. Arch. Derm., *104*:1, 1971.

Warr, W., Bates, J. H., and Stone, A.: The spectrum of pulmonary cryptococcosis. Ann. Int. Med., *69*:1109, 1968.

Histoplasmosis

Baum, G. L., Schwarz, J., Slot, W. J. B., and Straub, M.: Mucocutaneous histoplasmosis. Arch. Derm., *76*:4, 1957.

Binford, C. H.: Histoplasmosis. Tissue reactions and morphologic variations of the fungus. Am. J. Clin. Path., *25*:25, 1955.

Cramer, H. J.: Erythrodermatische Hauthistoplasmose. Dermatologica, *146*:249, 1973.

Curtis, A. C., and Grekin, J. N.: Histoplasmosis. J.A.M.A., *134*:1217, 1947.

Dumont, A., and Piché, C.: Electron microscopic study of human histoplasmosis. Arch. Path., *87*:168, 1969.

Ende, N., Pizzolato, P., and Ziskind, J.: Hodgkin's disease associated with histoplasmosis. Cancer, *5*:763, 1952.

Kligman, A. M., and Baldridge, G. D.: Morphology of *Sporotrichum schenckii* and *Histoplasma capsulatum* in tissue. Arch. Path., *51*:567, 1951.

Miller, H. E., Keddie, F. M., Johnstone, H. G., and Bostick, W. L.: Histoplasmosis. Arch. Derm. Syph., *56*:715, 1947 (review of cutaneous lesions).

Nejedly, R. F., and Baker, L. A.: Treatment of localized histoplasmosis with 2-hydroxystilbamidine. Arch. Intern. Med., *95*:37, 1955.

Reddy, P., Gorelick, D. F., Brasher, C. A., and Larsh, H.: Progressive disseminated histoplasmosis as seen in adults. Am. J. Med., *48*:629, 1970.

Rippon, J. W.: Medical Mycology. p. 323. Philadelphia, W. B. Saunders, 1974.

Rubin, H., Furculow, M. L., Yates, J. L., and Brasher, C. A.: The course and prognosis of histoplasmosis. Am. J. Med., *27*:278, 1959.

Samovitz, M., and Dillon, T. K.: Disseminated histoplasmosis presenting as exfoliative erythroderma. Arch. Derm., *101*:216, 1970.

Sarosi, G. A., Voth, D. W., Dahl, B. A., et al.: Disseminated histoplasmosis: result of long-term follow-up. Ann. Int. Med., *75*:511, 1971.

Symmers, W. S. C.: Localized cutaneous histoplasmosis. Brit. Med. J., *2*:790, 1956.

Tosh, F. E., Balhuizen, J., Yates, J. L., and Brasher, C. A.: Primary cutaneous histoplasmosis. Arch. Intern. Med., *114*:118, 1964.

Yates, J. L.: Course and prognosis of untreated histoplasmosis. J.A.M.A., *177*:292, 1961.

Sporotrichosis

Baum, G. L., Donnerberg, R. L., Stewart, D., et al.: Pulmonary sporotrichosis. New Eng. J. Med., *280*:410, 1969.

Cawley, E. P.: Sporotrichosis, a protean disease, with report of a disseminated subcutaneous gummatous case of the disease. Ann. Intern. Med., *30*:1287, 1949.

Collins, W. T.: Disseminated ulcerating sporotrichosis with widespread visceral involvement. Arch. Derm. Syph., *56*:523, 1947.

Fetter, B. F.: Human cutaneous sporotrichosis. Arch. Path., *71*:416, 1961.

Fetter, B. F., and Tindall, J. F.: Cutaneous sporotrichosis. Arch. Path., *78*:613, 1964.

Geraci, J. E., Dry, T. J., Ulrich, J. A., et al.: Experiences with 2-hydroxystilbamadine in systemic sporotrichosis. Arch. Intern. Med., *96*:478, 1955.

Itani, Z.: Die Sporotrichose. Hautarzt, *22*:110, 1971.

Krause, H.: Kasuistischer Beitrag zur Sporotrichose. Hautarzt, *19*:428, 1968.

Lurie, H. I.: Histopathology of sporotrichosis. Arch. Path., *75*:421, 1963.

Lynch, P. J., Voorhees, J. J., and Harrell, E. R.: Systemic sporotrichosis. Ann. Int. Med., *73*:23, 1970 (review).

Maberry, J. D., Mullins, J. F., and Stone, O. J.: Sporotrichosis with demonstration of hyphae in human tissue. Arch. Derm., *93*:65, 1966.

Male, O.: Diagnostische und therapeutische Probleme bei der kutanen Sporotrichose. Z. Haut, *49*:505, 1974.

Moore, M., and Ackerman, L. V.: Sporotrichosis with radiate formation in tissue. Arch. Derm. Syph., *52*:253, 1946.

Parker, J. D., Sarosi, G. A., and Tosh, F. E.: Treatment of extracutaneous sporotrichosis. Arch. Int. Med., *125*:858, 1970.

Pinkus, H., and Grekin, J. N.: Sporotrichosis with asteroid tissue forms. Arch. Derm. Syph., *61*:813, 1950.

Seabury, J. H., and Dascomb, H. E.: Experience with amphotericin B for the treatment of systemic mycoses. Arch. Int. Med., *102*:960, 1958.

Stroud, J. D.: Sporotrichosis presenting as pyoderma gangrenosum. Arch. Derm., *97*:667, 1968.

Wilson, D. E., Mann, J. J., Beanett, J. E., and Utz, J. P.: Clinical features of extracutaneous sporotrichosis. Medicine, *46*:265, 1967.

Actinomycosis

Fry, G. R., Martin, W. J., Dearing, W. H., and Culp, C. E.: Primary actinomycosis of the rectum. Proc. Mayo Clin., *40*:296, 1965.

Graybill, J. R., and Silverman, B. D.: Sulfur granules. Arch. Int. Med., *123*:430, 1969.

McQuown, A. L.: Actinomycosis and nocardiosis. Am. J. Clin. Path., *25*:2, 1965.

Zaias, N., Taplin, D., and Rebell, G.: Mycetoma. Arch. Derm., *99*:215, 1969.

Nocardiosis

Peabody, J. W., and Seabury, J. H.: Actinomycosis and nocardiosis. Am. J. Med., *28*:99, 1960.

Robboy, S. J., and Vickery, A. J., Jr.: Tinctorial and morphological properties distinguishing actinomycosis and nocardiosis. New Eng. J. Med., *282*:593, 1970.

Welsh, J. D., Rhoades, E. R., and Jaques, W.: Disseminated nocardiosis involving spinal cord. Arch. Intern. Med., *108*:73, 1961.

Mycetoma and Maduromycosis

Butz, W. C., and Ajello, L.: Black grain mycetoma. Arch. Derm., *104*:197, 1971.

Heyd, H., Krempl-Lamprecht, L., and Wilhelm, K.: Zur Kasuistik des Mycetoms. Hautarzt, *22*:218, 1971.

Khandhari, K. C., Mohapatra, L. N., Sehgal, V. N., and Gugnani, H. C.: Black grain mycetoma of foot. Arch. Derm., *89*:867, 1964.

Mahvi, T. A.: Disseminated nocardiosis caused by *Nocardia brasiliensis.* Arch. Derm., *89*: 426, 1964.

Montes, L. F., Freeman, R. G., and McClarin, W.: Maduromycosis due to *Madurella grisea.* Arch. Derm., *99*:74, 1969.

Vasarinsh, P.: Primary cutaneous nocardiosis. Arch. Derm., *98*:489, 1968.

Zaias, N., Taplin, D., and Rebell, G.: Mycetoma. Arch. Derm., *99*:215, 1969.

19

Diseases Caused by Protozoa

Three different diseases are caused by *Leishmania*: oriental leishmaniasis, caused by *Leishmania tropica*; American leishmaniasis caused by *Leishmania brasiliensis*; and Kala-azar, caused by *Leishmania donovani*. These three types of leishmania cannot be differentiated morphologically. However, they differ immunologically.

ORIENTAL LEISHMANIASIS

Oriental leishmaniasis, also called cutaneous leishmaniasis, is endemic in many countries of the Middle East, of Central Asia and of Africa, especially in Turkey, Syria and India. It is a benign, though often disfiguring disease that remains limited to the skin. It is transmitted by sandflies of the genus *Phlebotomus,* most commonly by *P. papatasii.*

The clinical manifestations of oriental leishmaniasis can be divided into acute leishmaniasis, chronic leishmaniasis, and leishmaniasis recidivans (Farah and Malak).

Acute leishmaniasis designates primary lesions lasting one year or less. Ordinarily, a single lesion is seen. Multiple lesions occur occasionally and are the result of multiple infective bites by the sandfly (Farah and Malak). The lesions start as papules that grow into nodules that usually ulcerate and heal with a depressed scar.

Chronic leishmaniasis refers to primary lesions lasting longer than one year, and, possibly, for several years. This occurs in 3 to 10 per cent of the cases (Hart et al.).

One, and occasionally several, red, raised, nonulcerated plaques are present. In their clinical appearance the lesions of chronic leishmaniasis greatly resemble those of lupus vulgaris.

Leishmaniasis recidivans shows circinate papules at or near the periphery of scars of previously healed primary lesions. It represents a reactivation, rather than a reinfection.

Histopathology. In acute leishmaniasis, during the first few months, the dermal infiltrate consists predominantly of large macrophages filled with great numbers of leishmania organisms (Fig. 19-1). In addition, lymphoid cells and a few plasma cells are present. When ulceration sets in, a secondary infiltration with neutrophils occurs. Although the leishmania organisms are present mainly within macrophages, often they are found also extracellularly (Kurban et al.). The parasitized macrophages measure 20 to 30 μm in diameter. Primary lesions, after several months' duration, gradually show the development of a tuberculoid infiltrate with a considerable diminution in the number of macrophages (Lagerholm et al.). As the number of macrophages diminishes, the number of organisms decreases correspondingly. In the stage of healing no organisms may be detectable so that the diagnosis can be made only by means of culture or skin-testing.

In chronic leishmaniasis, one finds a tuberculoid infiltrate that often is indistinguishable from that of lupus vulgaris. However,

333

the lack of caseation necrosis and the sparsity of plasma cells in the infiltrate may help in the distinction (Kurban et al.). A few leishmania organisms can be found occasionally on careful searching (Kurban et al.; Farah and Malak).

In leishmaniasis recidivans the histologic changes combine features of both the acute and the chronic forms. The dermis shows an infiltrate of macrophages, lymphoid cells and some plasma cells as well as tuberculoid granulomas. Leishman bodies are rarely seen (Farah and Malak).

The leishmania organisms, which represent a protozoon, appear in sections as round to oval bodies from 2 to 4 μm in size. They have no capsule. Within the body there is a relatively large, deeply basophilic, round nucleus, about 1 μm in diameter, and, in addition, a small rodlike paranucleus, or kinetoplast. Although visible in routine stains, leishmania organisms are seen best when a Giemsa stain is used. With this stain the nucleus and the kinetoplast appear bright red.

Histogenesis. On electron microscopy, leishmania tropica is surrounded by a trilaminar membrane. The nucleus is located in the posterior portion of the organism (Pham et al.). The kinetoplast, located in the center, has an amorphous structure. The flagellum is located in a pocket or sheath that communicates with the surface of the organism. The flagellum is attached at its base to the kinetoplast (Nicolay and Bourlond-Reinert). When the parasite changes into its flagellate form outside the human body, either in the animal host or in the culture medium, the flagellum, as it increases in size, is released into the extracellular space near the anterior pole of the parasite.

Differential Diagnosis. The leishmania organisms can easily be differentiated from other parasites by the presence of a nucleus and a kinetoplast within the organism.

In addition to leishmaniasis, three other cutaneous diseases are characterized by an infiltrate containing large parasitized macrophages. They are rhinoscleroma and granuloma inguinale, which are caused by bacteria, and histoplasmosis, caused by a fungus. In spite of great similarities, these four diseases have points of differentiation that in most instances make a histologic diagnosis possible (see Table 19-1).

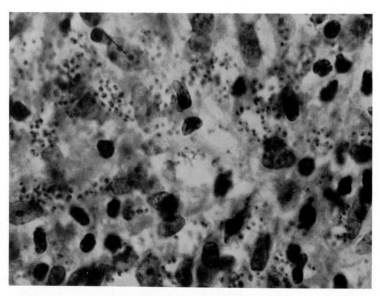

FIG. 19-1. **Oriental leishmaniasis, acute type.** Numerous leishmania organisms are present within macrophages and free in the tissue. Leishmania organisms possess a nucleus and a small paranucleus or kinetoplast. ($\times$600)

TABLE 19-1. Points of Differentiation of Four Cutaneous Diseases Showing Parasitized Macrophages

Disease	Distinctive Features in the Histologic Appearance of the Infiltrate	Size of the Organism (Micrometers)	Appearance of the Organism in the Tissue
Rhinoscleroma	Mikulicz cells, on the average, are larger than the parasitized macrophages in the other three diseases. There are more plasma cells than in the other three diseases. Russell bodies are present.	2-5	Encapsulated round or oval bodies.
Granuloma inguinale	Small abscesses composed of neutrophils are scattered through the infiltrate.	1-2 (smaller than in the other three diseases)	Encapsulated round or oval bodies.
Histoplasmosis	Foci of necrosis are common.	2-4	Round or oval bodies surrounded by a clear halo.
Leishmaniasis		2-4	Not encapsulated round or oval bodies containing a nucleus and a paranucleus.

AMERICAN LEISHMANIASIS

American leishmaniasis, also called mucocutaneous leishmaniasis, is caused by *Leishmania brasiliensis*. It occurs in South America, especially in Brazil and Peru, and less frequently in Central America. It is transmitted by flies of the genus *Phlebotomus*.

The initial lesion has the same appearance as in oriental leishmaniasis, but instead of healing after some months, the initial lesion increases greatly in size and becomes either ulcerated or papillomatous. In addition, new nodules and ulcers develop as the result of lymphatic or hematogenous dissemination. After several years, destructive mucosal lesions form in about 25 per cent of the patients, particularly in the nose, the mouth, and the pharynx. They are referred to as "espundia."

A variant of American leishmaniasis with very extensive skin lesions is the disseminated anergic form in which nodules, plaques and ulcerated lesions are widely scattered. Involvement of mucous membranes either is absent (Convit et al.) or consists of minimal lesions of the nasal mucosa (Convit and Kerdel-Vegas; Simpson et al.).

Histopathology. In early lesions one observes, just as in oriental leishmaniasis, macrophages containing leishmania organisms. However, the number of organisms is as a rule smaller than in oriental leishmaniasis. Usually, a few tuberculoid granulomas are also present (Snow et al.). The ulcerative mucosal lesions show predominantly a nonspecific inflammatory infiltrate. There are only a few leishmania organisms within macrophages and few or no tuberculoid formations (Fasal). In the presence of only a few organisms the diagnosis can be established by indirect immunofluorescent testing of the patient's serum for specific antibodies and by culture of aspirates from the lesions on 15 per cent rabbit-blood agar (Walton et al.).

In the disseminated anergic form of American leishmaniasis, on the other hand, the lesions contain numerous macrophages with abundant cytoplasm that is filled with numerous leishmania organisms. The presence of such large numbers of leishmania organisms is the result of an anergic state, as is shown by a negative intradermal test with leishmanin (Convit et al.; Simpson et al.).

POST-KALA-AZAR DERMAL LEISHMANIASIS

Kala-azar, caused by *Leishmania donovani,* is characterized by chronic, irregular fever, anemia, weight loss, and marked enlargement of the spleen and often also of the liver. Several years after apparent recovery there may occur, especially in India, three types of lesions: hypopigmented macular lesions, erythematous lesions, and nodular lesions (Gupta and Bhattacharjee). The hypopigmented macules are found predominantly on the trunk, and the erythematous lesions as patches on the face, often in a butterfly distribution (Yesudian and Thambiah). The nodules, which are asymptomatic and rarely larger than 1 cm in diameter, occur predominantly on the face and to a lesser extent also on the trunk and extremities (Frain-Bell).

Histopathology. The hypopigmented lesions show a decrease in the amount of melanin in the epidermis. The dermis shows a mild cellular infiltrate of macrophages, lymphoid cells, and a few plasma cells. Small numbers of leishmania organisms may be found in some of the macrophages.

The erythematous lesions also show a decrease in melanin in the epidermis. The cellular infiltrate is more pronounced than in the hypopigmented lesions and contains a larger proportion of plasma cells. Leishmania organisms are somewhat more numerous than in the hypopigmented lesions (Gupta and Bhattacharjee).

The nodular lesions show, separated from the epidermis by a narrow zone of normal collagen and extending into the subcutaneous fat, a compact cellular infiltrate composed largely of macrophages and epithelioid cells intermingled with lymphoid cells (Yesudian and Thambiah). In addition, there may be numerous plasma cells (Frain-Bell). Occasionally, a few giant cells are present. The number of leishmania organisms present within the macrophages is small, but usually some can be found (Gupta and Bhattacharjee). In cases in which they are difficult to find, cultures will confirm the diagnosis.

BIBLIOGRAPHY

Oriental Leishmaniasis

Farah, F. S., and Malak, J. A.: Cutaneous leishmaniasis. Arch. Derm., *103*:467, 1971.

Hart, M., Livingood, C. S., Goltz, R. W., and Totonchy, M.: Late cutaneous leishmaniasis. Arch. Derm., *99*:455, 1969.

Kurban, A. K., Malak, J. A., Farah, F., and Chaglassian, H. T.: Histopathology of cutaneous leishmaniasis. Arch. Derm., *93*:396, 1966.

Lagerholm, B., Gip, L., and Lodin, A.: The histopathological and cytological diagnosis of cutaneous leishmaniasis in two cases of *Leishmania tropica.* Acta dermatoven., *48*:60, 1968.

Nicolay, M., and Bourlond-Reinert, L.: Une leishmaniose cutanée. Arch. belges derm., *29*:327, 1973.

Pham, T. D., Azar, H. A., Moscovic, E. A., and Kurban, A. K.: The ultrastructure of *Leishmania tropica* in the oriental sore. Ann. Trop. Med. Parasitol., *64*:1, 1970.

American Leishmaniasis

Convit, J., and Kerdel-Vegas, F.: Disseminated cutaneous leishmaniasis. Arch. Derm., *91*:439, 1965.

Convit, J., Reyes, O., and Kerdel-Vegas, F.: Disseminated anergic cutaneous leishmaniasis. Arch. Derm., *76*:213, 1957.

Fasal, P.: American leishmaniasis or leishmaniasis mucocutanea. *In* Simons, R. D. G. P. (ed.): Handbook of Tropical Dermatology and Medical Mycology. vol. 1, p. 375. Amsterdam, Elsevier Publishing Co., 1952.

Simpson, M. H., Mullins, J. F., and Stone, O. J.: Disseminated anergic cutaneous leishmaniasis. Arch. Derm., *97*:301, 1968.

Snow, J. S., Satulsky, E. M., and Kean, B. H.: American cutaneous leishmaniasis. Arch. Derm. Syph., *57*:90, 1948.

Walton, B. C., Paulson, J. E., Arjona, M. A., and Petersen, C. A.: American cutaneous leishmaniosis. J.A.M.A., *228*:1256, 1974.

Post-Kala-Azar Dermal Leishmaniasis

Frain-Bell, W.: Symposium on tropical diseases. Trans. St. John's Hosp. Derm. Soc., *42*:1, 1959.

Gupta, P. C., and Bhattacharjee, B.: Histopathology of post-kala-azar dermal leishmaniasis. J. Trop. Med. Hyg., *56*:110, 1953.

Yesudian, P., and Thambiah, A. S.: Amphotericin B therapy in dermal leishmanoid. Arch. Derm., *109*:720, 1974.

20

Diseases Caused by Viruses

INTRODUCTION

Viruses are obligatory intracellular parasites that differ from the larger microorganisms, such as bacteria, in that they are not cells (White). They lack organelles, such as ribosomes and mitochondria, hence have no metabolism of their own, and consequently must use the organelles, the energy, and many of the enzymes of the host cell for their replication. In doing so, viruses disturb the metabolism of the host cell irreversibly and thus act as pathogens (Luger).

Viruses are composed of a central core of nucleoprotein called the nucleoid that contains either deoxyribonucleic acid (DNA) or ribonucleic acid (RNA). The core is surrounded by the capsid whose subunits, called capsomeres, contain the major antigenic components of the virus. The core and the capsid form the essential part of the virus or virion. Viruses that replicate in the nucleus, when leaving the nucleus, may acquire an outer coat derived from the nuclear membrane, while virions that replicate in the cytoplasm may derive an outer coat from the plasma membrane (E.M. No. 31).

Before viruses can enter a cell they must be able to attach themselves to specific receptors of the plasma membrane and thus are species-specific. Viruses enter the cytoplasm of a cell by a process akin to phagocytosis, namely, by becoming enveloped by the plasma membrane of the cell as an outer coat. The viruses, once inside the cell, induce the synthesis of an "uncoating" protein in the host cell. As their outer coat and their capsid are being digested by the "uncoating" protein, the uncoated nucleoids lose their characteristic structure. The viruses now are in "eclipse" and are not apparent until replication has taken place and new virions or viruses, each composed of a core and a capsid, have been

formed. During the process of replication the proteins of the cell follow the genetic code of the specific virus nucleic acid, and the proteins that are formed are characteristic of the virus rather than of the cell. The first proteins that are formed after the "uncoating" are specific enzymes needed for the replication of the virus nucleic acids. Also, the proteins constituting the capsid are synthesized (Luger). Thousands of viruses may be released from an infected cell.

The diameter of viruses infecting the skin varies from 20 nm for the echoviruses to 300 nm for the poxviruses. The latter group of viruses under favorable conditions may be recognizable with the light microscope—for example, variola viruses as Paschen bodies. As a rule, however, viruses can be seen with the light microscope only when aggregated into inclusion bodies.

In many instances, recognition of inclusion bodies is not adequate for a diagnosis and other methods are needed to prove the existence of a specific virus infection, as for instance, inoculation of laboratory animals or of cell cultures. Also, in some instances, direct immunofluorescent staining of viral antigen is used, employing specific antibody conjugates (Liu and Llanes-Rodas). Also serologic tests may be of value, particularly if an increase in antibody titer has occurred in the course of a disease. The titer of antibodies may be determined either by complement fixation or by neutralization (Artenstein and Demis). There are, however, two viral infections of the skin in which none of the above-mentioned methods can be applied, and histologic examination of tissue is the only method to prove the existence of the viral infections. They are molluscum contagiosum, and warts.

The electron microscope has been of great value in studying the anatomy of the various viruses and also the replication of viruses in tissue; but its use is rarely practical for the purpose of diagnosis (Blank et al.).

HERPES SIMPLEX

The primary infection with *Herpesvirus hominis* takes place subclinically in childhood in over 90 per cent of cases. Clinically evident primary infection can, however, occur either in childhood or in later life in one of the following locations: the oral cavity, the genitals, the skin, the cornea, the lungs, or the brain; and on rare occasions it may be systemic. In exceptional cases the infection takes place prior to birth in the uterus.

A primary infection of the oral cavity, the genitals, or the skin differs from recurrent infections in these areas by being more pronounced and by regularly showing regional lymphadenopathy. Antibodies are absent in the serum of the patient in the beginning and are formed during the disease. Primary infections are always caused by infection from another person. The incubation period in the case of genital herpes simplex varies between 3 and 14 days and on the average is 5 days (Chang et al.).

Recurrent infections of the oral cavity, the genitals, or the skin can be due either to reactivation of a latent infection or to a new infection. Antibodies are present in the patient's serum at the onset, and the titer may or may not rise. If at any time the titer falls to very low levels or zero, a patient may again react to a new infection as to a primary infection.

Both primary and recurrent herpes simplex show one or several groups of vesicles on an inflamed base. Healing usually takes place within one to three weeks. It is noteworthy that in women with herpes simplex of the vulva virus-positive cultures can be regularly obtained also from the cervix uteri (Chang et al.).

Special forms of cutaneous herpes simplex are the following: *Kaposi's varicelliform eruption* (eczema herpeticum), which is discussed on page 345. *Herpetic folliculitis of the bearded region* is a benign eruption of grouped vesiculofollicular lesions, healing within a few weeks (Izumi et al.). *Chronic cutaneous herpes simplex with ulceration* shows persistent crusted ulcers, usually on the face. The reason for the slow healing is impairment of the cellular immune system either through the existence of lymphoma or through treatment with immunosuppressive drugs (Logan et al.; Muller et al.).

Herpes simplex pneumonia usually is fatal. It may occur in children as well as in adults and probably is an aspiration infection, since it usually follows a herpes simplex infection of the mouth, the esophagus, or the trachea (Herout et al.; Nash and Foley).

Herpes simplex encephalitis represents the most frequent and devastating of the acute viral infections of the brain in the United States today. It has a high mortality and those who survive often have severe residual cerebral damage. Most patients are adults. It is not associated with cutaneous herpes simplex (Leider et al.; Nolan et al.).

Systemic herpes simplex infection associated with viremia and usually fatal may occur in the newborn as the result of a genital herpes simplex infection of the mother. The infection reaches the newborn either through the placenta, by ascending into the uterus, or through direct contact in the birth canal (Catalano et al.). In addition, fatal systemic herpes simplex infections have been observed, although rarely, in children and adults (1) with congenital defective cell-mediated immunity, as seen in the Wiskott-Aldrich syndrome or in dysplasia or aplasia of the thymus (Sutton et al.; Joseph and Vogt); (2) with lymphoma; (3) receiving immunosuppressive therapy; and (4) with severe burns (Foley et al.). This may be associated with widespread herpes simplex lesions on the skin of the newborn (Golden et al.) or of the adult (Sutton et al.).

Prenatal herpes simplex infection may occur in an unborn child in the uterus and cause congenital malformations, especially of the brain and the eyes (Florman et al.).

Histopathology. The characteristic lesion in herpes simplex of the skin is an intraepidermal vesicle produced by profound degeneration of epidermal cells, resulting in marked acantholysis. The degeneration of the epidermal cells occurs in two forms: ballooning degeneration and reticular degeneration. These degenerative changes are

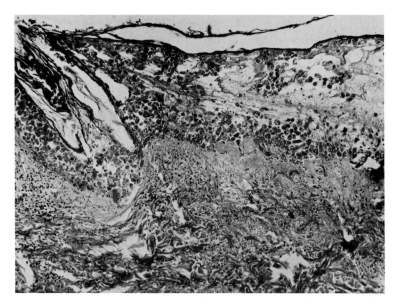

FIG. 20-1. **Herpes simplex.** Low magnification. There is marked ballooning degeneration of the cells at the floor of the vesicle. The cells of a hair follicle, shown at the left, likewise show ballooning degeneration. Reticular degeneration, observed at the top of the vesicle, is only slight. (×100)

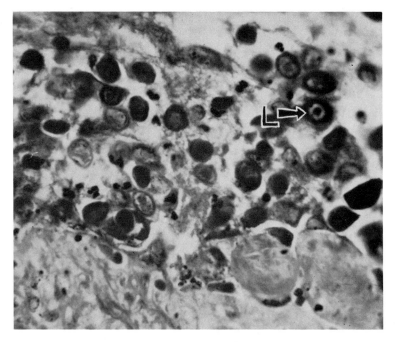

FIG. 20-2. **Herpes simplex.** High magnification of Figure 20-1. Balloon cells at the floor of a vesicle are shown. On the right, an inclusion body (which is eosinophilic) lies in the center of a balloon cell (L). The inclusion body is surrounded by a halo. (×400)

typical of viral vesicles and make the viral vesicle histologically distinct from the vesicles seen in other vesiculobullous diseases (see Classification of Bullae, p. 96). However, as in all vesiculobullous diseases, it is important that an early lesion be selected for biopsy; otherwise, secondary changes, especially invasion of inflammatory cells, may obscure the diagnostic features.

Ballooning degeneration causes marked swelling of epidermal cells. Such swollen balloon cells have a homogeneous, eosinophilic cytoplasm (Figs. 20-1 and 20-2). They may have one nucleus or may be multinucleated. Because the balloon cells lose their intercellular bridges, acantholysis occurs: the cells become separated from one another and unilocular vesicles result. The process of ballooning degeneration occurs mainly at the base of viral vesicles, leading to a dissolution of the lower epidermis, so that ultimately the vesicle that formed intraepidermally has a subepidermal location in many places. Ballooning degeneration can also affect the epithelial cells of hair follicles and sebaceous glands.

Reticular degeneration represents a process in which the epidermal cells become greatly distended by intracellular edema, so that the cell wall bursts. Through coalescence of neighboring, similarly affected cells, a multilocular vesicle results, the septa of which are formed by the resistant cellular walls (Fig. 20-3). Reticular degeneration occurs mainly in the upper portion and at the periphery of viral vesicles. In older vesicles the cellular walls no longer are resistant and disappear. In this way, the originally multilocular portions of the vesicle become unilocular. It may be pointed out that, in contrast to ballooning degeneration, reticular degeneration is not specific for viral vesicles, since it also occurs in the vesicles of dermatitis (see p. 98).

The upper dermis of virus vesicles shows an inflammatory infiltrate, the density of which depends on the severity of the reaction. In severe reactions, as they occur especially in primary infections with *H. hominis,* the dermis may show a severe vasculitis characterized by the presence of fibrinoid deposits and a dense inflammatory infiltrate

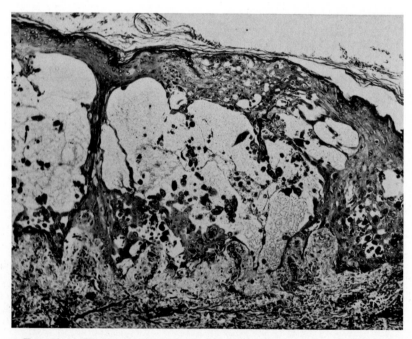

FIG. 20-3. **Herpes simplex.** Reticular degeneration is present, especially at the top of the vesicle, resulting in a multilocular vesicle. In addition, ballooning degeneration is present at the floor of the vesicle. (×200)

with many neutrophils both within and around the capillary walls. In addition, there may be extravasation of erythrocytes, fragmentation of the nuclei of neutrophils, and, occasionally also, fibrinoid thrombi resulting in necrosis (Cheatham et al.; Grimmer).

Viral inclusion bodies are seen quite frequently in the center of the enlarged, round nuclei of balloon cells. The inclusion bodies are eosinophilic and usually are surrounded by a clear space or halo (Fig. 20-2). They measure from 3 to 8 μm in diameter.

Herpetic folliculitis of the bearded region shows pronounced changes in the outer root sheath of the affected hair follicles with ballooning degeneration and formation of multinucleated epithelial giant cells. The heavy inflammatory perifollicular infiltrate can cause destruction of some of the hair follicles (Izumi et al.).

Chronic cutaneous herpes simplex with ulceration may be impossible to diagnose as being of viral genesis in specimens that are devoid of epidermis. Viral changes may be seen, however, in the epidermis at the margin of the ulcer, including typical intranuclear inclusions (Logan et al.; Muller et al.). Viral cultures may represent the best way to prove the diagnosis.

VISCERAL LESIONS. In *herpes simplex pneumonia,* the alveolar lining cells show eosinophilic inclusion bodies in their nuclei as the most characteristic feature (Herout et al.; Nash and Foley).

In *herpes simplex encephalitis,* the brain shows extensive areas of hemorrhagic necrosis, particularly of the medial surfaces of the temporal lobes. Eosinophilic intranuclear inclusion bodies may be present in the cerebral cortex (Leider et al.).

In *systemic herpes simplex of the newborn,* autopsy reveals characteristic small foci of necrosis in the liver and the adrenals, and often also in the lungs and the brain with the presence of intranuclear eosinophilic inclusion bodies (Catalano et al.; Patrizi et al.).

TZANCK SMEAR. For a rapid, though preliminary diagnosis cytologic examination is often useful. It is carried out on a smear that is taken from the floor of an early, freshly opened vesicle and is stained with Giemsa's stain. As a rule, many acantho-

lytic, balloon cells with either one or several nuclei are seen (Graham et al.). The presence of so many balloon cells is due to the fact that the smear is taken from the floor of the blister where ballooning degeneration is most pronounced.

VIRAL IDENTIFICATION. The virus can be directly identified either by culture or by the direct immunofluorescent test. For the culture, material from the floor of a blister or other infected material is inoculated on cell cultures consisting of HeLa cells or primary human amnion cells. The virus has a cytopathogenic effect on the cells of the culture. This effect is specifically inhibited, or neutralized, by prior addition to the cell culture of a serum containing *H. hominis* antibodies (Luger). The direct immunofluorescent examination for the presence of the viral antigen present in cells infected with *H. hominis* is carried out on smears of such cells to which is added, first, rabbit serum containing *H. hominis* antibody, and then fluorescein-conjugated anti-rabbit serum globulin of mice (Liu and Llanes-Rodas). For the determination of the antibody level in the patient's serum the complement fixation reaction can be used.

Histogenesis. On electron microscopy, *Herpesvirus hominis* is a spherical virus. Its DNA-containing core measures approximately 40 nm in diameter. The virion has a diameter of about 100 nm, while the virion together with its outer coat measures around 135 nm in size (Morecki and Becker). Ultrastructurally, the virion of *H. hominis* is indistinguishable from that of *H. varicellae* (Bastian et al.), for its description, see page 344.

The nature of the *eosinophilic nuclear inclusion bodies* seen by light microscopy in herpes simplex, as well as in herpes zoster and varicella, is still problematical. In the first place, these inclusion bodies are Feulgen-negative and thus do not contain DNA, as do viruses, such as *H. hominis,* that replicate in the nucleus of cells; and, in the second place, they cannot be visualized by electron microscopy (Southam et al.). It is assumed that they represent a residuum left after the escape of virus from the nucleus (Crouse et al.). According to Scott and McLeod, during viral replication areas of Feulgen-positive, i.e., DNA-containing, material appear between strands of condensed chromatin in the nucleus. These areas coalesce to form a basophilic, Feulgen-positive, homogenous body which fills most of the nucleus, compressing the chromatin to the margin. Later, after most virions have left the nucleus, this body shrinks, becomes Feulgen-negative and eosinophilic, and lies separated from the marginated chromatin, seemingly surrounded by a halo.

Herpesvirus hominis includes two different types, Types 1 and 2. They differ not only in their antigenicity, since each type is preferentially neutralized by its specific antiserum, but also in their effects on tissue cultures and in their growth characteristics on the chorioallantoic membrane of chick embryos (Nahmias and Dowdle). Type 1 usually affects the skin and the oral mucosa, while Type 2 affects the genital mucosa and adjoining skin. However, Chang et al. in their study of genital herpes simplex found both types with about the same frequency, attributing the high incidence of Type 1 to orogenital contact. Virus isolated from the skin of infants with neonatal infection is usually Type 2 (Zavoral et al.). Several studies have shown an association between antibodies of Type 2 *H. hominis* and cancer of the cervix (Allen and Cole). It seems, however, that often the atypia precedes the herpesvirus infection so that a causal relationship is doubtful (Amstey et al.).

Inadequacy in the cell-mediated immune response results in impaired delayed hypersensitivity and thus predisposes to various viral infections, including infection with herpes simplex. This has become particularly apparent in patients receiving immunosuppressive treatment, for instance after a renal transplant (Muller et al.), and in patients with the Wiskott-Aldrich syndrome (St. Geme et al.). Also infants with thymic aplasia fail to develop delayed hypersensitivity and are unable to cope with various infections, including infections with *H. hominis* (Glasgow).

Differential Diagnosis. Even though *Herpesvirus hominis* and *H. varicellae* are indistinguishable by light microscopy and electron microscopy and the viral vesicles produced by these two viruses on the skin or the mucous membranes look alike, they differ in their antigenicity and in their growth in culture (see p. 344). For differentiation of herpes simplex from variola, see page 344.

Herpes simplex vesicles must be differentiated from those of pemphigus vulgaris. Even though the blisters of pemphigus vulgaris show, as do viral vesicles, acantholysis and degeneration of epidermal cells, differentiation usually is quite easy because the ballooning degeneration in viral vesicles represents a far more profound degeneration than that occurring in the blisters of pemphigus vulgaris. Furthermore, viral vesicles never are seen in suprabasal location, since

the viral degeneration causes lysis of the basal layer from the dermis. The presence of eosinophilic nuclear inclusion bodies in the viral vesicles further aids in differentiation.

VARICELLA AND HERPES ZOSTER

Varicella and herpes zoster are produced by the same virus, *Herpesvirus varicellae*. Varicella results from contact of the nonimmune host with this virus, whereas herpes zoster occurs in a host that is partially immune as the result of previously having had varicella either clinically or subclinically. Although varicella not infrequently develops in children exposed to herpes zoster, reinfection does not play a significant role in acquiring herpes zoster. In most instances in which herpes zoster was reported to have been acquired through exposure to varicella or herpes zoster the patients had a defect of cellular immunity (Rogers and Tindall). As a rule, herpes zoster is caused by reactivation of a latent virus infection which originally took place in either spinal or cranial sensory ganglia as the result of hematogenous dissemination during the initial varicella infection. On reactivation the virus spreads from the single ganglion or from several adjoining ganglia along the corresponding sensory nerve or nerves to the skin (Muller and Winkelmann).

Varicella. In varicella, a generalized eruption is seen. The lesions begin as small papules which develop into vesicles. In mild cases most vesicles become crusted without changing into pustules. A slightly hemorrhagic base to the vesicles may be seen in severe cases. New lesions continue to develop in varicella for several days so that, in contrast to variola, lesions in different stages of development can be observed.

Varicella pneumonia occurs occasionally in adults as a primary disease without cutaneous lesions. Usually, it runs a fairly mild course and ends in recovery (Weinstein and Meade). However, it may be severe and even fatal (Frank).

Systemic varicella with widely disseminated systemic lesions is a rare, fatal disease and may occur in the newborn (Lucchesi et al.), as well as in children and in adults (Cheatham et al.; Eisenbud). Such fatalities have been observed particularly in patients who had defects in the cell-mediated immune response (Berg et al.) or were receiving corticosteroid treatment.

Herpes Zoster. In herpes zoster the eruption consists of groups of vesicles situated on an inflammatory base and arranged along the course of one or several adjoining sensory nerves. The base of the lesions frequently appears hemorrhagic, and some of the lesions may become necrotic and ulcerate. Not infrequently, in addition to the localized eruption, there are a few scattered lesions elsewhere and, rarely, a generalized eruption indistinguishable from that of varicella (Rado et al.). Such generalized herpes zoster is apt to occur particularly in patients with immunologic defects, particularly in lymphoma (see p. 344). Rarely, in adult patients with a severe immunologic defect, varicella develops in place of a generalized herpes zoster (Nasemann et al.).

Systemic lesions may occur in patients with generalized herpes zoster. The presence of widely scattered cutaneous lesions in such patients is indicative of a hematogenous dissemination of the virus. Among the systemic manifestations are pneumonia (Kain et al.) and encephalitis (Appelbaum et al.).

Histopathology. The cutaneous lesions of varicella and herpes zoster are histologically indistinguishable from those seen in herpes simplex (see p. 338). The same type of intranuclear eosinophilic inclusion bodies are seen in all three diseases. Frequently, however, the inflammatory reaction, including the degree of vasculitis and hemorrhage, are more pronounced in varicella and, particularly, in herpes zoster than in herpes simplex. In severe cases of varicella eosinophilic inclusion bodies have been observed also in the dermis within the nuclei of histiocytes (Nasemann et al.).

VISCERAL LESIONS. The visceral lesions caused by hematogenous dissemination in varicella and herpes zoster are indistinguishable from one another and from those produced by herpes simplex. On the other hand, the neural lesions in herpes zoster are quite specific for that disease (see below).

In fatal cases of *pneumonia due to varicella or herpes zoster,* the autopsy reveals intranuclear eosinophilic inclusion bodies in bronchiolar epithelial cells and alveolar cells (Frank).

In *systemic varicella or herpes zoster,* one finds in various organs areas of focal necrosis containing intranuclear eosinophilic inclusion bodies, especially in the liver, the kidneys, the adrenals, and the lungs. As evidence of hematogenous dissemination, intranuclear eosinophilic inclusion bodies are seen in the vascular endothelium (Berg et al.). In contrast with herpes zoster, varicella does not show intranuclear eosinophilic inclusion bodies in dorsal root ganglia (Cheatham et al.).

The *neural lesions in herpes zoster* begin with a severe inflammatory infiltrate in one or several adjoining dorsal root ganglia or a cranial nerve ganglion, extending from there to the associated sensory spinal or cranial nerves (Cheatham). The inflammation leads to destruction of nerve cells within the affected ganglia. The affected ganglia in herpes zoster have been shown to contain intranuclear eosinophilic inclusion bodies, on light microscopy (Cheatham), on electron microscopy (Ghatak and Zimmerman), and on culturing with monkey kidney cells (Bastian et al.). Degenerative changes extend from the involved ganglia along the sensory nerves to the skin. In addition, there may be a unilateral, segmental poliomyelitis in the posterior columns of the spinal cord and a localized leptomeningitis (Denny-Brown and Adams).

In the dermatomes affected by herpes zoster the dermal nerve network appears significantly reduced, as shown by staining with the acetylcholinesterase method (Muller and Winkelmann). This reduction can be regarded as being due to the presence of the causative virus because (1) eosinophilic inclusion bodies have been demonstrated within neurilemmal cells of the small nerves in the dermis underlying the vesicles (Cheatham); and (2) virions have been found by electron microscopy in the axons of unmyelinated dermal nerves, together with severe destruction of unmyelinated nerve fibers (Hasegawa).

Asymptomatic upward extension of the virus along the spinal cord from the dorsal root ganglion to the brain apparently is not too uncommon in view of the fact that about half of the patients with herpes zoster have pleocytosis of the spinal fluid (Appelbaum et al.) and *H. varicellae* occasionally can be isolated from the spinal fluid of such patients (Gold). However, fatal cases of encephalomyelitis (Rose et al.) or encephalitis (Appelbaum et al.) are rare in herpes zoster.

TZANCK SMEAR. Cytologic examination, useful as a preliminary diagnostic test, is carried out in the same way as in herpes simplex (see p. 341).

VIRAL IDENTIFICATION. *Herpesvirus hominis* and *H. varicellae* are morphologically indistinguishable (Bastian et al.). However, in contrast with *H. hominis, H. varicellae* does not grow in ordinary tissue cultures, although it will grow in tissue cultures containing human fetal diploid kidney cells or monkey kidney cells (Weller et al.). Also, whereas *H. hominis* is a pathogen for several laboratory animals such as the rabbit, *H. varicellae* is not pathogenic for any animal (Gold). Furthermore, *H. hominis* and *H. varicellae* differ in their antigenicity so that, on serologic testing for *H. hominis* antibodies, an increase in antibody titer during the disease occurs only in herpes simplex (see p. 341).

Histogenesis. On electron microscopic examination, round virus particles, or virions, are seen primarily in the nucleus in infections with *H. varicellae,* just as in infections with *H. hominis.* If present in sufficient numbers, the virions may lie partially in crystalloid aggregates. Some virus particles consist only of a hollow coat, or "capsid," while others show within the capsid a DNA-containing core, or "nucleoid" (Bastian et al.). The nucleoid averages 40 nm in diameter, and the capsid 100 nm (Morecki and Becker). On leaving the nucleus for the cytoplasm most virions are enveloped by an outer coat that is derived from the nuclear membrane, increasing the size of the virus particle from about 100 nm to about 150 nm (E.M. No. 31). In the presence of many virions they may be seen in crystalloid arrangement also in the cytoplasm (Nasemann). It is worth noting that both *H. hominis* and *H. varicellae* often can be identified by electron microscopy even in tissue that has not been specifically prepared for electron microscopy but was routinely fixed in formalin and embedded in paraffin (Morecki and Becker).

As in infections with *Herpesvirus hominis,* defects in cellular immunity often are an eliciting or an aggravating factor in infections with *H. varicellae* (see p. 342).

VARIOLA

Variola shows a generalized eruption that at first consists of papules. After two or three days the papules are transformed into vesicles that characteristically are umbilicated. After three more days the vesicles change into pustules. In severe cases the lesions may have a purpuric base. It is typical of variola that all lesions are at the same stage of development.

Histopathology. In variola reticular degeneration is prominent, especially in the early stage of vesiculation. Therefore, early vesicles are multilocular. Balloon cells are few in number and small in size, and they rarely are multinucleated (Michelson and Ikeda).

Even though in herpes simplex, varicella, and herpes zoster ballooning degeneration predominates, and multinucleated balloon cells are commonly seen, the histologic structure of the vesicle is no reliable criterion for the differentiation of variola from the other three diseases since older vesicles of variola that are in the suppurative stage, through rupture of the septa, often become unilocular; furthermore, in occasional instances of the other three diseases reticular degeneration is more pronounced than usual.

Only the demonstration of intracytoplasmic inclusion bodies definitely differentiates variola from herpes simplex, varicella, and herpes zoster. The intracytoplasmic inclusion bodies of variola are eosinophilic and Feulgen-positive. Often they are surrounded by an unstained halo. Occasionally, more than one intracytoplasmic inclusion body are present in one cell. In addition, intranuclear eosinophilic inclusion bodies are often seen in older lesions. The latter are thought to be the result of a toxic degeneration and not viral in origin (Nasemann).

In addition to variola, also vaccinia and milkers' nodules show eosinophilic, Feulgen-positive intracytoplasmic inclusion bodies; and milkers' nodules, like variola, may show also intranuclear inclusion bodies (see p. 346).

VISCERAL LESIONS. In variola visceral lesions rarely are prominent. However, vesicles occur not only on the palate and in the pharynx but also in the trachea and the esophagus. The pulmonary lesions usually are bacterial in type by the time that they are observed, but they probably have a viral basis (Blank and Rake). Encephalitis occurs occasionally, but it is immunologic in origin, just as in postvaccinial encephalitis, since variola organisms have never been found (Blank and Rake).

Histogenesis. Variola is caused by one of the poxviruses. The poxviruses, on the basis of their morphology, can be divided into two classes: First, viruses that are rectangular ("brick-shaped"), have DNA cores in the shape of biconcave disks, and measure approximately 250 by 300 nm in diameter, comprising the viruses of variola, vaccinia, cowpox, and molluscum contagiosum; and second, viruses that are cylindrical and measure approximately 140 by 300 nm, comprising the virus of paravaccinia, causing milkers' nodules, and the virus causing orf (Davis and Musil).

ECZEMA HERPETICUM, ECZEMA VACCINATUM (KAPOSI'S VARICELLIFORM ERUPTION)

Eczema herpeticum and eczema vaccinatum, both of which often are referred to as Kaposi's varicelliform eruption, occur only in patients with a pre-existing dermatosis. Usually, this pre-existing dermatosis is atopic dermatitis (Barton and Brunsting). Occasionally, however, other forms of dermatitis, such as seborrheic dermatitis, or other dermatoses, such as Darier's disease (Loeffel and Meyer), pemphigus foliaceus (Silverstein and Burnett) and ichthyosis vulgaris (Verbow et al.) may provide the "soil" on which Kaposi's varicelliform eruption develops. Eczema herpeticum is produced by the accidental inoculation on the skin of the virus of herpes simplex, usually of Type 1 of *Herpesvirus hominis*; whereas eczema vaccinatum results from the accidental inoculation of the vaccinia virus.

Clinically, the two diseases look alike. They show a more or less extensive eruption composed of vesicles and pustules that may be umbilicated. They are situated chiefly on the areas of the pre-existing dermatosis, but

also on otherwise normal skin. The face usually is the site of severest involvement and may show marked edema. There are fever and prostration, and occasionally the disease ends fatally, especially in infants.

Histopathology. On histologic examination both eczema herpeticum and eczema vaccinatum show vesicles and pustules of the viral type. Even though the pustules show in their center only necrotic epidermis, one may still see at their periphery reticular and ballooning degeneration (Lynch; Lausecker). In instances of eczema herpeticum, but not in eczema vaccinatum, multinucleated epithelial giant cells often are present (Lausecker; von Weiss et al.). Because of the presence of innumerable inflammatory cells, especially neutrophils, the demonstration of inclusion bodies often is difficult. If they are found, they are located exclusively in the cytoplasm in eczema vaccinatum, and exclusively within the nucleus in eczema herpeticum.

Differential Diagnosis. Since eczema herpeticum and eczema vaccinatum look alike clinically, and since the histologic similarity is great in the absence of inclusion bodies and of multinucleated epithelial cells, differentiation of the two diseases may have to depend on nonhistologic means, such as a history of possible exposure to the vaccinia virus and a number of laboratory tests.

Among the tests are: (1) inoculation of HeLa cell or primary human-amnion-cell cultures, without and with the addition of sera containing antibodies to *Herpesvirus hominis* and to the vaccinia virus, respectively, for the purpose of neutralization; (2) direct immunofluorescent examination for the presence of viral antigen (see p. 341); and (3) the complement fixation reaction, or the viral neutralization reaction, which, if carried out during the course of the disease, will reveal in the patient's serum an increase in the antibody titer either with herpes simplex antigen or with vaccinia antigen (Marchionini and Nasemann; von Weiss et al.).

MILKERS' NODULES

Milkers' nodules are acquired from cows whose udders are infected with pseudocowpox or paravaccinia, a disease that, in contrast to cowpox or vaccinia, does not provide cross immunity to variola.

Clinically, infected individuals show, usually on their fingers, one to three and, occasionally, more nodules, measuring 1 to 2 cm in diameter. The nodules are bluish-red, semiglobular, and usually painless. The center of the nodules may appear vesicular or crusted. Spontaneous healing takes place within one or two months.

Histopathology. The epidermis shows hyperkeratosis with parakeratosis, as well as acanthosis with marked elongation of the rete ridges. The dermis shows a nonspecific, chronic inflammatory infiltrate of varying density. There often is a striking increase in the number of capillaries showing dilatation of their lumina (Nomland and McKee).

The epidermis in some instances shows multilocular vesicles as evidence of reticular degeneration and also may show some balloon cells (Evins et al.). In other instances there is merely spongiosis and intracellular edema (Katzenellenbogen).

In some cases one can find fairly numerous eosinophilic inclusion bodies in the cytoplasm of vacuolated epidermal cells (Katzenellenbogen; Marchionini and Nasemann; Evins et al.). Like the inclusion bodies in variola and in vaccinia, they are surrounded by a halo and are Feulgen-positive. In addition, there may be, just as in variola, intranuclear eosinophilic inclusion bodies (Evins and Leavell). In other cases, no inclusion bodies can be demonstrated (Nomland and McKee). However, even in the absence of inclusion bodies, the virus may be demonstrable in tissue sections by electron microscopy (Davis and Musil).

Histogenesis. On electron microscopy, the paravaccinia virus is cylindrical in shape and has convex ends. It consists of a dense DNA core surrounded by a less dense, wide capsid. The virus measures, on the average, 140 by 300 nm. Mature virus particles are generally located in the stratum corneum (Davis and Musil). The paravaccinia virus, like the vaccinia virus, can be propagated on tissue culture cells of bovine origin; but, in contrast to the vaccinia virus, it does not grow on cell lines of monkey or human origin (Friedman-Kien et al.).

ECTHYMA CONTAGIOSUM (ORF)

Ecthyma contagiosum, or orf, is a benign, self-limited viral infection contracted by handling infected sheep. Clinically, the lesions in infected humans appear on exposed surfaces and vary in number from one to several. They begin as papules, and become vesicular and then pustular, and finally crusted. They heal in about five weeks.

Histopathology. One observes intraepidermal vesiculation with reticular degeneration and areas of intracellular edema suggestive of ballooning degeneration (Wheeler et al.). Marked acanthosis and a severe inflammatory infiltrate in the dermis are also seen. Inclusion bodies have not been found in the lesions by light microscopy.

Histogenesis. Electron microscopic examination reveals in the cytoplasm of epidermal cells viral particles in various stages of maturation. Mature viruses are cylindrical in shape and have convex ends and thus resemble the paravaccinia virus (Leavell et al.). Like all pox virus, the virus of orf has a central dense DNA core and a wide, laminated capsid. Its size varies, depending on the maturity of the virus, and averages 200 by 300 nm. Occasionally, markedly elongated virions reach a length of 400 to 500 nm (Yeh and Soltani). The orf virus can be cultured on human-amnion-cell culture and on primary rhesus-monkey kidney-cell cultures (Naggington and Whittle).

MOLLUSCUM CONTAGIOSUM

This disorder consists of a variable number of small, discrete, waxy, skin-colored, dome-shaped papules, usually 2 to 4 mm in size and having an umbilicated center. When fully developed, a small amount of a curd-like substance can be expressed from the center of the lesion. In occasional instances some of the lesions and the surrounding skin appear inflamed. The lesions ultimately involute spontaneously by discharging the central curdlike material.

Histopathology. In molluscum contagiosum the epidermis grows down into the dermis as multiple, closely packed pear-shaped lobules. Many epidermal cells contain large, intracytoplasmic inclusion bodies (Fig. 20-4). The intracytoplasmic inclusion bodies, the so-called molluscum bodies, first appear as single minute ovoid eosinophilic structures in the lower cells of the stratum malpighii at a level one or two layers above the basal cell layer. The basal cell layer itself does not contain molluscum bodies (Lutzner). The molluscum bodies increase considerably in size as the infected cells move toward the surface. At the level of the midepidermis the size of the molluscum bodies already exceeds the original size of the invaded cells. The molluscum body displaces and compresses the nucleus of the invaded cells, so that the nucleus appears as a thin crescent at the periphery of the cell. At the level of the granular layer the staining reaction of molluscum bodies changes from eosinophilic to basophilic (Mescon et al.). In the horny layer numerous large basophilic molluscum bodies measuring up to 35 μm in diameter lie enmeshed in a network of eosinophilic horny fibers (see Plate 2, facing p. 250). In the center of the lesion the horny fibers break, releasing the molluscum bodies. Thus, a central crater forms.

The surrounding dermis usually shows little or no inflammatory reaction, except in rare instances when the lesion of molluscum contagiosum ruptures and discharges molluscum bodies and horny material into the dermis. This results in a pronounced inflammatory infiltrate containing lymphoid cells, neutrophils, macrophages, and often also a few foreign-body giant cells (Henao and Freeman).

The molluscum inclusion bodies contain, embedded in a protein matrix, myriads of molluscum contagiosum viruses. The virus of molluscum contagiosum belongs to the poxvirus group (see p. 345). Analogous to the inclusion bodies of other poxviruses, the inclusion bodies of molluscum contagiosum, as they form in the stratum malpighii, are eosinophilic and Feulgen-positive. The occasionally observed negative or weakly positive Feulgen reaction in some of the inclusion bodies is caused by a predominance of the protein matrix. In such instances expo-

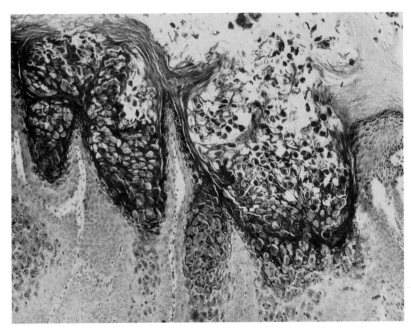

Fig. 20-4. **Molluscum contagiosum.** Numerous intracytoplasmic inclusion bodies, the so-called molluscum bodies, are seen forming in the lower epidermis. They grow in size as they move toward the surface. (×100)

sure of the section to pepsin results in a positive Feulgen reaction, as the pepsin digests the protein matrix that surrounds the virus particles (Nasemann and Stanka).

Histogenesis. Electron microscopic examination (E.M. No. 32) has revealed the virus of molluscum contagiosum, like the viruses of variola, vaccinia and cowpox, to be "brick-shaped" and to measure approximately 300 × 240 nm. It consists of an electron-dense nucleoid, approximately 230 nm in length, which appears dumbbell-shaped in profile (E.M. No. 32, *inset*) and rectangular in front view. The nucleoid is composed of interwoven filaments measuring approximately 6 nm in diameter and representing the fibrous DNA. The nucleoid is surrounded by a medium electron-dense amorphous coat, about 16 nm in width, representing the capsid (E.M. No. 32, *inset*). Peripheral to this is a thin trilaminar outer membrane (Robinson et al.; Hasegawa et al.).

The virus of molluscum contagiosum does not grow in tissue cultures. In an attempt to explain this failure to grow, Robinson et al. inoculated tissue cultures of chick embryo cells with extracts from skin lesions of patients with molluscum contagiosum. Even though the viral particles were adsorbed to the cell surface and phagocytized by these cells, and also the thin outer membrane of the viral particles was lysed, the viral coat nevertheless failed to rupture. Thus, the viral DNA was not extruded into the cytoplasm and replication of the virus was blocked. The authors postulate that the viral coat remained present around the nucleoid because the virus of molluscum contagiosum fails to induce the synthesis of "uncoating" protein in the host cells (see p. 337).

VERRUCA

There are four types of verrucae: verruca vulgaris, verruca plana, verruca plantaris, and condyloma acuminatum. All four are caused by the same virus, and differences in appearance are the result of the location of the wart and of the degree of reactivity of the host (Oriel and Almeida).

VERRUCA VULGARIS

Verrucae vulgares are circumscribed, firm elevated growths having a papillomatous, hyperkeratotic surface. Verrucae vulgares may occur anywhere on the skin, and in rare instances they occur also on the oral mucosa, especially the buccal mucosa (see Oral Florid

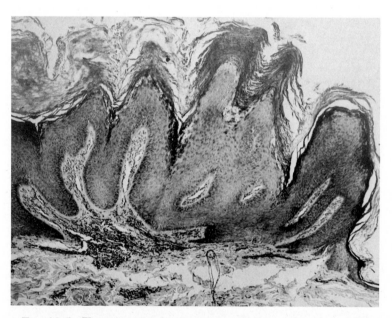

FIG. 20-5. **Verruca vulgaris.** Low magnification. There are hyperkeratosis, acanthosis, and papillomatosis. The rete ridges are elongated and bent inward at both margins and thereby appear to point radially to the center. (×100)

Papillomatosis, p. 472). The fingers are the most common site of verrucae vulgares.

Histopathology. Verrucae vulgares show acanthosis, papillomatosis, and hyperkeratosis with interspersed areas of parakeratosis. The rete ridges are elongated, and at the periphery of the verruca they often are bent inward so that they appear to point radially toward the center (Fig. 20-5). The characteristic feature that distinguishes verruca vulgaris from other papillomas (see p. 451) is the presence of large vacuolated cells in the upper stratum malpighii and in the granular layer (Fig. 20-6). However, such cells are present regularly only in young verrucae and may be absent in older ones. The large vacuolated cells possess round, deeply basophilic nuclei that are surrounded by a clear zone (Fig. 20-6). These cells contain few or no keratohyaline granules, even when they are located in the granular layer. In contrast, heavy clumps of keratohyaline granules often are present in nonvacuolated granular cells among them. The thickened horny layer contains many parakeratotic cells, often

arranged in vertical tiers overlying the crests of papillomatous elevations of the rete malpighii. The nuclei of the parakeratotic cells, in comparison with ordinary parakeratotic nuclei, are larger and more deeply basophilic and appear rounded rather than elongated (Fig. 20-7) (Blank et al.). Comparative histologic and electron microscopic studies have shown that the deeply basophilic, rounded nuclei present in the vacuolated cells of the upper stratum malpighii and in the parakeratotic cells of the stratum corneum contain numerous viral particles (Almeida et al.; Nasemann and Georgiewa; Gianotti et al.).

Occasionally, the epidermal cells of verrucae vulgares contain, especially when they are only a few weeks old, round eosinophilic bodies located mainly within vacuolated nuclei but also in the cytoplasm (Fig. 20-8). Because of their resemblance to the eosinophilic inclusion bodies seen in viral vesicles they were regarded in the past by some authors as viral inclusion bodies (Strauss et al.). However, electron microscopic studies

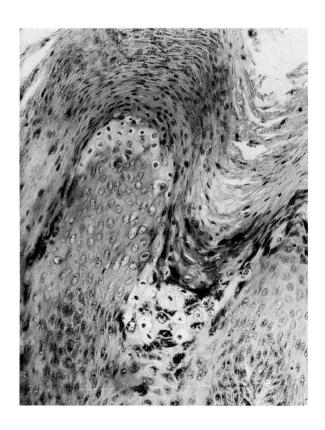

FIG. 20-6. **Verruca vulgaris.** High magnification of Figure 20-5. Groups of large vacuolated cells lie in the upper stratum malpighii and in the granular layer. A tier of parakeratotic cells lies over the crest of a papillomatous elevation. (×400)

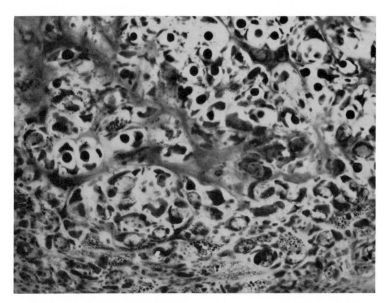

FIG. 20-7. **Verruca vulgaris.** In the lower portion of the illustration
the nuclei of the epidermal cells are vacuolated. In the upper portion
many of the nuclei are round and very deeply basophilic, and are
surrounded by a clear zone. The deeply basophilic nuclei have been
shown by electron microscopy to contain numerous virus particles.
(×200)

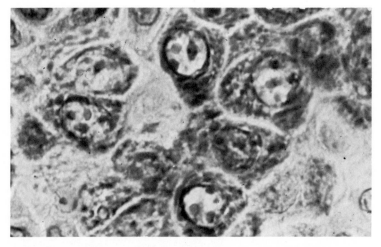

FIG. 20-8. **Verruca vulgaris.** The epidermal cells have large vacuolated nuclei. Five of the nuclei contain a round eosinophilic body,
formerly thought to represent an inclusion body but actually representing a degeneration product. The darker basophilic particles in the
nuclei are nucleoli. (×600)

have shown these bodies to be large, homogeneous, very electron-dense structures that bear no resemblance to viral particles, and also show in their distribution no direct relationship to the virus (Almeida et al.). They probably represent a degeneration product.

Histogenesis. The wart virus is a DNA virus belonging to the papova group. The virus particles are spherical bodies with a diameter of about 50 nm. Each particle consists of an electron-dense nucleoid with a stippled appearance surrounded by a less dense capsid (Gianotti et al.; Rajagopalan et al.). The wart virus replicates in the nucleus where the viral particles often are arranged as dense aggregates in a semicrystalloid arrangement (E.M. No. 33) (Cornelius et al.). A few viral particles may be located in the cytoplasm after having left the nucleus through pores in the nuclear membrane (Nasemann and Georgiewa). The wart virus does not grow in tissue cultures and is not pathogenic for any animal.

Differential Diagnosis. Difficulties may arise in differentiating between the "granular degeneration" (or "epidermolytic hyperkeratosis") seen occasionally in epidermal nevi (see p. 452) and the "vacuolar changes" seen in verruca vulgaris, since in both conditions one may find perinuclear vacuolization and irregular clumping of the keratohyaline granules (Shapiro and Baraf). Generally, however, the "vacuolar changes" in verruca vulgaris are limited to the upper epidermis, while the "granular degeneration" in epidermal nevi extends nearly through the entire epidermis. Furthermore, parakeratosis, caused in verruca vulgaris by the presence of viral particles in the nuclei, is absent in the "granular degeneration" in epidermal nevi.

For differentiation of verruca vulgaris from other papillomas, see page 451.

VERRUCA PLANA

Verrucae planae are slightly elevated, flat, smooth papules. They may be the color of normal skin, but usually they have a brownish hue. The face and the dorsa of the hands are affected most commonly.

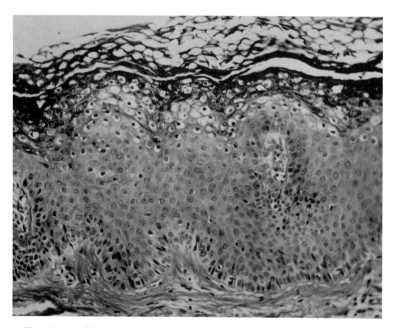

Fig. 20-9. **Verruca plana.** There are hyperkeratosis and acanthosis but no papillomatosis or parakeratosis. Numerous vacuolated cells lie in the upper stratum malpighii, including the granular layer. The horny layer has a pronounced basket-weave appearance resulting from the vacuolization of the horny cells. (×200)

Verrucae planae may occur as a very extensive eruption and then involve, in addition to the face and the dorsa of the hands, also the trunk and the extremities. Often several members of a family are affected (Rajagopalan et al.). The term *epidermodysplasia verruciformis of Lewandowsky and Lutz* is applied to this condition. Of particular interest is the fact that in a considerable number of patients with such an extensive eruption of verrucae planae a change of some of the lesions into solar keratosis, Bowen's disease, or squamous cell carcinoma has been observed (Jablonska et al., 1970; Ruiter and van Mullem; Schellender and Fritsch; Delescluse et al.).

Histopathology. Verrucae planae show hyperkeratosis and acanthosis but, in contrast with verrucae vulgares, they have no papillomatosis, only slight elongation of the rete ridges and no areas of parakeratosis. Furthermore, there is much more extensive vacuolization of the cells in the upper epidermis than in verruca vulgaris.

In the upper stratum malpighii, including the granular layer, many of the cells are vacuolated (Fig. 20-9). Some of the vacuolated cells are twice their normal size. The nuclei of the vacuolated cells lie in the center of the cell and some of them appear deeply basophilic. The granular layer is uniformly thickened, and the stratum corneum has a pronounced basket-weave appearance, resulting from the vacuolization of the horny cells. The dermis appears normal.

EPIDERMODYSPLASIA VERRUCIFORMIS shows the same histologic picture as verruca plana. Evidence that epidermodysplasia verruciformis represents an extensive eruption of verrucae planae includes: (1) successful autoinoculation and heteroinoculation experiments (Lutz, 1946; Jablonska and Formas); and (2) demonstration by electron microscopy of intranuclear viral particles having the same appearance as the wart virus (Jablonska et al., 1970; Ruiter and van Mullem). It can be concluded that both the extensive distribution of the warts and the rather frequent development of carcinoma within them are due to a special predisposition of the patients (Lutz, 1957; Grupper et al.).

Histogenesis. The occurrence of epidermodysplasia verruciformis in several members of a family is best explained on the basis of increased exposure and susceptibility to the wart virus rather than on a genetic basis, particularly since the assumed inheritance has been on a dominant basis in some families (Jablonska et al., 1968) and on a recessive basis in others (Rajagopalan et al.).

Malignant changes in lesions of epidermodysplasia verruciformis have been observed so far only in sun-exposed areas so that sun damage represents the major factor. The presence of the wart virus probably acts as an additional predisposing factor (Schellender and Fritsch). On electron microscopic examination, the wart virus can still be seen in areas of early in-situ malignant degeneration; but the wart virus is no longer present in well developed lesions of Bowen's disease or squamous cell carcinoma (Jablonska et al., 1970; Ruiter and van Mullem; Schellender and Fritsch; Delescluse et al.).

VERRUCA PLANTARIS

Verrucae plantares occur on the soles of the feet. Usually, they are covered with a thick callus. When the callus is removed, they become visible as soft, granular white or brownish tissue.

Histopathology. The histologic appearance of verruca plantaris resembles that of verruca vulgaris except that the horny layer is much thicker. There frequently is extensive parakeratosis with the presence of large, rounded, deeply basophilic nuclei in the horny layer. In early lesions the upper stratum malpighii and the stratum granulosum may contain numerous vacuolated epidermal cells showing deeply basophilic nuclei and, in some instances, also cells showing irregular clumping of their keratohyaline granules.

CONDYLOMA ACUMINATUM

Condylomata acuminata can occur on the penis, on the mucosal surfaces of the female genitals, and around as well as within the anus. They consist of fairly soft verrucous nodules that occasionally coalesce into cauliflowerlike masses.

Development of a carcinoma has been observed in rare instances in condylomata acuminata, in contrast with verruca vulgaris and verruca plantaris in which malignant

FIG. 20-10. **Condyloma acuminatum.** There is pronounced acanthosis. Many cells of the stratum malpighii appear vacuolated and have a round, hyperchromatic nucleus. (×50)

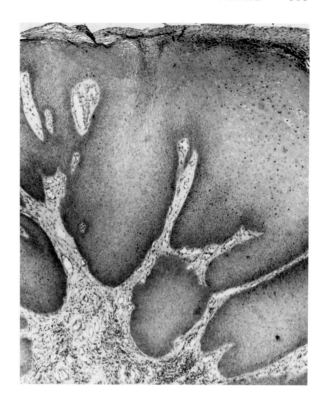

degeneration does not seem to take place. If carcinomatous transformation takes place, it may occur within a few months after the appearance of the condylomata acuminata (Kovi et al.), or many years later (Bauer and Friederich).

In rare instances condylomata acuminata can attain considerable size on the glans penis and foreskin of noncircumcised patients. They are known as *giant condylomata acuminata of Buschke and Loewenstein.* They can resemble carcinoma clinically not only by their large size but also by causing multiple fistulas extending into the urethra (Becker et al.). A few cases are known in which a carcinoma with regional lymph node metastases developed (Dawson et al.).

Analogous to the glans penis, giant condylomata acuminata can occur also in the anal region (Knoblich and Failing) and on the vulva (Judge). Development of a carcinoma in giant condylomata of the vulva has been observed in a few instances together with metastases (Sonck).

Histopathology. In condyloma acuminatum the stratum corneum is only slightly thickened and is composed, as it usually is on mucosal surfaces, of parakeratotic cells, with absence of the granular layer. The stratum malpighii shows papillomatosis and considerable acanthosis, with thickening and elongation of the rete ridges. The rete ridges branch to such a degree that the picture of pseudocarcinomatous hyperplasia may result. A considerable number of mitotic figures may be present. Usually, squamous cell carcinoma can be ruled out because the epithelial cells show an orderly arrangement, and the border between the epithelial proliferations and the dermis is sharp (Fig. 20-10). The most characteristic feature, important for the diagnosis, is the presence of areas in which the epithelial cells show distinct vacuolization. These vacuolated epithelial cells are relatively large and possess a clear cytoplasm and in their center a deeply hyperchromatic round nucleus. These nuclei resemble those seen in the upper portion of the epidermis in verrucae vulgares. It must be kept in mind, however, that vacuolization is a normal occurrence in the upper portion of all mucosal surfaces, so that vacuolization in condylomata acuminata can be regarded as being possibly of viral genesis only if it is associated with large, round, deeply basophilic nuclei in both the stratum malpighii and the stratum corneum.

The dermis in condylomata acuminata usually appears edematous and shows dilated capillaries and a moderately dense, chronic inflammatory infiltrate.

GIANT CONDYLOMATA ACUMINATA OF BUSCHKE AND LOEWENSTEIN. Although in ordinary condylomata acuminata the differentiation from squamous cell carcinoma usually is easy, it can be very difficult in cases of giant condylomata acuminata because the extreme degree of downgrowth of the epidermis with displacement of the underlying tissue seen in such cases mimics the invasion of tissue seen in squamous cell carcinoma (Machacek and Weakley). Multiple biopsies may be necessary to arrive at a decision. It is likely that lesions showing slow but relentless progression actually are not of viral genesis but represent from their inception a low-grade malignant process, a so-called verrucous carcinoma, a term used for carcinomas with slow, locally aggressive growth but without tendency to metastasis (Kraus and Perez-Mesa) (see p. 473).

In 4 instances of extensive and long-standing giant condylomata acuminata of the vulva Basset et al. found, on histologic examination, Bowen's disease which in 1 of the 4 patients had invaded the dermis. Although the authors have interpreted their findings as representing a "condylomatous form of Bowen's disease," it seems possible that the Bowen's disease had developed secondarily in giant condylomata acuminata, as observed by Kerl and Pickel.

HAND-FOOT-AND-MOUTH DISEASE

Hand-foot-and-mouth disease occurs in small epidemics, affecting mainly children. It takes a mild course and lasts less than a week. Small vesicles occur. They may be confined to the mouth where they result in small ulcers. If present on the skin, only a few vesicles are generally seen on the flexor aspects of the fingers and toes, and occasionally on the palms and soles. They have an erythematous base.

The disease is caused by an enterovirus of Coxsackie group A. Type A16 is most common, but several outbreaks have been due to types A5 or A10.

Histopathology. Early vesicles are intraepidermal, whereas older vesicles may be subepidermal in location. There is pronounced reticular degeneration of the epidermis, resulting in multilocular vesiculation (Miller and Tindall). In the deeper layers of the epidermis some ballooning degeneration may be found (Evans and Waddington). Neither inclusion bodies nor multinucleating giant cells are present. A nonspecific inflammatory infiltrate is present in the vesicles as well as in the underlying dermis.

Histogenesis. The coxsackie virus can be cultured from the stool, and occasionally also from the vesicles. The virus grows well on human-epithelial-cell cultures and on monkey kidney tissue cultures. It is pathogenic to suckling mice (Miller and Tindall).

CAT-SCRATCH DISEASE

Within a few days or weeks after having been scratched by a cat, a large, tender, visible swelling of a lymph node develops in the drainage area of the scratch. The cat scratch itself in some patients heals in a normal fashion, while in others it shows diffuse swelling or the presence of one or a few papules. Also, one or a few papules may appear on the skin in the vicinity of the scratch one or several months after the scratch.

Histopathology. The skin shows in the dermis one or several acellular areas of necrobiosis or necrosis. These areas are of various shapes, including round, triangular, or stellate. Surrounding the areas of necrobiosis one finds several layers of epithelioid cells, with the innermost layer of epithelioid cells showing a palisading arrangement. A few giant cells may be present among the epithelioid cells. The periphery of the epithelioid-cell reaction is surrounded by a zone of lymphoid cells (Johnson and Helwig).

The reaction in the lymph node is similar to that observed in the skin, except that in the center of epithelioid cell granulomas first abscesses of neutrophils appear that may have a stellate shape. Subsequently, the abscesses are replaced by areas of acellular necrosis. Around them are several layers of epithelioid cells and a peripheral mantle of lymphoid cells (Daniels and MacMurray).

Histogenesis. The agent causing cat-scratch disease is believed to belong to the same group as the agent causing lymphogranuloma venereum (see below).

Differential Diagnosis. For differentiation from lymphogranuloma venereum, see page 356.

LYMPHOGRANULOMA VENEREUM

Lymphogranuloma venereum, occasionally referred to also as lymphogranuloma inguinale, is a venereal disease. The organism causing it is one of the *Chlamydia* agents, which includes also the agents causing psittacosis and pneumonitis, and possibly also the agent causing cat-scratch disease. *Chlamydiae* resemble bacteria, especially the rickettsiae, more than they do viruses. *Chlamydiae* are large in comparison with viruses, measuring from 250 to 450 nm in diameter. The *Chlamydia* agent causing lymphogranuloma venereum can be cultured in the yolk sac of embryonated eggs, in mouse brain, and in some cell cultures (Philip et al.).

This disease begins about one week after exposure as a small initial papule on the genitals. This heals within a few days and may pass unnoticed. Within two to four weeks after exposure enlargement of the inguinal lymph nodes begins, usually on one side but occasionally bilaterally. This manifestation occurs in all heterosexual males infected with this disease but in only one third of the women. The involved inguinal lymph nodes at first are firm and tender but

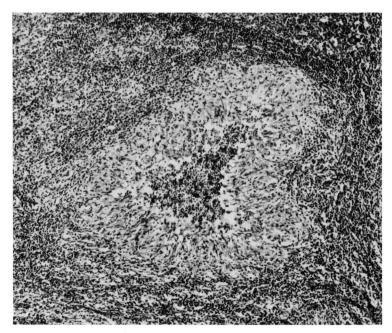

FIG. 20-11. **Lymphogranuloma venereum.** In the lymph node a stellate abscess is present. It is surrounded by epithelioid cells in palisade formation. (×100)

subsequently suppurate. The overlying skin then shows multiple draining sinuses.

In women in whom the infection begins in the lower two thirds of the vagina, drainage, rather than to inguinal lymph nodes, is to the iliac and ano-rectal lymph nodes, often leading to rectal stricture. Male homosexuals also may develop a rectal stricture if the primary lesion is in the perianal region (Sonck).

Histopathology. The changes in the initial papule are nonspecific. In the lymph nodes so-called stellate abscesses represent the characteristic lesion and, although not specific for lymphogranuloma venereum, are highly suggestive.

The earliest change in the lymph nodes consists of the formation of small islands of epithelioid cells scattered through the lymph nodes. Often, a few giant cells are found among the epithelioid cells. As the islands of epithelioid cells increase in size they become embedded in a chronic granulation tissue containing many plasma cells. With further increase in size, the centers of the epithelioid cell islands undergo necrosis and become filled with numerous neutrophils, as well as some macrophages (Sheldon and Heyman). These central abscesses tend to have a triangular or a quadrangular shape with elongated corners, resulting in the stellate appearance (Fig. 20-11). The epithelioid cells surrounding the abscesses show a palisading arrangement. As the abscesses enlarge gradually, they coalesce and lose their stellate appearance. No organisms have been identified in histologic sections so far (Sheldon and Heyman).

In the late stage of the disease the lymph nodes show areas of acellular necrosis, rather than abscesses as in the early stage of the disease. In addition, the lymph nodes contain numerous plasma cells (Jørgensen).

Differential Diagnosis. Lymphogranuloma venereum and cat-scratch disease may show identical reactions in the affected lymph nodes: either abscesses, some of them stellate, or areas of necrosis surrounded by epithelioid cells and a round-cell infiltrate. Clinical data may be required, therefore, for their differentiation.

BIBLIOGRAPHY

Introduction

Artenstein, M. S., and Demis, D. J.: Recent advances in the diagnosis and treatment of viral diseases of the skin. New Eng. J. Med., *270*:1101, 1964 (review).

Blank, H., Davis, C., and Collins, D.: Electron microscopy for the diagnosis of cutaneous viral infections. Brit. J. Derm., *83*:69, 1970.

Liu, C., and Llanes-Rodas, R.: Application of the immunofluorescent technic to the study of pathogenesis and rapid diagnosis of viral infections. Am. J. Clin. Path., *57*:829, 1972.

Luger, A.: Verlauf und Behandlung der Infektionen mit dem *Herpesvirus hominis*. II. Therapie. Z. Haut, *46*:399, 1971.

White, D. O.: Viral infections of the skin. Austral. J. Derm., *11*:5, 1970 (review).

Herpes Simplex

Allen, D. W., and Cole, P.: Viruses and human cancer. New Eng. J. Med., *286*:70, 1972.

Amstey, M. S., Patten, S. F., and Turk, M.: Herpesvirus cervicitis and cervical neoplasia. Cancer, *32*:1321, 1973.

Bastian, F. O., Rabson, A. S., Yee, C. L., and Tralka, T. S.: *Herpesvirus varicellae*. Arch. Path., *97*:331, 1974.

Catalano, L. W., Jr., Safley, G. H., Muscles, M., and Jarzynski, O. J.: Disseminated herpesvirus infection in a newborn infant: virologic, serologic, coagulation and interferon studies. J. Pediat., *79*:393, 1971.

Chang, T. W., Fiumara, N. J., and Weinstein, L.: Genital herpes. J.A.M.A., *229*:544, 1974.

Cheatham, W. J., Weller, T. H., Dolan, T. F., and Dower, J. C.: Varicella report of two fatal cases with necropsy, virus isolation, and serologic studies. Am. J. Path., *32*:1015, 1956.

Crouse, H. V., Coriell, L. L., Blank, H., and Scott, T. F. M.: Cytochemical studies on the intranuclear inclusion of herpes simplex. J. Immun., *65*:119, 1950.

Florman, A. L., Gershon, A. A., Blackett, P. R., and Nahmias, A. J.: Intrauterine infection with herpes simplex virus. J.A.M.A., *225*: 129, 1973.

Foley, F. D., Greenawald, K. A., Nash, G., and Pruitt, B. A., Jr.: Herpes virus infection in burned patients. New Eng. J. Med., *282*: 652, 1970.

Glasgow, L. A.: Cellular immunity in host resistance to viral infections. Arch. Int. Med., *126*:125, 1970.

Golden, B., Bell, W. E., and McKee, A. P.: Disseminated herpes simplex with encephalitis in a newborn. J.A.M.A., *209*:1219, 1969.

Graham, J. H., Bingul, O., and Burgoon, C. B., Jr.: Cytodiagnosis of inflammatory dermatoses. Arch. Derm., *87*:118, 1963.

Grimmer, H.: Zoster. Z. Haut, *45*:(29), 1970.

Herout, V., Vortel, V., and Vondrackova, A.: Herpes simplex involvement of the lower respiratory tract. Am. J. Clin. Path., *46*:411, 1966.

Izumi, A. K., Kim, R., and Arnold, H., Jr.: Herpes sycosis. Arch. Derm., *106*:372, 1972.

Joseph, T. J., and Vogt, P. J.: Disseminated herpes with hepatoadrenal necrosis in an adult. Am. J. Med., *56*:735, 1974.

Leider, W., Magoffin, R. L., Lennette, E. H., and Leonards, L. N. R.: Herpes-simplex-virus encephalitis. New Eng. J. Med., *273*:341, 1965.

Liu, C., and Llanes-Rodas, C.: Application of the immunofluorescent technic to the study of pathogenesis and rapid diagnosis of viral infections. Am. J. Clin. Path., *57*:829, 1972.

Logan, W. S., Tindall, J. P., and Elson, M. L.: Chronic cutaneous herpes simplex. Arch. Derm., *103*:606, 1971.

Luger, A.: Verlauf und Behandlung der Infektionen mit dem *Herpesvirus hominis*. I. Epidemiologie, Klinik und Serologie. Z. Haut *46*:387, 1971.

Muller, S. A., Herrmann, E. C., Jr., and Winkelmann, R. K.: Herpes simplex infections in hematologic malignancies. Am. J. Med., *52*:102, 1972.

Nahmias, A. J., and Dowdle, W. R.: Antigenic and biologic differences in *Herpesvirus hominis*. Progr. Med. Virol., *10*:110, 1968.

Nash, G., and Foley, F. D.: Herpetic infection of the middle and lower respiratory tract. Am. J. Clin. Path., *54*:857, 1970.

Nolan, D. C., Carruthers, M. M., and Lerner, M.: *Herpesvirus hominis* encephalitis in Michigan. New Eng. J. Med., *282*:10, 1970.

Patrizi, G., Middlekamp, J. N., and Reed, C. A.: Fine structure of herpes simplex virus in hepatoadrenal necrosis in the newborn. Am. J. Clin. Path., *49*:325, 1968.

St. Geme, J. W., Jr., Prince, J. T., Burke, B. A., *et al.*: Impaired cellular resistance to herpes-simplex virus in Wiskott-Aldrich syndrome. New Eng. J. Med., *273*:229, 1965.

Scott, T. F. M., and McLeod, D. L.: Cellular responses to infection with strains of herpes simplex virus. Ann. N.Y. Acad. Sci., *81*:118, 1959.

Southam, J. C., Colley, I. T., and Clarke, N. G.: Oral herpetic infection in adults. Brit. J. Derm., *80*:248, 1968.

Sutton, A. L., Smithwick, E. M., and Kim, D.: Fatal disseminated *Herpesvirus hominis* Type 2 infection in an adult with associated thymic dysplasia. Am. J. Med., *56*:545, 1974.

Zavoral, J. H., Ray, W. L., Kinnard, P. G., and Nahmias, A. J.: Neonatal herpetic infection. J.A.M.A., *213*:1492, 1970.

Varicella and Herpes Zoster

Appelbaum, E., Kreps, S. I., and Sunshine, A.: Herpes zoster encephalitis. Am. J. Med., *32*: 25, 1962.

Bastian, F. O., Rabson, A. S., Yee, C. L., and Tralka, T. S.: *Herpesvirus varicellae*. Arch. Path., *97*:331, 1974.

Berg, R., Hansson, O., Nordbring, F., *et al.*: Fatal varicella generalisata in a child with immunopathy and hereditary neurological syndrome. Virchows Arch. (Abt. A. Path. Anat.), *346*:103, 1969.

Cheatham, W. J.: The relation of heretofore unreported lesions to pathogenesis of herpes zoster. Am. J. Path., *29*:401, 1953.

Cheatham, W. J., Weller, T. H., Dolan, T. F., and Dower, J. C.: Varicella: report of two fatal cases with necropsy, virus isolation, and serologic studies. Am. J. Path., *32*:1015, 1956.

Denny-Brown, D., and Adams, R. D.: Pathologic features of herpes zoster. Arch. Neurol. Psychiat., *51*:216, 1944.

Eisenbud, M.: Chickenpox with visceral involvement. Am. J. Med., *12*:740, 1952.

Frank, L.: Varicella pneumonitis. Arch. Path., *50*:450, 1950.

Ghatak, N. R., and Zimmerman, H. M.: Spinal ganglion in herpes zoster. A light and electron microscopic study. Arch. Path., *95*:411, 1973.

Gold, E.: Serologic and virus-isolation studies of patients with varicella or herpes-zoster infection. New Eng. J. Med., *274*:181, 1966.

Hasegawa, T.: Further electron microscopic observations of herpes zoster virus. Arch. Derm., *103*:45, 1971.

Kain, H. K., Feldman, C. A., and Cohn, L. H.: Herpes zoster generalisatus pneumonia. Arch. Intern. Med., *110*:98, 1962.

Lucchesi, P. F., La Boccetta, A. C., and Peale, A. R.: Varicella neonatorum. Am. J. Dis. Child., *73*:44, 1947.

Morecki, R., and Becker, N. H.: Human herpesvirus infection. Its fine structure identification in paraffin-embedded tissue. Arch. Path., *86*: 292, 1968.

Muller, S. A., and Winkelmann, R. K.: Cutaneous nerve changes in zoster. J. Invest. Derm., *52*:71, 1969.

Nasemann, T., Menzel, I., and Schaeg, G.: Generalisierte Varicellen bei Morbus Hodgkin. Licht- und elektronenoptische Beobachtungen. Hautarzt, *24*:530, 1973.

Rado, J. P., Tako, J., Geder, L., and Jeney, E.: Herpes zoster house epidemic in steroid-treated patients. Arch. Intern. Med., *116*:329, 1965.

Rogers, R. S., III, and Tindall, J. P.: Herpes zoster in children. Arch. Derm., *106*:204, 1972.

Rose, F. C., Brett, E. M., and Burston, J.: Zoster encephalomyelitis. Arch. Neurol., *11*:155, 1964.

Weinstein, L., and Meade, R. H.: Respiratory manifestations of chicken pox. Arch. Intern. Med., *98*:91, 1956.

Weller, T. H., Witton, H. M., and Bell, E. J.: The etiologic agents of varicella and herpes zoster. Isolation, propagation, and cultural characteristics in vitro. J. Exp. Med., *108*:843, 1958.

Variola

Blank, H., and Rake, G.: Viral and Rickettsial Diseases of the Skin, Eye, and Mucous Membranes of Man. pp. 9 and 105. Boston, Little, Brown & Co., 1955.

Davis, C. M., and Musil, G.: Milker's nodule. Arch. Derm., *101*:305, 1968.

Michelson, H. E., and Ikeda, K.: Microscopic changes in variola. Arch. Derm. Syph., *15*:138, 1927.

Nasemann, T.: Die Viruskrankheiten der Haut. *In* Marchionini, A. (ed.): Handbuch der Haut- und Geschlechtskrankheiten, Ergänzungswerk, vol. IV/2, p. 129. Berlin, Springer Verlag, 1961.

Eczema Herpeticum, Eczema Vaccinatum

Barton, R. L., and Brunsting, L. A.: Kaposi's varicelliform eruption. Arch. Derm. Syph., *50*:99, 1944.

Lausecker, H.: Kaposis varicelliforme Eruption-Ekzema herpetiforme. Arch. f. Derm. u. Syph., *196*:183, 1953.

Loeffel, E. D., and Meyer, J. S.: Eczema vaccinatum in Darier's disease. Arch. Derm., *102*:451, 1970.

Lynch, F. W.: Kaposi's varicelliform eruption. Arch. Derm. Syph., *51*:129, 1945.

Marchionini, A., and Nasemann, T.: Zur Diagnostik der durch Viren der Pockengruppe hervorgerufenen Erkrankungen des Menschen. Arch. klin. exp. Derm., *202*:69, 1955.

Silverstein, E. A., and Burnett, J. W.: Kaposi's varicelliform eruption complicating pemphigus foliaceus. Arch. Derm., *95*:214, 1967.

Verbov, J., Munro, D. D., and Miller, A.: Recurrent eczema herpeticum associated with ichthyosis vulgaris. Brit. J. Derm., *86*:638, 1972.

von Weiss, J. F., Kibrick, S., and Lever, W. F.: Eczema herpeticum as complication of Darier's disease. Ann. Intern. Med., *62*:1293, 1965.

Milkers' Nodules

Davis, C. M., and Musil, G.: Milker's nodule. Arch. Derm., *101*:305, 1968.

Evins, S., Leavell, U. W., Jr., and Phillips, J. A.: Intranuclear inclusions in milker's nodules. Arch. Derm., *103*:91, 1971.

Friedman-Kien, A. E., Rowe, W. P., and Banfield, W. G.: Milkers' nodules: Isolation of a poxvirus from a human case. Science, *140*:1335, 1963.

Katzenellenbogen, I.: Studies on milkers' nodules. Dermatologica, *105*:69, 1952.

Marchionini, A., and Nasemann, T.: Zur Diagnostik der durch Viren der Pockengruppe hervorgerufenen Erkrankungen des Menschen. Arch. klin. exp. Derm., *202*:69, 1959.

Nomland, R., and McKee, A. P.: Milkers' nodules. Arch. Derm. Syph., *65*:663, 1952.

Ecthyma Contagiosum (Orf)

Leavell, U. W., Jr., McNamara, M. J., Muelling, R., *et al.*: Orf. J.A.M.A., *204*:657, 1968.

Naggington, J., and Whittle, C. H.: Human orf: isolation of virus by tissue culture. Brit. Med. J., *2*:1324, 1961.

Wheeler, C. E., Cawley, E. P., and Johnson, J. H.: Ecthyma contagiosum (orf). Arch. Derm. Syph., *71*:481, 1955.

Yeh, H. P., and Soltani, K.: Ultrastructural studies in human orf. Arch. Derm., *109*:390, 1974.

Molluscum Contagiosum

Hasegawa, T., Fujiwara, E., Ametani, T., and Tsuruhara, T.: Further electron microscopic observation of molluscum contagiosum virus. Arch. klin. exp. Derm., *235*:319, 1969.

Henao, M., and Freeman, R. G.: Inflammatory molluscum contagiosum. Arch. Derm., *90*:479, 1964.

Lutzner, M. A.: Molluscum contagiosum, verruca and zoster viruses. Arch. Derm., *87*:436, 1963.

Mescon, H., Gray, M., and Moretti, G.: Molluscum contagiosum. J. Invest. Derm., *23*:293, 1954.

Nasemann, T., and Stanka, P.: Darstellung der Einschlusskörper des Molluscum contagiosum durch Pepsin-Hydrolyse und anschliessende Feulgen-Reaktion. Derm. Wschr., *140*:747, 1959.

Robinson, H. J., Jr., Prose, P. H., Friedman-Kien, A. E., *et al.*: The molluscum contagiosum virus in chick embryo cell cultures: an electron microscopic study. J. Invest. Derm., *52*:51, 1969.

Verruca

Almeida, J. D., Howatson, A. F., and Williams, M. G.: Electron microscope study of human warts; sites of virus production and nature of the inclusion bodies. J. Invest. Derm., *38*: 337, 1962.

Basset, A., Maleville, J., Grosshans, E., et al.: La forme condylomateuse de la maladie de Bowen vulvaire. Semaine hôp. Paris, *48*: 1343, 1972.

Bauer, K. M., and Friederich, H. C.: Peniscarcinom auf dem Boden vorbehandelter Condylomata acuminata. Z. Haut Geschlechtskr., *39*:150, 1965.

Becker, F. T., Walder, H. J., and Larson, D. M.: Giant condylomata acuminata. Arch. Derm., *100*:184, 1969.

Blank, H., Buerk, M., and Weidman, F.: The nature of the inclusion body of verruca vulgaris: a histochemical study of the nucleotids. J. Invest. Derm., *16*:19, 1951.

Cornelius, C. E., Witkowski, J. A., and Wood, M. G.: Viral verruca, human papova virus infection. Arch. Derm., *98*:377, 1968.

Dawson, D. F., Duckworth, J. K., Bernhardt, H., and Young, J. M.: Giant condyloma and verrucous carcinoma of the genital area. Arch. Path., *79*:225, 1965.

Delescluse, C., Pruniéras, M., Regnier, M., *et al.*: Epidermodysplasia verruciformis. Arch. Derm. Forsch., *242*:202, 1972.

Gianotti, F., Caputo, R., and Califano, A.: Ultrastructural study of epidermodysplasia verruciformis Lewandowsky and Lutz. Arch. klin. exp. Derm., *235*:161, 1969.

Goldstein, M. B.: Besondere Verlaufsformen der rein papillomatösen Geschwülste des Penis. Hautarzt, *13*:25, 1962.

Grupper, C., Pruniéras, M., Delescluse, C., *et al.*: Épidermodysplasie verruciforme: étude ultrastructurale et autoradiographique. Ann. derm. syph., *98*:33, 1971.

Jablonska, S., Biczysko, W., Jakubowicz, K., and Dabrowski, J.: On the viral etiology of epidermodysplasia verruciformis Lewandowsky-Lutz. Dermatologica, *137*:113, 1968.

Jablonska, S., Biczysko, W., Jakubowicz, K., and Dabrowski, H.: The ultrastructure of transitional states to Bowen's disease and invasive Bowen's carcinoma in epidermodysplasia verruciformis. Dermatologica, *140*:186, 1970.

Jablonska, S., and Formas, I.: Weitere positive Ergebnisse mit Auto- und Heteroinokulation bei Epidermodysplasia verruciformis Lewandowsky-Lutz. Dermatologica, *118*:86, 1959.

Judge, J. R.: Giant condyloma acuminatum involving vulva and rectum. Arch. Path., *88*: 46, 1969.

Kerl, H., and Pickel, H.: Maligne Umwandlung von Condylomata acuminata der Vulva. Z. Haut, *46*:[155], 1971.

Knoblich, R., and Failing, J. F., Jr.: Giant condyloma acuminatum (Buschke-Loewenstein tumor) of the rectum. Am. J. Clin. Path., *48*:389, 1967.

Kovi, J., Tillman, L., and Lee, S. M.: Malignant transformation of condyloma acuminatum. Am. J. Clin. Path., *61*:702, 1974.

Kraus, F. T., and Perez-Mesa, C.: Verrucous carcinoma. Cancer, *19*:26, 1966.

Lutz, W.: A propos de l'épidermodysplasie verruciforme. Dermatologica, *92*:30, 1946.

Lutz, W.: Zur Epidermodysplasia verruciformis. Dermatologica, *115*:309, 1957.

Machacek, G. F., and Weakley, D. R.: Giant condylomata acuminata of Buschke and Lowenstein. Arch. Derm., *82*:41, 1960.

Nasemann, T., and Georgiewa, S.: Elektronenoptische Schnittuntersuchungen bei Virusacanthomen von Mensch und Tier. Hautarzt, *18*:52, 1967.

Oriel, J. D., and Almeida, J. D.: Demonstration of virus particles in human genital warts. Brit. J. Ven. Dis., *46*:37, 1970.

Rajagopalan, K., Bahru, J., Loo, D. S. C., *et al.*: Familial epidermodysplasia verruciformis of Lewandowsky and Lutz. Arch. Derm., *105*: 73, 1972.

Ruiter, M., and van Mullem, P. J.: Behavior of virus in malignant degeneration of skin lesions in epidermodysplasia verruciformis. J. Invest. Derm., *54*:324, 1970.

Schellender, F., and Fritsch, P.: Epidermodysplasia verruciformis. Neue Aspekte zur Symptomatologie und Pathogenese. Dermatologica, *140*:251, 1970.

Shapiro, L., and Baraf, C. S.: Isolated epidermolytic acanthoma. Arch. Derm., *101*:220, 1970.

Sonck, C. E.: Condylomata acuminata mit Übergang in Karzinom. Z. Haut, *46*:273, 1971.

Strauss, M. J., Bunting, H., and Melnick, J. L.: Virus-like particles and inclusion bodies in skin papillomas. J. Invest. Derm., *15*:433, 1950.

Hand-Foot-and-Mouth Disease

Evans, A. D., and Waddington, E.: Hand, foot and mouth disease in South Wales, 1964. Brit. J. Derm., *79*:309, 1967.

Miller, G. D., and Tindall, J. P.: Hand-foot-and-mouth disease. J.A.M.A., *203*:827, 1968.

Cat-Scratch Disease

Daniels, W. B., and MacMurray, F. G.: Cat-scratch disease. Arch. Int. Med., *88*:736, 1951.

Johnson, W. T., and Helwig, E. B.: Cat-scratch disease. Histopathologic changes in the skin. Arch. Derm., *100*:148, 1969.

Lymphogranuloma Venereum

Jørgensen, L.: Lymphogranuloma venereum. Acta path. microbiol. scand., *47*:113, 1959.

Philip, R. N., Hill, D. A., Greaves, A. B., *et al.*: Study of *Chlamydiae* in patients with lymphogranuloma venereum and urethritis attending a venereal disease clinic. Brit. J. Vener. Dis., *47*:114, 1971.

Sheldon, W. H., and Heyman, A.: Lymphogranuloma venereum. Am. J. Path., *23*:653, 1947.

Sonck, C. E.: Lymphogranuloma inguinale. Klinische, epidemiologische and immunologische Aspekte. Hautarzt, *23*:280, 1972.

21

Lipidoses

The term lipidoses may be applied to a group of diseases in which the lesions, due to a generalized or local disturbance of the lipid metabolism, contain lipid substances.

The lipidoses can be divided into the following four groups:

1. *Systemic Lipidoses With Altered Serum Lipoprotein Values*
   Hyperlipoproteinemia, Types I to V
   Tangier Disease
2. *Tissue Storage Lipidoses*
   Niemann-Pick disease
   Gaucher's disease
   Angiokeratoma corporis diffusum
   (Fabry)
   Lipogranulomatosis
   (Farber's disease)
3. *Histiocytosis*
4. *Predominantly Cutaneous Lipidoses*
   Diffuse normolipemic plane
   xanthoma
   Juvenile xanthogranuloma
   Reticulohistiocytosis
   Generalized eruptive histiocytoma

HYPERLIPOPROTEINEMIA

The division of hyperlipoproteinemia into five types, as proposed by Fredrickson et al., is based on the paper electrophoretic separation of the plasma lipoproteins in barbital buffer pH 8.6 containing 1 per cent of albumin (Lees and Hatch). Four fractions are thus obtained, which are, in order of decreasing electrophoretic mobility: chylomicrons, beta lipoproteins, prebeta lipoproteins, and alpha lipoproteins. These four fractions correlate well with those obtained by fractionation of the lipoproteins by means of analytic ultracentrifugation, whereby the ultracentrifugal flotation rate is expressed in Svedberg flotation units (S_f). The chylomicrons, having an ultracentrifugal flotation rate in excess of S_f 400, contain about 81 per cent of triglycerides and 9 per cent of cholesterol; the prebeta lipoproteins with an S_f of from 20 to 400 contain approximately 52 per cent of triglycerides and 22 per cent of cholesterol; and the beta lipoproteins with an S_f of 0 to 20 have only about 9 per cent of triglycerides but 47 per cent of cholesterol (Fleischmajer, 1971). The beta lipoprotein molecules, in contrast to the prebeta lipoprotein molecules and chylomicrons, are of such small size that they cause no turbidity of the plasma. The five types of hyperlipoproteinemia (Table 21-1) are:

Type I: *Hyperchylomicronemia.* First described by Bürger and Grütz, this condition is recessively inherited and begins in infancy. It is very rare. It is always associated with hepatosplenomegaly and abdominal cramps (Holt et al.). There is a deficiency in lipoprotein lipase activity in the plasma as well as in the tissue (Ferrans et al.).

Type II: *Hyperbetalipoproteinemia.* This condition is dominantly inherited. In the homozygous the disease is apt to be severe, with development of xanthomas in childhood and death from coronary occlusion at a rather early age (Lever et al.; Maher et al.).

Type III: *Broad-beta Lipoproteinemia.*

TABLE 21-1. Biochemical and Clinical Data in Hyperlipoproteinemia

Type	Plasma Electrophoresis			Plasma Lipids		Appearance of Serum After Standing		Type of Xanthomas					Association With		
	Chylo-micron	Pre-beta	Beta	Choles-terol	Tri-glyc	Super-natant	Infra-natant	Erup-tive	Tuber-ous	Tendi-nous	Xan-thel-asma	Plane	Athero-sclero-sis	Dia-betes	Hepato-megaly Pancre-atitis
I	↑			(+)	+++	cream	clear	+							yes
II			↑	++		clear			+	+	+	+	yes		
III		↑	↑	+	+	turbid		+	+	+	+	+	yes	yes	(yes)
IV		↑		+	++	milky		+	(+)				yes	yes	(yes)
V	↑	↑		+	+++	cream	turbid	+						yes	yes

This shows an increase in both beta and prebeta lipoproteins. It is biochemically and also clinically intermediate between Types II and IV (Polano et al.). It is recessively transmitted (Fleischmajer, 1969). Usually it does not start until adult life (Holimon and Wasserman).

Type IV: *Hyperprebetalipoproteinemia.* It usually is dominantly inherited (Schreibman et al.). It is the most common of the five types of hyperlipoproteinemias.

Type V: *Mixed Prebeta and Chylomicronemia.* Biochemically, it is a combination of Types I and IV. There occasionally is a deficiency of lipoprotein lipase activity in plasma and tissue, similar to that seen in Type I (Schreiber and Shapiro; Fleischmajer, 1971).

Although, as a rule, the five types of hyperlipoproteinemia are well defined entities, some relationship exists between Types IV and V since there are instances in which the Type IV electrophoretic pattern can be converted into Type V by minor dietary measures; and in families of Type V probands, relatives can be found with Type IV pattern (Borrie and Slack).

The hyperlipoproteinemias in their idiopathic form can evoke several other diseases, such as atherosclerosis, diabetes, or pancreatis (see under Systemic Lesions, and Table 21-1). In addition, rather than occurring as a primary disorder, several types of hyperlipoproteinemia may occur secondary to other diseases. Thus, hyperlipoproteinemia Type II may be induced by myxedema, biliary cirrhosis, or nephrosis; hyperlipoproteinemia of Type IV may be brought on by diabetes, or by von Gierke's disease (also called Cori Type I glycogenosis); and hyperlipoproteinemia of Type V may develop in myxedema, nephrosis, diabetes, or pancreatitis (Roberts et al.; Fleischmajer, 1971).

Cutaneous lesions may occur in all five types of hyperlipoproteinemia (Table 21-1). They may be divided into eruptive xanthomas, tuberous xanthomas, tendon xanthomas, xanthelasmata, and plane xanthomas.

Eruptive xanthomas are typical of triglyceridemia or hyperlipemia and, therefore, may occur in all four types of hyperlipoproteinemia that are associated with an increase in the concentration of either chylomicrons or prebeta lipoproteins in the plasma (Types I, III, IV, V). Eruptive xanthomas consist of small, soft, yellowish papules with a predilection for the buttocks and the posterior aspects of the thighs. They come and go with fluctuations of the concentration of the triglycerides in the plasma (Lever et al.; Cornelius).

Tuberous xanthomas are found predominantly in cases with an increase in the beta lipoproteins, i.e., in Types II and III, and rarely in Type IV. They are large nodes or plaques, located most commonly on the elbows, knees, fingers, and the buttocks.

Tendon xanthomas occur in patients with excessive plasma levels of beta lipoproteins, i.e., in Types II and III. The Achilles tendons and the extensor tendons of the fingers are most frequently affected.

Xanthelasmata is the term used for slightly raised, yellowish, soft plaques on the eyelids. Although xanthelasmata are the commonest of the cutaneous xanthomas in Types II and III hyperlipoproteinemia, they also occur in individuals with normal lipoprotein levels. It is estimated that two thirds of individuals with xanthelasma palpebrarum have normal lipid levels in their serum (Polano; Pedace and Winkelmann).

Plane xanthomas develop in skin folds and, especially, in the palmar creases. They occur in Type III hyperlipoproteinemia, and in biliary cirrhosis producing Type II.

Systemic diseases that can be evoked by the idiopathic hyperlipoproteinemias include atherosclerosis, diabetes, and hepatosplenomegaly with pancreatitis (Table 21-1). Atherosclerosis is associated mainly with elevated beta lipoprotein values and, to a lesser degree, with elevated prebeta lipoprotein values. Whereas atherosclerotic coronary heart disease occurs mainly in Types II and III, and occasionally in Type IV, occlusive peripheral vascular disease, particularly of the lower extremities, can occur in Type III. Diabetes occurs most commonly with elevated prebeta lipoprotein values in Types III to V. Hepatosplenomegaly and pancreatitis causing severe abdominal cramps are found mainly in association with chylomicronemia (Types I and V), and less commonly with elevated prebeta lipoprotein values (Type IV, rarely Type III).

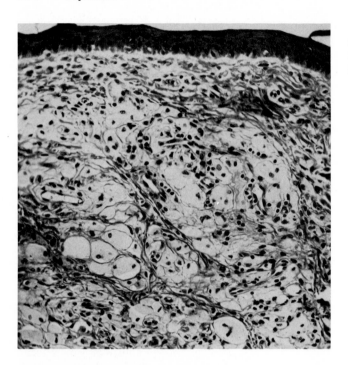

FIG. 21-1. **Xanthoma tuberosum, early lesion.** Numerous xanthoma cells (foam cells) are present. Fibrosis is slight. (×200)

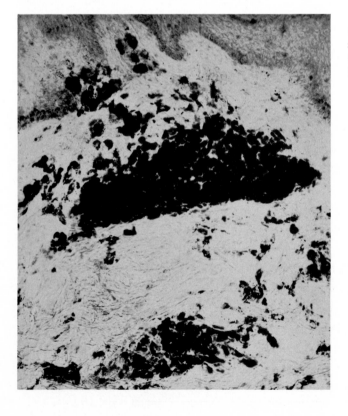

FIG. 21-2. **Xanthoma tuberosum, early lesion.** Scarlet red stain for fat. The xanthoma cells are filled with lipid material. (×100)

Histopathology. The histologic appearance of xanthomas of the skin and the tendons is characterized by the presence of xanthoma or foam cells. Foam cells are macrophages that, because of their ability to phagocytize, have become filled with lipid droplets. In routine sections xanthoma cells have a reticulated or foamy cytoplasm (Fig. 21-1), because the lipid droplets have dissolved and have been extracted from the cytoplasm during the automatic processing carried out on routine specimens. However, the lipid droplets can be seen when frozen or formalin-fixed sections are stained with fat stains, such as scarlet red or Sudan red (Fig. 21-2).

Xanthoma cells usually have only one nucleus, although they may have several. In multinucleated xanthoma cells either the nuclei are irregularly distributed, as in foreign-body giant cells, or they lie near the center of the cell grouped around a small island of nonfoamy cytoplasm and are surrounded by foamy cytoplasm. The latter type is called a Touton giant cell (Fig. 21-3). Only minor differences exist in the histologic appearance and chemical composition of the various types of xanthoma.

Eruptive xanthomas, which usually are of recent origin, often show a considerable admixture of nonfoamy cells, among them lymphoid cells, histiocytes and neutrophils, whereas the number of well-developed foam cells may still be small (Fig. 21-4). Eruptive xanthomas, in comparison with tuberous xanthomas, contain more free fatty acids and triglycerides and less cholesterol esters than the other types of xanthoma (Baes et al.). Like the subcutaneous fat and the lipid in the sebaceous glands, they stain orange-red with scarlet red and usually the lipid within them is not doubly refractile on polariscopic examination of frozen sections.

Tuberous xanthomas consist of large and small aggregates of xanthoma or foam cells. In early lesions there usually is a slight admixture of nonfoamy cells, among them lymphoid cells, histiocytes and neutrophils. In

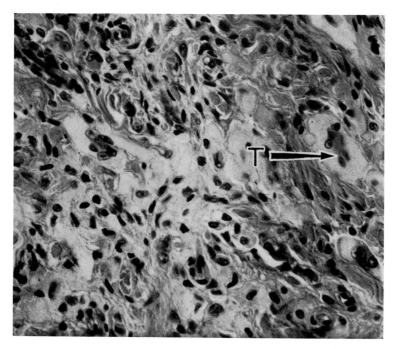

FIG. 21-3. **Xanthoma tuberosum, late lesion.** In addition to xanthoma cells, many fibroblasts are present. On the right side there is a typical Touton giant cell (T). In the Touton cell the nuclei lie near the center of the cell, grouped around a small island of nonfoamy cytoplasm and surrounded by foamy cytoplasm. (×400)

well developed lesions the infiltrate is composed almost entirely of foam cells (Fig. 21-1). In older lesions fibroblasts appear (Fig. 21-3). Ultimately, collagen bundles replace many of the foam cells. Tuberous xanthomas, in comparison with eruptive xanthomas, contain more cholesterol esters. The foam cells of tuberous xanthomas, therefore, stain brownish-red rather than orange-red with Sudan red or scarlet red and, on polariscopic examination, they are doubly refractile.

Tendon xanthomas are identical with tuberous xanthomas in their histologic appearance and chemical composition.

Xanthelasmata located on the eyelids differ from tuberous xanthomas by the fairly superficial location of the foam cells and the nearly complete absence of fibrosis.

Plane xanthomas, located usually in the palmar creases, also lack fibrosis. Similar to tuberous and tendon xanthomas and to xanthelasmata, plane xanthomas stain brownish-red with Sudan red or scarlet red and show double refraction on polariscopic examination.

SYSTEMIC LESIONS. Atherosclerosis of the coronary arteries is accelerated and extensive in patients with hyperlipoproteinemia of the Types II, III and IV. The peripheral arteries often are excessively atheromatous in Type III. The bone marrow, lymph nodes, liver and spleen often contain foam cells in Types I, IV and V, their number generally being dependent on the degree of hypertriglyceridemia (Roberts et al.). The number of foam cells in the liver and spleen is particularly high in patients with hepatosplenomegaly and pancreatitis, as seen especially in Types I and V, with the liver showing, in addition, extensive fatty degeneration, and the pancreas fibrosis (Bruton and Kanter). In contrast with Types I, IV and V, Type III generally shows no foam cells in the liver, the lymph nodes, and the bone marrow, but they may be found in the spleen and in the mesangium of the renal glomeruli (Amatruda et al.).

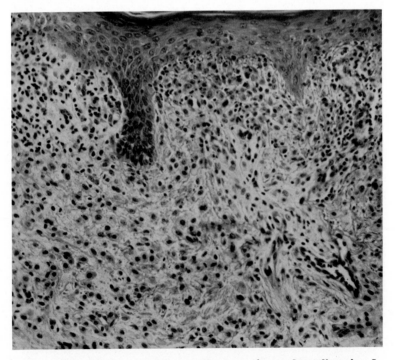

FIG. 21-4. **Papular, eruptive xanthoma, primary hyperlipemia.** In this early lesion the foam cells are fairly small. There is an admixture of inflammatory cells. (×200)

The Type IV hyperlipoproteinemia observed secondary to von Gierke's disease, now often referred to as Cori Type I glycogenosis, is a result of a deficiency of glucose-6-phosphatase. The inability of the patient to dephosphorylate glucose-6-phosphate to glucose leads to hepatomegaly as the result of glycogen storage, and to hyperlipoproteinemia as a result of an increased fat synthesis, predominantly of long chain triglycerides (Cuttino et al.). Eruptive xanthomas form as a consequence of the hyperprebetalipoproteinemia.

Of interest are the findings in the liver in patients having hyperlipoproteinemia Type II secondary to biliary cirrhosis. Such patients have pronounced jaundice, and the jaundice precedes the appearance of xanthomatous lesions often by several years. The blood serum is clear, but due to its high content of bilirubin it is intensely green. The cutaneous lesions consist of xanthelasmata and often also of plane xanthomas in the palmar creases. The biliary cirrhosis, which is responsible for the hyperbetalipoproteinemia, is produced in the great majority of cases by a pericholangiolitis that leads to an obliteration of the interlobular bile ducts (Ahrens et al.). In rare instances the biliary cirrhosis is produced by an obstruction of extrahepatic bile ducts (Ahrens et al.), or, in infants, by a congenital hypoplasia of the interlobular bile ducts (Ito et al.).

Histogenesis. Electron microscopic examination of the foam cells or xanthoma cells shows them to have an irregular cytoplasmic border typical of macrophages. Early foam cells show scattered rounded lipid vacuoles that are without limiting membrane. In addition, their cytoplasm contains numerous organelles, including lysosomes. Older foam cells are filled with many large lipid vacuoles surrounded by lysosomes including many residual bodies containing myelin figures, indicating that the macrophages have attempted to digest the lipid vacuoles but have failed to accomplish this (Zemel; Wolff and Braun-Falco).

In patients with eruptive xanthomas due to hypertriglyceridemia electron microscopic examination reveals many lipid droplets extracellularly in the vicinity of capillaries, allowing the conclusion that the lipid droplets originate from the plasma lipids. The lipid particles are not phagocytized by the endothelial cells but by the pericytes and by pericapillary macrophages. The macrophages contain, in addition, numerous lysosomes, including residual bodies (Parker and Odland).

TANGIER DISEASE

In this recessively inherited disease the plasma alpha lipoproteins are greatly decreased. This is associated with reduced concentrations of cholesterol and phospholipids in the plasma. In contrast to the low plasma cholesterol level the cholesterol ester concentration in many tissues, including the skin, is increased.

Clinically, patients with hypoalphalipoproteinemia have markedly enlarged tonsils that show orange-yellow striations. There may be hypersplenism. The skin usually is free of lesions (Krebs and Kuske). In one patient, however, numerous scattered papules were noted, mainly on the trunk (Waldorf et al.).

Histopathology. Irrespective of whether the skin has papular lesions or appears normal, the dermis shows extensive deposits of cholesterol esters both within foamy macrophages and extracellularly (Waldorf et al.; Krebs and Kuske). The lipid material stains positively with the Schultz stain, indicating the presence of cholesterol or cholesterol esters. It is markedly birefringent under the polarizing microscope, indicating the presence of cholesterol esters.

Deposits similar to those in the skin are found in the tonsils, as well as in the liver, the spleen, the lymph nodes, and the thymus.

Histogenesis. It is assumed that the deficiency of alpha lipoproteins disturbs the lipid transport function of chylomicrons, possibly by rendering the chylomicrons relatively unstable so that cholesterol esters coming from the intestines bound to chylomicrons are prematurely released and are deposited in various tissues and thus do not reach the plasma (Waldorf et al.).

NIEMANN-PICK DISEASE

Niemann-Pick disease, like Gaucher's disease and Fabry's disease, represents a sphingolipidosis. The metabolic error is intracellular and consists of a diminution of sphingomyelinase activity (Brady). As a result of this defect, sphingomyelin and cholesterol accumulate in various tissues, mainly in the macrophages of lymphoid tissue, such as the lymph nodes, the spleen and the thymus, in the Kupffer cells and parenchymal cells of the liver, in the alveolar cells of the lungs, and in the ganglion cells and the glial cells of the brain. The skin, however, is spared.

The usual infantile form of Niemann-Pick disease leads to death, generally within a few years. There are massive enlargement of the liver and spleen and severe central nervous system manifestations. In association with cachexia, a diffuse yellow-brown pigmentation of the skin occurs. Some patients show also papular eruptive xanthomas in association with a secondary hyperlipemia (Crocker and Farber).

In the rare adult form the prognosis is much better than in the infantile form, since there is only mild visceral and no central nervous system involvement (Lynn and Terry).

Histopathology. On histologic examination the brownish discoloration of the skin is found to be due to the presence of increased amounts of melanin in the basal layer of the epidermis. The eruptive xanthomas show the histologic features already described (see p. 365).

The characteristic cell of Niemann-Pick disease is a large foam cell, 20 to 100 μm in diameter. The lipids within this cell stain with scarlet red and Sudan black B and are doubly refractile.

Histogenesis. The sphingomyelinase activity is greatly reduced and in one patient studied by Brady it was only 7 per cent of the normal activity in the liver and not measurable in the kidney. Electron microscopic study shows in the foam cells, as the result of the enzymatic defect, numerous lipid vacuoles and lysosomes. The latter either are engorged with lipids or are present as laminated residual bodies, so-called myelin bodies, resembling those seen in Fabry's disease (Lynn and Terry). This is suggestive of a deficiency of enzymatic activity within the lysosomes.

GAUCHER'S DISEASE

The metabolic error in Gaucher's disease consists of an intracellular deficiency of glucocerebrosidase (Brady et al.). As a result of this defect, glucocerebrosides accumulate, mainly in the macrophages or reticuloendothelial cells of the spleen, the liver, the lymph nodes, and the bone marrow. The skin, however, is spared. The serum lipids are normal.

Gaucher's disease may start in infancy, in childhood or in adult life. When starting in early life it is fatal, whereas cases starting in later life take a chronic course. There are hepatosplenomegaly and rarefaction and cortical thickening of the long bones. Frequently, the bulbar conjunctiva shows wedge-shaped pigmentation next to the cornea. In the chronic or adult form the skin may show yellow-brown pigmentation, especially on the face and the shins.

Histopathology. The pigmented skin merely shows increased amounts of melanin in the basal layer of the epidermis.

The characteristic cell of Gaucher's disease, as found in the liver, the spleen, and the bone marrow, is a large cell, 20 to 100 μm in diameter, containing numerous thin, wavy fibrils. This gives the cytoplasm a striated, granular appearance, which is in contrast with the vacuolated appearance of the Niemann-Pick cell. The cells, in addition to staining positively for lipids, contain abundant iron as the result of the phagocytosis of erythrocytes.

Histogenesis. The activity of glucocerebrosidase is markedly diminished not only in the spleen but also in leukocyte suspension (Kampine et al.). On electron microscopic examination, the Gaucher cell contains within lysosomes tubular structures with a diameter of 20 to 30 nm in which filaments, about 8 nm wide, lie in a spiral arrangement. These filaments probably represent aggregated glucocerebroside molecules (Lee et al.). Marked acid phosphatase activity is present within the intertubular matrix of small, young lysosomes. On the other hand, little or no activity is seen within large, matured lysosomes, since, as residual bodies, they no longer are active (Hibbs et al.).

ANGIOKERATOMA CORPORIS DIFFUSUM (FABRY)

Fabry's disease, like Niemann-Pick disease and Gaucher's disease, represents a sphingolipidosis. As the result of a deficiency of alpha-galactosidase, or ceramide

FIG. 21-5. **Angiokeratoma corporis diffusum (Fabry).** Superficial capillaries, some of them completely enclosed by the hyperplastic epidermis, are dilated, as are some of the more deeply situated vessels. (×100)

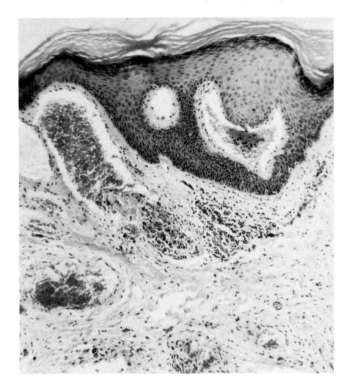

trihexosidase, the glycolipid or ceramide trihexoside galactosylgalactosylglucosylceramide cannot be cleaved (Klint). Consequently, it is deposited in many types of cells and in many organs, including the endothelial cells and pericytes of blood vessels throughout the body. In addition, smooth muscle cells, ganglion cells, nerves, the epithelial cells of the cornea, the kidney, the skin, and many other organs may be affected (Sagebiel and Parker). Recently, a clinical picture resembling that of Fabry's disease has been reported as a result of a severely reduced alpha-L-fucosidase activity (Epinette et al.).

The cutaneous eruption in most instances of Fabry's disease consists of innumerable small "angiomas," usually only 1 to 2 mm in size. The greatest number of lesions is located on the lower trunk. The first lesions, as a rule, begin to appear in late childhood. The angiomas of angiokeratoma corporis diffusum, in contrast with those of angiokeratoma of Mibelli (see p. 594), show little or no hyperkeratosis. In occasional in-stances, cutaneous lesions are absent (Urbain et al.). A few angiomas may be present in the mouth.

Systemic manifestations include the gradual development of renal insufficiency as the result of lipid deposits in the glomeruli. Death usually occurs in the fourth or fifth decade of life as the result of renal failure (Ruiter, 1957). In other patients death may occur as the result of myocardial infarction or of a cerebrovascular accident (Wise et al.). Early symptoms of the disease are paresthesias of the hands and feet subsequent to changes in the temperature.

Histopathology. In routine sections of the skin one merely observes dilatation of the superficial capillaries and occasionally also of the more deeply situated vessels (Fig. 21-5). Whereas the lipid deposits in the heart muscle, the kidneys, and the bone marrow macrophages generally can be suspected even with routine fixation and staining because of the presence of swelling and vacuolization within affected cells, the amount of lipid in the skin is too small to be detected in routinely fixed and stained sections. One must resort to special fixation and lipid-staining technics (Tarnowski and Hashimoto, 1969).

For the demonstration of the lipid deposits in the skin one either fixes the specimen in a solution containing 1 per cent calcium chloride in addition to 10 per cent formalin (Pittelkow et al.) or exposes the specimen first to 10 per cent formalin for two days and then to a 3 per cent solution of potassium bichromate for one week (Ruiter, 1954). Staining with Sudan black B, which demonstrates the lipids particularly well, is preferable to staining with scarlet red. Since the lipid material is doubly refractile, it can be demonstrated by means of polariscopic examination of formalin-fixed frozen sections. Staining of unfixed frozen sections with PAS or Sudan black B also reveals the lipid granules (Frost et al.). Lipid deposits are not restricted to the cutaneous areas showing angiomas but are present also in normal-appearing skin (de Groot).

Lipid deposits in the skin are seen particularly in the endothelial cells and pericytes of the cutaneous capillaries (Fig. 21-6), but also in many fibroblasts and in the arrector pilorum muscles (Ruiter, 1954; Pittelkow et al.; Tarnowski and Hashimoto, 1969). The dilatation of the blood vessels is the result of damage caused to them by the lipid deposits in the vascular wall. Thus, the cutaneous lesions represent not true angiomas but angiectases (von Gemmingen et al.).

SYSTEMIC LESIONS. On routine fixation and staining the aorta and the large blood vessels show considerable thickening of their media as the result of a marked vacuolization in their muscle bundles. Similar changes are seen in the heart muscle (Ruiter, 1957). In the kidneys marked vacuolization is seen not only in the walls of the large blood vessels but especially also in the glomerular endothelium, the epithelium of Bowman's capsule, the loops of Henle, and the distal tubules. In patients who have died of uremia there is marked fibrosis of the kidney, particularly of the glomeruli. The glomerular changes have been shown by means of renal biopsies to be present even in patients with still normal renal function (Wallace; Wachtel and Mattei). Generally, in such instances there is, however, proteinuria; and the urinary sediment shows both intra- and extracellular lipid globules that are birefringent and thus show Maltese crosses under polarized light. A bone marrow biopsy also shows varying numbers of lipid-filled macrophages (von Gemmingen et al.).

Histogenesis. The disease is inherited as a sex-linked recessive trait carried on the X chromosome (Wallace). There is complete penetrance in the homozygous male, and only

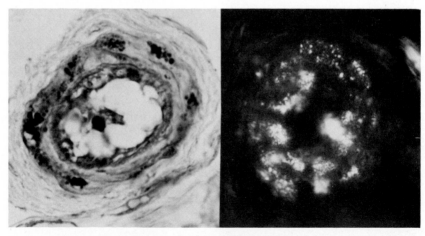

FIG. 21-6. **Angiokeratoma corporis diffusum (Fabry).** Cutaneous capillary. (*Left*) Staining with sudan black B reveals lipid granules in the endothelial cells and pericytes. (*Right*) Frozen section in polarized light shows the lipid granules to be doubly refractile. (×800) (M. Ruiter, M.D.)

occasional and usually mild penetrance in the heterozygous female (Burda and Winder). The affected male transmits the defective gene to all his daughters; and in the heterozygous female each conception carries a 50 per cent probability of transmittal of the defective gene: to a male child as disease, or to a female child as trait or mild disease (von Gemmingen et al.). Patients with this disease and also female carriers of the disease show an asymptomatic opacity of the cornea due to dystrophy of the corneal epithelium that is visible only by slit-lamp examination (von Gemmingen et al.; Wallace).

On *electron microscopic examination,* the lipid deposits present in endothelial cells (E.M. No. 34), pericytes and fibroblasts of the skin are situated within greatly enlarged lysosomes. Most of the lysosomes show acid phosphatase activity, with the exception of large matured lysosomes which as residual bodies often show laminated myelin figures (E.M. No. 34, *inset*) (Hashimoto et al.; Tarnowski and Hashimoto, 1968; Sagebiel and Parker). It seems likely that the greatly engorged lysosomes form on the basis of a genetic deficiency of a lysomal enzyme essential for the digestion of the lipid material.

Patients with Fabry's disease, as the result of their ceramide trihexosidase deficiency, show no ceramide trihexosidase activity but increased levels of ceramide trihexoside in their serum and excrete large amounts of ceramide trihexoside in their urine. After intravenous injections of placental ceramide trihexosidase the level of ceramide trihexoside in the plasma decreases (Brady et al.). Also, after a renal transplant patients show in the plasma a rise in the alpha galactosidase or ceramide trihexosidase activity (Philippart et al.).

LIPOGRANULOMATOSIS
(FARBER'S DISEASE)

This rare disorder, first described by Farber in 1952, shows nodular swellings caused by histiocytic granulomas in the skin, the subcutaneous tissue, the tendon sheaths, and the synovial membrane. Similar granulomas are present in the viscera in varying degrees. Some of the patients, especially those in whom the disease is rapidly fatal, show, in addition, involvement of the central nervous system, including motor weakness, hypotonia and chronic respiratory insufficiency (Battin et al.). In such patients glycolipid accumulations are found in distended neurons (Farber et al.).

Histopathology. The histiocytic granulomas in the skin, the periarticular regions and the viscera show accumulations of histiocytes (Zetterström). Some of them have a foamy cytoplasm giving a weakly positive reaction for lipid and carbohydrate (Battin et al.). In addition to histiocytes and foam cells, there is an admixture of inflammatory cells.

HISTIOCYTOSIS

Histiocytosis is a disease of unknown cause and is characterized by a proliferation of histiocytes. Three clinical forms are recognized: Letterer-Siwe disease, Hand-Schüller-Christian disease, and eosinophilic granuloma. The three conditions are not demarcated sharply from each other and, therefore, transitional cases among these three forms are common. In general, if the histiocytosis occurs during the first year of life, it is characterized by major and often fatal visceral involvement (Letterer-Siwe disease). During early childhood the disease is expressed predominantly in osseous lesions associated with usually minor visceral involvement (Hand-Schüller-Christian disease). In older children and adults the histiocytosis, as a rule, is localized and appears most commonly as one or several lesions of a bone (eosinophilic granuloma). Cutaneous lesions are very commonly encountered in Letterer-Siwe disease, and occur occasionally in the two other forms.

Transformation of some of the histiocytes into lipid-laden foam cells occurs in some of the cases. It may be seen in both the acute and the chronic forms of histiocytosis, and thus it is not a time-related phenomenon. Usually, the formation of foam cells, if it occurs, is limited to a few organs, especially the dura mater, the bones, and the skin; whereas the histiocytic infiltrations located in the liver, the spleen, the lungs, and the lymph nodes do not show a tendency to lipidization. It appears likely that, as Thannhauser first expressed it, there is an inhibition of an enzyme within lipidized histiocytes that prevents them from adequately digesting phagocytized lipids (see also under Histogenesis). The values for serum lipids are within normal limits in histiocytosis.

LETTERER-SIWE DISEASE usually occurs in infants and, unless treated with alkylating agents, is almost inevitably fatal within a few months to a year. The most common manifestations are fever, anemia, enlargement of the liver and the spleen, lymphadenopathy, and pulmonary infiltrations. Osseous infiltrations are most common in the temporal bones, but they may occur elsewhere also. In most cases cutaneous and oral lesions are present. The cutaneous lesions usually consist of petechiae and papules. In some cases one observes numerous closely set, brownish papules covered with scales or crusts. This type of eruption may be extensive and involve particularly the scalp, the face, and the trunk. The resemblance of this eruption to seborrheic dermatitis or Darier's disease often is striking (Laymon and Sevenants; Concilla et al.).

In HAND-SCHÜLLER-CHRISTIAN DISEASE, diabetes insipidus, exophthalmos, and multiple defects of the bones, especially of the cranium, represent the classical triad. However, any one or even all three of the cardinal symptoms may be absent, and involvement may occur in entirely different organs. For example, enlargement of the liver, the spleen, and the lymph nodes may be found. A rather common manifestation is a granulomatous infiltration of the temporal bones, causing a chronic type of otitis media. Hand-Schüller-Christian disease takes a chronic course, usually extending over years. The mortality without treatment is about 30 per cent.

Cutaneous lesions occur in about one third of the cases (Curtis and Cawley). They may be of four types: (1) Most commonly, one finds an extensive eruption of coalescing, scaling or crusted papules, as is seen also in Letterer-Siwe disease (Freeman). (2) One may observe infiltrated plaques undergoing ulceration, especially in the axillae, the anogenital region, and the mouth, as seen also in eosinophilic granuloma (Curtis and Cawley). (3) Numerous small yellowish-brown xanthomata with a tendency to coalesce may be present, especially on the face, the neck, the axillae, and the sides of the trunk. The term *xanthoma disseminatum* often is used for this type of eruption (Braun-Falco and Braun-Falco; Altman and Winkelmann, 1962; Kalz et al.). As a rule, xanthomata

disseminata occur in rather mild cases of Hand-Schüller-Christian disease in association with diabetes insipidus. (4) In very rare instances only, one observes small, scattered, soft, raised yellowish xanthomata that clinically and histologically are indistinguishable from those seen in juvenile xanthogranuloma (see p. 378). Diabetes insipidus is present in some instances (Jausion et al.; Altman and Winkelmann, 1963), and lytic bone lesions and diffuse lymphadenopathy in others (Thannhauser). In most of these cases the course is benign; but a fatal outcome has been observed by Thelander and by Crocker.

EOSINOPHILIC GRANULOMA represents the third and least severe disease in this group. The lesions are either solitary or few in number. Most common are lesions of the bones, but occasionally the skin or the oral mucosa is involved. In some cases diabetes insipidus also is present (Kierland et al.; Koch and Panscherewski; Cohen and Ehrenfeld). The cutaneous lesions may be of two types: (1) They may consist of an extensive eruption of crusted papules, as seen also in Letterer-Siwe and Hand-Schüller-Christian disease (Lever and Leeper). (2) There may be one or several erythematous infiltrated plaques with a tendency to ulceration, as seen also in Hand-Schüller-Christian disease (Curtis and Cawley; McCreary). The two types of cutaneous lesions may be present simultaneously.

Histopathology. Not only clinically but also histologically, a close relationship exists among the three forms of histiocytosis. Generally, three types of histologic reactions can occur in histiocytosis: a proliferative, a granulomatous, and a xanthomatous reaction, in all three of which the histiocyte is the basic cell type. Several authors have pointed out that these three types of reaction may occur as subsequent stages, the proliferative reaction being the first stage, the granulomatous reaction being the second, and the xanthomatous reaction being the third (Engelbreth-Holm et al.). However, each of the three types of reaction may arise as such, and healing can occur during any one of them.

A definite relationship exists between the type of histologic reaction and clinical type of disease. In general, the proliferative reaction with its almost purely histiocytic infiltrate is typical of Letterer-Siwe disease, the granulomatous reaction of eosinophilic granuloma, and the xanthomatous reaction of Hand-Schüller-Christian disease; although in Hand-Schüller-Christian disease lipid deposits often are present only in a few organs, especially the dura mater, while other involved organs, including the skin, may instead show the proliferative or the granulomatous type of reaction (Laymon and

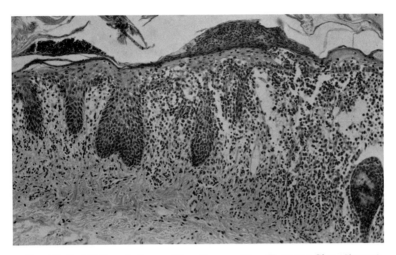

FIG. 21-7. **Histiocytosis, proliferative reaction (Letterer-Siwe disease).** Low magnification. The upper portion of the dermis contains an infiltrate composed almost entirely of loosely aggregated histiocytes. The infiltrate has invaded the epidermis in many areas. (×100)

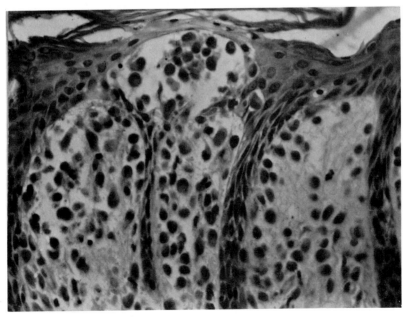

FIG. 21-8. **Histiocytosis, proliferative reaction (Letterer-Siwe disease).** High magnification. The histiocytes of the infiltrate possess irregularly shaped nuclei and abundant cytoplasm. In the center the infiltrate has invaded the epidermis. (×400)

Sevenants; Altman and Winkelmann, 1963). Thus, lipid-containing cells need not be present in the skin lesions of Hand-Schüller-Christian disease.

The histologic reaction present in the skin depends on the type of skin lesion. Since occasionally more than one type of skin lesion is present, different types of histologic reactions may be found in the same patient.

The *proliferative reaction* is encountered in the skin in petechiae, in hemorrhagic and nonhemorrhagic papules, in the seborrheic-like dermatitis, and occasionally in the often extensive eruption of scaling and crusting papules, entirely independently of whether the lesions occur in Letterer-Siwe disease, Hand-Schüller-Christian disease, or eosinophilic granuloma.

Histologically, the proliferative reaction is characterized in the skin by the presence of an extensive infiltrate of histiocytes. The infiltrate usually lies close to the epidermis and invades the epidermis (Fig. 21-7). It may even destroy the epidermis, resulting in ulceration. The histiocytes composing the infiltrate appear as large cells with irregularly shaped vesicular nuclei and abundant, slightly eosinophilic cytoplasm (Fig. 21-8). In some areas these cells are outlined distinctly and even separated by edema, whereas in other areas their cytoplasm is confluent (Sweitzer and Laymon; Ruch). A few scattered lymphoid cells and varying numbers of eosinophils may be present. Extravasated erythrocytes frequently lie within the aggregates of histiocytes. Occasionally, some of the histiocytes have a foamy cytoplasm and stain positive with fat stains. In older lesions one may find within the histiocytic infiltrate a few multinucleated histiocytes, indicating a transition to the granulomatous reaction (Eberhartinger and Santler).

The *granulomatous reaction* is found in the skin not only in the infiltrated plaques in the genital area, axillary region, or on the scalp, but also occasionally in the extensive eruption of scaling or crusted papules occurring in Hand-Schüller-Christian disease or eosinophilic granuloma.

Histologically, the granulomatous reaction

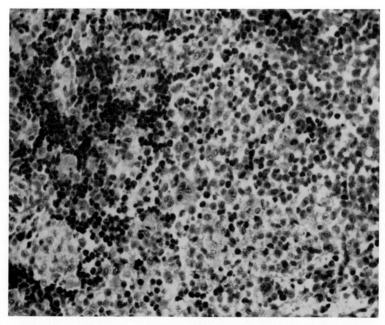

FIG. 21-9. **Histiocytosis, granulomatous reaction (eosinophilic granuloma).** This biopsy, taken from an infiltrated plaque, contains rather large histiocytes and eosinophils. The eosinophils show a tendency to lie in aggregates. (×200)

shows extensive aggregates of histiocytes often extending deep into the dermis. Eosinophils are present in various quantities. Generally they lie in clusters instead of being diffusely scattered (Fig. 21-9). Irregularly shaped, multinucleated giant cells are seen frequently (Fig. 21-10). In addition, neutrophils, lymphoid cells, and plasma cells may be present. Frequently extravasations of erythrocytes are found. True foam cells are usually absent. Occasionally, however, some of the histiocytes possess a vacuolated cytoplasm, and, on staining for fat, they reveal small amounts of lipids (Farber; Curtis and Cawley; McCreary; Lever and Leeper).

The *xanthomatous reaction* is encountered in the skin in xanthoma disseminatum lesions and also in the rarely occurring yellow nodular xanthoma lesions of Hand-Schüller-Christian disease.

Histologically, the xanthomatous reaction reveals in the dermis numerous foam cells, as well as varying numbers of histiocytes and some eosinophils (Fig. 21-11). Multinucleated giant cells are frequently present. They are mainly of the foreign body type but occasionally have the appearance of Touton giant cells (lipid-containing giant cells). Thus, the histologic picture usually is more polymorphous than that seen in the tuberous xanthomas associated with the various types of hyperlipoproteinemia, and represents a xanthogranuloma rather than a true xanthoma (Thannhauser; Altman and Winkelmann, 1962).

Visceral Lesions. The visceral lesions seen in histiocytosis show the same three types of reactions just described for the skin. The organs most commonly affected are the spleen, the liver, the lungs, the lymph nodes, and the bones (Engelbreth-Holm et al.; Sweitzer and Laymon; Thannhauser). In the triad occasionally seen in Hand-Schüller-Christian disease, the diabetes insipidus is caused by granulomatous infiltration of the posterior pituitary gland, the tuber cinereum, or the hypothalamus; the exophthalmos, by retro-orbital accumulations of granulomatous tissue; and the multiple defects in the skull by the osteolytic effect of granulomatous infiltrations (Avioli et al.).

Histogenesis. On electron microscopic examination, about one half of the histiocytes present in the cutaneous and visceral lesions of all

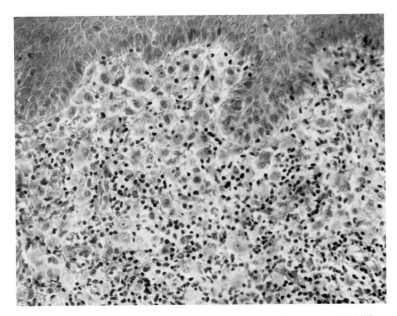

FIG. 21-10. **Histiocytosis, granulomatous reaction (Hand-Schüller-Christian disease).** The dermis contains, in addition to large histiocytes, several giant cells and an inflammatory infiltrate. (×200)

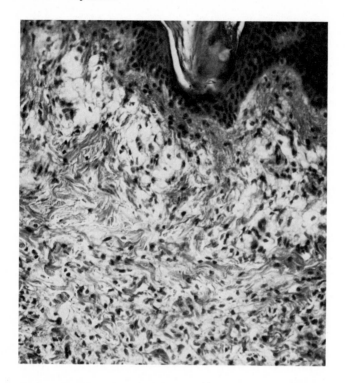

FIG. 21-11. **Histiocytosis, xanthomatous reaction (Hand-Schüller-Christian disease).** Groups of foam cells are present in the upper dermis. The lower dermis contains histiocytes. (×200)

three forms of histiocytosis contain in their cytoplasm so-called Langerhans granules (Basset and Nezelof; Tarnowski and Hashimoto; de Man; Gianotti and Caputo; Wolff and Braun-Falco). These granules, which are absent in normal histiocytes, are morphologically indistinguishable from the Langerhans granules present in normal epidermal Langerhans cells (see p. 20). In both the epidermal Langerhans cells and the histiocytes of histiocytosis the Langerhans granules are lined by a trilaminar membrane and contain a central lamella with a periodicity of approximately 6 nm. However, only the Langerhans granules in epidermal Langerhans cells show positive staining of the periodic striation of the central lamella on fixation with osmium zinc iodide (Niebauer et al.). This difference between the Langerhans granules in epidermal Langerhans cells and those in the histiocytes of histiocytosis makes a relationship between these two types of cells somewhat questionable.

In addition to Langerhans granules, varying in size from 0.1 to 1 μm, the histiocytes of histiocytosis contain a variable number of lysosomes, 0.3 to 0.5 μm in diameter (Niebauer et al.).

The foam cells are histiocytes, or macrophages, containing numerous clear lipid vacuoles of varying sizes without any definite limiting membrane. Surrounding the lipid vacuoles are numerous lysosomes filled with small vacuoles and granules. It is possible that the lipid accumulates in the histiocytes as a result of an impaired lysosomal degradation (Zemel et al.).

DIFFUSE NORMOLIPEMIC PLANE XANTHOMA

In this rather rare disorder one observes patches or, more commonly, diffuse areas of orange-yellow discoloration of the skin. While patchy areas have a recognizable border and often have a slight degree of palpable infiltration, the diffuse areas have a poorly defined border. The face, particularly the periorbital areas, and the upper trunk are sites of predilection. The lesions usually persist indefinitely.

Some cases of diffuse normolipemic plane xanthoma can be regarded as idiopathic, not being associated with any other illness. Others, however, are preceded by erythroderma either on the basis of atopic dermatitis (Walker and Sneddon) or on the basis of lymphoma (Lynch and Winkelmann).

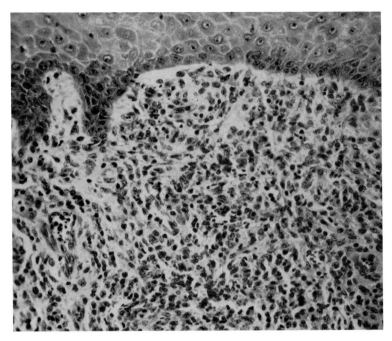

FIG. 21-12. **Juvenile xanthogranuloma (nevoxantho-endothelioma), early lesion.** There is a uniform infiltrate of histiocytes or macrophages. Lipid infiltration is absent. (×200)

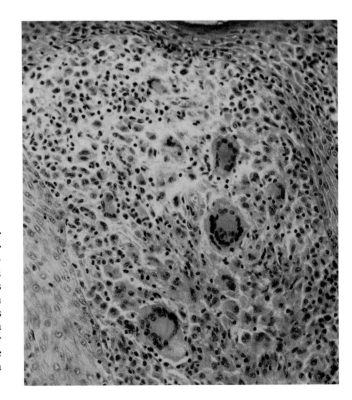

FIG. 21-13. **Juvenile xantho-granuloma (nevoxantho-endothelioma), mature lesion.** Many histiocytes or macrophages show a vacuolated cytoplasm and thus have the appearance of foam cells. Several giant cells possess a perfect "wreath" of nuclei, a feature that is quite typical for juvenile xanthogranuloma. The giant cell in the lower field is a Touton giant cell. (×200)

The most common association, however, is with multiple myeloma (Moschella). Interestingly, the plane xanthomatosis usually antedates the multiple myeloma by many years, as long as 18 years (Thannhauser) or 27 years (Levin et al.). In patients with the association of plane xanthoma and multiple myeloma hyperlipoproteinemia is not uncommon (Moschella).

Histopathology. Histologic examination reveals diffusely scattered throughout the dermis large sheets and clusters of foam cells, as well as foam cells singly and in small groups. In some areas the foam cells lie in thin streaks between collagen bundles, whereas in others they show a perivascular arrangement (Fleischmajer et al.). There may be an admixture of histiocytes and lymphoid cells; and rarely Touton giant cells are seen (Walker and Sneddon). There is no fibrosis. Fat stains reveal droplets of lipid in the foam cells.

JUVENILE XANTHOGRANULOMA

Juvenile xanthogranuloma, a designation that gradually has replaced the old term nevoxantho-endothelioma, generally is a benign disorder in which one or several and occasionally numerous, small, soft, raised yellowish cutaneous nodules are present. The lesions may be present already at birth (Helwig and Hackney), but usually they arise in early infancy; and occasionally they do not arise until childhood or even early adult life (Gartmann and Tritsch). They involute spontaneously, usually within a year.

In rare instances one may find, in association with juvenile xanthogranuloma, nodular lesions of the iris (Blank et al.) or of the epibulbar area (Cogan et al.). Lesions of the iris may lead to hemorrhages into the anterior chamber of the eye and to glaucoma. In a few instances ocular lesions have been present without cutaneous lesions (Sanders). In several cases of juvenile xanthogranuloma there were pulmonary infiltrations (Lamb and Lain; Nödl; Lottsfeldt and Good; Schmid and Usener), hepatosplenomegaly (Lamb and Lain; Nödl; Lever), swelling of a testis (Helwig and Hackney; Nödl) or pericardial infiltration (Webster et al.).

Histopathology. Early lesions may show large accumulations of histiocytes or macrophages without any lipid infiltration intermingled with only a few lymphoid cells and eosinophils (Nödl; Gartmann and Tritsch) (Fig. 21-12). Usually, however, some degree of lipidization is present, even in very early lesions. One finds then that many of the histiocytes or macrophages have a pale, vacuolated cytoplasm staining positive with fat stains (Esterly et al.). In mature lesions a granulomatous infiltrate is present, containing, in addition to histiocytes, lymphocytes, and eosinophils, foam cells, foreign-body giant cells, and Touton giant cells. The presence of giant cells showing a perfect "wreath" of nuclei is quite typical for juvenile xanthogranuloma (Gartmann and Tritsch; Webster et al.) (Fig. 21-13). Older regressing lesions show proliferation of fibroblasts and fibrosis.

Histogenesis. Electron microscopy has revealed the lesion to be composed of macrophages with complex pseudopodia. In mature lesions one finds in the macrophages abundant lysosomal structures containing lipid, but most lipid material is found as vacuoles not bound by membranes (E.M. No. 35) (Gonzalez-Crussi and Campbell).

Juvenile xanthogranuloma now is generally regarded as an independent entity, as a reactive granuloma of unknown cause (Helwig and Hackney; Nödl; Gartmann and Tritsch). In the past, the view that juvenile xanthogranuloma represents an abortive, monosymptomatic, purely cutaneous form of Hand-Schüller-Christian disease was considered by several authors (Crocker; Nilsby; Thannhauser). As points in favor of a relationship between juvenile xanthogranuloma and Hand-Schüller-Christian disease the following resemblances were cited: (1) Clinically, both diseases have their onset early in life and tend to involute spontaneously. (2) Histologically, both have histiocytes as the basic cell type and, with aging of the lesions, show progressive lipidization and formation of giant cells. (3) Internal lesions of the same type as those seen in Hand-Schüller-Christian disease occur occasionally in cases of juvenile xanthogranuloma (see above). (4) In rare instances even fatal cases of Hand-Schüller-Christian disease had at their onset cutaneous lesions that were indistinguishable from those seen in juvenile xanthogranuloma (Thelander; Crocker). A strong argument against any relationship between juvenile xanthogranuloma and Hand-

Schüller-Christian disease is, however, the absence of Langerhans granules in the histiocytes of juvenile xanthogranuloma upon electron microscopic examination. (Gonzalez-Crussi and Campbell; Esterly et al.), whereas in all three forms of histiocytosis approximately half of the histiocytes show these characteristic organelles (see p. 376).

Differential Diagnosis. In spite of their close histologic resemblance, juvenile xanthogranuloma differs from Hand-Schüller-Christian disease in certain features. In its early stage it differs by the monomorphous appearance of the massively aggregated histiocytes, and in its granulomatous stages by the slighter inflammatory reaction with fewer eosinophils and by the wreath-shaped giant cells that are rarely seen in the xanthomatous lesions of Hand-Schüller-Christian disease in which irregularly shaped giant cells of the foreign body type predominate. A differentiation from dermatofibroma with lipid-ization also can be made usually through the presence of the wreath-shaped giant cells in juvenile xanthogranuloma. Furthermore, dermatofibroma does not show eosinophils and frequently has a hyperplastic epidermis.

RETICULOHISTIOCYTOSIS

Two types of reticulohistiocytosis are recognized: reticulohistiocytic granuloma, and multicentric reticulohistiocytosis. Both types occur almost exclusively in adults. The histologic picture is the same in both types.

In *reticulohistiocytic granuloma* one observes usually a single nodule and occasionally a few nodules, most commonly on the head and neck. The nodules are smooth and measure from 0.5 to 2.0 cm in diameter (Zak; Purvis and Helwig; Davies and Wood; Nödl). They usually involute spontaneously.

In *multicentric reticulohistiocytosis* one finds, in addition to numerous papules and

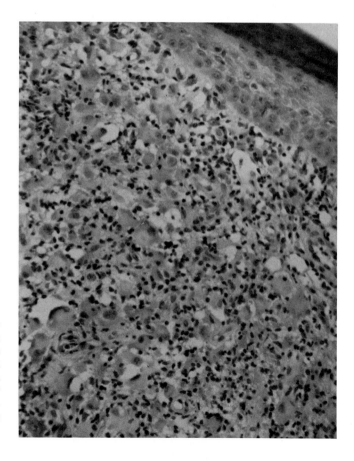

FIG. 21-14. **Reticulohistiocytosis.** The histiocytes with "ground-glass" cytoplasm in this case are largely mononuclear, in contrast with those shown in Fig. 21-15, which are largely multinuclear. A rather pronounced inflammatory infiltrate is present. (×200)

FIG. 21-15. **Reticulohistiocytosis.** Numerous large, multinucleated giant cells with pale, finely granular "ground-glass" cytoplasm are present. (×200) (Joseph Albert, M.D.)

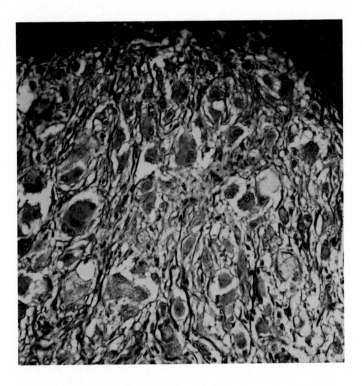

small nodules, a polyarthritis which may either precede or follow the cutaneous lesions. The cutaneous papules and nodules are present in many areas of the skin, with a predilection for the face and hands. In about half of the patients nodules are present also in the oral or nasal mucosa (Barrow and Holubar). The polyarthritis may be mild or severe. If severe, it may be mutilating, especially on the hands, through destruction of articular cartilage and of subarticular bone (Orkin et al.). In most instances, the disease gradually loses its activity after several years (Barrow and Holubar).

Histopathology. The characteristic histologic feature in both reticulohistiocytic granuloma and multicentric reticulohistiocytosis is the presence of numerous large histiocytes showing an abundance of eosinophilic, homogeneous to finely granular cytoplasm having a "ground-glass" appearance. The cytoplasm is sharply, though often irregularly demarcated. The histiocytes have either one nucleus (Fig. 21-14) or numerous irregularly distributed nuclei (Fig. 21-15) (Purvis and Helwig; Davies and Wood; Orkin et al.). Although in some cases the number of mul-

tinucleated giant cells is small (Flam et al.), they nevertheless are regularly present and are a prerequisite for the diagnosis (Barrow and Holubar).

The large histiocytes are embedded in a stroma that in early lesions shows a rather pronounced inflammatory infiltrate composed largely of lymphoid cells and plasma cells (Orkin et al.). In older lesions the inflammatory reaction is replaced more or less by fibrous tissue surrounding almost every large histiocyte (Fig. 21-15) (Davies and Wood).

The contents of the large and partly multinucleated histiocytes with "ground-glass" cytoplasm is somewhat variable except that in all cases the cytoplasm is strongly PAS-positive, and diastase-resistant. In some cases the PAS-positive material is extractable by lipid solvents, such as chloroform or acetone, indicating that the PAS-positive polysaccharide is attached to a lipid and represents a glycolipid (Albert et al.; Anderson et al.). In other cases the PAS reactivity is not abolished after extraction with lipid solvents, indicating the presence of a glycoprotein rather than a glycolipid (Davies et al.). Lipids are regularly present in small amounts in the "ground glass" cytoplasm of the large histiocytes (Barrow and Holubar). The presence of phospholipids is indicated by a positive reaction with Baker's acid hematein (Davies et al.), and of neutral fat by positive staining with scarlet red (Albert et al.; Orkin et al.). On the other hand, cholesterol is regularly absent in view of a negative Schultz reaction, as are cholesterol esters since there is no birefringence (Anderson et al.). Because of the regular presence of lipids the term *lipoid dermatoarthritis* used by some authors (Ehrlich et al.) appears justified.

The polyarthritis present in all instances of multicentric reticulohistiocytosis is caused by the same type of infiltrate as is found in the cutaneous lesions. In early or mild cases the granulomatous infiltrate is confined to the synovia (Albert et al.; Orkin et al.). In patients with mutilating arthritis the granulomatous infiltrate is found also in the subarticular bone, leading to fragmentation and degeneration of bone (Montgomery et al.).

Systemic lesions usually are absent in patients who have died of unrelated diseases. In one case, however, granulomatous nodules were found in bronchial lymph nodes and in the endocardium (Warin et al.).

Histogenesis. Electron microscopic examination has revealed within the large histiocytes numerous electron-dense lysosomes, including also residual bodies with a lamellar, myelinlike structure. Their osmiophilia and internal structure suggest the presence of phospholipids (Ebner and Gebhart). In some cells occasional lipid vacuoles are seen (Flam et al.). No definite Langerhans organelles are present (Flam et al.), although Ebner and Gebhart found in a few cells cross sections of rods resembling Langerhans organelles.

Differential Diagnosis. Juvenile xanthogranuloma, which hardly ever occurs in adults, differs from reticulohistiocytosis by the different appearance of the histiocytes. In juvenile xanthogranuloma, the cytoplasm of the histiocytes does not have a "ground-glass" appearance, and, except in very early lesions, abundant lipids are present in many histiocytes, giving them a foamy appearance. If giant cells are present in juvenile xanthogranuloma, some of them show a regular arrangement of their nuclei near the periphery, often in a wreathlike fashion.

GENERALIZED ERUPTIVE HISTIOCYTOMA

This rare dermatosis is characterized by the presence of innumerable flesh-colored to reddish papules developing in crops and involuting spontaneously. All patients so far have been adults (Winkelmann and Muller).

Histopathology. Histologic examination reveals a monomorphous infiltrate composed of histiocytes having a large, pale nucleus and abundant pale cytoplasm (Winkelmann and Muller; Baccaredda-Boy; Cramer). Histochemical studies reveal the absence of lipids. On electron microscopic examination the histiocytes contain numerous lysosomes but only occasionally a few lipid droplets (Muller et al.).

Differential Diagnosis. As pointed out by Winkelmann and Muller, the histologic picture is indistinguishable from the earliest stage of juvenile xanthogranuloma; but the failure of the lesions to progress to lipidization and the occurrence in adults sets generalized eruptive histiocytoma apart from juvenile xanthogranuloma. The absence of ground-glass cytoplasm and of giant cells distinguishes it from reticulohistiocytosis.

BIBLIOGRAPHY

Hyperlipoproteinemia

Ahrens, E. H., Jr., *et al.*: Primary biliary cirrhosis. Medicine, *29*:299, 1950.

Amatruda, J. M., Margolis, S., and Hutchins, G. M.: Type III hyperlipoproteinemia. Arch. Path., *98*:51, 1974.

Baes, H., van Gent, C. M., and Pries, C.: Lipid composition of various types of xanthoma. J. Invest. Derm., *51*:286, 1968.

Borrie, P., and Slack, J.: A clinical syndrome characteristic of primary Type IV-V hyperlipoproteinemia. Brit. J. Derm., *90*:245, 1974.

Bruton, O. C., and Kanter, A. J.: Idiopathic familial hyperlipemia. Am. J. Dis. Child., *82*:153, 1951.

Cornelius, C. E.: Disappearance of eruptive xanthoma following carbohydrate restriction. Arch. Derm., *96*:45, 1967.

Cuttino, J. T., Jr., Summer, G. K., and Hill, H. D.: Treatment of eruptive xanthomas in Cori Type I glycogenosis. Arch. Derm., *101*:469, 1970.

Ferrans, V. J., Buja, L. M., Roberts, W. C., and Fredrickson, D. S.: The spleen in Type I hyperlipoproteinemia. Am. J. Path., *64*:67, 1971.

Fleischmajer, R.: Familial hyperlipoproteinemia Type III. Arch. Derm., *100*:401, 1969.

————: Diagnosis and treatment of familial lipoproteinemias. Internat. J. Derm., *10*:251, 1971 (review).

Fredrickson, D. S., Levy, R. I., and Lees, R. S.: Fat transport in lipoproteins: an integrated approach to mechanisms and disorders. New Eng. J. Med., *276*:34, 1967.

Holimon, J. L., and Wasserman, A. J.: Autopsy findings in Type 3 hyperlipoproteinemia. Arch. Path., *92*:415, 1971.

Ito, J., Sugai, T., and Saito, T.: Atresia of the intrahepatic bile ducts with xanthomatosis. Arch. Derm., *96*:53, 1967.

Lees, R. S., and Hatch, F. T.: Sharper separation of lipoprotein species by paper electrophoresis in albumin-containing buffer. J. Lab. Clin. Med., *61*:518, 1963.

Lever, W. F., Smith, P. A. J., and Hurley, N. A.: Idiopathic hyperlipemia and primary hypercholesteremic xanthomatosis. I. Clinical data and analysis of the plasma lipids. J. Invest. Derm., *22*:33, 1954.

Maher, J. A., Epstein, F. H., and Hand, E. A.: Xanthomatosis and coronary heart disease. Arch. Int. Med., *102*:437, 1958.

Parker, F., and Odland, G. F.: Electron microscopic similarities between experimental xanthoma and human eruptive xanthomas. J. Invest. Derm., *52*:136, 1969.

Pedace, F. J., and Winkelmann, R. K.: Xanthelasma palpebrarum. J.A.M.A., *193*:893, 1965.

Polano, M. K.: Die Xanthelasmatosen der Haut. Arch. f. Derm. u. Syph., *181*:139, 1940.

Polano, M. K., Baes, H., Hulsmans, H. A. M., et al.: Xanthomata in primary hyperlipoproteinemia. Arch. Derm., *100*:387, 1969.

Roberts, W. C., Levy, R. I., and Fredrickson, D. S.: Hyperlipoproteinemia. Arch. Path., *90*:46, 1970.

Schreiber, M. M., and Shapiro, S. I.: Secondary eruptive xanthoma. Type V hyperlipoproteinemia. Arch. Derm., *100*:601, 1969.

Schreibman, P. H., Wilson, D. E., and Arky, R. A.: Familial Type IV hyperlipoproteinemia. New Eng. J. Med., *281*:981, 1969.

Wolff, H. H., and Braun-Falco, O.: Die Ultrastruktur des Xanthelasma palpebrarum. Arch. klin exp. Derm., *238*:308, 1970.

Zemel, H., Decken, J., Asel, N., and Packer, J.: The ultrastructural features of normolipemic plane xanthoma. Arch. Path., *89*:111, 1970.

Tangier Disease

Krebs, A., and Kuske, H.: Familiäre Analphalipoproteinämie ("Tangier disease"). Dermatologica, *138*:196, 1969.

Waldorf, D. S., Levy, R. I., and Fredrickson, D. S.: Cutaneous cholesterol ester deposition in Tangier disease. Arch. Derm., *95*:161, 1967.

Niemann-Pick Disease

Brady, R. O.: The sphingolipidoses. New Eng. J. Med., *275*:312, 1966.

Crocker, A. C., and Farber, S.: Niemann-Pick disease: A review of eighteen patients. Medicine, *37*:1, 1958.

Lynn, R., and Terry, R. D. L.: Lipid histochemistry and electron microscopy in adult Niemann-Pick disease. Am. J. Med., *37*:987, 1964.

Gaucher's Disease

Brady, R. O., Kanfer, J. W., Bradley, R. M., and Shapiro, D.: Demonstration of a deficiency of glucose-cerebroside-cleaving enzyme in Gaucher's disease. J. Clin. Invest., *45*:112, 1966.

Hibbs, R. G., Ferrans, V. J., Cipriano, P. R., and Tardiff, K. J.: A histochemical and electron microscopic study of Gaucher cells. Arch. Path., *89*:137, 1970.

Kampine, J. P., Brady, R. O., and Kanfer, J. W.: Diagnosis of Gaucher's disease and Niemann-Pick disease with small samples of venous blood. Science, *155*:86, 1967.

Lee, R. E., Balcerzak, S. P., and Westerman, M. P.: Gaucher's disease: a morphologic study and measurement of iron metabolism. Am. J. Med., *42*:891, 1967.

Angiokeratoma Corporis Diffusum (Fabry)

Brady, R. O., Tallman, J. F., Johnson, W. G., et al.: Replacement therapy for inherited enzyme deficiency. New Eng. J. Med., *289*:9, 1973.

Burda, C. D., and Winder, P. R.: Angiokeratoma corporis diffusum universale (Fabry's disease) in female subjects. Am. J. Med., *42*:293, 1967.

de Groot, W. P.: Angiokeratoma corporis diffusum Fabry. Dermatologica, *128*:321, 1964.

Epinette, W. W., Norins, A. L., Drew, A. L., et al.: Angiokeratoma corporis diffusum with alpha-L-fucosidase deficiency. Arch. Derm., *107*:754, 1973.

Frost, P., Tanaka, Y., and Spaeth, G. L.: Fabry's disease: Glycolipid lipidosis. Am. J. Med., *40*:618, 1966.

Hashimoto, K., Gross, B. G., and Lever, W. F.: Angiokeratoma corporis diffusum (Fabry). Histochemical and electron microscopic studies of the skin. J. Invest. Derm., *44*:119, 1965.

Kint, J. A.: Fabry's disease: α-galactosidase deficiency. Science, *167*:1268, 1970.

Philippart, M., Franklin, S. S., and Gordon, A.: Reversal of an inborn sphingolipidosis (Fabry's disease) by kidney transplantation. Ann. Int. Med., *77*:195, 1972.

Pittelkow, R. B., Kierland, R. R., and Montgomery, H.: Polariscopic and histochemical studies in angiokeratoma corporis diffusum. Arch. Derm., *76*:59, 1957.

Ruiter, M.: Histologic investigation of the skin in angiokeratoma corporis diffusum in particular with regard to the associated disturbance of phosphatid metabolism. Dermatologica, *109*:273, 1954.

————: Some further observations on angiokeratoma corporis diffusum. Brit. J. Derm., *69*:137, 1957 (review).

Sagebiel, R. W., and Parker, F.: Cutaneous lesions of Fabry's disease: glycolipid lipidosis. J. Invest. Derm., *50*:208, 1968.

Tarnowski, W. M., and Hashimoto, K.: Lysosomes in Fabry's disease. Acta dermatoven., *48*:143, 1968.

————: New light microscopic findings in Fabry's disease. Acta dermatoven., *49*:386, 1969.

Urbain, G., Philippart, M., and Peremans, J.: Fabry's disease with hypogammaglobulinemia and without angiokeratoma. Arch. Int. Med., *124*:72, 1969.

von Gemmingen, G., Kierland, R. R., and Opitz, J. M.: Angiokeratoma diffusum (Fabry's disease). Arch. Derm., *91*:206, 1965.

Wachtel, H. L., and Mattei, I. R.: Angiokeratoma corporis diffusum universale. Arch. Intern. Med., *114*:805, 1964.

Wallace, H. J.: Anderson-Fabry disease. Brit. J. Derm., *88*:1, 1973 (review).

Wise, D., Wallace, H. J., and Jellinek, E. H.: Angiokeratoma corporis diffusum. Quart. J. Med., *31*:177, 1962.

Lipogranulomatosis (Farber's disease)

Battin, J., Vital, C., and Azanza, X.: Une neurolipidose rare avec lésions nodulaires sous-cutanées et articulaires: La lipogranulomatose disseminée de Farber. Ann. derm. syph., *97*: 241, 1970.

Farber, S.: A lipid metabolic disorder: disseminated "lipogranulomatosis." A syndrome with similarity to, and important difference from Niemann-Pick, and Hand-Schüller-Christian disease. Am. J. Dis. Child., *84*:499, 1952.

Farber, S., Cohen, J., and Uzman, L. L.: Lipogranulomatosis: a new lipo-glyco-protein storage disease. J. Mount Sinai Hosp. New York, *24*:816, 1957.

Zetterström, R.: Disseminated lipogranulomatosis (Farber's disease). Acta Paediat., *47*: 501, 1958.

Histiocytosis

Altman, J., and Winkelmann, R. K.: Xanthoma disseminatum. Arch. Derm., *86*:582, 1962.

Altman, J.: Xanthomatous cutaneous lesions of histiocytosis X. Arch. Derm., *87*:164, 1963.

Avioli, L. V., Lasersohn, J. T., and Lopresti, J. M.: Histiocytosis X (Schüller-Christian disease): a clinicopathologic survey. Medicine, *42*:119, 1963.

Basset, F., and Nezelof, C.: Présence en microscopie électronique de structures filamenteuses originales dans les lésions pulmonaires et osseuses de l'histiocytose X. Etat actuel de la question. Bull. Soc. méd. Hôp. Paris, *117*:413, 1966.

Braun-Falco, O., and Braun-Falco, F.: Zum Syndrom "Diabetes insipidus und disseminierte Xanthome." Z. Laryng. Rhinol. Otol., *36*:378, 1957.

Cohen, H. A., and Ehrenfeld, E. N.: Granulome éosinophile de la peau et des muqueuses associé au diabète insipide. Ann. derm. syph., *89*:602, 1962.

Concilla, P. A., Lahey, M. E., and Carnes, W. H.: Cutaneous lesions of Letterer-Siwe disease. Cancer, *20*:1986, 1967.

Crocker, A. C.: Skin xanthomas in childhood. Pediatrics, *8*:573, 1951.

Curtis, A. C., and Cawley, E. P.: Eosinophilic granuloma of bone with cutaneous manifestations. Arch. Derm. Syph., *55*:810, 1947.

de Man, J. C. H.: Rod-like tubular structures in the cytoplasm of histiocytes in "histiocytosis X." J. Path., *95*:123, 1968.

Eberhartinger, C., and Santler, R.: Reticulose vom Typ der Abt-Letterer-Siweschen Erkrankung. Arch. klin. exp. Derm., *208*:367, 1959.

Engelbreth-Holm, J., Teilum, G., and Christensen, E.: Eosinophil granuloma of bone; Schüller-Christian's disease. Acta med. scand., *118*:292, 1944.

Farber, S.: The nature of "solitary or eosino-philic granuloma" of bone. Am. J. Path., *17*: 625, 1941.

Freeman, S.: A benign form of Letterer-Siwe disease. Austral. J. Derm., *12*:165, 1971.

Gianotti, F., and Caputo, R.: Skin ultrastructure in Hand-Schüller-Christian disease. Arch. Derm., *100*:342, 1969.

Jausion, H., Roussel, A., and Bellalune, A.: Curieuse évolution d'une xanthomatose érup-tive, avec diabète insipide. Bull. Soc. franç. Derm. Syph., *61*:469, 1954.

Kalz, F., Hoffman, M., and Lafrance, A.: Xan-thoma disseminatum. Dermatologica, *140*: 129, 1970.

Kierland, R. B., Epstein, J. G., and Weber, W. E.: Eosinophilic granuloma of skin and mucous membranes. Arch. Derm., *75*:45, 1957.

Koch, H., and Panscherewski, D.: Das eosino-phile Granulom in Bereich der Mundschleim-haut. Hautarzt, *14*:173, 1963.

Laymon, C. W., and Sevenants, J. J.: Systemic reticuloendothelial granuloma. Arch. Derm. Syph., *57*:873, 1948.

Lever, W. F., and Leeper, R. W.: Eosinophilic granuloma of the skin. Arch. Derm. Syph., *62*:85, 1950.

McCreary, J. H.: Eosinophilic granuloma of the skin. Arch. Derm. Syph., *58*:372, 1948.

Niebauer, G., Krawczyk, W., and Wilgram, G. F.: Über die Langerhans-Zellorganelle bei Morbus Letterer-Siwe. Arch. klin. exp. Derm., *239*:125, 1970.

Ruch, D. M.: Cutaneous manifestations of Letterer-Siwe's disease. Arch. Derm., *75*:88, 1957.

Sweitzer, S. E., and Laymon, C. W.: Letterer-Siwe disease. Arch. Derm. Syph., *59*:549, 1949.

Tarnowski, W. M., and Hashimoto, K.: Langer-hans' cell granules in histiocytosis X. Arch. Derm., *96*:298, 1967.

Thannhauser, S. J.: Lipidoses. ed. 3, p. 408. New York, Grune & Stratton, 1958.

Thelander, H. E.: Xanthomatosis. J. Pediat., *34*:490, 1949.

Wolff, H. H., and Braun-Falco, O.: Zur Diag-nostik und Therapie des Morbus Hand-Schüller-Christian. Hautarzt, *23*:163, 1972.

Zemel, H., Deeken, J., Asel, N., and Packer, J.: The ultrastructural features of normolipemic plane xanthoma. Arch. Path., *89*:111, 1970.

Diffuse Normolipemic Plane Xanthoma

Fleischmajer, R., Hyman, A. B., and Weidman, A. I.: Normolipemic plane xanthomas. Arch. Derm., *89*:319, 1964.

Levin, W. C., Aboumrad, M. H., Ritzmann, S. E., *et al.*: Gamma-type I myeloma and xan-thomatosis. Arch. Int. Med., *114*:688, 1964.

Lynch, P. I., and Winkelmann, R. K.: General-ized plane xanthoma and systemic disease. Arch. Derm., *93*:639, 1966.

Moschella, S. L.: Plane xanthomatosis associated with myelomatosis. Arch. Derm., *101*:683, 1970.

Thannhauser, S. J.: Atypical clinical cases of disseminated xanthoma. *In* Lipidoses. ed. 3, p. 360. New York, Grune & Stratton, 1958.

Walker, A. E., and Sneddon, I. B.: Skin xan-thoma following erythroderma. Brit. J .Derm., *80*:580, 1968.

Juvenile Xanthogranuloma

Altman, J., and Winkelmann, R. K.: Xanthoma-tous cutaneous lesions of histiocytosis X. Arch. Derm., *87*:164, 1963.

Blank, H., Eglick, P. G., and Beerman, H.: Nevoxanthoendothelioma with ocular involve-ment. Pediatrics, *4*:349, 1949.

Cogan, D. G., Kuwabara, T., and Parke, D.: Epibulbar nevoxanthoendothelioma. Arch. Ophthal., *59*:717, 1958.

Crocker, A. C.: Skin xanthomas in childhood. Pediatrics, *8*:573, 1951.

Esterly, N. B., Sahihi, T., and Medenica, M.: Juvenile xanthogranuloma. An atypical case with study of ultrastructure. Arch. Derm., *105*:99, 1972.

Gartmann, H., and Tritsch, H.: Klein- und grossknotiges Naevoxanthoendotheliom. Arch. klin. exp. Derm., *215*:409, 1963.

Gonzalez-Crussi, F., and Campbell, R.: Juve-nile xanthogranuloma. Ultrastructural study. Arch. Path., *89*:65, 1970.

Helwig, E. B., and Hackney, V. C.: Juvenile xanthogranuloma (nevoxanthoendothelioma). Am. J. Path., *30*:625, 1954.

Lamb, J. H., and Lain, E. S.: Nevo-xantho-endothelioma. Its relation to juvenile xan-thoma. Southern Med. J., *30*:585, 1937.

Lever, W. F.: Histiocytosis. Arch. Derm., *79*: 608, 1959.

Lottsfeldt, F. I., and Good, R. A.: Juvenile xanthogranuloma with pulmonary lesions. Pediatrics, *33*:233, 1964.

Nilsby, J.: Juvenile xanthoma. Acta Paediat., *41*:373, 1952.

Nödl, F.: Systematisierte grossknotige Naevo-xanthoendotheliome. Arch. klin. exp. Derm., *208*:601, 1959.

Sanders, T. E.: Intraocular juvenile xantho-granuloma (Nevoxantho-endothelioma). Am. J. Ophthal., *53*:455, 1962.

Schmid, A. H., and Usener, M.: Grossknotiges Naevoxanthoendotheliom mit Lungenbeteiligung. Arch. klin. exp. Derm., *228*:239, 1967.

Thannhauser, S. J.: Juvenile xanthoma. Its relation to, and variation from, the skin lesions of eosinophilic xanthomatous granuloma. *In* Lipidoses. ed. 3, p. 362. New York, Grune & Stratton, 1958.

Thelander, H. E.: Xanthomatosis. J. Pediat., *34*:490, 1949.

Webster, S. B., Reister, H. C., and Harman, L. E., Jr.: Juvenile xanthogranuloma with extracutaneous lesions. Arch. Derm., *93*:71, 1966.

Reticulohistiocytosis

Albert, J., Bruce, W., Allen, A. C., and Blank, H.: Lipoid dermato-arthritis. Reticulohistiocytoma of the skin and joints. Am. J. Med., *28*:661, 1960.

Anderson, T. E., Carr, A. J., Chapman, R. S., *et al.*: Myositis and myotonia in a case of multicentric reticulohistiocytosis. Brit. J. Derm., *80*:39, 1968.

Barrow, M. V., and Holubar, K.: Multiple reticulohistiocytosis. A review of 33 patients. Medicine, *48*:287, 1969.

Davies, E. J., Roenigk, H. H., Hawk, W. A., and O'Duffy, J. D.: Multicentric reticulohistiocytosis. Arch. Derm., *97*:543, 1968.

Davies, B. T., and Wood, S. R.: The so-called reticulohistiocytoma of the skin. Brit. J. Derm., *67*:205, 1955.

Ebner, H., and Gebhart, W.: Zur Ultrastruktur der multizentrischen Reticulohistiocytose. Arch. Derm. Forsch., *240*:259, 1971.

Ehrlich, G. E., Young, I., Nosheny, S. Z., and Katz, W. A.: Multicentric reticulohistiocytosis (lipoid dermatoarthritis). Am. J. Med., *52*: 830, 1972.

Flam, M., Ryan, S. C., Mah-Poy, G. L., *et al.*: Multicentric reticulohistiocytosis. Am. J. Med., *52*:841, 1972.

Montgomery, H., Polley, H. F., and Pugh, D. G.: Reticulohistiocytoma (reticulohistiocytic granuloma). Arch. Derm., *77*:61, 1958.

Nödl, F.: Zur Histogenese der riesenzelligen Reticulohistiocytome. Arch. klin. exp. Derm., *207*:275, 1958.

Orkin, M., Goltz, R. W., Good, R. A., *et al.*: A study of multicentric reticulohistiocytosis. Arch. Derm., *89*:640, 1964.

Purvis, W. E., and Helwig, E. B.: Reticulohistiocytic granuloma ("reticulohistiocytoma") of the skin. Am. J. Clin. Path., *24*:1005, 1954.

Warin, R. P., Evans, C. D., Hewitt, M., *et al.*: (Reticulohistiocytosis lipoid dermatoarthritis). Brit. Med. J., *1*:1387, 1957.

Zak, F. G.: Reticulohistiocytoma ("ganglioneuroma") of the skin. Brit. J. Derm., *62*:351, 1950.

Generalized Eruptive Histiocytoma

Baccaredda-Boy, A.: Paraxanthomatöse (thesaurotische) System-Histiocytose. Hautarzt, *11*: 58, 1960.

Cramer, H. J.: Multiple Reticulohistiocytome der Haut ohne nachweisbare Zweiterkrankung. Hautarzt, *14*:297, 1963.

Muller, S. A., Wolff, K., and Winkelmann, R. K.: Generalized eruptive histiocytoma. Arch. Derm., *96*:11, 1967.

Winkelmann, R. K., and Muller, S. A.: Generalized eruptive histiocytoma. Arch. Derm., *88*: 586, 1963.

22

Metabolic Diseases

AMYLOIDOSIS

Three forms of amyloidosis occur: primary systemic amyloidosis, secondary systemic amyloidosis, and localized amyloidosis. Primary systemic amyloidosis, which involves mainly mesenchymal tissue, is frequently associated with cutaneous lesions. In contradistinction, secondary systemic amyloidosis, which occurs secondarily to chronic inflammatory diseases and shows amyloid deposits mainly in the parenchymal organs, shows no cutaneous lesions. Localized amyloidosis may occur in the skin in three variants: lichen amyloidosus, macular amyloidosis, and nodular amyloidosis. In addition, amyloid is found on rare occasions in the stroma of certain cutaneous tumors without, however, causing clinical symptoms. This may occur, for instance, in basal cell epithelioma and in Bowen's disease (Brownstein and Helwig, 1970, II).

In histologic sections stained with hematoxylin and eosin amyloid often can be recognized, provided that it is present in sufficiently large aggregates. It then appears as homogeneous, slightly eosinophilic masses that contain clefts as the result of shrinkage of the amyloid during the process of fixation and dehydration. Three staining methods are mainly used for the demonstration of amyloid: crystal violet, Congo red, and thioflavine T. As pointed out by Hashimoto et al. (1965), better results are obtained when crystal violet, which causes reddish metachromasia, or Congo red are used on unfixed, frozen sections rather than on paraffin-embedded sections. The method regarded as most reliable for the demonstration of amyloid consists of staining paraffin-embedded sections with alkaline Congo red, followed by studying the sections in polarized light, according to the method of Puchtler et al. The amyloid then shows greenish birefringence (Shapiro et al.). This method is superior to staining paraffin-embedded sections with thioflavine T and examining them with a fluorescence microscope, because greenish fluorescence is seen occasionally as a false-positive reaction in a variety of conditions (Brownstein and Helwig 1970, II). However, it must be realized that greenish birefringence following staining with alkaline Congo red is frequently found also in the other three diseases with a similarly disturbed collagen synthesis in dermal fibroblasts, namely in colloid milium, hyalinosis cutis et mucosae, and porphyria. Fortunately, clinical differentiation of these three diseases from amyloidosis causes difficulties only rarely.

PRIMARY SYSTEMIC AMYLOIDOSIS

Primary systemic amyloidosis, in which mesenchymal tissues rather than parenchymal organs are involved, shows amyloid deposits principally in the smooth and striated musculature, in the connective tissue, and in the walls of blood vessels. In this way nearly every organ can be affected. However, myocardial insufficiency and gastro-intestinal bleeding most commonly cause clinical symptoms and, ultimately, death (Brandt et al.). Macroglossia is present in about 40 per cent of the cases, and cutaneous lesions in about 25 per cent (Rukawina et al.). In the absence of macroglossia and skin lesions biopsy of the rectal mucosa or of the gingiva has been recommended. Recently, it has become evident that either biopsy of normal-appearing skin including the subcutaneous fat or multiple fine-needle aspirations of subcutaneous abdominal fat are useful procedures (Brownstein and Helwig, 1970, III; Westermark and Stenkvist). (For details, see under Secondary Systemic Amyloidosis, p. 389.)

Clinically, the cutaneous lesions consist of discrete and coalescing papules and nodules. They usually have a waxy color but may be bluish red as the result of hemorrhage into them. Frequently, petechiae are seen in the vicinity of the papules and nodules, and occasionally ecchymoses. The face is affected predominantly, especially the eyelids and periorbital region (Natelson et al.). In rare instances one observes firm subcutaneous nodules and plaques (Binkley) or areas of

induration of the skin resembling morphea (Miescher; Brownstein and Helwig, 1970, III).

Histopathology. Examination of cutaneous lesions reveals faintly eosinophilic, amorphous, often fissured masses of amyloid deposited in the dermis as well as in the subcutaneous tissue. Quite frequently, accumulations of amyloid are deposited close to the epidermis. They may or may not be separated from the overlying epidermis by a narrow zone of collagen (Fig. 22-1). In addition, deposits of amyloid may be seen in the membrana propria surrounding the sweat glands as well as around and within the walls of blood vessels. The involvement of the walls of blood vessels is responsible for the frequent presence of extravasated erythrocytes. In most instances no inflammatory reaction is present, although in some cases one finds focal accumulations of lymphoid cells, plasma cells, and foreign-body giant cells (Pearson et al.).

In the subcutaneous tissue one may find, in addition to large aggregates of amyloid and to amyloid infiltration of the walls of the blood vessels, so-called amyloid rings, formed by the deposition of amyloid around

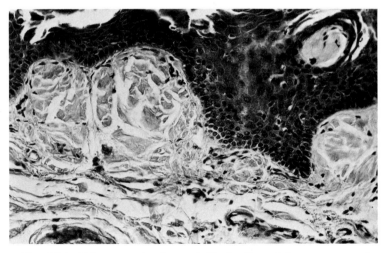

FIG. 22-1. **Primary systemic amyloidosis.** Round, homogeneous, fissured masses of amyloid are present in the uppermost dermis. A moderate number of fibroblasts is present within the amyloid. The amyloid material greatly resembles that seen in colloid milium (see Fig. 22-4). (×200)

individual fat cells (Fig. 22-2) (Pearson et al.). The fat cells then may appear as if cemented together by the amyloid substance.

SYSTEMIC LESIONS. Not only in the skin and in the subcutaneous tissue but also throughout the body the small arteries and veins may show amyloid deposits, often replacing entirely the media and adventitia, while the intima is usually spared (Brownstein and Helwig, 1970, III). The skeletal muscles, the tongue, the heart muscle, and the smooth musculature of the gastrointestinal and the urinary tracts often are severely affected. Not infrequently, deposits of amyloid are found in renal glomeruli (Eisen). Occasionally, therefore, a patient with primary systemic amyloidosis may die of renal failure (Brandt et al.). In many cases the liver and the spleen, in addition to vascular involvement, also show some parenchymatous involvement (Rukawina et al.).

Relationship to Multiple Myeloma. In about 20 per cent of the cases primary systemic amyloidosis is associated with multiple myeloma (Brunsting and MacDonald). Generally in such instances the multiple myeloma shows no IgA or IgG myeloma globulin in the serum but only micromolecular components, i.e., abnormal light chains representing Bence Jones protein.

Usually, Bence Jones protein can be demonstrated easily by electrophoresis in the urine, whereas serum electrophoresis shows only a decrease in the gamma globulins. However, the Bence Jones protein can be demonstrated in the serum by immunoelectrophoresis with anti-human sera directed against type K Bence Jones protein or the FAB-fragment of IgG (Herrmann et al.). In some cases of primary systemic amyloidosis without evidence of Bence Jones protein either elevations or depressions in the serum levels of IgG, IgA, or IgM are encountered as an indication of participation of the immune mechanism (Cathcart et al.). However, the view once expressed by Osserman et al., that primary systemic amyloidosis was a plasma cell dyscrasia in which abnormal proteins are produced by plasma cells, has been abandoned. The presence of abnormal immunoglobulins, such as Bence Jones light chains in the serum, are not a prerequisite for the development of primary systemic amyloidosis. (For further details, see under Histogenesis.)

SECONDARY SYSTEMIC AMYLOIDOSIS

Secondary systemic amyloidosis occurs secondarily to chronic inflammatory diseases, among which tuberculosis, lepromatous lep-

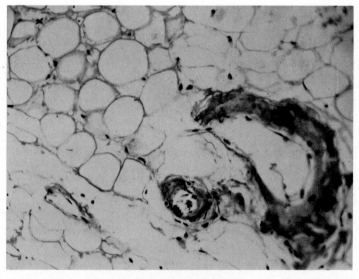

FIG. 22-2. **Primary systemic amyloidosis.** Subcutaneous fat. Amyloid is deposited in the walls of two blood vessels and also around fat cells, forming so-called amyloid rings. ($\times 400$)

rosy, rheumatoid arthritis, and osteomyelitis are the most common. Also, certain chronic cutaneous diseases, such as stasis ulcer, hidradenitis suppurativa and dystrophic epidermolysis bullosa, can lead to secondary systemic amyloidosis (Brownstein and Helwig, 1970, I). It is generally assumed that secondary systemic amyloidosis represents an aberrant response following prolonged antigenic stimulation.

Clinically, hepatomegaly and proteinuria are the initial manifestations, followed by nephrosis and uremia. The skin is free of lesions.

Histopathology. The parenchymatous organs, such as the kidneys, the liver, the spleen ("sago spleen"), and the adrenals, are predominantly involved, beginning with deposits in the walls of the arterioles.

Up to the present time the preferred procedure for the diagnosis of secondary, as well as of primary, systemic amyloidosis has been biopsy of the rectal mucosa. Lately, biopsy of normal skin including the subcutaneous fat (Westermark) or multiple fine-needle aspirations of subcutaneous abdominal fat (Westermark and Stenkvist) have been recommended, instead.

When a biopsy of normal skin is routinely processed and stained with alkaline Congo red, and is then examined for green birefringence in a microscope with polarizing equipment, amyloid may be seen as thin rings around some of the sweat glands, and in some cases also around some of the sebaceous glands, hair follicles, and fat cells (Westermark).

For fine-needle biopsy of subcutaneous abdominal fat multiple aspirations are performed with a syringe and needle having a diameter of 0.7 mm and a length of 50 mm. The aspirated material is spread on a glass slide, allowed to air-dry, and then stained without prior fixation with alkaline Congo red. After this, the slide is dipped into concentrated (99.6%) ethanol and into xylene, mounted, and examined in a polarizing microscope. A positive result consists of finding clear green double refraction in the fragments of fatty tissue (Westermark and Stenkvist).

LICHEN AMYLOIDOSUS

In localized amyloidosis of the skin which, in addition to lichen amyloidosus, also includes macular amyloidosis and nodular amyloidosis, only cutaneous lesions occur. In lichen amyloidosus lesions are seen most commonly on the legs, but they may occur elsewhere. They consist of closely set, discrete, conical or flat, brownish-red papules that resemble the papules of lichen planus. The papules may have a translucent appearance. In some instances through coalescence of papules plaques form that may have a verrucous surface and then resemble lichen simplex chronicus. Usually, the lesions of lichen amyloidosus itch severely, in contrast to those of primary systemic amyloidosis.

Histopathology. The amyloid deposits are much smaller than those found in primary systemic amyloidosis and are limited to the papillary dermis, as a rule. In very early lesions several small angular aggregates may be seen in the involved papillae. As they increase in size, the amyloid deposits coalesce and gradually occupy some of the dermal papillae entirely, and by further increase in size they can greatly extend the involved papillae. Ultimately, some neighboring papillae may coalesce. While at first the accumulations of amyloid are separated from the overlying epidermis by a narrow zone of normal collagen, ultimately the amyloid lies in direct apposition to the epidermis.

The amyloid consists of a fissured, homogeneous material. It stains only faintly eosinophilic with hematoxylin and eosin, less so than the surrounding collagen. Elastic tissue stains reveal the absence of elastic fibers within the accumulations of amyloid. A moderate number of fibroblasts and capillaries are seen within the amyloid. In some cases a mild, chronic inflammatory infiltrate will be seen beneath the amyloid-filled dermal papillae in the subpapillary dermis (Dostrovsky and Sagher). Occasionally, small amyloid particles are seen in the overlying thickened epidermis, indicating the elimination of amyloid through the epidermis (Anekoji and Irisawa).

Differential Diagnosis. Colloid milium greatly resembles lichen amyloidosus in sections stained with hematoxylin and eosin, since both appear as homogeneous, pale pink aggregates containing clefts; and no reliable differentiation is possible by histochemical methods (see under Colloid Milium, p. 393).

MACULAR AMYLOIDOSIS

Macular amyloidosis is characterized by moderately pruritic, symmetrically distributed, brownish, reticulated macules. Although macular amyloidosis may occur anywhere on the trunk or the extremities, the upper back is a fairly common site (Shanon and Sagher). The eruption is easily passed off as postinflammatory hyperpigmentation by those unfamiliar with the condition (Brownstein and Hashimoto). Occasionally, in addition to macules, there are micropapules that are smaller in size than the papules of lichen amyloidosus (Black and Wilson Jones). Macular amyloidosis in a few instances has been seen in association with lichen amyloidosus (Kurban et al.; Brownstein and Hashimoto).

Histopathology. The amyloid deposits in the dermal papillae are small and can easily be overlooked without special staining. In some cases amyloid has been found only after a repeat biopsy (Black and Wilson Jones). The amyloid in sections stained with hematoxylin and eosin is present either as fairly small angulated globules that are similar in size to the hyaline bodies found in lichen planus or as larger aggregates of homogeneous material (Black and Wilson Jones). Although the amyloid deposits usually are separated from the basal layer of the epidermis by a narrow band of uninvolved collagen, in some areas the amyloid lies in direct contact with the basal cells. This impingement upon the basal cells is the apparent reason for the pigmentary incontinence and the presence of melanophages in the papillary and subpapillary dermis (Brownstein and Hashimoto). The pigmentary incontinence usually is associated with a slight degree of chronic inflammatory infiltration.

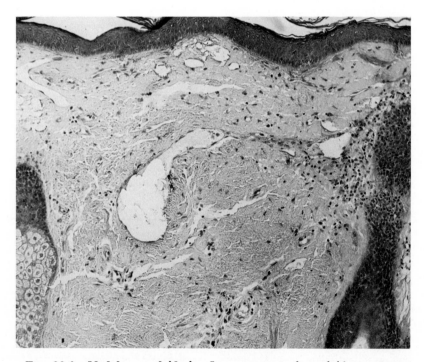

FIG. 22-3. **Nodular amyloidosis.** Large masses of amyloid are present throughout the dermis. The nuclei and the cutaneous appendages are well preserved. (×100)

Although the amyloid deposits usually are smaller in macular amyloidosis than in lichen amyloidosus a differentiation of the two conditions on the basis of the amount of amyloid present usually is not possible, since the amount is variable in both conditions in different papillae (Brownstein and Hashimoto).

NODULAR AMYLOIDOSIS

In this rare condition one or several nodules or plaques are encountered, most commonly on the legs (Potter and Johnson), but occasionally elsewhere, as for instance on the trunk (Rodermund) or on the glans penis (Weitzner). In the center of the nodule the skin may appear atrophic as a result of involution of the amyloid.

Histopathology. Large masses of amyloid are present (Fig. 22-3). They extend through the entire dermis into the subcutaneous fat. Amyloid deposits are found also within the walls of vessels, in the membrana propria of the sweat glands and around fat cells (Lindemayr and Partsch). A chronic inflammatory infiltrate may be present within and around the masses of amyloid, containing in some instances an admixture of plasma cells (Brownstein and Helwig, 1970, II) or foreign body giant cells (Rodermund).

On a histologic basis a differentiation from primary systemic amyloidosis is not possible.

Histogenesis of Amyloid. It has long been known that amyloid deposits can form in response to prolonged antigenic stimulation. Thus, extensive amyloidosis, corresponding in distribution to systemic secondary amyloidosis, can be experimentally produced in many species of animals by repeated injections of various antigenic substances, of which casein is the most widely used for experimental purposes (Janigan).

It was, therefore, natural to assume that all amyloid formed as a result of an antigen-antibody interaction and, since in many cases of both primary and secondary systemic amyloidosis a significant proliferation of plasma cells is found, it was assumed that amyloid was a product of antigenically stimulated plasma cells. The discovery that amyloid was a filamentous protein suggested a relationship with the light chains present in immunoglobulins.

The theory of identity of amyloid with light chains seemed to be strengthened by the finding that the amino acid sequence of purified amyloid fibril protein is similar to that of the variable region of the light chains of homogeneous immunoglobulins (Glenner et al., 1971, II; 1972). Observations indicating that precipitated lambda light chains of Bence Jones proteins have a green birefringence on alkaline Congo red staining and such precipitated light chains have a diameter of 7 to 8 nm and a length between 110 to 200 nm, very similar to amyloid filaments, seemed to be additional proof of a close relationship (Glenner et al., 1971, I).

The identification of amyloid with light chains of immunoglobulins, as justified as it may seem on the basis of Glenner's biochemical findings, cannot be applied to all cases of amyloidosis: in the first place, there is no evidence that plasma cells, which are the only source of immunoglobulins, are active participants in localized amyloidosis, in secondary systemic amyloidosis, or even in every case of primary systemic amyloidosis (Cathcart et al.); and in the second place, several instances of secondary amyloidosis on the basis of chronic infections have been observed in patients with primary agammaglobulinemia, none of whom had humoral immunoglobulins, and some did not even have plasma cells (Mawas et al.).

The main argument against identifying amyloid with plasma-cell-derived immunoglobulins rests on the *electron microscopic findings* which have shown the fibroblast to be the only cell in the skin to produce amyloid. The production of amyloid by fibroblasts was first demonstrated in a case of lichen amyloidosus by Hashimoto et al. in 1965, and in a case of primary systemic amyloidosis by Gafni et al. in 1966. Gafni et al. have postulated that in cases of primary systemic amyloidosis associated with multiple myeloma plasma cells synthesize the myeloma proteins and fibroblasts produce the amyloid, indicating that plasma cells and fibroblasts stand in a certain relationship with one another. Thus, a single stimulus can cause alterations in the metabolism of both cells, resulting in the synthesis of an abnormal product in either cell.

The elaboration of amyloid in the skin by fibroblasts has since been confirmed by many authors, e.g., by Ebner in nodular amyloidosis; by Rodermund and Klingmüller, and by Shapiro et al. in lichen amyloidosus; by Brownstein and Hashimoto in macular amyloidosis; and by Piérard and Kint, and by Goodman et al. in primary systemic amyloidosis.

In all instances of amyloid formation in the skin, the fibroblasts show a well-developed rough endoplasmic reticulum as evidence of active protein synthesis. The cisternae of the rough endoplasmic reticulum are dilated and contain amorphous material and some thin, straight, nonbranching filaments, 6 to 8 nm in diameter, resembling in their size the small variety of amyloid filament. Amorphous material and amyloid filaments are present also in the cytoplasm of the fibroblasts and are being discharged into the extracellular space by means of secretory vesicles. In the vicinity of the fibroblasts amyloid filaments are seen arranged as islands of various sizes. The amyloid islands often are surrounded by cytoplasmic processes of the fibroblasts. Thus, the pattern of amyloid deposition greatly resembles that of collagen formation. Most of the amyloid filaments measure from 6 to 10 nm in diameter, and are straight and nonbranching. Some filaments, however, are thicker, up to 25 nm in diameter (Brownstein and Hashimoto). In addition, mature collagen fibrils are present between the amyloid islands, in the vicinity of some fibroblasts, and also in small numbers within the amyloid islands (Hashimoto and Onn). Special emphasis is placed by Hashimoto and Onn on their observation that the filaments of amyloid are straight and nonbranching, a feature regarded by them as specific for amyloid, since in colloid and hyalin the filaments are wavy and show anastomosing and branching (see p. 397). Nevertheless, all three materials

form as the result of a disturbed collagen synthesis within fibroblasts and in the extracellular space outside of fibroblasts.

Differential Diagnosis. Although clinically the differentiation between amyloidosis and colloid milium, as a rule, is easy, on histologic and histochemical examination amyloid and colloid may be indistinguishable. Further electron microscopic studies are necessary to establish the significance of the differences in appearance between amyloid and colloid filaments, described by Hashimoto and Onn. (For a detailed discussion of colloid, see below.)

COLLOID MILIUM

Colloid milium is characterized by numerous round, brownish, waxy papules of the skin, 1 to 2 mm in size. Although in some areas the papules are so closely set that they form plaques, it still can be recognized that the plaques are composed of individual papules. The lesions occur only in areas exposed to the sun, most commonly on the

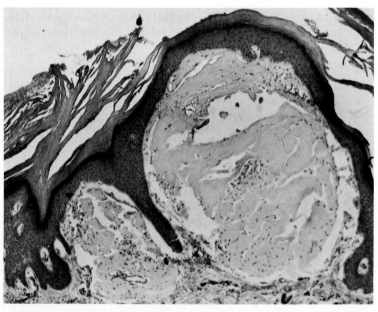

Fig. 22-4. **Colloid milium.** Two round, homogeneous, fissured masses of colloid are present in the uppermost dermis. A moderate number of fibroblasts is present within the colloid. The colloid material greatly resembles the material seen in amyloid. (See Fig. 22-2).

face and the dorsa of the hands. Although the disorder often starts in childhood (Percival and Duthie; Woolridge and Frerichs; Miedzinski et al.), in other cases the onset is in adolescence (Agius), or in early adult life (Graham and Marques).

A few cases have been described in which smooth nodules or plaques of "colloid degeneration" were present in various areas, such as the face (Sullivan and Ellis; Bienvenu and Lever) or the trunk (Reuter and Becker). Such cases are best classified, as suggested by Brownstein and Helwig, as instances of nodular amyloidosis (see p. 391).

Histopathology. On histologic examination colloid milium, like amyloid, shows homogeneous, fissured aggregates, staining faintly eosinophilic, and occupying most or all of the involved dermal papillae (Fig. 22-4). Although the aggregates of colloid contain no elastic fibers, considerable amounts of elastotic material may be present in the underlying dermis as a result of chronic sun exposure (Graham and Marques). In several cases of colloid milium all

stains regarded as specific for amyloid have been positive (Woolridge and Frerichs; Graham and Marques) (see below, under Histogenesis).

Histogenesis. Not only the histologic findings but also histochemical studies show that colloid and amyloid deposits have identical characteristics (Graham and Marques). The well known variability of staining reactions with crystal violet and Congo red applies equally to colloid and to amyloid; but, when frozen sections are used in place of formalin-fixed, paraffin-embedded material, positive staining is obtained with crystal violet for both colloid and amyloid (Hashimoto et al.). In addition, both substances show greenish birefringence after staining with alkaline Congo red according to the method recommended by Puchtler et al.; and both substances show greenish fluorescence after staining with thioflavine T (Graham and Marques).

Electron microscopic examination by Hashimoto et al. has revealed that colloid, like amyloid, is produced by fibroblasts that show dilated cisternae of their rough-surfaced endoplasmic reticulum as evidence of active protein synthesis. The colloid is released from fibroblasts as filaments and amorphous material by means of

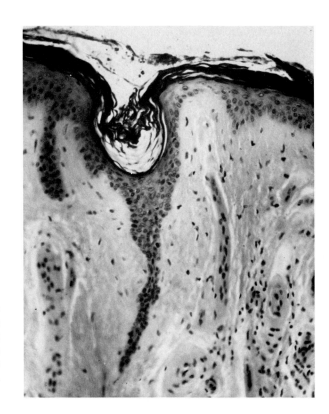

FIG. 22-5. **Hyalinosis cutis et mucosae.** The hyaline material consists of thick, homogeneous bundles that extend perpendicularly to the skin surface. In addition, thick hyaline mantles surround the blood vessels. (×200)

secretory vesicles. Islands of colloid, like those of amyloid, are separated from one another partially by fibroblasts and their processes and partially by collagen. The islands contain amorphous material, tropocollagen filaments, 2 nm wide, and larger filaments varying from 5 to 10 nm in width. The larger filaments show curving, branching, or anastomoses with each other. Hashimoto et al. contrast this with the appearance of the filaments of amyloid which, although similar in width, are straight and nonbranching. Also, colloid differs from amyloid by the presence of considerable amounts of amorphous material (see p. 392).

HYALINOSIS CUTIS ET MUCOSAE (LIPOID PROTEINOSIS)

In this recessively inherited disorder there are rather widespread depositions of a hyaline material. The skin, the oral mucosa, and the larynx show the most pronounced involvement. Not infrequently the hyaline material, largely a glycoprotein, also has a lipid component so that also the term *lipoid proteinosis* is being used for this disease.

Clinically, one observes papular and nodular lesions on the face, and areas of diffuse infiltration associated with hyperkeratosis on the elbows, knees, hands, and occasionally elsewhere. The papules and nodules on the face may cause pitted scars, giving the skin a pigskin-leather appearance. Beads of small nodules may be present along the free margin of the eyelids. The tongue is firm because of diffuse infiltration; and the presence of laryngeal lesions causes hoarseness since birth. The occurrence of convulsive seizures is not uncommon (Holtz and Schulze; Caplan).

Histopathology. The earliest change consists of a thickening of the capillary walls due to a deposition of hyaline material within and around the basement membrane (van der Walt and Heyl). In well developed lesions the skin presents a striking and diagnostic picture. Beneath a hyperkeratotic and occasionally papillomatous epidermis a homogeneous, eosinophilic, hyaline mantle surrounds the vessels throughout the dermis and similarly the sweat glands, the epithelium of which becomes atrophic. The dermis, which usually is thickened considerably, consists in its upper portion also of hyaline

material arranged in homogeneous bundles, staining a pale pink with hematoxylin and eosin. In areas of papillomatosis these bundles often run perpendicularly to the skin surface (Fig. 22-5). In the lower dermis the hyaline changes are focal and do not involve all of the connective tissue, as in the upper dermis. In the hyaline areas the nuclei of the fibroblasts and the vascular endothelium are well preserved. Similar hyaline mantles, as seen around the vessels and sweat glands, often surround the hair follicles (Fleischmajer et al.). In addition, the smooth muscle of the arrectores pilorum shows marked infiltration with hyaline material (Caplan).

The hyaline material is strongly PAS-positive and diastase-resistant, indicating the presence of neutral mucopolysaccharides. Staining for acid mucopolysaccharides with alcian blue is negative at pH 0.9, but is slightly positive at pH 2.9. The fact that the staining with alcian blue at pH 2.9 is no longer positive after prior exposure to hyaluronidase indicates that the acid mucopolysaccharides are largely hyaluronic acid (Fleischmajer et al.). Staining with Congo red and crystal violet may give slightly positive results (Fleischmajer et al.).

Lipid stains have given varying results. Although lipids are present in most instances, occasionally there is no reaction to lipid stains (Grosfeld et al.; Rasiewicz et al.); or in the same patient one lesion may contain lipids, while another contains none (Fleischmajer et al.). Of the various lipids neutral fat is present most commonly, as shown by a positive reaction to staining to Sudan III or IV (Wood et al.; Ungar and Katzenellenbogen; Eberhartinger and Niebauer; McCusker and Caplan). The neutral fat is distributed as numerous small droplets throughout the hyaline material, particularly around the blood vessels (Fig. 22-6). The fact that in most instances the staining with Sudan is dark orange rather than bright orange red indicates that neutral fat is not the only lipid present (Wood et al.). As shown by a positive Schultz reaction, cholesterol is often present (Wood et al.; Eberhartinger and Niebauer; McCusker and Caplan), but only as free cholesterol and not as cholesterol ester since the lipid material in

Fig. 22-6. **Hyalinosis cutis et mucosae.** Scarlet red stain for fat. Numerous small lipid droplets are seen throughout the hyaline material particularly around the blood vessels. (×100)

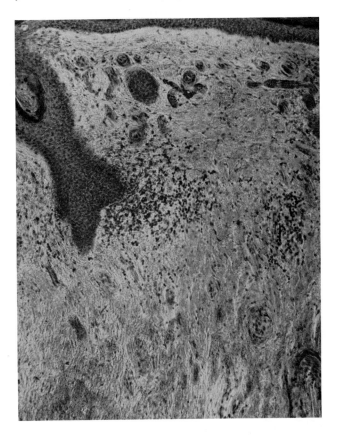

frozen sections is not bifringent (Ramos e Silva; Wood et al.). Phospholipids are absent or present in only small amounts since the test most specific for phospholipids, i.e., Baker's acid hematein test, is either negative (Wood et al.; Ungar and Katzenellenbogen; McCusker and Caplan) or only weakly positive (Eberhartinger and Niebauer).

SYSTEMIC LESIONS. Intracranial calcification has been noted quite frequently by x-ray examination in patients with hyalinosis cutis et mucosae, and it has been held responsible for the occurrence of convulsive seizures (Holtz and Schulze; Laymon and Hill). Autopsy findings by Holtz have established that the calcium is deposited within the walls of capillaries located in the hippocampal gyri of the temporal lobes. Holtz was able to prove that the capillaries had been hyalinized prior to calcification because after decalcification a mantle of PAS-positive material was seen around the endothelium of these vessels.

The very widespread distribution of the pericapillary hyaline deposits has been established by biopsies and autopsies. Thus, deposits have been found not only in the submucosa of the upper respiratory and digestive tracts, but also in the submucosa of the stomach, the jejunum, the rectum, and the vagina, in the retina between the vitreous membrane and the pigment epithelium, and also in the testes, the pancreas, the lungs, the kidneys, as well as elsewhere (Holtz; Caplan).

Histogenesis. PAS-positive neutral mucopolysaccharides are a characteristic component of the hyaline material. Since this PAS-positive material disappears following digestion with pepsin, it can be concluded that it is bound to a protein and thus represents a glycoprotein (Fleischmajer et al.). Lipids are not an essential feature of the disease. If they are present they can be removed with lipid solvents without damage to the protein-carbohydrate complex. This suggests that the lipids are either free or loosely bound to the hyaline material (McCusker and Caplan).

TABLE 22-1. Classification of the Porphyrias

	Type	Onset	Cutaneous Manifestations	Extracutaneous Manifestations	Urine	Feces	Erythrocytes
Congenital erythropoietic porphyria	erythropoietic	infancy; recessive	blisters; scarring	red teeth; hemolytic anemia	uro I	copro I	uro I; stable fluorescence
Erythrohepatic protoporphyria	erythropoietic and hepatic	childhood; dominant	burning; edema; thickening; rarely blisters	decreased liver function	*neg.*	protoporphyrin continuously	protoporphyrin continuously; transient fluorescence
Acute intermittent porphyria (AIP)	hepatic	young adults; dominant	*neg.*	abdominal pain; neuropathy; psychoses	ALA, PBG; continuously	*neg.*	*neg.*
Variegate porphyria	hepatic	young adults; dominant	like PCT	like AIP	ALA, PBG; during attacks	protoporphyrin continuously	*neg.*
Porphyria cutanea tarda (PCT)	hepatic	middle age; dominant	blisters; thickening; hypertrichosis	decreased liver function; slight iron overload	uro III; stable fluorescence	often *neg.*	*neg.*

ALA = delta-aminolevulinic acid
PBG = porphobilinogen

On *electron microscopic examination* the hyaline material is shown to be composed mainly of filaments that are secreted by fibroblasts. The fibroblasts show in their dilated cisternae both amorphous and filamentous material. Outside the fibroblasts hyalin, like colloid, consists of tropocollagen filaments, 1 to 2 nm wide, as well as of larger filaments, 5 to 10 nm wide, and of amorphous material. The filaments composing the hyaline material more closely resemble the filaments of colloid than of amyloid, since amyloid filaments are straight and nonbranching, whereas the filaments of colloid and of the hyaline material in hyalinosis cutis et mucosae are wavy and anastomose (Hashimoto et al.). A feature that is typical of the hyaline material and is found neither in amyloid nor in colloid is the close relationship of the filaments to the capillaries (Kint; Rodermund and Klingmüller). A network of filaments forms a wide coat around the dermal capillaries. Several layers of capillary basal lamina that are concentrically arranged around the capillaries are embedded in this network of hyaline filaments (Rodermund and Klingmüller). Peripheral to the layers of basal lamina one observes, in addition to the thin filaments, thicker striated filaments, up to 30 nm in diameter, and collagen fibrils that are thinner than mature collagen fibrils and probably represent young collagen fibrils. (The average diameter of mature collagen fibrils is 100 nm; see p. 34.) The hyaline filaments are seen not only around capillaries and as islands in the dermis but also diffusely throughout the dermis between normal appearing collagen fibrils (Kint).

Differential Diagnosis. Erythrohepatic (or erythropoietic) protoporphyria shows hyaline changes in the collagen around the superficial dermal capillaries indistinguishable from the hyaline changes seen in hyalinosis cutis et mucosae. There is, however, no involvement in the deeper dermis, particularly not around the sweat glands (see below).

PORPHYRIA

Five types of porphyria are recognized (Table 22-1). The light sensitivity in the four types with cutaneous lesions is caused by wavelengths that are absorbed by the porphyrin molecule, i.e., by visible light with a wavelength above 400 nm, rather than by ultraviolet light (Rimington et al.).

In *congenital erythropoietic porphyria,* a very rare disease, blisters followed by ulceration and severe scarring are observed in exposed areas (Haining et al.).

In *erythrohepatic protoporphyria* (erythropoietic protoporphyria) the usual reaction to light is edema followed by thickening of the skin. In some patients, however, there are vesicles on the face resembling those seen in hydroa aestivale (Horkay et al.) or in hydroa vacciniforme (Suurmond et al.). Both the bone marrow and the liver show fluorescence (Cripps and MacEachern). Cirrhosis of the liver causes death in some of the patients (Donaldson et al.).

In *porphyria variegata* cutaneous manifestations similar to those of porphyria cutanea tarda may be combined with the internal manifestations of acute intermittent porphyria (Baxter and Permowicz).

In *porphyria cutanea tarda* blisters occur mainly on the dorsa of the hands through a combination of light exposure and trauma, but they may occur also on the face. The skin of the face and of the dorsa of the hands often is thickened. The liver shows fluorescence (Ennerböck and Lundvall). Often, there is a mild degree of iron overload (Sauer and Funk).

Histopathology. The blisters arise subepidermally in all four types of porphyria in which they may occur. However, as a result of regeneration of the epidermis, older bullae may be located partially or entirely within the epidermis. Also, hyaline deposits are found in all four types of porphyria with cutaneous lesions in varying degrees, depending on the type and severity of the porphyria. The hyaline material may show green birefringence in polarized light after staining with alkaline Congo red (Epstein et al.), just as it is seen in amyloidosis, colloid milium, and hyalinosis cutis et mucosae.

CONGENITAL ERYTHROPOIETIC PORPHYRIA. Extensive deposits of PAS-positive, diastase-resistant hyalin are present throughout the upper dermis but are most pronounced in the thickened walls of capillaries (Bhutani et al.).

ERYTHROHEPATIC PROTOPORPHYRIA. Areas of the skin that have become thickened from many years' exposure to light show amorphous, strongly PAS-positive, diastase-resistant material around the capillaries

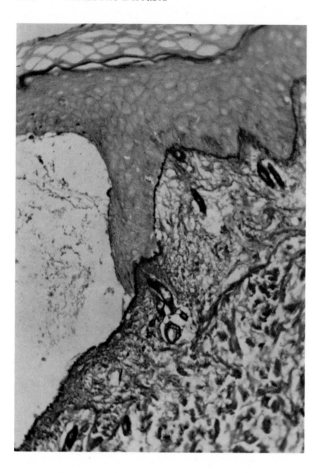

FIG. 22-7. **Porphyria cutanea tarda.** On staining with the PAS reaction after diastase digestion the PAS-positive basement zone is seen at the floor of the blister. PAS-positive hyalin is present in the wall of capillaries in the upper dermis. ($\times 100$)

in the upper third of the dermis. In severe cases extensive hyalinization is present throughout the upper dermis (Suurmond). The pericapillary hyalin usually contains, like the hyalin in hyalinosis cutis et mucosae, lipids since it stains with Sudan IV (Ryan and Madill).

PORPHYRIA CUTANEA TARDA. It is regarded as quite characteristic of the bullae of porphyria cutanea tarda that often the dermal papillae rise irregularly from the floor of the bulla into the bulla cavity. This is referred to as festooning of the base of the bulla (Feldaker et al.). This phenomenon can be explained by the rigidity of the upper dermis induced by the presence of PAS-positive, diastase-resistant hyalin around the capillaries in the papillae and the upper dermis (Fig. 22-7). However, in contrast with erythrohepatic protoporphyria and hyalinosis cutis et mucosae, the hyaline deposits

of porphyria cutanea tarda contain no lipids (Kint).

Histogenesis. The actual enzyme defect is known so far in only two types of porphyria. In congenital erythropoietic porphyria, uroporphyrinogen III cosynthetase is decreased so that much of the porphyrins is "sidetracked" to the isomer type I (Romeo and Levin); and in acute intermittent porphyria, uroporphyrinogen I synthetase is decreased, resulting in a decreased inhibition of hepatic ALA (delta-aminolevulinic acid) synthetase (Meyer et al.) and thus in an increased production of ALA.

On electron microscopic examination the hyaline material observed in the upper third of the dermis in erythrohepatic protoporphyria, in porphyria cutanea tarda, and in porphyria variegata appears indistinguishable from the filamentous material seen in hyalinosis cutis et mucosae (Kint et al). Like the hyalin in hyalinosis cutis et mucosae, the hyalin seen in porphyria is produced by active fibroblasts with abundant rough endoplasmic reticulum (Charles et al.). One observes multiplication of the basal lamina of the capillaries and accumulation of hyaline filaments between the multiple layers of the basal lamina (Kint; Epstein et al.). According to Anton-Lamprecht and Meyer, the filaments of the hyaline material and of the capillary basal lamina have a similar ultrastructure. Peripheral to the basal lamina hyaline filaments are found intermingled with small collagen fibrils that show cross striation but possess an average thickness of only 35 nm, rather than of 100 nm like mature collagen (Kint). Deposits of IgG around capillaries and at the dermal-epidermal junction are regularly present; but, since deposits of complement are only occasionally seen, it is likely that the deposits are not related to immune responses (Epstein et al.).

Differential Diagnosis. For the histologic differentiation between porphyria and hyalinosis cutis et mucosae, see p. 397.

CALCINOSIS CUTIS

Four forms of calcinosis cutis exist: metastatic calcinosis, dystrophic calcinosis, idiopathic calcinosis, and subepidermal calcified nodules.

METASTATIC CALCINOSIS CUTIS

Metastatic calcification develops as the result of either hypercalcemia or hyperphosphatemia. Hypercalcemia may be the result either of primary hyperparathyroidism, excessive intake of vitamin D, or excessive intake of milk and alkali, or of extensive destruction of bone through osteomyelitis or metastases of a carcinoma (Mulligan). Hyperphosphatemia occurs in chronic renal failure and is associated with hypocalcemia. The low level of ionized calcium in the serum stimulates parathyroid secretion, leading to resorption of calcium and phosphorus from bone and to secondary hyperparathyroidism. The demineralization of bone causes both osteodystrophy and metastatic calcification (Katz et al.).

Metastatic calcification affects mainly the media of blood vessels, the kidneys, and the subcutaneous tissue located in the vicinity of the large joints. Rarely the lungs, the myocardium, the spleen or the skin show calcium deposits (Katz et al.).

Instances of metastatic calcification of the skin or the subcutaneous tissue have been

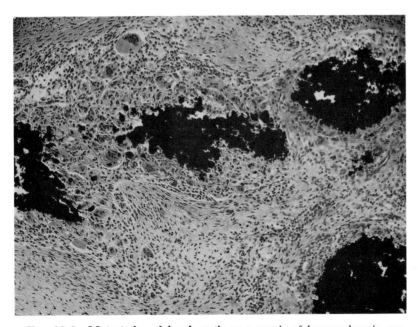

FIG. 22-8. **Metastatic calcinosis cutis** as a result of hypercalcemia produced by prolonged and excessive intake of vitamin D. Von Kossa stain for calcium. Irregular masses of calcium surrounded by a foreign-body giant cell reaction are present in the subcutaneous fat. ($\times 100$)

reported occasionally in hypervitaminosis D (Wilson et al.), and as the result of excessive intake of milk and alkali (Wermer et al.); but most reports have been in patients with renal osteodystrophy and secondary hyperparathyroidism (Putkonen and Wangel; Eisenberg and Bartholow; Posey and Ritchie; Kolten and Pedersen). The cutaneous lesions may consist of firm, white papules (Posey and Ritchie), of papules in linear arrangement (Putkonen and Wangel), of symmetrical infiltrated nodular plaques (Kolten and Pedersen), or of papules and nodules from which a granular, whitish substance can be expressed (Eisenberg and Bartholow). In addition, calcification of vessels in the deep dermis or in the subcutaneous tissue may occur in primary or secondary hyperparathyroidism and may lead to occlusion of these vessels and to infarctive ulcerations, especially on the legs (Winkelmann and Keating).

Histopathology. Calcium deposits are recognized easily in histologic sections, since they stain deep blue with hematoxylin and eosin. They stain black with von Kossa's stain for calcium. The calcium occurs as a rule as massive deposits when located in the subcutaneous fat (Fig. 22-8), whereas in the dermis it is found usually as granules and small deposits. Larger deposits of calcium often evoke a foreign-body reaction, so that giant cells, an inflammatory infiltrate, and fibrosis may be present around them (Kolten and Pedersen).

In areas of infarctive necrosis as a result of calcification of dermal or subcutaneous vessels, the involved vessels show calcification of their walls and intravascular fibrosis with attempts at recanalization of the obstructed lumina (Winkelmann and Keating).

DYSTROPHIC CALCINOSIS CUTIS

In dystrophic calcinosis cutis the calcium is deposited in previously damaged tissue. The values for serum calcium and phosphorus are normal. The internal organs are spared. There may be numerous large deposits of calcium (calcinosis universalis) or only a few deposits (calcinosis circumscripta).

Calcinosis universalis, as a rule, occurs in patients with dermatomyositis. Large deposits of calcium are found in the skin and subcutaneous tissue, and often also in muscles and tendons (Wheeler et al.; Reich). If the patient survives, the nodules of dystrophic calcinosis gradually resolve.

Calcinosis circumscripta, as a rule, occurs in patients with systemic scleroderma. Generally, in the presence of calcinosis, systemic scleroderma is a rather mild disease and has a good prognosis. It is referred to as the CRST syndrome since the manifestations consist of calcinosis cutis, Raynaud's phenomenon, sclerodactylia, and telangiectasias (Carr et al.) (see also p. 442). Lupus erythematosus only rarely is associated with dystrophic calcinosis (Kabir and Malkinson).

Aside from the connective tissue diseases, dystrophic calcinosis is seen often in subcutaneous fat necrosis of the newborn, and rarely in the subcutaneous nodules occurring in Ehlers-Danlos disease.

Histopathology. As in metastatic calcinosis cutis, the calcium in dystrophic calcinosis cutis usually is present as granules or small deposits in the dermis and as massive deposits in the subcutaneous tissue. A foreign-body giant cell reaction often is found around the large deposits of calcium (Reich). The calcium deposits usually are located in areas where the collagen or the fatty tissue appears degenerated as a result of the disease preceding the calcinosis.

IDIOPATHIC CALCINOSIS CUTIS

Even though in some instances of dystrophic calcinosis cutis the underlying connective tissue disease may be mild and can be overlooked unless specifically searched for, there remain cases of idiopathic calcinosis cutis where no underlying disease can be found. Thus, Haim and Friedman-Birnbaum have reported two very similar cases of circumscribed calcinosis cutis, one of which was an obvious case of scleroderma, whereas the second was apparently idiopathic.

There are two entities that are generally regarded as idiopathic calcinosis cutis: tumoral calcinosis and idiopathic calcinosis of the scrotum.

Tumoral calcinosis consists of numerous large subcutaneous calcified masses that may be associated with papular and nodular skin lesions of calcinosis (Whiting et al.). The disease usually is familial and is associated with hyperphosphatemia (Mozaffarian et al.). The resemblance of tumoral calcinosis to the dystrophic calcinosis universalis seen with dermatomyositis is great.

Idiopathic calcinosis of the scrotum consists of multiple asymptomatic nodules of the scrotal skin. The nodules begin to appear in childhood or in early adult life, increase in size and number, and sometimes break down to discharge chalky contents (Shapiro et al.).

Histopathology. Tumoral calcinosis shows large masses of calcium surrounded by a foreign-body reaction.

In regard to idiopathic calcinosis of the scrotum, Shapiro et al. emphasize that histologically the nodules represent not cysts but areas of calcinosis, even though clinically they may suggest cysts.

Histogenesis. Two authors have studied by electron microscopy lesions of "idiopathic" calcinosis cutis (Paegle; Cornelius et al.). These authors agree that the deposits consist of pleomorphic calcium phosphate (apatite) crystals. However, whereas Paegle thought that the earliest deposits of calcium were situated in the

ground substance, Cornelius et al. saw the earliest calcium deposits within collagen fibrils. As the calcium deposits grow in size, they produce degeneration of the collagen.

SUBEPIDERMAL CALCIFIED NODULE

In this disorder usually a single small, raised, hard nodule is present. In one reported case, however, there were two nodules (Woods and Kellaway), and in another nine nodules (Shmunes and Wood). In some individuals the nodule is present at birth (Winer), whereas in others it forms later in life (Steigleder and Elschner). In most instances the surface of the nodule is verrucous, but it may be smooth. The most common locations are the extremities and the face.

Histopathology. The calcified material is located predominantly in the uppermost dermis, although in larger nodules it may extend into the deeper layers of the dermis. The calcium is present as irregular granules and globules. Occasionally, the calcium globules lie in nests, and nuclei are still recognizable

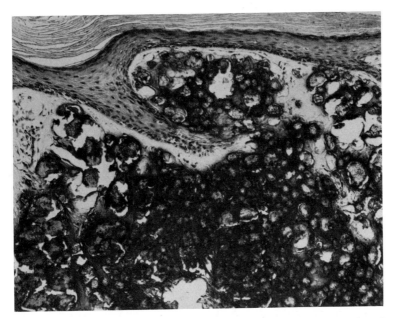

FIG. 22-9. **Subepidermal calcified nodule.** Granules and globules of calcium are located beneath the epidermis. There is some tendency to nesting of the globules of calcium, suggesting that the calcification occurred in nevus cell nests. (×200)

within the calcified material (Woods and Kellaway). Macrophages and foreign-body giant cells may be seen arranged around the larger deposits (Fig. 22-9). The epidermis often is hypertrophic. Calcium granules may be seen within the epidermis (Duperrat and Goetschel).

Histogenesis. It is impossible to state with certainty which structures have undergone calcification. Winer believes that the tumor is a calcified hamartoma of sweat duct origin. This view is supported by Shmunes and Wood on the basis that in syringoma calcific deposits are commonly encountered within the lumen of the ductal structures; but Shmunes and Wood admit that they could not identify a pre-existing epithelial structure in the two nodules examined by them. Steigleder and Elschner believe that in their cases the calcification arose in the nevus cells of a nevus. The development from a nevus appears quite likely because of the nest-like arrangement of the calcium globules near the epidermis.

GOUT

In the early stage of gout there usually are irregularly recurring attacks of acute arthritis. In the late stage deposits of monosodium urate form within and around various joints, leading to chronic arthritis with destruction in the joints and the adjoining bone. During this late stage urate deposits, called tophi, may occur in the subcutaneous tissue, most commonly on the helix of the ears, in the bursae of the elbows, and on the fingers and toes (Sorensen). They may attain a diameter of several centimeters. When large, tophi may discharge a chalky material. In rare instances, intracutaneous tophi are seen as firm yellowish nodules, usually only 3 to 5 mm in size (Gottron and Korting).

Histopathology. For the histologic examination of tophi, fixation in alcohol is preferable to fixation in formalin, because formalin destroys the characteristic urate crystals and merely leaves amorphous material (Lichtenstein et al.).

On fixation in alcohol tophi are seen to consist of variously sized, sharply demarcated aggregates of needle-shaped urate crystals lying closely packed in the form of bundles or sheaves. The crystals often have a brownish color and are doubly refractile on polariscopic examination. The aggregates of urate crystals are surrounded by a granulomatous infiltrate containing many foreign-

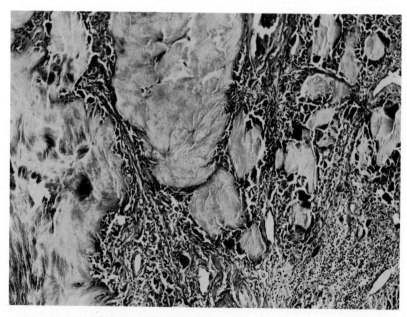

Fig. 22-10. **Gout.** Deposits of urate are surrounded by a foreign-body giant cell reaction. On the left the urate is present as needle-shaped crystals. (×100)

body giant cells (Gottron and Korting). As a secondary phenomenon, calcification may take place in the sodium urate aggregates.

Even when the specimen has been fixed in formalin, the diagnosis of gout can be made without difficulty because of the characteristic rim of foreign-body giant cells and macrophages surrounding the aggregates of amorphous material (Fig. 22-10).

Histogenesis. Gout, a dominantly inherited disorder, is characterized by hyperuricemia. An asymptomatic stage of hyperuricemia precedes the development of gouty arthritis by many years. The hyperuricemia in some patients is the result of a diminished renal excretion of uric acid, whereas in others it is the result of an excessive production of uric acid through an increased synthesis of purines (Sorensen). According to Pagliari and Goodman, about half of the patients with gout show a significant elevation of the plasma glutamate level, indicative of an overproduction of purines. Seegmiller et al. believe that most patients with gout have both an excessive synthesis of uric acid and a decreased renal excretion of uric acid.

OCHRONOSIS

In ochronosis, over the course of many years, homogentisic acid accumulates in many tissues, especially in the cartilage of the joints, of the ears, and of the nose, in ligaments and tendons, and in the sclerae. This results in osteoarthritis, in blackening of cartilages, ligaments, and tendons, and in patchy pigmentation of the sclerae. Occasionally, homogentisic acid accumulates also in the dermis, causing patchy brownish pigmentation of the skin.

Histopathology. The ochronotic pigment, as present in the dermis, is of a light-brown color. It does not stain with silver nitrate as melanin does, but it becomes black when stained with cresyl violet or methylene blue (Laymon). The skin may show ochronotic pigment as fine granules in the endothelial cells of blood vessels, in the basement membrane and the secretory cells of sweat glands, and within scattered macrophages (Lichtenstein and Kaplan). In rare instances only, the ochronotic pigment is found within collagen bundles, causing homogenization and swelling of the affected collagen bundles. Some collagen bundles assume a bizarre shape (Fig. 22-11) (Friderich and Nikolowski; Laymon). In addition, ochronotic pigment can be found within elastic fibers (Bazex and Dupré), and also as irregular, homogeneous, light-brown clumps free in the tissue (Teller and Winkler). There may be scattered multinucleated giant cells showing ochronotic pigment in their cytoplasm (Teller and Winkler).

Histogenesis. In ochronosis, because of an inborn lack of homogentisic acid oxidase, the two amino acids tyrosine and phenylalanine cannot be catabolized beyond homogentisic acid. Most of the homogentisic acid is excreted in the urine. The urine on standing, or after the addition of

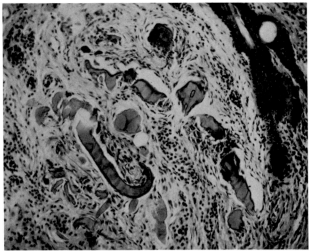

Fig. 22-11. **Ochronosis.** The ochronotic pigment is present within homogenized and swollen collagen bundles, most of which appear broken up. It is present also free in the tissue as irregularly shaped clumps. (×160) (Friderich, H., and Nikolowski, W.: Endogene Ochronose. Arch. f. Derm. u. Syph., *192*: 273, Figure 7, 1951)

sodium hydroxide, turns black (alkaptonuria), since homogentisic acid through oxidation and polymerization is converted into a dark-colored insoluble product. Some of the homogentisic acid gradually accumulates in certain tissues. It is bound irreversibly to collagen fibers as a polymer, after oxidation to benzoquinoneacetic acid (Zannoni et al.).

On electron microscopic examination electron-dense deposits of ochronotic pigment can be seen in some areas within individual collagen fibrils. In most areas, however, the ochronotic pigment lies as irregular aggregates measuring up to 700 nm in diameter throughout areas of degenerating collagen fibrils that no longer show any periodicity (Teller and Winkler; Kutty et al.). Aggregates up to 1 μm in diameter are found within elastic fibers (Teller and Winkler). In addition, large homogeneous electron-dense plaques, measuring up to 100 μm in diameter, lie free in the tissue, partially surrounded by long processes of macrophages. Ochronotic pigment is seen also within macrophages (Teller and Winkler).

MYXEDEMA

Three types of myxedema occur: generalized myxedema, pretibial myxedema, and lichen myxedematosus. Generalized myxedema is a manifestation of hypothyroidism. Pretibial myxedema usually is associated with thyrotoxicosis but occasionally occurs in nonthyrotoxic thyroid disease. In nearly all cases of pretibial myxedema the presence of an immunoglobulin of the IgG class called LATS (long-acting thyroid stimulator) can be demonstrated in the blood serum. Lichen myxedematosus is not associated with any disturbance of thyroid function; but it also is regularly associated with the presence of an abnormal IgG type of immunoglobulin that is very basic and has light chains only of one type, usually of the lambda or L type.

The mucin present in the dermis in these three diseases represents an increase of the mucin that is normally present in the ground substance of the dermis. The mucin consists of proteins bound to hyaluronic acid, an acid mucopolysaccharide (Johnson and Helwig). As a result of the great water-binding capacity of hyaluronic acid, the mucin contains a considerable amount of water. This water is largely removed during the process of dehy-

dration of the specimen; consequently, in routine sections the mucin because of its marked shrinkage appears largely as threads and granules.

The mucin present in the three types of myxedema stains a light blue in sections stained with hematoxylin and eosin. It stains with colloidal iron. It is alcian-blue-positive at pH 2.5 but negative at pH 0.4, and shows metachromasia with toluidine blue at pH 3.0 but absence of metachromasia below pH 2.0. It is PAS-negative (indicating the absence of neutral mucopolysaccharides), and aldehyde-fuchsin-negative (indicating the absence of sulfated acid mucopolysaccharides). The mucin is completely removed on incubation of histologic sections with testicular hyaluronidase for one hour at 37°C. (Johnson and Helwig).

GENERALIZED MYXEDEMA

Clinically, the entire skin appears swollen, dry, pale, and waxy. It is firm to the touch. In spite of its edematous appearance, the skin does not pit on pressure. There often is a characteristic facial appearance: The nose is broad, the lips are swollen, and the eyelids are puffy.

Histopathology. Usually, routinely stained sections show no abnormality, except in severe cases, in which one may observe swelling of the collagen bundles with splitting up of the bundles into individual fibers and some bluish threads and granules of mucin (Reuter). However, on using histochemical stains, such as alcian blue or toluidine blue, it is possible in most cases to demonstrate small amounts of mucin. It is found mainly in the vicinity of the blood vessels and hair follicles (Gabrilove and Ludwig).

PRETIBIAL MYXEDEMA

Usually, the lesions are limited to the anterior aspects of the legs, but they may extend to the dorsa of the feet. They consist of raised, nodular, yellow waxy plaques with prominent hair follicles.

Histopathology. Mucin in large amounts is present in the dermis, particularly in the middle and lower thirds of the dermis. As a result of this, the dermis is greatly thickened.

FIG. 22-12. **Pretibial myxedema.** Considerable amounts of mucin are present, especially in the middle portion of the dermis, separating the collagen bundles as well as individual collagen fibers. The empty spaces are caused by shrinkage of the mucin during the process of fixation and dehydration. (×200)

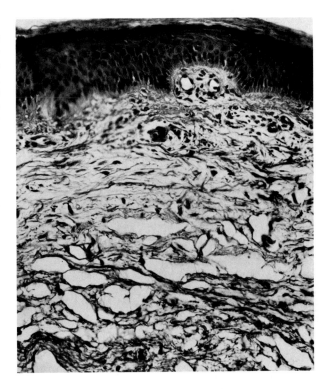

The mucin occurs not only as individual threads and granules but also as extensive deposits causing wide separation of the collagen fibers (Fig. 22-12). The number of fibroblasts is not increased as a rule, but some of them show in areas where there is much mucin a stellate shape (Cawley et al.; Wodniansky).

Histogenesis. On electron microscopic examination two types of cells can be recognized: stellate mucoblasts and fibroblasts (Korting et al.). The mucoblasts have numerous long, branching and intertwining processes. The cisternae of their rough endoplasmic reticulum are greatly dilated and filled with granular material. The entire cell is surrounded by the same granular material. No filaments are formed by these cells. The fibroblasts also appear as actively synthesizing cells; they contain and are surrounded by filamentous material.

Pretibial myxedema usually occurs in association with thyrotoxicosis and not infrequently becomes more pronounced after treatment of the thyrotoxicosis. It nearly always occurs in association with exophthalmos. Rarely, pretibial myxedema, with or without exophthalmos, occurs in nonthyrotoxic thyroid disease, such as chronic lymphocytic thyroiditis, with the patient being either euthyroid or hypothyroid (Lynch et al.).

Of interest is the almost invariable presence of LATS (long-acting thyroid stimulator) in the serum of patients with pretibial myxedema. However, LATS is found in about 80 per cent of patients having thyrotoxicosis without pretibial myxedema and thus it cannot be regarded as the cause of pretibial myxedema (Schermer et al.). It appears likely that the IgG LATS represents an autoantibody that is produced by lymphocytes in thyroid disease, especially in thyrotoxicosis, and is a reflection of, rather than a cause for, the underlying disease (Lynch et al.).

LICHEN MYXEDEMATOSUS

Lichen myxedematosus, or papular mucinosis, is characterized by a more or less extensive eruption of asymptomatic soft papules, usually 2 to 3 mm in diameter, which, though densely grouped, do not coalesce. The face and arms are most commonly affected.

A variant of lichen myxedematosus is *scleromyxedema,* in which one observes, in addition to a generalized eruption of papules as in lichen myxedematosus, diffuse thickening of the skin associated with erythema. There is marked accentuation of the skin folds, particularly on the face. In contrast with scleroderma, the thickened skin is freely movable.

Histopathology. In lichen myxedematosus fairly large amounts of mucin are present (Fig. 22-13). In contrast with pretibial myxedema, however, the mucinous infiltration is found only in circumscribed areas, is most pronounced in the upper dermis, and is associated with an increase in fibroblasts and collagen (Dalton and Seidell; Tappeiner). The collagen bundles may show a rather irregular arrangement.

SCLEROMYXEDEMA. The histologic picture found in the papules resembles that seen in lichen myxedematosus. In the diffusely thickened skin one finds extensive proliferation of fibroblasts throughout the dermis associated with irregularly arranged bundles of collagen. In many areas the collagen bundles are split up into individual fibers by mucin. As a rule, the amount of mucin is greater in the upper half than in the lower

half of the dermis (Rudner et al.). Histochemical examination reveals the acid mucopolysaccharides present in the mucin to be hyaluronic acid, since they are hyaluronidase-labile, alcian-blue-positive at pH 2.5 but negative at pH 0.4, and metachromatic with toluidine blue at pH 3.0 (Feldman et al.).

Autopsy examination of patients with scleromyxedema so far has not shown any mucinous deposits in any internal organs (Montgomery and Underwood; Rudner et al.; Braun-Falco and Weidner). In one patient the autopsy was thought to reveal the coexistence of scleromyxedema and multiple myeloma (Proppe et al.) (see below, under Histogenesis).

Histogenesis. Electron microscopic examination of scleromyxedema reveals an increase in the number of fibroblasts. They show considerable activity, as indicated by the presence of a markedly dilated rough endoplasmic reticulum and long cytoplasmic processes. These fibroblasts produce both collagen and ground substance. The presence of many collagen fibrils with re-

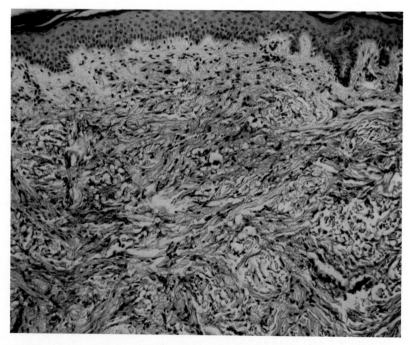

FIG. 22-13. **Lichen myxodematosus (scleromyxedema).** In addition to fairly large amounts of mucin there is extensive proliferation of fibroblasts associated with irregularly arranged bundles of collagen. (×100)

duced diameter, similar to scleroderma, indicates that it is young collagen. In many areas one observes rather small bundles of young collagen fibrils, with each fibril richly coated with ground substance (Hardmeyer and Vogel, 1970, I and II).

The abnormal IgG that is regularly present in the serum of patients with lichen myxedematosus and scleromyxedema is a very basic protein and in most instances migrates more slowly than gamma globulin on electrophoresis. In instances in which it migrates with the same speed as gamma globulin immunoelectrophoresis is required for its recognition (Piper et al.). The IgG of lichen myxedematosus differs from the IgG of multiple myeloma not only by usually showing slower electrophoretic migration but also by the fact that its IgG. molecules nearly always possess light chains of the lambda type, since in only one instance the light chains were of the kappa type (Lai A Fat et al.). In contrast, in multiple myeloma with elevated values for IgG only about one third of the reported cases with IgG molecules have lambda light chains and the other two thirds have kappa light chains (James et al.). In addition to this abnormal IgG, most cases of lichen myxedematosus show a hyperplasia of plasma cells in the bone marrow (Perry et al.; Piper et al.; Feldman et al.; Braun-Falco and Weidner) which are the source of the abnormal IgG. In regard to the patient reported by Proppe et al. as having multiple myeloma in association with scleromyxedema, it is unlikely that this patient had multiple myeloma, since the autopsy revealed no atypical plasma cells in the bone marrow (Braun-Falco and Weidner).

The role of the abnormal IgG in lichen myxedematosus is still not clarified. Since this IgG has been demonstrated to be present in the dermal mucin by direct immunofluorescence (McCarthy et al.), it has been speculated that it might stimulate fibroblasts to increased activity (Piper et al.); but it seems more likely that it represents an autoantibody and, like the IgG LATS in pretibial myxedema, is a consequence rather than the cause of lichen myxedematosus (Lawrence et al.).

SCLEREDEMA (BUSCHKE)

Scleredema, often also called scleredema adultorum even though it may occur in children (Greenberg et al.), is characterized by diffuse nonpitting swelling and induration of the skin. Its cause is unknown, but it is noteworthy that frequently it follows an infectious disease such as influenza or tonsillitis. Usually, it begins on the face and extends from there to the neck and upper trunk. In about three quarters of the patients complete resolution takes place within a few months, whereas in the remaining fourth the disease may persist for many years and may be present even after forty years (Fleischmajer et al.). Although visceral lesions may occur, only one instance of death from scleredema has been recorded (see below).

Diabetes is commonly associated with persistent scleredema and in most of these instances the diabetes is quite resistant to antidiabetic therapy (Fleischmajer et al.; Cohn et al.). It has been suggested that the association of persistent scleredema with maturity-onset diabetes be recognized as a special form of scleredema (Krakowski et al.).

Histopathology. The dermis is about three times thicker than normal. The collagen bundles are thickened and separated by clear spaces, resulting in "fenestration" of the collagen. The secretory coils of the sweat glands, surrounded by fat tissue, are located in the upper or middermis, rather than, as normally, in the lower dermis or at the junction of the dermis with the subcutaneous fat. Since the distance between the epidermis and the sweat glands is unchanged, it can be concluded that in scleredema much of the subcutaneous fat has been replaced by dense collagenous bundles (Fleischmajer et al.). No increase in the number of fibroblasts is noted in association with the hyperplasia of the collagen.

In most instances, especially in early cases, histochemical staining reveals the presence of hyaluronic acid between the bundles of collagen, particularly in the areas of fenestration. The hyaluronic acid, an acid mucopolysaccharide, can best be demonstrated with the colloidal iron stain (Cohn et al.). Staining with toluidine blue usually reveals metachromasia which is most evident at pH 7.0, weaker at pH 5.0, and absent at pH 1.5, indicating the presence of only nonsulfated acid mucopolysaccharides (Holubar and Mach). Similarly, staining with alcian blue usually is positive at pH 4.0, is either weakly positive or negative at pH 2.5, and is negative at pH 0.5 (Cohn et al.). Digestion with hyaluronidase removes the material that stains metachromatically with toluidine blue (Holubar and Mach).

In some instances staining with toluidine blue at pH 7.0 is more intense if unfixed cryostat sections are used in place of formalin-fixed material (Niebauer and Ebner). However, in some cases even frozen sections fail to stain with alcian blue or toluidine blue (Curtis and Shulak). It may be postulated that in cases of long standing in which the disease has reached a steady stage of collagen turnover staining for hyaluronic acid may give negative results (Fleischmajer et al.).

SYSTEMIC LESIONS. Occasionally, the tongue and skeletal muscle are involved; and on histologic examination the muscle bundles show edema and loss of striation (Reichenberger). In a few cases pleural and pericardial effusions were present (Vallee; Curtis and Shulak). In one such case the disease terminated in death, and autopsy revealed in addition to pleural and pericardial effusions, diffuse edema of the heart, the liver, and the spleen (Leinwand).

Differential Diagnosis. It can be difficult to differentiate between scleroderma and scleredema. As a rule, however, in scleroderma the collagen in the subcutaneous tissue appears homogenized and hyalinized and stains only lightly with eosin and with Masson's trichrome stain, whereas in scleredema the collagen bundles in the subcutaneous tissue are thickened without being hyalinized and stain normally with eosin and the trichrome stain (Fleischmajer and Perlish) (see p. 440).

HURLER'S AND HUNTER'S SYNDROMES

Of the six genetic mucopolysaccharidoses (MPS) two show on histologic examination characteristic cutaneous changes. They are MPS I, or Hurler's syndrome; and MPS II, or Hunter's syndrome. Both are lysosomal deficiency diseases in which heparitin sulfate and chondroitin sulfate B are not adequately degraded (see below, under Histogenesis).

Hurler's syndrome and Hunter's syndrome have in common coarse facial features with hirsutism, dwarfism, skeletal deformities, hepatosplenomegaly, and progressive mental deterioration with premature death from cardiorespiratory complications. Hurler's syndrome, the more severe of the two diseases,

is inherited as an autosomal recessive and has as additional features corneal clouding and a lumbar gibbus, with death usually occurring before the age of 10. Hunter's syndrome, inherited as an X-linked recessive, runs a milder course, so that some patients survive until adult life (Gerich).

Histopathology. Biopsy specimens of the skin, irrespective of the area from which the biopsy was obtained, show, on staining with Giemsa's stain, bluish fibrillar mucinous material between the collagen bundles, and bluish granules within the cytoplasm of some of the fibroblasts (Levin). Staining with toluidine blue reveals the material between the collagen bundles and within fibroblasts to be metachromatic (Hambrick and Scheie).

In the epidermis some of the basal cells and squamous cells show diffuse vacuolization, while others show a large perinuclear vacuole, or the nucleus appears displaced to the margin of the cell by a large vacuole (Hambrick and Scheie). Generally, the number of vacuolated cells in the epidermis does not exceed 20 per cent of the epidermal cells (Belcher, 1970, II). Similarly vacuolated cells as seen in the epidermis are found also in the outer root sheath of hair follicles (Hambrick and Scheie), and also in some of the secretory and ductal cells of eccrine glands (Belcher, 1973). The vacuoles in the epithelial cells contain, like the fibroblasts, metachromatic mucinous material demonstrable with Giemsa's stain or toluidine blue.

Histogenesis. Both Hurler's and Hunter's syndrome are caused by the absence of a lysosomal enzyme, namely alpha-L-iduronidase. Consequently, there is a reduced degradation of the two acid mucopolysaccharides heparitin sulfate ("heparan sulfate") and chondroitin sulfate B ("dermatan sulfate") (Bach et al.). This results in the intracellular lysosomal storage of these two substances. In addition, these two substances accumulate extracellularly in certain tissues and also are excreted in the urine in excessive amounts (Dekaban and Patton). Intracellularly, the two mucopolysaccharides are present as metachromatic granules in the cytoplasm of circulating lymphocytes, a fact that often facilitates the diagnosis of Hurler's or Hunter's syndrome (McKusick et al.). By staining for acid phosphatase activity and by electron microscopy these metachromatic granules have been identified as lysosomes containing acid mucopolysaccharides which the lysosomes are unable to degrade (Belcher, 1972, I). Also, deposition of gangliosides occurs in the brain as a result of a deficiency of the lysosomal enzyme betagalactosidase, leading to mental deterioration through degeneration and loss of neurons (McKusick).

Electron microscopic examination of the skin reveals within the fibroblasts large numbers of greatly dilated lysosomes. Most of these lysosomes have a clear content, but some contain lamellar inclusions, representing residual bodies (DeCloux and Friederici). In addition, from 5 to 20 per cent of the epidermal cells contain lysosomal vacuoles with acid phosphatase activity varying from a solitary vacuole to 20 or 30 vacuoles per cell. Also, gangliosides are found as laminated membranous structures ("zebra bodies") in Schwann cells and Merkel cells of the skin (Belcher, 1972, II).

ACANTHOSIS NIGRICANS

Four types of acanthosis nigricans exist: the malignant, the inherited, the endocrine, and the idiopathic type (Brown and Winkelmann). The malignant type differs from the three benign types by showing more extensive and more pronounced lesions as a rule. The histologic picture is essentially the same in all four types.

The *malignant* type is associated with a malignant tumor, usually an adenocarcinoma (Curth et al.). However, in rare instances it may be a lymphoma, such as Hodgkin's disease (Ackerman and Lantis), or an osteogenic sarcoma (Garrott). The *inherited* type may have its onset during infancy, childhood or adult life. The *endocrine* type is associated most commonly with a pituitary tumor, usually manifesting itself as acromegaly. In other instances the endocrine disorder consists of diabetes, Addison's disease, or the Stein-Leventhal syndrome. Obesity may or may not be present in the endocrine type (Brown and Winkelmann; Hollingsworth and Amatruda). In the *idiopathic* type, the most common type, there is no associated malignancy, endocrine disorder or genetic predisposition. Obesity is often present but without clear-cut evidence for its being of endocrine genesis (Hollingsworth and Amatruda).

Clinically, all four types of acanthosis nigricans present papillomatous brownish patches, predominantly in the intertriginous areas such as the axillae, the neck, and the genital and the submammary regions.

Histopathology. Histologic examination reveals a moderate degree of hyperkeratosis and papillomatosis (Fig. 22-14). Slight and irregular acanthosis is present in most instances, whereas hyperpigmentation usually

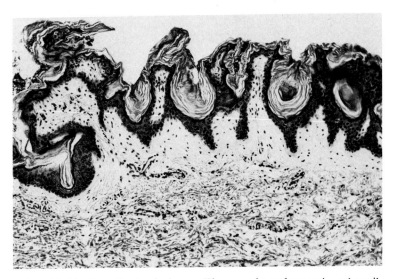

Fig. 22-14. **Acanthosis nigricans.** There are hyperkeratosis and papillomatosis. Several papillae project upward as fingerlike projections. As is usually the case, acanthosis and hyperpigmentation are slight. (×100)

is absent. Thus, the term acanthosis nigricans has little histologic justification.

In a typical lesion the papillae project upward as fingerlike projections. The valleys between the papillae show mild to moderate acanthosis and are filled with keratotic material. On the other hand, the stratum malpighii at the tips of the papillae, and often also on the sides of the protruding papillae, appears thinned. The rete ridges as a rule are poorly developed.

Slight hyperpigmentation of the basal layer is demonstrable with silver nitrate staining in some cases but not in others (Brown and Winkelmann). The brownish color of the lesions thus is caused by hyperkeratosis, rather than by melanin.

Differential Diagnosis. Differentiation of acanthosis nigricans from other benign papillomas often is impossible, particularly from epidermal nevi and from the hyperkeratotic type of seborrheic keratosis. As a rule, however, epidermal nevi show more marked acanthosis than acanthosis nigricans and often considerable elongation of the rete ridges.

CONFLUENT AND RETICULATED PAPILLOMATOSIS

This disorder, originally described by Gougerot and Carteaud, probably represents a variant of acanthosis nigricans, either of the inherited or of the idiopathic type (Kesten and James).

The lesions in confluent and reticulated papillomatosis consist of slightly hyperkeratotic, pigmented papules in a reticulated arrangement. The lesions occur largely in the sternal, epigastric and interscapular regions. Thus, the eruption differs from acanthosis nigricans mainly by its location and by its reticulated appearance.

Histopathology. Mild hyperkeratosis and papillomatosis are present, as well as focal acanthosis limited largely to the valleys between elongated papillae (Kesten and James). Some lesions also show hyperpigmentation (Baden). Thus, the histologic changes are similar to, but milder than those of acanthosis nigricans.

IDIOPATHIC HEMOCHROMATOSIS

In idiopathic hemochromatosis large amounts of iron are deposited in various organs of the body, especially in the parenchymal cells of the liver and the pancreas and in the myocardial fibers. The classical tetrad of idiopathic hemochromatosis consists of hepatic cirrhosis, diabetes, hyperpigmentation of the skin, and cardiac failure.

Pigmentation of the skin is present in about 90 per cent of the patients with idiopathic hemochromatosis at the time the diagnosis is made (Cawley et al.). The pigmentation is most pronounced in exposed areas, especially on the face. Its color usually is brown or bronze but it may be bluish. The pigmentation is caused by melanin and not by iron.

Histopathology. Histologic examination of pigmented skin shows melanin to be present in increased amounts in the basal layer of the epidermis and occasionally also within melanophages in the upper dermis. Hemosiderin can be demonstrated in the skin of most cases with the aid of an iron stain, such as Perls' stain. It is found as blue-staining granules mainly around blood vessels, both extracellularly and within macrophages, and in the basement membrane of the sweat glands (Perdrup and Poulsen). In addition, some iron may be present in the epidermis, particularly in the basal cell layer, and in the epithelial cells of the sweat glands (Weintraub et al.).

In selecting a site for biopsy it is not necessary to choose a pigmented area, because if deposits of iron are present in the skin, they are not limited to the areas of pigmentation. It is important, however, not to take a specimen from the legs, where deposits of iron are frequently found in association with even minor venous stasis or as a consequence of a preceding inflammation that may no longer be evident.

A skin biopsy no longer represents the most important test for establishing the diagnosis of idiopathic hemochromatosis; it is merely of confirmatory value. Determination of the quantity of serum iron and of the degree of saturation of the serum transferrin has replaced the skin biopsy in importance (Finch and Finch).

Liver biopsies are of value in determining the quantity of iron present, the degree of fibrosis, and the distribution of the iron. Presence of iron predominantly in the parenchymal cells is found both in idiopathic hemochromatosis and in alcoholic cirrhosis, whereas in cases of iron overload most of the iron is in the Kupffer cells. In deciding between idiopathic hemochromatosis and alcoholic cirrhosis the rule holds: If the iron deposition is mild in comparison with the fibrotic changes, alcoholic cirrhosis is more likely; but if the deposition of iron is out of proportion to the degree of fibrosis, idiopathic hemochromatosis is probable. If both are advanced, on a statistical basis, secondary hemochromatosis developing in the course of cirrhosis is more likely than idiopathic hemochromatosis, since the latter is much rarer than the former (Kent and Popper).

Histogenesis. The general view is that idiopathic hemochromatosis is an inborn error of metabolism in which there is, as shown by Heilmeyer through the oral administration of radioactive iron, an increased rate of intestinal absorption of iron. Through this increased rate of absorption the iron-binding capacity of transferrin is almost completely saturated in idiopathic hemochromatosis. Consequently, not all of the iron passing from the intestinal tract can be bound to transferrin, and iron is deposited in a variety of organs (Heilmeyer). Iron accumulates particularly in the parenchyma of the liver and the pancreas, and in the myocardium; and, by damaging the cells in which it accumulates, it causes hepatic cirrhosis, diabetes, and cardiac insufficiency.

As has been pointed out in describing the findings in liver biopsies, a histologic differentiation between idiopathic hemochromatosis and secondary hemochromatosis developing in alcoholic cirrhosis may be impossible. However, the view held by MacDonald that idiopathic hemochromatosis does not exist as an entity has not found many adherents. MacDonald believes that all cases regarded as idiopathic hemochromatosis in reality are instances of hepatic cirrhosis with excessive iron intake and that the iron deposits as such do not damage tissue. There are, however, too many cases on record in which idiopathic hemochromatosis has caused death in young adults who had no history of alcohol intake or iron overloading (Charlton et al.). Also, as proof that idiopathic hemochromatosis is a genetically determined disease, Sinniah was able to show

that the mean serum iron level and the degree of plasma transferrin saturation are higher in family members related by blood to patients with idiopathic hemochromatosis than they are in normal control persons and in family members not related by blood to the patients. Is is likely, as Scheinberg believes, that idiopathic hemochromatosis develops in individuals who are homozygous for a pair of abnormal autosomal genes, whereas the much more common secondary hemochromatosis develops in heterozygous carriers of one such abnormal gene whose livers have been damaged exogenously, generally by alcohol.

Two observations prove that the cutaneous pigmentation in idiopathic hemochromatosis is due solely to melanin and not to hemosiderin. The first observation concerned a patient who, in addition to idiopathic hemochromatosis, had vitiligo. The areas of vitiligo were fully depigmented in spite of the fact that on histologic examination they contained just as much iron as the deeply pigmented areas (Perdrup and Poulsen). The second observation was made in a Negro patient with idiopathic hemochromatosis who had three epidermal cysts. Although no change in skin color had been noted by the patient he had observed progressive darkening of the cysts; and histologic examination revealed considerable amounts of melanin both in the wall of the cysts and in their keratinous center (Leyden et al.).

The increase in the amount of melanin in the skin in patients with hemochromatosis is brought about by the presence of iron in the skin. The iron stimulates melanocytic activity either by increasing oxidative processes (Robert and Zürcher) or by reacting with epidermal sulfhydryl groups and reducing their inhibitory effect on the enzyme system governing melanin synthesis (Buckley). (See also under argyria, p. 244.)

VITAMIN A DEFICIENCY (PHRYNODERMA)

Deficiency of vitamin A is very rare in the United States and occurs mainly in Asia and Africa. It produces cutaneous changes to which the name *phrynoderma* has been given. These changes consist of dryness and roughness of the skin and the presence of follicular hyperkeratosis. In addition to cutaneous changes, deficiency of vitamin A may cause night blindness, xerophthalmia, and keratomalacia.

Histopathology. The skin shows moderate hyperkeratosis with marked distention of the upper part of the hair follicles by large horny plugs (Fasal). The sebaceous gland lobules are greatly reduced in size. In addition, one may find evidence of atrophy of the sweat glands, such as flattening of the secretory cells (Frazier and Hu). In severe cases the sweat glands may undergo keratinizing metaplasia (Bessey and Wolbach).

Differential Diagnosis. Histologic differentiation of phrynoderma from dominant ichthyosis vulgaris and keratosis pilaris is impossible, except in very severe cases of phrynoderma, in which the sweat glands and the sebaceous glands show keratinizing metaplasia. Pityriasis rubra pilaris differs from phrynoderma by showing, in addition to hyperkeratosis and follicular plugging, spotted parakeratosis, irregular acanthosis, and an inflammatory infiltrate in the upper dermis.

PELLAGRA

Pellagra is caused by a deficiency of nicotinic acid (niacin) or its precursor, the essential amino acid tryptophan. As a dietary deficiency disease it may occur in chronic alcoholics. In addition, it may occur in patients with the carcinoid syndrome, since the tumor cells divert tryptophan towards serotonin, thus depressing the endogenous niacin production (Castiello and Lynch) (see p. 568). In regard to the association of pellagra with Hartnup's disease, see below.

Besides cutaneous lesions, pellagra usually presents also a stomatitis associated with a red, swollen and painful tongue. In addition, gastrointestinal symptoms and mental changes may be present, resulting in the triad of the three D's: dermatitis, diarrhea, and dementia.

The cutaneous lesions are precipitated by damage to the skin, either through sunburn in the exposed areas, or through maceration and friction in intertriginous areas (Harber and Baer). Thus, the dorsa of the hands, wrists and forearms, the face, the nape of the neck, and the inguinal region are predominantly involved. In the early stage there is erythema, which usually is sharply demarcated; in severe cases it may be accompanied by vesicles. Later, the skin becomes thickened, scaling and pigmented.

Histopathology. The histologic changes of the skin are nonspecific. Early lesions present a chronic inflammatory infiltrate in the upper dermis. Vesicles, if present, are usually located at the dermal-epidermal junction (Moore et al.).

In older lesions one observes hyperkeratosis with areas of parakeratosis. The amount of melanin in the basal layer of the epidermis is increased. The dermis may show fibrosis, in addition to chronic inflammation (Moore et al.).

HARTNUP DISEASE

This recessively inherited disease first manifests itself in early childhood and often improves with advancing age. A photosensitivity eruption is present that usually is indistinguishable from pellagra (Halvorsen and Halvorsen; Kimmig). In other cases the cutaneous reaction to sun exposure resembles poikiloderma atrophicans vasculare (Clodi et al.) or, because of the prominence of vesicles, hydroa vacciniforme (Ashurst). In addition, there may be cerebellar ataxia and mental retardation.

Histopathology. The cutaneous eruption in Hartnup disease shows the same histologic changes as pellagra (see above). In patients with poikilodermalike changes one observes flattening of the epidermis and presence of a chronic inflammatory infiltrate and of melanophages in the upper dermis (Clodi et al.).

Histogenesis. The sun sensitivity eruption with its resemblance to pellagra is caused by a defect in the transport of tryptophan and the resultant decrease in the endogenous production of niacin. The defect in tryptophan transport consists of both an intestinal defect in tryptophan absorption and a renal tubular defect resulting in inadequate reabsorption of amino acids, including tryptophan. Thus, chromatographic study of the urine shows a constant aminoaciduria. Fecal amino acids, particularly tryptophan and tyrosine, also are increased (Halvorsen and Halvorsen; Clodi et al.; Ashurst; Barrett-Connor).

BIBLIOGRAPHY

Amyloidosis

Anekoji, K., and Irisawa, K.: Five cases of lichen amyloidosus. Arch. Derm., *84*:759, 1961.

Binkely, G. W.: Primary systemic amyloidosis. Arch. Derm. Syph., *37*:330, 1938.

Black, M. M., and Wilson Jones, E.: Macular amyloidosis. Brit. J. Derm., *84*:199, 1971.

Brandt, K., Cathcart, E. S., and Cohen, A. S.: A clinical analysis of the course and prognosis of forty-two patients with amyloidosis. Am. J. Med., *44*:955, 1968.

Brownstein, M. H., and Hashimoto, K.: Macular amyloidosis. Arch. Derm., *106*:50, 1972.

Brownstein, M. H., and Helwig, E. B.: Systemic amyloidosis complicating dermatoses. Arch. Derm., *102*:1, 1970 (I).

————: The cutaneous amyloidoses. I. Localized forms. Arch. Derm., *102*:8, 1970 (II).

————: The cutaneous amyloidoses. II. Systemic forms. Arch. Derm., *102*:20, 1970 (III).

Brunsting, L. A., and MacDonald, I. D.: Primary systemic amyloidosis with macroglossia: a syndrome related to Bence Jones proteinuria and myeloma. J. Invest. Derm., *8*:145, 1947.

Cathcart, E. S., Ritchie, R. F., Cohen, A. S., and Brandt, K.: Immunoglobulins and amyloidosis. Am. J. Med., *52*:93, 1972.

Dostrovsky, A., and Sagher, F.: Localized amyloidosis of the skin. Arch. Derm. Syph., *44*:891, 1941.

Ebner, H.: Licht- und elektronenmikroskopische Untersuchungen über das Amyloid der Haut. Z. Haut, *43*:833, 1968.

Eisen, H. N.: Primary systemic amyloidosis. Am. J. Med., *1*:144, 1946.

Gafni, I., Merker, H., and Heller, H.: On the origin of amyloid. Ann. Int. Med., *65*:1031, 1966.

Glenner, G. G., Ein, D., Eanes, E. D., et al.: Creation of "amyloid" fibrils from Bence Jones proteins in vitro. Science, *174*:712, 1971 (I).

Glenner, G. G., Ein, D., and Terry, W. D.: The immunoglobulin, origin of amyloid. Am. J. Med., *52*:141, 1972.

Glenner, G. G., Terry, W. D., Harada, M., *et al.*: Amyloid fibril proteins: proof of homology with immunoglobulin light chains by sequence analyses. Science, *172*:1150, 1971 (II).

Goodman, T. F., Jr., Abele, D. C., and West, C. S., Jr.: Electron microscopy in the diagnosis of amyloidosis. Arch. Derm., *106*:393, 1972 (review).

Hashimoto, K., Gross, B. G., and Lever, W. F.: Lichen amyloidosus. Histochemical and electron microscopic studies. J. Invest. Derm., *45*:204, 1965.

Hashimoto, K., and Onn, L. L. Y.: Lichen amyloidosus. Electron microscopic study of a typical case and a review. Arch. Derm., *104*:648, 1971.

Herrmann, W. P., Gartmann, H., and Zach, J.: Systematisierte Paramyloidose der Haut bei sog. Bence-Jones-Plasmocytom. Hautarzt, *19*:357, 1968.

Janigan, D. T.: Experimental amyloidosis. Am. J. Path., *47*:159, 1965.

Kurban, A. K., Malak, J. A., Afifi, A. K., and Mire, J.: Primary localized macular cutaneous amyloidosis: histochemistry and electron microscopy. Brit. J. Derm., *85*:52, 1971.

Lindemayr, W., and Partsch, H.: Plattenartiginfiltrierte lokalisierte Hautamyloidose. Hautarzt, *21*:104, 1970.

Mawas, C., Sors, C., and Bernier, J. J.: Amyloidosis associated with primary agammaglobulinemia, severe diarrhea, and familial hypogammaglobulinemia. Am. J. Med., *46*:624, 1969.

Miescher, G.: Beitrag zur Klinik der Paramyloidose (Pseudomyxoedema paramyloidosum). Dermatologica, *91*:177, 1945.

Natelson, E. A., Duncan, W. C., Macossay, C. R., and Fred, H. L.: Amyloidosis palpebrarum. Arch. Int. Med., *125*:304, 1970.

Osserman, E. F., Takatsuki, K., and Talal, N.: The pathogenesis of amyloidosis. Seminars Hemat., *1*:1, 1964.

Pearson, B., Rice, M. M., and Dickens, K. LaV.: Primary systemic amyloidosis. Arch. Path., *32*:1, 1941.

Piérard, J., and Kint, A.: Amyloide. Arch. belg. derm. syph., *27*:153, 1971.

Potter, B. S., and Johnson, W. C.: Primary localized amyloidosis cutis. Arch. Derm., *103*:448, 1971.

Puchtler, H., Sweat, F., and Levine, M.: On the binding of Congo red by amyloid. J. Histochem. Cytochem., *10*:355, 1962.

Rodermund, O. E.: Zur Amyloidosis cutis nodularis atrophicans (Gottron 1950). Arch. klin. exp. Derm., *230*:153, 1967.

Rodermund, O. E., and Klingmüller, G.: Zur submikroskopischen Struktur des Amyloid. Arch. klin. exp. Derm., *236*:147, 1970.

Rukawina, J. G., Block, W. D., Jackson, C. E., *et al.*: Primary systemic amyloidosis. Medicine, *35*:239, 1956 (review).

Shanon, J., and Sagher, F.: Interscapular cutaneous amyloidosis. Arch. Derm., *102*:195, 1970.

Shapiro, L., Kurban, A. K., and Azar, H. A.: Lichen amyloidosus. A histochemical and electron microscopic study. Arch. Path., *90*:499, 1970.

Weitzner, S., Keen, P. E., and Doughty, W. E.: Primary localized amyloidosis of glans penis. Arch. Derm., *102*:463, 1970.

Westermark, P.: Skin involvement in secondary amyloidosis. Acta path. microbiol. scand., *79A*:79, 1971.

Westermark, P., and Stenkvist, B.: A new method for the diagnosis of systemic amyloidosis. Arch. Int. Med., *132*:522, 1973.

Colloid Milium

Agius, J. R. G.: Colloid pseudomilium. Brit. J. Derm., *75*:55, 1963.

Bienvenu, L., and Lever, W. F.: Colloid degeneration (colloid milium) of the skin. Arch. Derm., *78*:115, 1958.

Brownstein, M. H., and Helwig, E. B.: The cutaneous amyloidoses. I. Localized forms. Arch. Derm., *102*:8, 1970.

Graham, J. H., and Marques, A. S.: Colloid milium: a histochemical study. J. Invest. Derm., *49*:497, 1967.

Hashimoto, K., Miller, F., and Bereston, E. S.: Colloid milium. Histochemical and electron microscopic studies. Arch. Derm., *105*:684, 1972.

Miedzinski, F., Kozakiewicz, J., and Szarmach, H.: Zur Klinik des Pseudomilium colloidale. Derm. Wschr., *142*:927, 1960.

Percival, B. H., and Duthie, D. A.: Notes on a case of colloid pseudomilium. Brit. J. Derm., *60*:399, 1948.

Puchtler, H., Sweat, F., and Levine, M.: On the binding of Congo red by amyloid. J. Histochem. Cytochem., *10*:355, 1962.

Reuter, M. J., and Becker, S. W.: Colloid degeneration (collagen degeneration) of the skin. Arch. Derm. Syph., *46*:695, 1942.

Sullivan, M., and Ellis, F. A.: Facial colloid degeneration in plaques. Arch. Derm., *84*:816, 1961.

Woolridge, W. E., and Frerichs, J. B.: Amyloidosis; a new clinical type. Arch. Derm., *82*:230, 1960.

Hyalinosis Cutis et Mucosae

Caplan, R. M.: Visceral involvement in lipoid proteinosis. Arch. Derm., *95*:149, 1967.

Eberhartinger, C., and Niebauer, G.: Beitrag zur Kenntis der Lipoidproteinose Urbach-Wiethe. Hautarzt, *10*:54, 1959.

Fleischmajer, R., Nedwich, A., and Ramos e Silva, J.: Hyalinosis cutis et mucosae. J. Invest. Derm., *52*:495, 1969.

Grosfeld, J. C. M., Spaas, J., van de Staak, W. J. B. M., and Stadhouders, A. M.: Hyalinosis cutis et mucosae. Dermatologica, *130*:239, 1965.

Hashimoto, K., Klingmüller, G., and Rodermund, O. E.: Hyalinosis cutis at mucosae. Acta dermatoven., *52*:179, 1972.

Holtz, K. H.: Über Gehirn- und Augenveränderungen bei Hyalinosis cutis et mucosae (Lipoidproteinose) mit Autopsiebefund. Arch. klin. exp. Derm., *214*:289, 1962.

Holtz, K. H., and Schulze, W.: Beitrag zur Klinik und Pathogenese der Hyalinosis cutis et mucosae (Lipoid-Proteinose Urbach-Wiethe). Arch. f. Derm. u. Syph., *192*:206, 1950.

Kint, A.: A comparative electron microscopic study of the perivascular hyaline from porphyria cutanea tarda and from lipoid proteinosis. Arch. klin. exp. Derm., *239*:203, 1970.

Laymon, C. W., and Hill, E. M.: An appraisal of hyalinosis cutis et mucosae. Arch. Derm., *75*:55, 1957.

McCusker, J. J., and Caplan, R. M.: Lipoid proteinosis (lipoglycoproteinosis). Am. J. Path., *40*:599, 1962.

Ramos e Silva, S.: Lipoid proteinosis. Arch. Derm. Syph., *47*:30, 1943.

Rasiewicz, W., Rubisz-Brzezineka, J., and Konecki, J.: Hyalinosis cutis et mucosae Urbach-Wiethe. Dermatologica, *130*:145, 1965.

Rodermund, O. E., and Klingmüller, G.: Elektronenmikroskopische Befunde des Hyalins bei Hyalinosis cutis et mucosae. Arch. klin. exp. Derm., *236*:238, 1970.

Ungar, H., and Katzenellenbogen, I.: Hyalinosis of skin and mucous membranes. Arch. Path., *63*:65, 1957.

Van der Walt, J. J., and Heyl, T.: Lipoid proteinosis and erythropoietic protoporphyria. Arch. Derm., *104*:501, 1971.

Wood, M. G., Urbach, F., and Beerman, H.: Histochemical study of a case of lipoid proteinosis. J. Invest. Derm., *26*:263, 1956.

Porphyria

Anton-Lamprecht, I., and Meyer, B.: Zur Ultrastruktur der Haut bei Protoporphyria. Dermatologica, *141*:76, 1970.

Baxter, D. L., and Permowicz, S. E.: Variegate porphyria (mixed porphyria). Arch. Derm., *96*:98, 1967.

Bhutani, L. K., Sood, S. K., Das, P. K., et al.: Congenital erythropoietic porphyria. Arch. Derm., *110*:427, 1974.

Charles, R. C., Beidler, J. G., and Johnson, B. L.: Erythropoietic protoporphyria. Arch. Path., *97*:79, 1974.

Cripps, D. J., and MacEachern, W. N.: Hepatic and erythropoietic protoporphyria. Arch. Path., *91*:497, 1971.

Donaldson, E. M., McCall, A. J., Magnus, I. A., et al.: Erythropoietic protoporphyria: two deaths from hepatic cirrhosis. Brit. J. Derm., *84*:14, 1971.

Ennerböck, L., and Lundvall, O.: Properties and distribution of liver fluorescence in porphyria cutanea tarda (PCT). Virchows Archiv (Abt. A., Path. Anat.), *350*:293, 1970.

Epstein, J. H., Tuffanelli, D. L., and Epstein, W. L.: Cutaneous changes in the porphyrias. Arch. Derm., *107*:689, 1973.

Feldaker, M., Montgomery, H., and Brunsting, L. A.: Histopathology of porphyria cutanea tarda. J. Invest. Derm., *24*:131, 1955.

Haining, R. G., Cowger, M. L., Shurtleff, D. B., and Labbe, R. F.: Congenital erythropoietic porphyria. Am. J. Med., *45*:624, 1968.

Horkay, J., Balogh, E., and Vitalis, S.: Protoporphia erythropoietica. Z. Haut, *43*:639, 1968.

Kint, A.: A comparative electron microscopic study of the perivascular hyaline from porphyria cutanea tarda and from lipoid proteinosis. Arch. klin. exp. Derm., *239*:203, 1970.

Kint, A., Gheorghin, G., and de Bersaques, J.: Étude comparative au microscope électronique de la substance hyaline dans divers types de porphyrie. Arch. belg. derm. syph., *27*:31, 1971.

Meyer, U. A., Strand, L. J., Doss, M., et al.: Intermittent acute porphyria—demonstration of a genetic defect in porphobilinogen metabolism. New Eng. J. Med., *286*:1277, 1972.

Rimington, C., Magnus, J. A., Ryan, E. A., and Cripps, D. J.: Porphyria and photosensitivity. Quart. J. Med., *36*:29, 1967.

Romeo, G., and Levin, E. Y.: Uroporphyrinogen III cosynthetase in human congenital erythropoietic porphyria. Proc. Nat. Acad. Sci., *63*:856, 1969.

Ryan, E. A., and Madill, G. T.: Electron microscopy of the skin in erythropoietic protoporphyria. Brit. J. Derm., *80*:561, 1968.

Sauer, G. F., and Funk, D. D.: Iron overload in cutaneous porphyria. Arch. Int. Med., *124*:190, 1969.

Suurmond, D.: Erythropoietic protoporphyria. Dermatologica, *131*:276, 1965.

Suurmond, D., van Steveninck, J., and Went, L. N.: Some clinical and fundamental aspects of erythropoietic protoporphyria. Brit. J. Derm., *82*:323, 1970.

Calcinosis Cutis

Carr, R. D., Heisel, E. B., and Stevenson, T. D.: CRST syndrome. Arch. Derm., *92*:519, 1965.

Cornelius, C. E., Tenenhouse, A., and Weber, J. C.: Calcinosis cutis. Arch. Derm., *98*:219, 1968.

Duperrat, B., and Goetschel, G.: Calcification nodulaire solitaire congénitale de la peau (Winer, 1952). Ann. derm. syph., *90*:283, 1963.

Eisenberg, E., and Bartholow, P. V., Jr.: Reversible calcinosis cutis. New Eng. J. Med., *268*:1216, 1963.

Haim, S., and Friedman-Birnbaum, R.: Two cases of circumscribed calcinosis. Dermatologica, *143*:111, 1971.

Kabir, D. J., and Malkinson, F. D.: Lupus erythematosus and calcinosis cutis. Arch. Derm., *100*:17, 1969.

Katz, A. I., Hampers, C. L., and Merrill, J. P.: Secondary hyperparathyroidism and renal osteodystrophy in chronic renal failure. Medicine, *48*:333, 1969 (review).

Kolten, B., and Pedersen, J.: Calcinosis cutis and renal failure. Arch. Derm., *110*:256, 1974.

Mozaffarian, G., Lafferty, F. W., and Pearson, O. H.: Treatment of tumoral calcinosis with phosphorus deprivation. Ann. Int. Med., *77*:741, 1972.

Mulligan, R. M.: Metastatic calcification. Arch. Path., *43*:177, 1947.

Paegle, R. D.: Ultrastructure of mineral deposits in calcinosis cutis. Arch. Path., *82*:474, 1966.

Posey, R. E., and Ritchie, E. B.: Metastatic calcinosis cutis with renal hyperparathyroidism. Arch. Derm., *95*:505, 1967.

Putkonen, T., and Wangel, G. A.: Renal hyperparathyroidism with metastatic calcification of the skin. Dermatologica, *118*:127, 1959.

Reich, H.: Das Teutschlaender-Syndrom. Hautarzt, *14*:462, 1963.

Shapiro, L., Platt, N., and Torres-Rodriguez, V. M.: Idiopathic calcinosis of the scrotum. Arch. Derm., *102*:199, 1970.

Shmunes, E., and Wood, M. G.: Subepidermal calcified nodules. Arch. Derm., *105*:593, 1972.

Steigleder, G. K., and Elschner, H.: Lokalisierte Calcinosis. Hautarzt, *8*:127, 1957.

Wermer, P., Kuschner, M., and Riley, E. A.: Reversible metastatic calcification associated with excessive milk and alkali intake. Am. J. Med., *14*:108, 1953.

Wheeler, C. E., Curtis, A. C., Cawley, E. P., et al.: Soft tissue calcification with special reference to its occurrence in the collagen diseases. Ann. Int. Med., *36*:1050, 1952.

Whiting, D. A., Simson, I. W., Kallmeyer, J. C., and Dannheimer, I. P. L.: Unusual cutaneous lesions in tumoral calcinosis. Arch. Derm., *102*:465, 1970.

Wilson, C. W., Wingfield, W. L., and Toone, E. C., Jr.: Vitamin D poisoning with metastatic calcification. Am. J. Med., *14*:116, 1953.

Winer, L. H.: Solitary congenital nodular calcification of the skin. Arch. Derm. Syph., *66*: 204, 1952.

Winkelmann, R. K., and Keating, F. R., Jr.: Cutaneous vascular calcification, gangrene and hyperparathyroidism. Brit. J. Derm., *83*:263, 1970.

Woods, B., and Kellaway, T. D.: Cutaneous calculi. Brit. J. Derm., *75*:1, 1963.

Gout

Gottron, H. A., and Korting, G. W.: Chronische Hautgicht. Arch. klin. exp. Derm., *204*:483, 1957.

Lichtenstein, L., Scott, H. W., and Levin, M. H.: Pathologic changes in gout. Am. J. Path., *32*: 871, 1956.

Pagliara, A. S., and Goodman, A. D.: Elevation of plasma glutamate in gout. New Eng. J. Med., *281*:767, 1969.

Seegmiller, J. E., Laster, L., and Howell, R. R.: Biochemistry of uric acid and its relation to gout. New Eng. J. Med., *268*:712, 764 and 821, 1963.

Sorensen, L. B.: The pathogenesis of gout. Arch. Int. Med., *109*:379, 1962.

Ochronosis

Bazex, A., and Dupré, A.: L'ochronose est-elle une maladie du tissu conjuctif? Ann. derm. syph., *89*:7, 1962.

Friderich, H., and Nikolowski, W.: Endogene Ochronose. Arch. f. Derm. u. Syph., *192*: 273, 1951.

Kutty, M. K., Igbal, Q. M., and Teh, E. C.: Ochronotic arthropathy. Arch. Path., *98*:55, 1974.

Laymon, C. W.: Ochronosis. Arch. Derm., *67*: 553, 1953.

Lichtenstein, L., and Kaplan, L.: Hereditary ochronosis. Am. J. Path., *30*:99, 1954.

Teller, H., and Winkler, K.: Zur Klinik und Histopathologie der endogenen Ochronose. Hautarzt, *24*:537, 1973.

Zannoni, V. G., Malawista, S. E., and La Du, B. N.: Studies on ochronosis. II. Studies on benzoquinone-acetic acid, a probable intermediate in the connective tissue pigmentation of alcaptonuria. Arthritis Rheum., *5*:547, 1962.

Myxedema

Braun-Falco, O., and Weidner, F.: Skleromyxödem Arndt-Gottron mit Knochenmarks-Plasmocytose und Myositis. Arch. belg. derm. syph., *26*:193, 1970.

Cawley, E. P., Lupton, C. H., Jr., Wheeler, C. E., and McManus, J. F. A.: Examination of normal and myxedematous skin. Arch. Derm., *76*:537, 1957.

Dalton, J. E., and Seidell, M. A.: Studies on lichen myxedematosus (papular mucinosis). Arch. Derm., *67*:194, 1953.

Feldman, P., Shapiro, L., Pick, A. I., and Slatkin, M. H.: Scleromyxedema. Arch. Derm., *99*:51, 1969.

Gabrilove, J. L., and Ludwig, A. W.: The histogenesis of myxedema. J. Clin. Endocrinol., *17*:925, 1957.

Hardmeier, T., and Vogel, A.: Electronenmikroskopische Befunde beim Skleromyxödem Arndt-Gottron. Arch. klin. exp. Derm., *237*: 722, 1970.

————: Scléromyxoedème avec paraprotéinémie familiale de type gamma-G. Dermatologica, *141*:183, 1970.

James, K., Fudenberg, H., Epstein, W. L., and Shuster, J.: Studies on a unique diagnostic serum globulin in papular mucinosis (lichen myxedematosus). Clin. Exp. Immunol., *2*: 153, 1967.

Johnson, W. C., and Helwig, E. B.: Cutaneous focal mucinosis. Arch. Derm., *93*:13, 1966.

Korting, G. W., Nürnberger, F., and Müller, G.: Zur Ultrastruktur der Bindegewebszellen beim Myxoedema circumscriptum praetibiale. Arch. klin. exp. Derm., *229*:381, 1967.

Lai A Fat, R. F. M., Suurmond, D., Radl, J., and van Furth, R.: Scleromyxedema (lichen myxedematosus) associated with a paraprotein, IgG_1 of the type kappa. Brit. J. Derm., *88*: 107, 1973.

Lawrence, D. A., Tye, M. J., and Liss, M.: Isolation and characterization of the basic, diagnostic IgG globulin in the rare gammopathy, papular mucinosis. Prep. Biochem., *1*:1, 1971.

Lynch, P. J., Maize, J. C., and Lisson, J. C.: Pretibial myxedema and nonthyrotoxic thyroid disease. Arch. Derm., *107*:107, 1973.

McCarthy, J. T., Osserman, E., Lombardo, P. C., and Takatsuki, K.: An abnormal serum globulin in lichen myxedematosus. Arch. Derm., *89*:446, 1964.

Montgomery, H., and Underwood, L. J.: Lichen myxedematosus (differentiation from cutaneous myxedemas or mucoid states). J. Invest. Derm., *20*:213, 1953.

Perry, H. O., Montgomery, H., and Stickney, J. M.: Further observations on lichen myxedematosus. Ann. Int. Med., *53*:955, 1060.

Piper, W., Hardmeier, T., and Schäfer, E.: Das Skleromyxödem Arndt-Gottron: eine paraproteinämische Erkrankung. Schweiz. med. Wschr., *97*:829, 1967.

Proppe, A., Becker, V., and Hardmeier, T.: Skleromyxödem Arndt-Gottron und Plasmocytom. Hautarzt, *20*:53, 1969.

Reuter, M. J.: Histopathology of the skin in myxedema. Arch. Derm. Syph., *24*:55, 1931.

Rudner, E. J., Mehregan, A., and Pinkus, H.: Scleromyxedema. Arch. Derm., *93*:3, 1966.

Schermer, D. R., Roenigk, H. H., Jr., Schumacher, O. P., and McKenzie, J. M.: Relationship of long-acting thyroid stimulator to pretibial myxedema. Arch. Derm., *102*:62, 1970.

Tappeiner, J.: Zur Pathogenese des Lichen myxoedematosus. Arch. klin. exp. Derm., *201*:160, 1955.

Wodniansky, P.: Über die Ätiologie und Pathogenese des Myxoedema circumscriptum praetibiale symmetricum. Arch. klin. exp. Derm., *205*:22, 1957.

Scleredema (Buschke)

Cohn, B. A., Wheeler, C. E., Jr., and Briggaman, R. A.: Scleredema adultorum of Buschke and diabetes mellitus. Arch. Derm., *101*:27, 1970.

Curtis, A. C., and Shulak, B. M.: Scleredema adultorum. Arch. Derm., *92*:526, 1965.

Fleischmajer, R., Faludi, G., and Krol, S.: Scleredema and diabetes mellitus. Arch. Derm., *101*:21, 1970.

Fleischmajer, R., and Perlish, J. S.: Glycosaminoglycans in scleroderma and scleredema. J. Invest. Derm., *58*:129, 1972.

Greenberg, L. M., Geppert, C., Worthen, H. G., and Good, R. A.: Scleredema "adultorum" in children. Pediatrics, *32*:1044, 1963.

Holubar, K., and Mach, K. W.: Scleredema (Buschke). Acta dermatoven., *47*:102, 1967.

Krakowski, A., Covo, J., and Berlin, C.: Diabetic scleredema. Dermatologica, *146*:193, 1973.

Leinwand, I.: Generalized scleredema; report with autopsy findings. Ann. Int. Med., *34*:226, 1951.

Niebauer, G., and Ebner, H.: Skleroedema (Buschke). Derm. Monatsschr., *156*:940, 1970.

Reichenberger, M.: Betrachtungen zum Skleroedema adultorum Buschke. Hautarzt, *15*:339, 1964.

Vallee, B. L.: Scleredema: a systemic disease. New Eng. J. Med., *235*:207, 1946.

Hurler's and Hunter's Syndromes

Bach, G., Friedman, R., Weissmann, B., and Neufeld, E. F.: The defect in the Hurler and Scheie syndromes: deficiency of alpha-L-iduronidase. Proc. Nat. Acad. Sci., *69*:2048, 1972.

Belcher, R. W.: Ultrastructure and cytochemistry of lymphocytes in the genetic mucopolysaccharidoses. Arch. Path., *93*:1, 1972 (I).

———: Ultrastructure of the skin in the genetic mucopolysaccharidoses. Arch. Path., *94*:511, 1972 (II).

———: Ultrastructure and function of eccrine glands in the mucopolysaccharidoses. Arch. Path., *96*:339, 1973.

DeCloux, R. J., and Friederici, H. H. R.: Ultrastructural studies of the skin in Hurler's syndrome. Arch. Path., *88*:350, 1969.

Dekaban, A. S., and Patton, V. M.: Hurler's and Sanfilippo's variants of mucopolysaccharidoses. Arch. Path., *91*:434, 1971.

Gerich, J. E.: Hunter's syndrome: beta-galactosidase deficiency in skin. New Eng. J. Med., *280*:799, 1969.

Hambrick, G. W., Jr., and Scheie, H. G.: Studies of the skin in Hurler's syndrome. Arch. Derm., *85*:455, 1962.

Levin, S.: A specific skin lesion in gargoylism. Am. J. Dis. Child., *99*:444, 1960.

McKusick, V. A.: The nosology of the mucopolysaccharidoses. Am. J. Med., *47*:730, 1969.

McKusick, V. A., Kaplan, D., Wise, D., *et al.*: The genetic mucopolysaccharidoses. Medicine, *44*:445, 1965.

Acanthosis Nigricans, Confluent and Reticulated Papillomatosis

Ackerman, A. B., and Lantis, L. R.: Acanthosis nigricans associated with Hodgkin's disease. Arch. Derm., *95*:202, 1967.

Baden, H. F.: Familial cutaneous papillomatosis. Arch. Derm., *92*:394, 1965.

Brown, J., and Winkelmann, R. K.: Acanthosis nigricans: a study of 90 cases. Medicine, *47*:33, 1968 (review).

Curth, H. O., Hilberg, A. W., and Machacek, G. F.: The site and histology of the cancer associated with malignant acanthosis nigricans. Cancer, *15*:364, 1962.

Garrott, T. C.: Malignant acanthosis nigricans associated with osteogenic sarcoma. Arch. Derm., *106*:384, 1972.

Hollingsworth, D. R., and Amatruda, T. T., Jr.: Acanthosis nigricans and obesity. An endocrine abnormality? Arch. Int. Med., *124*:481, 1969.

Kesten, B. M., and James, H. D.: Pseudoatrophoderma colli, acanthosis nigricans, and confluent and reticular papillomatosis. Arch. Derm., *75*:525, 1957.

Idiopathic Hemochromatosis

Buckley, W. R.: Localized argyria. Arch. Derm., *88*:531, 1963.

Cawley, E. P., Hsu, Y. T., Wood, B. T., and Weary, P. E.: Hemochromatosis of the skin. Arch. Derm., *100*:1, 1969.

Charlton, R. W., Abrahams, C., and Bothwell, T. H.: Idiopathic hemochromatosis in young subjects. Arch. Path., *83*:132, 1967.

Finch, S. C., and Finch, C. A.: Idiopathic hemochromatosis, an iron storage disease. Medicine, *34*:381, 1955.

Heilmeyer, L.: Pathogenesis of hemochromatosis. Medicine, *46*:209, 1967 (review).

Kent, G., and Popper, H.: Liver biopsy in diagnosis of hemochromatosis. Am. J. Med., *44*: 837, 1968.

Leyden, J. L., Lockshin, N. A., and Kriebel, S.: The black keratinous cyst. A sign of hemochromatosis. Arch. Derm., *106*:379, 1972.

MacDonald, R. A.: Tissue iron and hemochromatosis. Arch. Path., *84*:543, 1967.

Perdrup, A., and Poulsen, H.: Hemochromatosis and vitiligo. Arch. Derm., *90*:34, 1964.

Robert, P., and Zürcher, H.: Pigmentstudien. I. Mitteilung. Über den Einfluss von Schwermetallverbindungen, Hämin, Vitaminen, mikrobiellen Toxinen, Hormonen und weiteren Stoffen auf die Dopamelaninbildung in vitro und die Pigmentbildung in vivo. Dermatologica, *100*:217, 1950.

Scheinberg, I. H.: The genetics of hemochromatosis. Arch. Int. Med., *132*:126, 1973.

Sinniah, R.: Environmental and genetic factors in idiopathic hemochromatosis. Arch. Int. Med., *124*:455, 1969.

Weintraub, L. R., Demis, D. J., Conrad, M. E., and Crosby, W. H.: Iron excretion by the skin. Selective localization of iron[59] in epithelial cells. Am. J. Path., *46*:121, 1965.

Vitamin A Deficiency

Bessey, O. A., and Wolbach, S. B.: Vitamin A, physiology and pathology. J.A.M.A., *110*: 2072, 1938.

Fasal, P.: Clinical manifestations of vitamin deficiencies as observed in the Federated Malay States. Arch. Derm. Syph., *50*:160, 1944.

Frazier, C. N., and Hu, C.: Nature and distribution according to age of cutaneous manifestations of vitamin A deficiency. Arch. Derm. Syph., *33*:825, 1936.

Pellagra, Hartnup Disease

Ashurst, P. J.: Hydroa vacciniforme occurring in association with Hartnup disease. Brit. J. Derm., *81*:486, 1969.

Barrett-Connor, E.: The etiology of pellagra and its significance for modern medicine. Am. J. Med., *42*:859, 1967.

Castiello, R. J., and Lynch, P. J.: Pellagra and the carcinoid syndrome. Arch. Derm., *105*: 574, 1972.

Clodi, P. H., Deutsch, E., and Niebauer, G.: Krankheitsbild mit poikilodermieartigen Hautveränderungen, Aminoacidurie und Indolaceturie. Arch. klin. exp. Derm., *218*:165, 1964.

Halvorsen, L., and Halvorsen, S.: Hartnup disease. Pediatrics, *31*:29, 1963.

Harber, L. C., and Baer, R. L.: Pathogenic mechanisms of drug-induced photosensitivity. J. Invest. Derm., *58*:327, 1972.

Kimmig, J.: Stoffwechselstörungen bei polymorphen Lichtdermatosen und neuere Untersuchungsergebnisse im Zusammenhang mit dem Hartnup-Syndrom. Arch. klin. exp. Derm., *219*:753, 1964.

Moore, R. A., Spies, T. D., and Cooper, Z. K.: Histopathology of the skin in pellagra. Arch. Derm. Syph., *46*:100, 1942.

23

Pigmentary Disorders

ADDISON'S DISEASE

Addison's disease, caused by a hypofunction of the adrenal cortex, is characterized by weakness, hypotension, and hyperpigmentation of the skin and oral mucosa.

The hyperpigmentation is most pronounced in areas of the skin exposed to the sun, at sites of pressure, and on the genitalia. Pigmentation of the oral mucosa usually is patchy.

Histopathology. The histologic picture is not diagnostic. The hyperpigmentation is the result of an increased activity of the melanocytes, without an increase in their number (Szabo). Increased amounts of melanin are present in the epidermis and often also in the upper dermis. In the epidermis the melanin is present chiefly in the basal cells, but it may be found also in the upper layers of the stratum malpighii. In the upper dermis a moderate number of melanin-laden macrophages (melanophages) may be present (Montgomery and O'Leary).

Histogenesis. The blood plasma shows decreased levels of cortisol and increased levels of corticotropin (ACTH). In addition, the concentration of serum sodium is decreased, and that of serum potassium is increased. In early cases, a subnormal increment in the plasma cortisol level following the injection of ACTH establishes the diagnosis.

The hyperpigmentation of Addison's disease is caused by increased concentrations of beta-MSH (melanocyte-stimulating hormone) in the serum. The overproduction of the beta-MSH in Addison's disease is due to a common mechanism controlling the synthesis and release of ACTH and beta-MSH (Abe et al.). The reason for the increased output of ACTH by the pituitary gland lies in the fact that in Addison's disease the damaged adrenal glands respond weakly to the stimulation by ACTH; and, as a compensatory phenomenon, the pituitary gland increases its output of ACTH.

Differential Diagnosis. A diagnosis of Addison's disease cannot be made from histologic sections, because the same histologic picture is observed in nonspecific hyperpigmentation of the skin and in individuals with naturally dark skin.

ALBINISM

Albinism, also referred to as oculocutaneous albinism, shows a generalized lack of pigmentation of the skin and the hair since birth. In addition, the eyes show lack of pigmentation of their fundi, translucent irides, and nystagmus. It is recessively inherited. In rare instances, oculocutaneous albinism is associated with congenital deafness (Ziprkowski and Adam).

There are two types of albinism: a "tyrosinase-positive" type in which the melanocytes are dopa-positive in vitro, and a "tyrosinase-negative" type. The two types are easily distinguished by incubating plucked hair bulbs in a solution of tyrosine or dopa. In the "tyrosinase-positive" type the hair bulbs will darken on incubation (Kugelman and Van Scott). In the other type the melanocytes are dopa-negative in vitro as well as in vivo (Witkop et al.; Jung and Anton-Lamprecht). Patients with in vitro dopa-positive melanocytes in the course of their lives acquire a slight capacity for pigmentation in vivo, whereas patients with in vitro dopa-negative melanocytes fail to form pigment throughout their lives (Jung and Anton-Lamprecht).

Histopathology. Histologic examination shows in albinism basal "clear cells" to be present; but silver stains fail to show any melanin. In patients with the dopa-positive type of albinism the melanocytes will form pigment if sections of skin are incubated in solutions of either tyrosine or dopa (Kugelman and Van Scott); whereas in patients with the dopa-negative type of albinism the melanocytes will not form pigment.

Histogenesis. Electron microscopic examination reveals in albinism normally structured melanocytes in which the melanosomes appear normal except that they show no evidence of melanization. The Langerhans cells also appear normal (Mishima).

Jung and Anton-Lamprecht were able to demonstrate that in a patient with "tyrosinase-negative" albinism the melanocytes can be stimulated in vivo by ultraviolet light in every way except melanin production. After daily ultraviolet irradiation for four weeks, electron microscopic examination revealed an increase in the number of melanocytes in the epidermis and evidence of stimulation within individual melanocytes. The melanocytes showed an increase in the various types of organelles, including an increase in the number of melanin-free melanosomes. Some melanin-free melanosomes were seen within keratinocytes as a result of pigment transfer.

The failure of the melanosomes in albinism to form melanin in vivo may be due either to the presence of an endogenous tissue inhibitor of tyrosinase, or to a membrane defect of the melanosomes (Kugelman and Van Scott).

PIEBALDISM
(PATTERNED LEUKODERMA)

In this autosomally dominant disorder one finds irregularly shaped areas without pigmentation that are present since birth and usually are associated with a white forelock. The cutaneous areas lacking in pigmentation have a predilection for the ventral skin, i.e., the center of the face, the ventral chest, and the abdomen. Formerly called partial albinism, this term is no longer used because of the difference in pathogenesis between oculocutaneous albinism and piebaldism.

A variant of piebaldism is the *Waardenburg syndrome,* also dominantly inherited, in which one observes a white forelock, lateral displacement of the inner canthi of the eyes, heterochromia of the irides, and congenital deafness (Reed et al.).

Histopathology. The areas without pigmentation show absence of melanin. Suprabasal clear cells, however, can be recognized (Comings and Odland).

Histogenesis. Electron microscopic examination, according to Comings and Odland, reveals in skin lacking pigmentation absence of melanocytes, while Langerhans cells are present. Thus, the findings are like those in vitiligo (see p. 421) and differ from those in oculocutaneous albinism.

The electron microscopic findings obtained by Breathnach et al. from the skin of the scalp within the region of the white forelock were like those obtained by Comings and Odland. On the other hand, the nonpigmented skin of the forearm showed some melanocytes; but their melanosomes were either nonmelanized or only partially melanized, and some were morphologically abnormal. Grupper et al. found in the nonpigmented areas of his case the melanocytes to be absent, as described by Comings and Odland; whereas in areas of pigmented skin located near nonpigmented areas they observed defective melanocytes resembling those described by Breathnach et al. These melanocytes contained small and irregularly outlined melanosomes.

VITILIGO

Vitiligo represents an acquired patchy loss of pigment of the skin. The patches are sharply though irregularly demarcated and often are surrounded by hyperpigmented skin. The areas may slowly increase in size. The scalp hair and eyelashes are only rarely affected.

In the *Vogt-Koyanagi syndrome* patches of vitiligo involving the skin and frequently also the eyelashes and scalp hair are found in association with uveitis, and often also with dysacousia and alopecia areata (Johnson).

Histopathology. The essential process in vitiligo is a destruction of melanocytes. When using silver staining or the dopa reaction long-standing lesions of vitiligo show no melanocytes. In early lesions appearing hypopigmented rather than completely depigmented a few dopa-positive melanocytes and some melanin granules in the basal layer are still present (Birbeck et al.). At the border of the patches of vitiligo the melanocytes often appear large and possess long dendritic processes filled with melanin granules.

Histogenesis. Electron microscopic studies have confirmed the absence of melanocytes in areas of long-standing vitiligo (Birbeck et al.; Zelickson and Mottaz). In regard to the Langerhans cells, it was thought at first that their concentration in the epidermis was increased in areas of vitiligo, although there were some discrepancies in the reported findings. Thus, increases in the concentration of Langerhans cells were observed with the gold chloride technic by Birbeck et al., with the adenosine triphosphatase method by Riley, and with the electron microscope by Birbeck et al., by Zelickson and Mottaz, and by Mishima and Kawasaki. However, in contrast with Birbeck et al. and with Mishima and Kawasaki who saw an increase only in the basal Langerhans cells, Riley found the increase to be among the suprabasal Langerhans cells. In a thorough evaluation of the role of the Langerhans cell in vitiligo Brown et al. used adenosine triphosphatase activity for the demonstration of Langerhans cells and compared in epidermal sheets their concentration in vitiliginous skin with that in nonvitiliginous skin from the same anatomic region. They found no increase in the concentration of Langerhans cells in areas of vitiligo. Brown et al. point out not only that the concentration of Langerhans cells varies greatly in different anatomic regions but also that in regions of thin epidermis Langerhans cells frequently occupy a position close to or even on the basement membrane in both normal and vitiliginous skin.

CHEDIAK-HIGASHI SYNDROME

Chediak-Higashi syndrome, a recessively inherited disease characterized by defective giant lysosomes in the granulocytes and monocytes, leads to death usually before the age of 10 through severe viral and bacterial infections.

The skin of patients with this syndrome is very fair and the eyes show translucency of the irides with nystagmus, causing a considerable clinical resemblance to oculocutaneous albinism.

Histopathology. The epidermis shows, even in sections stained with hematoxylin and eosin but better still in sections stained with silver, sparse, irregularly shaped, large melanin granules scattered through its lower portion (Moran and Estevez). The same type of large, irregularly shaped melanin granules is seen scattered through the upper dermis within melanophages (Bedoya). Similarly, the hairs contain large, clumped, sparse melanin granules.

Blood smears reveal, on staining with Wright's or Giemsa's stain, in the neutrophils and monocytes numerous coarse granules, representing giant lysosomes (Moran and Estevez).

Histogenesis. Electron microscopic examination reveals within melanocytes giant particles arising from defective melanosomes either through fusion or through continued growth of melanosomes. The giant melanosomes thus formed ultimately degenerate. In addition, normal melanosomes are present in the melanocytes and are transferred to keratinocytes, but there they are packaged into abnormally large phagolysosomes (Zelickson et al.). Similar abnormally large membrane-bound phagolysosomes are found in the hair (Blume and Wolff). It is likely that the giant melanosomes in melanocytes and the giant phagolysosomes in keratinocytes form because of a defect in their membranes (Zelickson et al.). The hypopigmentation is caused by the fact that within keratinocytes the melanosomes, rather than being dispersed, lie within relatively few large phagolysosomes.

The giant primary lysosomes present in neutrophils and monocytes also form as a result of a membrane defect. Even though microorganisms are phagocytized in a normal fashion by neutrophils and monocytes, their inactivation is delayed since the giant primary lysosomes because of their membrane defect are unable to discharge their enzymes into the phagocytic vacuoles in a normal manner (Stossel et al.).

BIBLIOGRAPHY

Addison's Disease

Abe, K., Nicholson, W. E., Liddle, G. W., *et al.*: Radioimmunoassay of beta-MSH in human plasma and tissues. J. Clin. Invest., *46*:1609, 1967.

Montgomery, H., and O'Leary, P. A.: Pigmentation of the skin in Addison's disease, acanthosis nigricans and hemochromatosis. Arch. Derm. Syph., *21*:970, 1930.

Szabo, G.: Quantitative histological investigations on the melanocyte system of the human epidermis. *In* Pigment Cell Biology. p. 99. New York, Academic Press, 1959.

Albinism

Jung, E. G., and Anton-Lamprecht, I.: Untersuchungen über Albinismus. Arch. Derm. Forsch., *240*:123, 1971.

Kugelman, T. P., and Van Scott, E. J.: Tyrosinase activity in melanocytes of human albinos. J. Invest. Derm., *37*:73, 1961.

Mishima, Y.: Macromolecular changes in pigmentary disorders. Arch. Derm., *91*:519, 1965.

Witkop, C. J., Jr., White, J., and Nance, W. E.: Heterogeneity in human albinism. J. Invest. Derm., *54*:100, 1970.

Ziprkowski, L., and Adam, A.: Recessive albinism and congenital deaf-mutism. Arch. Derm., *89*:151, 1964.

Piebaldism

Breathnach, A. S., Fitzpatrick, T. B., and Wyllis, L. M. A.: Electron microscopy of melanocytes in human piebaldism. J. Invest. Derm., *45*:28, 1965.

Comings, D. E., and Odland, G. F.: Partial albinism. J.A.M.A., *195*:519, 1966.

Grupper, C., Pruniéras, M., Hincky, M., and Garelly, E.: Albinisme partiel familial (piebaldisme): Étude ultrastructurale. Ann. derm. syph., *97*:267, 1970.

Reed, W. B., Stone, V. M., Boder, E., and Ziprkowski, L.: Pigmentary disorders in association with congenital deafness. Arch. Derm., *95*:167, 1967.

Vitiligo

Birbeck, M. S., Breathnach, A. S., and Everall, J. D.: An electron microscope study of basal melanocytes and high-level clear cells (Langerhans cells) in vitiligo. J. Invest. Derm., *73*:51, 1961.

Brown, J., Winkelmann, R. K., and Wolff, K.: Langerhans cells in vitiligo. J. Invest. Derm., *49*:386, 1967.

Johnson, W. C.: Vogt-Koyanagi-Harada syndrome. Arch. Derm., *88*:146, 1963.

Mishima, Y., and Kawasaki, H.: Dendritic cell dynamics in progressive depigmentation. J. Invest. Derm., *54*:93, 1970.

Riley, R. A.: A study of the distribution of epidermal dendritic cells in pigmented and unpigmented skin. J. Invest. Derm., *48*:28, 1967.

Zelickson, A. S., and Mottaz, J. H.: Epidermal dendritic cells. Arch. Derm., *98*:652, 1968.

Chediak-Higashi Syndrome

Bedoya, V.: Pigmentary changes in Chediak-Higashi syndrome. Brit. J. Derm., *85*:336, 1971.

Blume, R. S., and Wolff, S. M.: The Chediak-Higashi syndrome: Studies in four patients and a review of the literature. Medicine, *51*: 247. 1972 (review).

Moran, T. J., and Estevez, J. M.: Chediak-Higashi disease. Arch. Path., *88*:329, 1969.

Stossel, T. P., Root, R. K., and Vaughan, M.: Phagocytosis in chronic granulomatous disease and the Chediak-Higashi syndrome. New Eng. J. Med., *286*:120, 1972.

Zelickson, A. S., Windhorst, D. B., White, J. G., and Good, R. A.: The Chediak-Higashi syndrome: Formation of giant melanosomes and the basis of hypopigmentation. J. Invest. Derm., *49*:575, 1967.

24

Connective Tissue Diseases

LUPUS ERYTHEMATOSUS

Two types of lupus erythematosus are recognized: discoid lupus erythematosus (DLE) and systemic lupus erythematosus (SLE). In DLE the lesions are limited to the skin, and serologic and hematologic abnormalities are slight. On the other hand, in SLE visceral lesions dominate the clinical picture, and serologic and hematologic abnormalities are pronounced. Although the transition of a well established case of DLE to one of SLE with fatal outcome is rare, such transitions do occur (Scott and Rees; Storck and Berzups). In some instances it is difficult to decide on a clinical basis whether an individual patient has DLE or SLE, and only the further course of the disease will decide the issue (Pohle and Tuffanelli). On a histologic basis, a differentiation between DLE and SLE generally is not possible, since early lesions of DLE resemble those of SLE, and lesions having the histologic appearance of DLE can occur in SLE.

DISCOID LUPUS ERYTHEMATOSUS (DLE)

Characteristically, the cutaneous lesions of DLE consist of well defined, erythematous, slightly infiltrated, "discoid" patches that often show adherent thick scales and follicular plugging. In older lesions one often sees atrophic scarring, associated occasionally with verrucous hyperkeratosis at the periphery of the lesions. On the other hand, involution of the lesions without scarring can occur (Bielicky and Trapl).

In many instances the discoid cutaneous lesions are limited to the face, where the malar areas and the nose are affected predominantly. However, the scalp, the ears, the upper extremities, the chest, the upper back, and the oral mucosa also may be involved. Although discoid cutaneous lesions are typical of DLE they may occur in SLE also (Haim and Shafrir).

A second type of lesion that may be found in DLE, although it is associated more commonly with SLE, consists of erythematous, slightly edematous patches that show little or no scaling and no evidence of atrophy. Usually, they are not sharply demarcated. In rare instances small vesicles may be seen within some of the patches.

Histopathology. In most instances of *discoid lesions* a diagnosis of lupus erythematosus is possible on the basis of a combination of histologic findings. The five important changes in the skin are: (1) hyperkeratosis with keratotic plugging; (2) atrophy of the stratum malpighii; (3) hydropic degeneration of the basal cells; (4) a patchy, chiefly lymphoid cell infiltrate with a tendency to arrangement about the cutaneous appendages (Fig. 24-1); and (5) edema, vasodilatation, and a slight extravasation of erythrocytes in the upper dermis. However, not all five changes are present in every case.

The epidermal changes usually develop after those in the dermis. Therefore, the hyperkeratosis may not be present until after the lesion is several weeks old. Parakeratosis, as a rule, is not conspicuous, and it may be absent. Keratotic plugs are found mainly in the follicular openings, but they may occur also independently of them. The follicles inside the dermis may contain concentric layers of keratin instead of hairs (Fig. 24-1). Focal hydropic degeneration of the basal layer, also referred to as liquefaction degeneration, represents the most significant histologic change in lupus erythematosus (Fig. 24-2). In its absence a histologic diagnosis of lupus erythematosus is difficult and often impossible (see below).

The epidermal changes encountered in discoid lesions vary in different types of lesions so that thinning and flattening of the stratum malpighii do not always predominate. In cases showing clinically verrucous hyperkeratosis the epidermis appears hyperplastic, papillomatous and hyperkeratotic, causing considerable resemblance to a hyperplastic solar keratosis (von Eickstedt and Hassenpflug). In lesions of DLE that clinically do not show adherent scaling or keratotic plugging, the epidermis may show few if any changes and, in particular, may show no hydropic changes in the basal layer (Bielicki and Trapl).

The dermis shows edema in its upper portion. Frequently, small foci of extravasated erythrocytes are seen in the edematous upper dermis. In dark-skinned persons melanin often is seen within melanophages in the upper dermis, since the hydropic degeneration in the basal cells causes them to lose their melanin (pigmentary incontinence). The capillaries and, in the lower dermis, also the larger vessels are dilated, and their walls may show edema; however, proliferative or obliterative changes are absent. Fibrinoid deposits in the dermis are encountered only rarely in discoid lesions, and then in early lesions. (For the description of the fibrinoid changes, see Systemic Lupus Erythematosus,

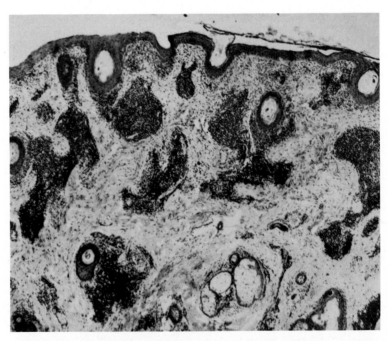

FIG. 24-1. **Discoid lupus erythematosus.** Low magnification. There is keratotic plugging, and the follicles inside the dermis contain, instead of hairs, concentric layers of keratin. The epidermis is atrophic and devoid of rete ridges. The inflammatory infiltrate is patchy and largely located in the vicinity of hair follicles. (×50)

p. 428). The inflammatory infiltrate in the dermis usually is distinctly patchy. In areas such as the face or scalp, where there are many pilosebaceous structures, the infiltrate is located mainly in the vicinity of the hair follicles and the sebaceous glands. Frequently, one can observe hydropic changes in the basal layer of the hair follicles. In the absence of hydropic changes in the epidermis this finding may have considerable diagnostic value. The infiltrate, by impinging upon the pilosebaceous structures, causes their gradual atrophy and disappearance. Not infrequently, the infiltrate extends into the subcutaneous fat (Pascher et al.). The infiltrate in DLE is composed predominantly of lymphoid cells but contains also a small number of plasma cells and histiocytes.

Not infrequently one sees in sections of DLE two types of hyaline or colloid bodies, referred to also as Civatte bodies (Ueki, 1969). They are round to ovoid, have an eosinophilic, homogeneous appearance and measure approximately 10 μm in diameter. One type forms through degeneration of epidermal cells and is present in the lower epidermis or in the papillary dermis. This type of hyaline body occurs also in lichen planus (see p. 149), and occasionally in other diseases with damage to the basal cells. The other type originates from the thickened basement membrane zone and occurs only in the uppermost dermis. It occurs also in dermatomyositis. Both types of hyaline bodies, when located in the dermis, are PAS-positive and diastase-resistant and, on direct immunofluorescent staining, contain immunoglobulins (IgG, IgM, IgA), complement and fibrin (Ueki; Copeman et al.).

Staining with the PAS reaction often shows broadening of the PAS-positive, diastase-resistant subepidermal basement membrane zone. Also the capillary walls show thickening, homogenization, and increase in the intensity of the PAS reaction (Stoughton and Wells; Beljaewa et al.). Thickening of the basement membrane zone is seen often also around hair follicles. However, in areas of pronounced hydropic degeneration of the basal cells the PAS-positive subepidermal

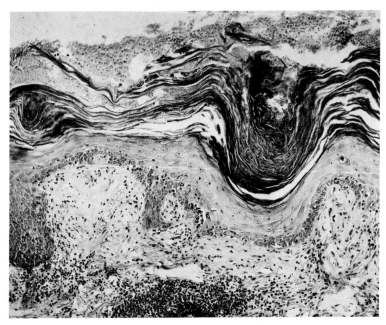

FIG. 24-2. **Discoid lupus erythematosus.** High magnification. There are hyperkeratosis and keratotic plugging, atrophy of the stratum malpighii, hydropic degeneration of the basal layer, edema of the upper dermis, and a patchy infiltrate composed of lymphoid cells. (×100)

basement zone may be fragmented and may even be absent (Ueki, 1968).

The histologic changes in the *erythematous, edematous lesions* differ only in degree from those seen in the discoid lesions. The hydropic degeneration of the basal cell layer, and the edema of the dermis are more pronounced than in the discoid lesions, whereas the hyperkeratosis and the inflammatory infiltrate are less prominent. Occasionally, the edema in the upper dermis and, with it, the hydropic degeneration of the basal cell layer are severe enough to result in the formation of clefts and even vesicles between the epidermis and the dermis (Fig. 24-3). (McCreight and Montgomery). Focal extravasations of erythrocytes are quite common. Also, there may be fibrinoid deposits in the dermis. (For a description of the fibrinoid deposits, see Systemic Lupus Erythematosus.)

Differential Diagnosis. The epidermal changes seen in the discoid lesions of lupus erythematosus must be differentiated from those of lichen planus, since both diseases may show hydropic degeneration of the basal cell layer (see p. 148). Yet, whereas in DLE hydropic degeneration persists, in lichen planus it is followed by a replacement of the basal cells by squamous cells. Also, the triangular elongation of the rete ridges seen as "saw-toothing" in lichen planus is not observed in DLE, in which the epidermis appears flattened, as a rule.

The dermal changes in DLE consisting of a patchy infiltrate must be differentiated from four other diseases in which the dermal infiltrate may also be patchy. The five diseases with a patchy dermal infiltrate (the "five L's" because they all begin with the letter L) are **L**upus erythematosus, lymphocytic **L**ymphoma, pseudo-**L**ymphoma of Spiegler-Fendt, polymorphous **L**ight eruption of the plaque type, and **L**ymphocytic infiltration of the skin of Jessner. Lupus erythematosus can easily be differentiated from the four other diseases if a significant degree of hydropic degeneration of the basal cell layer is present. Since, however, this degeneration is occasionally absent in lupus erythematosus, the following additional points of differentiation may be important.

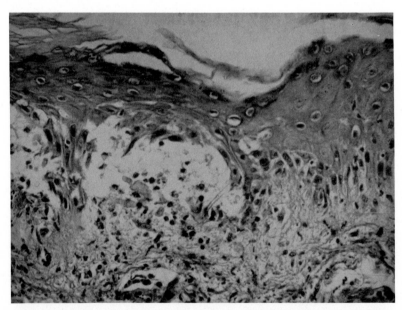

Fig. 24-3. **Discoid lupus erythematosus with erythematous, edematous lesions.** Edema of the upper dermis and pronounced hydropic degeneration of the basal layer have led to the formation of a subepidermal bulla. (×200)

In lymphocytic lymphoma (see p. 690) and in pseudolymphoma of Spiegler-Fendt (see p. 709), the infiltrate shows no tendency to arrangement around pilosebaceous structures. Furthermore, in lymphocytic lymphoma immature lymphocytes often are present and the cells of the infiltrate are more tightly packed than they are in an inflammatory infiltrate, whereas in pseudolymphoma of Spiegler-Fendt there usually are, in addition to lymphocytes, numerous histiocytes, and the infiltrate often is arranged in lymphoid follicles, with the light-staining nuclei of the histiocytes suggesting germinal centers.

In the other two diseases, the plaque type of polymorphous light eruption and Jessner's lymphocytic infiltration of the skin, the dermal infiltrate is indistinguishable from that seen in early, nonscarring lesions of lupus erythematosus. In the plaque type of polymorphous light eruption, which like lupus erythematosus responds well as a rule to therapy with antimalarial drugs of the 4-aminoquinoline group, such as chloroquine, differentiation from DLE is best accomplished by direct immunofluorescent testing of a skin biopsy specimen, since deposits of immunoglobulins and complement usually are found at the epidermal junction in DLE but not in polymorphous light eruption (Pohle and Tuffanelli; Chorzelski et al.) (see p. 432). In addition, phototesting with wave lengths shorter than 320 mn may be carried out, although it is not always reliable, since about one third of the patients with DLE also show a positive phototest (Fisher et al.). Testing for circulating antinuclear antibodies similarly is of limited usefulness: although it is nearly always negative in polymorphous light eruption, it is negative also in almost one half of the patients with DLE (Peterson and Fusaro; Fisher et al.) (see p. 431). For differentiating between DLE and Jessner's lymphocytic infiltration of the skin, see page 435.

SYSTEMIC LUPUS ERYTHEMATOSUS (SLE)

SLE is associated with systemic symptoms and leads to death within ten years in about one half of the patients (Kellum and Haserick; Estes and Christian). The demarcation of SLE from DLE and other connective tissue diseases is not always easy. A diagnosis of SLE is justified, according to Ropes, if a patient has at least three of the following four criteria: (1) a cutaneous eruption consistent with lupus erythematosus, (2) renal involvement, (3) serositis, and (4) joint involvement. Also the diagnosis is justified, according to Ropes, if the first two of these four criteria are present.

Cutaneous lesions often are lacking at first in SLE, and in about 20 per cent of the cases are absent throughout the course of the disease (Dubois and Tuffanelli; Estes and Christian). Usually, the cutaneous eruption consists of erythematous, slightly edematous patches without a significant degree of scaling and without atrophy. Usually, the patches are not sharply demarcated. The most common site of involvement is the malar region, but any area of the skin may be involved, particularly the palms and fingers. Occasionally, the lesions show a petechial, vesicular or ulcerative component. Well defined "discoid" lesions with atrophic scarring, as seen typically in DLE, occur in about 20 per cent of the patients with SLE (Haim and Shafrir). They may precede all other clinical manifestations of SLE and, if they do, are convincing evidence that a case is undergoing transition from DLE to SLE (Scott and Rees).

The visceral manifestations of SLE include arthralgia as the most common symptom. Renal involvement, referred to as lupus nephritis, if severe, may produce a nephrotic syndrome and ultimately uremia (Baldwin). In addition, there often are pleurisy and pericarditis as manifestations of serositis, and seizures and psychoses as evidence of central nervous system involvement. Irregular fever, malaise, and weakness are common. The laboratory findings include leukopenia, an elevated erythrocyte sedimentation rate, and hypergammaglobulinemia in almost every case; proteinuria and hematuria as common findings; and thrombocytopenia and hemolytic anemia as occasional findings. The LE cell phenomenon is found in about 85 per cent of the patients (Ropes). (For discussion of this phenomenon and other immunologic abnormalities see under Histogenesis.)

The coexistence of SLE with systemic

scleroderma has been repeatedly described (Dubois et al.). In addition, the existence of a "mixed connective tissue disease" has been recognized in which the skin lesions may resemble those of either lupus erythematosus, dermatomyositis or acrosclerosis (Sharp et al.). The systemic manifestations are largely those occurring in acrosclerosis, i.e., Raynaud's phenomenon and decreased motility of the esophagus. The prognosis of this "mixed connective tissue disease" is favorable.

Periarticular subcutaneous nodules indistinguishable from rheumatoid nodules may occur in patients with SLE without the coexistence of rheumatoid arthritis (Hahn et al.).

Concerning the induction of SLE by various drugs, see under Drug-Induced Lupus Erythematosus, page 241.

Histopathology. In early lesions of SLE of the erythematous, edematous type the histologic changes may be slight and nonspecific (Pruniéras and Montgomery). However, in well developed lesions the histologic changes correspond to those described for the erythematous, edematous lesions in DLE (see p. 426). In particular, the hydropic degeneration of the basal cell layer in association with edema of the upper dermis and extravasation of erythrocytes often facilitates the diagnosis of lupus erythematosus (Pruniéras and Montgomery). In well defined "discoid" lesions the findings are similar to those described for the discoid lesions in DLE (see p. 423). Hyperkeratosis and inflammatory changes may be quite pronounced in lesions of this type.

Fibrinoid deposits in the connective tissue of the skin may be seen in the erythematous, edematous lesions, especially in patients with SLE. Such fibrinoid deposits consist of the precipitation of fibrin in the ground substance. As a rule, the fibrinoid deposits are not as pronounced in the dermis as they are in the connective tissue of visceral organs, where they were first described by Klemperer et al. in 1941. Furthermore, fibrinoid deposits in the dermis are not specific for lupus erythematosus but occur also in several other unrelated dermatoses, especially in allergic vasculitis. As a result of the precipitation of

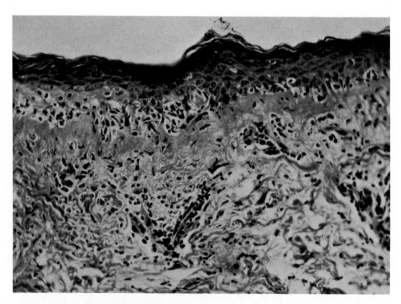

FIG. 24-4. **Systemic lupus erythematosus.** The epidermis is atrophic and shows marked liquefaction degeneration of the basal layer. Some of the collagen bundles appear thickened as a result of the precipitation of fibrinoid material on them. Only a mild perivascular inflammatory infiltrate is present. (×100)

fibrin, which is characterized by strong eosinophilia, homogeneous, strongly eosinophilic, "fibrinoid" material is deposited between and within the collagen bundles, so that the collagen fibers and bundles appear thickened and more deeply eosinophilic than normally (Fig. 24-4). The fibrinoid deposits are seen also in the walls of dermal capillaries. Thus, vascular changes, if present, are part of the connective tissue changes. In addition, fibrinoid deposits may be seen in the subepidermal basement membrane zone and often also within areas of edema in the upper dermis (Fig. 24-5).

The presence of the fibrinoid deposits, because of their homogenizing effect on the collagen and vascular walls, originally was interpreted as a process of collagen degeneration; but subsequently electron microscopic studies have revealed no damage to the collagen fibrils, and direct immunofluorescent studies carried out with fluorescein-labeled rabbit antisera against human fibrin have shown that the fibrinoid deposits consisted, at least in part, of fibrin (Gitlin et al.).

The fibrinoid deposits are strongly PAS-positive and diastase-resistant. In addition, one often finds in areas of fibrinoid deposits an increase in the amount of ground substance, particularly of hyaluronic acid, so that the areas in which there are fibrinoid deposits stain positive with alcian blue (Cawley et al.) and show metachromasia on staining with toluidine blue (Pruniéras and Montgomery).

The subcutaneous fat often is involved in SLE. It may show focal mucoid degeneration with a reactive lymphocytic infiltrate. The trabeculae of collagen separating the fat lobules may be increased in thickness and show edema and fibrinoid deposits similar to the collagen bundles of the dermis (Fig. 24-6). Although the histologic changes in the subcutaneous fat as just described produce no clinically apparent lesions, except for being much milder, they resemble the histologic changes that occur in lupus erythematosus profundus, also referred to as lupus erythematosus panniculitis (see p. 434).

SYSTEMIC LESIONS. Visceral involvement

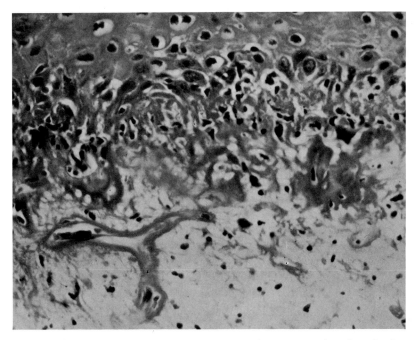

FIG. 24-5. **Systemic lupus erythematosus.** There are marked liquefaction degeneration of the basal layer and edema of the upper dermis. Precipitation of fibrinoid material can be seen in the zone of subepidermal edema and also around a capillary. (×200)

usually is widespread in patients who have died of SLE. Some of the lesions, however, are small so that they may be overlooked on gross inspection and are found only on histologic examination. The endocardium, the renal glomeruli, the serous membranes, the spleen, the cardiac and skeletal muscle, and the visceral fat deposits are affected most commonly.

The verrucous endocarditis of SLE, the so-called Libman-Sacks syndrome, occurs mainly on the mitral and tricuspid valves. One finds in the subendothelial connective tissue a chronic inflammatory infiltrate together with fibrinoid deposits followed by fibrosis and formation of small vegetations on the valve leaflets (Klemperer et al.).

The renal glomeruli are frequently involved. Depending on the extent of their involvement one may recognize: (1) a focal proliferative lupus nephritis in which only portions of some glomeruli are involved and progression to renal failure is a rare event; (2) a diffuse proliferative lupus nephritis in which all or nearly all glomeruli are involved and uremia often develops; and (3) a membranous lupus nephritis in which there is diffuse uniform thickening of the capillary walls in all glomeruli and uremia develops regularly (Baldwin et al.). In all three forms

one finds to a varying degree: (a) endothelial proliferation in the glomerular tufts, (b) thickening of the basement membrane, (c) deposits of fibrinoid material between the basement membrane and the endothelial cells of the capillary lumina, and (d) focal necroses within the glomeruli. The characteristic "wire loop" lesion results from the thickening of the basement membrane and the subendothelial deposits of fibrinoid material (Muehrke et al.; Everall et al.). The finding of a focal proliferative lupus nephritis on the initial renal biopsy does not necessarily indicate a good prognosis, since in the course of years the renal disease may become diffuse (Ginzler et al.).

The serous membranes, such as the pleura, the epicardium, and the peritoneum may show in their submucosa a chronic inflammatory infiltrate associated with fibrinoid deposits (Klemperer et al.).

In the spleen periarterial fibrosis around the follicular arteries is a common lesion in SLE and is highly characteristic of it. Thick, concentrically layered rings of sclerotic collagen fibers surround these arteries.

The myocardium and the skeletal muscles may show small foci of degeneration in the muscle bundles, usually associated with mild to moderately severe reactive inflammation

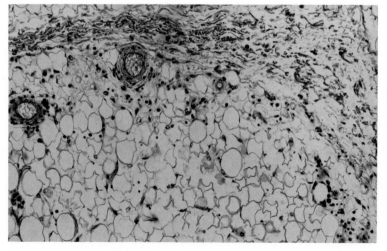

Fig. 24-6. **Systemic lupus erythematosus, subcutaneous layer.** The fat cells show mucoid degeneration. A scattered lymphocytic infiltrate is present. The collagen is increased in amount and shows precipitation of fibrinoid material. (×100)

in the interfascicular connective tissue. These changes are identical with those of dermatomyositis, though much milder (Klemperer; Erbslöh and Baedeker).

The visceral fat may show the same changes as those described for the subcutaneous fat (see p. 429).

Vascular changes usually are not conspicuous in SLE. In rare instances, however, there may be widespread vasculitis of the type seen in patients with periarteritis nodosa, causing rupture of some of the vessels and resulting in hemorrhage (Case Records of the Massachusettts General Hospital). It is probable that in these cases SLE and periarteritis nodosa are present simultaneously.

A highly specific structure, the so-called hematoxylin bodies, can be found in SLE in various organs, but only on autopsy and not in biopsy specimens. They form through the action of the LE factor, an IgG, on nuclei. However, the LE factor cannot penetrate into nuclei during life but only after the cell has suffered damage through death. The LE factor in penetrating the nucleus damages its chromatin pattern so that the nucleus swells and becomes homogeneous in appearance and stains reddish purple with hematoxylin-eosin (McDuffie). Hematoxylin bodies are found especially in the endocardium, the lumina of glomerular capillaries, the ovaries, and lymph nodes, and occasionally also in the skin (Worthington et al.). The hematoxylin bodies represent the counterpart in the tissue of the LE bodies found in the blood. LE bodies are formed in vitro through the action of the LE factor on dead nuclei which are then phagocytized by still viable neutrophils, constituting the LE cell phenomenon (see below).

Histogenesis. The presence of multiple antibodies in the serum and in the tissues of patients with SLE has led to the concept of LE as an autoimmune disorder. Among the antibodies present in the serum are, for instance, anti-DNA antibodies (Pincus et al.) and antinucleoprotein antibodies, the latter being used in two diagnostic tests, namely the LE cell test (McDuffie) and in the fluorescent antinuclear-antibody test (Carnabuci et al.). Among antibodies that are only occasionally present in the serum are those against red cells, causing hemolytic anemia; those against platelets, causing thrombocytopenia; and those causing false positive serologic tests of syphilis.

Comparing the fluorescent antinuclear-antibody test with the LE cell test, the fluorescent antinuclear-antibody test is more sensitive but also less specific. The antinuclear-antibody test, being an indirect immunofluorescent test, uses as substrate either frozen sections of rat liver or tumor imprints. On this are placed first the serum to be tested and then fluorescein-labeled antihuman gamma globulin (Burnham et al., 1969). This test is positive in nearly 100 per cent of the cases of SLE (Carnabuci et al.). However, it is positive quite frequently also in DLE (Petersen and Gokcen), in systemic scleroderma, and in rheumatoid arthritis (Pollack). The titer of the test is of diagnostic importance in that a titer higher than 1:64 is very suggestive of SLE or systemic scleroderma, and almost certainly rules out dermatomyositis and periarteritis nodosa (Rowell). With few exceptions, the titer is low also in patients with DLE having a positive antinuclear-antibody test. Thus, Carnabuci et al. found a positive antinuclear-antibody test with undiluted serum in 100 per cent of the patients with SLE, and in 57 per cent of the patients with DLE. However, at a dilution of 1:20 a positive test was obtained in 73 per cent of the patients with SLE, as compared with only 5 per cent of the patients with DLE. While the sera of both SLE and systemic scleroderma patients produce nuclear fluorescence, the patterns differ somewhat in that the sera of patients with SLE are apt to produce either homogeneous or peripheral fluorescence of the substrate nuclei, and the sera of patients with systemic scleroderma either speckled or nucleolar fluorescence (Burnham et al., 1969).

The LE cell test has high specificity and generally is postive only in SLE and thus represents an important test for it. However, being less sensitive than the fluorescent antinuclear-antibody test, it is positive in only about 85 per cent of the patients with SLE (Harvey et al.; Ropes). In rare instances only, a positive LE cell test has been observed in DLE (Marten and Blackburn), systemic scleroderma (Arnold and Tilden; Rowell), dermatomyositis (Christianson et al.), and rheumatoid arthritis (Friedman et al.). Quite frequently, a positive LE cell test is obtained in drug-induced lupus erythematosus (see p. 241). Very rarely, a positive LE cell test is seen in other kinds of drug eruption, for instance in a severe reaction to penicillin (Paull).

In carrying out the LE cell test the patient's serum is incubated with normal white blood cells. If the LE factor, an IgG, is present in the patient's serum, this factor penetrates into the nuclei of some of the normal white blood cells and causes nuclear damage. The damage varies from homogenization of the nucleus, manifesting itself as LE body or smoky body, to disintegration of the nucleus (see p. 431). The damaged nuclei, being leukotactic, are phagocytized by some of the neutrophils that have escaped damage. On making a smear of the incubated white blood cells and staining the smear with Wright's stain, one observes within some of the neutrophils the phagocytized nuclear material as a large, round, amorphous, smoky basophilic body of such large size that it presses the nucleus of the neutrophil against the cell membrane. This represents the so-called LE cell (Fig. 24-7) (Hargraves et al.; Weiss and Swift; McDuffie). In addition to LE cells, one observes so-called rosettes (Fig. 24-7). They consist of disintegrated nuclear material surrounded by neutrophils that are in the process of phagocytizing this material.

In addition to the fluorescent antinuclear-antibody test and the LE cell test, a third diagnostic test consists of submitting unfixed, frozen skin biopsy specimens to direct immunofluorescent testing for the presence of antigen-antibody-complement complexes at the epidermal-dermal junction. For this purpose sections are cut on a cryostat and are incubated with fluorescein-conjugated antisera; either with antihuman gamma globulin or separately with antihuman IgG, IgA, IgM, and complement (Pohle and Tuffanelli). Immunoglobulins, most commonly IgG and IgM, and complement are present in about 90 per cent of the specimens obtained from involved skin of patients with either SLE or DLE. In addition, about 50 per cent of the specimens obtained from uninvolved SLE skin are positive, whereas uninvolved DLE skin is regularly negative (Tuffanelli et al.; Chorzelski et al.; Burnham et al., 1970). The impression was gained by Burnham and Fine that patients with SLE showing immunoglobulin deposits in uninvolved skin generally have more severe disease than the patients not showing it. The method of direct immunofluorescent testing has resulted in very few positive results outside of LE, for instance in one case of systemic scleroderma (Pohle and Tuffanelli), and one of Jessner's lymphocytic infiltration (Burnham et al., 1970).

At one time the specificity of subepidermal fluorescence on direct immunofluorescent testing was questioned by several authors who had observed junctional fluorescent patterns with immunoglobulins and complement in the exposed skin of patients with either acne rosacea or facial telangiectasia (Baart de la Faille and Baart de la

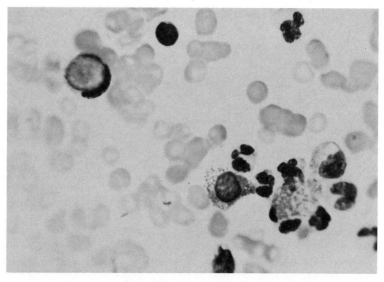

Fig. 24-7. **Systemic lupus erythematosus, L.E. cell test.** For the demonstration of the L.E. cell phenomenon normal white blood cells are incubated with the patient's serum. In this positive test an L.E. cell is seen in the left upper corner; it is a neutrophil containing a large smoky body. In the right lower corner a rosette is seen consisting of amorphous material surrounded by phagocytizing neutrophils. (×400)

Faille-Kuyper; Jablonska et al.). Subsequently, it became apparent, however, that this occasionally observed nonspecific junctional fluorescent band actually was an ill defined fibrillar pseudoband probably formed by the compression of the dermal connective tissue against the epidermis (Burnham and Fine, 1971 (II); Abell et al.).

The specific band seen in lupus erythematosus consists of coalescing clumps located subepidermally and in the uppermost dermis (Burnham and Fine, 1971 (I); Nebe and Barthelmes). This irregular band differs from that seen on direct immunofluorescent testing in bullous pemphigoid and occasionally also in cicatricial pemphigoid, which is narrow, tubular, and immediately subepidermal in location (Burnham and Fine, 1971, I).

The glomerular wire loops, similar to the subepidermal immunofluorescent band, contain antigen-antibody-complement complexes, and in addition contain fibrin (Koffler et al.):

Electron microscopic examination of the cutaneous lesions of both DLE and SLE shows marked changes in the basal cells and the basal lamina. The basal cells show vacuolization of their cytoplasm that may progress to disintegration and necrosis of the cytoplasm. In addition, the basal cells show numerous greatly elongated, narrow cytoplasmic projections into the dermis which, because of their irregular shape, often appear as cross sections (E.M. No. 36). The projections are surrounded by basal lamina, resulting in an irregular and extensive network of basal lamina. This network persists even in areas where the projections of the basal cells have disintegrated. The impression is thus gained that the basal cells are a primary site of damage in the cutaneous lesions of lupus erythematosus (Tuffanelli et al.).

The hyaline or colloid bodies that may be seen in the epidermis as well as in the dermis, on electron microscopy, are similar in appearance to those observed in lichen planus (see p. 151, and E.M. No. 28). They are finely filamentous to amorphous granular in appearance and do not possess a delimiting membrane (Haustein).

The exact electron microscopic location of the subepidermal immune complexes in lupus erythematosus has been studied after staining them with peroxidase-labeled antihuman gamma globulin. With this method the antigen-antibody complexes are seen as irregular aggregates in the uppermost dermis, beneath the basal lamina, located in the ground substance as well as on collagen fibrils, often masking their cross banding (Ueki et al.). The localization of the immune complexes in lupus erythematosus differs from their localization in bullous phemphigoid

where they are situated between the basal lamina and the basal cells (see p. 117).

The presence of structures resembling unenveloped nucleocapsids of paramyxovirus has been described in the cutaneous and renal lesions of SLE (Györkey et al.), and in the cutaneous lesions of DLE (Hashimoto and Thompson). The presence of these structures is, however, not specific for LE, since they have been observed also in the cutaneous and muscular lesions of dermatomyositis (Hashimoto and Thompson). They consist of tangled tubular formations measuring about 20 nm in diameter and are present in the cytoplasm of endothelial cells and fibroblasts (E.M. No. 37). If it is assumed that the formations are viral RNA strands, they exist in the host cells without being able to mature and to replicate, possibly because the virus is defective. According to Györkey et al., the pathogenesis of collagen or autoimmune diseases is compatible with the etiologic role of a defective virus.

Two recent observations have thrown doubt on the viral nature of the cytoplasmic tubules. In one study they were found within vascular endothelial cells of various epithelial tumors, such as seborrheic keratosis, basal cell epithelioma, and Bowen's disease (Maciejewski et al.). In the other study, cytoplasmic tubules were observed quite frequently in the visibly normal skin of patients with SLE, and rarely also in the normal skin of patients with DLE. Following a ten day course of ultraviolet irradiation to visibly normal skin the incidence of cytoplasmic tubules in the irradiated skin of patients with SLE or DLE increased significantly (Berk and Blank). These two cited observations would favor the interpretation of the cytoplasmic tubules as a cell reaction product.

LUPUS ERYTHEMATOSUS PROFUNDUS

In rare instances one observes one or several firm, asymptomatic, often fairly large subcutaneous nodules, usually as a manifestation of systemic lupus erythematosus, but occasionally also as a manifestation of discoid lupus erythematosus (Winkelmann; Tuffanelli). The nodules occur most commonly on the head and arms, and may either precede or follow the cutaneous lesions. The skin overlying the subcutaneous nodules often appears normal; but in some instances cutaneous lesions of lupus erythematosus are seen overlying the nodules (Fountain; Tuffanelli). On healing, the subcutaneous lesions may leave behind a cup-shaped depression. In place of lupus erythematosus profundus, the term lupus erythematosus panniculitis is now often used for the subcutaneous nodules.

Histopathology. The subcutaneous nodules may merely show a nonspecific panniculitis composed of lymphoid cells, plasma cells, and histiocytes. However, frequently one finds necrobiotic changes with fibrinoid deposits in the subcutaneous tissue (Fountain; Tuffanelli). Subsequent hyalinization of the collagen may result in broad septa subdividing the subcutaneous fat (Winkelmann). In some cases mucinous changes and foci of calcification are seen (Winkelmann). There may be severe vasculitis, but it represents involvement of the vessels in the inflammatory process rather than the cause of the changes (Fountain). The vessels thus affected show inflammatory infiltration and

thickening of their walls with narrowing of their lumina (Schirren and Eggert).

LYMPHOCYTIC INFILTRATION OF THE SKIN (JESSNER)

The lesions generally are described as asymptomatic, well demarcated, slightly infiltrated, reddish plaques. The lesions begin as papules and expand peripherally. There may be central clearing. The surface of the lesions appears normal and, in particular, shows no follicular plugging or atrophy. The most common locations of the lesions are the face, the neck, and the upper back. After having persisted for several months or even several years, they disappear without sequelae; but they may recur either at the previous sites or elsewhere. In some instances the eruption is precipitated or aggravated by sunlight (Gottlieb and Winkelmann). Antimalarial drugs of the 4-aminoquinoline

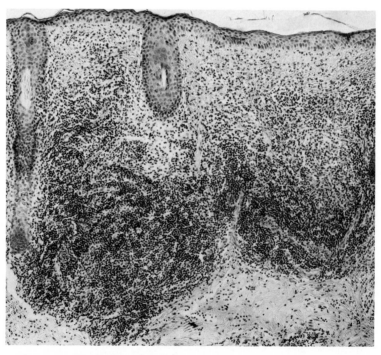

FIG. 24-8. **Lymphocytic infiltration of the skin.** The epidermis is normal. The dermis contains large, fairly well demarcated patches of an inflammatory infiltrate composed almost entirely of lymphocytes. (×100)

group, such as chloroquine, sometimes clear the eruption dramatically, but they do not do so consistently (Calnan).

Histopathology. The epidermis is normal, except that often it appears slightly flattened. In the dermis one observes large, fairly well circumscribed patches of a cellular infiltrate composed almost entirely of lymphoid cells (Fig. 24-8). In addition to the lymphoid cells, a few histiocytes and plasma cells are usually present. There often is a tendency to arrangement around cutaneous appendages and blood vessels. The infiltrate may extend into the subcutaneous fat (Jessner and Kanof).

Histogenesis. It is as yet undecided whether lymphocytic infiltration of the skin represents an entity, or an abortive or initial phase of any of the four other diseases with a patchy dermal infiltrate, i.e., discoid lupus erythematosus, the plaque type of polymorphous light eruption, pseudo-lymphoma of Spiegler-Fendt, and lymphocytic lymphoma (which form together the five diseases with an "L" as an initial, see p. 426).

Several authors favor recognition of lymphocytic infiltration of the skin as an entity because the lesions differ sufficiently from DLE: clinically by the absence of hyperkeratosis, by healing without atrophy, by an occasional lack of response to the antimalarial drugs, and by the fairly common occurrence of lesions on the back; and histologically by the absence of hydropic degeneration in the basal layer (Jessner and Kanof; Calnan; Bazex). To these criteria an additional criterion has lately been added: a negative result on direct immunofluorescent testing consisting of the absence of immunoglobulins at the dermal-epidermal border (Barthelmes and Sönnichsen; Chorzelski et al.). However, a positive test is obtained only in about 90 per cent of the patients with DLE (see p. 432); and aside from the 10 per cent of negative cases, the direct immunofluorescent test has been used in doubtful cases to decide whether a case should be regarded as DLE or as lymphocytic infiltration of the skin (Chorzelski et al.).

The apparently close relationship of at least some of the cases of lymphocytic infiltration of the skin to DLE has influenced some authors to regard a certain number of the cases reported as lymphocytic infiltration of the skin as instances of nonscarring DLE, but other cases as representing a separate entity (Cabré and Steigleder; Gottlieb and Winkelmann). A third group of authors holds the view that all cases of lympho-

cytic infiltration of the skin, on the basis of their clinical and histologic resemblance, the presence of photosensitivity, and response to antimalarial drugs, were instances of nonscarring DLE (Bielicky and Trapl; Burnham).

A fourth view, which appears to be the most likely, regards the cases reported as lymphocytic infiltration of the skin as a heterogeneous group, rather than an entity. Accordingly, lymphocytic infiltration of the skin may be used as a preliminary diagnostic term until a more definitive diagnosis is possible. There seems to be little doubt that, if followed long enough, most, if not all, cases of lymphocytic infiltration of the skin, unless the lesions subside spontaneously, can be reclassified, usually as DLE or the plaque type of polymorphous light eruption, and occasionally as pseudolymphoma or Spiegler-Fendt or as lymphocytic lymphoma, as in Calnan's case.

DERMATOMYOSITIS

In dermatomyositis the skin and skeletal muscles are affected predominantly. However, in some cases cutaneous lesions are absent (Vignos et al.). Dermatomyositis most commonly occurs either in late childhood or in middle age (Medsger).

The cutaneous lesions consist of erythematous to purplish patches that show slight edema. Through gradual extension fairly extensive areas of the skin may become involved. The face is most commonly affected, particularly the periorbital areas, and also the upper chest, the arms, the knuckles, and the distal portions of the fingers. Often the eruption greatly resembles the erythematous-edematous lesions seen in systemic lupus erythematosus; and, as in systemic lupus erythematosus, exposure to the sun may cause a flare-up. Not infrequently, the cutaneous lesions assume the appearance of poikiloderma atrophicans vasculare (see p. 438).

Involvement of the skeletal muscles causes progressive weakness, vague muscular pain and, later, atrophy of the muscles. The proximal muscles of the extremities and the anterior neck muscles often are the first to be involved. Involvement of the pharynx may result in dysphagia and aspiration of food; and involvement of the diaphragm and of the intercostal muscles may lead to respiratory failure. The prognosis of dermatomyositis, on the whole, is favorable, however, especially when treatment with corticosteroids is being used. Thus, the mortality has been between 5 per cent (Pearson) and 14 per cent (Rose and Walton) in recent series of cases.

Areas of subcutaneous and periarticular calcification may occur and, if extensive, are referred to as dystrophic calcinosis universalis (see p. 400). The nodules gradually resolve if the patient survives (Muller et al.). In rare instances, systemic scleroderma, especially acrosclerosis, occurs in association with dermatomyositis.

Histopathology. The erythematous-edematous lesions of dermatomyositis often show histologic changes that are indistinguishable from those seen in systemic lupus erythematosus (see p. 428). In particular, one observes atrophy of the epidermis, hydropic degeneration of the basal cell layer, edema of the upper dermis, a scattered inflammatory infiltrate, and often also hyaline, PAS-positive fibrinoid deposits at the dermal-epidermal junction and around the capillaries of the upper dermis (Janis and Winkelmann).

Older cutaneous lesions with the clinical appearance of poikiloderma atrophicans vasculare usually show a bandlike infiltrate under a flattened epidermis (for details see under poikiloderma atrophicans vasculare, p. 439).

Not infrequently, the dermis shows focal accumulations of mucin in the form of acid mucopolysaccharides, usually without an associated inflammatory infiltrate (Janis and Winkelmann).

The subcutaneous tissue may show focal areas of panniculitis associated with mucoid degeneration of the fat cells in early lesions (Wainger and Lever). Extensive areas of calcification may be present in the subcutis in the later stage (Reich) (see Calcinosis Cutis, p. 400).

In selecting a site for muscle biopsy it is advisable to choose a proximal muscle from an extremity, preferably one that is tender. Muscles merely showing weakness and atrophy are best avoided, since in this end stage the muscle fibers may have been replaced by fibrous connective tissue (Vignos et al.). Muscles that are actively involved show de-

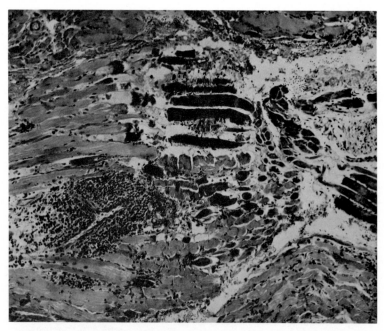

Fig. 24-9. **Dermatomyositis; muscle.** The muscle bundles show various degrees of degeneration. In addition, one sees edema and focal collections of inflammatory cells. (×100)

generative changes and inflammation. The degree of these changes varies not only in different muscles but also within each affected muscle. It has been suggested that the degenerative changes represent infarctions resulting from the occlusion of small perimysial and endomysial vessels by intimal hyperplasia and fibrin thrombi (Banker and Victor). Subsequent observers, however, have not found such pronounced vascular changes (Shafiq et al.; Mintz, et al.; Janis and Winkelmann); or, when present, they were regarded as part of the degenerative process rather than as its cause (Gonzalez-Angulo et al.).

In areas of mild degeneration the muscle bundles show loss of their transverse striation and hyalinization of the sarcoplasm, associated with a proliferation of sarcolemma nuclei. In areas of severe degeneration the muscle bundles may show, in addition, fragmentation of fibers, granular and vacuolar degeneration of groups of fibers, basophilic staining, and phagocytosis of degenerated muscle fragments by macrophages (Fig. 24-9). In areas of early degeneration inflammatory changes in the muscles usually are mild and often are absent. They can be regarded, therefore, as a reaction to the muscular damage (Shafiq; Janis and Winkelmann). If present, the inflammatory reaction consists of patchy, perivascular, interstitial infiltrations of lymphoid cells and a few plasma cells. In addition, edema usually separates the muscle bundles in areas of active degenerative changes.

SYSTEMIC LESIONS. Changes in organs other than the skin and the striated muscles occur only rarely, in contrast with systemic lupus erythematosus and systemic scleroderma. The myocardium may show changes identical with those in the skeletal muscle but less severe (Kinney and Maher; O'Leary and Waisman; Wainger and Lever). Ulcerative lesions in the gastrointestinal tract as the result of vascular occlusions have been described (Horn; Wainger and Lever; Banker and Victor).

Association of Dermatomyositis With Malignant Tumors. This occasional association has been much commented upon in recent years. The figures about the frequency of this occurrence vary. Williams, in a review of the literature up to 1959, found reports on 590 patients with dermatomyositis. Among them 92 persons, or 16 per cent, had an associated malignant tumor. Individual series show considerable variations. Thus, Curtis et al. observed among 45 patients with dermatomyositis 8, or 18 per cent, with malignant disease. Arundel et al. noted this occurrence in 12 of 23 adult patients, amounting to 52 per cent; whereas Christianson et al. found among 270 patients only 18, or 6.7 per cent, with malignancy. The latter authors, because of the low incidence, doubted that a relationship existed between dermatomyositis and malignancy. A similar view was expressed by Logan et al. who among 43 adult patients with dermatomyositis had 8, or 18.6 per cent, with malignancy. Logan et al. had doubts about an etiologic relationship because in 3 of their 8 patients the malignant tumor preceded the dermatomyositis, whereas in the other 5 patients the malignancy developed several months or years after the onset of the dermatomyositis. Similarly, Degos et al., observing the association of dermatomyositis with cancer in 7 of 31 adult patients (22.6%), found the cancer to precede the dermatomyositis in 3 patients and to follow it in 4 patients. This variance in the relationship between dermatomyositis and cancer weakens the theory proposed by Weston and Thorne that a profound T lymphopenia existing in dermatomyositis lowered the patient's immunologic defenses against cancer and predisposed him to cancer.

Histogenesis. Electron microscopic examination revealed that the degeneration of the muscle fibers in dermatomyositis shows many similarities to the degenerative changes found in other diseases of muscle (Shafiq et al.). The earliest change seen by electron microscopy seems to consist of focal disintegration of myofilaments and myofibrils resulting in areas of vacuolization and in the accumulation of lipid globules and lysosomes within muscle cells (Gonzalez-Angulo et al.; Hashimoto et al.).

Paramyxoviruslike structures can be found in the skin lesions and muscular lesions of dermatomyositis, just as in lupus erythematosus (see p. 433). These structures are located mainly in the cytoplasm of endothelial cells of all types of blood vessels in the skin and in the muscle, and also in dermal fibroblasts (Hashimoto et al.). (Concerning the possible significance of these structures, see p. 433.)

POIKILODERMA ATROPHICANS VASCULARE

In three genodermatoses cutaneous lesions with the appearance of poikiloderma atrophicans vasculare occur. They are: (a) poikiloderma congenitale (see p. 68), with the lesions of poikiloderma limited to the face, the extremities, and the buttocks; (b) Bloom's syndrome (see p. 69), with poikilodermalike lesions limited to the face, the forearms and the dorsa of the hands; and (c) dyskeratosis congenita (see p. 63), in which there may be extensive netlike pigmentation of the skin suggestive of poikiloderma atrophicans vasculare.

An extensive eruption greatly resembling poikiloderma atrophicans vasculare is seen in parapsoriasis variegata (see p. 145). This may be regarded as the prototype of idiopathic poikiloderma atrophicans vasculare. It should be kept in mind, however, that some cases of parapsoriasis variegata eventually are shown to have lymphoma.

It probably simplifies the concept of poikiloderma atrophicans vasculare if cases described as idiopathic poikiloderma atrophicans vasculare, such as the cases of Dowling and Freudenthal, Downing et al., and Steig-leder, are regarded as identical with parapsoriasis variegata, as suggested by Janis and Winkelmann.

In the great majority of cases, however, poikiloderma atrophicans vasculare occurs not as an idiopathic disease but secondarily to two groups of diseases. One group is represented by dermatomyositis and systemic lupus erythematosus, whereby dermatomyositis is much more commonly seen as the primary disease than is lupus erythematosus, and the association with dermatomyositis often is referred to as poikilodermatomyositis (Guy et al.; Horn). The other group is represented by the lymphomas, particularly mycosis fungoides (see p. 696). Although as a rule the lymphoma is well established by the time the cutaneous lesions assume the appearance of poikiloderma atrophicans vasculare, occasionally an apparently idiopathic poikiloderma atrophicans vasculare is the forerunner of lymphoma, as pointed out above.

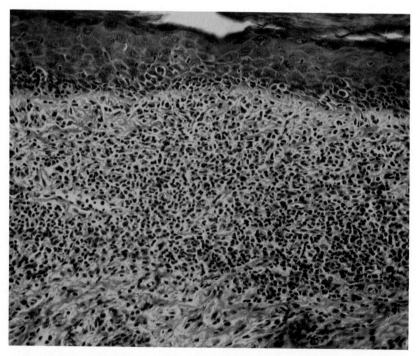

FIG. 24-10. **Poikilodermatomyositis, early stage.** The epidermis appears flattened and shows hydropic degeneration of the basal cells. The upper dermis contains a bandlike infiltrate, which in places invades the epidermis. (×200)

Clinically, poikiloderma atrophicans vasculare presents large ill-defined areas, usually in symmetrical distribution, which in the early stage show erythema with slight, superficial scaling, a mottled pigmentation, and telangiectases. In the late stage the skin appears atrophic, the erythema is less pronounced than in the early stage, but the mottled pigmentation and the telangiectases are more pronounced. The clinical picture then resembles chronic radiodermatitis.

Histopathology. In the idiopathic form of poikiloderma and in poikiloderma associated with dermatomyositis or lupus erythematosus, the histologic changes are identical. In the early erythematous stage the epidermis shows moderate atrophy of the stratum malpighii, effacement of the rete ridges, and hydropic degeneration of the basal cells (Fig. 24-10). In the upper dermis one finds a bandlike infiltrate, which in places invades the epidermis. The infiltrate consists mainly of lymphoid cells but contains also a few histiocytes. Melanophages also are found within the infiltrate. There is edema in the upper dermis, and the superficial capillaries are dilated (Horn).

In the late stage the epidermis is atrophic and the basal cells still show hydropic degeneration of the basal cells. The dermal infiltrate, however, is much less pronounced than in the early stage, although melanophages, edema of the upper dermis, and capillary dilatation are still present (Janis and Winkelmann).

In poikiloderma atrophicans vasculare associated with mycosis fungoides or other types of lymphoma the dermal infiltrate is much more pronounced than it is in idiopathic poikiloderma atrophicans vasculare or in poikiloderma atrophicans vasculare associated with dermatomyositis or with systemic lupus erythematosus. In addition, atypical cells characteristic of lymphoma are present (see p. 700).

SCLERODERMA

Two types of scleroderma exist: circumscribed scleroderma (morphea) and systemic scleroderma. In morphea the lesions usually are limited to the skin and to the subcutaneous tissue beneath the cutaneous lesions; but occasionally the underlying muscles are also affected. In systemic scleroderma, in addition to extensive involvement of the skin and the subcutaneous tissue, visceral lesions are present, leading to death in about one half of the patients.

Although morphea may be associated with arthralgia and in rare instances with Raynaud's phenomenon (see below), generally accepted instances of transition from morphea to systemic scleroderma with visceral involvement have not been reported so far. Cases that have been regarded by their authors as having undergone this transition can be interpreted either as instances of generalized morphea, including the cases reported by Stava (case 1) and by Grabner; or as having been systemic scleroderma from the beginning, including the cases reported by Stava (case 2) and by Weidner and Braun-Falco (case 1).

MORPHEA

Morphea, also referred to as circumscribed scleroderma, may be divided into five types: the guttate, the plaque, the linear, the segmental and the generalized types.

Guttate lesions occur almost always in association with lesions of the plaque type. Guttate lesions are small and superficial; they resemble the lesions of lichen sclerosus et atrophicus, but they do not show hyperkeratosis or follicular plugging.

Lesions of the plaque type are round or oval, but through coalescence they may assume an irregular configuration. They are indurated, have a smooth surface, and show an ivory color. As long as they are enlarging, they may show a violaceous border, the so-called lilac ring.

Lesions of the linear type occur predominantly on the extremities and on the anterior scalp (Dilley and Perry).

Segmental morphea can occur on the face, where it results in hemiatrophy, or on one or several extremities, where it produces, in addition to induration of the skin, marked atrophy of the subcutaneous fat and of the muscles, resulting in contractures of muscles and tendons, and ankyloses of joints on the hands and feet (Hickman and Sheils).

Generalized morphea refers to very extensive cases showing a combination of the four types just described (Christianson et al.; Driessen et al.).

Segmental or generalized morphea frequently is accompanied by arthralgia in the involved extremities (Christianson et al.), and occasionally by Raynaud's phenomenon (Lawrence; Christianson et al.; Weidner and Braun-Falco). Also, in patients with extensive morphea lesions of lichen sclerosus et atrophicus may be found to coexist (see p. 260).

Histopathology. An early inflammatory and a late sclerotic stage exist. Most sections obtained routinely show a histologic picture intermediate to the two stages. It is of great importance that the specimen for biopsy include adequate amounts of subcutaneous tissue, since most of the diagnostic alterations are seen there.

In the early inflammatory stage, found particularly at the violaceous border of enlarging lesions, the dermis shows closely packed, thick collagen bundles and a fairly mild inflammatory infiltrate, predominantly lymphocytic, between the collagen bundles and around the blood vessels (Fig. 24-11). A much more pronounced inflammatory infiltrate than that seen in the dermis involves the subcutaneous fat and its upward projections toward the eccrine glands. The trabeculae subdividing the subcutaneous fat are thickened because of the presence of an inflammatory infiltrate and the deposition of new collagen. Large areas of the subcutaneous fat are being replaced by newly formed collagen that is composed of fibers rather than of bundles and stains only faintly with hematoxylin and eosin (Fig. 24-12) (Fleischmajer and Nedwich).

In the late sclerotic stage, as seen in the center of older lesions, the inflammatory infiltrate has disappeared almost completely, except in some areas of the subcutis. The epidermis is normal. The dermal collagen appears thickened and closely packed, even in its uppermost portion, including the papillary layer, where normally it is loosely arranged. It stains more eosinophilic than normal. The eccrine glands appear markedly atrophic and the fatty tissue normally surrounding them is greatly reduced in amount

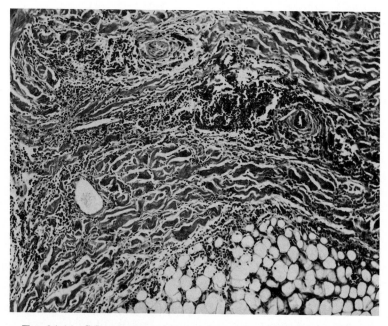

FIG. 24-11. **Scleroderma, early stage.** A rather pronounced inflammatory infiltrate is present in the lower dermis and in the subcutaneous fat where new collagen is being deposited; part of the collagen appears as closely packed, thick collagen bundles. (×100)

FIG. 24-12. **Scleroderma, early stage, subcutaneous fat.** The trabeculae subdividing the subcutaneous fat are thickened. Large areas of subcutaneous fat are replaced by newly formed collagen fibers that show only faint staining. (×100)

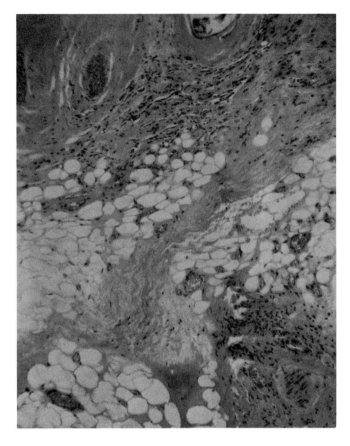

or absent. Instead, they are surrounded by newly formed collagen and appear tightly "bound down" by this newly formed collagen. Also, instead of lying, as they normally do, near the cutaneous-subcutaneous border, the sweat glands seem to lie well inside the dermis as the result of the replacement of most of the subcutaneous fat by newly formed collagen. The newly formed collagen throughout the subcutaneous tissue shows at first very fine, wavy collagen fibers and numerous fibroblasts and an increase in reticulum fibers (Fleischmajer and Nedwich). Ultimately, however, the collagen consists of thick, pale, sclerotic, homogeneous or hyalinized bundles with fewer fibroblasts than normally, giving the newly formed collagen in the subcutis an "empty look" (Fig. 24-13). Only few blood vessels are seen within the sclerotic collagen, often having a fibrotic wall and a narrowed lumen. Only a few short elastic fibers are seen throughout the

newly formed collagen in the subcutaneous tissue (Fleischmajer and Nedwich).

The striated muscles underlying lesions of morphea are affected only in the linear and segmental types. The muscle fibers appear vacuolated and separated from one another by edema and focal collections of inflammatory cells (Hickman and Sheils).

SYSTEMIC SCLERODERMA

In systemic scleroderma the indurated lesions of the skin are not sharply demarcated or "circumscribed," as in morphea; although in occasional cases of systemic scleroderma a few well demarcated morphealike patches may be seen (Black et al.).

The cutaneous involvement may start centrally on the trunk or it may start peripherally on the hands and on the face as so-called acrosclerosis, in which case it is associated with Raynaud's phenomenon. The indurated

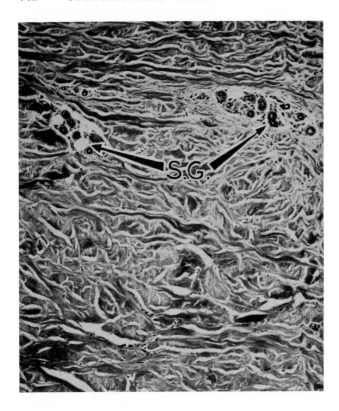

Fig. 24-13. **Scleroderma, late stage.** Two groups of sweat glands (S.G.) appear markedly atrophic and are tightly "bound down" by newly formed collagen. Below the sweat glands, where formerly subcutaneous fat was located, the collagen consists of thick, closely packed, hyalinized bundles with only few fibroblasts. There is no longer any inflammatory infiltrate. (×100)

skin as a result of a diffuse fibrosis of the subcutaneous fat becomes firmly bound to the underlying structures. Ulcerations may occur, most commonly on the tips of the fingers. The involved skin may show hyperpigmentation or numerous small patches of telangiectasia. Calcinosis cutis occurs occasionally and is observed most commonly on the extremities in association with acrosclerosis (Muller et al.). The skeletal musculature is invariably affected, resulting in weakness and atrophy. Contractures of the muscles and tendons and ankyloses of the joints may develop, especially on the hands.

Involvement of *internal organs* is usually present, but varies greatly in extent and degree. Lesions in the esophagus may cause difficulties in deglutition; in the intestinal tract symptoms of malabsorption or, late in the disease, ileus (Korting and Lachner); in the lungs dyspnea and right-sided heart failure secondary to cor pulmonale (D'Angelo et al.); and in the kidneys uremia (Fisher and Rodnan). A peculiar clinical feature of the renal involvement in sclero-

derma is the rapidity with which either renal failure or "malignant" hypertension may develop. Renal failure and the cardiac complications of "malignant" hypertension are the most common causes of death in scleroderma (Cannon et al.). In quite a few patients the disease ultimately comes to a standstill. Among the 309 patients followed by Medsger et al. the 7-year survival rate was 35 per cent; and among the 267 patients followed by Tuffanelli and Winkelmann the 10-year survival rate was 47 per cent (or when only the traced patients were considered 59 per cent).

A rather mild form of systemic scleroderma is the Thibierge-Weissenbach syndrome, also referred to as the CRST syndrome, consisting of calcinosis cutis, Raynaud's phenomenon, sclerodactyly, and telangiectasias (Carr et al.). Involvement of the esophagus may occur, but death from visceral lesions of scleroderma is rare, and among the 14 patients with the CRST syndrome followed by Medsger death occurred in only 1 patient so that the 7-year survival rate was 93 per cent.

Histopathology. The histologic appearance of the skin lesions in systemic scleroderma is similar to that seen in morphea, so that a histologic differentiation of the two types is not possible. However, in the early lesions the inflammatory reaction is much less pronounced in systemic scleroderma than in morphea, so that only a mild cellular infiltrate is present around the dermal vessels, around the eccrine coils, and in the subcutaneous tissue. On the other hand, in the late stage, systemic scleroderma shows more pronounced vascular changes in the subcutis than does morphea, consisting of a paucity of blood vessels and of thickening and hyalinization of their walls and narrowing of the lumen (O'Leary et al.; Fleischmajer et al.). In the late stage of systemic scleroderma the epidermis may show, in contrast with morphea, atrophy with disappearance of the rete ridges. Also, in the late stage aggregates of calcium may be seen within areas of sclerotic, homogeneous collagen of the subcutaneous tissue (Kanee) (see also Calcinosis Cutis, p. 400).

Histologic examination of skeletal muscle shows changes that are indistinguishable from those of dermatomyositis, although as a rule the degenerative changes are less pronounced and atrophy and fibrosis predominate.

SYSTEMIC LESIONS. Deposits of homogeneous, hyalinized collagen may be extensive on autopsy, since they can occur wherever connective tissue exists normally (Piper and Helwig). Unless the involvement in a given organ is severe, it may be asymptomatic.

The primary role of obliterative vascular changes in producing the visceral lesions of systemic scleroderma has been emphasized by several recent authors, especially in regard to the lesions of the gastrointestinal tract, the lungs, and the kidneys (Alpert and Warner; Norton and Nardo; Toth and Alpert). The vessels primarily involved are the precapillary arterioles which in the earliest stage show endothelial proliferation and perivascular inflammation. This then is followed by mucoid intimal proliferation with narrowing of the lumen. However, in rare instances only does the vascular disease in systemic scleroderma progress into a necro-tizing arteriolitis, thus terminating as periarteritis nodosa (Toth and Alpert).

In the gastrointestinal tract widespread arteriolitis has been described as preceding the replacement of the smooth musculature by fibrous tissue (Alpert and Warner).

In the lungs also, intimal thickening in the arterioles often seems to precede the development of interstitial fibrosis. In addition, pulmonary hypertension may develop, leading to congestive heart failure. Cardiac insufficiency in systemic scleroderma usually is secondary to pulmonary fibrosis or hypertension, rather than the result of myocardial fibrosis which rarely is severe enough to produce clinical symptoms (D'Angelo et al.). Severe interstitial fibrosis of the lungs may lead to degeneration of alveolar septa and to formation of large and small cystic spaces, resulting in a so-called honeycomb lung (Getzowa). In several cases secondary development of a pulmonary carcinoma has been reported. In most instances the pulmonary carcinoma has been an alveolar cell or bronchiolar adenocarcinoma (Collins et al.); but also bronchogenic squamous cell carcinoma (Tomkin) and oat cell carcinoma (Haggani and Holti) have been observed.

The histologic changes found in the kidneys in scleroderma are quite characteristic and differ from those of hypertensive disease. A primary distinguishing feature of renal scleroderma is the presence of adventitial fibrosis around the interlobar, the arcuate and the interlobular arteries. Secondly, the interlobular arteries are the site of the most advanced vascular changes, whereas in hypertensive disease these vessels are normal and the smaller arteries and arterioles are the site of pathologic changes (Cannon et al.). Characteristically, in renal scleroderma the interlobular arteries show, regardless of whether the patients have a normotensive or hypertensive history, marked mucoid thickening of their intima leading to narrowing or occlusion of their lumina (Fisher and Rodnan; Cannon et al.). The resulting cortical infarcts are larger, as a rule, in patients with scleroderma than in those with hypertensive disease (Cannon et al.).

Histogenesis. Two factors are recognized in the etiology of scleroderma: it is both a vascular disease and an autoimmune disorder (Rosenthal and Sack). In favor of an autoimmune etiology are (a) its occasional association with other connective tissue diseases, occurring either in association with systemic lupus erythematosus or as "mixed connective tissue disease" (see p. 428), and (b) the frequent presence of antinuclear antibodies in the serum, according to Rowell and Beck, in 67 per cent of the cases of systemic scleroderma. The pattern most commonly evoked by the antinuclear antibodies in systemic scleroderma is either a speckled or a nucleolar fluorescence (Burnham et al.).

On the basis of the histologic findings indicating a replacement of much of the subcutaneous fat by collagen, an increased collagen synthesis in scleroderma has been postulated. This has been borne out by enzymatic and electron microscopic studies.

Enzymatic studies have revealed that the skin of systemic scleroderma (1) has a significantly higher protocollagen proline hydroxylase activity than normal skin (Keiser et al.), and (2) shows an increased rate of in vitro formation of ^{14}C-hydroxyproline from ^{14}C-proline (Uitto et al.).

Electron microscopic examination of the skin in scleroderma has revealed the presence of highly active fibroblasts with dilated cisternae filled with amorphous material. In addition, there is a decided increase in the proportion of thin collagen fibrils. Thus, Hayes and Rodman found that 38 per cent of the collagen fibrils had a diameter of less than 50 nm, whereas in the normal adult the diameter of collagen fibrils varies between 70 and 140 nm, with the average width being at 100 nm. This preponderance of thin fibrils is not specific for scleroderma but is merely indicative of recently deposited collagen and a consequence of increased collagen synthesis. Kobayasi and Asboe-Hansen, in confirming these findings, stated that the decrease in the thickness of the collagen fibrils was generally more pronounced in the deep dermis than in the upper layers of the dermis. In addition, they found, on staining ultrathin sections with ruthenium red, a high content of acid glycosaminoglycans in the sclerodermic dermis and thus confirmed earlier histochemical studies by Braun-Falco which had indicated an increase in acid mucopolysaccharides in early lesions of scleroderma.

ATROPHODERMA OF PASINI AND PIERINI

In this disorder, described by Pasini in 1923 and by Pierini in 1936, one observes, usually on the trunk and particularly on the back, several areas in which the skin appears slightly depressed and has a slate-gray color but shows no other surface changes. The lesions are sharply but often irregularly demarcated and measure from 1 to 10 cm in diameter. They often show a "cliff-drop" border, which is largely an optical effect of the slate-gray discoloration. In older lesions the center of the depressed area may feel slightly indurated.

Histopathology. The histologic changes in early lesions usually are slight and nonspecific, consisting of some thickening of the collagen bundles and a mild, scattered chronic inflammatory infiltrate (Quiroga and Woscoff; Weiner and Gant). Older lesions may show in the deeper layers of the dermis collagen bundles that are not only thickened but also appear tightly packed (Jablonska and Szczepanski). Indurated areas may show, in addition, homogeneous, hyalinized collagen bundles (Miller).

Since the collagen bundles in the skin of the back normally are rather thick, it may be difficult to determine whether or not the collagen shows any changes. It is desirable, therefore, to take a biopsy specimen not only from the lesion but also from normal skin, either from an area nearby or from the opposite side. Naturally, subcutaneous fat should be included in the biopsy specimens.

Histogenesis. Some authors believe that atrophoderma of Pasini and Pierini is a disease entity, as suggested by the original describers. Among them are Canizares et al., who regard the late induration occurring in some lesions as a pseudosclerosis. Weiner has pointed out that in atrophoderma the atrophy comes first and possibly later the sclerosis, whereas in morphea the sequence of events is reversed: the sclerosis comes first and the atrophy later. On the other hand, it has been pointed out by authors favoring the identification of atrophoderma of Pasini Pierini with morphea that there are in some instances clinical similarities between morphea and atrophoderma: morphealike induration may not only follow atrophoderma (Miller) but may also precede it (Rupec), or morphea may develop later in other areas of the skin (Kee et al.).

Pierini et al., in reviewing the evidence on hand, have recently suggested that there are two types of atrophoderma: an idiopathic type of atrophoderma, and an atropho-scleroderma secondary to morphea.

Although this compromise may be acceptable to some, the impression remains that the two types proposed by Pierini et al. are one and the same disease. It may be pointed out that an atrophic form of morphea was first described by Gougerot in 1932 as a *forme lilacée non indurée*. However, even though the atrophoderma of Pasini and Pierini probably represents morphea, the term should not be abandoned because of the typical clinical picture it presents.

BIBLIOGRAPHY

Lupus Erythematosus

Abell, E., Black, M. M., and Marks, R.: Immunoglobulin and complement deposits in the skin in inflammatory dermatoses, an immunofluorescence study. Brit. J. Derm., *91*:281, 1974.

Arnold, H. L., Jr., and Tilden, I. L.: Fatal scleroderma with L.E. phenomenon. Arch. Derm., *76*:427, 1957.

Baart de la Faille, H., and Baart de la Faille-Kuyper, E. H.: Immunofluorescent studies of the skin in rosacea. Dermatologica, *139*:49, 1969.

Baldwin, D. S., Lowenstein, J., Rothfield, N. F., *et al.*: The clinical course of the proliferative and membranous forms of lupus nephritis. Ann. Int. Med., *73*:929, 1970.

Barthelmes, H., and Sönnichsen, N.: Differentialdiagnostische Untersuchungen zwischen Lupus erythematodes chronicus discoides und lymphocytärer Infiltration Jessner-Kanof mit Hilfe der Immunofluoreszenz-Histologie. Arch. klin. exp. Derm., *232*:384, 1968.

Bazex, A., Salvador, R., Dupré, A., *et al.*: Ist es berechtigt, die lymphozytäre Infiltration der Haut von Jessner und Kanof als nosologische Einheit anzusehen? Hautarzt, *16*:250, 1965.

Beljaewa, H. F., Smelov, N. S., Sjitsch, L. I., and Trofimova, L. J.: Hautgefässe bei verschiedenen Formen des Lupus erythematosus im Laufe der Behandlung. Derm. Wschr., *154*:631, 1968.

Berk, S. H., and Blank, H.: Ultraviolet light and cytoplasmic tubules in lupus erythematosus. Arch. Derm., *109*:364, 1974.

Bielicky, T., and Trapl, J.: Nichtvernarbender chronischer Erythematodes. Arch. klin. exp. Derm., *217*:438, 1963.

Burnham, T. K.: *In* discussion of Krieger, B. L.: Lymphocytic infiltration of the skin (Jessner). Arch. Derm., *100*:247, 1969.

Burnham, T. K., and Fine, G.: The immunofluorescent "band" test for lupus erythematosus. Arch. Derm., *103*:24, 1971 (I).

————: The immunofluorescent "band" test for lupus erythematosus. Brit. J. Derm., *84*:176, 1971 (II).

Burnham, T. K., Fine, G., and Neblett, T. R.: Immunofluorescent "band" test for lupus erythematosus. Arch. Derm., *102*:42, 1970.

Burnham, T. K., Neblett, T. R., Fine, G., and Bank, P.: The immunofluorescent tumor imprint technique. Arch. Derm., *99*:611, 1969.

Cabré, J., and Steigleder, G. K.: Das Krankheitsbild der lymphozytären Infiltration (Lymphocytic Infiltration) im Sinne von Jessner und Kanof. Arch. klin. exp. Derm., *212*:525, 1961.

Calnan, C. D.: Lymphocytic infiltration of the skin (Jessner). Brit. J. Derm., *69*:169, 1957.

Carnabuci, G. I., Luscombe, H. A., and Stoloff, I. L.: ANA titers in lupus erythematosus and certain chronic dermatoses. Arch. Derm., *95*:247, 1967.

Case Records of the Massachusetts General Hospital, Case 18-1969. New Eng. J. Med., *280*:1009, 1969.

Cawley, E. P., McManus, J. F. A., Lupton, C. H., Jr., and Wheeler, C. E.: An examination of skin from patients with collagen disease utilizing the combined alcian blue–periodic acid Schiff stain. J. Invest. Derm., *27*:389, 1956.

Chorzelski, T., Jablonska, S., and Blaszczyk, M.: Diagnostischer und differentialdiagnostischer Wert der immunpathologischen Untersuchungen bei Erythematodes chronicus. Arch. klin. exp. Derm., *233*:211, 1968.

Christianson, H. B., Brunsting, L. A., and Perry, H. O.: Dermatomyositis. Arch. Derm., *74*:581, 1956.

Copeman, P. W. M., Schroeter, A. L., and Kierland, R. R.: An unusual variant of lupus erythematosus or lichen planus. Brit. J. Derm., *83*:269, 1970.

Dubois, E. L., Chandor, S., Friou, G. J., and Bischel, M.: Progressive systemic sclerosis (PSS) and localized scleroderma (morphea) with positive LE cell test and unusual systemic manifestations compatible with systemic lupus erythematosus (SLE). Medicine, *50*:199, 1971.

Dubois, E. L., and Tuffanelli, D. L.: Clinical manifestations of systemic lupus erythematosus. J.A.M.A., *190*:104, 1964.

Erbslöh, E., and Baedeker, W. D.: Lupus Myopathie. Deutsch. Med. Wschr., *87*:2464, 1962.

Estes, D., and Christian, C. L.: The natural history of systemic lupus erythematosus by prospective analysis. Medicine, *50*:85, 1971.

Everall, J. D., Heptinstall, R. H., and Jockes, A. M.: An early renal lesion in systemic lupus erythematosus. Brit. J. Derm., *70*:44, 1958.

Fisher, D. A., Epstein, J. H., Kay, D. N., and Tuffanelli, D. L.: Polymorphous light eruption and lupus erythematosus. Arch. Derm., *101*:458, 1970.

Fountain, R. B.: Lupus erythematosus profundus. Brit. J. Derm., *80*:571, 1968.

Friedman, I. A., et al.: The L.E. phenomenon in rheumatoid arthritis. Ann. Int. Med., *46*:1113, 1957.

Ginzler, E. M., Nicastri, A. D., Chen, C. K., et al.: Progression of mesangial and focal to diffuse lupus nephritis. New Eng. J. Med., *291*:693, 1974.

Gitlin, D., Craig, J. M., and Janeway, C. A.: Studies on the nature of fibrinoid in the collagen diseases. Am. J. Path., *33*:55, 1957.

Gottlieb, B., and Winkelmann, R. K.: Lymphocytic infiltration of skin. Arch. Derm., *86*: 626, 1962.

Györkey, F., Sinkovics, J. G., Min, K. W., and Györkey, P.: A morphologic study on the occurrence and distribution of structures resembling viral nucleocapsids in collagen diseases. Am. J. Med., *53*:148, 1972.

Hahn, B. H., Yardley, J. H., and Stevens, M. B.: "Rheumatoid" nodules in systemic lupus erythematosus. Ann. Int. Med., *72*:49, 1970.

Haim, S., and Shafrir, A.: The nature of discoid lupus erythematosus. Acta dermatoven., *50*: 86, 1970.

Hargraves, M. M., Richmond, H., and Morton, R. J.: Presentation of two bone marrow elements: the "tart" cell and the "L.E." cell. Proc. Mayo Clin., *23*:25, 1948.

Harvey, A. M., Shulman, L. E., Tumulty, P. A., et al.: Systemic lupus erythematosus: Review of the literature and clinical analysis of 138 cases. Medicine, *33*:291, 1954.

Hashimoto, K., and Thompson, D. F.: Discoid lupus erythematosus. Electron microscopic studies of paramyxovirus-like structures. Arch. Derm., *101*:565, 1970.

Haustein, U. F.: Membranlose fibrilläre und amorph-granuläre Körper bei Lupus erythematodes. Derm. Wschr., *159*:185, 1973.

Jablonska, S., Chorzelski, T., and Maciejowska, E.: The scope and limitations of the immunofluorescence method in the diagnosis of lupus erythematosus. Brit. J. Derm., *83*:242, 1970.

Jessner, M., and Kanof, N. B.: Lymphocytic infiltration of the skin. Arch. Derm., *68*:447, 1953.

Kellum, R. E., and Haserick, J. R.: Systemic lupus erythematosus: statistical evaluation of mortality based on consecutive series of 299 patients. Arch. Int. Med., *113*:200, 1964.

Klemperer, P., Pollack, A. D., and Baehr, G.: Pathology of disseminated lupus erythematosus. Arch. Path., *32*:569, 1941 (review of the pathology of visceral lesions).

Koffler, D., Agnello, V., Carr, R. I., and Kunkel, H. G.: Variable patterns of immunoglobulins and complement deposition in the kidneys of patients with systemic lupus erythematosus. Am. J. Path., *56*:305, 1969.

Lester, R. S., Burnham, T. K., Fine, G., and Murray, K.: Immunologic concepts of light reactions in lupus erythematosus and polymorphous light eruptions. Arch. Derm., *96*:1, 1967.

Maciejewski, W., Dabrowski, J., Jablonska, S., and Jakubowicz, K.: Virus-like tubular cytoplasmic inclusions in epithelial tumors. Dermatologica, *146*:141, 1973.

Marten, R. H., and Blackburn, E. K.: Lupus erythematosus. Arch. Derm., *73*:1, 1953.

McCreight, W. G., and Montgomery, H.: Cutaneous changes in lupus erythematosus. Arch. Derm. Syph., *61*:1, 1950.

McDuffie, F. C.: Twenty years of the lupus erythematosus cell. Ann. Int. Med., *70*:413, 1969.

Muehrke, R. C., Kark, R. M., Pirani, C. L., and Pollak, V. E.: Lupus nephritis; a clinical and pathologic study based on renal biopsies. Medicine, *36*:1, 1957.

Nebe, H., and Barthelmes, H.: Über den diagnostischen Wert der subepidermalen Immunoglobulin- und Komplementablagerungen beim Lupus erythematodes. Derm. Monatsschr., *159*:594, 1973.

Pascher, F., Sims, C. F., and Pensky, N.: Lupus erythematosus profundus (Kaposi-Irgang). J. Invest. Derm., *25*:347, 1955.

Paull, A. M.: Occurrence of the "L.E." phenomenon in a patient with a severe penicillin reaction. New Eng. J. Med., *252*:128, 1955.

Petersen, W. C., Jr., and Fusaro, R. M.: Antinuclear factor in light sensitivity and lupus erythematosus. Arch. Derm., *87*:563, 1963.

Petersen, W. C., Jr., and Gokcen, M.: Antinuclear factors in chronic discoid lupus erythematosus. Arch. Derm., *86*:783, 1962.

Pincus, T., Schur, P. H., Rose, J. A., et al.: Measurement of serum DNA-binding activity in systemic lupus erythematosus. New Eng. J. Med., *281*:701, 1969.

Pohle, E. L., and Tuffanelli, D. L.: Study of cutaneous lupus erythematosus. Arch. Derm., *97*:520, 1968.

Pollack, V. E.: Antinuclear antibodies in families of patients with systemic lupus erythematosus. New Eng. J. Med., *271*:165, 1964.

Pruniéras, M., and Montgomery, H.: Histopathology of cutaneous lesions in systemic lupus erythematosus. Arch. Derm., *74*:177, 1956 (review).

Ropes, M.: Observations on the natural course of disseminated lupus erythematosus. Medicine, *43*:387, 1964.

Rowell, N. R.: Laboratory abnormalities in the diagnosis and management of lupus erythematosus. Brit. J. Derm., *84*:210, 1971.

Schirren, C. G., and Eggert, D.: Beitrag zum Erythematodes profundus (Kaposi-Irgang). Arch. klin. exp. Derm., *216*:541, 1963.

Scott, A., and Rees, E. G.: The relationship of systemic lupus erythematosus and discoid lupus erythematosus. Arch. Derm., *79*:422, 1959.

Sharp, G. C., Irwin, W. S., Tan, E. M., *et al.*: Mixed connective tissue disease, an apparently distinct rheumatic disease syndrome associated with a specific antibody to an extractable nuclear antigen (ENA). Am. J. Med., *52*: 148, 1972.

Storck, H., and Berzups, S.: Über Lupus erythematodes unter besonderer Berücksichtigung des Überganges von lokalisierten in generalisierte Formen. Dermatologica, *124*: 142, 1962.

Stoughton, R., and Wells, G.: A histochemical study on polysaccharides in normal and diseased skin. J. Invest. Derm., *14*:37, 1950.

Tuffanelli, D. L.: Lupus erythematosus panniculitis (profundus). Arch. Derm., *103*:231, 1971.

Tuffanelli, D. L., Kay, D., and Fukuyama, K.: Dermal-epidermal junction in lupus erythematosus. Arch. Derm., *99*:652, 1969.

Ueki, H.: The application of the fluorescent antibody technique in dermatology. Jap. J. Derm., Series B, *78*:367, 1968.

————: Hyaline bodies in subepidermal papillae. Arch. Derm., *100*:610, 1969.

Ueki, H., Wolff, H. H., and Braun-Falco, O.: Cutaneous localization of human gammaglobulins in lupus erythematosus. Arch. derm. Forsch., *248*:297, 1974.

von Eickstedt, U. M., and Hassenpflug, K. H.: Zur Kenntnis des Lupus erythematodes hypertrophicus (et profundus) Bechet. Arch. klin. exp. Derm., *214*:471, 1962.

Weiss, R. S., and Swift, S.: The significance of a positive L.E. phenomenon. Arch. Derm., *72*: 103, 1955.

Winkelmann, R. K.: Panniculitis and systemic lupus erythematosus. J.A.M.A., *211*:472, 1970.

Worthington, J. M., Baggenstoss, A. H., and Hargraves, M. M.: Significance of hematoxylin bodies in the necropsy diagnosis of systemic lupus erythematosus. Am. J. Path., *35*:955, 1959.

Dermatomyositis, Poikiloderma Atrophicans Vasculare

Arundel, F. D., Wilkinson, R. D., and Haserick, J. R.: Dermatomyositis and malignant neoplasms in adults. Arch. Derm., *82*:164, 1960.

Banker, B. Q., and Victor, M.: Dermatomyositis (systemic angiopathy) of childhood. Medicine, *45*:261, 1966.

Christianson, H. B., Brunsting, L. A., and Perry, H. O.: Dermatomyositis. Arch. Derm., *74*: 581, 1956.

Curtis, A. C., Blaylock, H. C., and Harrell, E. R., Jr.: Malignant lesions associated with dermatomyositis. J.A.M.A., *150*:844, 1952.

Degos, R., Civatte, J., Belaich, S., and Delarue, A.: The prognosis of adult dermatomyositis. Trans. St. John's Hosp. Derm. Soc., *57*:98, 1971.

Dowling, G. B., and Freudenthal, W.: Dermatomyositis and poikiloderma atrophicans vasculare: a clinical and histological comparison. Brit. J. Derm., *50*:519, 1938.

Downing, J. G., Edelstein, J. M., and Fitzpatrick, T. B.: Poikiloderma vasculare atrophicans. Arch. Derm. Syph., *56*:740, 1947.

Gonzalez-Angulo, A., Fraga, A., and Mintz, G.: Submicroscopic alterations in capillaries of skeletal muscles in polymyositis. Am. J. Med., *45*:873, 1968.

Guy, W. H., Grauer, R. C., and Jacob, F. M.: Poikilodermatomyositis. Arch. Derm. Syph., *40*:867, 1939.

Hashimoto, K., Robinson, L., Velayos, E., and Niizuma, K.: Dermatomyositis. Electron microscopic, immunologic, and tissue culture studies of paramyxovirus-like inclusions. Arch. Derm., *103*:120, 1971.

Horn, R. C., Jr.: Poikilodermatomyositis. Arch. Derm. Syph., *44*:1086, 1941.

Janis, J. F., and Winkelmann, R. K.: Histopathology of the skin in dermatomyositis. Arch. Derm., *97*:640, 1968.

Kinney, T. D., and Maher, M. M.: Dermatomyositis. Am. J. Path., *16*:561, 1940.

Logan, R. G., Bandera, J. M., Mikkelsen, W. M., and Duff, I. F.: Polymyositis: a clinical study. Ann. Int. Med., *65*:996, 1966.

Medsger, T. A., Jr., Dawson, W. N., Jr., and Masi, A. T.: The epidemiology of polymyositis. Am. J. Med., *48*:715, 1970.

Mintz, G., Gonzalez-Angulo, A., and Fraga, A.: Ultrastructure of muscle in polymyositis. Am. J. Med., *44*:216, 1968.

Muller, S. A., Winkelmann, R. K., and Brunsting, L. A.: Calcinosis in dermatomyositis. Arch. Derm., *79*:669, 1959.

O'Leary, P. A., and Waisman, M.: Dermatomyositis: A study of forty cases. Arch. Derm. Syph., *41*:1001, 1940 (review).

Pearson, C. M.: Treatment of polymyositis and dermatomyositis. Mod. Treatment, *49*:789, 1966.

Reich, H.: Das Teutschlaender-Syndrom. Hautarzt, *14*:462, 1963.

Rose, A. L., and Walton, J. N.: Polymyositis: A survey of 89 cases with particular reference to treatment and prognosis. Brain, *89*:747, 1966.

Shafiq, S. A., Milhorat, A. T., and Gorycki, M. A.: Electron microscope study of muscular degeneration and vascular changes in polymyositis. J. Path., *94*:139, 1967.

Steigleder, G. K.: Die Poikilodermien—Genodermien und Genodermatosen? Arch. f. Derm. u. Syph., *194*:461, 1952.

Vignos, P. J., Bowling, G. F., and Watkins, M. P.: Polymyositis. Arch. Int. Med., *114*:263, 1964.

Wainger, C. K., and Lever, W. F.: Dermatomyositis: a report of three cases with postmortem observations. Arch. Derm. Syph., *59*:196, 1949.

Weston, W. L., and Thorne, E. G.: Profound T lymphopenia in dermatomyositis with cancer. New Eng. J. Med., *291*:208, 1974.

Williams, R. C.: Dermatomyositis and malignancy: a review of the literature. Ann. Int. Med., *50*:1174, 1959.

Scleroderma

Alpert, L. I., and Warner, R. R. P.: Systemic sclerosis. Am. J. Med., *45*:468, 1968.

Black, M. M., Bottoms, E., and Shuster, S.: Skin collagen content and thickness in systemic sclerosis. Brit. J. Derm., *83*:552, 1970.

Braun-Falco, O.: Über das Verhalten der interfibrillären Grundsubstanz bei Sklerodermie. Derm. Wschr., *136*:1085, 1957.

Burnham, T. K., Neblett, T. R., and Fine, G.: The immunofluorescent tumor imprint technic. III. The diagnostic and prognostic significance of the "speckle"-inducing antinuclear antibody. Am. J. Clin. Path., *50*:683, 1968.

Canizares, O., Sachs, P. M., Jaimovich, L., and Torres, V. M.: Idiopathic atrophoderma of Pasini and Pierini. Arch. Derm., *77*:42, 1958.

Cannon, P. J., Hassar, M., Case, D. B., et al.: The relationship of hypertension and renal failure in scleroderma (progressive systemic sclerosis) to structural and functional abnormalities of the renal cortical circulation. Medicine, *53*:1, 1974.

Carr, R. D., Heisel, E. B., and Stevenson, T. D.: CRST syndrome. Arch. Derm., *92*:519, 1965.

Christianson, H. B., Dorsey, C. S., O'Leary, P. A., and Kierland, R. R.: Localized scleroderma. Arch. Derm., *74*:629, 1956.

Collins, D. H., Darke, C. S., and Dodge, O. G.: Scleroderma with honeycomb lungs and bronchiolar carcinoma. J. Path. Bact., *76*:531, 1958.

D'Angelo, W. A., Fries, J. F., Masi, A. T., and Shulman, L. E.: Pathologic observations in systemic sclerosis (scleroderma). Am. J. Med., *46*:428, 1969.

Dilley, J. J., and Perry, H. O.: Bilateral linear scleroderma en coup de sabre. Arch. Derm., *97*:688, 1968.

Driessen, W., Hornstein, O., and Orfanos, K.: Morphea systematisata mit Hemiatrophie. Derm. Wschr., *152*:75, 1966.

Fisher, E. R., and Rodnan, G. P.: Pathologic observations concerning the kidney in progressive systemic sclerosis. Arch. Path., *65*:29, 1958.

Fleischmajer, R., Damiano, V., and Nedwich, A.: Alteration of subcutaneous tissue in systemic scleroderma. Arch. Derm., *105*:59, 1972.

Fleischmajer, R., and Nedwich, A.: Generalized morphea. I. Histology of the dermis and subcutaneous tissue. Arch. Derm., *106*:509, 1972.

Getzowa, S.: Cystic and compact pulmonary sclerosis in progressive scleroderma. Arch. Path., *40*:99, 1945.

Gougerot, H.: Sclérodermie atypique. La forme lilacée non indurée en plaques ou en bandes. Bull. Soc. franç. derm. syph., *39*:1667, 1932.

Grabner, K.: Zur Frage der Übergangsformen zwischen Morphaea und progressiver Sklerodermie. Derm. Wschr., *154*:625, 1968.

Haggani, M. T., and Holti, G.: Systemic sclerosis with pulmonary fibrosis and oat cell carcinoma. Acta Dermatoven., *53*:369. 1973.

Hayes, R. L., and Rodnan, G. P.: The ultrastructure of skin in progressive sclerosis (scleroderma). Am. J. Path., *63*:433, 1971.

Hickman, J. W., and Sheils, W. S.: Progressive facial hemiatrophy. Arch. Int. Med., *113*:716, 1964.

Jablonska, S., and Szczepanski, A.: Atrophoderma Pasini-Pierini: is it an entity? Dermatologica, *125*:226, 1962.

Kanee, B.: Scleropoikiloderma with calcinosis cutis, Raynaud-like syndrome and atrophoderma. Arch. Derm. Syph., *50*:254, 1944.

Kee, C. E., Brothers, W. S., and New, W.: Idiopathic atrophoderma of Pasini and Pierini with coexistent morphea. Arch. Derm., *82*:100, 1960.

Keiser, H. R., Stein, H. D., and Sjoerdsma, A.: Increased protocollagen proline hydroxylase activity in sclerodermatous skin. Arch. Derm., *104*:57, 1971.

Kobayasi, T., and Asboe-Hansen, G.: Ultrastructure of generalized scleroderma. Acta dermatoven., *52*:81, 1972.

Korting, G. W., and Lachner, H.: Sclerodermia malabsorptiva. Hautarzt, *23*:12, 1972.

Lawrence, H.: Scleroderma, circumscribed. Arch. Derm., *54*:363, 1946.

Medsger, T. A., Masi, A. T., Rodnan, G. P., *et al.*: Survival with systemic sclerosis (scleroderma). Ann. Int. Med., *75*:369, 1971.

Miller, R. F.: Idiopathic atrophoderma. Arch. Derm., *92*:653, 1965 (review).

Muller, S. A., Brunsting, L. A., and Winkelmann, R. K.: Calcinosis cutis: its relationship to scleroderma. Arch. Derm., *80*:15, 1959.

Norton, W. L., and Nardo, J. M.: Vascular disease in progressive systemic sclerosis (scleroderma). Ann. Int. Med., *73*:317, 1970.

O'Leary, P. A., Montgomery, H., and Ragsdale, W. E.: Dermatohistopathology of various types of scleroderma. Arch. Derm., *75*:78, 1957 (review).

Pasini, A.: Atrofodermia idiopatica progressiva. G. Ital. Derm. Sif., *58*:785, 1923.

Pierini, L. E., Abulafia, J., and Mosto, S. J.: Atrophodermie idiopathique progressive et états voisins. Ann. derm. syph., *97*:391, 1970.

Pierini, L. E., and Vivoli, D.: Atrofodermia idiopatica progressiva (Pasini). G. Ital. Derm. Sif., *77*:403, 1936.

Piper, W. N., and Helwig, E. B.: Progressive systemic sclerosis. Arch. Derm., *72*:535, 1955.

Quiroga, M. I., and Woscoff, A.: L'atrophodermie idiopathique progressive (Pasini-Pierini) et la sclérodermie atypique lilacée non indurée (Gougerot). Ann. Derm. Syph., *88*:507, 1961.

Rowell, N. R., and Beck, J. S.: The diagnostic value of an antinuclear antibody test in clinical dermatology. Arch. Derm., *96*:290, 1967.

Rupec, M.: Über die Beziehungen der zirkumskripten Sklerodermie zum Morbus Pasini-Pierini. Z. Haut Geschlechtskr., *33*:114, 1962.

Rosenthal, D. S., and Sack, B.. Autoimmune hemolytic anemia in scleroderma. J.A.M.A., *216*:2011, 1971.

Stava, Z.: Zirkumskripte Sklerodermie. Derm. Wschr., *139*:513, 1959.

Tomkin, G. H.: Systemic sclerosis associated with carcinoma of the lung. Brit. J. Derm., *81*:213, 1969.

Toth, A., and Alpert, L. I.: Progressive systemic sclerosis terminating as periarteritis nodosa. Arch. Path., *92*:31, 1971.

Tuffanelli, D. L., and Winkelmann, R. K.: Systemic scleroderma. Arch. Derm., *84*:359, 1961.

Uitto, J., Helin, G., Helin, P., and Lorenzen, I.: Connective tissue in scleroderma. Acta dermatoven., *51*:401, 1971.

Weidner, F., and Braun-Falco, O.: Gleichzeitiges Vorkommen von Symptomen der circumscripten und progressiven Sklerodermie. Hautarzt, *19*:345, 1968.

Weiner, M.: *In* discussion to Eshelman, O. M.: Idiopathic atrophoderma of Pasini and Pierini. Arch. Derm., *92*:737, 1965.

Weiner, M. A., and Gant, J. Q., Jr.: Idiopathic atrophoderma of Pasini and Pierini in two brothers. Arch. Derm., *80*:195, 1959.

25

Tumors and Cysts of the Epidermis

CLASSIFICATION OF TUMORS OF THE EPIDERMIS

Epidermal tumors can be divided into tumors of the surface epidermis and tumors of the epidermal appendages. In each of the two classes benign and malignant tumors occur.

Benign tumors in general are characterized by (1) uniformity in the appearance of the tumor cell nuclei; (2) architectural order in the arrangement of the tumor cell nuclei; (3) restraint in the ratio of growth; and (4) absence of metastases.

Malignant tumors, on the other hand, are characterized by (1) atypicality in the appearance of the tumor cell nuclei that is evident as pleomorphism, i.e., great variability in size and shape, and anaplasia, i.e., hyperplasia and hyperchromasia, (2) architectural disorder in the arrangement of the tumor cell nuclei with loss of polarity; (3) rapid growth with presence of mitoses, including atypical mitoses; and (4) potentiality to give rise to metastases.

Of the four criteria of malignancy just cited only the potentiality to give rise to metastases is decisive evidence for the malignancy of a tumor. For metastases to form, the tumor cells must possess a degree of autonomy that nonmalignant cells do not have. This autonomy enables malignant tumor cells to induce foreign tissue to furnish the necessary stroma in which they can multiply.

In addition to malignant tumors one finds in the surface epidermis so-called premalignant tumors, better referred to as tumors located largely in situ. Thus, even though they are cytologically malignant, they are biologically still benign.

The tumors of the surface epidermis may be classified as follows:

1. Benign Tumors
   Localized linear epidermal nevus
   Inflammatory linear epidermal nevus
   Systematized linear epidermal nevus
   Oral epithelial nevus
   Seborrheic keratosis
   Clear cell acanthoma
   Epidermal, pilar, and dermoid cysts
   Steatocystoma multiplex
   Warty dyskeratoma
   Keratoacanthoma
2. Precancerous Tumors
   (located largely in situ)
   Solar keratosis
   Leukoplakia
   Oral florid papillomatosis
   Bowen's disease
   Erythroplasia of Queyrat
3. Carcinomas
   Squamous cell carcinoma
   Paget's disease

LOCALIZED LINEAR EPIDERMAL NEVUS

There are three types of linear epidermal or verrucous nevi: the localized type, with a histologic picture of a papilloma, the inflam-

FIG. 25-1. **Linear epidermal nevus.** There are hyperkeratosis, papillomatosis, and acanthosis with elongation of the rete ridges.

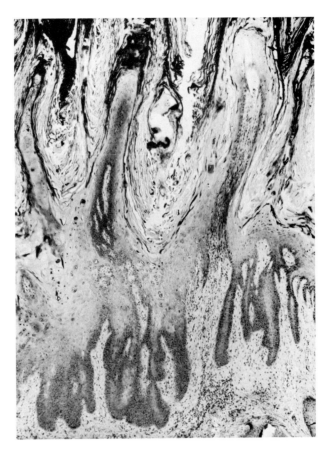

matory type, with a "dermatitic" histologic appearance; and the extensive or systematized type, in which the histologic picture may be that of a papilloma although often it shows "granular degeneration" of the epidermis indistinguishable from that seen in the dominant or bullous type of congenital ichthyosiform erythroderma. All three types of linear epidermal nevus either are present at birth or appear in early childhood.

In the localized type of linear epidermal nevus only one linear lesion is present as a rule. It consists of closely set, papillomatous, hyperkeratotic papules. It may be located anywhere: on the head, the trunk, or the extremities. Being located on only one side of the patient it often is referred to as *nevus unius lateris*.

Histopathology. The localized type of linear epidermal or verrucous nevus shows hyperkeratosis, papillomatosis, and acanthosis with elongation of the rete ridges (Fig.

25-1). Thus, the histologic picture is that of a papilloma (Pack and Sunderland).

The papillomatous changes seen in the localized type of linear epidermal nevus may be found in association with nevus sebaceus or syringocystadenoma papilliferum, especially in lesions located on the scalp or face (Haber).

Differential Diagnosis. The histologic picture of the localized type of linear epidermal nevus must be differentiated from that of other papillomas, i.e., solar keratosis, seborrheic keratosis, verruca vulgaris and acanthosis nigricans. These five diseases show hyperkeratosis and papillomatosis. In typical cases differentiation is easy, but occasionally one is unable to make a diagnosis any more specific in these diseases than papilloma.

In typical instances solar keratosis differs from the localized type of linear epidermal nevus by showing atypicality and disorder of the epidermal cells, and often also irregular downward budding of the epidermis. Seborrheic keratosis in most cases shows, in addition to typical squamous cells, accumulations of small basophilic cells resembling the basal cells of the basal layer of the epidermis, so-called basaloid cells. Furthermore, the epidermis often contains pseudohorncysts as well as horncysts. Verruca vulgaris usually shows groups of large vacuolated cells in the upper stratum malpighii and granular layer, and also intermittent areas of parakeratosis. Acanthosis nigricans as a rule shows less acanthosis and less elongation of the rete ridges than the localized type of linear epidermal nevus.

NEVUS COMEDONICUS

Nevus comedonicus, like localized linear epidermal nevus, usually has a linear configuration and occurs as a single lesion, although occasionally it shows bilateral linear lesions (Fritsch and Wittels), or randomly distributed rather than linear lesions (Paige and Mendelson). It consists of closely set, slightly elevated papules that have in their center a dark, firm, hyperkeratotic plug resembling a comedo.

Histopathology. Each comedo is represented by a wide and deep invagination of the epidermis filled with keratin. These invaginations resemble dilated hair follicles and, as evidence that the invaginations actually do represent rudimentary hair follicles, one occasionally finds at their base one or even several hair shafts (Fritsch and Wittels). Also one or two small sebaceous gland lobules may be seen opening into the lower pole of the invaginations (Paige and Mendelson).

INFLAMMATORY LINEAR EPIDERMAL NEVUS

This persistent linear, pruritic lesion is composed of red, scaling, often slightly verrucous papules arranged in one or several lines. The usual time of onset is early childhood. The most common location is one of the lower extremities.

Histopathology. The histologic picture is essentially that of a nonspecific chronic dermatitis. One observes hyperkeratosis with foci of parakeratosis, moderate to marked acanthosis, elongation of the rete ridges, and occasionally slight spongiosis (Kaidbey and Kurban; Altman and Mehregan). The dermis shows a chronic inflammatory infiltrate.

Differential Diagnosis. Although the inflammatory linear epidermal nevus resembles lichen striatus in its clinical appearance, it differs from it by its persistence. Histologically it differs from lichen striatus by the presence of acanthosis (Kaidbey and Kurban).

SYSTEMATIZED LINEAR EPIDERMAL NEVUS

Papillomatous hyperkeratotic papules in a linear configuration are present, as in localized linear epidermal nevus; but instead of one linear lesion there are many linear lesions. On the trunk they often show a parallel arrangement. The linear lesions may be limited to one side of the patient or may show a bilateral, symmetrical distribution, in which case the designation *ichthyosis hystrix* is often applied.

Systematized linear epidermal nevus frequently is associated with skeletal deformities and central nervous system disease, such as mental retardation, epilepsy, and neural deafness (Solomon et al.) (see also p. 501).

Histopathology. Most cases with unilateral systematized linear epidermal nevus and some cases of bilateral systematized linear nevus merely show hyperkeratosis, papillomatosis and acanthosis, just as is seen in localized linear nevus (Solomon et al.).

Frequently, however, in bilateral and occasionally also in unilateral systematized linear epidermal nevus one observes the rather striking histologic picture of "granular degeneration" of the epidermis, also referred to as "epidermolytic hyperkeratosis," as seen also in all cases of dominant or bullous congenital ichthyosiform erythroderma (see p. 60). The salient histologic features in formalin-fixed sections stained with hematoxylin and eosin are: (1) shrinking of the cytoplasm of epidermal cells resulting in perinuclear vacuolization; (2) indistinct cellular boundaries formed by lightly staining material and by keratohyaline granules; and (3) premature and excessive formation of irregularly shaped keratohyaline granules and hyperkeratosis (Zeligman and Pomeranz; Braun-Falco et al.).

It is of interest that the histologic picture of "granular degeneration" of the epidermis or of "epidermolytic hyperkeratosis" is seen occasionally also in the dominantly inherited keratosis palmo-plantaris circumscripta of Unna-Thost (Klaus et al.; Orbaneja et al.) (see p. 63) and occurs regularly in the solitary epidermolytic acanthoma (see below).

Histogenesis. A systematized linear epidermal nevus may be dominantly inherited. Also the occurrence in the same family of both an extensive systematized linear epidermal nevus and of the dominantly inherited bullous type of congenital ichthyosiform erythroderma has been reported (Barker and Sachs). This and the fact that the histologic picture is the same in both diseases suggests a relationship between them, even though bullous lesions do not occur in systematized linear epidermal nevi. The two diseases probably represent different expressions of a pleiotropic, dominant gene (Weibel and Schnyder).

Studies carried out by Braun-Falco et al. on cryostat sections and by electron microscopy have shown that shrinking of the cytoplasm and vacuolization of the epidermal cells seen in routinely processed sections of systematized linear epidermal nevi is largely an artifact, just as it is in dominant congenital ichthyosiform erythroderma (see p. 61). Frozen sections show merely widening of the intercellular spaces; and electron microscopy shows, as it does also in dominant congenital ichthyosiform erythroderma, premature aggregation of tonofilament bundles in which are embedded keratohyaline granules formed prematurely and in excess.

SOLITARY AND DISSEMINATED EPIDERMOLYTIC ACANTHOMA

Solitary epidermolytic acanthoma, histologically characterized by the presence of "epidermolytic hyperkeratosis," does not have a characteristic clinical appearance or location. It is a papillomatous lesion, usually less than 1 cm in diameter (Shapiro and Baraf). In addition, "epidermolytic hyperkeratosis" may occur as an incidental histologic finding in several different types of solitary lesions, such as seborrheic or solar keratosis (Ackerman) (see p. 470).

Disseminated epidermolytic acanthoma occurs as a randomly distributed eruption consisting of multiple elevated skin-colored verrucoid papules, 2 to 6 mm in diameter (Hirone and Fukushiro).

Histopathology. In addition to hyperkeratosis and papillomatosis, there is pronounced "granular degeneration" or "epidermolytic hyperkeratosis" throughout the stratum malpighii, sparing only the basal layer, just as it is seen in systematized linear epidermal nevi. Routinely fixed sections show both intracellular and intercellular edema of the epidermal cells with keratohyaline granules being coarser than normal, and extending to a greater depth in the stratum malpighii (Shapiro and Baraf). The epidermis at the margins of the lesion may be raised like a wall or lip above the central keratin-filled crater (Gebhart and Kidd).

Differential Diagnosis. As pointed out by Shapiro and Baraf, verrucae vulgares may show a type of "granular degeneration" similar to that seen in epidermolytic hyperkeratosis. However, even though both show perinuclear vacuolization, epidermolytic acanthoma, like other dermatoses with epidermolytic hyperkeratosis, shows more pronounced intercellular edema than verruca vulgaris, extending to a greater depth in the stratum malpighii. Furthermore, it lacks the large parakeratotic nuclei commonly present in verrucae.

ORAL EPITHELIAL NEVUS

This condition, described by Cannon in 1935 as "white spongy nevus of the oral mucosa," often is dominantly inherited. It may be present at birth or may appear in childhood. It reaches its full extent in adolescence. Extensive areas of the oral mucosa and sometimes the entire oral mucosa have a thickened, folded, creamy white appearance. In some instances, also the rectal mucosa (Cannon), the vagina (Zegarelli et al.), the nasal mucosa (Witkop and Gorlin), or the esophagus (Haye and Whitehead) is involved. Malignant degeneration is not known to occur.

The oral lesions seen in pachyonychia congenita are indistinguishable from an oral epithelial nevus both clinically and histologically (Witkop and Gorlin) (see p. 63).

Histopathology. The oral epithelium shows hyperplasia with much more pronounced hydropic swelling of the epithelial cells than is normal for the oral mucosa. The swelling often is focal (Cooke and Morgan). It extends into the rete ridges but spares the basal layer (Stüttgen et al.). The surface shows parakeratosis, as the normal oral mucosa does; and only rarely are there small accumulations of keratohyaline granules (Zegarelli et al.).

Differential Diagnosis. Differentiation from oral leukoplakia is generally easy because in leukoplakia, in contrast with oral epithelial nevus, the epithelial cells show loss of polarity, the nuclei show evidence of atypicality, and furthermore the dermis shows a fairly pronounced inflammatory reaction. Differentiation from oral florid papillomatosis may be difficult, although as a rule oral florid papillomatosis shows a papillomatous rather than a smooth surface and a fairly pronounced inflammatory infiltrate beneath the epithelium.

LINGUA GEOGRAPHICA

The dorsum of the tongue shows irregularly shaped red patches surrounded by a whitish, raised border a few millimeters wide. The patches change their configuration from day to day.

Histopathology. Whereas the dorsum of the tongue normally shows a stratum corneum (see p. 13), this is largely absent in the red patches of lingua geographica. Along the whitish border the epithelium is permeated with neutrophils. In the upper portion of the epithelium the neutrophils have accumulated within the interstices of a sponge-like network formed by degenerated and thinned epithelial cells (Dawson). The histologic picture thus shows Kogoj's spongiform pustules that are indistinguishable from those seen in pustular psoriasis.

Although O'Keefe et al. believe that there is some clinical resemblance between lingua geographica and the lesions on the tongue in severe pustular psoriasis, the evidence is not sufficient, aside from the spongiform pustule, to support a relationship between lingua geographica and psoriasis.

SEBORRHEIC KERATOSIS

Seborrheic keratoses are a very common lesion. They are seen, often in large number, on the trunk, the face, and the extremities with the exception of the palms and soles. Seborrheic keratoses, though dominantly inherited, usually do not appear before middle

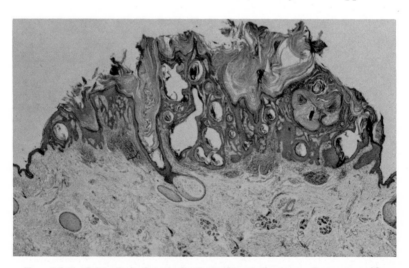

Fig. 25-2. **Seborrheic keratosis, hyperkeratotic type.** Low magnification. The lower border of the tumor in general follows a straight line that could be drawn from the normal epidermis at one end of the tumor to the normal epidermis at the other end. (×25)

age. They are sharply demarcated, brownish in color and slightly raised so that they look as if stuck on the surface of the skin. Most of them have a verrucous surface, with the verrucous covering having a soft, friable consistency. Some, however, have a smooth surface but characteristically show keratotic plugs. Although most lesions measure only a few millimeters in diameter, occasionally a lesion may reach a size of several centimeters. Crusting and an inflammatory base are found if the lesion has been subjected to irritation.

Histopathology. Seborrheic keratoses occur in three histologic types: hyperkeratotic, acanthotic, and adenoid (Braun-Falco and Kint). Often more than one type is found in the same lesion. In addition to these three types, the histologic appearance of the irritated seborrheic keratosis deserves separate mention, since it differs from that of a non-irritated seborrheic keratosis. In addition, there are two clinical variants of seborrheic keratosis that will be described subsequently. They are: dermatosis papulosa nigra, and stucco keratosis.

The three histologic types of seborrheic keratosis have in common hyperkeratosis, acanthosis, and papillomatosis. The acanthosis is due entirely to the upward growth of epidermal cells. Thus, the lower border of the tumor is even and lies on a straight line that may be drawn from the normal epidermis at one end of the tumor to the normal epidermis at the other end (Fig. 25-2). Two types of cells are seen in the acanthotic epidermis: squamous cells and basaloid cells. The former have the appearance of the squamous cells normally found in the epidermis, whereas the basaloid cells are small and uniform in appearance and have a relatively large nucleus. In areas of slight intercellular edema intercellular bridges can be easily recognized (Andrade and Steigleder). Thus, they resemble the basal cells found normally in the basal layer of the epidermis.

In the *hyperkeratotic type* of seborrheic keratosis, hyperkeratosis and papillomatosis are pronounced, while acanthosis is less conspicuous. In some lesions the upward extension of papillae lined with epidermis causes

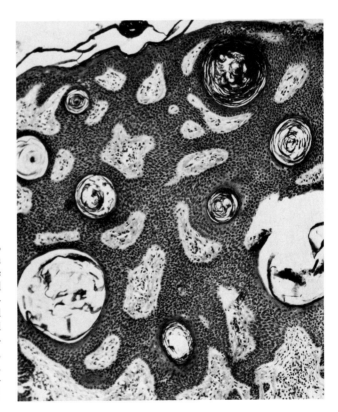

FIG. 25-3. **Seborrheic keratosis, acanthotic type.** Thick interwoven tracts of epidermal cells compose the tumor. Most of the epidermal cells have the appearance of epidermal basal cells. They are referred to as basaloid cells. Interspersed are cystic inclusions of horny material representing either horn cysts, when they form within the tumor, or pseudohorncysts, when they represent horny invaginations. (×100)

circumscribed elevations of the epidermis, resembling church spires. This histologic picture is identical with that seen in acrokeratosis verruciformis of Hopf (see p. 76). In other lesions of the hyperkeratotic type the greatly thickened horny layer invaginates the epidermis in some areas. Because of the tortuosity of these invaginations, they often appear in histologic sections as cystic inclusions of horny material. They are known as pseudohorncysts (Fig. 25-3). The epidermis consists largely of squamous cells, although here and there small aggregates of basaloid cells are seen.

In the *acanthotic type,* hyperkeratosis and papillomatosis often are slight, but the epidermis is greatly thickened. Although in some cases only narrow papillae are included in the thickened epidermis, one can see in other lesions a retiform pattern composed of thick, interwoven tracts of epithelial cells surrounding islands of connective tissue (Fig. 25-3). Horny invaginations that on cross sections appear as pseudohorncysts are numerous. In addition there also are true horn cysts showing, like the pseudohorncysts, sudden and complete keratinization. The true horn cysts begin as foci of orthokeratosis within the substance of the lesion (Sanderson). In time they enlarge and by the current of epidermal cells are carried toward the surface of the lesion where the

horn cysts unite with the invaginations of surface keratin. In the greatly thickened epidermis basaloid cells usually outnumber the squamous cells. Not infrequently, well defined nests of basaloid cells may be seen within the epidermis surrounded by squamous cells. In such cases the histologic picture has been erroneously interpreted in the past by some authors as representing an intraepidermal basal cell epithelioma of Borst-Jadassohn (Mehregan and Pinkus) (see p. 547).

In the *adenoid type* of seborrheic keratosis numerous thin tracts of epidermal cells extend from the epidermis and show branching and interweaving in the dermis. Most of the tracts are composed of a double row of basaloid cells (Fig. 25-4). Horn cysts and pseudohorncysts are absent in purely adenoid formations; but, since the adenoid type often also shows areas of the acanthotic type, horn cysts and pseudohorncysts are commonly seen in areas of the latter type.

The amount of melanin is variable. In lesions of the adenoid type pigmentation usually is pronounced, whereas lesions of the hyperkeratotic type often lack excess amounts of pigment. Lesions of the acanthotic type may or may not show hyperpigmentation. In a series of cases comprising all three histologic types, Becker found hyperpigmentation in 32 per cent of specimens

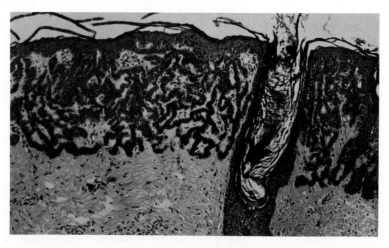

FIG. 25-4. **Seborrheic keratosis, adenoid type.** Thin interwoven tracts composed of a double row of epidermal basal cells compose the tumor. No cystic inclusions of horny material are present. (×100)

stained with hematoxylin and eosin, whereas Lennox on staining with silver found it in 67 per cent of his cases. On staining with dopa, melanocytes are found to be located largely between the basal cells, but in about 30 per cent of the specimens melanocytes are found also in a suprabasal position (Molokhia and Portnoy). In most pigmented seborrheic keratoses nearly all the melanin is found to be present in the keratinocytes, analogous to the situation in the normal epidermis (Lund; Molokhia and Portnoy). In one rather rare histologic variant of seborrheic keratosis, however, referred to as *melanoacanthoma* by Mishima and Pinkus, one finds numerous large, richly dendritic melanocyts distributed throughout the lesion and containing great amounts of melanin, whereas the keratinocytes contain hardly any melanin. Since the melanin in ordinary seborrheic keratoses is found predominantly within the tumor cells, Mishima and Pinkus believe that melanoacanthoma

represents a different entity. However, it appears likely from the histologic description that melanoacanthomas usually are irritated seborrheic keratoses (see below). It could then be assumed that, on account of the transformation of most basaloid cells into squamous cells, the transfer of melanin to the keratinocytes is blocked.

Seborrheic keratoses apparently do not change into basal cell epithelioma. The few cases in which this event has been reported either were, in reality, instances of fibro-epithelioma (Pinkus, 1953) or represented an intrusion of a basal cell epithelioma into a pre-existing seborrheic keratosis (Balabanow and Angelow).

IRRITATED SEBORRHEIC KERATOSIS. Although occasionally, in the past, authors (e.g., Becker in 1951) emphasized the rather frequent occurrence of "squamous anaplasia" in seborrheic keratoses, this phenomenon has been generally appreciated only in recent years. That it is the result of

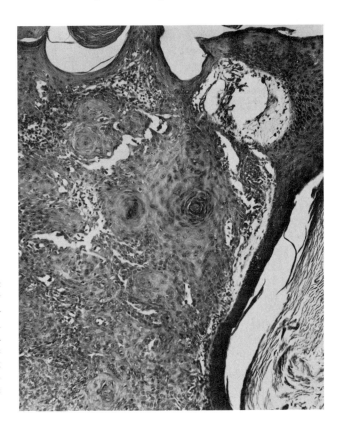

FIG. 25-5. **Irritated seborrheic keratosis.** Numerous whorls or eddies resembling poorly differentiated horn pearls give the lesion an appearance resembling that of a squamous cell carcinoma. The presence of a large pseudohorncyst on the right side aids in the recognition of the lesion as a seborrheic keratosis. (×100)

irritation could be proved experimentally by excising the lesion either after a previous biopsy (Morales and Hu) or after irritation with croton oil (Mevorah and Mishima). It was shown in these experiments that irritation of a seborrheic keratosis causes a differentiation of many of the basaloid cells into squamous cells and arrangement of the squamous cells in numerous whorls or eddies resembling poorly differentiated horn pearls. In some instances the squamous cell proliferation may reach the proportions of a pseudocarcinomatous hyperplasia (Rowe), and it may be difficult indeed to differentiate this proliferation from a true squamous cell carcinoma (Fig. 25-5) (Braun-Falco).

It is now widely accepted that the *basosquamous cell acanthoma* described by Lund represents an irritated seborrheic keratosis, since its histologic features have been induced experimentally in seborrheic keratoses (Morales and Hu; Mevorah and Mishima). It also is likely that the *inverted follicular keratosis,* first described by Helwig and later by Mehregan and by Duperrat and Mascaro, belongs in this category, since its major features are seen also in irritated seborrheic keratoses. These features are: a papillomatous surface, one or several invaginations that have been interpreted as hair follicles, and fingerlike tumor masses showing at their periphery small basal-cell-like cells and in their center small concentric formations of squamous cells referred to as squamous eddies.

Histogenesis. Electron microscopic examination has confirmed the impression that the small basaloid cells seen in seborrheic keratoses are related to the cells of the epidermal basal cell layer more closely than to the basalioma cells of basal cell epithelioma. They possess a fair number of desmosomes and also a moderate number of tonofilaments that differ from those present in the cells of the epidermal basal cell layer by showing less orientation (Braun-Falco et al.).

The basaloid cells in seborrheic keratoses, in contrast with the cells of the epidermal basal cell layer, multiply without tendency to differentiation, although they possess the potential to become mature squamous cells and to keratinize (Mehregan and Pinkus). To a certain extent they behave like the basaloid cells present in eccrine poroma, which also multiply without differentiation although they have the potential to develop into intraepidermal sweat duct cells.

Differential Diagnosis. The differentiation of an irritated seborrheic keratosis from a

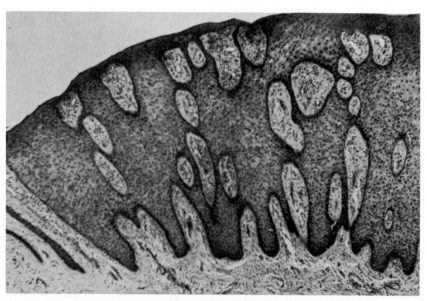

Fig. 25-6. **Clear cell acanthoma.** The cells within the thickened epidermis appear strikingly clear because of the presence of large amounts of glycogen. (×100)

solar keratosis or a squamous cell carcinoma can be difficult at times. As a rule, however, one still can find in an irritated seborrheic keratosis remnants of horn cysts or pseudo-horncysts, and also the straight line of demarcation at the base of the tumor, that is so typical of seborrheic keratoses. Furthermore, the apparent anaplasia is seen largely in the inner portions of the tumor, whereas the periphery still shows fairly numerous basaloid cells. Although solar keratoses also may show tracts composed of a double row of cells, in solar keratoses these cells have nuclei with an anaplastic appearance, in contrast with seborrheic keratoses. For a differentiation of the acanthotic type of seborrheic keratosis from eccrine poroma, see page 532.

DERMATOSIS PAPULOSA NIGRA

The condition is found in about 35 per cent of all adult Negroes, and often has its onset at the time of adolescence (Hairston et al.). The lesions are located predominantly on the face, especially in the malar regions, but they may occur in addition on the upper trunk. They consist of small smooth pigmented papules.

Histopathology. The lesions have the histologic appearance of seborrheic keratoses, except that they are smaller in size. Most lesions are of the acanthotic type and show thick interwoven tracts of epithelial cells. The cells are largely squamous in appearance, with only a few basaloid cells (Hairston et al.). Horncysts are quite common. An occasional lesion shows an adenoid pattern in which the tracts are composed of a double row of basaloid cells. Melanin pigmentation is pronounced.

STUCCO KERATOSIS

Stucco keratoses are small grayish-white seborrheic keratoses, 1 to 3 mm in diameter, located in symmetrical arrangement on the distal portions of the extremities, especially on the ankles. They can easily be scraped off, without any resulting bleeding.

Histopathology. Stucco keratoses have the appearance of the hyperkeratotic type of seborrheic keratosis showing the "church-spire" pattern of upward-extending papillae (Willoughby and Soter). Horn cysts and basaloid cells are either absent or inconspicuous (Kocsard and Carter).

CLEAR CELL ACANTHOMA

This tumor which both clinically and histologically is quite distinct was first described by Degos et al. in 1962. By 1970 more than one hundred cases had already been reported (Degos and Civatte).

In most instances the lesion is solitary and is located on the legs. Usually, the lesion consists of a slowly growing, dome-shaped, sharply delineated, red nodule, 1 to 2 cm in diameter. The smooth surface may show dilated capillaries and exude some moisture. A fringe of fine scaling may be seen at the periphery. According to Fine and Chernosky, the lesion appears stuck on, like a seborrheic keratosis, and is vascular, like a granuloma pyogenicum.

Histopathology. Within a sharply demarcated area of the epidermis, all epidermal cells, but least so the cells of the basal cell layer appear strikingly clear and slightly enlarged (Fig. 25-6). The nuclei of the clear epidermal cells appear normal. Upon staining with the PAS reaction, the presence of large amounts of glycogen is revealed within the cells (Degos et al.; Zak et al.).

Slight spongiosis is present between the clear cells. The rete ridges are elongated and may show intertwining (Delacrétaz). The surface shows parakeratosis with few or no granular cells. The acrosyringium and acrotrichium within the tumor retain their normal stainability (Zak and Girerd). There is absence of melanin within the tumor cells; but sparsely scattered, weakly dopa-positive melanocytes are present, and melanin can be seen within the melanocytes and their dendritic processes on silver staining (Wells and Wilson Jones).

In most lesions one observes neutrophils scattered throughout the epidermis of the tumor, often forming tiny microabscesses at all levels of the epidermis (Wilson Jones and Wells). Dilated capillaries are seen in the elongated papillae and often also in the dermis underlying the tumor (Wells and

Wilson Jones). In addition, a mild to moderately severe cellular infiltrate composed largely of lymphoid cells is present in the dermis.

Some cases have shown beneath the tumor hyperplasia of sweat ducts (Wilson Jones and Wells), or syringomalike proliferations (Cramer).

Histogenesis. Electron microscopy reveals the tumor cells to be filled with glycogen granules that obscure most of the cellular organelles. Although the melanocytes are filled with melanosomes, hardly any melanosomes are present within the tumor cells, indicating a blockage in the transfer of melanosomes from the melanocytes to the tumor cells (Hu and Sisson).

EPIDERMAL CYST

Epidermal cysts are slowly growing, elevated, round, firm, intradermal or subcutaneous tumors that cease growing after having reached a size of from 1 to 5 cm in diameter. They occur most commonly on the face, the scalp, the neck and the trunk. Usually, a patient has only one or a few epidermal cysts, rarely many. In Gardner's syndrome, however, numerous epidermal cysts occur, especially on the scalp and face (see p. 579).

Milia which histologically differ from epidermal cysts only in size, are whitish, globoid, firm lesions, generally only 1 to 2 mm in size. They may arise spontaneously, especially on the face, in which case they represent a keratinizing type of benign tumor (Epstein and Kligman). Milia, however, may form as a result of trauma or in the course of bullous diseases, such as epidermolysis bullosa and porphyria cutanea tarda. They represent retention cysts in such instances caused by the occlusion of the orifice of a pilosebaceous follicle (Love and Montgomery).

Histopathology. Epidermal cysts have a wall composed of true epidermis, as seen on the skin surface and in the infundibulum of hair follicles; the infundibulum being the

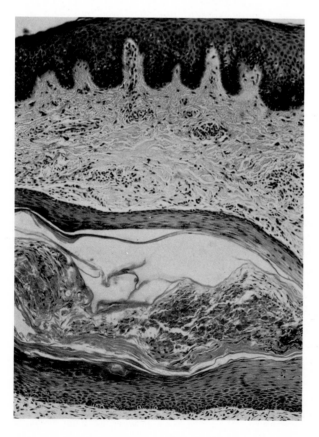

Fig. 25-7. **Epidermal cyst.** The wall of the cyst is composed of true epidermis, i.e., squamous, granular and horn cells. The cyst is filled with horny material arranged in laminated layers. (×100)

uppermost part of the hair follicle that extends down to the entry of the sebaceous duct. In young epidermal cysts usually several layers of squamous and granular cells can be recognized (Fig. 25-7). In older epidermal cysts, however, the wall often is markedly atrophic either in some areas or in the entire cyst, and the wall then consists of only one or two rows of greatly flattened cells. The cyst is filled with horny material arranged in laminated layers. Melanocytes and melanin pigmentation of keratinocytes can be seen only rarely in epidermal cysts of Caucasoids, but are seen frequently in epidermal cysts of Negroids (McGavran and Binnington).

When an epidermal cyst ruptures and the contents of the cyst are released into the dermis, a considerable foreign-body reaction with numerous multinucleated giant cells results. The foreign-body reaction usually causes disintegration of the cyst wall. On the other hand, it may lead to a pseudo-carcinomatous proliferation in remnants of the cyst wall, simulating a squamous cell carcinoma (Raab and Steigleder).

MALIGNANT DEGENERATION in epidermal cysts is rare. If it occurs it is in the direction of a low-grade squamous cell carcinoma that does not metastasize (Fig. 25-8). It is obvious now that in the past some cases were regarded as malignant degeneration of epidermal cysts that now are interpreted either as pseudocarcinomatous hyperplasia in a ruptured epidermal cyst (Raab and Steigleder) or as a pilar tumor of the scalp (Wilson-Jones) (see p. 521).

Histogenesis. Electron microscopically, the keratinization in epidermal cysts is identical with that in the surface epidermis and in the pilo-sebaceous infundibulum, since it consists of the aggregation of tonofilaments and the formation of an interfilamentous matrix by keratohyaline granules. The cyst content consists of fully

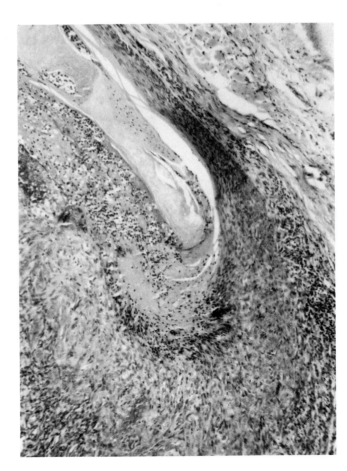

FIG. 25-8. **Epidermal cyst with squamous cell carcinoma.** The squamous cell carcinoma present in the wall of the cyst is walled off by an inflammatory infiltrate. (×100)

keratinized cells which have a markedly flattened and elongated appearance and are surrounded by a thick marginal band rather than a plasma membrane (see p. 15). The intercellular spaces between the fully keratinized cells is filled with moderately electron dense material, with desmosomes no longer present (McGavran and Binnington).

PILAR CYST

Pilar cysts are clinically indistinguishable from epidermal cysts. They differ, however, from epidermal cysts in their frequency and their distribution. In the first place, they are much less common than epidermal cysts, comprising only about 15 per cent of the combined material; and, in the second place, 90 per cent of pilar cysts occur on the scalp (McGavran and Binnington).

Histopathology. Pilar cysts have a wall composed of epithelial cells that possess no clearly visible intercellular bridges. The peripheral layer of cells shows a distinct palisade arrangement, which is not seen in epidermal cysts. The epithelial cells close to the cystic cavity appear swollen because of an increase in the amount of cytoplasm and possess no sharp cell boundaries. These swollen cells do not produce a granular layer but seem to float off into the lumen (Kligman). Although usually they lose their nucleus abruptly on entering the lumen, in a few cells nuclear remnants are retained. The content of the cysts consists of homogenous eosinophilic material (Fig. 25-9). In contrast with epidermal cysts in which focal calcification of the cyst content does not occur, foci of calcification are seen in ap-

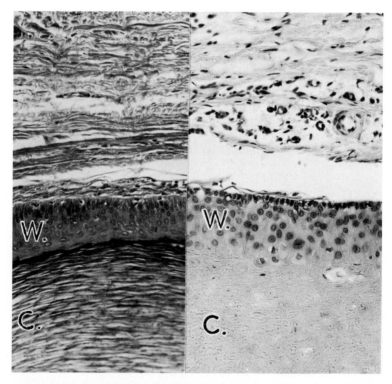

FIG. 25-9. **Comparison of epidermal cyst** (*left*) **with pilar cyst** (*right*). The wall (W.) of the epidermal cyst is composed of epidermis; the cystic cavity (C.) contains horny material arranged in laminated layers. The wall (W.) of the pilar cyst is composed of cells that possess no clearly visible intercellular bridges. Many cells near the cystic cavity (C.) appear swollen. The content of the cyst consists of amorphous material. (×200)

Fig. 25-10. **Calcified pilar cyst.** The palisading of the basal layer makes it evident that this is a pilar cyst. It has ruptured, and fibrous tissue has proliferated into the lumen. (×100)

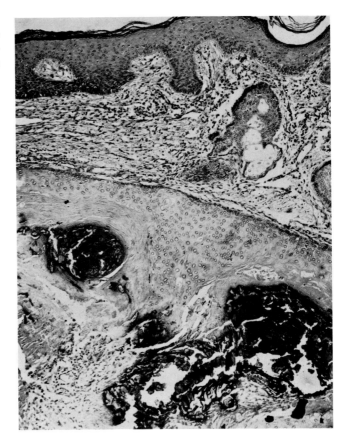

proximately 25 per cent of pilar cysts (Fig. 25-10). As in epidermal cysts a considerable foreign-body reaction results when the wall of a pilar cyst ruptures and the cyst may then undergo partial or complete disintegration.

Histogenesis. Pilar cysts originally were called sebaceous cysts; the name was changed to pilar when it became apparent that differentiation within them is toward hair keratin (Kligman). Pinkus has demonstrated that the keratinization in pilar cysts is analogous to the keratinization process taking place in that portion of the outer root sheath that is referred to as the follicular isthmus. The follicular isthmus is limited at its lower end by the zone of sloughing of the inner root sheath and at its upper end by the opening of the sebaceous duct. The sloughing of the inner root sheath exposes the outer root sheath, or trichilemma, which in its exposed portion undergoes a specific type of homogeneous keratinization without interposition of a granular layer. This type of trichilemmal keratinization can take place whenever the trichilemma is not

covered by the inner root sheath, as, for instance, in the sac surrounding the catagen hair after the latter has lost its inner root sheath (see p. 31). Since pilar cysts show this type of keratinization, Pinkus has designated them as trichilemmal cysts.

Electron microscopic examination of the epithelial lining of pilar cysts shows that on their way from the peripheral layer toward the center the epithelial cells show in their cytoplasm an increasing number of filaments and these filaments aggregate to fibrils. The transition from nucleate to anucleate cells is associated with the loss of all cytoplasmic organelles. The keratinized cells, in contrast to those in epidermal cysts, retain their desmosomal connections (McGavran and Binnington).

STEATOCYSTOMA MULTIPLEX

Steatocystoma multiplex often is dominantly inherited. One observes numerous small, rounded, moderately firm, cystic nodules that are adherent to the overlying skin. They usually measure from 1 to 3 cm in diameter. On puncturing, the cysts discharge an oily fluid and, in some instances, also small hairs (Contreras and Costello). They are found most commonly in the axillae, in the sternal region and on the arms.

Histopathology. Histologic examination reveals an intricately folded cyst wall consisting of several layers of epithelial cells. In areas of atrophy of the cyst wall only two or three layers of flat cells may be present. Elsewhere there is a basal layer in palisade arrangement, above which there are two or three layers of swollen cells without recognizable intercellular bridges. Centrally to these cells there is a thick, homogeneous, eosinophilic horny layer that protrudes irregularly into the lumen in a fashion simulating the decapitation secretion of apocrine glands (Fig. 25-11) (Hashimoto et al.).

A very characteristic feature of steatocystoma multiplex is the presence of flattened sebaceous gland lobules either within or close to the cyst wall (Oyal and Nikolowski). Also, in some cysts invaginations resembling hair follicles extend from the cyst wall into the surrounding stroma; and in rare instances true hair shafts are seen within them, indicating that the invaginations represent the outer root sheath of a hair. In occasional cysts the lumen contains clusters of hair, mainly of lanugo size but some of intermediate character (Kligman and Kirschbaum). On staining with the PAS reaction, the cells of the cyst wall are found to be rich in glycogen.

Histogenesis. Electron microscopic examination has shown that the cyst wall consists of keratinizing cells. The innermost layer of the cyst wall consists everywhere of several layers of flattened, very elongated horny cells. It appears likely that the differentiation in the cyst wall is in the direction of the outer root sheath of hair because (1) the cells of the cyst wall contain abundant glycogen and amylophosphorylase; (2) sebaceous glands are present within or near the cyst wall; (3) the cyst wall may form invaginations containing a hair; and (4) the homogeneous eosinophilic horny layer lining the cyst wall greatly resembles the cyst content of pilar, or trichilemmal, cysts (Hashimoto et al.).

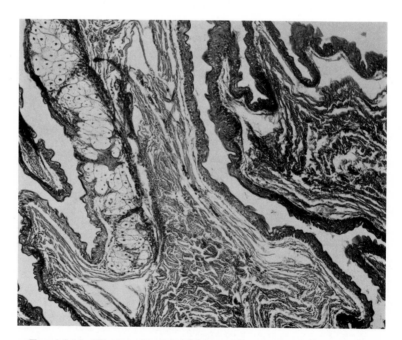

FIG. 25-11. **Steatocystoma multiplex.** The cyst wall shows intricate folding. The lining of the cyst consists of a homogeneous horny layer that protrudes irregularly into the lumen. On the left, flattened sebaceous gland lobules lie within, or close to, the cyst wall. (×100)

FIG. 25-12. **Warty dyskeratoma.** Low magnification. The lesion shows a large central invagination containing keratinous material in its upper portion and numerous villi in its lower portion. (×25) (Armed Forces Institute of Pathology, No. 57-6202)

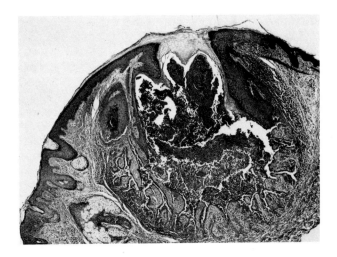

DERMOID CYSTS

Dermoid cysts are subcutaneous cysts usually present at birth. They occur most commonly on the face, mainly around the eyes. There they often are adherent to the periosteum. Usually they measure between 1 and 4 cm in size.

Histopathology. Dermoid cysts are lined by an epidermis that, in contrast with epidermal cysts, possesses various epidermal appendages. These appendages are as a rule fully matured. Hair follicles containing hairs that project into the lumen of the cyst are regularly present. In addition, the dermis of dermoid cysts nearly always contains

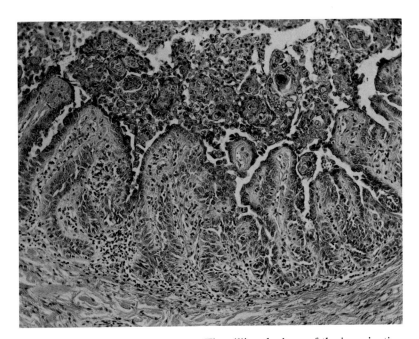

FIG. 25-13. **Warty dyskeratoma.** The villi at the base of the invagination are covered with a single layer of epidermal cells. Acantholytic, dyskeratotic cells lie above the villi. (×100) (Armed Forces Institute of Pathology, No. 57-6203)

sebaceous glands, often also eccrine glands, and occasionally apocrine glands. The latter were noted by Brownstein and Helwig in 9 of 50 dermoid cysts.

Histogenesis. Dermoid cysts are the result of the sequestration of skin along lines of embryonic closure.

WARTY DYSKERATOMA

Warty dyskeratoma occurs nearly always as a solitary lesion, most commonly on the scalp, face or neck. In several instances it has been reported to occur in areas not customarily exposed to the sun; and on one occasion it was observed on the oral mucosa (Gorlin and Peterson). Although its clinical appearance is not always distinctive, it often occurs as a slightly elevated papule or nodule with a keratotic umbilicated center (Tanay and Mehregan). The lesion, after having reached a certain size, persists indefinitely.

Histopathology. The center of the lesion is occupied by a large, cup-shaped invagination containing keratinous material in its upper portion and numerous acantholytic, dyskeratotic cells in its lower portion (Fig. 25-12). Numerous villi lined often with only a single layer of basal cells project upward from the base of the cup-shaped invagination (Fig. 25-13). In some cases one observes between and beneath the upward-growing villi an irregular downward growth of epidermal strands, often as a double row of cells, with a narrow lumen separating the two rows of cells (Szymanski; Graham and Helwig; Nikolowski; Delacrétaz). Typical corps ronds can usually be seen in the granular layer of the epidermis just below the entrance to the invagination (Fig. 25-14) (Furtado and Szymanski). The entrance to the invagination itself shows marked hypergranulosis (Tanay and Mehregan). Dyskeratotic changes are absent in this area.

Histogenesis. The central cup-shaped depression is believed by many observers to represent a greatly dilated hair follicle, since in early lesions a hair follicle or sebaceous gland often is seen to be connected with the cup-shaped invagination (Graham and Helwig; Delacrétaz; Furtado and Szymanski). Occasionally, two or three adjoin-

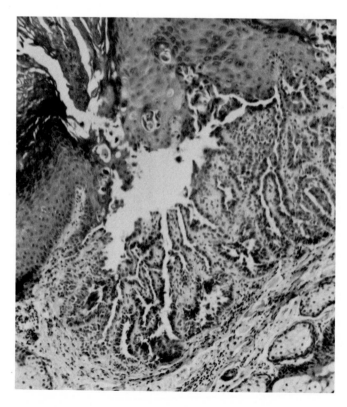

FIG. 25-14. **Warty dyskeratoma.** Typical corps ronds are seen in the granular layer of the epidermis just below the entrance into the invagination. (×100)

ing follicles seem to be involved (Tanay and Mehregan).

Although no full agreement exists in regard to the nature of the lesion, most likely it represents a distinct tumor entity with no relation to either Darier's disease or solar keratosis.

In regard to a possible relationship with Darier's disease, warty dyskeratoma shows no clinical resemblance to it. Although Kellum and Haserick reported that in one patient with localized linear Darier's disease later on a warty dyskeratoma developed, this occurrence may have been coincidental. Histologically, it is true that Darier's disease and warty dyskeratoma are the only two diseases that show a pronounced formation of corps ronds. Nevertheless, they differ in that Darier's disease is not known to show such a deep invagination as is seen in warty dyskeratoma.

A possible relationship with solar keratosis is suggested by the occasional presence of dyskeratosis and acantholysis in solar keratosis (Jablonska and Chorzelski; Metz and Schröpl). However, the following observations speak against a relationship: (1) warty dyskeratoma occasionally occurs in areas that are not exposed to the sun; (2) warty dyskeratoma not infre-quently occurs in Negroes, whereas solar keratosis of Negro skin is practically unknown (Tanay and Mehregan); (3) warty dyskeratoma develops within a cup-shaped depression into which solar rays are unlikely to penetrate; and (4) in contrast with solar keratosis, malignant changes have not been observed in warty dyskeratoma.

SOLAR KERATOSIS

Solar keratoses are seen as single but more often as multiple lesions on sun-exposed areas of the skin in persons in or past middle life having a fair complexion. They are seen most commonly on the face, the dorsa of the hands, the bald portions of the scalp in men, and on the dorsa of the forearms in women. Prolonged exposure to sunlight and inadequate protection against it are the essential predisposing factors.

Usually, the lesions measure less than 1 cm in diameter. They are erythematous, often are covered by adherent scales, and show little or no infiltration. Occasionally,

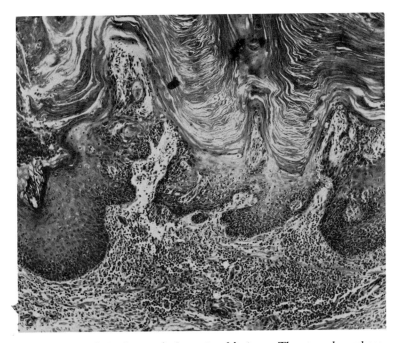

Fig. 25-15. **Solar keratosis, hypertrophic type.** There are hyperkeratosis and papillomatosis. The stratum malpighii shows areas of atrophy as well as areas of irregular downward proliferation in which the epidermal cells show a disorderly arrangement. The upper dermis shows a rather pronounced chronic inflammatory infiltrate. (×100)

lesions show marked hyperkeratosis and then have the clinical aspect of a cutaneous horn (see below). A lesion analogous to solar keratosis occurs on the vermilion border of the lower lip as solar cheilitis and may show areas of erosion and of hyperkeratosis (Koten et al.; Mashkillejson).

Development of a solar keratosis into squamous cell carcinoma can occur. However, its incidence is difficult to determine because the borderline between solar keratosis and squamous cell carcinoma is not clear-cut (see under Histopathology). It has been estimated that in 20 per cent of patients with solar keratoses, squamous cell carcinoma develops in one or more of the lesions (Montgomery and Dörffel). As a rule, however, squamous cell carcinomas arising either in solar keratoses or as such in sun-damaged skin do not metastasize, as shown by Lund, who found that only 0.5 per cent of them caused metastases.

Histopathology. The best definition that may be given to solar keratosis is that of "squamous cell carcinoma, grade ½." This definition is preferable to its designation as a precancerosis because morphologically anaplastic cells are present. However, biologically the lesion still is benign, since invasion into the dermis, if present at all, is limited to the most superficial portion of the dermis.

Three types of solar keratosis can be recognized histologically: the hypertrophic, the atrophic, and bowenoid types (Pinkus; Woringer). Transitions among these three types occur. Recently, a fourth type of solar keratosis has been described, the solitary lichen-planus-like keratosis or solitary lichenoid solar keratosis (see below).

In the *hypertrophic type* hyperkeratosis is pronounced and usually is intermingled with areas of parakeratosis. Mild or moderate papillomatosis may be present. The epidermis is atrophic in some areas and thickened in other areas. In the latter areas it shows irregular downward proliferation which, however, is limited to the uppermost dermis and thus does not represent frank invasion (Fig. 25-15). The cells of the entire stra-

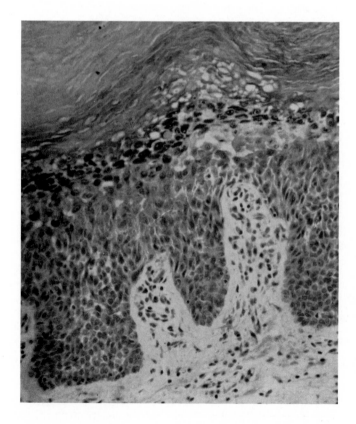

FIG. 25-16. **Solar keratosis, hypertrophic type, showing epidermolytic hyperkeratosis.** In addition to disorderly arrangement and anaplasia of the nuclei in the lower epidermis, epidermolytic hyperkeratosis is present in the upper epidermis. In epidermolytic hyperkeratosis, referred to also as granular degeneration, one observes clear spaces around the nuclei and a thickened granular layer with large, irregularly shaped keratohyaline granules. (×200)

FIG. 25-17. **Solar keratosis, atrophic type.** Hyperkeratosis is mild. The epidermis is atrophic. The nuclei of the basal cells are anaplastic and appear closely crowded together. Anaplastic basal cells also line a hair follicle as a cell mantle. (×200)

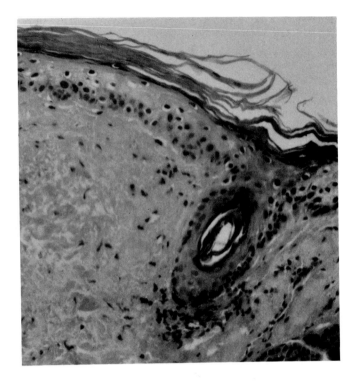

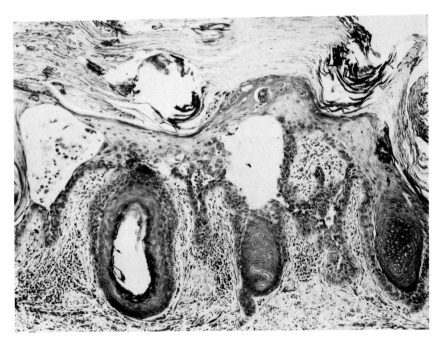

FIG. 25-18. **Solar keratosis, atrophic type.** Hyperkeratosis is present. The epidermis on the whole appears atrophic. Cellular atypicality is most pronounced in the basal layer, which proliferates into the dermis as short ductlike structures. Suprabasal clefts and lacunae are present containing a few acantholytic cells. (×150)

tum malpighii present a disorderly arrangement. Some of these cells show pleomorphism and anaplasia of their nuclei which
appear large, irregular and hyperchromatic.
Often, the nuclei in the basal layer are
closely crowded together. In areas of
crowded, hyperchromatic nuclei irregular
branches of atypical epidermal cells may
extend into the upper dermis. In rare instances, one finds in a solar keratosis of
the hypertrophic type, in addition to anaplastic nuclei in the lower epidermis, epidermolytic hyperkeratosis in the upper epidermis (Fig. 25-16). These changes are like
those seen in dominant congenital ichthyosiform erythroderma (see p. 60). In epidermolytic hyperkeratosis, referred to also
as granular degeneration, one observes in
the upper epidermis clear spaces around
the nuclei and a thickened granular layer
with large, irregularly shaped keratohyaline
granules (Ackerman and Reed).

In the *atrophic type* of solar keratosis
hyperkeratosis usually is slight. The epidermis on the whole is atrophic. Atypicality of the cells is found predominantly in the
basal cell layer, which consists of cells with
large hyperchromatic nuclei that lie close
together (Fig. 25-17). The atypical basal
layer may proliferate into the dermis as
buds and ductlike structures. Also, it may
surround as cell mantles the upper portion
of pilosebaceous follicles and sweat ducts,
the epithelium of which otherwise appears
normal (Fig. 25-18) (Halter; Pinkus). Not
infrequently in this type of solar keratosis
one observes immediately above the atypical
basal layer clefts or lacunae similar to those
seen in Darier's disease (see p. 72). These
clefts form as the result of anaplastic
changes in the lowermost epidermis, resulting in dyskeratosis and in a loss of the intercellular bridges. A few acantholytic cells
may be present within the clefts. Above the
clefts the epidermis may show little or no
atypicality. This can be explained by the
fact that the normal adnexal epithelium proliferates in the manner of an umbrella over
the anaplastic lower epidermis (Pinkus).

In the *bowenoid type* of solar keratosis
the histologic picture is indistinguishable
from that of Bowen's disease. Within the
epidermis one observes, just as in Bowen's

disease, a carcinoma in situ that is sharply
demarcated against the dermis but within
the epidermis shows considerable disorder
in the arrangement of the nuclei, as well as
clumping of nuclei, and dyskeratosis (see
p. 473).

In all three types of solar keratosis the
upper dermis usually shows solar, or basophilic, degeneration of the collagen and a
fairly dense, chronic inflammatory infiltrate
composed predominantly of lymphoid cells
but often containing also plasma cells. Solar
cheilitis more frequently than solar keratosis
of the skin shows an inflammatory infiltrate
in which plasma cells predominate (Koten
et al.).

In instances in which the histologic diagnosis is solar keratosis but the clinical diagnosis is squamous cell carcinoma, it is
advisable to section deeper into the block
of tissue, because actual progression into
squamous cell carcinoma may have taken
place in another area. Because no sharp
line of demarcation exists between the two
conditions it is not always possible to decide
definitely whether a lesion can still be regarded as a solar keratosis or should be classified as an early squamous cell carcinoma.
Such situations arise, for instance, when
irregular branches of atypical cells descend
from a hypertrophic solar keratosis fairly
deep into the dermis; or when mantles of
atypical cells extend quite deep along hair
follicles in an atrophic solar keratosis (Fig.
25-18). However, as already pointed out,
this decision is not a vital one, as it may be
in the case of malignant melanoma in situ
versus invasive malignant melanoma, since
squamous cell carcinoma arising in a solar
keratosis rarely causes metastases.

SOLITARY LICHENOID SOLAR KERATOSIS

In this condition an erythematous, asymptomatic, small, keratotic lesion is seen in a
sun-exposed area such as the upper chest,
the forearm, the dorsum of the hand, or the
face.

Histopathology. The histologic resemblance to lichen planus is such that Lumpkin
and Helwig who originally described this lesion in 1966 regarded it as solitary lichen

planus. Its possible relationship to solar keratosis was suspected by Shapiro and Ackerman when they reported 18 such cases in the same year. They emphasized, however, in their report the absence of any anaplasia. Subsequently, however, Hirsch and Marmelzat described in five lesions the histologic features of lichen planus, but they noted, in addition, some atypicality. The atypicality was manifested by dyskeratosis, loss of polarity, and pleomorphism of the squamous cells.

CORNU CUTANEUM

Cornu cutaneum is the clinical term for a circumscribed, conical, markedly hyperkeratotic lesion in which the height of the keratotic mass amounts to at least one half of its largest diameter (Bart et al.).

Histopathology. On histologic examination a variety of lesions can be seen at the base of the conical hyperkeratosis of a cornu cutaneum. Most commonly a solar keratosis is encountered (Cramer and Kahlert). In

other instances, a filiform verruca, a seborrheic keratosis, or a squamous cell carcinoma are found (Bart et al.); and in rare instances a basal cell epithelioma (Sandbank).

LEUKOPLAKIA

Leukoplakia is the term that is used for early anaplastic lesions on the oral mucosa and the vulva, whereas leukokeratosis is the term applied to benign hyperkeratotic lesions in these locations (McAdams and Kistner). It is realized that this usage is at variance with the terminology used by oral pathologists who designate both conditions as leukoplakia and distinguish between a simple and a premalignant variety of leukoplakia (Shklar). The reason generally given for using the term leukoplakia for both conditions is that as a rule one cannot distinguish between the two on clinical grounds but only on histologic grounds. In the development of oral leukokeratosis and leukoplakia chemical irritation through tobacco, or mechanical irritation through dental stumps or

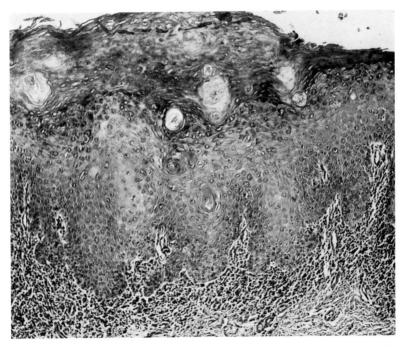

FIG. 25-19. **Leukoplakia of the oral mucosa.** There is hyperkeratosis and irregular acanthosis. In addition to disorder in the arrangement of the cells, there is cellular atypicality. The latter is a prerequisite for the histologic diagnosis of leukoplakia. (×200)

ill-fitting dentures plays a role. While leuko-keratosis usually reverts to normal when the irritation is removed, leukoplakia is irrevers-ible and may progress to invasive squamous cell carcinoma. Vulvar leukokeratosis and leukoplakia usually develop as a result of involutional atrophy of the vulva.

Clinically, the lesions of leukokeratosis and leukoplakia on the oral mucosa and on the vulva consist of one or several white patches that may not be raised and then appear ill defined. On the other hand, if they are slightly elevated they appear sharply demarcated with irregular outline.

It should be realized that the presence of whitish lesions on the oral or vulvar mucosa does not necessarily indicate leukokeratosis or leukoplakia. Any hyperkeratotic lesion in these locations may appear whitish as the result of hydration of a thickened horny layer. Thus, on the vulva a chronic derma-titis and, in particular, lichen sclerosus et atrophicus may appear whitish through hy-perkeratosis; and in the oral cavity many chronic inflammatory diseases, such as lupus erythematosus and lichen planus, and also chronic hyperplastic candidiasis (Cawson and Lehner) may appear as whitish lesions.

Histopathology. Leukokeratosis of the oral cavity or the vulva shows either hyper-keratotic or parakeratotic thickening of the horny layer, acanthosis, and a chronic in-flammatory infiltrate. Evidence of anaplasia of the epithelium is absent (Cooke).

Leukoplakia of the oral cavity or of the vulva shows epithelial changes that greatly resemble those of the hypertrophic type of solar keratosis of the skin (see p. 468). Thus, there is irregular acanthosis with varying degrees of cellular atypicality and disorder in the arrangement of the cells (Fig. 25-19). The horny layer shows either parakeratotic or hyperkeratotic thickening.

Differential Diagnosis. A decision as to whether or not epithelial anaplasia is present and in case of its presence, whether or not it has progressed to invasive squamous cell carcinoma, may require step sections throughout the biopsy specimen, and possi-bly examination of additional biopsy speci-mens. The decision in respect to whether or not invasive squamous cell carcinoma has developed from a leukoplakia is of consider-

able importance. In comparison with squa-mous cell carcinoma of the skin that has developed from a solar keratosis, squa-mous cell carcinoma of the oral mucosa or the vulva that has developed from a leuko-plakia has a much greater tendency to metastasize.

ORAL FLORID PAPILLOMATOSIS

Papillomas arising on the adult oral mu-cosa may occur in two clinically distinct pat-terns: (1) as a solitary papilloma, and (2) as multiple growth or oral florid papillomato-sis. The more common solitary oral papil-loma has been reported in several instances to give rise to squamous cell carcinoma (Shklar; Rose).

The rare condition known as oral florid papillomatosis at first was thought to remain benign in all instances. Lately, however, two instances have been reported in which squamous cell carcinoma supervened (Samitz et al.; Kanee).

Clinically, oral florid papillomatosis shows multiple cauliflowerlike lesions extending over large areas of the oral mucosa. The lesions usually arise late in life, gradually extend, and coalesce. They frequently recur after excision or electrodesiccation.

Histopathology. In oral florid papilloma-tosis one observes papillomatous hyperplasia of the oral epithelium (Samitz et al.). The epithelial cells in the superficial layers show marked vacuolization with little or no kera-tinization. In the lower layers a moderate loss of polarity, as well as hyperchromatic nuclei and many mitotic figures may be seen; but atypical nuclei and frank invasion are absent at first (Wechsler and Fisher). A moderately severe chronic inflammatory infiltrate is present beneath the epithelium. In cases in which squamous cell carcinoma has developed atypical nuclei and invasion are evident (Samitz et al.; Kanee).

Histogenesis. At first, oral florid papilloma-tosis was regarded as a form of benign hyper-plasia (Wechsler and Fisher). However, since the potential for the development of a frank squamous cell carcinoma has been shown to exist, it seems best to regard oral florid papillo-matosis as a "verrucous carcinoma" from the very beginning (Kraus and Perez-Mesa). "Verrucous carcinoma" has been defined as a distinctive, slowly growing, fungating tumor representing a well differentiated squamous cell carcinoma in which metastases arise very late or not at all. Other manifestations of verrucous carcinoma are the so-called giant condylomata acuminata of Buschke and Loewenstein (see p. 354), and "epithelioma cuniculatum" of the foot, a fungating low-grade carcinoma occurring on the sole of the foot (Aird et al.).

BOWEN'S DISEASE

Bowen's disease usually but not always consists of a solitary lesion. It may occur on exposed or on nonexposed skin. On exposed skin it may be caused by exposure to the sun, and on nonexposed skin by the ingestion of arsenic (see below, under Histogenesis).

Bowen's disease manifests itself as a slowly enlarging erythematous patch of sharp but irregular outline, showing little or no infiltration. Within the patch there generally are areas of crusting. Although Bowen's disease may resemble a superficial basal cell epithelioma it differs from it by the absence of a fine pearly border and by

not showing any tendency to central healing.

Lesions of Bowen's disease can occur on the glans penis, the vulva, or the oral mucosa. Lesions in these locations generally are referred to as erythroplasia of Queyrat (see p. 475).

Histopathology. Bowen's disease is an intraepidermal squamous cell carcinoma, referred to also as squamous cell carcinoma in situ. Thus it represents only biologically but not morphologically a "precancerous dermatosis," under which title it was described originally by Bowen in 1912.

The epidermis shows acanthosis with elongation and thickening of the rete ridges, often to such a degree that the papillae located between them are reduced to thin strands. The thickened horny layer consists largely of parakeratotic cells. Throughout the epidermis the cells lie in complete disorder. Many of them appear highly atypical, showing large and hyperchromatic nuclei. Multinucleated epidermal cells containing clusters of nuclei are often present (Fig. 25-20) (Montgomery).

A common and rather characteristic feature is the presence of cells showing individ-

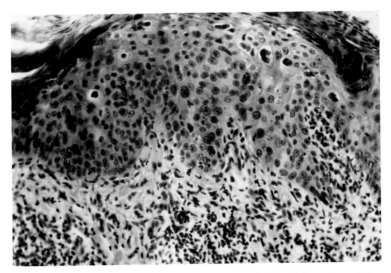

FIG. 25-20. **Bowen's disease.** The epidermis is thickened, and the border between the epidermis and dermis appears sharp. The stratum corneum shows parakeratosis, and the cells of the stratum malpighii lie in complete disorder, and many of them are atypical, showing large and hyperchromatic nuclei. Several multinucleated epidermal cells are present. (×200)

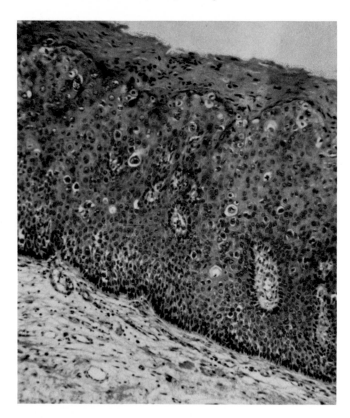

FIG. 25-21. **Bowen's disease.** In addition to the changes described for Figure 25-20, there are within the stratum malpighii scattered cells showing individual cell keratinization, or dyskeratosis. (×200)

ual cell keratinization (Fig. 25-21). Such dyskeratotic cells are large and round, and have a homogeneous, strongly eosinophilic cytoplasm, and a pyknotic nucleus. Occasionally actual horn pearls are seen within the acanthotic epidermis. In some cases of Bowen's disease marked vacuolization of the cells is present, especially in the upper portions of the epidermis (Montgomery and Waisman).

Even though the marked atypicality of the epidermal cells includes the cells of the basal layer, the border between the epidermis and dermis everywhere appears sharp; and, on staining with the PAS reaction, the PAS-positive basement zone is intact. The upper dermis usually shows a moderate amount of a chronic inflammatory infiltrate.

In a small percentage of cases, according to Graham and Helwig in 11 per cent of the patients, usually after many years' duration, an invasive squamous cell carcinoma develops. The invasive tumor retains the cytologic characteristics of the intraepidermal tumor.

Invasion may occur at first in only a limited area. In order not to miss such an area it is advisable to examine representative sections throughout the entire tissue block. As soon as invasion has taken place, the prognosis changes. So long as Bowen's disease remains in its intraepidermal stage metastases do not occur. However, once invasion of the dermis has occurred, the likelihood of regional and even visceral metastases is rather great (Graham and Helwig).

Histogenesis. Of significance in regard to the etiology of Bowen's disease is the association with visceral carcinoma in a fairly high percentage of patients with Bowen's disease. The first authors to point out an association between Bowen's disease and visceral cancer were Graham and Helwig in 1959. Subsequently, however, Peterka et al. showed that this association applied only to those patients in whom the lesions of Bowen's disease were located in areas not exposed to the sun. It can be assumed that at least some of the Bowen lesions in nonexposed areas, as well as the associated visceral cancer, are caused by the ingestion of arsenic. (For further details, see under Arsenical Keratosis and Carcinoma, p. 245).

Electron microscopic examination of lesions of Bowen's disease has demonstrated the presence of many dyskeratotic cells. In these dyskeratotic cells the perinuclear aggregation and condensation of tonofilaments is similar to but more pronounced than in the dyskeratotic cells of Darier's disease (Seiji and Mizuno). Some of the markedly dyskeratotic cells disintegrate and portions of such cells are phagocytized by other epidermal cells which then contain, in addition to the phagocytized dyskeratotic material, also within their cytoplasm phagocytized desmosomes (Seiji and Mizuno; Olsen et al., 1969). In other instances, the intracellularly located desmosomes were not phagocytized but were drawn into the dyskeratotic cells of Bowen's disease together with aggregating tonofilaments (Sato and Seiji). The phenomenon of intracytoplasmic desmosomes, however, is specific neither for Bowen's disease nor for dyskeratotic cells. For instance, intracytoplasmic desmosomes have been observed within the dyskeratotic cells of squamous cell carcinoma (Klingmüller et al.) and keratoacanthoma (Fisher et al.) and within nondyskeratotic keratinocytes of 2 cases of keratosis palmaris et plantaris and 1 case of malignant melanoma (Klug and Haustein). It is likely that in cells without dyskeratosis some of the desmosomes have come into the cytoplasm through invaginations of the plasma membrane, while others have formed within the cytoplasm after the plasma membrane has invaginated.

Two types of epidermal giant cells can be recognized in Bowen's disease: In one type an entire dyskeratotic cell has been "cannibalized" by another keratinocyte and is located within the cytoplasm of the phagocytizing cell (Olsen et al., 1968). In the second type of giant cell multiple nuclei lie in the center of the cell surrounded by dyskeratotic tonofilaments. It seems that the dyskeratotic tonofilaments by becoming entangled with the spindles of the mitotic apparatus interfere with the normal division of the cell so that, even though nuclear division can take place, cellular division cannot (Seiji and Mizuno; Olsen et al., 1969).

Differential Diagnosis. No histologic difference exists between bowenoid solar keratosis and Bowen's disease. They merely differ in size, with the bowenoid solar keratosis smaller in size than Bowen's disease.

Paget's disease may share with Bowen's disease the presence of vacuolated cells; but, in contrast with Bowen's disease, shows no dyskeratosis. In addition, Paget cells, in contrast with the vacuolated cells in Bowen's disease, often contain PAS-positive, diastase-resistant material.

ERYTHROPLASIA OF QUEYRAT

Erythroplasia of Queyrat is the term used for carcinoma in situ situated either on the glans penis (Blau and Hyman; Graham and Helwig), the vulva (Abell and Gosling), or the oral mucosa (Hornstein and Pape). The glans penis is by far the most common site. The lesion on the glans penis occurs as a single, red, velvety area that occasionally is elevated, papillary or ulcerated (Graham and Helwig).

Histopathology. Erythroplasia of Queyrat has the same histologic appearance as Bowen's disease. Progression into an invasive squamous cell carcinoma and development of metastases, however, is seen in a much higher percentage of cases with erythroplasia of the vulva and the oral mucosa than with Bowen's disease of the skin (Abell and Gosling; Hornstein and Pape). On the other hand, erythroplasia of the glans penis is about equivalent to Bowen's disease, according to Graham and Helwig, in regard to the development of invasive squamous cell carcinoma, which they observed in 10 of 100 patients, with metastases in 2 patients.

Differential Diagnosis. A clinical diagnosis of erythroplasia of Queyrat requires histologic examination for confirmation, since a reliable differentiation from balanitis or vulvitis circumscripta plasmacellularis on a clinical basis is not possible.

BALANITIS OR VULVITIS CIRCUMSCRIPTA PLASMACELLULARIS

The disorder occurs on the glans penis or on the inner surfaces of the labia majora or minora. The clinical appearance may be the same as in erythroplasia of Queyrat, although in some instances the patches of balanitis or vulvitis circumscripta plasmacellularis appear shiny and smooth, rather than velvety and granular, as do most of the lesions of erythroplasia of Queyrat (Grimmer). In some instances erosions with a

tendency to bleeding are present (Eberhartinger and Bergmann).

Histopathology. The epithelium often appears thinned and may be even partially
absent. The upper dermis contains an inflammatory infiltrate composed largely of
plasma cells (Zoon; Hyman and Leider). In
addition, the capillaries are dilated, and
there may be deposits of hemosiderin (Nödl;
Grimmer).

Histogenesis. Although several authors believe
balanitis and vulvitis circumscripta plasmacellularis to be an entity, it is regarded by others as a
nonspecific inflammation. It has been pointed
out that any chronic inflammation occurring on
the glans penis or the vulva, as well as on the
lips, is prone to show a fairly large admixture
of plasma cells (Korting and Theisen).

SQUAMOUS CELL CARCINOMA

Squamous cell carcinoma may occur anywhere on the skin as well as on the mucous
membranes. It rarely arises from normal
appearing skin. Most commonly it arises in
sun-damaged skin, either as such or from
a solar keratosis. Carcinomas arising in sun-
damaged skin have a very low propensity to
metastasize, amounting only to about 0.5
per cent (Lund), as compared with a rate
of about 2 per cent for all squamous cell
carcinomas of the skin (Epstein et al.).
Carcinomas arising in other types of pre-
existing lesions, such as chronic leg ulcers,
burn scars, or sinuses of osteomyelitis, have
a much higher rate of metastasis than those
arising in sun-damaged skin. Thus, Sedlin
and Fleming found a rate of metastasis of
31 per cent among 71 cases of squamous
cell carcinoma in osteomyelitic sinuses col-
lected by them from the literature. The rate
of metastasis is rather high also in squamous
cell carcinomas arising in areas of radiodermatitis, with an incidence varying from
20 to 26 per cent (Hueper), and in squamous cell carcinomas arising without a pre-
existing lesion, with an incidence of 18 per
cent (Graham and Helwig). Furthermore,
carcinomas arising from modified skin, such
as the lips, glans, and vulva, and from the
oral mucosa have a rather high rate of metastasis unless they are recognized and adequately treated in their early stage.

Clinically, squamous cell carcinoma of the
skin most commonly consists of a shallow
ulcer surrounded by a wide, elevated, and
indurated border. Often, the ulcer is covered
by a crust that conceals a red granular base.
Occasionally raised, fungoid, verrucous lesions without ulceration occur.

A rare variant of squamous cell carcinoma is the so-called *verrucous carcinoma*
(Kraus and Perez-Mesa). It occurs on the
oral mucosa as *oral florid papillomatosis*
(see p. 472); on the penis, and, in very rare
instances, also in the anal region and the
vulva, as *giant condylomata acuminata of
Buschke and Loewenstein* (see p. 354); and
as *epithelioma cuniculatum* on the sole of
the foot (see p. 473). Verrucous carcinoma
is a slowly growing, fungating tumor that
may penetrate deep into the tissue but
causes metastases only very late or not at
all. Because of its high degree of histologic
differentiation it often is not recognized as
a carcinoma for a long time.

Histopathology. Squamous cell carcinoma
is a true, invasive carcinoma of the surface
epidermis. On histologic examination one
finds the tumor to consist of irregular masses
of epidermal cells that proliferate downward
and invade the dermis. The invading tumor
masses are composed in varying proportions
of normal squamous cells and of atypical
(pleomorphic, anaplastic) squamous cells
(see p. 450). The more malignant the
tumor, the greater is the number of atypical
squamous cells. Atypicality of squamous
cells expresses itself in such changes as great
variation in the size and the shape of the
cells, hyperplasia and hyperchromasia of the
nuclei, absence of intercellular bridges, keratinization of individual cells, and the presence of atypical mitotic figures.

Differentiation in squamous cell carcinomas is in the direction of keratinization.
Keratinization often takes place in the form
of horn pearls, which are very characteristic
structures composed of concentric layers of
squamous cells showing gradually increasing
keratinization toward the center. The center shows usually incomplete and only rarely
complete keratinization. Keratohyaline granules within the horn pearls are sparse or
absent.

GRADING AND GRADES. Broders intro-

FIG. 25-22. **Squamous cell carcinoma, Grade 1.** There is invasion of the dermis by epidermal masses. The cells of the invading epidermal masses are predominantly mature squamous cells showing relatively slight atypicality. Several horn pearls are present. The dermis shows a marked inflammatory reaction. (×100)

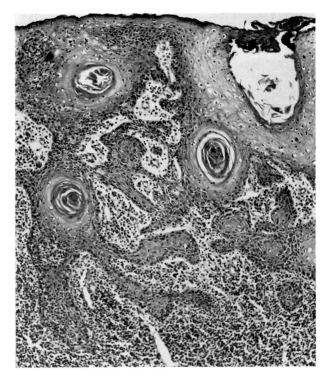

duced a system of grading squamous cell carcinoma. He established four grades according to the proportion of maturing (differentiating) cells present. In Grade 1, more than 75 per cent of the cells are differentiating; in Grade 2, more than 50 per cent; in Grade 3, more than 25 per cent; and in Grade 4, less than 25 per cent. Since differentiation is in the direction of keratinization, the degree of keratinization represents the essential feature in Broder's system of grading. However, it is now generally recognized that, in addition to the number of differentiating cells, the degree of atypicality of the tumor cells and the depth of penetration of the lesion are important factors in grading. It also must be kept in mind that different degrees of malignancy may be present in different fields of the same tumor. Therefore, it is advisable to examine several sections of every tumor that is to be graded and then grade according to the least differentiated portion (Edmundson).

In squamous cell carcinoma, Grade 1 (Fig. 25-22) the tumor masses have not penetrated below the level of the sweat glands. They still show in some areas an intact basal layer at their periphery. In other areas, however, the basal layer has become disorganized and may no longer be present. In such areas the cell masses appear poorly demarcated from the surrounding stroma. The cells of the invading cell masses are predominantly squamous cell with well developed intercellular bridges differentiating toward horny cells. Nevertheless, some of the squamous cells are atypical. Horn pearls are present in fairly large number. Some are well developed and have fully keratinized centers; others, however, show only partial keratinization of their centers, and the concentric arrangement of the cells is not distinct. Besides horn pearls, sheets of partially keratinized cells may be present. The dermis often shows a rather marked inflammatory reaction. It is noteworthy that in solar keratosis and squamous cell carcinoma, Grade 1, the inflammatory reaction in the dermis usually is much more pronounced than in the more malignant forms of squamous cell carcinoma. This phenomenon, which may well represent an immune reaction, indicates that tissue, when invaded by carcinomatous cells, is able to react against the tumor cells to some extent, provided that the cells are only moderately malignant. (The same observation can be made also in malignant melanoma and mycosis fungoides; see pp. 673 and 702.)

In squamous cell carcinoma, Grade 2 (Fig. 25-23), the invading cell masses as a rule are poorly demarcated from the surrounding stroma. Keratinization is much less evident than in Grade 1. There are only a few horn pearls, and those present show incompletely keratinized centers. A fairly large number of the squamous cells are atypical.

In squamous cell carcinoma, Grade 3 (Fig. 25-24), keratinization is absent in many areas. Horn pearls are not found. Instead, keratinization occurs in small cell groups, in which the cells possess a slightly eosinophilic cytoplasm and a few intercellular bridges. In addition, one finds individual cell keratinization, in which the dyskeratotic cells are large and round, have a deeply eosinophilic cytoplasm, and a pyknotic nucleus. The majority of the tumor cells are atypical. Mitotic figures are conspicuous, and many of them are atypical.

In squamous cell carcinoma, Grade 4 (Fig. 25-25), keratinization is almost completely absent. Nearly all tumor cells are atypical and devoid of intercellular bridges. Thus, it is often difficult to arrive at the correct diagnosis so long as individual fields only are studied. The tumor then may suggest a malignant melanoma in some instances and a fibrosarcoma in others. The latter diagnosis may be particularly difficult to rule out when the cells are spindle-shaped, as in the so-called spindle-celled squamous cell carcinoma (Brooks; Underwood et al.). If, however, sections are studied thoroughly, evidence of origin from the epidermis or the presence in a few areas of cells showing intercellular bridges and beginning keratinization usually establishes the diagnosis. Squamous cell carcinoma, Grade 4, is relatively rare in the skin. Many of the reported cases of spindle-celled squamous cell carcinoma occurred in areas of radiodermatitis. In this connection it may be pointed out that most cases reported as postradiation sarcomas in the literature represent squamous cell carcinomas of the spindle cell type (Sims and Kirsch) (see p. 584).

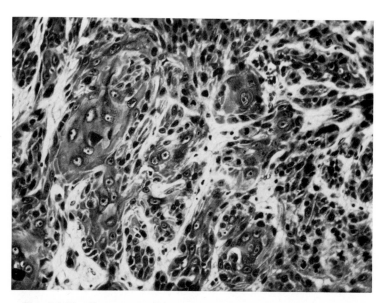

FIG. 25-23. **Squamous cell carcinoma, Grade 2.** The cell masses show much less keratinization than in Grade 1. There are only a few horn pearls, and those present show incompletely keratinized centers. Atypical cells are conspicuous. (×200)

FIG. 25-24. **Squamous cell carcinoma, Grade 3.** No horn pearls are present. Keratinization occurs only in small cell groups. Many cells are atypical and devoid of prickles. To the right, a cell shows individual cell keratinization (I.K.). (×200)

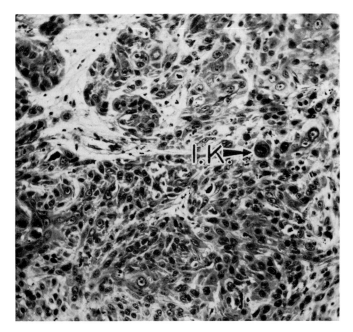

THE INCIDENCE OF METASTASIS largely depends on the type of skin or the type of skin lesion on which the squamous cell carcinoma has arisen (see p. 476). Squamous cell carcinomas producing metastases show as a rule extensive invasion but not necessarily pronounced anaplasia (Lund). Nevertheless, the more anaplastic a squamous cell carcinoma is, the more likely it is to give rise to metastases. The regional lymph nodes are the first site to be invaded by metastases.

Histogenesis. Squamous cell carcinomas show in areas of invasion, as evidence of a disturbed interaction between the tumor cells and the stroma, absence of the PAS-positive basement membrane zone on light microscopy, and either partial or complete absence of the basal lamina on electron microscopy (Kobayasi). The fact that also in Bowen's disease, in which there is no invasion of the tumor, the basal lamina shows discontinuities casts doubt on the hypothesis that the basal lamina is important in restraining the invasion of cancer cells into the connective tissue (Olsen et al.).

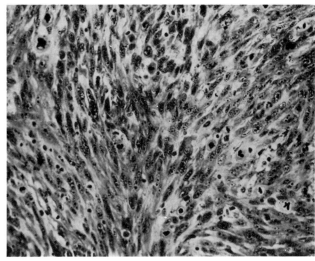

FIG. 25-25. **Squamous cell carcinoma, Grade 4.** Evidence of keratinization is absent. The tumor cells appear atypical and without recognizable intercellular bridges. Because many tumor cells are elongated the tumor suggests a fibrosarcoma more than a carcinoma. (×200)

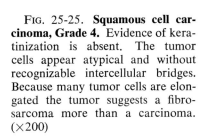

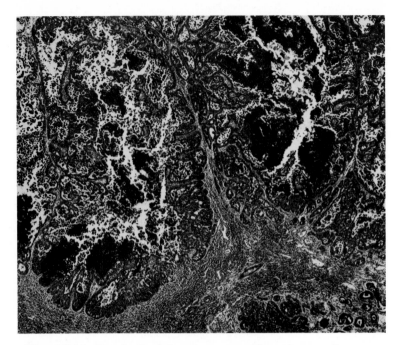

FIG. 25-26. **Pseudoglandular squamous cell carcinoma.** Low magnification. The tumor contains large alveolar spaces into which papillary projections protrude. The alveolar spaces are filled with desquamated, acantholytic cells, many of which are partially or completely keratinized. (×50)

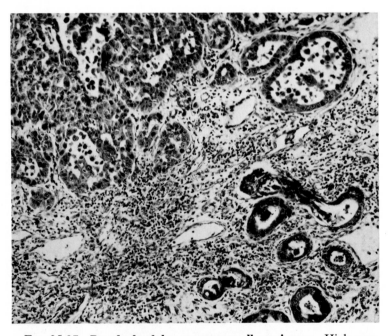

FIG. 25-27. **Pseudoglandular squamous cell carcinoma.** High magnification of the base of the tumor shown in Figure 25-26. The tubular lumina of the tumor contain acantholytic cells. The sweat glands in the right lower corner show some epithelial proliferation, probably induced by the inflammatory infiltrate. (×200)

Electron microscopy furthermore shows a reduction in the number of desmosomes on the cell surface. In their place microvilli extend into the widened intercellular spaces. Desmosomes can be seen within the cytoplasm of some of the tumor cells, either by themselves or attached to bundles of tonofilaments (E.M. No. 38) (Klingmüller et al.). It is as yet not clear whether their intracytoplasmic location is the result of phagocytosis, of infolding, or of intracytoplasmic new formation. It is not, however, a specific finding for squamous cell carcinoma since similar intracytoplasmic desmosomes have been observed in keratoacanthoma (see p. 484) and in Bowen's disease, as well as in several unrelated epidermal proliferations (see p. 475).

Differential Diagnosis. The diagnosis of squamous cell carcinoma, although easily made in typical cases, may be difficult at times. Squamous cell carcinoma must be differentiated from solar keratosis, pseudocarcinomatous hyperplasia, keratoacanthoma, and basal cell epithelioma.

The differences between squamous cell carcinoma and solar keratosis lie in the degree rather than in the type of changes. In both conditions one finds atypicality of cells with dyskeratosis of individual cells and downward proliferation of the epidermis. However, in squamous cell carcinoma actual invasion of the dermis is present, and the invading tumor masses may contain horn pearls. No sharp line of demarcation exists between the two conditions, and it is not infrequent to find in a lesion that in general has the histologic appearance of solar keratosis, when step sectioning is carried out, one or several areas in which the changes have progressed to squamous cell carcinoma.

For differentiation from pseudocarcinomatous hyperplasia, see page 482; from keratoacanthoma, see page 485; and from basal cell epithelioma, see page 550.

PSEUDOGLANDULAR SQUAMOUS CELL CARCINOMA

Occasionally on histologic examination, squamous cell carcinomas as a result of dyskeratosis and subsequent acantholysis show tubular and alveolar formations. Clinically, such pseudoglandular squamous cell carcinomas occur almost exclusively in sun-damaged skin of elderly patients, especially on the face and ears; although in rare instances they have been found on non-exposed skin (Lasser et al.). On sun-exposed skin they may arise as such, or they may develop from a solar keratosis (Chorzelski; Johnson and Helwig). In most instances they do not differ in their clinical appearance from the usual type of squamous cell carcinoma and thus commonly show a central ulceration surrounded by a raised, indurated border. Occasionally they greatly resemble a keratoacanthoma in their clinical appearance (Muller et al.). Metastases are rare but were observed on 3 occasions in a series of 213 lesions (Johnson and Helwig).

Histopathology. Pseudoglandular squamous cell carcinomas show tubular and alveolar lumina lined with one or several layers of epithelium (Fig. 25-26). In areas where the lumina are lined with a single layer of epithelium, the epithelial cells resemble glandular cells; but in areas with several layers of epithelium, squamous and partially keratinized cells usually form the inner layers. The lumina are filled with desquamated, acantholytic cells, many of which are partially or fully keratinized. In addition, there are solid areas with the appearance of squamous cell carcinoma (Delacrétaz et al.; Muller et al.; Johnson and Helwig). In some cases eccrine glands and ducts having a somewhat atypical appearance are present at the periphery of these tumors (Fig. 25-27) (Lever).

Histogenesis. These tumors represent squamous cell carcinomas of lobular growth in which there is considerable dyskeratosis with individual cell keratinization, resulting in acantholysis in the center of the lobular formations. This process is analogous to the suprabasal clefts seen in some solar keratoses (Muller et al.). The somewhat atypical appearance of some of the eccrine glands and ducts probably is the result of an epithelial proliferation induced in them by the inflammatory reaction accompanying the tumor and does not represent a neoplastic process (Delacrétaz et al.).

PSEUDOCARCINOMATOUS HYPERPLASIA

A considerable proliferation of the epidermis, which clinically as well as histologically may suggest carcinoma, occurs occasionally (1) in chronic proliferative inflammatory

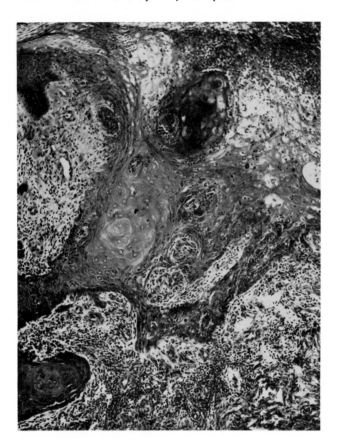

Fig. 25-28. **Pseudocarcinomatous hyperplasia in bromoderma.** There is downward proliferation of the epidermis analogous to squamous cell carcinoma, Grade 1. In the field shown it is impossible to rule out carcinoma. Note, however, the permeation of the epidermis in many areas by inflammatory cells. (×100)

processes, such as bromoderma, blastomycosis, or granuloma inguinale, and (2) at the edges of chronic ulcers, such as occur after burns or in stasis dermatitis, basal cell epithelioma, lupus vulgaris, scrofuloderma, gumma and pyoderma gangrenosum. In addition, granular cell myoblastoma is known to evoke quite frequently a pseudocarcinomatous hyperplasia.

Histopathology. Histologically, one observes in pseudocarcinomatous hyperplasia an epithelial hyperplasia that often closely resembles squamous cell carcinoma, Grade 1 or 2. Although squamous cell carcinoma may develop at the edges of chronic ulcers, it is likely that some of the cases that have been regarded as such in the past represented in reality pseudocarcinomatous hyperplasia. On the other hand, a lesion starting out as pseudocarcinomatous hyperplasia at the edge of an ulcer may eventually develop into a squamous cell carcinoma and even metastasize (Ju).

The histologic picture of pseudocarcinomatous hyperplasia shows irregular invasion of the dermis by epidermal cell masses and strands with horn-pearl formation and often numerous mitotic figures (Fig. 25-28). Irregular proliferations of the epidermis may extend even below the level of the sweat glands, where they appear in sections as isolated islands of epidermal tissue (Sommerville). However, the squamous cells usually are well differentiated, and atypicalities, such as individual cell keratinization and nuclear hyperplasia and hyperchromasia, are absent. Furthermore, in pseudocarcinomatous hyperplasia one often sees invasion of the epithelial proliferations by leukocytes and disintegration of some of the epidermal cells, findings that usually are absent in squamous cell carcinoma (Winer). But even when all these criteria are taken into account, it may still be difficult to differentiate squamous cell carcinoma from pseudocarcinomatous hyperplasia by the study of histologic sections alone (Sommerville). Multiple biopsies and detailed clinical data may be necessary for differentiation.

It is worthwhile to study the inflammatory infiltrate in every section in which one contemplates a diagnosis of squamous cell carcinoma, Grade 1 or 2, for the possible presence of tuberculosis, or of one of the granulomatous mycoses. If such evidence is found, one may be dealing with pseudocarcinomatous hyperplasia instead of squamous cell carcinoma.

KERATOACANTHOMA

Two types of keratoacanthoma exist: the solitary type, and the multiple type.

SOLITARY KERATOACANTHOMA

Only since 1950, subsequent to the publications by Rook and Whimster and by Musso and Gordon, has this fairly common lesion been accepted as an entity and differentiated from squamous cell carcinoma, which it resembles both clinically and histologically. Solitary keratoacanthoma occurs in older persons usually as a single lesion; but occasionally there are several lesions, or subsequently new lesions develop. The lesion consists of a firm dome-shaped nodule, 1 to 2 cm in diameter, which in its center has a horn-filled crater. The sites of predilection are exposed areas, where about 90 per cent of solitary keratoacanthomas occur (Ghadially et al.), but they may occur on any hairy cutaneous site. They have not been reported as occurring on the palms, the soles, or the mucous surfaces. The nodule reaches its full size within a few weeks and involutes spontaneously within a few months, generally in less than 6 months. Healing takes place with a slightly depressed scar.

It has become apparent that some keratoacanthomas, especially those located on the lip where they usually involve both the skin and the vermilion border, have a ten-

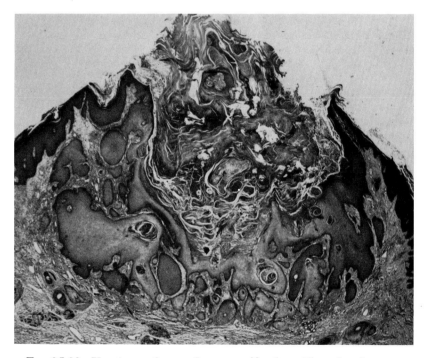

Fig. 25-29. **Keratoacanthoma.** Low magnification. There is a large, central, keratin-filled crater. On the right, the epidermis extends like a lip over the side of the crater. Irregular proliferations of the epidermis extend into the dermis at the base of the crater. (×25)

dency to increase in size for longer than 2 months. They may reach a size of 4 to 5 cm and may take 12 months or more to involute. While increasing in size they show a sharply marginated raised border. Keratoacanthomas of this type may be more difficult to differentiate histologically from squamous cell carcinoma than the usual type of keratoacanthoma, and have a tendency to recur after treatment (Silberberg et al.; Belisario). Occasionally, rather large and destructive keratoacanthomas have been observed on the nose (Burge and Winkelmann) and on the eyelids (Obermayer). It is doubtful, however, that a keratoacanthoma ever changes into a squamous cell carcinoma, as maintained by some authors, e.g., by Belisario and by Burge and Winkelmann. It appears more likely that in such instances a squamous cell carcinoma existed from the beginning (see under Differential Diagnosis).

Histopathology. Inasmuch as in a keratoacanthoma the architecture of the lesion is as important as the cellular characteristics in arriving at the diagnosis, it is advisable, if the lesion cannot be excised in its entirety, to excise for the purpose of biopsy a fusiform specimen from the center of the lesion including the edge on both sides (Popkin et al.). In the early proliferative stage a horn-filled invagination of the epidermis is seen, from which strands of epidermis protrude into the dermis. These strands in many areas are poorly demarcated from the surrounding stroma and contain cells of atypical appearance and many mitotic figures. Also dyskeratotic cells, i.e., cells showing individual cell keratinization, may be seen in areas otherwise not showing advanced keratinization. However, even at this early stage some of the tumor areas show a fairly pronounced degree of keratinization, giving them an eosinophilic "glassy" appearance. In the dermis a rather pronounced inflammatory infiltrate is present (de Moragas et al.; Milewski and Chorzelski).

A fully developed lesion shows in its center a large, irregularly shaped crater filled with keratin (Fig. 25-29). The epidermis extends like a "lip" or a "buttress" over the sides of the crater. At the base of the crater irregular epidermal proliferations extend both upward into the crater and downward from the base of the crater. These proliferations still appear somewhat atypical, but less so than in the initial stage: the keratinization is extensive and fairly advanced, with only a thin shell of one or two layers of basophilic, nonkeratinized cells at the periphery of the proliferations, while the cells within this shell appear eosinophilic and glassy as the result of keratinization (Fig. 25-30). There are many horn pearls, most of which show complete keratinization in their center. A rather dense inflammatory infiltrate is present at the base of the lesion (Levy et al.; Lapière).

In the involuting stage proliferation has ceased, and most cells at the base of the crater have undergone keratinization. Gradually, the crater flattens and finally disappears during the process of healing.

Histogenesis. It is generally agreed that the lesion starts with hyperplasia of one or of several adjoining hair follicles and with squamous metaplasia of the attached sebaceous glands (Calnan and Haber). This is thought to be the mode of formation also of keratoacanthomas involving the vermilion border of the lips, since probably they arise from a hair follicle in the adjacent skin (Silberberg et al.). The application of cutaneous carcinogens to the skin of animals frequently produces, among other tumors, lesions having the histologic appearance of keratoacanthomas, and these tumors take their origin from the infundibulum of one or several hair follicles, with the infundibulum representing that portion of the hair follicle situated above the entry of the sebaceous duct (Ghadially).

The cause of keratoacanthoma is not known. The theory of a viral genesis has not been confirmed. The electron microscopic findings are largely nonspecific. It is of interest, however, that keratoacanthomas, like squamous cell carcinomas and lesions of Bowen's disease, often show the presence of intracytoplasmic desmosomes. Whereas Takaki et al. found them only within dyskeratotic cells, von Bülow and Klingmüller observed them also in keratinizing and in keratinized cells of keratoacanthomas. They were seen most frequently in involuting keratoacanthomas in which from 1 to 5 per cent of the keratinocytes in the middle and upper cell layers contained intracytoplasmic desmosomes. Their intracytoplasmic location was regarded by von Bülow and Klingmüller as being caused by invaginations of the plasma membrane and the attachment of two intracytoplasmic half-desmosomes to one another.

Differential Diagnosis. In the early stage, differentiation from squamous cell carcinoma is difficult and at times impossible even when central sections through a fully excised lesion are available, allowing a study of the architecture of the lesion. Aside from the architecture, the high degree of keratinization, manifested by the eosinophilic, glassy appearance of many of the cells, is the most important diagnostic feature. In addition, clinical data are of great value: rapid development of a lesion showing a central, horn-filled crater speaks for keratoacanthoma rather than for squamous cell carcinoma. The greatest difficulties in the differentiation of a keratoacanthoma from a squamous cell carcinoma are encountered in very early lesions, since, on the one hand, a horn-filled invagination may be seen in squamous cell carcinoma and, on the other hand, cells with an atypical appearance can occur in early keratoacanthoma. Whereas cells showing individual cell keratinization can occur in keratoacanthoma it is highly doubtful whether pseudoglandular formations caused by extensive dyskeratosis and acantholysis can occur in keratoacanthomas, as described by Stevanovic. Since it is generally agreed that squamous cell carcinomas can masquerade as keratoacanthomas not only clinically but occasionally also histologically (Muller et al.; Nikolowski), it is best to err on the safe side and in case of doubt to proceed on the assumption that the lesion is a squamous cell carcinoma.

MULTIPLE KERATOACANTHOMA

There are two variants of multiple keratoacanthoma: the multiple self-healing epitheliomas of the skin, and eruptive keratoacanthomas. Both variants are rare in contrast with solitary keratoacanthoma.

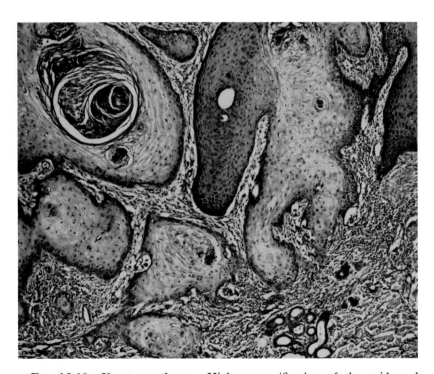

FIG. 25-30. **Keratoacanthoma.** Higher magnification of the epidermal proliferations at the base of the crater shows their resemblance to squamous cell carcinoma. However, there is more keratinization than is usually seen in squamous cell carcinoma, giving the tumor islands a glassy appearance. (×100)

In multiple self-healing epitheliomas of the skin there is a continual appearance of new lesions on any part of the skin, including the palms and soles, but especially on the face and the extremities. The lesions start as papules, develop into nodules having a central, horn-filled crater, and after a few months heal with a depressed scar. In some patients the condition is inherited (Sommerville and Milne).

In eruptive keratoacanthoma thousands of lesions are present consisting largely of follicular papules from 2 to 3 mm in diameter. The oral mucosa and the larnyx may be involved (Rossman et al.; Winkelmann and Brown).

Histopathology. The histologic appearance of multiple keratoacanthoma is similar to that of solitary keratoacanthoma except that crater formation and accumulation of keratin in the crater usually are less pronounced (Rook and Moffat; Rossman et al.).

Histogenesis. It appears likely that multiple keratoacanthoma basically represents the same condition as solitary keratoacanthoma, and that predisposition or genetic factors are responsible for the greater number of lesions (Rook and Moffat). As in solitary keratoacanthoma, lesions arising in hair-bearing parts of the skin have their onset in the upper portion of a hair follicle, whereas in lesions arising on the palms, the soles, and the mucous membranes the site of origin is not apparent (Rossman et al.).

PAGET'S DISEASE

Paget's disease of the breast occurs almost exclusively in women on and around the nipple. Only a few instances of its occurrence on the male breast have been described (Chrichlow and Czernobilsky). The lesion is always unilateral. The cutaneous lesion in Paget's disease of the breast begins either on the nipple or the areola of the breast and extends slowly to the surrounding skin. It consists of a sharply defined, slightly infiltrated area of erythema showing scaling, oozing and crusting. There may or may not be retraction of the nipple.

The cutaneous lesion is regularly associated with carcinoma of the breast; and in

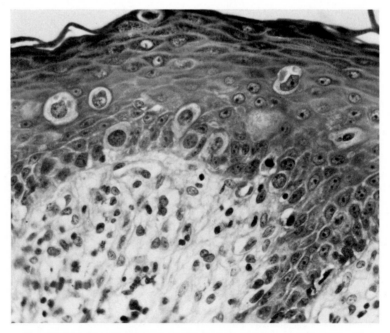

Fig. 25-31. **Paget's disease of the breast.** High magnification. Only a few Paget cells are scattered through the epidermis. They are large, rounded cells devoid of intercellular bridges, with ample, pale-staining cytoplasm. (×400)

FIG. 25-32. **Paget's disease of the breast.** Low magnification. The epidermis is permeated with numerous Paget cells lying singly and in groups. There is no invasion of the dermis by Paget cells. Flattened basal cells lie between the tumor cells and the dermis in many places, a finding that aids in the differentiation of Paget's disease from malignant melanoma in situ. (×200)

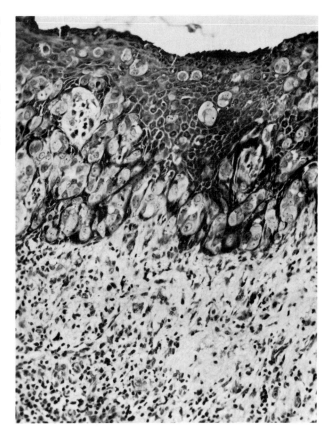

more than half of the patients a mass can be felt on palpation of the breast. Metastases in the axillary lymph nodes are found in about two thirds of the patients with a palpable mass, and in one third of those without a palpable mass (Ashikari et al.).

Histopathology. In early lesions of Paget's disease of the breast, the epidermis usually shows only a few scattered Paget cells (Fig. 25-31). They are large, rounded cells devoid of intercellular bridges and containing a large nucleus and ample cytoplasm that stains much lighter than the cytoplasm of the adjacent squamous cells (Fig. 25-32). As the number of Paget cells increases, they compress the squamous cells to such an extent that the squamous cells may form merely a network, the meshes of which are filled with Paget cells lying singly and in groups. In particular, one often observes flattened basal cells lying between Paget cells and the underlying dermis (Fig. 25-32). In many lesions one observes Paget cells that stain positive with the PAS reaction (Fig. 25-33). This reaction is diastase-resistant, an indication that the positive reaction is caused mainly by neutral mucopolysaccharides, rather than by glycogen (Fisher and Beyer). Often, however, neutral mucopolysaccharides can be shown to be present in only some of the Paget cells (Hopsu-Havu and Sonck); and in occasional cases neutral mucopolysaccharides are completely absent (Pinkus and Mehregan, 1963). In some cases in which the Paget cells contain neutral mucopolysaccharides they also stain with alcian blue, but only at pH 2.5 and not at pH 0.4 and fail to show metachromasia on staining with methylene blue or thionin (Fisher and Beyer). Such cells contain sialomucin, a nonsulfated, hyaluronidase-resistant acid mucopolysaccharide (Lattanand et al.). Not infrequently, Paget cells contain some melanin (Culberson and Horn); but they are dopa-negative (Helwig and Graham).

The dermis in Paget's disease shows a moderately severe chronic inflammatory re-

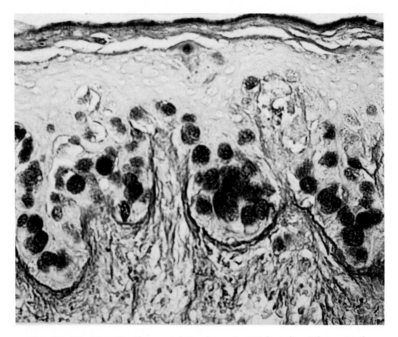

FIG. 25-33. **Paget's disease of the breast.** PAS stain. The cytoplasm of the Paget cells gives a positive PAS reaction, which is diastase-resistant. (×200)

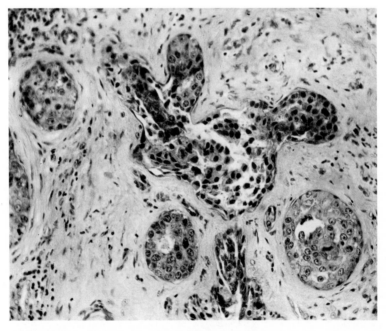

FIG. 25-34. **Paget's disease of the breast.** Intraductal carcinoma is present in the mammary ducts. (×200)

action. Although Paget cells do not invade the dermis from the epidermis, they may be seen extending from the epidermis into the epithelium of hair follicles.

Histologic examination of the mammary ducts and glands nearly always shows malignant changes in some of them. At first the carcinoma is confined within the walls of the ducts and glands (Fig. 25-34), but ultimately the tumor cells invade the connective tissue. From then on, lymphatic spread and metastases occur, just as in other types of mammary carcinoma.

Histogenesis. The divergent views concerning the Paget cell in mammary and extramammary Paget's disease that were based on light microscopic findings and their interpretations have not yet been resolved by the electron microscopic findings even though more than a dozen electron microscopic studies have been published. However, only one enzyme histochemical study has appeared (Belcher, 1972).

In regard to the light microscopic findings concerning the Paget cell in mammary Paget's disease, a few authors have maintained the view that the intraepidermal Paget cell represents a modified keratinocyte (Montgomery). Most authors, however, regard the intraepidermal Paget cell as a mammary gland cell, either ductal or secretory in nature. In favor of the view that the Paget cell is a mammary gland cell and the epidermal involvement in Paget's disease of the breast is due to the presence of an "epidermotropic mammary carcinoma" (Pinkus and Mehregan) are the following observations: (1) Paget cells act like foreign cells in the epidermis and, therefore, do not invade from the epidermis into the underlying dermis, whereas they do so from the mammary glands into the surrounding tissue, and (2) Paget cells, similar to apocrine and mammary gland cells, frequently contain neutral mucopolysaccharides (Fisher and Beyer; Greenwood and Minkowitz). It is likely that the initial lesion in Paget's disease of the breast is an intraductal carcinoma arising in one or several mammary ducts. The primary ductal carcinoma extends from its site of origin downward within the epithelium of the mammary ducts and glands and also upward into the epidermis, where it causes the cutaneous lesion (Muir).

Electron microscopic study of Paget's disease of the breast has led to various interpretations. Often, the Paget cells show relatively little differentiation, so that their identification with any mature cell type is difficult. Sagebiel's view that the intraepidermal Paget cells are epidermal cells is based largely on the presence of desmosomes between Paget cells and between Paget cells and epidermal cells. However, in his conclusions he did not consider the fact that desmosomes are found normally between the ductal cells of both apocrine and eccrine glands (Hashimoto et al.). Ebner favored the origin of the Paget cell from the luminal cells of mammary ducts because Paget cells tend to form lumina in the epidermis and microvilli are seen extending into these lumina, two observations that incidentally had been made also by Sagebiel. Belcher has shown in Paget's disease of the breast the presence of an apocrine enzymatic pattern in the intraepidermal Paget cells, namely a strong reactivity for acid phosphatase and esterase and only weakly positive reactions for aminopeptidase and succinic dehydrogenase. This finding, in Belcher's opinion, is in favor of the view that Paget's disease of the breast is a mammary gland tumor, since the mammary gland is a modified apocrine gland.

Differential Diagnosis. Paget's disease of the breast must be differentiated from Bowen's disease and the "pagetoid type" of malignant melanoma in situ. Although vacuolated cells may occur in both Paget's disease and Bowen's disease one observes clear-cut transitions between the vacuolated cells and epidermal cells only in Bowen's disease. Furthermore, one may observe in Bowen's disease, but not in Paget's disease, clumping of nuclei within multinucleated epidermal cells and individual cell keratinization. In addition, even though the PAS reaction is often positive both in Paget cells and in Bowen's disease, this reaction is abolished by diastase digestion only in Bowen's disease (Fisher and Beyer).

In the pagetoid type of malignant melanoma in situ one observes, as in the epidermis of Paget's disease of the breast, large and vacuolated cells scattered through the epidermis (Stout; Hopsu-Havu and Sonck). The difficulty in distinguishing between the two types of cells may be enhanced by the fact that Paget cells occasionally also contain melanin (Culberson and Horn). The most important points in differentiating the two types of cells are as follows: (1) Paget cells in many areas are separated from the dermis by flattened basal cells, whereas melanoma cells border directly on the dermis; (2) Paget cells do not invade the dermis, whereas melanoma cells often do so; (3) in many Paget cells the PAS reaction is positive and diastase-resistant and often also the alcian blue stain is positive, whereas in malignant melanoma these staining reactions are almost invariably negative (Fisher and Beyer; Helwig and Graham; Jacobsen and Haavelsrud); and (4) Paget cells are dopa-negative, in contrast with melanoma cells.

EXTRAMAMMARY PAGET'S DISEASE

Three types of extramammary Paget's disease occur: One arises in the axillary, genital or perianal region without being associated with a subjacent adnexal carcinoma; the second type arises in the axillary, genital or perianal region and is associated with a subjacent carcinoma of either apocrine or eccrine glands; and the third type arises in the perianal region in association with a subjacent adenocarcinoma of the rectum.

In extramammary Paget's disease the clinical picture shows, as in the mammary type, a slowly enlarging reddish patch with oozing and crusting that resembles an eczematous lesion except for having a sharp border. Only a wide excision of the lesion will show whether a subjacent carcinoma is present or not. In about 40 per cent of the patients no involvement of underlying structures is found in extramammary Paget's disease of the genital region (Bowman and Hartman), of the axillae (Kawatsu and Miki) or of the perianal region (Fisher and Beyer). It can be assumed that in such instances the tumor arises in the poral portion of a gland (Pinkus and Mehregan, 1969). In patients without involvement of underlying glands the prognosis is quite good after adequate excision (Murrell and McMullan). However, in patients with involvement of underlying apocrine glands (Becker et al.; Holleran and Schmutzer) or eccrine glands (Koss and Brockunier) the prognosis is generally poor because of the likelihood of metastases not only to regional lymph nodes but also to visceral organs. The prognosis is poorest in patients with an underlying adenocarcinoma of the rectum (Yoell and Price; Graham and Helwig).

Histopathology. In extramammary Paget's disease of the genital and axillary regions, the histologic picture is the same as that of Paget's disease of the breast, showing Paget cells scattered through the epidermis; and, as in Paget's disease of the breast, a large percentage of the Paget cells are PAS-positive and diastase-resistant, and occasionally also contain sialomucin.

In Paget's disease of the perianal region associated with an adenocarcinoma of the rectum the Paget cells that are found scattered through the epidermis regularly contain sialomucin, a nonsulfated acid mucopolysaccharide. This material (1) is PAS-positive and diastase-resistant, (2) stains with alcian blue at pH 2.5 but not at pH 0.4, (3) does not stain metachromatically with methylene blue, toluidine blue, or thionin, and (4) is hyaluronidase-resistant (Fisher and Beyer; Helwig and Graham; Mendoza and Helwig).

A decision as to whether a carcinoma of subjacent apocrine or eccrine glands exists is not always easy. Generally, as long as Paget cells are confined to the epidermis and to the outer root sheath of hairs extending not farther down than to the entrance of the sebaceous duct, the tumor can be regarded as a carcinoma in situ. If, however, Paget cells extend into ductal structures, an adnexal carcinoma exists.

Histogenesis. Even though extramammary Paget's disease of the genital and axillary regions greatly resembles Paget's disease of the breast histologically and histochemically and, furthermore, occurs exclusively in areas where apocrine glands are normally present, an apocrine derivation of genital and axillary Paget's disease is by no means evident in all cases on the basis of electron microscopic and enzyme histochemical studies.

An epidermal derivation of the cells in genital Paget's disease was postulated by Piérard and Kint, and by Medenica and Sahihi on the basis of their electron microscopic findings, largely because cells intermediate to keratinocytes and Paget cells were seen. Caputo and Califano regarded the genital Paget cells as being apocrine secretory cells because of the presence of electron-dense secretory granules and of macromitochondria. Similarly, Demopoulos regarded the Paget cells as secretory cells and as related to apocrine rather than eccrine secretory cells because of the absence of intercellular canaliculi.

Koss and Brockunier as well as Belcher, on the other hand, assumed that the Paget cells in genital Paget's disease were eccrine secretory cells. Koss and Brockunier regarded the Paget cells as eccrine because they could recognize two types of cells, one of them with secretory granules, and also intercellular canaliculi. Belcher, even though he could confirm these findings, pointed out the difficulties of differentiating between apocrine and eccrine secretory cells in malignant tumors by electron microscopy and attributed greater value to his enzyme histochemical studies. With this method he found in his case of genital Paget's disease the Paget cells to show strongly positive reactions for eccrine enzymes, especially amylophosphorylase and leucine aminopeptide, and minimal to absent reactions to apocrine enzymes, such as esterase, NADH diaphorase, beta-glucuronidase and acid phosphatase. This observation by Belcher contrasts with his finding a prevalence of apocrine enzymes in mammary Paget cells (see p. 489).

Differential Diagnosis. Extramammary Paget's disease, like Paget's disease of the breast, must be differentiated from Bowen's disease and especially from pagetoid malignant melanoma in situ. (See under Paget's disease of the breast, Differential Diagnosis.)

BIBLIOGRAPHY

Localized Linear Epidermal Nevus

Fritsch, P., and Wittels, W.: Ein Fall von bilateralem Naevus comedonicus. Hautarzt, *22*: 409, 1971.

Haber, H.: Verrucous naevi. Trans. St. John's Hosp. Derm. Soc., *34*:20, 1955.

Pack, G. T., and Sunderland, D. A.: Naevus unius lateris. Arch. Surg., *43*:341, 1941.

Paige, T. N., and Mendelson, C. G.: Bilateral nevus comedonicus. Arch. Derm., *96*:172, 1967.

Inflammatory Linear Epidermal Nevus

Altman, J., and Mehregan, A. H.: Inflammatory linear verrucose epidermal nevus. Arch. Derm., *104*:385, 1971.

Kaidbey, K. H., and Kurban, A. K.: Dermatitic epidermal nevus. Arch. Derm., *104*:166, 1967.

Systematized Linear Epidermal Nevus

Ackerman, A. B.: Histopathologic concept of epidermolytic hyperkeratosis. Arch. Derm., *102*:253, 1970.

Barker, L. P., and Sachs, W.: Bullous congenital ichthyosiform erythroderma. Arch. Derm. Syph., *67*:443, 1953.

Braun-Falco, O., Petzoldt, D., Christophers, E., and Wolf, H. H.: Die granulöse Degeneration bei Naevus verrucosus bilateralis. Arch. klin. exp. Derm., *235*:115, 1969.

Gebhart, W., and Kidd, R. L.: Das solitäre epidermolytische Akanthom. Z. Haut, *47*:(1), 1972.

Hirone, T., and Kukushiro, R.: Disseminated epidermolytic acanthoma. Acta dermatoven., *53*:393, 1973.

Klaus, S., Weinstein, G. D., and Frost, P.: Localized epidermolytic hyperkeratosis. A form of keratoderma of the palms and soles. Arch. Derm., *101*:272, 1970.

Orbaneja, J. G., Lozano de Sosa, J. L. S., and Huarte, P. S.: Hiperqueratosis palmoplantar diffusa y circunscrita (tipo Thost-Unna) con degeneracion reticular del cuerpo mucoso. Internat. J. Derm., *11*:96, 1972.

Shapiro, L., and Baraf, C. S.: Isolated epidermolytic acanthoma. Arch. Derm., *101*:220, 1970.

Solomon, L. M., Fretzin, D. F., and Dewald, R. L.: The epidermal nevus syndrome. Arch. Derm., *97*:273, 1968.

Weibel, E. R., and Schnyder, U. W.: Zur Ultrastruktur und Histochemie der granulösen Degeneration bei bullöser Erythrodermie congénitale ichthyosiforme. Arch. klin. exp. Derm., *225*:286, 1966.

Zeligman, J., and Pomeranz, J.: Variations of congenital ichthyosiform erythroderma. Arch. Derm., *91*:120, 1965.

Oral Epithelial Nevus

Cannon, A. B.: White nevus of the mucosa (naevus spongiosus albus mucosae). Arch. Derm. Syph., *31*:365, 1935.

Cooke, B. E. D., and Morgan, J.: Oral epithelial nevi. Brit. J. Derm., *71*:134, 1959.

Dawson, T. A. J.: Microscopic appearance of geographic tongue. Brit. J. Derm., *81*:827, 1969.

Haye, K. R., and Whitehead, F. I. H.: Hereditary leukokeratosis of the mucous membranes. Brit. J. Derm., *80*:529, 1968.

O'Keefe, E., Braverman, I. M., and Cohen, I.: Annulus migrans: Identical lesions in pustular psoriasis, Reiter's syndrome, and geographic tongue. Arch. Derm., *107*:240, 1973.

Stüttgen, G., Berres, H. H., and Will, W.: Leuko-
plakische epitheliale Naevi der Mundschleim-
haut. Arch. klin. exp. Derm., *221*:433, 1965.

Witkop, C. J., Jr., and Gorlin, R. J.: Four hereditary mucosal syndromes. Arch. Derm., *84*:
762, 1961.

Zegarelli, E. V., Everett, F. G., Kutscher, A. H.,
et al.: Familial white folded dysplasia of the
mucous membranes. Arch. Derm., *80*:59,
1959.

Seborrheic Keratosis

Andrade, R., and Steigleder, G. K.: Contribution
à l'étude histologique et histochimique de la
verrue seborrhéique (papillome basocellu-
laire). Ann. derm. syph., *86*:495, 1959.

Balabanow, K., and Angelow, N.: Ein Fall von
Verruca seborrhoica mit Übergang in Epitheliom. Derm. Wschr., *150*:683, 1964.

Becker, S. W.: Seborrheic keratosis and verruca
with special reference to the melanotic variety.
Arch. Derm. Syph., *63*:358, 1951.

Braun-Falco, O.: Frage der Entartung von
Verrucae seborrhoicae seniles. Hautarzt, *15*:
645, 1964.

Braun-Falco, O., and Kint, A.: Zur Histogenese
der Verruca seborrhoica. I. Mitteilung. Arch.
klin. exp. Derm., *216*:615, 1963.

Braun-Falco, O., Kint, A., and Vogell, W.: Zur
Histogenese der Verruca seborrhoica. II. Mit-
teilung. Elektronenmikroskopische Befunde.
Arch. klin. exp. Derm., *217*:627, 1963.

Duperrat, B., and Mascaro, J. M.: Une tumeur
développée aux dépens de l'acrotrichium ou
partie intraépidermique du follicule pilaire:
porome folliculaire. Dermatologica, *126*:291,
1963.

Hairston, M. A., Jr., Reed, R. J., and Derbes, V.
J.: Dermatosis papulosa nigra. Arch. Derm.,
89:655, 1964.

Helwig, E. B.: "Inverted follicular keratosis." *In*
Seminar on the Skin: Neoplasms and Dermatoses. Proceedings, 20th Seminar, Am. Soc.
Clinical Pathologists. International Congress
of Clinical Pathology, Washington, D.C.,
1954. Am. Soc. Clin. Pathologists, 1955, p. 38.

Kocsard, E., and Carter, J. J.: The papillomatous
keratoses. The nature and differential diagnosis of stucco keratosis. Austral. J. Derm.,
12:80, 1971.

Lennox, B.: Pigment patterns in epithelial tumors
of the skin. J. Path. Bact., *61*:587, 1949.

Lund, H. Z.: Tumors of the Skin, Atlas of Tumor
Pathology, sec. 1, fasc. 2, p. 42. Washington,
D.C., Armed Forces Institute of Pathology,
1957.

Mehregan, A. H.: Inverted follicular keratosis.
Arch. Derm., *89*:229, 1964.

Mehregan, A. H., and Pinkus, H.: Intraepidermal
carcinoma: a critical study. Cancer, *17*:609,
1964.

Mevorah, B., and Mishima, Y.: Cellular response
of seborrheic keratosis following croton oil
irritation and surgical trauma. Dermatologica,
131:452, 1965.

Mishima, Y., and Pinkus, H.: Benign mixed
tumor of melanocytes and malpighian cells.
Arch. Derm., *81*:539, 1960.

Molokhia, M. M., and Portnoy, B.: A study of
dendritic cells in seborrheic warts. Brit. J.
Derm., *85*:254, 1971.

Morales, A., and Hu, F.: Seborrheic verruca and
intraepidermal basal cell epithelioma of Jadassohn. Arch. Derm., *91*:342, 1960.

Pinkus, H.: Premalignant fibroepithelial tumors
of the skin. Arch. Derm. Syph., *67*:598, 1953.

Rowe, L.: Seborrheic keratosis. I. "Pseudo-
epitheliomatous hyperplasia" (Weidman). J.
Invest. Derm., *29*:165, 1957.

Sanderson, K. F.: The structure of seborrheic
keratoses. Brit. J. Derm., *80*:588, 1968.

Willoughby, C., and Soter, N. A.: Stucco keratosis. Arch. Derm., *105*:859, 1972.

Clear Cell Acanthoma

Cramer, H. J.: Klarzellenakanthom (Degos) mit
syringomatösen und naevus-sebaceus-artigen
Anteilen. Dermatologica, *143*:265, 1971.

Degos, R., and Civatte, J.: Clear-cell acanthoma:
experience of 8 years. Brit. J. Derm., *83*:248,
1970.

Degos, R., Delort, J., Civatte, J., and Poiares
Baptista, A.: Tumeur épidermique d'aspect
particulier: acanthome à cellules claires. Ann.
derm. syph., *89*:361, 1962.

Delacrétaz, J.: Acanthome à cellules claires.
Dermatologica, *129*:147, 1964.

Fine, R. M., and Chernosky, M. E.: Clinical
recognition of clear-cell acanthoma (Degos).
Arch. Derm., *100*:559, 1969.

Hu, F., and Sisson, J. K.: The ultrastructure of
pale cell acanthoma. J. Invest. Derm., *52*:185,
1969.

Wells, G. C., and Wilson Jones, E.: Degos'
acanthoma (acanthome à cellules claires).
Brit. J. Derm., *79*:249, 1967.

Wilson Jones, E., and Wells, G. C.: Degos'
acanthoma (acanthome à cellules claires).
Arch. Derm., *94*:286, 1966.

Zak, F. G., and Girerd, R. J.: Das blasszellige
Akanthom (Degos). Hautarzt, *19*:559, 1968.

Zak, F. G., Martinez, M., and Statsinger, A. L.:
Pale cell acanthoma. Arch. Dermat., *93*:674,
1966.

Epidermal Cyst

Epstein, W., and Kligman, A. M.: The pathogenesis of milia and benign tumors of the skin. J. Invest. Derm., *26*:1, 1956.

Love, W. R., and Montgomery, H.: Epithelial cysts. Arch. Derm. Syph., *47*:185, 1943.

McGavran, M. H., and Binnington, B.: Keratinous cysts of the skin. Arch. Derm., *94*:499, 1966.

Raab, W., and Steigleder, G. K.: Fehldiagnosen bei Horncysten. Arch. klin. exp. Derm., *212*: 606, 1961.

Wilson Jones, E.: Proliferating epidermoid cysts. Arch. Derm., *94*:11, 1966.

Pilar Cysts

Kligman, A. M.: The myth of the sebaceous cyst. Arch. Derm., *89*:253, 1964.

McGavran, M. H., and Binnington, B.: Keratinous cysts of the skin. Arch. Derm., *94*:499, 1966.

Pinkus, H.: "Sebaceous cysts" are trichilemmal cysts. Arch. Derm., *99*:544, 1969.

Steatocystoma Multiplex

Contreras, M. A., and Costello, M. J.: Steatocystoma multiplex with embryonal hair formation. Arch. Derm., *76*:720, 1957.

Hashimoto, K., Fisher, B. K., and Lever, W. F.: Steatocystoma multiplex. Hautarzt, *15*:299, 1964.

Kligman, A. M., and Kirschbaum, J. D.: Steatocystoma multiplex: a dermoid tumor. J. Invest. Derm., *42*:388, 1964.

Oyal, H., and Nikolowski, W.: Sebocystomatosen. Arch. klin. exp. Derm., *204*:361, 1957.

Dermoid Cysts

Brownstein, M. H., and Helwig, E. B.: Subcutaneous dermoid cysts. Arch. Derm., *107*: 237, 1973.

Warty Dyskeratoma

Delacrétaz, J.: Dyskératomes ' verruqueux et kératoses séniles dyskératosiques. Dermatologica, *127*:23, 1963.

Furtado, T. A., and Szymanski, F. J.: Étude histologique du dyskératose verruqueux. Ann. derm. syph., *88*:633, 1961.

Gorlin, R. J., and Peterson, W. C., Jr.: Warty dyskeratoma. A note concerning its occurrence in the oral mucosa. Arch. Derm., *95*: 292, 1967.

Graham, J. H., and Helwig, E. B.: Isolated dyskeratosis follicularis. Arch. Derm., *77*:377, 1958.

Jablonska, S., and Chorzelski, T.: Dyskeratoma and epithelioma (carcinoma) dyskeratoticum segregans. Dermatologica, *123*:24, 1961.

Kellum, R. E., and Haserick, J. R.: Localized linear keratosis follicularis. Arch. Derm., *86*: 450, 1962.

Metz, J., and Schröpl, F.: Zur Nosologie des Dyskeratoma segregans ("Warty dyskeratoma"). Arch. klin. exp. Derm., *238*:21, 1970.

Nikolowski, W.: Dyskeratosis follicularis isolata. Arch. klin. exp. Derm., *208*:174, 1959.

Szymanski, F. J.: Warty dyskeratoma. Arch. Derm., *75*:567, 1957.

Tanay, A., and Mehregan, A. H.: Warty dyskeratoma. Dermatologica, *138*:155, 1969 (review).

Solar Keratosis

Ackerman, A. B., and Reed, R. J.: Epidermolytic variant of solar keratosis. Arch. Derm., *107*:104, 1973.

Bart, R. S., Andrade, R., and Kopf, A. W.: Cutaneous horn. Acta dermatoven., *48*:507, 1968.

Cramer, H. J., and Kahlert, G.: Das Cornu cutaneum. Selbständiges Krankheitsbild oder klinisches Symptom? Derm. Wschr., *150*:521, 1964.

Halter, K.: Ueber ein wenig beachtetes histologisches Kennzeichen des Keratoma senile. Hautarzt, *3*:215, 1952.

Hirsch, P., and Marmelzat, W. L.: Lichenoid actinic keratosis. Derm. Internat., *6*:101, 1967.

Koten, J. W., Verhagen, A. R. H. B., and Frank, G. L.: Histopathology of actinic cheilitis. Dermatologica, *135*:465, 1967.

Lumpkin, L. R., and Helwig, E. B.: Solitary lichen planus. Arch. Derm., *93*:54, 1966.

Lund, H. Z.: How often does squamous cell carcinoma of the skin metastasize? Arch. Derm., *92*:635, 1965.

Mashkillejson, A. L.: Über die Vorkrebserkrankung der Lippen. Derm. Monatsschr., *155*: 103, 1969.

Montgomery, H., and Dörffel, J.: Verruca senilis und Keratoma senile. Arch. Derm. Syph., *166*:286, 1932.

Pinkus, H.: Keratosis senilis. Am. J. Clin. Path., *29*:193, 1958.

Sandbank, M.: Basal cell carcinoma at the base of cutaneous horn (cornu cutaneum). Arch. Derm., *104*:97, 1971.

Shapiro, L., and Ackerman, A. B.: Solitary lichen planus-like keratosis. Dermatologica, *132*: 386, 1966.

Woringer, F.: De la kératose sénile à l'épithélioma. Dermatologica, *122*:349, 1961.

Leukoplakia

Cawson, R. A., and Lehner, T.: Chronic hyperplastic candidiasis: candidal leukoplakia. Brit. J. Derm., *86*:9, 1968.

Cooke, B. E. D.: Leukoplakia buccalis and oral epithelial naevi. Brit. J. Derm., *68*:151, 1956.

McAdams, A. J., Jr., and Kistner, R. W.: The relationship of chronic vulvar disease, leukoplakia, and carcinoma in situ to carcinoma of the vulva. Cancer, *11*:740, 1958.

Shklar, G.: Oral leukoplakia—studies in enzyme histochemistry. J. Invest. Derm., *48*:153, 1967.

Oral Florid Papillomatosis

Aird, I., Johnson, H. D., Lennox, B., and Stansfeld, A. G.: Epithelioma cuniculatum: A variety of squamous carcinoma peculiar to the foot. Brit. J. Surg., *42*:245, 1954.

Kanee, B.: Oral florid papillomatosis complicated by verrucous squamous carcinoma. Arch. Derm., *99*:196, 1969.

Kraus, F. T., and Perez-Mesa, C.: Verrucous carcinoma. Cancer, *19*:26, 1966.

Rose, H. P.: Papillomas of the oral cavity. Oral Surg., *20*:542, 1965.

Samitz, M. H., Ackerman, A. B., and Lantis, L. R.: Squamous cell carcinoma arising at the site of oral florid papillomatosis. Arch. Derm., *96*:286, 1967.

Shklar, G.: The precancerous oral lesion. Oral Surg., *20*:58, 1965.

Wechsler, H. L., and Fisher, E. R.: Oral florid papillomatosis. Arch. Derm., *86*:480, 1962.

Bowen's Disease

Bowen, J. T.: Precancerous dermatosis. J. Cutan. Dis., *30*:241, 1912; *33*:787, 1915.

Fisher, E. R., McCoy, M. M., II, and Wechsler, H. L.: Analysis of histopathologic and electron microscopic determinants of keratoacanthoma and squamous cell carcinoma. Cancer, *29*:1387, 1972.

Graham, J. H., and Helwig, E. B.: Bowen's disease and its relationship to systemic cancer. Arch. Derm., *80*:133, 1959.

Klingmüller, G., Klehr, H. U., und Ishibashi, Y.: Desmosomen im Cytoplasma entdifferenzierter Keratinocyten des Plattenepithelcarcinoms. Arch. klin. exp. Derm., *238*:356, 1970.

Klug, H., und Haustein, U. F.: Vorkommen von intrazytoplasmatischen Desmosomen in Keratinozyten. Dermatologica, *148*:143, 1974.

Montgomery, H.: Precancerous dermatosis and epithelioma in situ. Arch. Derm. Syph., *39*: 387, 1939.

Montgomery, H., and Waisman, M.: Epithelioma attributable to arsenic. J. Invest. Derm., *4*:365, 1941.

Olsen, R. L., Nordquist, R., and Everett, M. A.: An electron microscopic study of Bowen's disease. Cancer Res., *28*:2078, 1968.

———: Dyskeratosis in Bowen's disease. Brit. J. Derm., *81*:676, 1969.

Peterka, E. S., Lynch, F. W., and Goltz, R. W.: An association between Bowen's disease and internal cancer. Arch. Derm., *84*:623, 1961.

Sato, A., and Seiji, M.: Electron microscopic observations of malignant dyskeratosis in leukoplakia and Bowen's disease. Acta dermatoven., *53* (suppl. 73): 101, 1973.

Seiji, M., and Mizuno, F.: Electron microscopic study of Bowen's disease. Arch. Derm., *99*:3, 1969.

Erythroplasia of Queyrat, Balanitis Circumscripta

Abell, M. R., and Gosling, J. R. G.: Intraepithelial and infiltrative carcinoma of the vulva: Bowen's type. Cancer, *14*:318, 1961.

Blau, S., and Hyman, A. B.: Erythroplasia of Queyrat. Acta dermatoven., *35*:341, 1955.

Eberhartinger, C., and Bergmann, M.: Balanoposthitis chronica circumscripta plasmacellularis Zoon und Phimose. Z. Haut, *46*:251, 1971.

Graham, J. H., and Helwig, E. B.: Erythroplasia of Queyrat: a precancerous dermatosis. *In* Jadassohn, W., and Schirren, C. B. (eds.): XIII Congressus Internationalis Dermatologiae, Munich, 1967. p. 89. Berlin, Springer, 1968.

Grimmer, H.: Vulvitis chronica plasmacellularis. Z. Haut, *42*:(12), 1967.

Hornstein, O., and Pape, H. D.: Morbus Bowen der Schleimhaut. Dermatologica, *131*:325, 1965.

Hyman, A. B., and Leider, M.: Erythroplasia of the female genitalia. Arch. Derm., *84*:381, 1961.

Korting, G. W., and Theisen, H.: Circumscripte plasmacelluläre Balanoposthitis und Conjunctivitis bei derselben Person. Arch. klin. exp. Derm., *217*:495, 1963.

Nödl, F.: Zur Klinik und Histologie der Balanoposthitis chronica circumscripta benigna plasmacellularis. Arch. f. Derm. u. Syph., *198*: 557, 1954.

Zoon, J. J.: Balanoposthite chronique circonscrite bénigne à plasmocytes. Dermatologica, *105*:1, 1952.

Squamous Cell Carcinoma

Broders, A. C.: Practical points on the microscopic grading of carcinoma. N.Y. J. Med., *32*:667, 1932.

Brooks, S. M.: Carcinoma which resembles sarcoma. Arch. Path., *36*:144, 1943.

Chorzelski, T.: Ein Fall von Übergang einer Keratosis senilis mit Dyskeratose vom Typ des Morbus Darier in ein dyskeratotisches Spinaliom. Hautarzt, *14*:37, 1963.

Delacrétaz, J., Madjedi, A. S., and Loretan, R. M.: Epithelioma spino-cellulare segregans. Über die sogenannten "Adenoacanthome der Schweissdrüsen" (Lever). Hautarzt, *8*:512, 1957.

Edmundson, W. F.: Microscopic grading of cancer and its practical implication. Arch. Derm. Syph., *57*:141, 1948.

Epstein, E., Epstein, N. N., Bragg, K., and Linden, G.: Metastases from squamous cell carcinoma of the skin. Arch. Derm., *97*:245, 1968.

Graham, J. H., and Helwig, E. B.: Cutaneous premalignant lesions. *In* Advances in Biology of the Skin. Vol. 7. Carcinogenesis. New York, Pergamon Press, 1966.

Hueper, W. C.: Occupational Tumors and Allied Diseases. Springfield, Ill., Charles C Thomas, 1942.

Johnson, W. C., and Helwig, E. B.: Adenoid squamous cell carcinoma (adenoacanthoma). Cancer, *19*:1639, 1966.

Ju, D. M. C.: Pseudoepitheliomatous hyperplasia of the skin. Dermat. Internat., *6*:82, 1967.

Klingmüller, G., Klehr, H. U., and Ishibashi, Y.: Desmosomen im Cytoplasma entdifferenzierter Keratinocyten des Plattenepithelcarcinoms. Arch. klin. exp. Derm., *238*:356, 1970.

Kobayasi, T.: Dermo-epidermal junction in invasive squamous cell carcinoma. Acta dermatoven., *49*:445, 1969.

Kraus, F. T., and Perez-Mesa, C.: Verrucous carcinoma. Cancer, *19*:26, 1966.

Lasser, A., Cornog, J. L., and Morris, J. McL.: Adenoid squamous cell carcinoma of the vulva. Cancer, *33*:224, 1974.

Lever, W. F.: Adenoacanthoma of sweat glands. Arch. Derm. Syph., *56*:157, 1947.

Lund, H. Z.: How often does squamous cell carcinoma of the skin metastasize? Arch. Derm., *92*:635, 1965.

Muller, S. A., Wilhelmj, C. M., Jr., Harrison, E. G., Jr., and Winkelmann, R. K.: Adenoid squamous cell carcinoma (adenoacanthoma of Lever). Arch. Derm. *89*:589, 1964.

Olsen, R. L., Nordquist, R., and Everett, M. A.: An electron microscopic study of Bowen's disease. Cancer Res., *28*:2078, 1968.

Sedlin, E. D., and Fleming, J. L.: Epidermoid carcinoma arising in osteomyelitic foci. J. Bone Joint Surg., *45*:827, 1963.

Sims, C. F., and Kirsch, N.: Spindle cell epidermoid epithelioma simulating sarcoma in chronic radiodermatitis. Arch. Derm. Syph., *57*:63, 1948.

Sommerville, J.: Pseudo-epitheliomatous hyperplasia. Acta dermatoven., *33*:236, 1953.

Underwood, L. J., Montgomery, H., and Broders, A. C.: Squamous-cell epithelioma that simulates sarcoma. Arch. Derm. Syph., *64*:149, 1951.

Winer, L. H.: Pseudoepitheliomatous hyperplasia. Arch. Derm. Syph., *42*:856, 1940.

Keratoacanthoma

Belisario, J. C.: Brief review of keratoacanthoma and description of keratoacanthoma centrifugum marginatum. Austral. J. Derm., *8*:65, 1965.

Burge, K. M., and Winkelmann, R. K.: Keratoacanthoma. Association with basal and squamous cell carcinoma. Arch. Derm., *100*:306, 1969.

Calnan, C. D., and Haber, H.: Molluscum sebaceum. J. Path. Bact., *69*:61, 1955.

de Moragas, J. M., Montgomery, H., and McDonald, J. R.: Keratoacanthoma versus squamous-cell carcinoma. Arch. Derm., *77*:390, 1957.

Ghadially, F. N.: The role of the hair follicle in the origin and evolution of some cutaneous neoplasms of man and experimental animals. Cancer, *14*:801, 1961.

Ghadially, F. N., Barton, B. W., and Kerridge, D. F.: The etiology of keratoacanthoma. Cancer, *16*:603, 1963.

Lapière, S.: Über Kerato-Acanthome. Hautarzt, *6*:38, 1955.

Levy, E. J., Cahn, M. M., Shaffer, B., and Beerman, H.: Keratoacanthoma. J.A.M.A., *155*:562, 1954.

Milewsky, B., and Chorzelski, T.: Vergleichende histologische und histochemische Untersuchungen von Keratoakanthomen und höher differenzierten spinozellulären Epitheliomen. Hautarzt, *13*:7, 1962.

Muller, S. A., Wilhelmj, C. M., Jr., Harrison, E. G., Jr., et al.: Adenoid squamous cell carcinoma (adenoacanthoma of Lever). Arch. Derm., *89*:589, 1964.

Musso, L., and Gordon, H.: Spontaneous resolution of molluscum sebaceum. Proc. Roy. Soc. Med., *43*:838, 1950.

Nikolowski, W.: Zur Problematik des Keratoakanthoms. Derm. Monatsschr., *156*:148, 1970.

Obermayer, M. E.: Das Keratoakanthom: seine zur Gewebsdestruktion führende Wachstumskapazität. Hautarzt, *15*:628, 1964.

Popkin, G. L., Brodie, S. J., Hyman, A. B., *et al.*: A technique of biopsy recommended for keratoacanthoma. Arch. Derm., *94*:191, 1966.

Rook, A., and Moffat, J. L.: Multiple self-healing epithelioma of Ferguson Smith type. Arch. Derm., *74*:525, 1956.

Rook, A., and Whimster, I. W.: Le kératoacanthome. Arch. belg. derm. syph., *6*:137, 1950.

Rossman, R. E., Freeman, R. G., and Knox, J. M.: Multiple keratoacanthomas. Arch. Derm., *89*:374, 1964.

Silberberg, I., Kopf, A., and Baer, R. L.: Recurrent keratoacanthoma of the lip. Arch. Derm., *86*:44, 1962.

Sommerville, J., and Milne, J. A.: Familial primary self-healing squamous epithelioma of the skin (Ferguson Smith type). Brit. J. Derm., *62*:485, 1950.

Stevanovic, D. V.: Keratoacanthoma dyskeratoticum and segregans. Arch. Derm., *92*:666, 1965.

Takaki, Y., Masutani, M., and Kawada, A.: Electron microscopic study of keratoacanthoma. Acta dermatoven., *51*:21, 1971.

von Bülow, M., and Klingmüller, G.: Elektronen-mikroskopische Untersuchungen des Keratoakanthoms. Arch. Derm. Forsch., *241*:292, 1971.

Winkelmann, R. K., and Brown, J.: Generalized eruptive keratoacanthoma. Arch. Derm., *97*:615, 1968.

Paget's Disease

Ashikari, R., Park, K., Huvos, A. G., and Urban, J. A.: Paget's disease of the breast. Cancer, *26*:680, 1970.

Becker, S. W., Jr., Brennan, B., and Weichselbaum, P. K.: Genital Paget's disease. Arch. Derm., *82*:857, 1960.

Belcher, R. W.: Extramammary Paget's disease. Enzyme histochemical and electron microscopic study. Arch. Path., *94*:59, 1972.

Bowman, H. E., and Hartman, F. W.: Extramammary Paget's disease of the vulva. Arch. Path., *58*:304, 1954.

Caputo, R., and Califano, A.: Ultrastructural features of extramammary Paget's disease. Arch. klin. exp. Derm., *236*:121, 1970.

Chrichlow, R. W., and Czernobilsky, B.: Paget's disease of the male breast. Cancer, *24*:1031, 1969.

Culberson, J. D., and Horn, R. C., Jr.: Paget's disease of the nipple. Arch. Surg., *72*:224, 1956.

Demopoulos, R. I.: Fine structure of the extramammary Paget's cell. Cancer, *27*:1202, 1971.

Ebner, H.: Zur Ultrastruktur des Morbus Paget mamillae. Z. Haut, *44*:297, 1969.

Fisher, E. R., and Beyer, F., Jr.: Differentiation of neoplastic lesions characterized by large vacuolated intraepidermal (pagetoid) cells. Arch. Path., *67*:140, 1959.

Graham, J. H., and Helwig, E. B.: Extramammary Paget's disease. *In* Graham, J. H., Johnson, W. C., and Helwig, E. B. (eds.): Dermal Pathology, p. 606. Hagerstown, Md., Harper and Row, 1972.

Greenwood, S. M., and Minkowitz, S.: Paget's disease in metastatic breast carcinoma. Arch. Derm., *104*:312, 1971.

Hashimoto, K., Gross, B. G., and Lever, W. F.: An electron microscopic study of the adult human apocrine duct. J. Invest. Derm., *46*:6, 1966.

————: Electron microscopic study of the human adult eccrine gland. I. The duct. J. Invest. Derm., *46*:172, 1966.

Helwig, E. B., and Graham, J. H.: Anogenital (extramammary) Paget's disease; a clinicopathologic study. Cancer, *16*:387, 1963.

Holleran, W. M., and Schmutzer, K. J.: Paget's disease of the groin. J.A.M.A., *193*:965, 1965.

Hopsu-Havu, V. K., and Sonck, C. E.: The problem of extramammary Paget's disease. Report of four cases with "pagetoid" cells. Z. Haut, *46*:41, 1971.

Jacobsen, K. B., and Haavelsrud, O. J.: Extramammary Paget's disease. Acta dermatoven., *49*:87, 1969.

Kawatsu, T., and Miki, V.: Triple extramammary Paget's disease. Arch. Derm., *104*:316, 1971.

Koss, L. G., and Brockunier, A.: Ultrastructural aspects of Paget's disease of the vulva. Arch. Path., *87*:592, 1969.

Lattanand, A., Johnson, W. C., and Graham, J. H.: Mucous cyst (mucocele): Arch. Derm., *101*:673, 1970.

Medenica, M., and Sahihi, T.: Ultrastructural study of a case of extramammary Paget's disease of the vulva. Arch. Derm., *105*:236, 1972.

Mendoza, S., and Helwig, E. B.: Mucinous (adenocystic) carcinoma of the skin. Arch. Derm., *103*:68, 1971.

Montgomery, H.: Dermatopathology. vol. 2, p. 1007. New York, Hoeber Medical Division, 1967.

Muir, R.: Further observations on Paget's disease of the nipple. J. Path. Bact., *49*:299, 1939.

Murrell, T. W., Jr., and McMullan, F. H.: Extra-mammary Paget's disease. Arch. Derm., *85*: 600, 1962.

Piérard, J., and Kint, A.: Maladie de Paget extra-mammaire. Étude d'un cas en microscopie électronique. Arch. belg. derm., *24*:335, 1968.

Pinkus, H., and Mehregan, A. H.: Epidermo-tropic eccrine carcinoma. A case combining features of eccrine poroma and Paget's derma-tosis. Arch. Derm., *88*:597, 1963.

————: A Guide to Dermatohistopathology.

p. 470. New York, Appleton-Century-Crofts, 1969.

Sagebiel, R. W.: Ultrastructural observations on epidermal cells in Paget's disease of the breast. Am. J. Path., *57*:49, 1969.

Stout, A. P.: The relationship of malignant amelanotic melanoma (naevocarcinoma) to extramammary Paget's disease. Am. J. Cancer, *33*:196, 1938.

Yoell, J. H., and Price, W. G.: Paget's disease of the perianal skin with associated adenocar-cinoma. Arch. Derm., *82*:986, 1960.

26

Tumors of the Epidermal Appendages

CLASSIFICATION OF THE APPENDAGE TUMORS

The benign tumors differentiating in the direction of epidermal appendages can be divided into four groups: those differentiating toward hair, toward sebaceous glands, toward apocrine glands, and toward eccrine glands.

Besides the benign tumors differentiating toward epidermal appendages, there are carcinomas of epidermal appendages. Three types of carcinoma are recognized: carcinoma of sebaceous glands, of eccrine sweat glands, and of apocrine glands.

Classification of the Benign Appendage Tumors. The four groups of benign appendage tumors with differentiation toward hair, sebaceous glands, apocrine glands, or eccrine glands can be divided, according to the decreasing degree of differentiation observed in them, into four subgroups: hyperplasias, adenomas, benign epitheliomas, and primordial epitheliomas or basal cell epitheliomas (Table 26-1).

Of the four subgroups into which the benign appendage tumors can be divided, the hyperplasias are composed of mature or nearly mature structures. The adenomas show less differentiation than the hyperplasias; nonetheless, well developed glandlike structures are present. In the benign epitheliomas there is a further step-down in regard to the degree of differentiation, and it is usually difficult to recognize the type of structure that the tumor is attempting to form. The primordial epitheliomas, or basal cell epitheliomas, are the least differentiated of the benign appendage tumors. According to the concept set forth here, basal cell epitheliomas are not carcinomas, since they are composed of immature rather than of anaplastic cells (see p. 450).

Although most of the benign appendage tumors fit well into one of the entities listed in Table 26-1, occasional tumors in an intermediate stage of differentiation are encountered. Also, because of differentiation in more than one direction, combinations of several tumor types occur, so that one may find within the same tumor, for instance, differentiation toward sebaceous as well as apocrine structures (Wechsler and Fisher).

Histogenesis of the Benign Appendage Tumors. In 1948 one of the authors (W. F. L.) advanced the thesis that the tumors differentiating toward hair, sebaceous glands, or apocrine glands developed from primary epithelial germ cells and, as such, were primary epithelial germ tumors; and further, that the hyperplasias, the adenomas, and the benign epitheliomas arose from primary epithelial germ cells that prior to the onset of neoplasia had attained a certain degree of differentiation, whereas the basal cell epitheliomas arose from primary epithelial germ cells that had attained little or no differentiation.

In the case of benign appendage tumors that are present at birth, such as the nevus sebaceus, one can assume that such tumors actually are derived from embryonic primary epithelial germ cells. In all other instances it is likely that the benign appendage tumors arise from pluripotential cells that have formed during life and possess

TABLE 26-1. Classification of the Benign Appendage Tumors

	Hair Differentiation	Sebaceous Differentiation	Apocrine Differentiation	Eccrine Differentiation
Hyperplasias (hamartomas)		Nevus sebaceus Sebaceous hyperplasia Fordyce condition	Apocrine nevus or hyperplasia	Eccrine nevus or hyperplasia
Adenomas	Trichofolliculoma	Sebaceous adenoma	Apocrine hidrocystoma Hidradenoma papilliferum Apocrine syringo-cystadenoma papilliferum	Eccrine hidrocystoma Syringoma Eccrine syringo-cystadenoma papilliferum
Benign epitheliomas	Trichoepithelioma Pilomatrixoma Pilar tumor Trichilemmoma	Sebaceous epithelioma	Cylindroma	Clear cell hidradenoma Eccrine poroma Eccrine spiradenoma Mixed tumor
Primordial epitheliomas	Keratotic basal cell epithelioma	Cystic basal cell epithelioma	Adenoid basal cell epithelioma	Basal cell epithelioma with eccrine differentiation

the potentiality, just as do primary epithelial germ cells, of differentiating into tumors with hair, sebaceous gland, or apocrine structures (Pinkus). Similarly, eccrine sweat gland tumors arise from pluripotential cells forming during adult life and possessing the potentiality of differentiating into tumors with eccrine gland structures. In genetically determined appendage tumors, such as cylindroma, trichoepithelioma, and the nevoid basal cell epithelioma syndrome, one may assume that the genes regulating the development of pluripotential cells into cutaneous appendages are abnormal and sooner or later modify the growth of pluripotential cells into appendage tumors rather than mature appendages. It appears unlikely, however, that any of the benign appendage tumors arise from mature structures. For this reason it is useless to search for any connection between, for instance, a benign eccrine gland tumor and a pre-existing eccrine gland.

In the original classification of the appendage tumors presented in 1948 several tumors were classified as apocrine tumors that are now regarded as eccrine, as for instance, syringoma. The reason for this lies in the fact that enzyme histochemical and electron microscopic methods that were not yet available in 1948 have proved of great value in distinguishing eccrine from apocrine differentiation (Hashimoto and Lever).

Terminology. The terms nevus and epithelioma used in the classification of the benign appendage tumors require definition.

NEVUS. The term *nevus* is used in the literature in two different ways, referring (a) to a tumor composed of nevus cells (nevocellular nevus, pigmented nevus); or (b) to a lesion present at birth and composed of mature or nearly mature structures (connatal hyperplasias, such as nevus sebaceus, eccrine nevus, nevus verrucosus, and nevus flammeus). In order to avoid confusion, it is advisable when referring to a connatal hyperplasia always to use the term *nevus* with a qualifying adjective, so that nevus without a qualifying adjective designates a tumor composed of nevus cells.

The term *hamartoma* would seem appropriate for those nevi that have no nevus cells and as congenital hyperplasias are composed of mature or nearly mature structures. Hamartoma, derived from the Greek word *hamartanein* (to fail, to err), was chosen by Albrecht as a designation for "tumorlike malformations showing a faulty mixture of the normal components of the organ in which they occur."

EPITHELIOMA. The term *epithelioma* is used by many authors as a synonym for car-cinoma. However, since the literal meaning of the word is tumor of the epithelium, the term may be employed, as was suggested by Jadassohn, as a designation of benign as well as malignant tumors of the epithelium, provided that a qualifying adjective is added. It would perhaps be best, as Becker has suggested, to reserve the term *epithelioma* for benign epithelial tumors and the term *carcinoma* for malignant epithelial tumors.

HYPERPLASIAS (HAMARTOMAS)

NEVUS SEBACEUS

Nevus sebaceus is located as a rule on the scalp or on the face as a single lesion and is present already at birth. In childhood it consists of a circumscribed, only slightly raised, hairless plaque. In puberty the lesion becomes verrucous and nodular (Mehregan and Pinkus).

In very rare instances nevus sebaceus consists of multiple and extensive plaques not necessarily limited to the head and also shows areas of linear distribution (Lentz

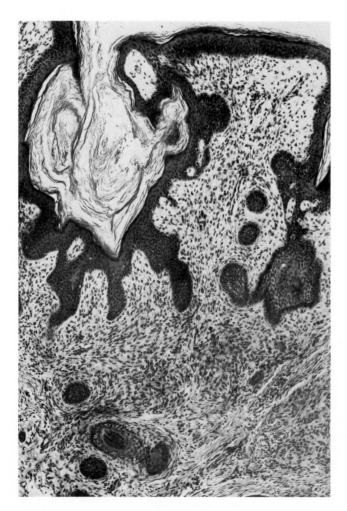

FIG. 26-1. **Nevus sebaceus from the scalp of an infant.** There are papillomatosis and hyperkeratosis. Numerous small epithelial protrusions, resembling primary epithelial germs, extend from the epidermis into the dermis. The dermis contains many young fibroblasts. One immature hair structure is located in the dermis, but sebaceous glands as yet are absent. (×100) (Benjamin K. Fisher, M.D.)

et al.). Some of the patients with extensive linear nevus sebaceus show, in addition, as evidence of a "neurocutaneous syndrome" epilepsy and mental retardation (Feuerstein and Mims; Marden and Venters), neurologic defects (Wauschkuhn and Rohde), or skeletal deformities (Hornstein and Knickenberg). In some patients the linear nevus is partly a linear nevus sebaceus and partly a linear epidermal nevus (Wauschkuhn and Rohde; Hornstein and Knickenberg). Thus, the "neurocutaneous syndrome" that is associated with nevus sebaceus overlaps with the abnormalities associated with systematized linear epidermal nevus. The abnormalities most commonly associated with systematized linear epidermal nevus consist, as described by Solomon et al., or skeletal deformities and central nervous system abnormalities (see p. 452).

Histopathology. During infancy and childhood the sebaceous glands in nevus sebaceus are underdeveloped and, therefore, are greatly reduced in size and number (Steigleder and Cortes; Lantis et al.). Thus, the diagnosis of nevus sebaceus may be missed (Fig. 26-1). However, the presence of incompletely differentiated hair structures is typical of this childhood stage of nevus sebaceus. There often are cords and buds of undifferentiated cells resembling primary epithelial germs or the embryonic stage of hair follicles (Mehregan and Pinkus).

At puberty the lesion assumes its diagnostic histologic appearance brought on by the presence of large numbers of mature or nearly mature sebaceous glands and by papillomatous hyperplasia of the epidermis. The hair follicles remain small and partly disappear. There often are buds of undifferentiated cells that resemble foci of basal cell epithelioma and represent malformed hair germs (Wilson Jones and Heyl). At puberty, and at times earlier, ectopic apocrine glands develop in about two thirds of the cases (Mehregan and Pinkus; Bourlond et al.; Wilson Jones and Heyl). They are located deep in the dermis beneath the masses of sebaceous gland lobules (Fig. 26-2).

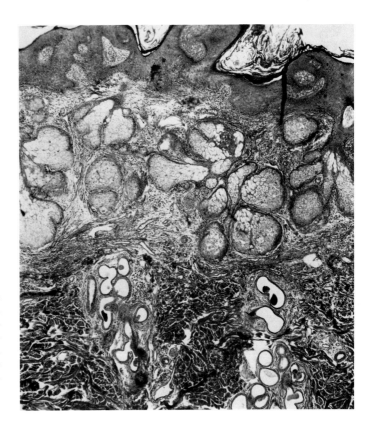

Fig. 26-2. **Nevus sebaceus from the scalp of an adult.** Hyperkeratosis and papillomatosis are present. Numerous mature sebaceous glands lie in the upper dermis. Mature apocrine glands are located in the lower dermis. (×50)

Quite commonly, various types of appendage tumors develop secondarily in lesions of nevus sebaceus. A syringocystadenoma papilliferum has been found in 8 to 19 per cent of the lesions (Wilson Jones and Heyl; Mehregan and Pinkus). Less commonly found appendage tumors include nodular hidradenoma, syringoma, and sebaceous epithelioma (Mehregan and Pinkus). A basal cell epithelioma has been observed in 7 to 14 per cent of the cases of nevus sebaceus (Fig. 26-3). In many instances such basal cell epitheliomas are small and have a slow evolution (Nikolowski); and it is not always possible to differentiate between "basaloid proliferations" in malformed hair germs and basal cell epithelioma (Wilson Jones and Heyl). In only rare instances a squamous cell carcinoma develops within a nevus sebaceus (Schirren and Pfirstinger; Wilson Jones and Heyl).

Histogenesis. The frequent association of nevus sebaceus with other appendage tumors as well as with apocrine glands suggests that nevus sebaceus is derived from the primary epithelial germ (Haber; Wilson Jones and Heyl). Also, a basal cell epithelioma develops in a nevus sebaceus not as a result of a "malignant degenera-

tion" (Michalowski) but because the primary epithelial germ cells present in the lesion show a decrease in the degree of differentiation and, associated with it, an increase in the rate of proliferation (Lever; Schirren and Pfirstinger).

SEBACEOUS HYPERPLASIA

Sebaceous hyperplasia, also called senile sebaceous nevi, occur on the face, chiefly on the forehead, in persons past middle life. Either one or, more commonly, several elevated, small, soft, yellowish, slightly umbilicated nodules are present. Their usual size is 2 to 3 mm in diameter.

Histopathology. Most lesions consist of a single greatly enlarged sebaceous gland composed of numerous lobules grouped around a centrally located, wide sebaceous duct (Fig. 26-4). Its opening to the surface corresponds to the central umbilication of the lesion. Serial sections show that all sebaceous lobules grouped around the central duct are connected with that duct (Gilman). Large lesions may consist of several enlarged sebaceous glands and contain several ducts, with sebaceous lobules grouped around each of them (Braun-Falco and

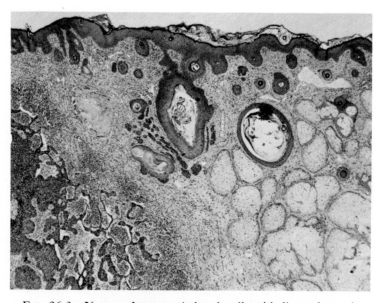

FIG. 26-3. **Nevus sebaceus.** A basal cell epithelioma has arisen within the lesion. The nevus sebaceus is on the right side; the basal cell epithelioma, on the left. (×25)

Thianprasit). Most sebaceous gland lobules appear fully matured, but some may show more than just one peripheral row of undifferentiated, generative cells.

Histogenesis. Since in sebaceous hyperplasia one observes an increase in the number of sebaceous gland lobules that are mature or nearly mature, this condition does not represent an adenoma, as the old designation senile sebaceous adenoma would imply, but rather a hyperplasia (Ramos e Silva and Portugal). The fact that, in contrast to rhinophyma, only one sebaceous gland or at the most a few sebaceous glands show this hyperplasia makes it appear likely that the lesion represents a hamartoma rather than a hypertrophy, as in rhinophyma.

Differential Diagnosis. In rhinophyma, which also shows large sebaceous glands and ducts, there is no "grapelike" grouping of the sebaceous lobules around the ducts, and the lesion is not sharply demarcated. In nevus sebaceus ductal structures are less apparent than in senile sebaceous hyperplasia, and also apocrine glands often are found beneath the sebaceous glands.

FORDYCE'S CONDITION

In this common condition groups of minute yellowish globoid lesions are observed on the vermilion border of the lips or on the oral mucosa. The incidence increases with age, so that among older adults 70 to 80 per cent show such lesions representing ectopic sebaceous glands (Miles).

Histopathology. Each globoid lesion consists of a group of small but mature sebaceous lobules situated around a small sebaceous duct leading to the surface epithelium (Chambers; Miles). Because of the small size of the sebaceous duct, serial sections may be required to demonstrate its presence.

APOCRINE NEVUS

Large numbers of mature apocrine secretory lumina frequently are present in scalp lesions of nevus sebaceus (see p. 501) and syringocystadenoma papilliferum (see p. 510). Pure apocrine nevi, however, are very rare. They show apocrine glands in a circumscribed area of the scalp without ac-

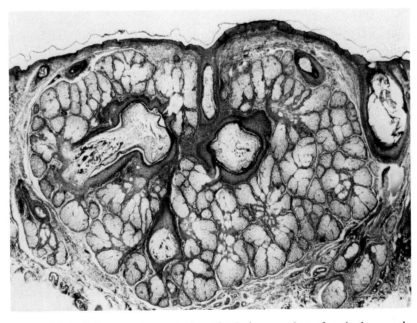

Fig. 26-4. **Sebaceous hyperplasia.** The lesion consists of a single, greatly enlarged sebaceous gland with a wide, branching sebaceous duct in the center. (×25)

companying pilosebaceous structures. However, basaloid proliferations of the epidermis may be present and can be so pronounced that they resemble basal cell epithelioma (Civatte et al.).

ECCRINE NEVUS

Eccrine nevi are very rare. They may show either one central pore (Herzberg), or numerous sweat-discharging pores (Goldstein). In the so-called eccrine angiomatous hamartoma one or several lesions are present having in most instances a clinical appear-

ance suggestive of an angioma. The lesion may show conspicuous hyperhidrosis (Hyman et al.; Zeller and Goldman).

Histopathology. Eccrine nevi show an increase in the size of the eccrine coil in cases with only one eccrine duct (Herzberg), or, in cases with multiple ducts, an increase in both the size and the number of coils (Goldstein).

Eccrine angiomatous hamartomas show, in addition to increased numbers of eccrine structures, numerous capillary channels surrounding the eccrine structures (Hyman et al.; Zeller and Goldman).

ADENOMAS

TRICHOFOLLICULOMA

Trichofolliculoma occurs in adults as a solitary lesion, usually on the face but occasionally on the scalp or neck. It consists of a small, skin-colored, dome-shaped nodule. Frequently, there is a central pore. If a central pore is present, a wool-like tuft of

immature, usually white hairs may be seen to emerge from it, a highly diagnostic clinical feature (Pinkus and Sutton).

Histopathology. On histologic examination the dermis contains a large cystic space that is lined by squamous epithelium and contains horny material and frequently also

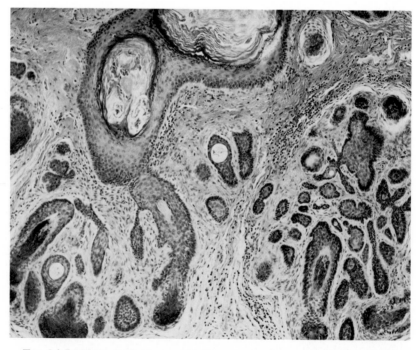

FIG. 26-5. **Trichofolliculoma.** At the top one sees part of a keratin-filled cyst lined with epidermis and representing a "primary" hair follicle. Grouped around the cyst are numerous small "secondary" hair follicles, some of which show, in addition to a hair and an outer root sheath, an inner root sheath with trichohyaline granules. (×100)

fragments of birefringent hair shafts (Gray and Helwig). In cases with a central pore, the large cystic space is continuous with the surface epidermis, an indication that it represents an enlarged, distorted hair follicle. In some cases one or two additional cystic spaces are present in the dermis. Radiating from the wall of these "primary" hair follicles, one sees many small but usually fairly well differentiated "secondary" hair follicles. Well developed "secondary" hair follicles often show a hair papilla. Furthermore, they usually show an outer and an inner root sheath, of which the latter may contain trichohyaline granules, and, located in the center, a fine hair (Fig. 26-5). These fine hairs are visualized best in areas where the "secondary" hair follicles appear in cross sections. Small groups of sebaceous gland cells may be embedded in the walls of the "secondary" hair follicles (Hyman and Clayman). In some of the more rudimentary "secondary" hair follicles one observes in place of a hair a central horn cyst, as is seen also in trichoepithelioma (Sanderson). The stroma is rich in fibroblasts and is oriented in parallel bundles of fibers that encapsulate the epithelial proliferations in a manner resembling the normal fibrous root sheath (Kligman and Pinkus). Just as in the outer root sheath of mature hair structures, large amounts of glycogen can be demonstrated in the outer root sheath of the "secondary" hair follicles (Gray and Helwig).

In all tumors there are epithelial strands interconnecting the secondary hair follicles. Since these epithelial strands differentiate in the direction of the outer root sheath, the peripheral cell row shows palisading and the cells within the strands appear large and vacuolated as the result of their content of glycogen.

Differential Diagnosis. If the large primary cavity is missed in histologic sections and the "secondary" hair follicles do not show any inner root sheath or central hair, the palisading at the periphery of the epithelial strands may suggest a trichoepithelioma or basal cell epithelioma. However, noting the vacuolated appearance of the cells within the epithelial strands which is due to the presence of glycogen within these cells,

facilitates the recognition of differentiation toward the outer root sheath, and establishes the diagnosis of trichofolliculoma.

SEBACEOUS ADENOMA

Sebaceous adenoma is a rare tumor if a strict definition of an adenoma is adhered to, namely, that it is an organoid tumor consisting of circumscribed proliferations of incompletely differentiated glandular structures. Many tumors described in the literature as sebaceous adenoma are in reality sebaceous nevi. Examples of sebaceous adenoma have been described by Woolhandler and Becker; Lever; Groterjahn; and Essenhigh et al., among others.

Solitary sebaceous adenoma occurs as a smooth, elevated, often slightly pedunculated tumor. In most of the reported cases the lesion was solitary, was located on the face or the scalp, and measured less than 1 cm in diameter.

Recently, the association of *multiple sebaceous neoplasms* of the skin with *multiple visceral carcinomas,* especially of the colon, has been described as a syndrome (Rulon and Helwig). The multiple sebaceous tumors of the skin most often involve the trunk and usually develop after the visceral carcinoma has been diagnosed. The sebaceous tumors of the skin are largely sebaceous adenomas (Sciallis and Winkelmann); but some have the histologic appearance of a sebaceous epithelioma or a sebaceous carcinoma (Leonard and Deaton). Even the tumors that are classified as sebaceous carcinoma on the basis of cellular atypicality remain localized and do not metastasize (Leonard and Deaton). The multiple visceral carcinomas also are generally of low-grade malignancy and with rare exceptions do not metastasize (Rulon and Helwig).

Histopathology. On histologic examination the tumor is sharply demarcated from the surrounding tissue. It is composed of lobules that are irregular in size and shape (Fig. 26-6). Two types of cells are present in the lobules. The cells of the first type are identical with the cells present at the periphery of normal sebaceous glands and represent undifferentiated, germinative cells.

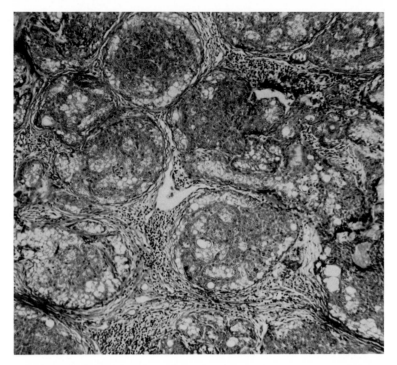

FIG. 26-6. **Sebaceous adenoma.** The tumor is composed of lobules of irregular size and shape. In the lobules two types of cells can be recognized: generative, and sebaceous. (×100)

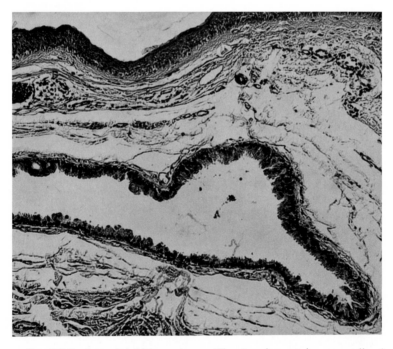

FIG. 26-7. **Apocrine hidrocystoma.** The dermis contains a cyst lined by a row of secretory cells showing secretion of the apocrine type, so-called decapitation secretion. Peripheral to the row of secretory cells, elongated myoepithelial cells are seen. (×100)

The cells of the second type are mature sebaceous cells. In addition, there often are some cells in a transitional stage between these two types of cells. The distribution of the germinative and the sebaceous cells within the lobules varies. Some lobules contain predominantly germinative cells and thus resemble basal cell epithelioma. Other lobules contain mainly sebaceous cells and resemble mature sebaceous lobules. In most lobules, however, the two types of cells occur in approximately equal proportions, often arranged in such a way that groups of sebaceous cells are surrounded by germinative cells. Fat stains reveal the presence of lipid material in the sebaceous and the transitional cells. Some large lobules contain cystic spaces in their center formed by the decomposition of mature sebaceous cells. Also, there may be foci of squamous epithelium with keratinization (Essenhigh et al.). They probably represent areas with differentiation toward sebaceous-duct structures or may be a manifestation of the keratinizing potentiality of the germinative cells.

APOCRINE HIDROCYSTOMA

The apocrine hidrocystoma occurs usually as a solitary translucent nodule of cystic consistency. Quite frequently, the lesion instead of being skin-colored has a bluish hue and then resembles a blue nevus. The usual location of the apocrine hidrocystoma is on the face, but occasionally it is seen on the ears, the scalp, or the prepuce (Ahmed and Jones).

Histopathology. The dermis contains several large cystic spaces into which often papillary projections extend. The inner surface of the wall and the papillary projections are lined by a row of secretory cells of variable height showing "decapitation" secretion suggestive of apocrine secretion (Fig. 26-7). Peripheral to the secretory cells most tumors show, at least in some areas, round to oval-shaped myoepithelial cells (Gross). Occasionally, however, no myoepithelial cells are present (Ahmed and Jones). In some cases, one finds in addition to the secretory lumina superficially located cysts lined by a double layer of ductal epithelium (Mehregan).

The stroma surrounding the cystic spaces usually is loosely woven and often contains accumulations of extravasated erythrocytes.

Histogenesis. The apocrine nature of the secretion of the luminal cells has been proven not only by the presence of numerous large PAS-positive, diastase-resistant granules in the secretory cells (Mehregan) but also by electron microscopic examination. The secretory cells, on electron microscopy, contain (1) many lysosomal secretory granules, (2) large and irregularly shaped mitochondria, and (3) stacks of annulate lamellae in much greater quantity than seen in normal apocrine secretory cells (Gross). The bluish color of some of the cysts is probably caused by the presence of small hemorrhages in the vicinity of the cysts.

The apocrine hidrocystoma can be regarded as an adenoma rather than as a retention cyst because (1) the secretory cells do not appear flattened, as they would be in a retention cyst, and (2) papillary projections extend into the lumen of the cystic spaces (Mehregan).

Differential Diagnosis. Eccrine hidrocystoma differs from apocrine hidrocystoma by the absence of "decapitation secretion," of PAS-positive granules, and of myoepithelial cells (see p. 512). However, those portions of an apocrine hidrocystoma in which the cystic spaces are lined by ductal epithelium have the same appearance as the cystic spaces seen in eccrine hidrocystoma, except that the latter usually consists of only a solitary cystic space (see p. 513).

HIDRADENOMA PAPILLIFERUM

This tumor occurs only in women, usually on the labia majora or in the perineal or perianal region, and rarely on the nipple (Tappeiner and Wolff). The tumor usually is covered by normal skin and measures only a few millimeters in diameter. Malignant changes have been reported in only one patient in whom a metastasizing, fatal squamous cell carcinoma developed within a perianally located hidradenoma papilliferum (Shenoy).

Histopathology. The tumor represents an adenoma with apocrine differentiation (Meeker et al.). It is located in the dermis surrounded by a fibrous capsule and shows no connections with the overlying epidermis. Some tumors have a peripheral epithelial

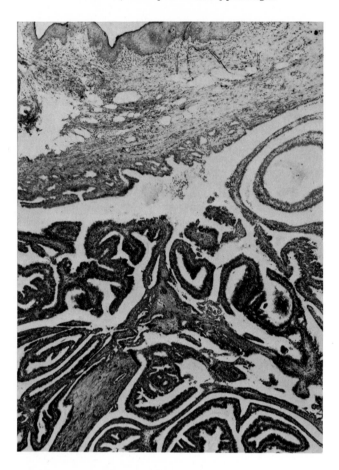

Fig. 26-8. **Hidradenoma papilliferum.** Low magnification. The tumor consists of a large cystic space. Numerous papillary folds project into the cystic lumen. (×50)

wall, showing keratinization (Hashimoto). Within the tumor one observes tubular and cystic structures (Fig. 26-8). Papillary folds project into the cystic spaces. The lumina are lined occasionally with only a single row of columnar cells that show an oval, pale-staining nucleus located near their base, a faintly eosinophilic cytoplasm, and active "decapitation" secretion, as seen in the secretory cells of apocrine glands (Fig. 26-9). Usually, however, the lumina are surrounded by a double layer of cells consisting not only of a luminal layer of secretory cells but also of an outer layer of small cuboidal cells with deeply basophilic nuclei, representing myoepithelial cells (Tappeiner and Wolff; Hashimoto).

Histogenesis. The apocrine nature of the secretion in hidradenoma papilliferum has been established by histochemical, enzyme histochemical, and electron microscopic examinations.

Histochemically, the luminal cells contain many large PAS-positive, diastase-resistant granules, as encountered in the secretory cells of apocrine glands. In addition, the luminal cells are positive for nonspecific esterase and acid phosphatase, the so-called apocrine enzymes, and negative for phosphorylase, a typical eccrine enzyme. Furthermore, the outer row of cells stains positive for alkaline phosphatase, as myoepithelial cells normally do (Tappeiner and Wolff).

Electron microscopic examination shows in the luminal cells two features that are regarded as characteristic of the secretory cells of apocrine glands: First, numerous membrane-limited, secretory granules of varying size and density and containing lipid droplets are present in the apical portion of these cells (Tappeiner and Wolff); and second, as evidence of decapitation secretion, portions of apical cytoplasm containing large secretory granules are being released into the lumen (Hashimoto). The peripheral layer of cells contains numerous myofilaments.

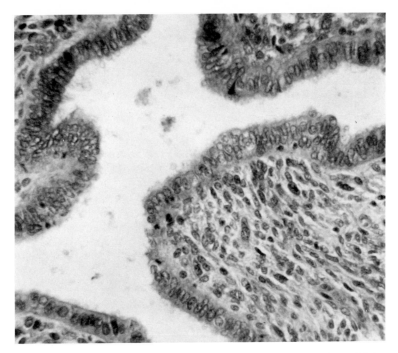

FIG. 26-9. **Hidradenoma papilliferum.** High magnification of Figure 26-8. The papillary folds are lined by one layer of high cylindric cells, which show evidence of active "decapitation" secretion like apocrine glands. (×400)

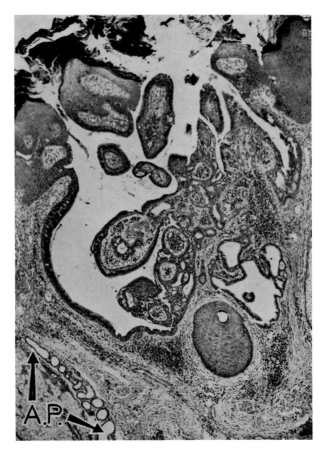

FIG. 26-10. **Syringocystadenoma papilliferum.** Low magnification. A cystic invagination extends downward from the epidermis. Numerous papillary projections extend into the lumen of the cystic invagination. A group of apocrine glands (A.P.) is present in the left lower corner. (×50)

SYRINGOCYSTADENOMA
PAPILLIFERUM

This lesion most commonly occurs on the scalp or the face where it arises around puberty in a nevus sebaceus that has been present since birth (see p. 502). However, in about one fourth of the cases it arises on the trunk or thigh during adolescence or adult life without a pre-existing lesion (Helwig or Hackney). The lesion consists most commonly of a fleshy nodule or plaque that may have a papillary, hyperkeratotic surface.

Histopathology. The epidermis shows varying degrees of papillomatosis. One or several cystic invaginations extend downward from the epidermis (Fig. 26-10). The upper portion of the invaginations, and in some instances large segments of the cystic invaginations are lined by squamous, keratinizing cells similar to those of the surface epidermis (Hashimoto). In the lower portion of the cystic invaginations numerous papillary projections extend into the lumina of the invag-

inations. The papillary projections and the lower portion of the invaginations are lined by glandular epithelium, often consisting of two rows of cells (Fig. 26-11). The luminal row of cells consists of high columnar cells with oval nuclei and faintly eosinophilic cytoplasm. Occasionally these cells show active "decapitation" secretion, and cellular debris is found in the lumina. The outer row of cells consists of small cuboidal cells with round nuclei and scanty cytoplasm. In some areas the cells of the luminal layer are arranged in multiple layers and form a lace-like pattern resulting in multiple small tubular lumina (Fig. 26-11) (Helwig and Hackney).

Beneath the cystic invaginations, deep in the dermis, one can find in many cases groups of tubular glands with large lumina (Fig. 26-12). The cells lining the large lumina often show evidence of active "decapitation" secretion (Fig. 26-13) and furthermore, according to Pinkus, may give a positive Turnbull blue reaction for iron, suggesting that they are apocrine glands

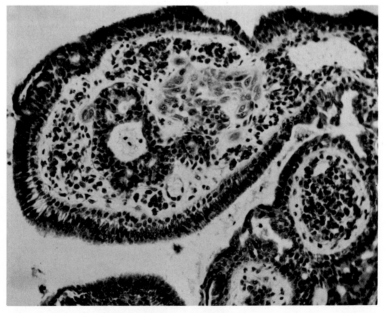

Fig. 26-11. **Syringocystadenoma papilliferum.** High magnification of Figure 26-10. The papillary projections are lined by two rows of cells. The luminal row of cells consists of columnar cells with evidence of active "decapitation" secretion like apocrine glands. The outer row of cells consists of small cuboidal cells. (×200)

FIG. 26-12. **Syringocystade-noma papilliferum.** Low magnification. In the upper dermis numerous papillary projections extend into cystic spaces. A marked inflammatory infiltrate containing many plasma cells is present around the cystic invaginations. The lower dermis contains numerous apocrine glands. (×50)

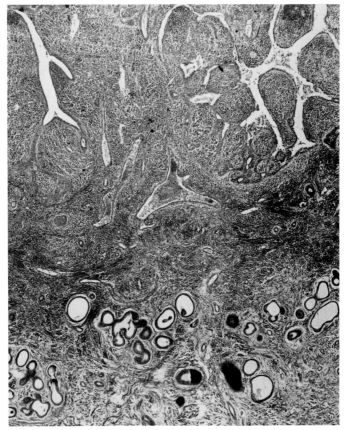

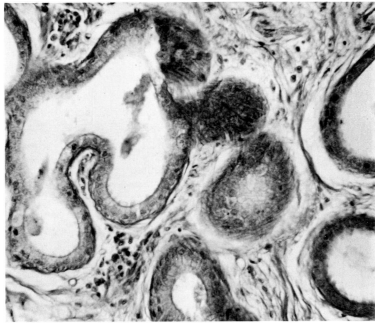

FIG. 26-13. **Syringocystadenoma papilliferum.** High magnification of the apocrine glands in Figure 26-12. The secretory cells of the apocrine glands show evidence of active "decapitation" secretion. (×400)

(Appel; Grund; Pinkus; Krinitz). Connections of the apocrine glands deep in the dermis with the cystic invaginations in the upper dermis can be traced when step sections are carried out (Krinitz).

A highly diagnostic feature is the almost invariable presence of a fairly dense cellular infiltrate composed almost entirely of plasma cells in the stroma of this tumor, especially in the papillary projections.

Frequently one finds in the lesions of syringocystadenoma papilliferum congenital abnormalities of the sebaceous glands and of the hair structures (Pinkus). In about one third of the cases syringocystadenoma papilliferum is associated with a nevus sebaceus; and, in about one tenth of the cases, a basal cell epithelioma develops within the lesion (Helwig and Hackney).

Histogenesis. There is no unanimity about the direction of differentiation in syringocystadenoma papilliferum. On the basis of light microscopic examinations alone many authors have concluded that it was an apocrine tumor because of the presence of decapitation secretion in some of the luminal cells and of tubular glands with large lumina beneath the tumor (Lever; Appel; Grund; Pinkus; Krinitz). Pinkus and Mehregan believe, however, that some lesions of syringocystadenoma papilliferum not associated with a nevus sebaceus and not showing apocrine glands in the deep dermis may be eccrine tumors. Helwig and Hackney, on the other hand, believe that all lesions of syringocystadenoma papilliferum are eccrine because in 90 per cent of the cases the lesion occurs on body surfaces where apocrine glands normally do not occur. However, this argument is not valid if it is assumed that syringocystadenoma papilliferum, rather than arising from mature structures, arises from pluripotential cells with the potential to develop into primary epithelial germ structures. It may be pointed out that apocrine hidrocystoma generally arises in an area where apocrine glands normally do not occur, namely the face.

So far, only two *electron microscopic and enzyme histochemical studies* have been published on syringocystadenoma papilliferum, with contradictory results. The tumor studied by Hashimoto, which had no underlying apocrine glands, proved to be eccrine in its differentiation. Although largely ductal in differentiation the secretory cells were of two types, light and dark, like the secretory cells of eccrine glands. The

secretory granules in the dark secretory cells, in contrast to apocrine secretory granules, were small and did not coalesce. None of the cuboidal cells showed myofilaments.

On the other hand, the tumor examined by Landry and Winkelmann had underlying apocrine glands. It showed differentiation largely toward apocrine secretory cells. Histochemically, phosphorylase, an eccrine enzyme, was absent, and indoxyl esterase and acid phosphatase, two apocrine enzymes, were present. Electron microscopically most luminal cells showed numerous membrane-bound secretory granules, some of which were of considerable size and contained many lipid droplets. Pinching off of cytoplasmic extensions was seen as evidence of "decapitation" secretion. In contrast to hidradenoma papilliferum, the peripheral cell layer contained no myofilaments.

In conclusion, the view expressed by Pinkus and Mehregan (see above) probably is correct that, although most lesions of syringocystadenoma papilliferum are apocrine in differentiation, some are eccrine. The differentiation in either case may be predominantly ductal or secretory.

ECCRINE HIDROCYSTOMA

In this condition usually one lesion, but occasionally a few, and rarely numerous lesions are present on the face (Smith and Chernosky). Just as in apocrine hidrocystoma, the lesion consists of a small, translucent, cystic nodule, 1 to 3 mm in diameter, and often has a bluish hue. In some patients with numerous lesions the number of cysts increases in warm weather and decreases during winter (Dostrovsky and Sagher).

Histopathology. Eccrine hidrocystoma usually shows only one cystic cavity located in the dermis, and rarely several. There usually are no papillary projections into the cystic cavity. The cyst wall generally consists of two layers of small, cuboidal epithelial cells, although in some areas there may be only one layer of epithelial cells (Smith and Chernosky). On serial sections one may find an eccrine duct leading from below into the cyst (Herzberg; Hashimoto and Lever).

Histogenesis. It is very likely that the so-called eccrine hidrocystoma is a ductal cyst,

FIG. 26-14. **Syringoma.** The dermis contains several small ducts. The walls of the ducts are lined predominantly by two rows of epithelial cells. Two of the ducts have commalike tails, giving them the appearance of tadpoles. (×200)

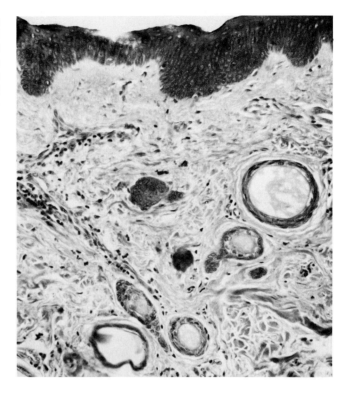

since usually there are two rows of epithelial cells, as seen in ducts, and myoepithelial cells are absent. In the presence of numerous lesions it can be assumed that the cysts are eccrine in nature. However, in the presence of a single cyst, or of a few cysts, it cannot be decided at present whether such cysts are derived from eccrine or from apocrine ducts (Smith and Chernosky).

Differential Diagnosis. For differentiation from apocrine hidrocystoma see page 507.

SYRINGOMA

Syringoma, according to histochemical and electron microscopic findings, represents an adenoma of intraepidermal eccrine ducts. It occurs predominantly in women at puberty or later in life. Although occasionally solitary, the lesions usually are multiple and may be present in great numbers. They are small, skin-colored or slightly yellowish, soft nodules, usually only 1 or 2 mm in size. In many patients the lesions are limited to the lower eyelids. Other sites of predilection are the cheeks, the axillae, the abdomen and the vulva. In the rare so-called eruptive hidradenoma or syringoma the lesions arise in large numbers in successive crops on the anterior trunk of young individuals (Hashimoto et al., 1967).

Histopathology. Embedded in a fibrous stroma one observes numerous small ducts (Fig. 26-14). The walls of the ducts are lined usually by two rows of epithelial cells. In most instances these cells are flat. Occasionally, however, the cells of the inner row appear vacuolated. The lumina of the ducts contain amorphous debris. Some of the ducts possess small commalike tails of epithelial cells, giving them the appearance of tadpoles. In addition, there are solid strands of basophilic epithelial cells independent of the ducts.

Near the epidermis there may be cystic ductal lumina filled with keratin and lined by cells containing keratohyaline granules (Fig. 26-15). These keratin cysts may rupture, whereupon they produce a marked foreign-body giant cell reaction that occasionally is followed by calcification (Hashimoto et al., 1967). In rather rare instances

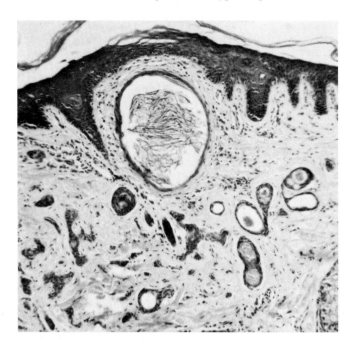

FIG. 26-15. **Syringoma.** Near the epidermis the lumen of a cystic duct is filled with keratin. (×100)

many of the tumor cells appear as clear cells as a result of glycogen accumulation (Headington et al.).

Histogenesis. The frequent onset at puberty, the rather common location in apocrine areas, and the interpretation of the amorphous material within the ducts as product of secretion had suggested differentiation toward apocrine structures in the past (Lever). However, enzyme histochemical and electron microscopic studies have established syringoma as a tumor with differentiation toward intraepidermal eccrine sweat ducts.

The enzyme pattern in the cells of syringoma shows a prevalence of eccrine enzymes, such as succinic dehydrogenase (Mustakallio), as well as phosphorylase and leucine aminopeptidase (Winkelmann and Muller). In contrast to apocrine structures, syringomas react only weakly to lysosomal, "apocrine" enzymes, such as acid phosphatase and beta-glucuronidase, except in a narrow lysosome-rich periluminal zone (Hashimoto et al., 1967).

Electron microscopic examination reveals the lumina of the small ducts to be lined by ductal rather than by secretory cells, showing numerous short microvilli, a periluminal band of tonofilaments, and many lysosomes (E.M. No. 39). In some tumor cells intracytoplasmic cavities are formed by lysosomal action. Coalescence of sev-eral such intracytoplasmic cavities to form an intercellular lumen is the mode by which the ductal lumina are formed in syringoma; and this is identical with the mode of formation of the embryonic as well as the regenerating intraepidermal eccrine duct (Hashimoto et al., 1966, 1967; Hashimoto and Lever) (see p. 7).

The finding of cystic ductal lumina filled with keratin near the epidermis is compatible with the natural keratinizing propensity of the luminal cells of the intraepidermal eccrine sweat duct toward the upper strata of the epidermis (Hashimoto et al., 1967).

Differential Diagnosis. The solid strands of basophilic epithelial cells embedded in a fibrous stroma have an appearance similar to that of the strands seen in fibrosing basal cell epithelioma (see p. 545). The latter tumor, however, lacks ductal structures containing amorphous material. The horn cysts near the epidermis resemble those occurring in trichoepithelioma, and their presence in syringoma was formerly misinterpreted as the occurrence of both types of tumors within the same lesion (Lever). While trichoepithelioma shows solid strands of basophilic epithelial cells and horn cysts, it lacks ductal structures.

BENIGN EPITHELIOMAS

TRICHOEPITHELIOMA

The name *trichoepithelioma* is preferable to the other designations, such as epithelioma adenoides cysticum and multiple benign cystic epithelioma, since it indicates that the differentiation in this tumor is directed toward hair structures. Trichoepithelioma usually occurs in multiple lesions, but occasionally it is seen as a solitary lesion.

Multiple trichoepithelioma is a dominantly inherited condition (Gaul). As a rule, the lesions begin to appear at adolescence and gradually increase in number and in size. One observes numerous rounded, skin-colored, firm nodules, usually between 2 and 8 mm in size, mainly on the face but occasionally also on the scalp, the neck, and the upper trunk. A few telangiectatic vessels often are present on the surface of the larger lesions. Ulceration of the lesions occurs very rarely, in contrast with basal cell epithelioma and the nevoid basal cell epithelioma syndrome; and change of the lesions into an expanding basal cell epithelioma does not seem to occur. The simultaneous presence of lesions of trichoepithelioma and cylindroma, which also is dominantly inherited, has been observed repeatedly (see Cylindroma, p. 524).

In solitary trichoepithelioma, which is not inherited, a firm, elevated, flesh-colored nodule is present, with onset usually in adult life. Most commonly, the lesion is seen on the face, but it may occur elsewhere. The presence within the same tumor of a solitary trichoepithelioma and an apocrine adenoma has been described (Müller-Hess and Delacrétaz).

Histopathology. On histologic examination the lesions of multiple trichoepithelioma appear well circumscribed as a rule. Horn cysts represent the characteristic histologic feature (Fig. 26-16). They consist of a fully keratinized center surrounded by a shell of flattened basophilic cells that have the same appearance as the cells in basal cell epithelioma ("basalioma cells"). The keratinization is abrupt and complete, not gradual and incomplete as in the horn pearls

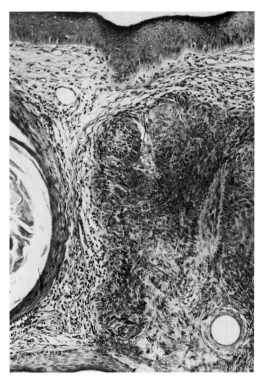

FIG. 26-16. **Trichoepithelioma.** The major components are horn cysts of varying sizes and formations resembling basal cell epithelioma and often showing an intricate, lacelike patterning of the cells, as shown here. (×200)

of squamous cell carcinoma. Occasionally, one sees eosinophilic cells with elongated nuclei arranged around some of the horn cysts (Gray and Helwig). Melanin granules often are present both in the cells surrounding the horn cysts and within the horn cysts. As the second major component of multiple trichoepitheliomas, besides the horn cysts, one finds tumor islands composed of basophilic cells of the same appearance as basalioma cells, arranged usually in a lacelike network but occasionally also as solid aggregates. These tumor islands show peripheral palisading of the cells and are indistinguishable from the tumor islands seen in basal cell epithelioma (Traenkle). The stroma of the tumor usually is quite cellular and often appears well demarcated from the surrounding stroma (Gray and Helwig).

Additional findings, observed in some but not in all multiple trichoepitheliomas, are the presence of a foreign-body giant cell reaction in the vicinity of ruptured horn cysts and of calcium deposits either within the foci of foreign-body reaction or within intact horn cysts (Gray and Helwig). Occasionally, lesions with a high degree of differentiation show abortive hair papillae and hair shafts (Fig. 26-17). Since hair papillae contain a high concentration of alkaline phosphatase, the presence of such abortive hair papillae in trichoepithelioma can be demonstrated by the use of the Gomori stain for alkaline phosphatase on unfixed frozen sections (Kopf).

Occasionally, some lesions in patients with multiple trichoepithelioma show relatively little differentiation toward hair structures. Then they contain only a few horn cysts but many areas with the appearance of basal cell epithelioma (Gray and Helwig). Such lesions are indistinguishable from a keratotic basal cell epithelioma, which may also show horn cysts (Fig. 26-18) (see p. 541). Thus, on a histologic basis no sharp line of demarcation can be drawn between multiple trichoepithelioma and basal cell epithelioma, and in order to arrive at a diagnosis in a given case it may be necessary to have knowledge of clinical data, such as the number and the distribution of the lesions and the presence of hereditary transmission.

SOLITARY TRICHOEPITHELIOMA is used as a histologic designation only for lesions showing a high degree of differentiation toward hair structures. Solitary lesions with relatively little differentiation toward hair structures are best classified as keratotic basal cell epithelioma. Thus, if a lesion is to qualify for the diagnosis of solitary trichoepithelioma, it should contain numerous horn cysts as well as abortive hair papillae and show only few areas with the appearance of basal cell epithelioma (Nikolowski; Zeligman).

Histogenesis. The horn cysts in trichoepithelioma represent immature hair structures. The abrupt and complete keratinization in the horn

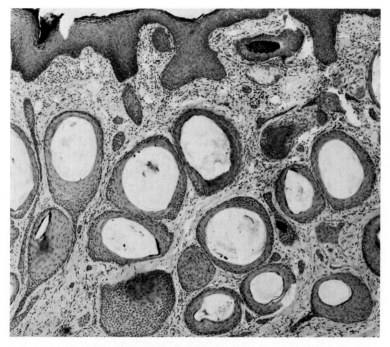

FIG. 26-17. **Trichoepithelioma.** This tumor is quite highly differentiated. It contains numerous horn cysts. In the center, near the epidermis, two rudimentary hairs can be seen. (×100)

cysts corresponds to the abrupt development of the horn cells of the hair from hair-matrix cells so that the basophilic cells surrounding the horn cysts are analogous to hair matrix cells, and the horn cysts represent attempts at hair-shaft formation. The eosinophilic cells seen occasionally around horn cysts probably represent cells with initial keratinization and are similar to the nucleated cells seen in normal hair shafts at the keratogenous zone.

The close relationship between trichoepithelioma and basal cell epithelioma can be explained by assuming that they have a common genesis from pluripotential cells that may develop toward hair structures, analogous to primary epithelial germ cells (Lever). Thus, the two types of tumors differ merely in the degree of maturity of their cells. Since cells of various degrees of maturity may occur in the same lesion, one may find in trichoepithelioma areas consistent with the histologic picture of basal cell epithelioma and vice versa.

The occasional association of multiple trichoepithelioma with cylindroma, an appendage tumor with differentiation probably toward apocrine structures (see p. 524), and of a solitary trichoepithelioma with an apocrine adenoma (see p. 515) also speaks in favor of a develop-ment of trichoepithelioma from immature cells with the potential to differentiate toward primary epithelial germ structures.

Differential Diagnosis. The difficulty of differentiating multiple trichoepithelioma from keratotic basal cell epithelioma on histologic grounds has been pointed out already and the need for clinical data has been stressed.

Just as difficult can be the differentiation of multiple trichoepithelioma from the nevoid basal cell epithelioma syndrome on histologic grounds. This too will require clinical data. Although both diseases are dominantly inherited and have multiple lesions, in trichoepithelioma the lesions are present mainly in the nasolabial fold, remain small and hardly ever ulcerate, whereas in the nevoid basal cell epithelioma syndrome the lesions are haphazardly distributed and, especially in the late "neoplastic phase," can grow to considerable size, ulcerate deeply, and show severely destructive growth. In addition, the patients with the nevoid basal cell epithelioma syndrome almost invariably

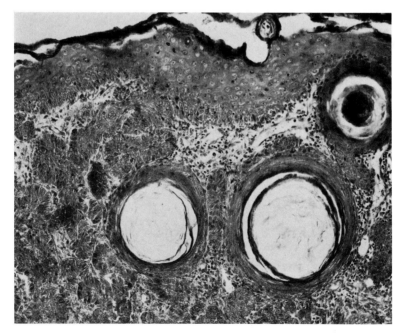

FIG. 26-18. **Basal cell epithelioma with horn cysts.** Histologically, this tumor is in an intermediate stage of differentiation between basal cell epithelioma and trichoepithelioma. Clinically, the lesion was a basal cell epithelioma. (×200)

show multiple skeletal and central nervous system anomalies, and frequently show multiple palmar and plantar pits. (See under Nevoid Basal Cell Epithelioma Syndrome, p. 538.)

PILOMATRIXOMA (CALCIFYING EPITHELIOMA)

Pilomatrixoma, or calcifying epithelioma of Malherbe, a tumor with differentiation toward hair cells, manifests itself as a firm, deep-seated nodule that is covered by normal skin. It occurs usually as a solitary lesion. The face and the upper extremities are the most common sites. Usually the size of the tumor varies from 0.5 to 3 cm, but it may be 5 cm. The tumor may arise at any age, but about 40 per cent of the tumors arise before the age of 10, and about 60 per cent in the first two decades (Moehlenbeck). It is not hereditary.

Histopathology. The tumor is sharply demarcated and often surrounded by a connective tissue capsule. It is located in the lower dermis and extends into the subcutaneous fat. Embedded in a rather cellular stroma, irregularly shaped islands of epithelial cells are present. As a rule, two types of cells, "basophilic cells" and "shadow cells," compose the islands (Fig. 26-19). In some tumors, however, basophilic cells are absent. The basophilic cells possess round or elongated, deeply basophilic nuclei and scanty cytoplasm, so that the nuclei lie close together. The cellular borders of the basophilic cells often are indistinct, so that it appears as if the nuclei were embedded in a symplasmic mass. The basophilic cells are arranged predominantly along the periphery of the tumor islands. The more mature cells, located toward the center of the islands, show a gradual loss of their nuclei ("transitional cells") and ultimately appear as

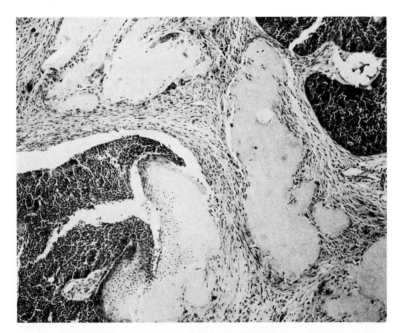

Fig. 26-19. **Pilomatrixoma (calcifying epithelioma).** The tumor consists of irregularly shaped islands embedded in a rather cellular stroma. Two types of cells compose the islands: "basophilic cells" and "shadow cells." The basophilic cells resemble hair matrix cells. The shadow cells show a central unstained shadow at the site of the lost nucleus. In the center of the field one can see transformation of the basophilic cells into shadow cells. The stroma contains numerous multinucleated giant cells. (×100)

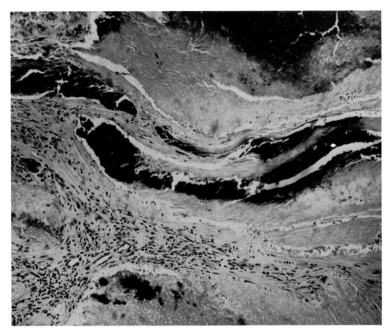

FIG. 26-20. **Pilomatrixoma (calcifying epithelioma).** Small and large areas of calcification are present within the lobules of "shadow cells." (×100)

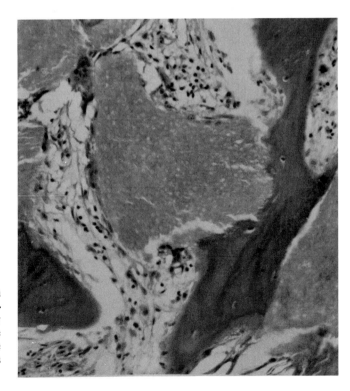

FIG. 26-21. **Pilomatrixoma (calcifying epithelioma), with ossification.** Elongated, irregularly shaped areas of ossification are present in the stroma. In the center an island of shadow cells is seen. (×200)

faintly eosinophilic, keratinized "shadow cells." The shadow cells have a distinct border and possess a central unstained area as a shadow of the lost nucleus. In tumors of recent origin numerous areas of basophilic cells usually are present. As the lesion ages, the number of basophilic cells decreases, owing to their development into shadow cells, and in tumors of long standing few or no basophilic cells remain.

In some tumors round eosinophilic structures representing immature hairs are seen. They may lie within areas of basophilic cells or within aggregates of shadow cells. In occasional instances melanin is present. It may be located in the basophilic cells, the shadow cells, or the stroma (Turhan and Krainer; Lever and Griesemer). The stroma of the tumor usually shows a considerable foreign-body giant cell reaction adjacent to the shadow cells.

On staining with hematoxylin and eosin calcium deposits are found in approximately three fourths of the tumors (Peterson and Hult). Most of the tumors containing calcium are composed largely of shadow cells. The calcium is seen either as fine basophilic granules within the cytoplasm of the shadow cells, or as large sheets of amorphous, basophilic material replacing the shadow cells (Fig. 26-20). On staining for calcium with the von Kossa stain, however, calcium deposits are readily recognized even in young tumors both in the tumor cells and in the connective tissue stroma (Geiser; Wiedersberg). Areas of ossification are seen in 15 to 20 per cent of the cases (Forbis and Helwig; Peterson and Hult). Ossification takes place in the stroma next to areas of shadow cells, probably through metaplasia of fibroblasts into osteoblasts (Fig. 26-21) (Geiser). Calcium-rich shadow cells act thereby as inducing factor (Wiedersberg). Malignant degeneration does not occur in lesions of pilomatrixoma.

Histogenesis. Originally described in 1880 by Malherbe and Chenantais as a calcified epithelioma of sebaceous glands, Turhan and Krainer in 1942 recognized that the cells in calcifying epithelioma differentiate in the direction of hair cortex cells, a view that electron microscopic studies subsequently have confirmed. The designation pilomatrixoma for calcifying epithelioma was suggested by Forbis and Helwig.

According to the view expressed by Turhan and Krainer, the basophilic cells represent hair-matrix cells, and the shadow cells immature hair-cortex cells. They regarded the small round foci of keratinization observed within aggregates of basophilic cells as cross sections of hair shafts, and the melanin present in some tumors as analogous to the melanin normally found in hair. It appears likely, however, that the basophilic cells are not mature hair-matrix cells but rather immature pluripotential cells that, analogous to primary epithelial germ cells, possess the potential to differentiate into hair-cortex cells; but, since they are less mature than hair-matrix cells, they produce not mature hair-cortex cells but irregular masses of immature hair-cortex cells represented by the shadow cells (Lever and Griesemer).

Histochemical studies have revealed in most tumor cells a strongly positive reaction for sulfhydryl or disulfide groups with the performic-acid-Schiff stain indicative of keratinization (Peterson and Hult; Hashimoto et al.). As evidence of keratinization the shadow cells show strong birefringence in polarized light (Lever and Hashimoto). A very similar birefringence is seen in the keratogenous zone of hair (Forbis and Helwig). Also, the regular occurrence of citrulline in the cells of pilomatrixoma is indicative of their forming hair keratin, rather than keratin of the type formed in the epidermis (Holmes) (see p. 549).

Electron microscopic examination has revealed in the areas of basophilic cells a few desmosomes and a moderate number of tonofilaments (McGavran). In cells that are in transition to shadow cells, numerous tonofilaments are seen in parallel alignment. They thus form keratin fibrils without the appearance of keratohyaline granules. A striking resemblance exists between the shadow cells and the cells in the keratogenous zone of normal hair, because both types of cells show thick keratin fibrils concentrically arranged around a hardly visible nucleus (Hashimoto et al.; Hashimoto and Lever).

Differential Diagnosis. The wall of pilar cysts also contains basophilic cells which, as they keratinize, gradually lose their nuclei and often undergo calcification. The peripheral layer of basophilic cells in pilar cysts, however, shows a palisading pattern which the basophilic cells of pilomatrixoma do not show. Furthermore, shadow cells characterized by a central unstained area at the site of the disintegrated nucleus are seen in no tumor other than pilomatrixoma.

PILAR TUMOR OF THE SCALP

This solitary tumor occurs on or near the scalp almost exclusively in elderly women. Starting as a subcutaneous nodule suggestive of a wen, it may grow into a large, elevated, nodular mass that may undergo ulceration. The tumor may occur in association with one or even several pilar cysts of the scalp (Holmes; Korting and Hoede). So far, there has been only one instance of a metastasis, observed in a preauricular lymph node (Holmes).

Histopathology. The tumor is composed of interlacing strands and lobules of squamous epithelium that undergo in their center an abrupt change into eosinophilic amorphous keratin (Fig. 26-22). This amorphous keratin is of the same type as that seen in the cavity of pilar cysts (Reed and Lamar). The squamous epithelium in many areas shows a slight degree of nuclear anaplasia, as well as horn pearl formation, and individual cell keratinization suggesting, at the first glance, a squamous cell carcinoma (Fig. 26-23) (Holmes; Dabska). The tumor differs, however, from a squamous cell carcinoma by its rather sharp demarcation from the surrounding stroma as well as by its abrupt mode of keratinization (Wilson Jones). Foci of calcification, although generally small, are often present in the areas of amorphous keratin (Fig. 26-23) (Wilson Jones; Korting and Hoede). Some tumors show extensive vacuolization, or clear-cell formation, of their tumor cells as the result of glycogen storage (Reed and Lamar; Holmes).

Histogenesis. According to Holmes, all pilar tumors are low-grade carcinomas because of the presence of nuclear anaplasia. However, the one case of regional metastasis observed by Holmes showed less anaplasia than some of his other cases of pilar tumor that did not metastasize.

Keratinization in the pilar tumor is of the same type as in pilar cysts, or trichilemmal cysts (see p. 462). In both pilar cyst and pilar tumor the keratinization is analogous to that of the outer root sheath, as seen at the follicular isthmus above the zone of sloughing of the inner root sheath (Pinkus) and especially in the sac surrounding the lower end of the telogen hair (Holmes; Pinkus). Analogous to the keratinization of the outer root sheath one observes in pilar tumors: (1) an abrupt change of squamous epithelium into amorphous keratin; (2) many vacuolated cells containing glycogen, similar to the cells of the outer root sheath; and (3) a prominent glassy layer of collagen surrounding many of the tumor formations (Reed and Lamar). Focal calcification within the amorphous keratin

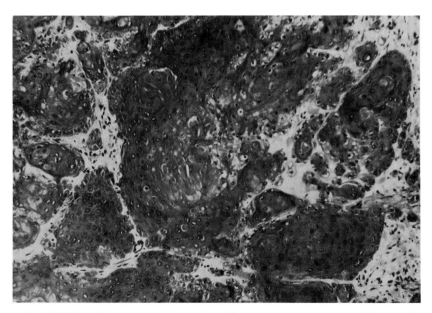

FIG. 26-22. **Pilar tumor of the scalp.** The tumor is composed of irregularly shaped lobules of squamous epithelium undergoing abrupt change into amorphous keratin. A large area of amorphous keratin is present in the center. (×200)

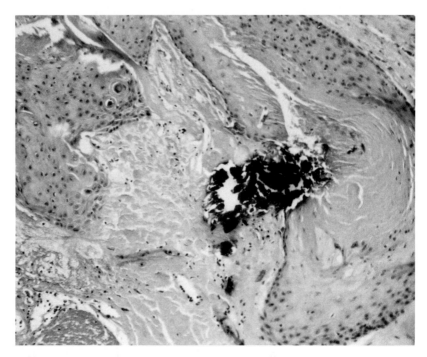

FIG. 26-23. **Pilar tumor of the scalp with calcification.** An area of calcification is present in the center. On the right side, an area of amorphous keratin is seen. On the left, two dyskeratotic cells are located in a lobule of squamous epithelium. (×200)

is a feature that pilar tumors of the scalp and pilar cysts have in common.

Differential Diagnosis. The presence of numerous sharply demarcated areas of amorphous eosinophilic material in the center of the tumor strands and lobules usually permits an easy differentiation from squamous cell carcinoma.

TRICHILEMMOMA

There are two variants of tumors that show differentiation toward the glycogen-rich clear cells normally found in the outer root sheath. Such tumors show·distinct palisading of the outer cell row. They have no characteristic clinical appearance.

Histopathology. In one variant of trichilemmoma, referred to as the *lobular variant of trichilemmoma,* the distinguishing histologic feature is the lobular architecture. The lesion occurs as a solitary, small tumor almost exclusively on the face. Histologically, one sees one or several lobules ori-

ented about a central hair follicle (Headington and French; Brownstein and Shapiro). The tumor through its localization around a hair follicle grows in close approximation to the epidermis (Fig. 26-24). In addition to a large proportion of clear cells there may be in the center of the lobules cells with a tendency to keratinization (Headington and French; Ingrish and Reed).

The second variant of trichilemmoma, referred to by Mehregan as *tumor of the follicular infundibulum,* occurs predominantly on the face either as a single growth (Mehregan) or as multiple small papules (Mehregan and Butler; Johnson and Hookerman). Histologically, one finds a platelike growth of epithelial cells in the upper dermis extending parallel to the epidermis and showing multiple connections with the lower margin of the epidermis. The peripheral cell layer of the tumor plate shows palisading, while the centrally located cells show a pale-staining to clear cytoplasm as the result of their content of glycogen. Small

FIG. 26-24, **Trichilemmoma**. The tumor shows lobular formations differentiating toward hair follicles, especially toward the outer root sheath. Thus, many cells appear clear because of their content of glycogen. (×50)

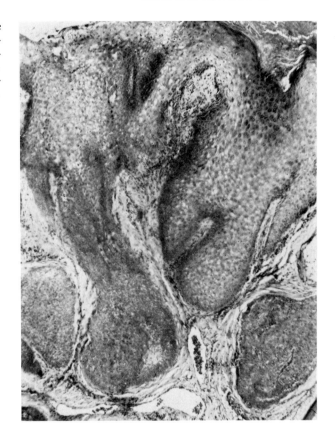

hair follicles with varying degrees of differentiation extend downward from the tumor plate, with some of the follicles showing a hair papilla (Johnson and Hookerman), or containing a hair (Mehregan).

Differential Diagnosis. For differentiation from clear cell hidradenoma, see page 530.

SEBACEOUS EPITHELIOMA

Clinically, sebaceous epitheliomas have the appearance of a basal cell epithelioma and may show ulceration. Some of the lesions possess a yellowish color. Usually, they occur on the face or the scalp as a solitary lesion. In one instance, however, the lesion was located on the sole of the foot (Raab). In addition to occurring as a primary lesion, sebaceous epitheliomas not infrequently arise within a nevus sebaceus (Zackheim; Mehregan and Pinkus; Wilson Jones and Heyl). Sebaceous epitheliomas may also be found among the multiple sebaceous neoplasms occurring in association with multiple visceral carcinomas (see p. 505).

Histopathology. In degree of differentiation sebaceous epithelioma stands between sebaceous adenoma, in which there are typical sebaceous lobules, and cystic basal cell epithelioma, in which there is only little differentiation toward sebaceous cells (see Table 26-1, p. 499).

Sebaceous epithelioma, in contrast to sebaceous adenoma, is not a well circumscribed tumor but grows in irregularly shaped cell masses (Fig. 26-25). Thus, it grows like a basal cell epithelioma, but its cells have undergone considerable differentiation toward sebaceous cells (McMullan). As a rule, the majority of cells are undifferentiated cells which, when arranged in a palisade fashion at the periphery of a cell mass, resemble the germinative cells of sebaceous glands but are indistinguishable from the cells of basal cell epithelioma when lying

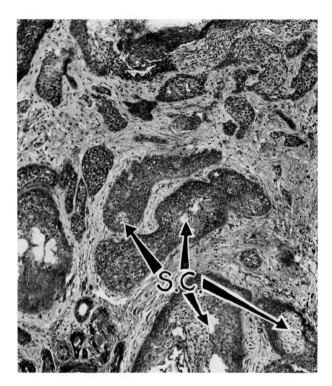

in aggregates (McMullan; Zackheim). In addition, there are a fairly large number of transitional cells showing beginning fatty vacuolization of their cytoplasm. Groups of mature sebaceous cells lie in the center of most cell masses. Cysts formed by the disintegration of cells and filled with amorphous material may be present in some of the tumor masses (Urban and Winkelmann).

Differential Diagnosis. For differentiation from sebaceous carcinoma, which, in contrast to sebaceous epithelioma, may cause metastases, see page 552.

CYLINDROMA

Cylindroma represents a tumor in which the differentiation probably is in the direction of apocrine structures. It occurs at least as commonly as a solitary lesion as it does as multiple lesions, its classical form (Crain and Helwig). Cases with multiple lesions are dominantly inherited and show numerous dome-shaped, smooth nodules of various sizes on the scalp. Occasionally, scattered nodules are present also on the face and, in rare instances, on the extremi-

ties (Kleine-Natrop; Baden). The lesions begin to appear in early adulthood and increase in number and size throughout life. They vary in size from a few millimeters to several centimeters. On the scalp the nodules may be present in such large numbers as to cover the entire scalp like a turban. For this reason they are referred to occasionally as turban tumors.

Cylindromas occasionally undergo malignant degeneration. Six cases are on record. In four of them autopsy revealed widespread metastases (Luger; Lausecker; Gertler; Korting et al.). In one patient the malignant degeneration led to invasion of the skull and a fatal hemorrhage (Zontschew), and in another to invasion of the brain and a fatal meningitis (Lyon and Rouillard).

The association of mutiple lesions of cylindroma with multiple lesions of trichoepithelioma is quite common (Lausecker; Kleine-Natrop; Guggenheim and Schnyder; Crain and Helwig; Bandmann et al.; Baden). In cases of such association the lesions of the scalp are cylindromas, and those elsewhere are partially cylindromas and partially trichoepitheliomas. The association of these two types of tumors, both of which are dominantly inherited, is of interest also in regard to their histogenesis (see below).

Solitary cylindromas are not inherited, they appear in adult life, and occur either on the scalp or the face. Their histologic appearance is the same as that of multiple cylindromas (Crain and Helwig).

Histopathology. The tumors of cylindroma are composed of numerous islands of epithelial cells. Varying considerably in size and shape and lying close together, separated often only by their hyaline sheath and a narrow band of collagen, the islands of epithelial cells seem to fit together like the pieces of a jigsaw puzzle (Fig. 26-26). The hyaline sheath surrounding the tumor islands like a cylinder is quite variable in thickness. In addition, droplets of hyalin are present in many islands, and some islands consist

largely of hyalin and contain only a few cells. The hyalin is PAS-positive, diastase-resistant and does not stain with alcian blue, indicating that it contains only neutral mucopolysaccharides (Fusaro and Goltz).

Two types of cells compose the islands: Cells with small, dark-staining nuclei are present predominantly at the periphery of the islands, often in palisade arrangement, whereas cells with large, light-staining nuclei lie in the center of the islands (Fig. 26-27). In addition, tubular lumina are present. They are quite numerous in some cases, whereas in others only a few lumina are found after a thorough search. The lumina may be lined by cells having the appearance of either secretory or ductal cells. Often amorphous material is found within the lumina, containing both neutral and acid mucopolysaccharides, since it stains positively both with

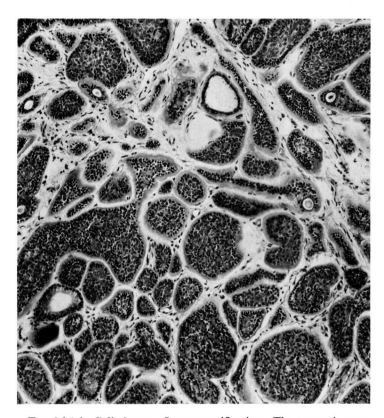

FIG. 26-26. **Cylindroma.** Low magnification. The tumor is composed of irregularly shaped islands fitting together like the pieces of a jigsaw puzzle. The islands are surrounded by a hyaline sheath. Several islands in the right lower quadrant contain droplets of hyalin. (×75)

the PAS reaction and with alcian blue (Fusaro and Goltz). In some instances, the luminal cells show active secretion, like the secretory cells of apocrine glands.

In the six reported cases of malignant degeneration occurring in lesions of cylindroma, the areas of malignant degeneration were characterized by islands of cells showing marked anaplasia and pleomorphism of the nuclei, many atypical mitotic figures, loss of the hyaline sheath, loss of palisading at the periphery, and invasion into the surrounding tissue.

Histogenesis. No agreement exists in regard to the direction of differentiation in cylindroma, whether it is eccrine or apocrine. Histochemical and enzyme histochemical examinations have not led to clear-cut conclusions, although electron microscopic findings are somewhat in favor of apocrine differentiation.

The fact that the amorphous material within the tubular lumina contains neutral as well as acid mucopolysaccharides allows no conclusion, since both the mucoid secretory cells of eccrine glands and the apocrine secretory cells excrete granules containing neutral and acid mucopolysaccharides.

Enzyme histochemical staining has revealed in cylindroma little or no phosphorylase activity, an "eccrine" type of enzyme. Of "apocrine" enzymes one finds weak reactions for acid phosphatase and beta glucuronidase, and a negative reaction for indoxyl esterase (Holubar and Wolff; Hashimoto and Lever). The absence of significant enzyme reactions may be due to the immaturity of the tumor cells.

Electron microscopic examination has revealed, analogous to the examination by light microscopy, two major types of cells: undifferentiated basal cells with small dark nuclei and differentiating cells with large pale nuclei. Most of the differentiating cells still appear quite immature as "indeterminate cells," but some of them show a certain degree of differentiation toward secretory or ductal cells and are arranged around lumina. The secretory cells contain two

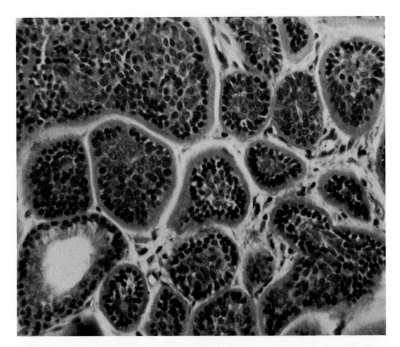

FIG. 26-27. **Cylindroma.** High magnification of Figure 26-26. Two types of epithelial cells compose the islands. There are cells with small dark nuclei, representing undifferentiated cells, and cells with large pale nuclei, representing cells with a certain degree of differentiation toward ductal or secretory cells. In the lower left corner there is a glandular lumen lined by two rows of cells. The cells of the inner row show active secretion, like the secretory cells of apocrine glands. (×200)

types of secretory granules similar to the secretory cells of apocrine glands: One type of secretory granule is large and contains lipid globules, while the other type of granule contains central cristae, suggesting origin from mitochondria (Hashimoto and Lever).

In addition to the electron microscopic findings, the common association of trichoepithelioma and cylindroma speaks in favor of an apocrine differentiation in cylindroma, since an origin from pluripotential cells with the potentiality of primary epithelial germ cells would explain the formation of both hair structures and apocrine structures.

The thick hyaline band surrounding the tumor islands of cylindroma shows two intermingled components: first, an amorphous material representing a greatly thickened basal lamina that is connected with the tumor cells by half-desmosomes, and, second, a fibrous component consisting of anchoring fibrils as well as collagen fibrils of varying maturity and thus varying in width and showing a range of periodicity from 15 to 68 nm, as found in tropocollagen, immature collagen, and mature collagen. The hyaline material within the tumor islands represents inclusions of the surrounding hyaline band into the tumor islands. One can assume that as the tumor islands extend peripherally, tumor cells encircle portions of the peripheral hyaline material and incorporate it into the tumor islands. The fibrous component of the hyaline material is produced by fibroblasts. The amorphous material, on the other hand, probably is secreted by the tumor cells (Hashimoto and Lever).

CLEAR CELL HIDRADENOMA

This tumor, referred to in the past as clear cell myoepithelioma (see Histogenesis), is presently called also nodular hidradenoma (Lund), eccrine sweat gland adenoma of the clear cell type (O'Hara et al., 1966; O'Hara and Bensch, 1967), solid-cystic hidradenoma (Winkelmann and Wolff, 1967, 1968) and eccrine acrospiroma (Johnson and Helwig).

Clear cell hidradenoma, now generally regarded as an eccrine sweat gland tumor on the basis of its enzyme histochemical and electron microscopic features, occurs as a solitary tumor in most instances; although occasionally several lesions are present (Efskind and Eker). The tumors present

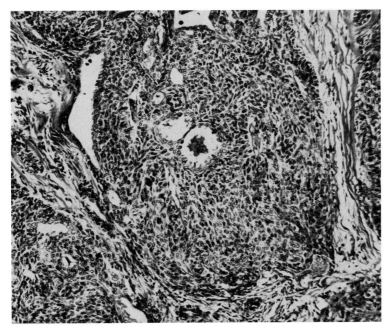

FIG. 26-28. **Clear cell hidradenoma.** The tumor consists of lobular masses composed of cells with clear cytoplasm. Small and large lumina are present lined either by cuboidal ductal cells or by columnar secretory cells. (×200)

themselves as firm intradermal nodules and in most instances measure between 0.5 and 2 cm in diameter, although they may be larger. Usually they are covered by intact skin, but some tumors show superficial ulceration (Winkelmann and Wolff, 1968) and discharge serous material (Lever and Castleman; Johnson and Helwig).

Histopathology. The tumor appears well circumscribed and often encapsulated. It is composed of lobulated masses located in the dermis and extending into the subcutaneous fat. Within the lobulated masses tubular lumina of various sizes are often present (Fig. 26-28). The tubular lumina often show branching. In addition, there often are cystic spaces which may be of considerable size and contain a faintly eosinophilic, homogeneous material (Fig. 26-29) (Winkelmann and Wolff, 1968). The tubular lumina are lined by cuboidal ductal cells or by columnar secretory cells. On the other hand, the wide, cystic spaces only rarely are lined by a single row of luminal cells and,

more frequently, are bordered by tumor cells that show no particular orientation and occasionally show degenerative changes (Lever and Castleman). This suggests that the cystic spaces form as a result of a degeneration of tumor cells.

In solid portions of the tumor two types of cells can be recognized (Lever and Castleman; Kersting; Hashimoto et al.; Winkelmann and Wolff, 1968). The proportion of these two types of cells varies considerably in different tumors. One type of cell is fusiform and has an elongated nucleus and basophilic cytoplasm (Fig. 26-30). The other type of cell is polygonal, has a round nucleus, and contains very clear cytoplasm so that the cell membrane is distinctly visible (Fig. 26-31). There also are cells transitional between these two varieties and such cells usually show a rather light, eosinophilic cytoplasm. The clear cells contain considerable amounts of glycogen; but they may show, in addition, significant amounts of diastase-resistant PAS-positive material

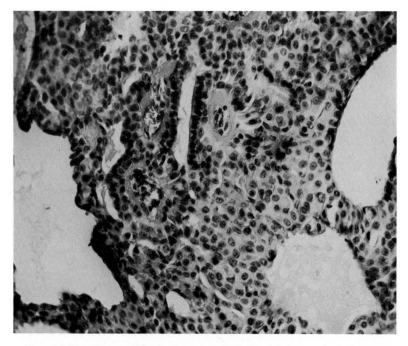

FIG. 26-29. **Clear cell hidradenoma.** Tubular lumina and cystic spaces are present within the tumor. The cystic spaces seem to form as a result of a degeneration of tumor cells. (×200)

along their periphery (Kersting). In some tumors keratinizing cells with formation of horn pearls are present (Lever and Castleman; O'Hara et al.). In other tumors groups of squamous cells are arranged around small lumina that are lined with a well-defined eosinophilic cuticle and thus resemble the intraepidermal portion of the eccrine duct (Kersting; Johnson and Helwig).

Although in most cases no connections of the tumor lobules with the surface epidermis are noted, in some instances the tumor replaces the epidermis centrally and merges with the acanthotic epidermis at the periph-

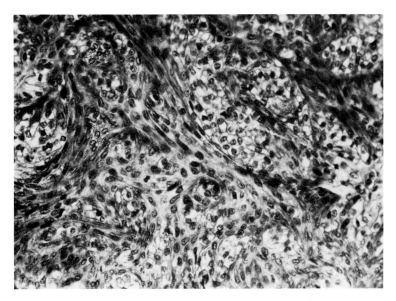

FIG. 26-30. **Clear cell hidradenoma.** This tumor contains, in addition to polygonal clear cells, also fusiform cells. (×200)

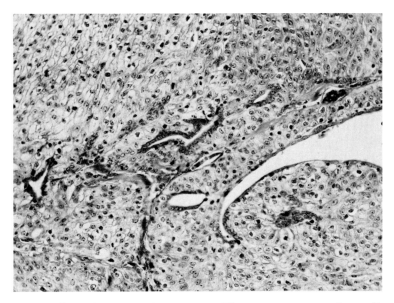

FIG. 26-31. **Clear cell hidradenoma.** There are numerous clear cells and, in addition, tubular lumina lined by a single layer of cuboidal ductal cells. (×200)

ery of the tumor (Lever and Castleman; O'Hara et al.; Johnson and Helwig).

Histogenesis. Originally the fusiform cells, because of their location peripheral to the luminal cells and because of their shape, had been regarded as cells differentiating in the direction of myoepithelial cells (Lever and Castleman; Efskind and Eker; Berger). However, the absence of alkaline phosphatase and, ultrastructurally, of myofilaments has disproved their relationship to myoepithelial cells.

Enzyme histochemical staining has established the presence of high concentrations of "eccrine" enzymes in clear cell hidradenoma, particularly of phosphorylase and of respiratory enzymes, including succinic dehydrogenase and diphosphopyridine nucleotide (DPNH) diaphorase (Hashimoto et al.; Winkelmann and Wolff, 1967).

Electron microscopic examination by Hashimoto et al. has shown in the fusiform cells a fair number of tonofilaments, and in the clear cells an abundance of glycogen. These two types of tumor cells resemble, in the opinion of Hashimoto et al., the tumor cells of eccrine poroma and, consequently, also resemble the cells composing the outer layers of the intraepidermal eccrine duct. In addition, four types of luminal cells were recognized by Hashimoto et al.: One type showed evidence of active secretion and, analogous to the secretory cells in the normal eccrine gland, cells of this type either were glycogen-rich or were glycogen-free and then contained a few small, dense secretory granules. The second type of luminal cell was regarded as dermal ductal in differentiation. The third type, by its content of lysosomes and keratohyaline granules, appeared to be epidermal ductal. Finally, the fourth type of luminal cell appeared to be immature and intermediate in differentiation, between a ductal and a secretory cell. Hashimoto et al. concluded that clear cell hidradenoma shows differentiation toward intraepidermal as well as intradermal eccrine structures ranging from the poral epithelium to the secretory segment, and thus ultrastructurally clear cell hidradenoma seems to be intermediate to eccrine poroma, with its largely intraepidermal ductal differentiation, and eccrine spiradenoma, with its dermal-ductal and secretory differentiation.

In contrast to Hashimoto et al., O'Hara and Bensch, on the basis of their ultrastructural study, believe that the clear cells of clear cell hidradenoma closely resemble the clear type of eccrine secretory cells not only by their high glycogen content but also by possessing a similar system of intracellular organelles and a similar complex intercellular canalicular system.

Differential Diagnosis. Clear cell hidradenoma shares with trichilemmoma the presence of clear cells rich in glycogen. Also foci of keratinization may be found in both. However, only clear cell hidradenoma shows the presence of large cystic spaces and usually also of tubular lumina.

Malignant Clear Cell Hidradenoma

Although clear cell hidradenomas usually are well demarcated and benign tumors, malignant clear cell hidradenomas occur occasionally. In some cases they have caused metastases to bones and lymph nodes and finally death (Keasby and Hadley). Such malignant clear cell hidradenomas show marked anaplasia of their clear cells, numerous atypical mitoses, and invasion into the surrounding tissue (Kersting; Santler and Eberhartinger). Atypical clear cells are encountered also in the metastases (Keasby and Hadley). Malignant clear cell hidradenomas that metastasize do not develop from benign clear cell hidradenomas but are malignant from their beginning (Keasby and Hadley; Santler and Eberhartinger).

ECCRINE POROMA

Eccrine poroma, first described by Pinkus et al. in 1956, is a fairly common solitary tumor. In about two thirds of the cases it is found on the sole or the sides of the foot (Hyman and Brownstein), occurring next in frequency on the hands and fingers. Eccrine poroma has also been observed in many other areas of the skin, such as the neck, the chest and the nose (Okun and Ansell; Penneys et al.). In the only instance of multiple eccrine poroma so far reported more than 100 tumors were present on the palms and soles (Goldner). Eccrine poroma generally arises in middle-aged or old persons. The tumor has a rather firm consistency, is raised and often slightly pedunculated, is asymptomatic, and usually measures less than 2 cm in diameter.

Histopathology. In its typical form, eccrine poroma arises within the epidermis from where it extends downward into the dermis as tumor masses that often consist of broad, anastomosing bands. The lateral border between epidermis and tumor is easily

FIG. 26-32. **Eccrine poroma.** The tumor consists of broad, anastomosing bands. The cells composing the tumor have a uniformly small, cuboidal appearance and are connected by intercellular bridges. A ductal lumen extends through the tumor in a vertical direction. It is lined by an eosinophilic cuticle and a single row of luminal cells. (×150)

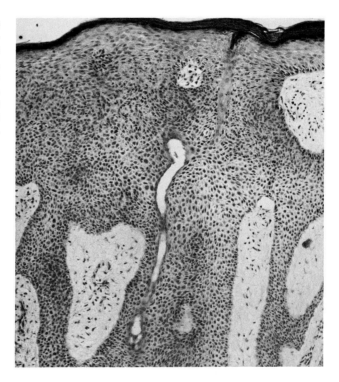

apparent because of the distinctive appearance of the tumor cells: they are smaller than squamous cells, have a uniform cuboidal appearance, have a round, deeply basophilic nucleus, and are connected by intercellular bridges (Fig. 26-32). These cells show no tendency to keratinization within the tumor, but they are able to keratinize on the surface of the tumor. Although the border between tumor formations and the stroma is sharp the tumor cells located at the periphery show no palisading.

As a characteristic feature the tumor cells contain significant amounts of glycogen, usually in an uneven distribution (Freeman et al.). Melanocytes and melanin often are absent (Pinkus et al.), although they may be present in tumors encountered in Negroes (Knox and Spiller), in Mongolians (Yasuda et al.), and occasionally even in Caucasians (Krinitz, 1967).

In most but not in all eccrine poromas, narrow ductal lumina and occasionally cystic spaces are found within the tumor bands (Freeman et al.). They are lined by an eosinophilic, PAS-positive, diastase-resistant cuticle similar to that lining the lumina of

eccrine sweat ducts and by a single row of luminal cells.

Poromas occasionally are located entirely within the epidermis where they appear as discrete aggregates. Such intraepidermal poromas were first described by Smith and Coburn under the designation *hidroacanthoma simplex* in 1956, the same year that Pinkus et al. described the eccrine poroma. A few ductal lumina lined by an eosinophilic cuticle can often be seen within the intraepidermal islands (Mehregan and Levson). On the other hand, eccrine poromas may be located largely or entirely within the dermis where they consist of variously shaped tumor islands containing ductal lumina (Winkelmann and McLeod).

Histogenesis. Enzyme histochemical staining has shown the prevalence of "eccrine" enzymes in eccrine poroma, particularly of phosphorylase but also of succinic dehydrogenase (Sanderson and Ryan; Hashimoto and Lever, 1964; Winkelmann and McLeod). The presence of large amounts of glycogen in many of the tumor cells is consistent with their being immature cells of the intraepidermal eccrine sweat duct, since these cells are rich in glycogen in the human embryo (Serri et al.).

On *electron microscopic examination* the tumor cells, except the luminal cells, contain a moderate number of tonofilaments and are connected with each other by desmosomes and appear identical to those cells that compose the outer layer of the intraepidermal eccrine duct (poral epithelial cells) (Hashimoto and Lever, 1964). The cells surrounding the lumina show extending into the lumen numerous tortuous microvilli coated with amorphous material which forms the eosinophilic cuticle seen by light microscopy. Small ductal lumina surrounded by numerous lysosomes are occasionally seen in the cytoplasm of tumor cells (Hashimoto and Lever, 1964; Mishima). Since it is characteristic of the embryonic as well as the regenerating intraepidermal eccrine duct to be located initially within the cytoplasm of cells (Hashimoto et al.), eccrine poroma can be regarded as a tumor differentiating in the direction of intraepidermal eccrine ducts. In a few areas, however, electron microscopic examination shows slitlike separation between tumor cells, resembling intradermal duct formation (Hashimoto and Lever, 1969). (For a description of the embryonic intraepidermal and dermal eccrine duct formation, see p. 7).

Differential Diagnosis. Eccrine poroma must be differentiated from basal cell epithelioma and seborrheic keratosis. In basal cell epithelioma the cells have no visible intercellular bridges, are more variable in size, often show peripheral palisading, and contain little or no glycogen. The cells of eccrine poroma greatly resemble the small basaloid cells of seborrheic keratosis, especially since they too possess clearly visible intercellular bridges. However, seborrheic keratoses have an even demarcation at their lower border and their cells have the potential to keratinize and in doing so form horn cysts. Also, both basal cell epithelioma and seborrheic keratosis lack lumina lined with an eosinophilic cuticle. Furthermore, it may be remembered that these two types of tumors hardly ever occur on the sole of the foot.

Malignant Eccrine Poroma

The first case of malignant eccrine poroma was reported by Pinkus and Mehregan in 1963 under the designation of epidermotropic eccrine carcinoma. In that case, which ended fatally, considerable metastatic spreading was found in the superficial lymphatic vessels of the skin. In innumerable areas the tumor cells had invaded the overlying epidermis so that sharply defined small and

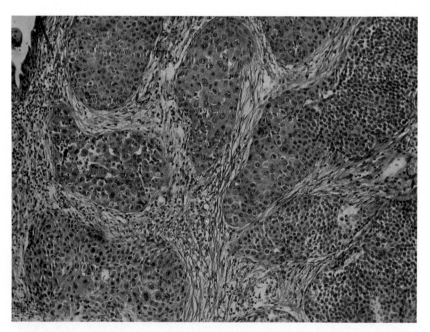

FIG. 26-33. **Malignant eccrine poroma.** On the right side, the tumor has an appearance similar to that of an eccrine poroma, whereas on the left side the tumor lobules are composed of cells showing anaplastic nuclei and dyskeratosis. (×100)

large nests of tumor cells were scattered through the epidermis in a "pagetoid" fashion. Such a "pagetoid" distribution of intraepidermal metastases was found also in the four subsequently reported cases of malignant eccrine poroma. In two of them most of the cutaneous metastases were intraepidermal rather than dermal (Mishima and Marioka; Ishikawa). In the other two cases the malignant eccrine paroma had arisen in a long-standing benign eccrine poroma. In addition to widespread metastases to lymph nodes and viscera, there were also cutaneous metastases. Although they were located largely in the dermis, some were intraepidermal in location (Miura; Krinitz, 1972).

Histopathology. Malignant eccrine poroma in areas of low malignancy resembles eccrine poroma except that scattered cells with anaplastic hyperchromatic nuclei are present (Ishikawa). In areas of higher malignancy the tumor cells are large and, in addition to having anaplastic nuclei, show a clear cytoplasm containing, on staining with the PAS reaction, large amounts of finely granular glycogen (Mishima and Marioka).

In addition, keratinization with horn pearl formation and dyskeratosis may be found (Fig. 26-33) (Krinitz, 1972).

ECCRINE SPIRADENOMA

Eccrine spiradenoma occurs usually as a solitary intradermal nodule, but occasionally there are several nodules (Hashimoto et al.; Munger et al.), and rarely more than one hundred (Nödl). In most instances, eccrine spiradenoma arises in early adult life. It has no characteristic location. The nodules are often tender, and occasionally painful.

Histopathology. The tumor may consist of one large, sharply demarcated lobule, but more commonly there are several such lobules located in the dermis without connections to the epidermis. The lobules are regularly and sharply demarcated and are encapsulated. On low magnification the tumor lobules often appear deeply basophilic because of the close aggregation of the nuclei (Fig. 26-34).

On higher magnification the epithelial cells within the tumor lobules are aggregated in clusters and in intertwining cords sepa-

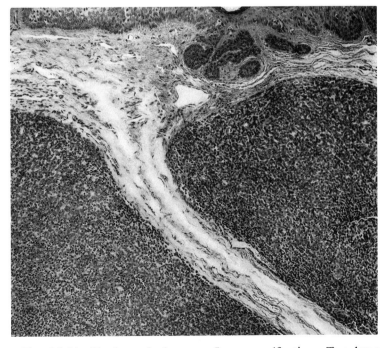

Fig. 26-34. **Eccrine spiradenoma.** Low magnification. Two large masses of tumor cells are shown. They are composed of two types of cells. (×100)

rated usually by rather thin connective tissue septa (Sheldon; Lever; Kersting and Helwig). Two types of epithelial cells are present, both of which possess only scant amounts of cytoplasm. The cells of the first type possess a small dark nucleus; they generally are located at the periphery of the cellular aggregates. The cells of the second type have a large pale nucleus; they are located in the center of the aggregates and may be arranged partly around small lumina (Fig. 26-35). In the absence of a lumen the cells with pale nuclei may show a rosettelike arrangement. The lumina frequently contain small amounts of a granular, eosinophilic material which is PAS-positive and diastase-resistant (Kersting and Helwig). Glycogen is absent in the tumor cells or is present in insignificant amounts.

In some cases of eccrine spiradenoma hyaline material is present in the stroma and also infiltrates between the tumor cells and may compress them (Munger et al.). The stroma surrounding the tumor lobules often shows lymphedema with greatly dilated blood or lymph capillaries (Kersting and Helwig).

Histogenesis. Enzyme histochemical staining has revealed a prevalence of "eccrine" enzymes, but the reactions are by far not as strong as in syringoma or eccrine poroma. The most characteristic "eccrine" enzyme, phosphorylase, was found by Hashimoto et al. only along the periphery of the tumor lobules, and Winkelmann and Wolff obtained a negative phosphorylase reaction. Respiratory enzymes however, such as succinic dehydrogenase and diphosphopyridine nucleotide (DPNH) diaphorase, found also largely in eccrine structures, are present. Stains for alkaline phosphatase are negative, indicating the absence of mature, functioning myoepithelial cells (Hashimoto et al.).

Electron microscopic examination has shown, similar to light microscopic examination, two types of cells: undifferentiated basal cells with small dark nuclei and differentiating cells with large pale nuclei. Even though most of the differentiating cells still are quite immature ("indeterminate cells"), some show evidence of

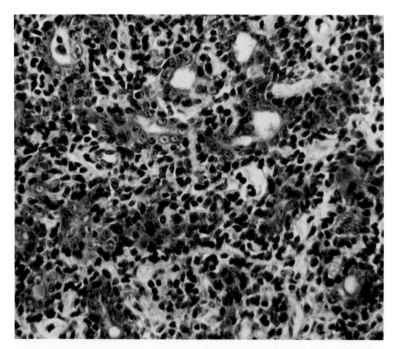

FIG. 26-35. **Eccrine spiradenoma.** High magnification. The epithelial cells are arranged in intertwining bands. Two types of cells can be seen. Cells with small dark nuclei lie at the periphery of the bands; they represent undifferentiated cells. Cells with large pale nuclei lie in the center of the bands and around small lumina. (×400)

differentiation toward intradermal eccrine ductal cells or toward eccrine secretory cells. As evidence of the immaturity of the tumor one may observe lumina lined by cells with different degrees and directions of differentiation. Thus, around the same lumen some cells may show numerous microvilli and a well developed periluminal zone of tonofilaments and thus resemble ductal cells, whereas other cells with only a few thin microvilli resemble secretory cells (Hashimoto et al.; Hashimoto and Lever). Some of the secretory cells show abundant ergastoplasmic sacs with endoplasmic reticulum, as seen in the mucoid cells of the eccrine secretory segment, but secretory granules are absent (Munger et al.). A few myoepithelial cells with typical myofilaments are present occasionally at the periphery of tubular structures (Hashimoto et al.).

It can be concluded that the direction of differentiation in eccrine spiradenoma is in the direction of both the dermal duct and the secretory segment of the eccrine sweat gland. However, the weakness and inconsistency of the enzyme histochemical reactions, the presence largely of undifferentiated and indeterminate cells, and the absence of secretory granules in the secretory cells indicate a rather low degree of differentiation. Certainly, the electron microscopic studies have disproved the original assumption, based on light microscopic examination, that all the cells peripheral to the luminal cells were cells differentiating toward myoepithelial cells and that the tumor thus was a myoepithelioma (Sheldon; Lever).

MIXED TUMOR OF THE SKIN

Mixed tumors of the skin are firm intradermal or subcutaneous nodules. Although the overlying skin may be attached to the tumor it otherwise appears normal. Mixed tumors occur most commonly on the head and neck (Hirsch and Helwig). Their usual size lies between 0.5 and 3.0 cm.

Histopathology. Histologically, two types of mixed tumors of the skin can be recognized: one with tubular and cystic, partially branching lumina, and the other with small tubular lumina (Headington).

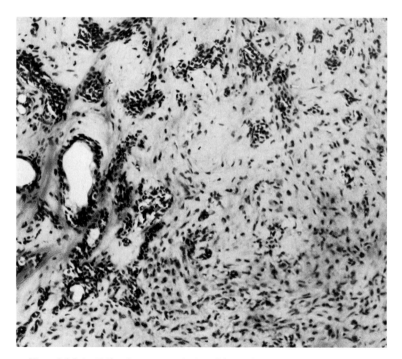

Fig. 26-36. **Mixed tumor of the skin, with tubular cystic lumina.** Embedded in an abundant stroma the tubular lumina are lined by two layers of cells: a luminar layer of cuboidal cells and a peripheral layer of flattened cells. Cells from the peripheral layer proliferate into the stroma. The stroma has a mucoid, faintly basophilic appearance. (×200)

Mixed tumors with tubular, branching lumina show marked variation in the size and shape of the tubular lumina, and in addition also cystic dilatation and branching (Fig. 26-36). Embedded in an abundant stroma the tubular lumina are lined by two layers of epithelial cells: a luminal layer of cuboidal cells and a peripheral layer of flattened cells (Kresbach). Furthermore, there are large and small aggregates of epithelial cells without lumina, and also single epithelial cells widely scattered through the stroma. One gains the impression that cells from the peripheral cell layer of the tubular structures and from the solid aggregates proliferate into the stroma (Hirsch and Helwig).

The abundant stroma in many areas has a mucoid, faintly basophilic appearance. As a result of shrinkage of the mucoid substance the nuclei that are scattered through it, both those of fibroblasts and of epithelial cells, are surrounded by a halo, resulting in an appearance of the stroma resembling that of cartilage. Since the mucoid stroma stains with alcian blue, mucicarmine, and aldehyde-fuchsin, and furthermore stains metachromatically with toluidine blue, the stroma contains acid mucopolysaccharides. In some tumors the intensity of staining with alcian blue and the metachromasia caused by staining with toluidine blue are not appreciably decreased by predigestion with hyaluronidase, indicating that the acid mucopolysaccharides are largely sulfated, i.e., chondroitin sulfate (Hirsch and Helwig). However, in other tumors incubation with hyaluronidase leads to a loss of the metachromasia, indicating that the acid mucopolysaccharides are largely nonsulfated, i.e., hyaluronic acid (Kresbach).

Mixed tumors with small tubular lumina show numerous small ducts as well as small groups of epithelial cells and solitary epithelial cells scattered through a mucoid stroma (Fig. 26-37). The tubular lumina are lined by only a single layer of flat epithelial cells from which small commalike proliferations often extend into the stroma (Headington). The mucoid stroma contains acid mucopolysaccharides that stain metachromatically with toluidine blue.

Histogenesis. The existence of two types of mixed tumors was first recognized by Headington. He postulated that the mixed tumors with tubular, branching lumina were apocrine in type,

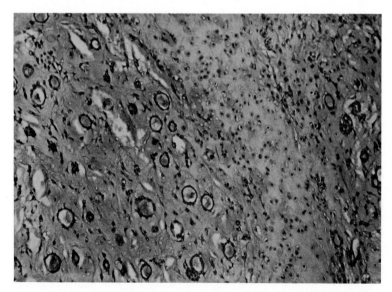

FIG. 26-37. **Mixed tumor of the skin, with small tubular lumina.** There are numerous small tubular lumina lined with a single layer of epithelial cells as well as small groups of epithelial cells and solitary epithelial cells. These epithelial structures are embedded in a mucoid stroma. (×100)

and the mixed tumors with small ductal lumina eccrine. However, most authors believe that also the mixed tumors with tubular, branching lumina are eccrine tumors (Nikolowski; Hirsch and Helwig; Kresbach). As a matter of fact, the mixed tumors with tubular, branching and occasionally cystic lumina greatly resemble clear cell hidradenomas, an eccrine type of tumor (see p. 527). Because of this resemblance Lund has grouped these two types of tumors together. It

is generally agreed that the epithelial cells of mixed tumors induce the mucinous changes in the stroma. Since these tumors thus are primarily epithelial tumors, the term *mucinous hidradenoma* would be preferable to the term *mixed tumor*. On the other hand, the term *chondroid syringoma*, chosen by Hirsch and Helwig, is apt to be misleading, since the stroma is not similar to cartilage and the epithelial portion does not resemble a syringoma.

PRIMORDIAL EPITHELIOMAS

BASAL CELL EPITHELIOMA

Basal cell epitheliomas occur almost exclusively on hair-bearing skin. Except in the nevoid basal cell epithelioma syndrome (see p. 538), their occurrence on the palms (Johnson; Hyman and Barsky) or on the soles (Hyman and Michaelides; Lewis et al.) is very rare. Their occurrence on the mucous membrane is doubted; and instances of basal cell epithelioma of the oral mucosa reported in the literature (Williamson et al.) probably are in reality ameloblastomas (Small and Waldron).

Basal cell epitheliomas usually occur as a single lesion, although the occurrence of several lesions either simultaneously or subsequently is not infrequent. Also, they generally occur in adults, even though in rare instances they may be seen in children (Murray and Cannon; Maron; Milstone and Helwig). However, in two rare forms of basal cell epithelioma, namely, the linear basal cell nevus and the nevoid basal cell epithelioma syndrome (see below), numerous lesions are present at birth and in childhood, respectively.

PREDISPOSING FACTORS. Although basal cell epitheliomas may arise without apparent reason, there are several predisposing factors. The most common of them is a light skin color in association with prolonged exposure to strong sun light (Gellin et al.). The predisposing effect of sun exposure is particularly evident in patients with xeroderma pigmentosum in whom both basal cell epithelioma and squamous cell carcinoma are common (see p. 65). Additional factors that predispose to the development

of both basal cell epithelioma and squamous cell carcinoma are large doses of x-irradiation (Anderson and Anderson; Sarkany et al.), and, less commonly, burn scars (Gaughan et al.; Margolis) and other scars (Wechsler et al.). On the other hand, nearly all, if not all, carcinomas of the skin caused by the prolonged administration of inorganic arsenic are squamous cell carcinomas, usually located in situ, analogous to Bowen's disease (Montgomery and Waisman; Hundeiker and Petres), rather than superficial basal cell epitheliomas, as had been thought at one time (Anderson) (see under Arsenical Keratosis and Carcinoma, p. 245).

OCCURRENCE OF METASTASES. As a rule, basal cell epitheliomas do not metastasize. However, there are exceptions to this rule. In a review published in 1974, Costanza et al. were able to collect from the literature a total of 90 cases. It was found that in most instances of metastasis the primary basal cell epithelioma was large, had been present for many years and had resisted several attempts at treatment (Assor). It is generally agreed that there are no histologic features that distinguish basal cell epitheliomas giving rise to metastases from those without metastasis (Assor).

In nearly two thirds of the reported cases metastasis was limited to the regional lymph nodes; viscera were involved in about one third of the cases, most commonly the lungs and pleura, the liver, and bone (Stell et al.). Concomitant metastases to lymph nodes and viscera have been reported only very rarely (Wermuth and Fajardo). Although in most reported cases the metastases were solitary, several instances of extensive visceral metastases were found on autopsy (Crawford and Joslin; Coletta et al.). Most metastases occurred in cachectic patients. It seems possible that cachetic patients have an immunologic deficit severe enough to tolerate distant implants of a tumor that ordinarily grows only in the skin (Wermuth and Fajardo).

Clinical Appearance. Clinically, seven types of basal cell epithelioma occur: (1) nodulo-ulcerative basal cell epithelioma, including rodent ulcer, by far the most common type; (2) pigmented basal cell epithelioma; (3) morphealike or fibrosing basal cell epithelioma; (4) superficial basal cell epithelioma; (5) fibroepithelioma; (6) the nevoid basal cell epithelioma syndrome; and (7) linear basal cell nevus and generalized follicular basal cell nevus, both very rare.

Nodulo-ulcerative basal cell epithelioma begins as a small waxy nodule that often shows on its surface a few small telangiectatic vessels. The nodule usually increases slowly in size and undergoes central ulceration. A typical lesion then consists of a slowly enlarging ulcer surrounded by a pearly, rolled border. This represents the so-called rodent ulcer.

Pigmented basal cell epithelioma differs from the nodulo-ulcerative type only by the brown pigmentation of the lesion.

Morphealike or fibrosing basal cell epithelioma manifests itself as an indurated yellowish plaque with an ill defined border. The overlying skin remains intact for a long time before finally ulceration occurs.

Superficial basal cell epithelioma consists of one or several erythematous, scaling, only slightly infiltrated patches that slowly increase in size by peripheral extension. The patches often are surrounded, at least in part, by a fine threadlike pearly border. The patches usually show small areas of superficial ulceration and crusting. In addition, their center may show smooth, atrophic scarring. Whereas the three types of basal cell epithelioma previously described commonly are situated on the face, superficial basal cell epithelioma occurs predominantly on the trunk.

Fibroepithelioma consists of one or several raised, moderately firm, often slightly

pedunculated nodules, covered by smooth, slightly reddened skin. Clinically, they resemble fibromas. The most common location is the back.

The nevoid basal cell epithelioma syndrome is an autosomal dominant disease with low penetration. During childhood and at the latest in puberty small nodules appear, of which there may be hundreds or thousands. During the "nevoid stage" the nodules slowly increase in number and size. They are haphazardly distributed over the face and body. Often during adult life many of the basal cell epitheliomas undergo ulceration, and in some patients during later life the disease enters into a "neoplastic stage" in which some of the basal cell epitheliomas, especially of the face, become invasive, destructive and mutilating. Occasionally, even death occurs as the result of invasion first of an orbit and, later on, of the brain (Taylor et al.; Berendes). There may be metastases to the lungs (Taylor et al.).

One half of the adult patients with the nevoid basal cell epithelioma syndrome show numerous palmar and plantar pits, 1 to 3 mm in diameter. They usually develop during the second decade of life and represent "formes frustes" of basal cell epithelioma (Howell and Mehregan) (see under Histopathology).

In nearly all patients there are, aside from the cutaneous lesions, multiple skeletal and central nervous system anomalies (Gorlin et al.). Among them are odontogenic jaw cysts, anomalies of the ribs, scoliosis, mental retardation and calcification of the dura. In several cases there was in addition a cerebellar medulloblastoma (Hermans et al.), or a fibrosarcoma of a mandible or maxilla (Reed). In the odontogenic jaw cysts an ameloblastoma may arise (Happle).

The linear and the generalized follicular basal cell nevi are extremely rare. In the linear basal cell nevus one observes an extensive unilateral linear eruption, usually present since birth, consisting of closely set nodules of basal cell epithelioma interspersed with comedones and epidermal cysts, and with striaelike areas of atrophy (Carney; Anderson and Best; Bleiberg and Brodkin). The lesions do not increase in size with aging of the patient. In the generalized follicular basal cell nevus there is a gradually extending hair loss, resulting from the damage inflicted on each hair follicle by gradually growing basal cell nevi (Brown et al.).

Histopathology. The characteristic cell of basal cell epithelioma, referred to by some as basalioma cell, has a large, oval or elongated nucleus and relatively little cytoplasm. Often, the cytoplasm of individual cells is poorly defined, so that it may appear as if the nuclei were embedded in a symplasmic mass. The nuclei resemble those of the basal cells of the epidermis, but basalioma cells differ from basal cells by not showing intercellular bridges on light microscopy. The nuclei in basal cell epitheliomas as a rule have a rather uniform and not an anaplastic appearance. Thus they do not show pronounced variation in size or in intensity of staining, and no abnormal mitoses, even in the rare instances of basal cell epithelioma with metastases. In the exceptional cases of basal cell epithelioma in which one finds, interspersed among the usual cells of basal cell epithelioma, cells with large hyperchromatic nuclei, with multiple nuclei, and with bizarre "star-burst" mitoses, the clinical course is not different from that of the usual basal cell epithelioma (Okun and Blumental; Rupec et al.).

The connective tissue stroma proliferates with the tumor and is arranged in parallel bundles around the tumor masses so that a mutual relationship seems to exist between the parenchyma of the tumor and its stroma (Pinkus). The stroma adjacent to the tumor masses often shows numerous young fibroblasts; and together with the proliferation of fibroblasts the stroma may appear mucinous and stain metachromatically due to the presence of large amounts of acid mucopolysaccharides (Fanger and Barker; Moore et al.). Since mucin shrinks during the process of fixation and dehydration of the specimen, frequently the stroma shows retraction from the tumor islands, so that in processed sections tumor islands may be partially or completely detached from the surrounding stroma (see Fig. 26-48). Although this retraction represents merely an artefact caused by shrinkage during the processing of the specimen, it is quite typical of basal cell epithelioma and may aid in its differentiation

from other tumors, such as squamous cell carcinoma. A mild inflammatory infiltrate is often seen in the stroma of nonulcerated basal cell epitheliomas, but it may be entirely lacking. If ulceration occurs, there usually is a rather pronounced inflammatory reaction.

From a histologic point of view, basal cell epitheliomas can be divided into two groups: undifferentiated and differentiated. Those of the latter group show differentiation toward the cutaneous appendages, i.e., hair, sebaceous glands, apocrine glands, or eccrine glands. A sharp dividing line between the two groups cannot be drawn, because many undifferentiated basal cell epitheliomas show differentiation in some areas, and most differentiated basal cell epitheliomas show areas lacking differentiation. By correlating the clinical with the histologic classification, it can be stated that the nodulo-ulcerative type of basal cell epithelioma, as well as the lesions of the nevoid basal cell epithelioma syndrome and of the two types of basal cell nevi, may either show differentiation or show no differentiation, whereas the other four types of basal cell epithelioma—pigmented basal cell epithelioma, fibrosing basal cell epithelioma, superficial basal cell epithelioma, and fibroepithelioma—usually show little or no differentiation.

Basal cell epitheliomas showing no differentiation are called solid basal cell epitheliomas. Those with differentiation toward hair structures are called keratotic; toward sebaceous glands, cystic; and toward apocrine or eccrine glands, adenoid basal cell epitheliomas. In many differentiated basal cell epitheliomas differentiation is directed toward more than one of these cutaneous appendages. For example, areas of keratinization may be found in a tumor that also shows adenoid structures.

Solid basal cell epithelioma, also called the primordial type of basal cell epithelioma (Foot), shows tumor masses of various sizes and shapes embedded in the dermis (Fig. 26-38). In more than 90 per cent of basal cell epitheliomas a connection between tumor cell formations and the surface epidermis can be shown to exist (Hundeiker and Berger). Occasionally, a tumor mass is found in contact with the external hair

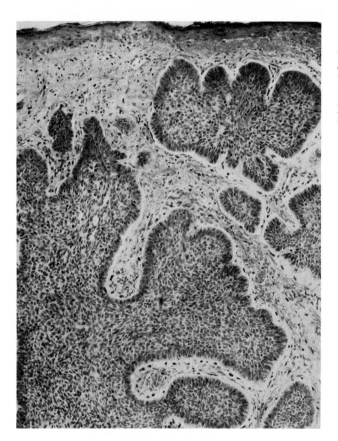

FIG. 26-38. **Solid basal cell epithelioma.** There are masses of various shapes and sizes composed of basal-cell-epithelioma cells, or basalioma cells. The peripheral cell layer of the tumor masses shows palisade arrangement of the nuclei. (×200)

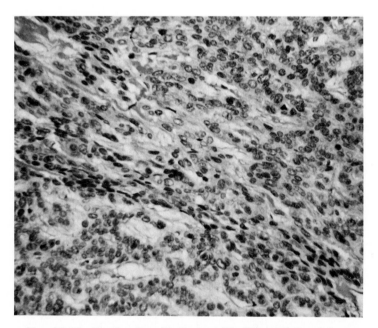

FIG. 26-39. **Basal cell epithelioma with differentiation into two types of cells.** One type of cell is large and has an oval, pale nucleus; the other type of cell is small and has an elongated, dark nucleus. (×400)

sheath. The peripheral cell layer of the tumor masses often shows palisade arrangement, whereas the nuclei of the cells inside lie in haphazard fashion.

Some basal cell epitheliomas, though they show little or no structural differentiation toward the epidermal appendages, nevertheless show two types of cells: a large cell with an oval, pale nucleus, and a small cell with an elongated, dark nucleus (Fig. 26-39) (Reidbord et al.).

Keratotic basal cell epithelioma, also called the pilar type (Foot), shows, in addition to undifferentiated cells, parakeratotic cells and horn cysts (Fig. 26-40). The parakeratotic cells possess an elongated nucleus and a slightly eosinophilic cytoplasm, in contrast to the deeply basophilic cytoplasm of the undifferentiated cells. The parakeratotic cells lie either in strands, or in concentric whorls, or around the horn cysts. It is likely that they are cells with initial keratinization somewhat similar to the nucleated cells in the keratogenic zone of normal hair shafts. The horn cysts, which are composed of fully keratinized cells, represent attempts at hair shaft formation (Foot). Just as normally the hair cells keratinize without the interposition of granular cells, so the horn cysts in keratotic basal cell epithelioma form directly from the parakeratotic cells.

Some keratotic basal cell epitheliomas possess large horn cysts (Fig. 26-41). They are like those observed in trichoepithelioma, so that at times it is difficult to decide whether a lesion represents a keratotic basal cell epithelioma or a trichoepithelioma (see p. 516). Clinical data may be necessary to arrive at a decision. Also the horn cysts must not be confused with the horn pearls that occur in squamous cell carcinoma (see Differential Diagnosis).

Cystic basal cell epithelioma shows cystic spaces in the center of the tumor masses. The cysts may form either by degeneration of the center of large tumor masses (Reidbord et al.) or by differentiation of the cells in the center of tumor masses toward sebaceous cells and subsequent disintegration

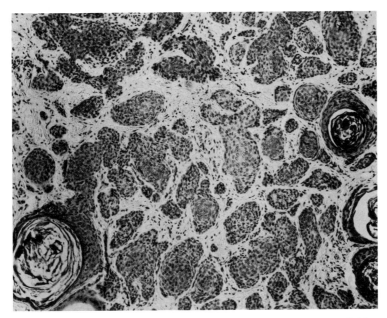

FIG. 26-40. **Keratotic basal cell epithelioma (pilar type).** In addition to undifferentiated tumor cells, there are parakeratotic cells and horn cysts. The parakeratotic cells possess an elongated nucleus and a slightly eosinophilic cytoplasm; they lie in strands, in concentric whorls, or around the horn cyst. (×100)

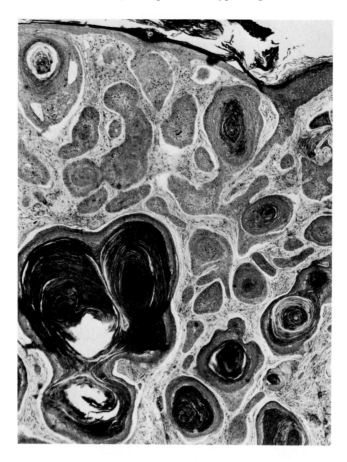

FIG. 26-41. **Keratotic basal cell epithelioma.** This tumor contains unusually large horn cysts. (×50)

analogous to the disintegration of sebaceous cells in the process of forming their secretion (Fig. 26-42). However, the latter mode of cyst formation in basal cell epithelioma is quite rare. If the cyst formation is due to sebaceous differentiation, some of the tumor cells in the vicinity of the cyst are vacuolated (Foot) or foamy (Piérard and Dupont), and there are lipid deposits within the cells (Wood et al.).

Adenoid basal cell epithelioma shows formations suggesting tubular glandlike structures. The cells are arranged in intertwining strands and radially around islands of connective tissue, resulting in a lacelike patterning of the tumor (Fig. 26-43). In some tumors one may find lumina surrounded by cells having the appearance of secretory cells (Fig. 26-44). The lumina may be filled with a colloidlike substance or with an amorphous granular material; but definite evidence of secretory activity of the cells

lining the lumina cannot be obtained, even with histochemical methods. Similarly, because of the low degree of differentiation of the cells, histochemical reactions that would indicate either apocrine or eccrine differentiation are negative (Wood et al.).

There is, however, one type of adenoid basal cell epithelioma, referred to as *eccrine epithelioma,* in which differentiation toward eccrine ductal structures is quite evident since, in the first place, the tumor, just like syringoma, is composed of ductal as well as cystic and commalike epithelial components. The difference from syringoma lies largely in the large size of the tumor and the depth of its invasion (Freeman and Winkelmann; Baer et al.). Furthermore, the tumor cells contain "eccrine" enzymes, such as phosphorylase and succinic dehydrogenase, and ultrastructurally resemble eccrine ductal cells (Freeman and Winkelmann).

NODULO-ULCERATIVE BASAL CELL EPI-

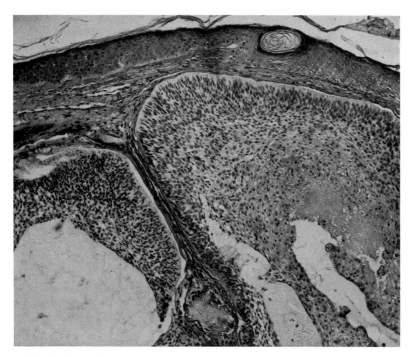

Fig. 26-42. **Cystic basal cell epithelioma.** The cyst on the right side has formed by disintegration of cells with sebaceous differentiation. (×100)

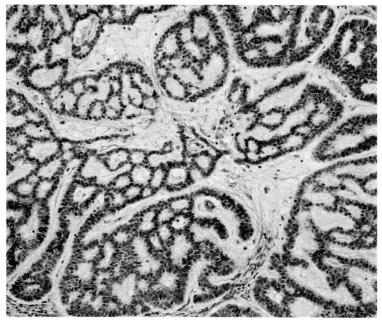

Fig. 26-43. **Adenoid basal cell epithelioma.** The strands of epithelial cells present a lacelike pattern. The stroma has a mucoid appearance. (×200)

THELIOMA. Nodulo-ulcerative basal cell epithelioma, clinically the most common type of basal cell epithelioma, on histologic examination may be solid, keratotic, cystic, or adenoid. The histologic descriptions given above for solid, keratotic, cystic, and adenoid basal cell epithelioma apply in general for the nodulo-ulcerative type of basal cell epithelioma.

PIGMENTED BASAL CELL EPITHELIOMA. Although the presence of melanin can be demonstrated by silver stains in about one third of all basal cell epitheliomas (Becker), large amounts are encountered only rarely. The presence of melanin in basal cell epitheliomas can be explained by the fact that melanocytes are present not only in the surface epidermis but also in the hair matrix and, therefore, also in tumors with pilar differentiation (see p. 29).

Basal cell epitheliomas with large amounts of melanin are shown to contain, on staining with silver, interspersed between the tumor cells, melanocytes that have in their cytoplasm, including their dendrites, numerous melanin granules (Streitmann). This contrasts with normal epidermal melanocytes, in which one finds as a rule only a few, rather small melanin granules (Zelickson et al.). The tumor cells contain very little melanin, but there are many melanophages in the connective tissue stroma surrounding the tumor masses (Sanderson). The reason for the presence of pigment-laden melanocytes and melanophages lies in the inability of the tumor cells to accept more than a small amount of melanin. (For details see under Electron Microscopy, p. 550.)

MORPHEALIKE OR FIBROSING BASAL CELL EPITHELIOMA. In this variant, connective tissue proliferation is much greater than in the other types of basal cell epithelioma. Embedded in a dense fibrous stroma, one observes innumerable groups of closely packed tumor cells arranged in elongated strands (Fig. 26-45) (Caro and Howell). Most of the strands are narrow, often only one layer of cells in thickness, so that they resemble the narrow strands of tumor cells seen in a metastatic, scirrhous carcinoma of the breast. Usually, however, on searching one finds at least a few larger aggregates of tumor cells as well as some strands of tumor cells showing branching. The strands of

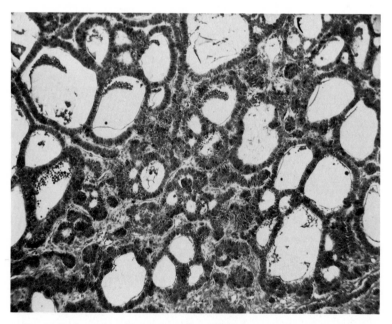

FIG. 26-44. **Adenoid basal cell epithelioma.** The tumor contains lumina surrounded by cells that have the appearance of glandular cells. (×200)

FIG. 26-45. **Morphealike or fibro-sing basal cell epithelioma.** Innumerable small groups of closely packed tumor cells, many of them arranged in elongated strands, are embedded in a dense fibrous stroma. (×100)

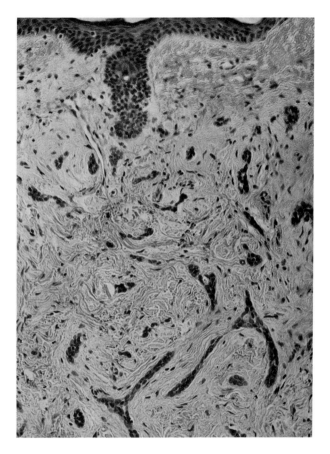

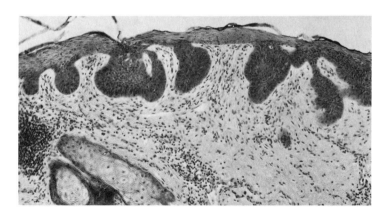

FIG. 26-46. **Superficial basal cell epithelioma.** The tumor shows buds and irregular proliferations of tumor tissue attached to the undersurface of the epidermis. Note the similarity between the tumor buds in this illustration and the primary epithelial germ buds in the embryonal skin shown in Figure 2-1. (×100)

tumor cells often extend deep into the dermis.

SUPERFICIAL BASAL CELL EPITHELIOMA. This type of basal cell epithelioma shows buds and irregular proliferations of tumor tissue attached to the undersurface of the epidermis (Fig. 26-46). The peripheral cell layer of the tumor formations often shows palisading. In most cases there is little penetration into the dermis. The overlying epidermis usually shows atrophy. Fibroblasts, often in a fairly large number, are arranged around the tumor cell proliferations. In addition, a mild to moderate amount of a nonspecific chronic inflammatory infiltrate is present in the upper dermis.

Some superficial basal cell epitheliomas, after having persisted as such for various lengths of time, become invasive basal cell epitheliomas. Since this change may be limited at first to a few areas, representative sections throughout the entire block should

be examined. For a discussion of the question whether superficial basal cell epithelioma is unicentric or multicentric in origin, see Histogenesis.

FIBROEPITHELIOMA. In this tumor long, thin, branching, and anastomosing strands of basal cell epithelioma are embedded in a fibrous stroma (Fig. 26-47) (Pinkus; Hornstein). Many of the strands show connections with the surface epidermis. Here and there small groups of dark-staining cells showing palisade arrangement of the peripheral cell layer may be seen along the epithelial strands, like buds on a branch. Usually, the tumor is quite superficial in location and is well demarcated at its lower border. According to Pinkus, who first described this variant of basal cell epithelioma, it combines features of the intracanalicular fibroadenoma of the breast, the reticulated type of seborrheic keratosis and superficial basal cell epithelioma. A change of fibroepitheli-

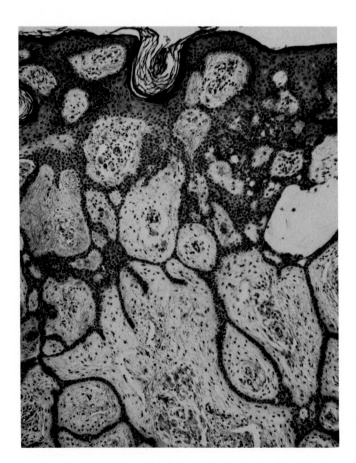

FIG. 26-47. **Fibroepithelioma.** Long, thin, branching, and anastomosing strands of basal cell epithelioma are embedded in a fibrous stroma. Here and there small buds of basophilic cells are seen along the epithelial strands. (×100)

oma into an invasive and ulcerating basal cell epithelioma can occur (Degos and Hewitt).

NEVOID BASAL CELL EPITHELIOMA SYNDROME. The multiple basal cell epitheliomas seen in this syndrome present no distinguishing features from ordinary basal cell epithelioma, even while they are still in their early "nevoid stage," and have not yet become invasive and destructive, as they may later in the "neoplastic stage" (Howell and Caro). All the diverse features of basal cell epithelioma can be seen in the lesions of the nevoid basal cell epithelioma syndrome, such as solid, adenoid, cystic, keratotic, and fibrosing formations (Mason et al.). Usually the histologic distinction from typical trichoepithelioma is easy, since in the latter keratotic cysts are more prominent. However, since some lesions of trichoepithelioma show relatively few horn cysts (see p. 516), a distinction in such cases may be impossible (Jablonska). Clinical data will then be necessary (see p. 517).

Histologic examination of the tiny palmar and plantar pits shows the pits to be present because of the absence of most of the horny layer. The epidermal rete ridges beneath the pits are crowded with basaliomalike cells, i.e., with cells resembling those of basal cell epithelioma. Overlying these rete ridges one finds a markedly thinned granular layer topped by a very thin layer of loose keratin (Howell and Mehregan). In some patients the pits actually show at their base the presence of small basal cell epitheliomas (Holubar et al.). In very rare instances only, a clinically visible basal cell epithelioma develops on the palms or soles in patients with palmar and plantar pits, presumably arising from a pit (Ward; Taylor and Wilkins).

The jaw cysts represent odontogenic cysts. They are lined by keratinizing squamous epithelium and contain laminated keratin. Each jaw cyst may consist of either one large cyst or multiple microcysts (Mason et al.).

LINEAR AND GENERALIZED FOLLICULAR BASAL CELL NEVI. The basal cell epitheliomas in linear basal cell nevus have a variable histologic appearance. The tumor formations may be solid, adenoid, or keratotic, or resemble fibroepithelioma (Carney; Anderson and Best). The walls of the comedones and epidermal cysts show numerous buds of basal cell epithelioma extending into the surrounding dermis (Carney; Bleiberg and Brodkin).

The generalized follicular basal cell nevus shows every hair follicle to be more or less distorted by the proliferation of islands of basal cell epithelioma extending downward either from the surface epidermis or from the outer root sheath. Horn cysts are commonly present in the tumor islands, causing a resemblance to trichoepithelioma (Brown et al.).

INTRAEPIDERMAL EPITHELIOMA OF BORST-JADASSOHN. This condition no longer is regarded as an entity. Rather, it includes all tumors showing within the epidermis well defined islands of cells that differ in their appearance from the surrounding epidermal cells (Mehregan and Pinkus). Originally, the Borst-Jadassohn tumor was thought to be an intraepidermal basal cell epithelioma because the cells composing the intraepidermal islands usually are small and have a deeply basophilic cytoplasm (Sims and Parker). Subsequently, however, it became evident on careful examination that the cells composing the intraepidermal islands possess intercellular bridges (Haber). It is now widely agreed that most of the cases described as intraepidermal epithelioma of Borst-Jadassohn either are seborrheic keratoses in which the small basaloid cells form circumscribed nests (Morales and Hu), or are intraepidermal poromas (Smith and Coburn; Mehregan and Levson). A few cases described as intraepidermal epithelioma in the past can be classified as representing either Bowen's disease or malignant melanoma (Tappeiner and Pfleger). The occurrence of an intraepidermal basal cell epithelioma is unlikely also because the close relationship existing between tumor and stroma in basal cell epithelioma excludes the formation of intraepidermal nests that would lack any contact with the stroma (Holubar and Wolff).

BASAL SQUAMOUS CELL EPITHELIOMA. The existence of basal cell epitheliomas with features of squamous cell carcinoma was postulated by Darier and Ferrand in 1922.

Two types of basal squamous cell epitheliomas were recognized by them: a mixed and an intermediary type. The mixed type was described by them as showing focal keratinization consisting of pearls with a colloidal or parakeratotic center; and the intermediary type as showing within a network of narrow strands two kinds of cells, namely, an outer row of dark-staining basal cells and an inner layer of cells appearing larger, lighter, and better defined than the basal cells and regarded as intermediate in character to basal and squamous cells. Several authors have accepted the existence of basal squamous cell epitheliomas. According to Montgomery (1928), they represent a transition from basal cell to squamous cell carcinoma. He stated that from 15 to 20 per cent of basal cell epitheliomas presented such changes, and that basal squamous cell carcinomas occasionally metastasize. Gertler distinguishes between "basaliomas" and "basal cell carcinomas" and classifies under the latter term about 8 per cent of the basal cell tumors examined by him. Borel, in a recently published study of 35 cases of basosquamous carcinoma, expressed the view that probably a continuum extends from basal cell carcinoma at one extreme to squamous cell carcinoma at the other. Three of his 35 cases of basosquamous carcinoma had caused metastases which in his opinion consisted primarily of poorly differentiated squamous cell carcinoma. Borel's review of the recent English language literature is interesting in that he could find descriptions of only 3 cases of basosquamous carcinoma since Montgomery's publication in 1928.

On the other hand, the existence of basal squamous cell epitheliomas is questioned by many (Welton et al.; Lennox and Wells; Smith and Swerdlow; Gottron; Holmes et al.; Pinkus and Mehregan). It would seem that the entirely different genesis of squamous cell carcinoma, a true anaplastic carcinoma of the epidermis, and of basal cell epithelioma, an appendage tumor composed of immature rather than anaplastic cells, makes the occurrence of transitional forms quite unlikely. It can be assumed that the so-called mixed type of basal squamous cell epithelioma represents a keratotic basal cell epithelioma (see Fig. 26-40), and the intermediate type, a basal cell epithelioma with

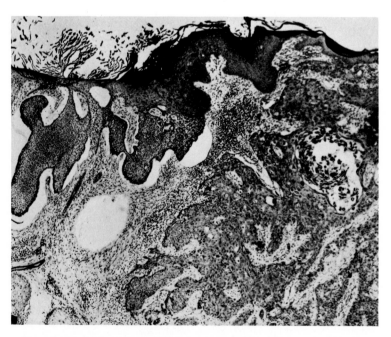

FIG. 26-48. **Mixed carcinoma.** A basal cell epithelioma (*left*) and a squamous cell carcinoma (*right*) lie side by side. (×50)

differentiation into two types of cells (see Fig. 26-39).

MIXED CARCINOMA. These tumors show a squamous cell carcinoma contiguous to a basal cell epithelioma (Fig. 26-48). It is likely that in most instances the squamous cell carcinoma develops secondary to the basal cell epithelioma. Like other chronic ulcerative lesions, such as burns and stasis ulcers, basal cell epithelioma may stimulate the development of a squamous cell carcinoma. Before making a diagnosis of mixed carcinoma, however, one must rule out the possibility of pseudocarcinomatous hyperplasia occurring in a basal cell epithelioma (see p. 481).

Histogenesis. Krompecher, the original describer of basal cell epithelioma, stated in 1903 that he regarded this tumor as a carcinoma of the basal cells of the epidermis and that those tumors that showed a tendency to gland formation imitated the potential of the basal cells to form the cutaneous glands. Krompecher's view is still supported by some (Montgomery, 1967; Teloh and Wheelock). According to Geschickter, only those basal cells with a potential to develop into glandular cells gave rise to basal cell epithelioma. He suggested the designation *appendage cell carcinoma*. Mallory held the opinion that basal cell epitheliomas were carcinomas of hair matrix cells. Foot, in 1947, expressed the view that basal cell epitheliomas were carcinomas that developed from distorted primordia of dermal adnexa rather than from ordinary epidermal basal cells. He stated that the tumors imitated the embryonal development of any one type or of all three types of adnexal primordia, i.e., hair, sebaceous gland, and sweat gland.

The first author to express doubts that basal cell epitheliomas were carcinomas was Adamson; in 1914 he stated that in his opinion basal cell epitheliomas were nevoid tumors originating "from latent embryonic foci aroused from their dormant state at a later period in life." He believed that the latent embryonic foci usually were embryonic pilosebaceous follicles but occasionally were embryonic sweat ducts. Several other authors have since reached similar conclusions, among them Wallace and Halpert who regarded basal cell epitheliomas as benign tumors either of the hair matrix or of the hair anlage and proposed the term *trichoma* for them.

In 1948 one of the authors (W.F.L.) expressed his belief that basal cell epitheliomas are not carcinomas and are not derived from basal cells, but are nevoid tumors, or hamartomas, derived from primary epithelial germ cells. In other words, basal cell epitheliomas originate from incompletely differentiated, immature cells and not from differentiated, anaplastic cells. They thus represent the least differentiated of the appendage tumors. (See Classification and Histogenesis of the Benign Appendage Tumors, p. 498; see also Table 26-1, p. 499.)

Originally, it was assumed, analogous to Adamson's view, that the primary epithelial germ cells giving rise to basal cell epithelioma were in all instances embryonic cells that had lain dormant until the onset of neoplasia. Even though this view applies to the linear and follicular basal cell nevi (see p. 538), it is likely that, as Pinkus has suggested, basal cell epitheliomas occurring in later life arise not from dormant embryonic primary epithelial germ cells but from pluripotential cells that form continuously during life and, like embryonic primary epithelial germ cells, have the potentiality of forming hair, sebaceous glands, and apocrine glands. The fact that basal cell epitheliomas may arise in sun-exposed areas and in areas of radiodermatitis supports the view expressed by Pinkus.

Pilar Differentiation. The differentiation in basal cell epithelioma is predominantly toward pilar keratin. The presence of citrulline in keratinized structures indicates the hair matrix origin of such keratin since epidermal keratin contains no citrulline (Holmes et al.). However, not all keratin of hair matrix origin contains citrulline. The hair cortex and hair cuticle do not contain it, whereas the medulla of the hair and the inner root sheath do. Also the outer root sheath, being of epidermal origin, is free of citrulline. Thus, citrulline is regularly present in pilomatrixoma (see p. 518), and is absent in pilar cysts and pilar tumors which are composed of outer root sheath cells (see p. 522). Keratotic basal cell epitheliomas contain both citrulline-positive and citrulline-negative keratin, reflecting the different lines of differentiation inherent in the hair matrix (Holmes et al.).

Eccrine Differentiation. Basal cell epitheliomas can arise not only from immature pluripotential cells differentiating toward primary epithelial germ structures but also from those differentiating toward eccrine glands. The occurrence of eccrine epitheliomas bears this out (see p. 542). The rarity of basal cell epitheliomas on the palms and soles would imply that cells with the potential to differentiate toward eccrine glands rarely participate in the formation of basal cell epithelioma. However, there is another possible explanation for the rare involvement of the palms and soles. The fact that the palmar and plantar pits of the nevoid basal cell epithelioma very rarely show a full-fledged basal cell epithelioma suggests that the palms and soles do not possess the stromal factor necessary for the formation of appendage tumor (Covo).

Stromal Factor. In addition to the rarity of basal cell epithelioma on the palms and soles, there is experimental evidence for the importance of the stromal factor in the development of basal cell epithelioma: Autotransplants of basal cell epitheliomas survive only when they include connective tissue stroma (Van Scott and Reinertson).

Lack of Autonomy. Basal cell epitheliomas when transplanted to the anterior chamber of the rabbit's eye together with their connective tissue stroma fail to grow, in contrast to squamous cell carcinoma (Gerstein). This observation suggests a lack of autonomy of the cells of basal cell epithelioma. Since autonomy of the tumor cell is a prerequisite for the formation of metastases and represents a characteristic feature of malignant tumors (Greene), the absence of autonomy in basal cell epithelioma indicates that it is not a true carcinoma.

Site of Origin. The usual site of origin of basal cell epithelioma is the surface epidermis (Hundeiker and Berger). Occasionally, however, it may originate from the outer root sheath of a hair follicle (Zackheim; Brown et al.).

Of particular interest is the manner of growth in the superficial basal cell epithelioma. Routine sectioning carried out perpendicular to the skin surface shows seemingly independent nests of basal cell epithelioma, suggestive at times of the growth of primary epithelial germs in the embryonic skin (see Fig. 2-1). Consequently, it had been widely assumed that the peripheral extension in superficial basal cell epithelioma was on the basis of a "multicentric" growth characterized by the formation of new buds of tumor tissue at the periphery. Madsen, however, on the basis of his findings in serial sections and wax reconstructions of superficial basal cell epitheliomas described in several publications (1941, 1955, 1965), has favored a "unicentric" origin. Madsen was able to show that the tumor strands are continuous but are attached to the undersurface of the epidermis, analogous to garlands, only at intervals. Madsen found not only in his wax reconstructions but also in sections cut parallel to the surface of the skin that the individual tumor islands were interconnected. Oberste-Lehn, using a technic of separating the epidermis from the dermis by maceration, could not find such interconnections; but it seems very likely, as Madsen has pointed out, that the interconnections had ruptured as a result of the maceration. It would seem that Madsen's "unicentric" concept serves best to explain the slow

peripheral extension that is clinically apparent in most superficial basal cell epitheliomas.

Electron Microscopy. The predominant cell in undifferentiated basal cell epithelioma is characterized by a large nucleus, poorly developed desmosomes, and rather sparse tonofilaments. Thus, the tumor cells differ from normal epidermal basal cells. They resemble the cells of the undifferentiated hair matrix (Zelickson), or the immature basal cells of the embryonic epidermis, particularly those of the primary epithelial germ (Lever and Hashimoto). In addition to the prevalent large, light cells, a few cells that are smaller, darker, and more irregularly shaped can be found (Lever and Hashimoto; Reidbord et al.). The darkness of these cells is due to the abundance of ribonucleoprotein particles in their cytoplasm.

Keratinization is commonly observed in basal cell epithelioma by electron microscopy. In addition to well developed desmosomes and many thick bundles of tonofilaments, dense clumps of homogeneous, dyskeratotic material are present in many keratinizing cells (E.M. No. 40). A small number of keratohyaline granules are often seen. They probably represent trichohyaline granules which occur in the process of keratinization of the inner root sheath and of its cuticle (Lever and Hashimoto).

Some basal cell epitheliomas may show areas of adenoid differentiation in which cells are grouped around glandlike lumina. Such cells may show pronounced infolding of the plasma membrane at their lateral borders, as seen normally in eccrine ductal cells (Reidbord et al.) (see p. 24).

In pigmented basal cell epitheliomas most of the melanin is found not within the tumor cells but within melanocytes of the tumor and in melanophages located in the connective tissue stroma. The reason for this distribution of melanin is the following: Although numerous melanosomes are present in the dendrites of the melanocytes, in general the tumor cells do not phagocytize the melanin-containing dendrites, resulting in a blockage of the transfer of melanin from melanocytes to the tumor cells (Zelickson, 1967; Miki). A similar situation of a blocked transfer from melanocytes to tumor cells is encountered in some pigmented seborrheic keratoses referred to as melanoacanthoma (see p. 457). Still, in occasional instances some transfer of melanosomes to the tumor cells takes place. The tumor cells then contain melanosomes, located largely as melanosome complexes within lysosomes (E.M. No. 41) (Lever and Hashimoto).

Differential Diagnosis. Differentiation of basal cell epithelioma from squamous cell carcinoma can be difficult at times, so difficult that some authors believe that intermediate forms (basal squamous cell epithelioma) occur. However, as a rule differentiation is fairly easy. One of the best points of differentiation is that most cells of basal cell epithelioma stain deeply basophilic, whereas most cells of squamous cell carcinoma, at least in Grades 1 and 2, have an eosinophilic tint due to partial keratinization. In squamous cell carcinomas, Grades 3 and 4, the cells, because of the absence of keratinization, may appear basophilic. However, they then differ from basal cell epithelioma by showing much greater atypicality of their nuclei and mitotic figures. It is important to remember that keratinization is not a prerogative of squamous cell carcinoma; it occurs also in basal cell epithelioma with differentiation toward hair structures. (See Keratotic Basal Cell Epithelioma, p. 541). Keratinization in basal cell epitheliomas may be partial and then result in parakeratotic bands and whorls, or it may be complete and result in horn cysts. The keratinization seen in the horn cysts differs from that seen in the horn pearls of squamous cell carcinomas by being abrupt and complete, rather than gradual and incomplete. The fairly common presence in basal cell epithelioma of areas of retraction of the tumor cell masses from the surrounding connective tissue (see p. 539) also aids in differentiating it from squamous cell carcinoma, since such areas of retraction are rarely found in the latter.

The differential diagnosis of basal cell epithelioma from trichoepithelioma already has been discussed (see p. 516).

CARCINOMA OF SEBACEOUS GLANDS

Carcinomas of the sebaceous glands are quite rare. They occur most frequently on the eyelids, where they originate from meibomian glands, which are modified sebaceous glands (Hartz). However, they may occur elsewhere on the skin. No characteristic clinical picture is associated with se-

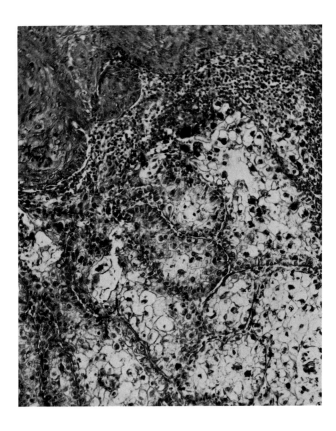

FIG. 26-49. **Carcinoma of sebaceous glands.** Irregular lobular formations are composed of sebaceous and undifferentiated cells showing considerable variation in the shape and size of their nuclei. The undifferentiated cells differ from the undifferentiated cells of sebaceous epithelioma by showing greater atypicality and an eosinophilic rather than a basophilic cytoplasm. (×200)

baceous carcinoma. As a rule, the lesion consists of an ulcerated nodule (Beach and Severance). Widespread metastases are common in cases of sebaceous carcinoma originating on the eyelids. On the other hand, sebaceous carcinomas arising elsewhere on the skin cause metastases only rarely (Rulon and Helwig). Also, the sebaceous carcinomas that may be found among the multiple sebaceous neoplasms occurring in association with multiple visceral carcinomas do not tend to metastasize (Leonard and Deaton) (see p. 505).

Histopathology. One observes irregular lobular formations with great variation in the size of the lobules (Fig. 26-49). Although many cells are undifferentiated, distinct sebaceous cells showing a foamy cytoplasm are present in the center of most lobules. Many undifferentiated cells and sebaceous cells appear atypical, showing considerable variation in the shape and the size of their nuclei. Also, many of the undifferentiated cells have an eosinophilic cytoplasm and, when fat stains are used on frozen sections, they contain fine lipid globules (Justi). Some of the larger lobules show areas composed of atypical keratinizing cells, as in squamous cell carcinoma (Urban and Winkelmann).

Differential Diagnosis. Sebaceous carcinomas must be differentiated from sebaceous epithelioma, which represents a basal cell epithelioma with considerable differentiation of the cells toward sebaceous gland cells (p. 523). Sebaceous carcinoma, in contrast with sebaceous epithelioma, shows no areas of basal cell epithelioma. The undifferentiated cells of sebaceous carcinoma differ from those of basal cell epithelioma by showing greater atypicality and a more eosinophilic cytoplasm (Beach and Severance).

CARCINOMA OF ECCRINE SWEAT GLANDS

Carcinoma of the eccrine glands has a high incidence of metastatic spread: of 39 cases reviewed in 1967 by Miller 28 had metastases. These carcinomas do not possess a characteristic clinical appearance or location. Although they may arise on the palms (Grant; Fresen; Hashimoto and Lever) or on the soles (Teloh et al.), more commonly they arise elsewhere.

Histopathology. It is difficult to differentiate carcinoma of the eccrine glands from metastatic adenocarcinoma. Therefore, this possibility always should be given serious consideration before deciding on a diagnosis of eccrine sweat gland carcinoma. So-called eccrine enzymes, such as amylophosphorylase and succinic dehydrogenase, may be present in moderate amounts and aid in the recognition of the tumors as eccrine (Hashimoto and Lever; Orbaneja et al.).

Several histologic types of eccrine sweat gland carcinoma are recognized. In addition to a "classical" type, there is a mucinous adenocarcinoma of eccrine glands (Mendoza and Helwig), and an undifferentiated type, referred to as trabecular carcinoma of the skin (Toker). It should also be pointed out here that the malignant eccrine poroma (see p. 532) as well as the malignant clear cell hidradenoma (see p. 530) are variants of eccrine sweat gland carcinoma, both characterized by the presence of significant amounts of glycogen in the tumor cells.

In the "classical" type of eccrine sweat gland carcinoma the histologic configuration varies from fairly well differentiated tubular structures in some areas to anaplastic carcinoma in other areas, not recognizable by itself as representing eccrine sweat gland structures (Teloh et al.). The glandular structures may be either single-layered (Fresen) or double-layered (Kay and Hall). The tubular structures usually show no branching and their lumina generally are small (Grant; Fresen). Occasionally, some tubular structures contain lumina lined with an eosinophilic PAS-positive, diastase-resistant cuticle analogous to eccrine ducts (Orbaneja et al.). Foci of squamous metaplasia may be present (Teloh et al.). The tumor cells frequently contain glycogen (Hashimoto and Lever; Dave) and in some instances also PAS-positive, diastase-resistant granules of neutral mucopolysaccharides (Miller).

In the mucinous adenocarcinoma of eccrine glands, a fairly benign variant with only one instance of regional lymph node metastasis among 14 cases reported by Mendoza and Helwig, the tumor is divided into numerous compartments by strands of fibrous tissue. In each compartment abundant amounts of mucinous material surround nests of moderately anaplastic epithelial cells some of which show a tubular lumen. Occasionally, also cystic spaces are present (Grossman and Izuno). The mucin is of the epithelial type. It consists of both neutral mucopolysaccharides and hyaluronidase-resistant, nonsulfated acid mucopolysaccharides, and thus it represents a sialomucin (Mendoza and Helwig; Grossman and Izuno).

In the undifferentiated type of sweat gland carcinoma, referred to as trabecular carcinoma of the skin (Toker), one finds solid cords of tumor cells with large, vesicular nuclei in the dermis showing no contact with the epidermis. Although distinct lumina are absent it can be assumed that the tumor is an eccrine sweat gland carcinoma, provided that the other possibility, that of metastatic carcinoma, has been excluded on the basis of clinical data.

CARCINOMA OF APOCRINE GLANDS

Carcinomas of apocrine glands have been described only rarely: according to Baes and Suurmond a total of 18 cases up to 1970. Their occurrence has been reported mainly in the axillae (Furtell et al.), but occasionally also in other areas endowed with apocrine glands, such as the nipples and the vulva, and also the eyelids and the external auditory meatus (Neldner), where Moll's glands and the ceruminal glands, respectively, are found as modified apocrine glands. The question naturally arises in cases described as apocrine carcinomas of the axillae or the nipples whether or not in reality they originated from aberrant mammary glands, which represent modified apocrine glands. Whereas some cases of carcinoma of apocrine glands show only local invasiveness without metastases (Neldner), others have widespread metastases (Baes and Suurmond).

Histopathology. The histologic picture is

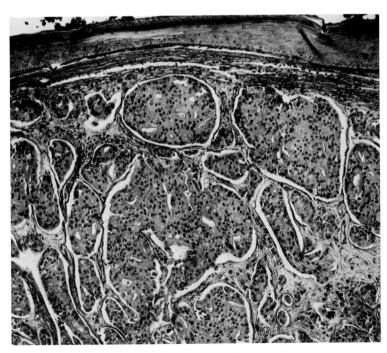

FIG. 26-50. **Apocrine carcinoma of vulva.** The tumor consists of atypical glandular cells with eosinophilic cytoplasm and active decapitation secretion. (×100)

that of an adenocarcinoma, with cells growing in sheets and cords and showing more or less well developed glandular lumina (Fig. 26-50). The lumina may be cystic and show branching. The cytoplasm of the tumor cells is strongly eosinophilic. Evidence of decapitation secretion is present in some instances (Furtell et al.), and absent in others (Baes and Suurmond). The cytoplasm of the tumor cells often also contains iron-positive granules (Kipkie and Haust) or PAS-positive, diastase-resistant granules (Elliot and Ramsay), but not in all cases. Actually, the best proof of an apocrine genesis lies in the histochemical demonstration of a strong activity of "apocrine" enzymes, such as acid phosphatase and nonspecific esterase, and of a low activity of "eccrine" enzymes, such as succinic dehydrogenase (Baes and Suurmond).

Extramammary Paget's disease, which in many instances represents an apocrine carcinoma, has already been discussed (see p. 490).

BIBLIOGRAPHY

Classification of the Appendage Tumors

Albrecht, E.: Über Hamartome. Verh. Deutsch. Ges. Path., *7*:153, 1904.

Becker, S. W.: Benign epidermal neoplasms. Arch. Derm. Syph., *26*:838, 1932.

Hashimoto, K., and Lever, W. F.: Appendage Tumors of the Skin. Springfield, Ill., Charles C Thomas, 1968.

Jadassohn, J.: Die benignen Epitheliome. Arch. f. Derm. u. Syph., *117*:577, 705, 833, 1913-1914.

Lever, W. F.: Pathogenesis of benign tumors of cutaneous appendages and of basal cell epithelioma. Arch. Derm. Syph., *57*:679, 1948.

Pinkus, H.: Premalignant fibroepithelial tumors of the skin. Arch. Derm. Syph., *67*:598, 1953.

Wechsler, H. L., and Fisher, E. R.: A combined polymorphic and adnexal tumor in nevus unius lateris. Dermatologica, *130*:158, 1964.

Nevus Sebaceus

Bourlond, A., Demeersman, E., and Fierens, F.: Polymorphisme clinique et histologique du naevus sébacé. Arch. belg. derm. syph., *25*:337, 1969.

Feuerstein, R., and Mims, L.: Linear nevus sebaceus with convulsions and mental retardation. Am. J. Dis., Child., *104*:675, 1962.

Haber, H.: Verrucous naevi. Trans. St. John's Hosp. Derm. Soc., *34*:20, 1955.

Hornstein, O. P., and Knickenberg, M.: Zur Kenntnis des Schimmelpenning-Feuerstein-Mims-Syndroms. Arch. derm. Forsch., *250*:33, 1974.,

Lantis, S., Leyden, J., Thew, M., and Heaton, C.: Nevus sebaceus of Jadassohn. Part of a new neurocutaneous syndrome. Arch. Derm., *98*:117, 1968.

Lentz, C. L., Altman, J., and Mopper, C.: Nevus sebaceus of Jadassohn. Arch. Derm., *97*:294, 1968.

Lever, W. F.: Pathogenesis of benign tumors of cutaneous appendages and of basal cell epithelioma. Arch. Derm. Syph., *57*:679, 1948.

Marden, P., and Venters, H.: A new neurocutaneous syndrome. Am. J. Dis. Child., *112*:79, 1966.

Mehregan, A. H., and Pinkus, H.: Life history of organoid nevi. Arch. Derm., *91*:574, 1965.

Michalowski, R.: Naevus sébacé de Jadassohn—un état précancéreux. Dermatologica, *124*:326, 1962.

Nikolowski, W.: Beitrag zur Klinik und Histologie der Talgdrüsen-Naevi und Carcinoma und deren Beziehungen zum sog. Basalzellen-Carcinom. Arch. f. Derm. u. Syph., *193*:340, 1951.

Schirren, C. G., and Pfirstinger, H.: Zur Entwicklung von Plattenepithelcarcinomen auf dem Boden des Naevus sebaceus (Jadassohn). Hautarzt, *14*:397, 1963.

Solomon, L. M., Fretzin, D. F., and Dewald, R. L.: The epidermal nevus syndrome. Arch. Derm., *97*:273, 1968.

Steigleder, G., and Cortes, A. C.: Verhalten der Talgdrüsen im Talgdrüsennaevus während des Kindesalters. Arch. klin. exp. Derm., *239*:323, 1971.

Wauschkuhn, J., and Rohde, B.: Systematisierte Talgdrüsen-, Pigment-, und epitheliale Naevi mit neurologischer Symptomatik; Feuerstein-Mimssches neuroektodermales Syndrom. Hautarzt, *22*:10, 1971.

Wilson Jones, E., and Heyl, T.: Naevus sebaceus. Brit. J. Derm., *82*:99, 1970.

Sebaceous Hyperplasia

Braun-Falco, O., and Thianprasit, M.: Über die circumscripte senile Talgdrüsenhyperplasie. Arch. klin. exp. Derm., *221*:207, 1965.

Gilman, R. L.: Adenomatoid sebaceous tumors with particular reference to adenomatoid hyperplasia. Arch. Derm. Syph., *35*:633, 1937.

Ramos e Silva, J., and Portugal, H.: Sur l'adénome sébacé sénile. Ann. derm. syph., *80*:121, 1953.

Fordyce's Condition

Chambers, S. O.: The structure of Fordyce's disease as demonstrated by wax reconstruction. Arch. Derm. Syph., *18*:666, 1928.

Miles, A. E. W.: Sebaceous glands in the lip and cheek mucosa of man. Brit. Dent. J., *105*:235, 1958.

Apocrine Nevus

Civatte, J., Tsoitis, G., and Préaux, J.: Le naevus apocrine. Ann. derm. syph., *101*: 251, 1974.

Eccrine Nevus

Goldstein, N.: Ephidrosis (local hyperhidrosis), nevus sudoriferus. Arch. Derm., *96*:67, 1967.

Herzberg, J. J.: Ekkrines Syringocystadenom. Arch. klin. exp. Derm., *214*:600, 1962.

Hyman, A. B., Harris, H., and Brownstein, M. H.: Eccrine angiomatous hamartoma. N.Y. State J. Med., *68*:2803, 1968.

Zeller, D. J., and Goldman, R. L.: Eccrine-pilar angiomatous hamartoma. Dermatologica, *143*: 100, 1971.

Trichofolliculoma

Gray, H. R., and Helwig, E. B.: Trichofolliculoma. Arch. Derm., *86*:619, 1962.

Hyman, A. B., and Clayman, S. J.: Hair follicle nevus. Arch. Derm., *75*:678, 1957.

Kligman, A. M., and Pinkus, H.: The histogenesis of nevoid tumors of the skin. Arch. Derm., *81*:922, 1960.

Pinkus, H., and Sutton, R. L., Jr.: Trichofolliculoma. Arch. Derm., *91*:46, 1965.

Sanderson, K. V.: Hair follicle naevus. Trans. St. John's Hosp. Derm. Soc., *47*:154, 1961.

Sebaceous Adenoma

Essenhigh, D. M., Jones, D., and Rack, J. H.: A sebaceous adenoma. Brit. J. Derm., *76*:330, 1964.

Groterjahn, A.: Die Talgdrüsengeschwülste mit besonderer Berücksichtigung des Talgdrüsenadenoms. Hautarzt, *1*:319, 1950.

Leonard, D. D., and Deaton, W. R., Jr.: Multiple sebaceous gland tumors and visceral carcinomas. Arch. Derm., *110*:917, 1974.

Lever, W. F.: Sebaceous adenoma, review of the literature and report of a case. Arch. Derm. Syph., *57*:102, 1948.

Rulon, D. B., and Helwig, E. B.: Multiple sebaceous neoplasms of the skin. An association with multiple visceral carcinomas, especially of the colon. Am. J. Clin. Path., *60*: 745, 1973.

Sciallis, G. F., and Winkelmann, R. K.: Multiple sebaceous adenomas and gastrointestinal carcinoma. Arch. Derm., *110*:913, 1974.

Woolhandler, H. W., and Becker, W. S.: Adenoma of sebaceous glands (adenoma sebaceum). Arch. Derm. Syph., *45*:734, 1942.

Apocrine Hidrocystoma

Ahmed, A., and Jones, A. W.: Apocrine cystadenoma. Brit. J. Derm., *81*:899, 1969.

Gross, B. G.: The fine structure of apocrine hidrocystoma. Arch. Derm., *92*:706, 1965.

Mehregan, A. H.: Apocrine cystadenoma. Arch. Derm., *90*:274, 1964.

Hidradenoma Papilliferum

Hashimoto, K.: Hidradenoma papilliferum. An electron microscopic study. Acta dermatoven., *53*:22, 1973.

Meeker, J. H., Neubecker, R. D., and Helwig, E. B.: Hidradenoma papilliferum. Am. J. Clin. Path., *37*:182, 1962.

Shenoy, Y. M. V.: Malignant perianal papillary hidradenoma. Arch. Derm., *83*:965, 1961.

Tappeiner, J., and Wolff, K.: Hidradenoma papilliferum. Eine enzymhistochemische und elektronenmikroskopische Studie. Hautarzt, *19*:101, 1968.

Syringocystadenoma Papilliferum

Appel, B.: Nevus syringadenomatosus papilliferus. Arch. Derm. Syph., *61*:311, 1950.

Grund, J. L.: Syringocystadenoma papilliferum and nevus sebaceus (Jadassohn) occurring as a single tumor. Arch. Derm. Syph., *65*:340, 1952.

Hashimoto, K.: Syringocystadenoma papilliferum. An electron microscopic study. Arch. derm. Forsch., *245*:353, 1972.

Helwig, E. B., and Hackney, V. C.: Syringadenoma papilliferum. Arch. Derm., *71*:361, 1955.

Krinitz, K.: Naevus syringocystadenomatosus papilliferus in linearer Anordnung. Hautarzt, *17*:260, 1966.

Landry, M., and Winkelmann, R. K.: An unusual tubular apocrine adenoma: histochemical and ultrastructural study. Arch. Derm., *105*:869, 1972.

Lever, W. F.: Pathogenesis of benign tumors of cutaneous appendages and of basal cell epithelioma. Arch. Derm. Syph., *57*:679, 1948.

Pinkus, H.: Life history of naevus syringadenomatosus papilliferus. Arch. Derm. Syph., *69*: 305, 1954.

Pinkus, H., and Mehregan, A. H.: A Guide to Dermatohistopathology. p. 435. New York, Appleton-Century-Crofts, 1969.

Eccrine Hidrocystoma

Dostrovsky, A., and Sagher, F.: Experimentally induced disappearance and reappearance of lesions of hidrocystoma. J. Invest. Derm., 5:167, 1942.

Hashimoto, K., and Lever, W. F.: Appendage Tumors of the Skin. p. 19. Springfield, Ill., Charles C Thomas, 1968.

Herzberg, J. J.: Ekkrines Syringocystadenom. Arch. klin. exp. Derm., 214:600, 1962.

Smith, J. D., and Chernosky, M. E.: Hidrocystomas. Arch. Derm., 108:676, 1973.

Syringoma

Hashimoto, K., Gross, B. G., and Lever, W. F.: Syringoma: Histochemical and electron microscopic studies. J. Invest. Derm., 46:150, 1966.

Hashimoto, K., DiBella, R. J., Borsuk, G. M., and Lever, W. F.: Eruptive hidradenoma and syringoma. Arch. Derm., 96:500, 1967.

Hashimoto, K., and Lever, W. F.: Histogenesis of skin appendage tumors. Arch. Derm., 100:356, 1969.

Headington, J. T., Koski, J., and Murphy, P. J.: Clear cell glycogenosis in multiple syringomas. Arch. Derm., 106:353, 1972.

Lever, W. F.: Pathogenesis of benign tumors of cutaneous appendages and of basal cell epithelioma. Arch. Derm. Syph., 57:679, 1948.

Mustakallio, K. K.: Succinic dehydrogenase activity of syringomas. Acta dermatoven., 39:318, 1959.

Winkelmann, R. K., and Muller, S. A.: Sweat gland tumors. Arch. Derm., 89:827, 1964.

Trichoepithelioma

Gaul, L. E.: Heredity of multiple benign cystic epithelioma. Arch. Derm. Syph., 68:517, 1953.

Gray, H. R., and Helwig, E. B.: Epithelioma adenoides cysticum and solitary trichoepithelioma. Arch. Derm., 87:102, 1963.

Kopf, A. W.: The distribution of alkaline phosphatase in normal and pathologic human skin. Arch. Derm., 75:1, 1957.

Lever, W. F.: Pathogenesis of benign tumors of cutaneous appendages and of basal cell epithelioma. Arch. Derm. Syph., 57:679, 1948.

Müller-Hess, S., and Delacrétaz, J.: Trichoepitheliom mit Strukturen eines apokrinen Adenoms. Dermatologica, 146:170, 1973.

Nikolowski, W.: "Tricho-adenom" (Organoides Follikel-Hamartom). Arch. klin. exp. Derm., 207:34, 1958.

Traenkle, H. L.: Epithelioma adenoides cysticum, trichoepithelioma and basal cell cancer. Arch. Derm. Syph., 42:822, 1940 (review).

Zeligman, I.: Solitary trichoepithelioma. Arch. Derm., 82:35, 1960.

Pilomatrixoma (Calcifying Epithelioma)

Forbis, R., Jr., and Helwig, E. B.: Pilomatrixoma (calcifying epithelioma). Arch. Derm., 83:606, 1961.

Geiser, J. D.: L'épithélioma calcifié de Malherbe. Ann. derm. syph., 86:383, 1959.

Hashimoto, K., and Lever, W. F.: Histogenesis of skin appendage tumors. Arch. Derm., 100:356, 1969.

Hashimoto, K., Nelson, R. G., and Lever, W. F.: Calcifying epithelioma of Malherbe. Histochemical and electron microscopic studies. J. Invest. Derm., 46:391, 1966.

Holmes, E. J.: A histochemical test for citrulline. Adaptation of the carbamidodiacetyl reaction to histologic sections with positive results in pilomatrixomas (calcifying epitheliomas). J. Histochem. Cytochem., 16:136, 1968.

Lever, W. F., and Griesemer, R. D.: Calcifying epithelioma of Malherbe. Arch. Derm. Syph., 59:506, 1949.

Lever, W. F., and Hashimoto, K.: Die Histogenese einiger Hautanhangstumoren im Lichte histochemischer und elektronenmikroskopischer Befunde. Hautarzt, 17:161, 1966.

Malherbe, A., and Chenantais, J.: Note sur l'épithéliome calcifié des glandes sebacées. Bul. Soc. anat. Paris, 5:169, 1880.

McGavran, M. H.: Ultrastructure of pilomatrixoma (calcifying epithelioma). Cancer, 18:1445, 1965.

Moehlenbeck, F.: Pilomatrixoma (calcifying epithelioma). Arch. Derm., 108:532, 1973.

Peterson, W. C., Jr., and Hult, A. M.: Calcifying epithelioma of Malherbe. Arch. Derm., 90:404, 1964.

Turhan, B., and Krainer, L.: Bemerkungen über die sogenannten verkalkenden Epitheliome der Haut und ihre Genese. Dermatologica, 85:73, 1942.

Wiedersberg, H.: Das Epithelioma calcificans Malherbe. Derm. Monatsschr., 157:867, 1971.

Pilar Tumor of the Scalp

Dabska, M.: Giant hair matrix tumor. Cancer, 28:701, 1971.

Holmes, E. J.: Tumors of lower hair sheath. The common histogenesis of certain so-called "sebaceous cysts," adenomas, and "sebaceous carcinomas." Cancer, 21:234, 1968.

Korting, G. W., and Hoede, N.: Zum sogenannten "Pilar Tumor of the Scalp." Arch. klin. exp. Derm., 234:409, 1969.

Pinkus, H.: "Sebaceous cysts" are trichilemmal cysts. Arch. Derm., 99:544, 1969.

Reed, R. J., and Lamar, L. M.: Invasive hair matrix tumors of the scalp. Arch. Derm., 94:310, 1966.

Wilson Jones, E.: Proliferating epidermoid cysts. Arch. Derm., 94:11, 1966.

Trichilemmoma

Brownstein, M. H., and Shapiro, L.: Trichilemmoma. Arch. Derm., *107*:866, 1973.

Headington, J. T., and French, A. J.: Primary neoplasms of the hair follicle. Arch. Derm., *86*:430, 1962.

Ingrish, F. M., and Reed, R. J.: Tricholemmoma. Dermat. Internat., *7*:182, 1968.

Johnson, W. C., and Hookerman, B. T.: Basal cell hamartoma with follicular differentiation. Arch. Derm., *105*:105, 1972.

Mehregan, A. H.: Tumor of follicular infundibulum. Dermatologica, *142*:177, 1971.

Mehregan, A. H., and Butler, J. D.: A tumor of follicular infundibulum. Arch. Derm., *83*: 924, 1961.

Sebaceous Epithelioma

McMullan, F. H.: Sebaceous epithelioma. Arch. Derm. Syph., *71*:725, 1955.

Mehregan, A. H., and Pinkus, H.: Life history of organoid nevi. Arch. Derm., *91*:574, 1965.

Raab, W.: Talgdrüsenepitheliom. Arch. klin. exp. Derm., *216*:325, 1963.

Urban, F. H., and Winkelmann, R. K.: Sebaceous malignancy. Arch. Derm., *84*:63, 1961.

Wilson Jones, E., and Heyl, T.: Naevus sebaceus. Brit. J. Derm., *82*:99, 1970.

Zackheim, H. S.: The sebaceous epithelioma. Arch. Derm., *89*:711, 1964.

Cylindroma

Baden, H.: Cylindromatosis simulating neurofibromatosis. New Eng. J. Med., *267*:296, 1962.

Bandmann, H. J., Hamburger, D., and Romiti, N.: Bericht zur Brooke-Spieglerschen Phakomatose. Hautarzt, *16*:450, 1965.

Crain, R. C., and Helwig, E. B.: Dermal cylindroma (dermal eccrine cylindroma). Am. J. Clin. Path., *35*:504, 1961.

Fusaro, R. M., and Goltz, R. W.: Histochemically demonstrable carbohydrates of appendageal tumors of the skin. J. Invest. Derm., *38*:137, 1962.

Gertler, W.: Spieglersche Tumoren mit Übergang in metastasierendes Spinaliom. Derm. Wschr., *128*:673, 1953.

Guggenheim, W., and Schnyder, U. W.: Zur Nosologie der Spiegler-Brooke'schen Tumoren. Dermatologica, *122*:274, 1961.

Hashimoto, K., and Lever, W. F.: Histogenesis of skin appendage tumors. Arch. Derm., *100*: 356, 1969.

Holubar, K., and Wolff, K.: Zur Histogenese des Cylindroms. Eine enzym-histochemische Studie. Arch. klin. exp. Derm., *229*:205, 1967.

Kleine-Natrop, H. E.: Gleichzeitige Generalisation gutartiger Basaliome der beiden Typen Spiegler und Brooke. Arch. klin. exp. Derm., *209*:45, 1959.

Korting, G. W., Hoede, N., and Gebhardt, R.: Kurzer Bericht über einen maligne entarteten Spiegler-Tumor. Derm. Monatsschr., *156*: 141, 1970.

Lausecker, H.: Beitrag zu den Naevo-epitheliomen. Arch. f. Derm. u. Syph., *194*:639, 1952.

Luger, A.: Das Cylindrom der Haut und seine maligne Degeneration. Arch. f. Derm. u. Syph., *188*:155, 1949.

Lyon, J. B., and Rouillard, L. M.: Malignant degeneration of turban tumour of scalp. Trans. St. John's Hosp. Derm. Soc., *46*:74, 1961.

Zontschew, P.: Cylindroma capitis mit maligner Entartung. Zentralbl. Chir., *86*:1875, 1961.

Clear Cell Hidradenoma

Berger, H.: Kasuistischer Beitrag zur Kenntnis myoepithelialer Schweissdrüsentumoren. Zbl. allg. Path., *103*:477, 1962.

Efskind, J., and Eker, R.: Myo-epitheliomas of the skin. Acta dermatoven., *34*:279, 1954.

Hashimoto, K., DiBella, R. J., and Lever, W. F.: Clear cell hidradenoma. Histologic, histochemical, and electron microscopic study. Arch. Derm., *96*:18, 1967.

Johnson, B. L., Jr., and Helwig, E. B.: Eccrine acrospiroma. Cancer, *23*:641, 1969.

Keasby, L. E., and Hadley, G. G.: Clear-cell hidradenoma; report of three cases with widespread metastases. Cancer, *7*:943, 1954.

Kersting, D. W.: Clear cell hidradenoma and hidradenocarcinoma. Arch. Derm., *87*:323, 1963.

Lever, W. F., and Castleman, B.: Clear cell myoepithelioma of the skin. Am. J. Path., *28*:691, 1952.

Lund, H. Z.: Tumors of the Skin. *In* Atlas of Tumor Pathology. section I, fascicle 2. Washington, D.C., Armed Forces Institute of Pathology, 1957.

O'Hara, J. M., and Bensch, K. G.: Fine structure of eccrine sweat gland adenoma, clear cell type. J. Invest. Derm., *49*:261, 1967.

O'Hara, J. M., Bensch, K., Ioannides, G., and Klaus, S. N.: Eccrine sweat gland adenoma, clear cell type. Cancer, *19*:1438, 1966.

Santler, R., and Eberhartinger, C.: Malignes Klarzellen-Myoepitheliom. Dermatologica, *130*:340, 1965.

Winkelmann, R. K., and Wolff, K.: Histochemistry of hidradenoma and eccrine spiradenoma. J. Invest. Derm., *49*:173, 1967.

————: Solid-cystic hidradenoma of the skin. Arch. Derm., *97*:651, 1968.

Eccrine Poroma

Freeman, R. G., Knox, J. M., and Spiller, W. F.: Eccrine poroma. Am. J. Clin. Path., *36*:444, 1961.

Goldner, R.: Eccrine poromatosis. Arch. Derm., *101*:606, 1970.

Hashimoto, K., Gross, B. G., and Lever, W. F.: The ultrastructure of the skin of human embryos. I. The intraepidermal eccrine sweat duct. J. Invest. Derm., *45*:139, 1965.

Hashimoto, K., and Lever, W. F.: Eccrine poroma. Histochemical and electron microscopic studies. J. Invest. Derm., *43*:237, 1964.

————: Histogenesis of skin appendage tumors. Arch. Derm., *100*:356, 1969.

Hyman, A. B., and Brownstein, M. H.: Eccrine poroma. An analysis of forty-five new cases. Dermatologica, *138*:29, 1969.

Ishikawa, K.: Malignant hidroacanthoma simplex. Arch. Derm., *104*:529, 1971.

Knox, J. M., and Spiller, W. F.: Eccrine poroma. Arch. Derm., *77*:726, 1958.

Krinitz, K.: Ein Beitrag zur Klinik und Histologie des ekkrinen Poroms. Hautarzt, *18*:504, 1967.

————: Malignes intraepidermales ekkrines Porom. Z. Haut, *47*:9, 1972.

Mehregan, A. H., and Levson, D. N.: Hidroacanthoma simplex. Arch. Derm., *100*:303, 1969.

Mishima, Y.: Epitheliomatous differentiation of the intraepidermal eccrine sweat duct. J. Invest. Derm., *52*:233, 1969.

Mishima, Y., and Marioka, S.: Oncogenic differentiation of the intraepidermal eccrine sweat duct: eccrine poroma, poroepithelioma and porocarcinoma. Dermatologica, *138*:238, 1969.

Miura, Y.: Epidermotropic eccrine carcinoma. Jap. J. Derm., Series B, *78*:226, 1968.

Okun, M. R., and Ansell, H. B.: Eccrine poroma. Arch. Derm., *88*:561, 1963.

Penneys, N. S., Ackerman, A. B., Indgin, S. N., and Mandy, S. H.: Eccrine poroma. Brit. J. Derm., *82*:613, 1970.

Pinkus, H., and Mehregan, A. H.: Epidermotropic eccrine carcinoma. Arch. Derm., *88*:597, 1963.

Pinkus, H., Rogin, J. R., and Goldman, P.: Eccrine poroma. Arch. Derm., *74*:511, 1956.

Sanderson, K. V., and Ryan, E. A.: The histochemistry of eccrine poroma. Brit. J. Derm., *75*:86, 1963.

Serri, F., Montagna, W., and Mescon, H.: Studies of the skin of the fetus and the child. II. Glycogen and amylophosphorylase in the skin of the fetus. J. Invest. Derm., *39*:199, 1962.

Smith, J. L. S., and Coburn, J. G.: Hidroacanthoma simplex. Brit. J. Derm., *68*:400, 1956.

Winkelmann, R. K., and McLeod, W. A.: The dermal duct tumor. Arch. Derm., *94*:50, 1966.

Yasuda, T., Kawada, A., and Yoshida, K.: Eccrine poroma. Arch. Derm., *90*:428, 1964.

Eccrine Spiradenoma

Hashimoto, K., Gross, B. G., Nelson, R. G., and Lever, W. F.: Eccrine spiradenoma. Histochemical and electron microscopic studies. J. Invest. Derm., *46*:347, 1966.

Hashimoto, K., and Lever, W. F.: Histogenesis of skin appendage tumors. Arch. Derm., *100*:356, 1969.

Kersting, D. W., and Helwig, E. B.: Eccrine spiradenoma. Arch. Derm., *73*:199, 1956.

Lever, W. F.: Myoepithelial sweat gland tumor: myoepithelioma. Report of three cases with a review of the literature. Arch. Derm. Syph., *57*:332, 1948.

Munger, B. L., Berghorn, B. M., and Helwig, E. B.: A light- and electron-microscopic study of a case of multiple eccrine spiradenoma. J. Invest. Derm., *38*:289, 1962.

Nödl, F.: Zur Histogenese der ekkrinen Spiradenome. Arch. klin. exp. Derm., *221*:323, 1965.

Sheldon, W. H.: The myoepithelium in sweat gland tumors. Arch. Path., *31*:326, 1941.

Winkelmann, R. K., and Wolff, K.: Histochemistry of hidradenoma and eccrine spiradenoma. J. Invest. Derm., *49*:173, 1967.

Mixed Tumor of the Skin

Headington, J. T.: Mixed tumors of the skin: eccrine and apocrine types. Arch. Derm., *84*:989, 1961.

Hirsch, P., and Helwig, E. B.: Chondroid syringoma. Arch. Derm., *84*:835, 1961.

Kresbach, H.: Ein Beitrag zum sogenannten Mischtumor der Haut. Arch. klin. exp. Derm., *221*:59, 1964.

Lund, H. Z.: Tumors of the Skin. *In* Atlas of Tumor Pathology. section I, fascicle 2, p. 108. Washington, D.C. Armed Forces Institute of Pathology, 1957.

Nikolowski, W.: Über sogenannte Mischtumoren der Haut. Arch. klin. exp. Derm., *209*:1, 1959.

Basal Cell Epithelioma

Adamson, H. G.: On the nature of rodent ulcer: its relationship to epithelioma adenoides cysticum of Brooke and to other tricho-epitheliomata of benign nevoid character; its distinction from malignant carcinoma. Lancet, *1*:810, 1914.

Anderson, N. P.: Bowen's precancerous dermatosis and multiple benign superficial epithelioma: evidence of arsenic as an etiologic agent. Arch. Derm. Syph., *26*:1052, 1932.

Anderson, N. P., and Anderson, H. E.: Development of basal cell epithelioma as a consequence of radiodermatitis. Arch. Derm. Syph., *63*:586, 1951.

Anderson, T. E., and Best, P. V.: Linear basal cell nevus. Brit. J. Derm., *74*:20, 1962.

Assor, D.: Basal cell carcinoma with metastasis to bone. Cancer, *20*:2125, 1967.

Baer, R. L., Robbins, P., Menn, H. W., and Andrade, R.: Ekkrines Epitheliom. Behandlung mittels Chemochirurgie nach Mohs. Hautarzt, *22*:241, 1971.

Becker, S. W.: Pigmented epitheliomas. Arch. Derm. Syph., *27*:981, 1933.

Berendes, U.: Die klinische Bedeutung des onkotischen Phase des Basalzellnaevus-Syndroms. Hautarzt, *22*:261, 1971.

Bleiberg, J., and Brodkin, R. H.: Linear unilateral basal cell nevus with comedones. Arch. Derm., *100*:187, 1969.

Borel, D. M.: Cutaneous basosquamous carcinoma. Review of the literature and report of 35 cases. Arch. Path., *95*:293, 1973.

Brown, A. C., Crounse, R. G., and Winkelmann, R. K.: Generalized hair-follicle hamartoma. Arch. Derm., *99*:478, 1969.

Carney, R. G.: Linear unilateral basal cell nevus with comedones. Arch. Derm. Syph., *65*:471, 1952.

Caro, M. R., and Howell, J. B.: Morphea-like epithelioma. Arch. Derm. Syph., *63*:53, 1951.

Coletta, D. F., Haentze, F. E., and Thomas, C. C.: Metastasizing basal cell carcinoma of the skin with myelophthisic anemia. Cancer, *22*: 879, 1968.

Costanza, M. E., Dayal, Y., Binder, S., and Nathanson, L.: Metastatic basal cell carcinoma. Cancer, *34*:230, 1974 (review).

Covo, J. A.: The pits in the nevoid basal cell carcinoma syndrome. Arch. Derm., *103*:568, 1971.

Crawford, H. J., and Joslin, C. A. F.: Metastasizing basal-cell carcinoma. J. Path. Bact., *87*:437, 1964.

Darier, J., and Ferrand, M.: L'épithéliome pavimenteux mixte et intermédiaire. Ann. derm. syph., *3*:385, 1922.

Degos, R., and Hewitt, J.: Tumeurs fibro-épithéliales prémalignes de Pinkus et épithélioma baso-cellulaire. Ann. derm. syph., *82*:124, 1955.

Fanger, H., and Barker, B. E.: Histochemical studies of some keratotic and proliferating skin lesions. Arch. Path., *64*:143, 1957.

Foot, N. C.: Adnexal carcinoma of the skin. Am. J. Path., *23*:1, 1947.

Freeman, R. G., and Winkelmann, R. K.: Basal cell tumor with eccrine differentiation. Arch. Derm., *100*:234, 1969.

Gaughan, L. J., Bergeron, J. R., and Mullins, J. F.: Giant basal cell epithelioma developing in acute burn site. Arch. Derm., *99*:594, 1969.

Gellin, G. A., Kopf, A. W., and Garfinkel, L.: Basal cell epithelioma. Arch. Derm., *91*:38, 1965.

Gerstein, W.: Transplantation of basal cell epithelioma to the rabbit. Arch. Derm., *88*:834, 1963.

Gertler, W.: Zur Epithelverbundenheit der Basaliome. Derm. Wschr., *151*:673, 1965.

Geschickter, C. F., and Koehler, H. P.: Ectodermal tumors of the skin. Am. J. Cancer, *23*:804, 1935.

Gorlin, R. J., Vickers, R. A., Keller, E., and Williamson, J. J.: The multiple basal-cell nevi syndrome. Cancer, *18*:89, 1965 (review).

Gottron, H. A.: Basaliomprobleme. Derm. Wschr., *150*:220, 1964.

Greene, H. S. N.: The heterologous transplantation of embryonic mammalian tissue. Cancer Res., *3*:809, 1943.

Haber, H.: Intraepidermal acanthoma. Recent observations on Borst-Jadassohn epithelioma. Dermatologica, *117*:304, 1958.

Happle, R.: Naevobasaliom und Ameloblastom. Hautarzt, *24*:290, 1973.

Hermans, E. H., Grosfeld, J. C. M., and Spaas, J. A. J.: The fifth phakomatosis. Dermatologica, *130*:446, 1965.

Holmes, E. J., Bennington, J. L., and Haber, S. L.: Citrulline-containing basal cell carcinomas. Cancer, *22*:663, 1968.

Holubar, K., Matras, H., and Smalik, A. V.: Multiple palmar basal cell epitheliomas in basal cell nevus syndrome. Arch. Derm., *101*: 679, 1970.

Holubar, K., and Wolff, K.: Intraepidermal eccrine poroma. Cancer, *23*:626, 1969.

Hornstein, O.: Über die Pinkussche Varietät der Basaliome. Hautarzt, *8*:406, 1957.

Howell, J. B., and Caro, M. R.: The basal cell nevus. Arch. Derm., *79*:67, 1959.

Howell, J. B., and Mehregan, A. H.: Pursuit of the pits in the nevoid basal cell carcinoma syndrome. Arch. Derm., *102*:586, 1970.

Hundeiker, M., and Berger, H.: Zur Morphogenese der Basaliome. Arch. klin. exp. Derm., *231*:161, 1968.

Hundeiker, M., and Petres, J.: Morphogenese und Formenreichtum der arseninduzierten Präkanzerosen. Arch. klin. exp. Derm., *231*: 355, 1968.

Hyman, A. B., and Barsky, A. J.: Basal cell epithelioma of the palm. Arch. Derm., *92*:571, 1965.

Hyman, A. B., and Michaelides, P.: Basal-cell epithelioma of the sole. Arch. Derm., *87*:481, 1963.

Jablonska, S.: Basaliome naevoider Abkunft. Hautarzt, *12*:417, 1961.

Johnson, D. E.: Basal-cell epithelioma of the palm. Arch. Derm., *82*:253, 1960.

Krompecher, E.: Der Basalzellenkrebs. Jena, Fischer, 1903.

Lennox, B., and Wells, A. L.: Differentiation in the rodent ulcer group of tumours. Brit. J. Cancer, 5:195, 1951.

Lever, W. F.: Pathogenesis of benign tumors of cutaneous appendages and of basal cell epithelioma. Arch. Derm. Syph., 57:679, 1948.

Lever, W. F., and Hashimoto, K.: Electron microscopic and histochemical findings in basal cell epithelioma, squamous cell carcinoma and some appendage tumors. XIII Congressus Internat. Dermat. Vol. I, p. 3. Berlin, Springer, 1968.

Lewis, H. M., Stensaas, C. O., and Okun, M. R.: Basal cell epithelioma of the sole. Arch. Derm., 91:623, 1965.

Madsen, A.: De l'épithélioma baso-cellulaire superficiel. Acta dermatoven., 22, Suppl. 7, 1941.

————: The histogenesis of superficial basal-cell epithelioma. Arch. Derm., 72:29, 1955.

————: Studies on basal-cell epithelioma of the skin. Acta path. microbiol., Suppl. 177, 1965.

Mallory, F. B.: Recent progress in the microscopic anatomy and differentiation of cancer. J.A.M.A., 55:1513, 1910.

Margolis, M. H.: Superficial multicentric basal cell epithelioma arising in thermal burn scar. Arch. Derm., 102:474, 1970.

Maron, H.: Basaliom bei Kindern. Derm. Wschr., 147:545, 1963.

Mason, J. K., Helwig, E. B., and Graham, J. H.: Pathology of the nevoid basal cell carcinoma syndrome. Arch. Path., 79:401, 1965.

Mehregan, A. H., and Levson, D. N.: Hidroacanthoma simplex. Arch. Derm., 100:303, 1969.

Mehregan, A. H., and Pinkus, H.: Intraepidermal epithelioma: a critical study. Cancer, 17:609, 1964.

Miki, Y.: Basal cell epithelioma among Japanese. Austral. J. Derm., 9:304, 1968.

Milstone, E. B., and Helwig, E. B.: Basal cell carcinoma in children. Arch. Derm., 108:523, 1973.

Montgomery, H.: Basal squamous cell epithelioma. Arch. Derm. Syph., 18:50, 1928.

————: Dermatopathology. p. 923. New York, Harper and Row, 1967.

Montgomery, H., and Waisman, M.: Epithelioma attributable to arsenic. J. Invest. Derm., 4:365, 1941.

Moore, R. D., Stevenson, J., and Schoenberg, M. D.: The response of connective tissue associated with tumors of the skin. Am. J. Clin. Path., 34:125, 1960.

Morales, A., and Hu, F.: Seborrheic verruca and intraepidermal basal cell epithelioma of Jadassohn. Arch. Derm., 91:342, 1965.

Murray, J. E., and Cannon, B.: Basal-cell cancer in children and young adults. New Eng. J. Med., 262:440, 1960.

Oberste-Lehn, H.: Zur Histogenese des Basalioms. Z. Haut und Geschlechtskr., 16:334, 1954.

Okun, M. R., and Blumental, G.: Basal cell epithelioma with giant cells and nuclear atypicality. Arch. Derm., 89:598, 1964.

Piérard, J., and Dupont, A.: Nodular epithelioma. Brit. J. Derm., 60:50, 1948.

Pinkus, H.: Premalignant fibroepithelial tumors of the skin. Arch. Derm. Syph., 67:598, 1953.

Pinkus, H., and Mehregan, A. H.: A Guide to Dermatohistopathology. p. 462. New York, Appleton-Century-Crofts, 1969.

Reed, J. C.: Nevoid basal cell carcinoma syndrome with associated fibrosarcoma of the maxilla. Arch. Derm., 97:304, 1968.

Reidbord, H. E., Wechsler, H. L., and Fisher, E. R.: Ultrastructural study of basal cell carcinoma and its variants with comments on histogenesis. Arch. Derm., 104:132, 1971.

Rupec, M., Vakilzadeh, F., and Korb, G.: Über das Vorkommen von mehrkernigen Riesenzellen in Basaliomen. Arch. klin. exp. Derm., 235:198, 1969.

Sanderson, K. V.: The architecture of basal-cell carcinoma. Brit. J. Derm., 73:455, 1961.

Sarkany, J., Fountain, R. B., Evans, C. D., et al.: Multiple basal cell epitheliomata following radiotherapy of the spine. Brit. J. Derm., 80:90, 1968.

Sims, C. F., and Parker, R. L.: Intraepidermal basal cell epithelioma. Arch. Derm. Syph., 59:45, 1949.

Small, I. A., and Waldron, C.: Ameloblastomas of the jaws. Oral Surg., 8:281, 1955.

Smith, J. L. S., and Coburn, J. G.: Hidroacanthoma simplex. Brit. J. Derm., 68:400, 1956.

Smith, O. D., and Swerdlow, M. A.: Histogenesis of basal-cell epithelioma. Arch. Derm., 74:286, 1956.

Stell, J. S., Moyer, D. G., and Dehne, E.: Basal cell epithelioma metastatic to bone. Arch. Derm., 93:338, 1966.

Streitmann, B.: Zur Klinik der pigmentierten Epitheliome. Z. Haut Geschlechtskr., 26:279, 1959.

Tappeiner, J., and Pfleger, L.: Das intraepitheliale Epitheliom Borst-Jadassohn. Hautarzt, 15:58, 1964.

Taylor, W. B., Anderson, D. E., Howell, J. B., and Thurston, C. S.: The nevoid basal cell carcinoma syndrome. Arch. Derm., 98:612, 1968.

Taylor, W. B., and Wilkins, J. W., Jr.: Nevoid basal cell carcinoma of the palm. Arch. Derm., *102*:654, 1970.

Teloh, H. A., and Wheelock, M. C.: Histogenesis of basal cell carcinoma. Arch. Path., *48*:447, 1949.

Van Scott, E. J., and Reinertson, R. P.: The modulating influence of stromal environment on epithelial cells studied in human autotransplants. J. Invest. Derm., *36*:109, 1961.

Wallace, S. A., and Halpert, B.: Trichoma: tumor of hair anlage. Arch. Path., *50*:199, 1950.

Ward, W. H.: Nevoid basal cell carcinoma associated with a dyskeratosis of the palms and soles. Austral. J. Derm., *5*:204, 1960.

Wechsler, H. L., Krugh, F. J., Domonkos, A. N., *et al.*: Polydysplastic epidermolysis bullosa and development of epidermal neoplasms. Arch. Derm., *102*:374, 1970.

Welton, D. G., Elliott, J. A., and Kimmelstiel, P.: Epithelioma. Arch. Derm. Syph., *60*:277, 1949.

Wermuth, B. M., and Fajardo, L. F.: Metastatic basal cell carcinoma. Arch. Path., *90*:458, 1970.

Williamson, J. J., Cohney, B. C., and Henderson, B. M.: Basal cell carcinoma of the mandibular gingiva. Arch. Derm., *95*:76, 1967.

Wood, M. G., Pranich, K., and Beerman, H.: Investigation of possible apocrine gland component in basal-cell epithelioma. J. Invest. Derm., *30*:273, 1958.

Zackheim, H. S.: Origin of the human basal cell epithelioma. J. Invest. Derm., *40*:283, 1963.

Zelickson, A. S.: An electron microscope study of the basal cell epithelioma. J. Invest. Derm., *39*:183, 1962.

————: The pigmented basal cell epithelioma. Arch. Derm., *96*:524, 1967.

Zelickson, A. S., Goltz, R. W., and Hartmann, J. F.: A histologic and electron microscopic study of a pigmenting basal cell epithelioma. J. Invest. Derm., *36*:299, 1961.

Carcinoma of Sebaceous Glands

Beach, A., and Severance, A. O.: Sebaceous gland carcinoma. Ann. Surg., *115*:258, 1942.

Hartz, P. H.: Carcinoma of meibomian gland. Am. J. Clin. Path., *25*:636, 1955.

Justi, R. A.: Sebaceous carcinoma. Arch. Derm., *77*:195, 1958.

Leonard, D. D., and Deaton, W. R., Jr.: Multiple sebaceous gland tumors and visceral carcinomas. Arch. Derm., *110*:917, 1974.

Rulon, D. B., and Helwig, E. B.: Cutaneous sebaceous neoplasms. Cancer, *33*:82, 1974.

Urban, F. H., and Winkelmann, R. K.: Sebaceous malignancy. Arch. Derm., *84*:63, 1961.

Carcinoma of Eccrine Sweat Glands

Dave, V. K.: Eccrine sweat gland carcinoma with metastases. Brit. J. Derm., *86*:95, 1972.

Fresen, O.: Über das Carcinom der Hautdrüsen am Beispiel eines Schweissdrüsenkrebses der Hóhlhand. Hautarzt, *11*:15, 1960.

Grant, R. A.: Sweat gland carcinoma with metastases. J.A.M.A., *173*:490, 1960.

Grossman, J. R., and Izuno, G. T.: Primary mucinous (adenocystrie) carcinoma of the skin. Arch. Derm., *110*:274, 1974.

Hashimoto, K., and Lever, W. F.: Appendage Tumors of the Skin. p. 150. Springfield, Ill., Charles C Thomas, 1968.

Kay, S., and Hall, W. E. B.: Sweat-gland carcinoma with proved metastases. Cancer, *7*:373, 1954.

Mendoza, S., and Helwig, E. B.: Mucinous (adenocystic) carcinoma of the skin. Arch. Derm., *103*:68, 1971.

Miller, W. L.: Sweat gland carcinoma. Am. J. Clin. Path., *47*:767, 1967.

Orbaneja, J. G., Yus, E. S., Diaz-Flores, L., and Moro, B. H.: Adenocarcinom der ekkrinen Schweissdrüsen. Hautarzt, *24*:197, 1973.

Teloh, H. A., Balkin, R. B., and Grier, J. P.: Metastasizing sweat gland carcinoma. Arch. Derm., *76*:80, 1957.

Toker, C.: Trabecular carcinoma of the skin. Arch. Derm., *105*:107, 1972.

Carcinoma of Apocrine Glands

Baes, H., and Suurmond, D.: Apocrine sweat gland carcinoma. Brit. J. Derm., *83*:483, 1970.

Elliot, G. B., and Ramsey, D. W.: Sweat gland carcinoma. Ann. Surg., *144*:99, 1956.

Furtell, J. W., Krueger, G. R., Chretien, P. B., and Ketcham, A. S.: Multiple primary sweat gland carcinoma. Cancer, *28*:686, 1971.

Kipkie, G. G., and Haust, M. D.: Carcinoma of apocrine glands. Arch. Derm., *78*:440, 1958.

Neldner, K. H.: Ceruminoma. Arch. Derm., *98*:344, 1968.

27

Metastatic Carcinoma and Carcinoid

INCIDENCE AND DISSEMINATION OF METASTATIC CARCINOMA

The incidence of the various tumors metastatic to the skin in men and women correlates well with the frequency of occurrence of the primary malignant tumor in each sex.

Brownstein and Helwig, in their large series of patients with cutaneous metastasis, found that in women, commensurate with the great frequency of carcinoma of the breast, 69 per cent of all cutaneous metastases had their origin in the breast. Carcinoma of the large intestine accounted for 9 per cent of cutaneous metastases, and carcinoma of the lungs, carcinoma of the ovary, and malignant melanoma for 4 to 5 per cent each. In contrast, among men with cutaneous metastases carcinoma of the lung was the primary tumor in 24 per cent of cases, carcinoma of the large intestine in 19 per cent, malignant melanoma in 13 per cent, carcinoma of the oral cavity in 12 per cent, and carcinoma of the kidney and of the stomach in 6 per cent each.

On account of their relative rarity, cutaneous metastases are encountered rather rarely in carcinomas of the prostate (Peison), of the testes (Schiff), of the bladder (Hollander and Grots), of the pancreas (Edelstein), and of the liver (Kahn et al.).

Dissemination may take place through the lymphatics or through the blood stream. In carcinoma of the breast and squamous cell carcinoma of the oral cavity metastases reach the skin largely through lymphatic channels and often are located in the overlying skin. On the other hand, cutaneous metastatic lesions in other carcinomas usually are the result of hematogenous dissemination and may appear in any area of the skin.

Whereas lymphatic dissemination usually is a late event, so that the primary tumor has been present for a long time, hematogenous dissemination not infrequently is an early event. This is true particularly of carcinoma of the lung and of the kidney, in which in over half of the cases with cutaneous metastases the existence of the primary carcinoma had not been known prior to the appearance of the cutaneous metastases (Ehlers and Krause; Brownstein and Helwig).

CUTANEOUS METASTASIS FROM CARCINOMA OF THE BREAST

Four types of cutaneous metastases occur in carcinoma of the breast by way of the lymphatics. A fifth, a rather rare type of metastasis takes place through the blood stream to the scalp.

The four types of cutaneous metastases through lymphatic dissemination are: inflammatory carcinoma, telangiectatic carcinoma, nodular carcinoma, and carcinoma en cuirasse. Several of these four types may be present in the same patient. If dissemination of metastases through the lymphatics proceeds rapidly, inflammatory carcinoma results in most instances and telangiectatic carcinoma in rare instances. If dissemination proceeds slowly, nodular carcinoma or cancer en cuirasse eventuates (Taylor and Meltzer).

In inflammatory carcinoma the skin of the affected breast and the adjoining skin present erythema and diffuse edema simulating erysipelas. In telangiectatic carcinoma the skin contains numerous purplish papules and hemorrhagic pseudovesicles resembling a hemolymphangioma. In nodular carcinoma asymptomatic firm nodules are located in the skin and in the subcutaneous tissue. Those located in the skin may cause ulceration of the skin. In cancer en cuirasse the skin of the breast affected by the carcinoma, and often also the surrounding skin, show diffuse, brawny induration.

In the case of hematogenous dissemination to the scalp one finds one or several patches of alopecia which at first appear atrophic because of the reduction in the number of hair follicles. In the course of time the patches may become elevated above the level of the surrounding skin (Cohen et al.).

This manifestation, referred to as alopecia neoplastica, does not always carry a poor prognosis, as borne out by the report on one patient who had had it for 28 years (Nelson).

Histopathology. In inflammatory carcinoma histologic examination of the skin reveals extensive invasion of the dermal lymphatics, especially of the subepidermal lymphatics, by groups and cords of tumor cells (Fig. 27-1) (Taylor and Meltzer). The tumor cells are similar to those of the primary growth, atypical in character, with large, pleomorphic, hyperchromatic nuclei. There is marked capillary congestion (which is the reason for the inflammatory appearance clinically). In addition, one observes edema and a slight perivascular lymphoid infiltrate in the dermis, but no fibrosis (Siegel).

In telangiectatic carcinoma the dilated lymphatics contain, in addition to groups of tumor cells, varying amounts of erythrocytes (Freeman and Lynch; Leavell and Tillotson). The location of many of these dilated lymphatics immediately beneath the epider-

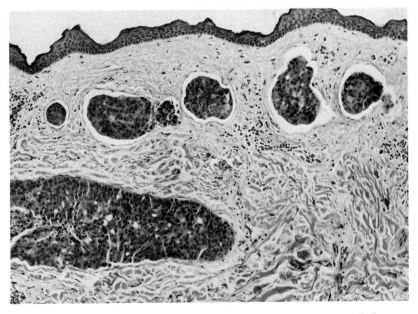

FIG. 27-1. **Cutaneous metastasis from carcinoma of the breast.** Inflammatory carcinoma. The dermal lymphatics are filled with clusters of tumor cells. (×100)

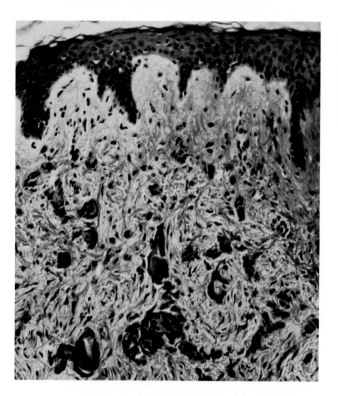

FIG. 27-2. **Cutaneous metastasis from carcinoma of the breast.** Nodular lesion. There are scattered islands of tumor cells and fibrosis of the dermis. Some of the tumor islands show a suggestive glandular arrangement of the tumor cells. (×200)

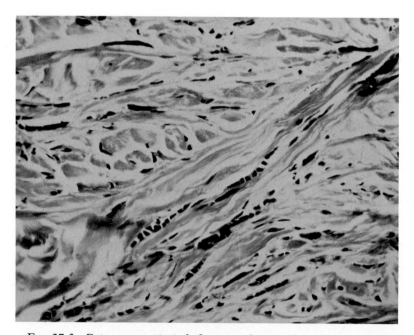

FIG. 27-3. **Cutaneous metastasis from carcinoma of the breast.** Cancer en cuirasse. Only a few tumor cells are present. They lie embedded between collagen bundles in single-row lines. Because of their small number and size, they may be overlooked easily. (×400)

mis causes the clinical resemblance of the lesions to vesicles.

In nodular carcinoma the nodules show large and small groups of tumor cells lying in the dermis and surrounded by fibrosis (Fig. 27-2) (Leavell and Tillotson). Some of the groups of tumor cells may show a glandular arrangement.

In cancer en cuirasse the indurated areas usually contain only a few tumor cells that may easily be overlooked because of their resemblance to fibroblasts. Like fibroblasts, the tumor cells have an elongated nucleus, but often their nucleus is larger, more angular, and more deeply basophilic than the nucleus of fibroblasts. Also, even though the tumor cells often lie singly, in some areas they lie in small groups or in single-row lines between thickened collagen bundles. This arrangement in single-row lines, "like Indians in a file," is of particular diagnostic importance (Fig. 27-3).

In alopecia neoplastica the histologic picture resembles that described for cancer en cuirasse, since one encounters cords of tumor cells between thickened collagen bundles (Cohen et al.). Elevated patches may show areas where the tumor cells show a glandular arrangement (Baran). The atrophy of the hair follicles is largely the result of the fibrosis (Cohen et al.).

CUTANEOUS METASTASIS FROM CARCINOMAS OTHER THAN BREAST CARCINOMA

In cutaneous metastases caused by hematogenous spread from a visceral carcinoma the appearance of the cutaneous lesions in a high percentage of the cases is an early event and often precedes the recognition of the primary tumor. In such instances not infrequently only one, or at the most only a few, cutaneous nodules are encountered (Winer and Wright; Kahn et al.). In patients in whom the cutaneous metastases appear late they often are multiple and may be numerous, and duration of life averages only three months after the appearance of the skin tumors (Reingold).

Histopathology. In cutaneous metastases caused by hematogenous dissemination large and small groups of anaplastic tumor cells are present in the dermis and often extend into the subcutaneous tissue. In most instances it is not possible to recognize from a histologic examination of the metastasis the organ in which the primary tumor is

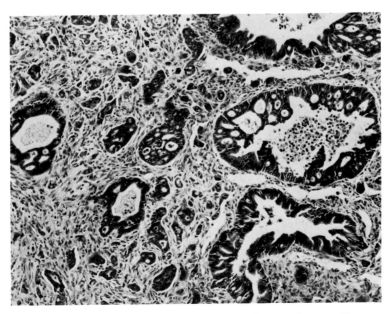

FIG. 27-4. **Cutaneous metastasis from an adenocarcinoma.** Numerous glandular lumina are present. (×100)

situated, and it is possible only to classify the metastatic carcinoma either as an adenocarcinoma, a squamous cell carcinoma, or an undifferentiated carcinoma. However, in three types of carcinoma it is often possible to recognize the site of the primary neoplasm from the histologic characteristics of the metastatic lesion in the skin. These three types are carcinoma of the gastrointestinal tract, of the kidney, and choriocarcinoma (see below).

As pointed out by several authors, the development of a solitary cutaneous metastasis, or of a few metastases, in a patient, especially a male, without known existence of a carcinoma, should immediately raise the suspicion of carcinoma of the lung (Ehlers and Krause; Brownstein and Helwig). The cutaneous metastases of a pulmonary carcinoma show a wide variety of histologic patterns, including squamous cell carcinoma and adenocarcinoma of varying degrees of differentiation, but most commonly, an undifferentiated carcinoma composed of small, closely packed "oat cells." Even if the initial examination reveals no evidence of pulmonary carcinoma because of the small size of

the tumor, further examinations, including bronchoscopy, are advisable.

In *carcinoma of the gastrointestinal tract* the tumor cells of the cutaneous metastases, like the primary tumor, often contain mucin (Winer and Wright). The mucin-containing cells present in the metastases may lie in glandular formations (Fig. 27-4); or they may be grouped irregularly as so-called signet-ring cells, i.e., as large round cells filled with mucin that presses the nucleus against the cellular wall (Fig. 27-5). The mucin, being epithelial mucin of the sialomucin type, contains both neutral and acid mucopolysaccharides. The mucin thus (1) is PAS-positive and diastase-resistant; (2) stains with alcian blue at pH 2.5 but not at pH 0.4, indicating that the acid mucopolysaccharides in the sialomucin are nonsulfated; (3) is hyaluronidase-resistant; and (4) shows no metachromasia on staining with toluidine blue or Giemsa stain (Winer and Wright; Cawley et al.; Mendoza and Helwig).

In *carcinoma of the kidney* the cutaneous metastases contain large polyhedral cells arranged in tubular, glandlike structures. The

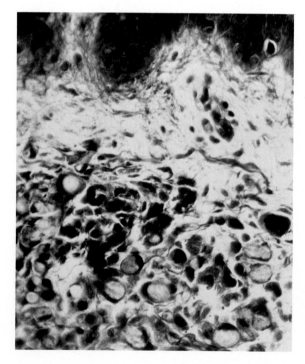

FIG. 27-5. **Cutaneous metastasis from carcinoma of the gastrointestinal tract.** Many of the tumor cells are so-called signet-ring cells, in which, because of the presence of mucin in the cytoplasm, the nucleus is pressed against the wall. (×400)

tumor cells have a light-staining, centrally located nucleus and abundant pale cytoplasm (Fig. 27-6). The pale appearance of the cytoplasm is due, at least in part, to the presence of glycogen (Rosenthal and Lever). The stroma of the metastases often is richly vascular, leading to the extravasation of erythrocytes into the lumina of the glandlike structures (Connor et al.).

In *choriocarcinoma* the cutaneous metastases show the two types of cells that arise from the fetal trophoblast; cytotrophoblasts and syncytiotrophoblasts. The cytotrophoblasts usually grow in clusters and the cells appear cuboidal, and have a large vesicular nucleus and a pale cytoplasm. The syncytiotrophoblasts, which have large and irregular nuclei and a basophilic cytoplasm, grow around the clusters of cytotrophoblasts in a plexiform pattern resembling chorionic villi (Cosnow and Fretzin). Patients with choriocarcinoma excrete large amounts of chorionic gonadotropin in their urine.

METASTATIC CUTANEOUS CARCINOID

The carcinoid syndrome develops, as a rule, only after a malignant carcinoid tumor has produced widely disseminated functioning metastases. In rare instances, a large nonmalignant carcinoid of the ovary may produce the manifestations of the carcinoid syndrome (Kierland et al.).

Malignant carcinoid tumors may originate in various locations, particularly in the intestinal and bronchial submucosa. The carcinoid syndrome is associated with an excessive production of 5-hydroxytryptamine (serotonin) in the tumor and the metastases. An excessive excretion of 5-hydroxyindoleacetic acid in the urine is diagnostic of the carcinoid syndrome. Clinically, the carcinoid syndrome is characterized by periodic attacks of flushing and of abdominal cramps associated with diarrhea. Since the functioning tumor and its metastases divert much tryptophan toward serotonin and thus away

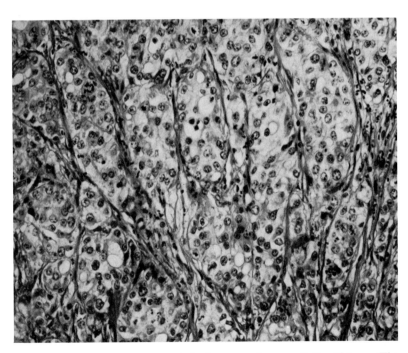

FIG. 27-6. **Cutaneous metastasis from carcinoma of the kidney.** The tumor cells possess abundant pale cytoplasm and are arranged in tubular, glandlike structures. (×400)

from niacin, the endogenous niacin production is depressed. If, in addition, diarrhea reduces the availability of exogenous niacin, pellagra, caused by niacin deficiency, may result (Castiello and Lynch). (For pellagra, see p. 412.)

The metastases caused by malignant carcinoid tumors are found most commonly in the regional lymph nodes and the liver, but may occur in many other organs, including the skin and the subcutaneous tissue. The cutaneous metastases consist of tender, hard, discrete nodules (Reingold and Escovitz). Subcutaneous metastases manifest themselves as one or several tender masses (Steele).

Histopathology. Carcinoid metastases in the skin and subcutaneous tissue consist of nests and sheets of small cuboidal cells having a small light-staining nucleus and pale cytoplasm. The cells are fairly uniform in size, although in some areas they may appear anaplastic and show numerous mitoses. The tumor nests may be separated from one another by fibrous septa. In some areas dilated vascular channels are seen near some of the tumor islands, and extravasated erythrocytes are seen among the tumor cells (Reingold and Escovitz).

Although the carcinoid tumors arising along the intestines and also their metastases contain argentaffin granules in their cells, such granules are few or absent in carcinoid tumors arising in areas other than the intestines (Reingold and Escovitz; Frank and Lieberthal).

Differential Diagnosis. Even though the cells of carcinoid tumors have a fairly characteristic appearance, being small, cuboidal, and pale, in the presence of dilated blood vessels and of hemorrhage a carcinoid tumor may resemble a malignant hemangioendothelioma. However, in carcinoid tumors the tumor cells do not line lumina. Dilated blood vessels and hemorrhages are seen also in the cutaneous metastases of renal cell carcinoma. In the latter condition, however, the tumor cells are larger than in carcinoid tumors, contain glycogen, and show a tubular, glandlike arrangement in at least some areas.

BIBLIOGRAPHY

Incidence and Dissemination of Metastatic Carcinoma

Brownstein, M. H., and Helwig, E. B.: Patterns of cutaneous metastasis. Arch. Derm., *105*: 862, 1972.

Edelstein, J. M.: Pancreatic carcinoma with unusual metastasis to the skin and subcutaneous tissue simulating cellulitis. New Eng. J. Med., *242*:779, 1950.

Ehlers, G., and Krause, W.: Über cutane Metastasen maligner Tumoren innerer Organe. Hautarzt, *21*:66, 1970.

Hollander, A., and Grots, I. A.: Oculocutaneous metastases from carcinoma of the urinary bladder. Arch. Derm., *97*:678, 1968.

Kahn, J. A., Sinhamohapatra, S. B., and Schneider, A. F.: Hepatoma presenting as a skin metastasis. Arch. Derm., *104*:299, 1971.

Peison, B.: Metastasis of carcinoma of the prostate to the scalp. Arch Derm., *104*:301, 1971.

Schiff, B. L.: Tumors of testis with cutaneous metastases to scalp. Arch. Derm. Syph., *71*: 465, 1955.

Cutaneous Metastases from Carcinoma of the Breast

Baran, R.: Les métastases alopéciantes scléro-atrophiques des cancers mammaires. Dermatologica, *138*:169, 1969.

Cohen, I., Levy, E., and Schreiber, H.: Alopecia neoplastica due to breast carcinoma. Arch. Derm., *84*:490, 1961.

Freeman, C. D., and Lynch, F. W.: Carcinoma of the breast with peculiar cutaneous metastases. Arch. Derm. Syph., *35*:643, 1937.

Leavell, U. W., Jr., and Tillotson, F. W.: Metastatic cutaneous carcinoma from the breast. Arch. Derm. Syph., *64*:774, 1951.

Nelson, C. T.: Alopecia neoplastica (possibly of 28 years' duration). Arch. Derm., *105*:120, 1972.

Siegel, J. M.: Inflammatory carcinoma of the breast. Arch. Derm. Syph., *66*:710, 1952.

Taylor, G. W., and Meltzer, A.: "Inflammatory carcinoma" of the breast. Am. J. Cancer, *33*: 33, 1938.

Cutaneous Metastasis from Carcinomas Other than Breast Carcinoma

Brownstein, M. H., and Helwig, E. B.: Patterns of cutaneous metastasis. Arch. Derm., *105*: 862, 1972.

Cawley, E. P., Hsu, Y. T., and Weary, P. E.: The evaluation of neoplastic metastases of the skin. Arch. Derm., *90*:262, 1964.

Connor, D. H., Taylor, H. B., and Helwig, E. B.: Cutaneous metastasis of renal cell carcinoma. Arch. Path., *76*:339, 1963.

Cosnow, I., and Fretzin, D. F.: Choriocarcinoma metastatic to skin. Arch. Derm., *109*: 551, 1974.

Ehlers, G., and Krause, W.: Über cutane Metastasen maligner Tumoren innerer Organe. Hautarzt, *21*:66, 1970.

Kahn, J. A., Sinhamohapatra, S. B., and Schneider, A. F.: Hepatoma presenting as a skin metastasis. Arch. Derm., *104*:299, 1971.

Mendoza, S., and Helwig, E. B.: Mucinous (adenocystic) carcinoma of the skin. Arch. Derm., *103*:68, 1971.

Reingold, I. M.: Cutaneous metastases from internal carcinoma. Cancer, *19*:162, 1966.

Rosenthal, A. L., and Lever, W. F.: Involvement of the skin in renal carcinoma. Arch. Derm., *76*:96, 1957.

Winer, L. H., and Wright, E. T.: Über den sekundären (metastatischen) Hautkrebs. Hautarzt, *11*:23, 1960.

Metastatic Cutaneous Carcinoid

Castiello, R. J., and Lynch, P. J.: Pellagra and the carcinoid syndrome. Arch. Derm., *105*: 574, 1972.

Frank, H. D., and Lieberthal, M. M.: Carcinoid syndrome originating in bronchial adenoma. Arch. Intern. Med., *110*:763, 1962.

Kierland, R. K., Sauer, W. G., and Dearing, W. H.: The cutaneous manifestations of the functioning carcinoid. Arch. Derm., *77*:86, 1958.

Reingold, I. M., and Escovitz, W. E.: Metastatic cutaneous carcinoid. Arch. Derm., *82*:971, 1960.

Steele, C. W.: Malignant carcinoid. Arch. Intern. Med., *110*:763, 1962.

28

Tumors of Fibrous Tissue

Among the tumors of fibrous tissue, both benign and malignant tumors occur. The malignant tumors are called fibrosarcomas. They usually occur as single tumors capable of producing metastases.

Fibrosarcomas are referred to also as spindle cell sarcomas. In addition, so-called round cell sarcomas exist. The latter occur in two varieties: lymphosarcoma and reticulum cell sarcoma. They are variants of lymphoma and as such, in contrast to fibrosarcomas, may arise in multiple foci (see p. 686).

DERMATOFIBROMA

Dermatofibromas occur in the skin as firm, indolent, single or multiple nodules. Usually, the nodules arise in adults. They are situated most commonly on the extremities, but they may be seen elsewhere. Although as a rule they are only a few millimeters in diameter, occasionally they measure 2 to 3 cm in size. Most lesions have a reddish color, but they may be reddish-brown because of hyperpigmentation of the overlying skin, or rarely bluish-black because of the presence of large amounts of hemosiderin within the tumor. In the latter case, the clinical appearance resembles that of a malignant melanoma. The lesions of dermatofibroma usually persist indefinitely although, in a few instances, spontaneous involution has been observed (Niemi).

Histopathology. Dermatofibromas are composed to varying degrees of fibroblasts, young collagen and mature collagen. They may be divided into "fibrous" and "cellular" tumors, depending on which component predominates, although in some tumors both components are present in about equal proportions. The majority of tumors are of the "fibrous" type and the volume of collagen clearly exceeds that of the fibroblasts.

In "fibrous" dermatofibromas, much of the collagen is young collagen and thus, instead of staining bright red with hematoxylin and eosin, it stains a pale blue; and further, instead of being assembled in firm bundles, the collagen in many areas lies in individual fibers (Plate 3, facing p. 586). The collagen, as a rule, is irregularly arranged in intertwining and anastomosing bands (Fig. 28-1). Occasionally, however, the fibroblasts and the collagen produced by them lie in whorls, which may have the appearance of cartwheels (Niemi). At both sides, the nodule shows poor demarcation so that the fibroblasts and the young collagen of the tumor extend between the collagen bundles of the dermis and surround them, thus trapping normal collagen bundles at the periphery of the nodule. At the lower border the demarcation usually is fairly sharp, but in some cases irregular penetration into the subcutaneous fat can be observed (Bandmann). At the upper border, the tumor usually, but not always, is separated from the overlying epidermis by a narrow band of collagen (Fig. 28-2). This band, if present, consists of young collagen composed of individual fibers rather than of bundles.

FIG. 28-1. **Dermatofibromas, fibrous type.** The collagen is irregularly arranged in intertwining and anastomosing bands. Some of the collagen, instead of being assembled in firm bundles, lies in individual fibers. A moderate increase in the number of fibroblasts is present. (×50)

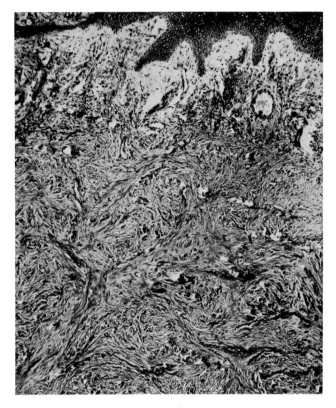

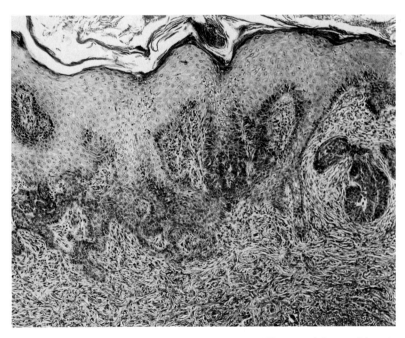

FIG. 28-2. **Dermatofibroma, fibrous type.** The overlying epidermis shows budding proliferations resembling a superficial basal cell epithelioma. (×100)

In "cellular" dermatofibromas, in contrast to those of the "fibrous" type, one finds numerous fibroblasts which, however, produce only small amounts of collagen. This collagen is present almost exclusively as individual fibers rather than as bundles (Fig. 28-3).

In both the "fibrous" type and the "cellular" type of dermatofibroma, scattered small capillaries with prominent endothelial cells are occasionally found, with fibroblasts arranged around the capillaries in a whorl-like pattern. Small areas of hemorrhage may be seen near the capillaries.

In about one third of all dermatofibromas, special staining reveals deposits of lipid or hemosiderin within the tumor cells (Cramer). Significant deposits are more apt to be found in "cellular" than in "fibrous" dermatofibromas. In routinely stained sections, the lipid-containing tumor cells, depending on the amount of lipid present, either have a pale, irregularly vacuolated cytoplasm or appear as true foam cells. In some instances, one also finds multinucleated giant cells. They may or may not contain lipid material. If they do, they may have the appearance of Touton giant cells (Frenk; Niemi).

A significant hyperplasia of the overlying epidermis in the center of the lesion occurs in more than 80 per cent of the lesions of dermatofibroma, irrespective of whether they are of the "fibrous" or of the "cellular" type (Steigleder et al.; Schoenfeld). The presence of such hyperplasia often has considerable value in the diagnosis of dermatofibroma. Most commonly, the hyperplasia consists of a regular elongation of the rete ridges, which may be associated with hyperpigmentation of the basal cell layer. In some cases the epidermal hyperplasia through the interlacing of thickened rete ridges is reminiscent of a seborrheic keratosis. Occasionally, downward proliferations are present that imitate the hair matrix to the point of having a connective tissue papilla (Steigleder et al.). In 2 to 5 per cent of the lesions, the downward proliferations are indistinguishable from those of a superficial basal epithelioma (Fig.

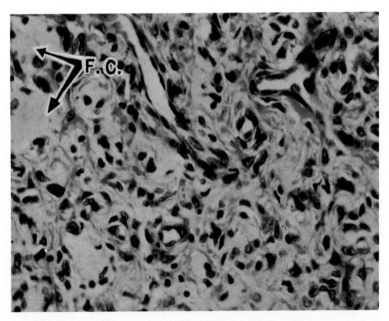

FIG. 28-3. **Dermatofibroma, cellular type.** Only small amounts of collagen are present, largely as individual fibers rather than as bundles. Many capillaries with prominent endothelial cells are present. Several fibroblasts have the appearance of foam cells; two particularly large foam cells (F.C.) can be seen in the left upper corner. (×400)

28-2) (Cramer and Cramer; Caron and Clink). Even though in most of these instances the proliferations are to be regarded as basal-cell-epithelioma-like, in rare instances a truly invasive basal cell epithelioma associated with ulceration develops (Halpryn and Allen; Thies and Hennies).

Histogenesis. Originally described as dermatofibroma, Woringer and Kviatkowski in 1932 showed that in some dermatofibromas phagocytizing cells were present, which they regarded as histiocytes. They proposed the term *histiocytoma* for tumors containing such phagocytizing cells. In 1936 Senear and Caro, on injecting colloidal iron under six dermatofibromas prior to excision, found that all of them phagocytized iron. They concluded, therefore, that all dermatofibromas were histiocytomas. Rentiers and Montgomery, on the other hand, regarded the presence of phagocytizing histiocytes within dermatofibromas as a secondary event "originating in response to hemorrhage, inflammatory changes and local tissue destruction in the nodules."

Even though no full agreement existed in regard to the relationship between histiocytes and fibroblasts, it became a widely accepted practice to refer to tumors composed predominantly of collagen fibers as dermatofibromas, and to tumors with significant deposits of lipids or hemosiderin in the tumor cells as histiocytomas (Niemi).

In recent years, several authors have stressed the essential unity of dermatofibroma and histiocytoma. Frenk came to the conclusion that even the tumors showing phagocytosis of iron or lipid were dermatofibromas, since phagocytosis lay within the functional potential of the fibroblast. Klaus and Winkelmann found acid phosphatase activity as evidence of a phagocytic potential within the cells of all nine dermatofibromas examined by them, irrespective of whether they showed predominance of stromal proliferation ("dermatofibromas") or were predominantly cellular ("histiocytomas").

Electron Microscopy. Electron microscopic examination of dermatofibromas has shown that even those lesions that show phagocytosis are composed of fibroblasts. Carrington and Winkelmann, on examining by electron microscopy two dermatofibromas with numerous lipid and hemosiderin inclusions, stated that the "histiocytes of this lesion resembled fibroblasts, having more of an oval nucleus, a prominent rough endoplasmic reticulum, and, in some, perinuclear fibrillar structures." Mihatsch-Konz et al., on examining eight dermatofibromas by electron microscopy,

found that fibroblasts were the essential cell and that the fibroblasts were engaged in both collagen production and lipid storage (E.M. No. 42). The intralesional injection of blood into one lesion 24 hours prior to excision demonstrated the ability of the fibroblasts to carry out phagocytosis since fragments of polymorphonuclear cells were seen within large phagolysosomes.

Neoplasm Versus Fibrosis. The view has been expressed that dermatofibromas were not tumors at all, but represented a reactive proliferation of fibroblasts subsequent to a trauma. Thus, Rentiers and Montgomery and also Klaus and Winkelmann refer to them as *nodular subepidermal fibrosis.* However, the fact that the lesions, with very few exceptions, show no tendency to regress but persist indefinitely speaks in favor of a neoplastic rather than a reactive, inflammatory genesis (Bandmann).

Dermatofibroma versus Sclerosing Hemangioma. The view expressed by Gross and Wolbach in 1943 that dermatofibromas actually were sclerosing hemangiomas still has adherents among general pathologists. According to Gross and Wolbach, early dermatofibromas show proliferating capillaries surrounded by fibroblasts and also proliferating endothelial cells with phagocytic ability that attempt to form new capillaries but do not always succeed and instead become engulfed by regressive fibrosis. Carstens and Schrodt in a recent electron microscopic study have made an attempt to support this theory. Naturally they found some endothelial cells, but not too many. So they stated that, even though the lining cells of some more or less obliterated vascular spaces had the ultrastructural characteristics of fibroblasts, endothelial cells "may obtain an ultrastructural similarity to fibroblasts." The mere fact that dermatofibromas do not regress but persist indefinitely speaks against the assumption that the fibrosis in dermatofibromas is a "regressive process."

Hyperplasia of the Epidermis. The hyperplasia of the epidermis overlying dermatofibromas can be explained by the presence of young collagen and of abundant amounts of metachromatic ground substance in the subepidermal region. This material, which resembles embryonic mesenchyme, stimulates the epidermis in a similar fashion as embryonic mesenchyme would do and thus causes the formation of immature hair structures and even of primary epithelial germs. Because the dermatofibroma prevents their downward growth, the immature hair structures, including the primary epithelial germ formations, proliferate in the narrow space between the epidermis and the tumor (Pinkus). The primary epithelial germ proliferations resemble basal cell epithelioma, and in rare instances even can give rise to a true basal cell epithelioma (Yanowitz and Goldstein; Thiess and Hennies; Halpryn and Allen).

Differential Diagnosis. In rare instances, dermatofibromas show a considerable number of nuclei. In such cases differentiation from fibrosarcomas, especially from dermatofibrosarcoma protuberans (see p. 583), may cause difficulties. However, the lack of atypicality in the appearance of the nuclei, the absence of mitotic figures, the absence of ulceration, and the presence of significant epidermal hyperplasia rule out fibrosarcoma (Michelson).

Dermatofibromas with many foam cells, in the absence of hemosiderin and foreign-body giant cells, may be indistinguishable from a xanthoma tuberosum in a regressive, fibrosing stage (Arnold and Tilden). In such cases clinical data, such as the number and location of the lesions and the presence or absence of elevated serum lipid values, are necessary to arrive at the correct diagnosis.

In the presence of foam cells and foreign-body giant cells and in the absence of hemo-siderin, a dermatofibroma may be difficult to distinguish from a lesion of Hand-Schüller-Christian disease or from a juvenile xanthogranuloma. In Hand-Schüller-Christian disease there usually is a more pronounced granulomatous reaction, and often eosinophils are present; and in a juvenile xanthogranuloma one usually finds wreath-shaped giant cells and some eosinophils, whereas capillary proliferation, which occasionally is seen in dermatofibroma, is absent.

SOFT FIBROMA

Soft fibromas, also called acrochordon or cutaneous tags, occur in two types: (1) as multiple filiform, smooth or furrowed soft papules, especially on the neck and in the axillae; and (2) as usually solitary soft, baglike, pedunculated growths on the trunk or extremities (Flegel and Tessmann).

Histopathology. The filiform soft fibromas show a hyperplastic epidermis characterized by papillomatosis, hyperkeratosis, and regular acanthosis (Fig. 28-4). The dermal connective tissue stalk enclosed in the epi-

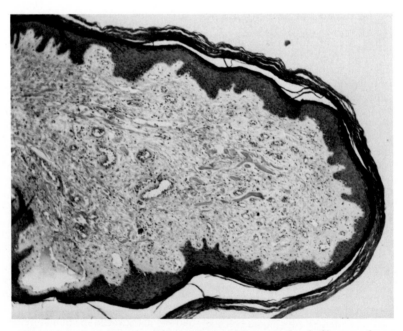

FIG. 28-4. **Soft fibroma, filiform type.** This type of soft fibroma shows a hyperplastic epidermis. The connective tissue stalk contains loosely arranged collagen fibers and many capillaries. (×50)

dermis is composed of loose collagen fibers and often contains numerous capillaries (Templeton; Flegel and Tessmann).

The baglike soft fibromas generally show a flattened epidermis. The dermis, like that of the filiform soft fibromas, is composed of loosely arranged collagen fibers. Mature fat cells often form the center. In some instances, the dermis is quite thin so that the fat cells compose a significant portion of the tumor which then may be regarded as a lipofibroma (Cramer).

INFANTILE DIGITAL FIBROMATOSIS

In this condition single or multiple fibrous nodules on the fingers or toes are present at birth or develop within the first few months of life. New lesions may appear during early childhood. The nodules involute spontaneously with scar formation (Wyatt and Cowan).

Histopathology. The dermis shows numerous proliferating fibroblasts and collagen bundles extending in different directions (Shapiro). There may be extension deeply into the subcutaneous tissue (Mehregan et al.). Thus, on purely histologic grounds a fibrosarcoma cannot be excluded (Shapiro). A valuable diagnostic feature is the presence of characteristic eosinophilic cytoplasmic inclusions within many of the fibroblasts. They measure from 3 to 10 μm in diameter and are best visualized with phosphotungstic acid-hematoxylin, staining it a deep purple (Shapiro). They are Feulgen-negative.

Histogenesis. Electron microscopic study of the cytoplasmic inclusions has shown them to consist of amorphous, granular material without a delimiting membrane (Mehregan et al.). It is most likely that the inclusion bodies are an accumulated abnormal by-product of metabolically deranged fibroblasts (McKenzie et al.). Viral studies have been consistently negative.

ACQUIRED DIGITAL FIBROKERATOMA

A solitary, rounded, firm, more or less hyperkeratotic projection is seen in the vicinity of either the proximal or the distal interphalangeal joint of a finger. The outgrowth is either elongated or dome-shaped and often is slightly pedunculated. In contrast to infantile digital fibromatosis, acquired digital fibrokeratoma occurs in adults.

Histopathology. The epidermis shows marked hyperkeratosis and acanthosis with thickened, often branching rete ridges. The core of the lesion is formed by thick, interwoven bundles of collagen (Bart et al.).

Histogenesis. Since the core of the lesion duplicates the normal dermis and since elastic tissue is present, it seems likely that the lesion is not a true fibroma but rather a protrusion of the dermis (Hare and Smith).

Differential Diagnosis. Although clinically acquired digital fibrokeratoma may resemble a rudimentary supernumerary digit, the latter is present since birth and contains numerous nerve bundles (Bart et al.).

TUBEROUS SCLEROSIS

Tuberous sclerosis, a dominantly inherited disorder, is characterized by the triad of mental deficiency, epilepsy, and angiofibromas of the face. The triad is not necessarily complete. The angiofibromas consist of numerous small, reddish, smooth papules in symmetrical distribution in the nasolabial folds, on the cheeks, and on the chin.

Additional cutaneous manifestations that may be present include the following: Asymmetrically arranged, large, raised, soft, brownish fibromas may be found scattered on the face and the scalp. Subungual and periungual fibromas may be present. There may be so-called shagreen patches, usually found in the lumbosacral region and consisting of slightly raised and slightly thickened areas of the skin. However, shagreen patches may occur also in the absence of tuberous sclerosis (see under Connective Tissue Nevus, p. 79).

Scattered hypopigmented leaf-shaped areas are present in more than one half of the patients with tuberous sclerosis. Their diagnostic importance lies in the fact that they either are present at birth or appear very early in life and thus are the earliest cutaneous sign of tuberous sclerosis (Fitzpatrick et al.).

Histopathology. In the past the symmetrically distributed small reddish angiofibromas of the face were mistakenly called *adenoma sebaceum of Pringle.* However, as

Nickel and Reed were able to show on the basis of 74 biopsies, the sebaceous glands are generally atrophic, and the main findings are dermal fibrosis and dilatation of some of the capillaries. In some lesions the fibrosis has a "glial" appearance, because the large size and stellate shape of the fibroblasts cause a resemblance to glial cells. In older lesions there may be perifollicular proliferation of collagen, leading to the compression of atrophic hair follicles by concentric layers of collagen. Elastic tissue is absent in the angiofibromas.

The larger asymmetrical fibromas on the face and the scalp show markedly sclerotic collagen arranged in thick concentric layers around atrophic pilosebaceous follicles. In contrast to the smaller lesions, dilated capillaries usually are absent (Fig. 28-5).

The ungual fibromas show fibrosis, usually without but occasionally with capillary dilatation. The areas of fibrosis may have a "glial" appearance due to the presence of large stellate fibroblasts (Nickel and Reed).

The shagreen patches show changes in the collagen and occasionally also in the elastic tissue. The collagen is increased in amount and the collagen bundles may appear thickened and homogenous (Nickel and Reed). The elastic fibers either appear essentially normal or are decreased or increased in amount (Raque and Wood) (see p. 80).

The hypopigmented leaf-shaped areas show with the dopa reaction a normal number of melanocytes but a reduction in the intensity of the reaction. On electron microscopy the melanosomes within the melanocytes and keratinocytes show a decrease in the degree of melanization and a diminution in size (Fitzpatrick et al.; Tilgen).

Systemic Lesions. Multiple tumors are commonly found in the brain, the retina, the heart, and the kidneys. The "tuberous" tumors of the brain, up to 3 cm in size, are gliomas; often they calcify in later life and then are visible on x-ray examination (Reed et al.). The retinal tumors also are gliomas. Because of their peripheral location, they cause no visual disturbances. They are either flat or extend as mulberrylike growths into the vitreous (Scheig and Bornstein). The cardiac tumors are rhabdomyomas in which the striated muscle cells appear markedly vacuolated as a result of the intracellu-

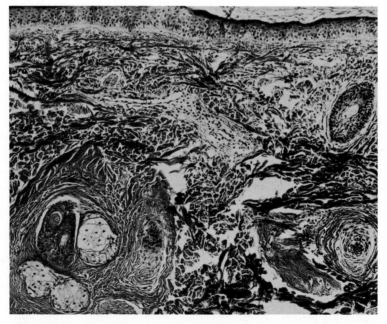

FIG. 28-5. **Tuberous sclerosis.** Markedly sclerotic collagen is arranged in thick concentric layers around atrophic pilosebaceous structures. (×100)

lar accumulation of glycogen (Morales). The renal tumors are angiomyolipomas which occur exclusively in tuberous sclerosis. They may be large or small, solitary or multiple, and they may be bilateral. Rarely, they may lead to renal failure by gradually replacing renal tissue (Farrow et al.). Histologically, there is a mixture of adipose tissue, blood vessels and smooth muscle. Even though there may be a slight degree of pleomorphism of some of the smooth muscle cells, the tumors always remain benign (Price and Mostofi).

HYPERTROPHIC SCAR AND KELOID

Both hypertrophic scars and keloids represent post-traumatic tissue proliferations. Initially, they have the same clinical appearance: They are red, raised, and firm, and possess a smooth and shiny surface. Whereas hypertrophic scars flatten spontaneously in the course of one or several years, keloids persist and may even extend beyond the site of the original injury.

Histopathology. Hypertrophic scars and keloids are indistinguishable from one another on histologic examination, since both show formation of whorls and nodules.

Whereas the whorls and nodules persist in keloid, they flatten out ultimately in hypertrophic scars (Linares et al.).

The difference between normal wound healing and healing with a hypertrophic scar or keloid lies not only in the length of time over which new collagen is being formed but also in the arrangement of the newly formed collagen. Normal wound healing proceeds through an early inflammatory stage to a "fibroblastic stage" in which one finds granulation tissue composed of numerous capillaries, fibroblasts and collagen fibers. The collagen fibers in the reticular dermis show a parallel, wavy orientation (Linares and Larson). Usually after five weeks, in the "hyaline stage," the number of capillaries and fibroblasts has decreased and the collagen lies as thick, hyaline bundles in parallel arrangement (Mancini and Quaife).

In hypertrophic scars and in keloids the formation of new collagen extends over a longer period of time than in normally healing wounds; but already in the early "fibroblastic stage" one can see that the collagen fibers in the granulation tissue are arranged in a whorl-like or nodular pattern (Linares and Larson). The nodules gradually increase in size and ultimately show thick,

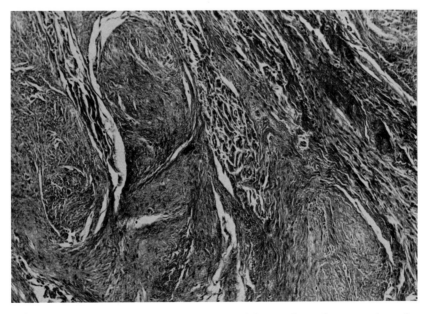

Fig. 28-6. **Keloid.** Highly compacted hyalinized collagen is present in nodular formations. (×50)

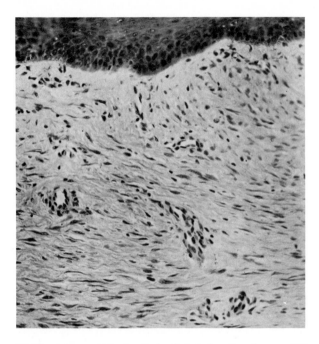

FIG. 28-7. **Hypertrophic scar.** In contrast to the nodular arrangement of the collagen in keloid and young hypertrophic scars, in a resolving hypertrophic scar the thick and hyalinized collagen bundles lie parallel to the free surface of the skin. (×200)

highly compacted, hyalinized bands of collagen lying in a concentric arrangement (Fig. 28-6) (Linares et al.).

Depending upon whether or not the nodular condensation of the collagen encroaches upon the papillary dermis, the epidermis appears either flattened or normal (Nikolowski).

Whereas in keloids the nodular condensation of the collagen persists indefinitely, in hypertrophic scars the thick and hyalinized collagen bundles in the nodules gradually straighten out and become thinner; and at the same time the orientation of the collagen bundles begins to parallel the free surface of the skin (Fig. 28-7).

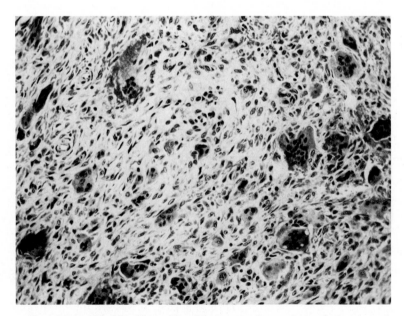

FIG. 28-8. **Giant cell epulis.** Numerous large, irregularly shaped, multinucleated giant cells are present. (×200)

GIANT CELL EPULIS

Giant cell epulis occurs as a solitary gingival tumor in children and young adults. It grows outward and thus does not invade the bone. It is found only in the vicinity of deciduous teeth, such as the bicuspids and the anterior teeth. The lesion is benign. It usually measures from 1 to 2 cm in diameter, is moderately firm and dark red in color, and has a smooth surface.

Histopathology. The lesion is well circumscribed but not encapsulated. It consists of dense accumulations of fibroblasts, scattered among which are numerous large multinucleated giant cells of the foreign-body type (Fig. 28-8). The giant cells possess ample amounts of homogenous, deeply basophilic cytoplasm and numerous irregularly arranged nuclei. Mitotic figures are few or absent (Sachs and Garbe).

Histogenesis. Because of the association of the giant cell epulis with deciduous teeth, it has been assumed that the giant cells within the tumor are derived from odontoclasts, which are multinucleated cells causing loosening of the deciduous teeth prior to their replacement by permanent teeth (Geschickter and Copeland).

DESMOID TUMOR

Desmoid tumors, also called fibromatosis, are benign fibrous neoplasms that arise from a muscular aponeurosis and tend to invade the muscle. They are firm, nontender masses. They may attain considerable size. They may be solitary or multiple.

Desmoid tumors may be present at birth, or may arise spontaneously in infancy, childhood, or adult life from a muscular aponeurosis of the neck, trunk or extremities (Fleischmajer et al.). However, the most common type of desmoid tumor arises in women from the rectus abdominis muscle either during or following a pregnancy. In some instances, desmoid tumors develop in a scar resulting from an abdominal operation.

In addition, desmoid tumors occur in the rare, dominantly transmitted *Gardner's syndrome.* This syndrome consists of (1) intestinal polyposis that is usually limited to the large intestine and is characterized by a high rate of malignant change into adenocarcinoma; (2) epidermal cysts, especially on the face and scalp; (3) osteomatosis with a predilection for the membranous bones of the head; and (4) fibrous tissue tumors consisting either of well demarcated fibromas located in the skin, the subcutaneous tissue or the abdominal cavity, or of desmoid tumors. The latter arise either in an abdominal scar following colectomy or at other sites spontaneously (Weary et al.).

Histopathology. Desmoid tumors are composed of fibroblasts that produce mature collagen. Although most desmoid tumors are quite cellular and show arrangement of their fibroblasts in interlacing bundles, atypical nuclei and atypical mitosis are absent (Fleischmajer et al.). Desmoid tumors show a great tendency to invasion of adjoining structures especially of muscle, where they may surround and entrap individual muscle bundles, ultimately leading to their destruction (Hunt et al.).

Desmoid tumors may contain areas of mucoid degeneration (Gonatas) or areas of calcification (Shapiro).

Histogenesis. Desmoid tumors are regarded as tumors by most authors, although some believe that they represent a hyperplasia of connective tissue analogous to keloids (Gonatas). They differ, however, from keloids by their location, their invasive tendency, their potential to occur without trauma, and their histopathologic appearance.

ATYPICAL FIBROXANTHOMA OF THE SKIN

Atypical fibroxanthoma of the skin, a fairly common lesion, was first described by Helwig in 1963. It is a benign, reactive lesion which paradoxically shows a highly malignant histologic picture.

Clinically, an intracutaneous, raised nodular lesion is seen in a sun-exposed area of the head or neck of an elderly person. In some instances x-irradiation had been given to the site at which the lesion arose (Samitz; Niemi).

In most instances, the nodule had been of recent origin, but in some reports the nodule had been present for several years (Levan et al.; Tapernoux et al.). Some lesions are covered by normal skin, whereas others show a crusted surface (Gordon) or superficial ulceration (Kempson and McGavran). Generally, the size of the lesion is less than 2 cm in diameter.

Histopathology. A very cellular dermal infiltrate extends to the epidermis or to the ulcerated surface of the lesion. It may also extend into the subcutaneous fat. The infiltrate is composed of cells with pleomorphic, often hyperchromatic nuclei that tend to be elongated or spindle-shaped. In addition, there are large, bizarre, multinucleated giant cells showing marked nuclear atypicality (Fig. 28-9) (Gordon; Kroe and Pitcock; Hudson and Winkelmann). Many mitoses are present, some of them atypical in appearance (Levan et al.). Only small amounts of collagen are seen.

The cytoplasm of some of the spindle-shaped cells and giant cells appears vacuolated so that they may resemble xanthoma cells. In the few cases in which fat stains could be carried out, sudanophilic material was demonstrable in the cytoplasm only in some instances and not in others (Kroe and Pitcock; Hudson and Winkelmann).

Histogenesis. This lesion with its highly malignant histologic appearance is regarded as non-neoplastic because of its limited growth potential and its tendency to involute even when inadequately excised. Thus, among the 101 patients reviewed by Fretzin and Helwig there were only 9 who had a recurrence after excision and none had metastases.

Differential Diagnosis. Atypical fibroxanthoma differs from dermatofibrosarcoma protuberans by the much smaller amount of collagen, by the greater pleomorphism of the spindle-shaped cells, and by the presence of a significant number of bizarre multinucleated giant cells. Unfamiliarity with this lesion would result in a diagnosis of a highly malignant fibrosarcoma. However, the limited extent and, especially, the superficial location differentiate the lesion from a true

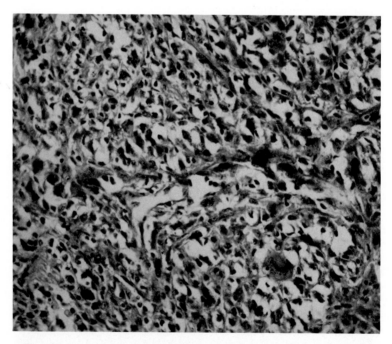

Fig. 28-9. **Atypical fibroxanthoma.** The lesion shows a dense infiltrate of highly pleomorphic, often hyperchromatic nuclei that tend to be elongated. As a characteristic feature, large bizarre, multinucleated giant cells are present. In addition, many atypical mitoses can be seen. The lesion is located in the dermis, in contrast to fibrosarcomas, which almost invariably arise in the subcutaneous layer or in fascial tissue. (×200)

fibrosarcoma, which arises almost invariably deep in the subcutaneous layer or in fascial tissue (Soule and Enriquez). In its morphologic details atypical fibroxanthoma otherwise shows great similarity with subcutaneous fibroxanthosarcoma, since considerable cellular pleomorphism, bizarre giant cells, and foam cells occur in both (see p. 585).

NODULAR PSEUDOSARCOMATOUS FASCIITIS

Although this subcutaneous nodular lesion is quite common, it was not recognized as an entity until Konwaler et al. described it in 1955. A considerable number of publications about this lesion have appeared since then, among which there are four dealing with more than 50 cases each (Price et al.; Soule; Stout; Hutter et al.).

The lesion is nearly always solitary. It consists of a rapidly developing subcutaneous nodule that reaches its ultimate size of 1 to 5 cm within 1 to 2 months. Often it is slightly tender. Although the arm is the most common site, the lesion may occur in any subcutaneous area. It is attached to the fascia, and the overlying skin is freely movable over it. The lesion is self-limited in duration, and thus, even if it is incompletely excised, it regresses (Soule; Hutter et al.).

The cause is unknown. Trauma does not seem to play a role. The general view is that nodular fasciitis represents a reactive fibroblastic and vascular proliferation.

Histopathology. The lesion is found to be partially attached to the fascia from which it arises. It is ill defined, and often, in addition to irregular extension into the subcutaneous fat, it may infiltrate into the underlying muscle. The extensions into the subcutaneous fat often are highly irregular, showing islands of fatty tissue and even individual fat cells enclosed by proliferating fibroblasts. The lesion may thus give the impression of being a highly infiltrating tumor (Mehregan).

The nodule consists of numerous large, pleomorphic fibroblasts growing haphazardly

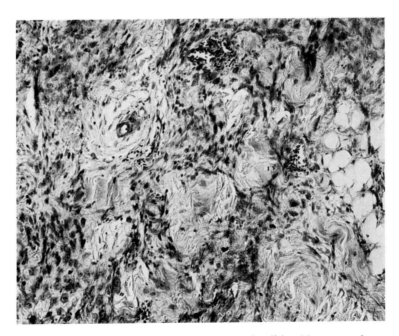

FIG. 28-10. **Nodular pseudosarcomatous fasciitis.** Numerous large pleomorphic fibroblasts are present. They are embedded in a mucoid ground substance on the right and are forming collagen on the left. A few fat cells of the invaded subcutaneous layer are still seen on the right. (×200)

in a stroma that often is highly vascularized and contains varying amounts of mucoid ground substance, of argyrophilic reticulum fibers, and of collagen fibers (Fig. 28-10) (Enterline et al.; Price et al.; Röckl and Schubert). The vascular component consists partially of well formed capillaries and partially of slitlike spaces. Erythrocytes are present not only in the capillaries and slitlike spaces, but also free in the tissue (Price et al.). The fibroblasts show a fair number of mitoses, but the mitoses do not appear atypical. In about one half of the cases, small spindle-shaped giant cells are found, representing young fibroblasts (Soule). A scattered chronic inflammatory infiltrate is often present, particularly at the periphery of the nodule (Mehregan).

Differential Diagnosis. Unfamiliarity with this lesion would result in a diagnosis of fibrosarcoma. Aside from clinical data, such as rapid growth and tenderness, the combination of fibroblastic and vascular proliferation is the most helpful diagnostic feature. Other findings suggesting the diagnosis of nodular fasciitis are the presence of a mucoid ground substance and of an inflammatory infiltrate, especially near the margin of the lesion.

DERMATOFIBROSARCOMA PROTUBERANS

Dermatofibrosarcoma protuberans represents a slowly growing tumor originating in the dermis. It usually begins an as indurated plaque in which subsequently multiple nodules arise. The nodules are reddish or bluish in color, firm in consistency and, as they slowly increase in size, they may ulcerate. The trunk is the most frequent location, followed by the extremities, particularly their proximal regions; whereas the scalp, neck and face are only rarely involved (Sauter and DeFeo).

Although the tumor is locally invasive, it gives rise to metastases only rarely and then generally only after many years' duration. McPeak et al. observed fatal metastases in 5 of 86 patients with dermatofibrosarcoma

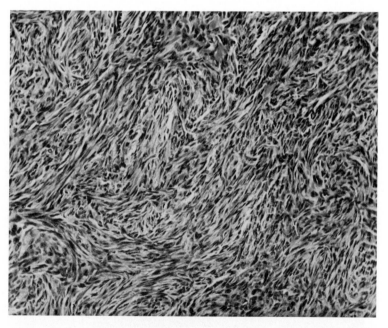

FIG. 28-11. **Dermatofibrosarcoma protuberans.** The nuclei of the fibroblasts lie in irregular strands and whorls. In some areas they form cartwheels, with the fibroblasts arranged radially about a small central hub of fibrous tissue. Some of the nuclei show a slight degree of atypicality. In contrast with the more malignant subcutaneous fibrosarcoma, formation of collagen is well in evidence. (×200)

protuberans. They involved the lungs, abdominal organs, the brain, or the bones. In rare instances metastases develop quite rapidly, as in a patient reported by Woolridge who died of pulmonary metastases 4 years after the onset of the tumor.

Histopathology. The histologic appearance of the tumor is that of a fairly well differentiated fibrosarcoma (Mopper and Pinkus). However, the degree of differentiation varies in different tumors and may vary even in different areas of the same tumor. Thus in some areas a dermatofibrosarcoma protuberans, because of the presence of large atypical nuclei and of atypical mitoses, may resemble a true subcutaneous fibrosarcoma, whereas in other areas it may show a degree of differentiation resembling that seen in dermatofibroma (Taylor and Helwig). In most areas formation of collagen is well in evidence. The fibroblasts lie in irregular, intertwining bands. Quite frequently, they also form whorls (Fig. 28-11). The whorls often show a cartwheel or storiform pattern in that fibroblastic nuclei are arranged radially about a small central hub of fibrous tissue (Taylor and Helwig). Giant cells are either absent or few in number. If present, the giant cells do not appear atypical or pleomorphic (Vargas-Cortes et al.). In some tumors the stroma contains mucoid areas (Binkley). Penetration of the tumor into the subcutaneous fat is common, and in rare instances tumor cells even infiltrate the fascia and the underlying muscle (Taylor and Helwig). The epidermis may show atrophy or ulceration (Fig. 28-12). Occasionally, the epidermis is mildly hypertrophic, but much less so than is commonly seen in dermatofibroma (Hashimoto et al.).

Histogenesis. On electron microscopic examination, the tumor cells in dermatofibrosarcoma protuberans show greatly elongated cytoplasmic processes, a markedly convoluted nucleus, rather scant rough-surfaced endoplasmic reticulum, and absence of phagolysosomes. As an unusual

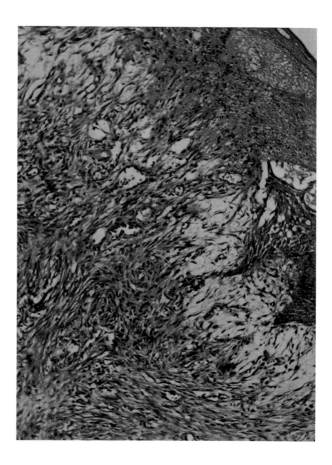

FIG. 28-12. **Dermatofibrosarcoma protuberans.** The tumor nuclei show only a mild degree of atypicality. However, the tumor cells are invading and destroying the epidermis, resulting in ulceration. ($\times 100$)

feature, many tumor cells show interrupted basal-lamina-like material along the plasma membrane. The presence of this material suggests that the tumor cells are modified fibroblasts possessing some features of neural supporting cells, such as perineural and endoneural cells (Hashimoto et al.).

Differential Diagnosis. For differentiation from dermatofibroma, see page 574; from atypical fibroxanthoma, see page 580.

Spindle-celled anaplastic tumors may arise within the dermis in areas of radiodermatitis. They are more pleomorphic than dermatofibrosarcoma protuberans. It is likely that most, if not all of them represent Grade 4 spindle-cell squamous cell carcinoma rather than fibrosarcoma (Sims and Kirsch; Gentele), even though some of them have been reported as fibrosarcoma (Kanaar and Oort).

SUBCUTANEOUS FIBROSARCOMA

True sarcomas almost invariably arise either deep in the subcutaneous layer or in fascial tissue. Aside from sarcomas developing from specialized structures, such as neurofibrosarcomas, liposarcomas, rhabdomyosarcomas, etc., which will be discussed elsewhere, fibrosarcomas have been subdivided on a histologic basis into pure fibrosarcomas, myxofibrosarcomas, epithelioid sarcomas, and fibroxanthosarcomas.

Subcutaneous fibrosarcomas, which occur most commonly on the extremities, at first grow in a nodular or multinodular fashion along fascial structures and tendons, and ultimately cause ulceration of the overlying skin. In the beginning, when only one nodule is present, clinical differentiation from nodular pseudosarcomatous fasciitis is often impossible.

Metastases usually occur only after extensive local infiltrating growth and may affect both regional lymph nodes and visceral organs (Frable et al.).

Histopathology. *Subcutaneous fibrosarcomas* usually are highly cellular. The nuclei are pleomorphic and thus vary greatly in size, shape, and staining intensity. However, at least some of the nuclei are spindle-shaped. Mitotic figures, including atypical mitoses, are present, often in large numbers.

The nuclei show an irregular, disorderly arrangement, and in some areas they lie in dense clusters. They may be arranged in bundles, and in some instances also in whorls and cartwheel formations, as seen typically in dermatofibrosarcoma protuberans. The crowding of nuclei may give the impression of multinucleated giant cells; but giant cells are absent in subcutaneous fibrosarcomas with the exception of fibroxanthosarcomas (see below) (Pritchard et al.). Subcutaneous fibrosarcomas usually contain some mature collagen bundles, but in highly cellular areas collagen bundles may be absent. However, in most such instances a reticulum stain will reveal the presence of rather numerous reticulum fibers (Gentele; Stout). Some subcutaneous fibrosarcomas show more or less extensive mucoid changes in their stroma. If the mucoid changes are extensive, the tumor can be classified as *myxofibrosarcoma* (See also myxosarcoma, p. 587).

Two histologic variants of subcutaneous fibrosarcoma have been described in recent years: epithelioid sarcoma by Enzinger in 1970, and fibroxanthosarcoma by Kempson and Kyriakos in 1972. In *epithelioid sarcoma* irregular nodular masses of large polygonal cells merge with spindle-shaped cells associated with large amounts of hyalinized collagen. The polygonal cells are suggestive of epithelioid cells and thus may falsely suggest a granulomatous process with reactive fibrosis. However, on electron microscopic examination, the polygonal or epithelioid cells have the appearance of fibroblasts (Fisher and Horvat).

In *fibroxanthosarcoma* one observes, in addition to spindle-shaped cells, cells with prominent vesicular nuclei, and, in addition, bizarre giant cells. In all tumors, the spindle-shaped cells are arranged in some areas in a cartwheel pattern. Some tumors contain clumps of foam cells, usually at the periphery of the tumor mass. Also, mucoid areas are seen in some tumors. The overall pattern is that of a highly pleomorphic sarcoma.

Differential Diagnosis. A highly malignant subcutaneous fibrosarcoma with no production of collagen may be difficult to differentiate from squamous cell carcinoma, Grade 4, amelanotic malignant melanoma, or reticulum cell sarcoma. On thorough inspection, however, one usually will find in squamous cell carcinoma, Grade 4, even in the presence of many spindle-shaped cells, some tendency to keratinization and connections of the tumor with the epidermis (p. 478); in malignant melanoma one will find "junctional activity" at the junction between the epidermis and the dermis (p. 671); and in reticulum cell sarcoma cells with round to oval nuclei predominate and spindle-shaped nuclei are absent (p. 693).

Subcutaneous fibroxanthosarcoma resembles atypical fibroxanthoma of the skin, since both lesions appear highly pleomorphic and contain bizarre giant cells and occasionally also foam cells. Since the former is malignant and the latter benign, differentiation is of great importance. The differentiation usually is easy, since atypical fibroxanthoma is a relatively small dermal lesion without tendency to uninhibited growth. In addition, it does not show the cartwheel formations that are seen regularly in subcutaneous fibroxanthosarcoma.

CUTANEOUS MYXOMA (FOCAL MUCINOSIS)

In cutaneous myxoma or focal mucinosis, a solitary, asymptomatic, flesh-colored nodule is found on the face, trunk, or extremities. The lesion does not occur on the fingers or toes. The nodule usually measures about 1 cm in diameter. Occasionally, there is some fluctuation.

Histopathology. Within a localized but not sharply circumscribed area of the dermis the collagen is largely replaced by homogeneous mucinous material in which scattered fibroblasts are seen. The number of fibroblasts is only slightly greater than normal. They are spindle-shaped or stellate. The mucinous stroma, in some instances, contains a small cavity. The mucinous material stains pale blue with hematoxylin and eosin. It also stains with alcian blue and shows a metachromatic staining reaction with toluidine blue before but not after exposure to hyaluronidase, indicating that the mucin consists largely of hyaluronic acid (Johnson and Helwig).

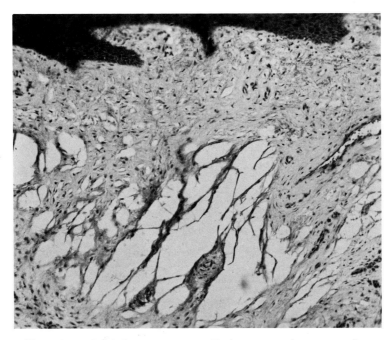

FIG. 28-13. **Digital mucous cyst.** Early stage, prior to actual cyst formation. The dermis contains much mucin. The cleftlike spaces, through coalescence, will later on form a large cystic space. (×200)

Differential Diagnosis. Lichen myxedematosus (papular mucinosis) differs from cutaneous myxoma by showing a larger number of fibroblasts, more collagen, less mucin, and no cleftlike spaces. Digital mucous cysts in their initial stage do not differ from cutaneous myxoma, but at a later stage they show a single large cavity, which does not occur in cutaneous myxoma.

DIGITAL MUCOUS CYST

This usually solitary lesion occurs most commonly on the distal phalanx of a finger near the base of a nail. Rarely, it is found on the dorsum of a toe. It consists of a small, semiglobular, translucent, slightly fluctuating nodule, usually less than 1 cm in size and slightly tender. When punctured, a clear mucinous fluid exudes. No tendency to spontaneous disappearance exists.

Histopathology. Very early lesions have the same histologic appearance as that of a cutaneous myxoma, namely, an ill defined area of mucinous material within which there is a slight increase in the number of fibroblasts. Subsequently, multiple cleftlike spaces form, which then coalesce to one large cystic space containing mucin (Fig. 28-13). The mucin stains pale blue with hematoxylin and eosin. It is composed largely of hyaluronic acid and thus stains with alcian blue at pH 2.5 but not at pH 0.4, and is PAS-negative (Johnson et al.). In early lesions the cystic space is separated from the epidermis by mucinous stroma, but in older lesions the cystic space is found in a subepidermal location and occasionally partly in an intraepidermal location (Bourns and Sanerkin).

Histogenesis. It is widely assumed that digital mucous cysts result from an overproduction of hyaluronic acid by fibroblasts, associated with a decreased or absent collagen formation (Götz and Koch; Johnson et al.). The old theory that they were synovial cysts, first expressed by MacKee and Andrews in 1922, has been largely abandoned, especially since radiographs after the injection of contrast fluid into the cyst had failed to show any contrast fluid to diffuse into

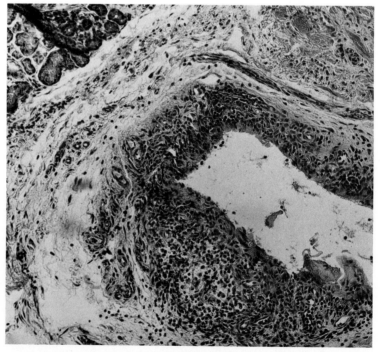

FIG. 28-14. **Mucous cyst of the lip.** The cyst, which results from the rupture of a salivary duct, possesses a wall composed of granulation tissue. Part of a salivary gland is seen in the upper left corner. (×100)

PLATE 3

Dermatofibroma. Most of the collagen is young, and stains faintly basophilic instead of deeply eosinophilic as mature collagen does. There are numerous spindle-shaped fibroblasts. Several capillaries lined by prominent endothelial cells are present. (×175).

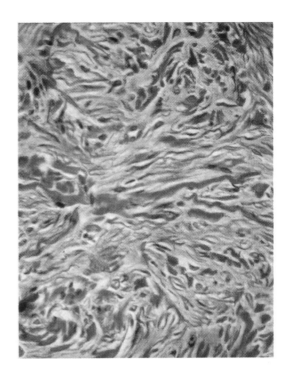

Kaposi's sarcoma. A fibroblastic area is shown. In addition to numerous fibroblasts there are narrow vascular slits filled with erythrocytes and areas of extravasation of erythrocytes. (×100)

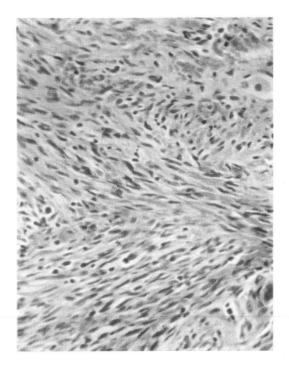

the distal interphalangeal joint space (Götz and Koch). Recently, however, Newmeyer et al. have shown in 20 consecutive patients with digital mucous cysts that, after the injection of methylene blue into the volar aspect of the distal interphalangeal joint space, the digital mucous cyst regularly contained the dye, suggesting that digital mucous cysts communicate with the joint space by a pedicle and thus are synovial cysts.

MUCOUS CYST OF ORAL MUCOSA

Mucous cysts of the oral mucosa occur as a solitary asymptomatic lesion, usually on the mucous surface of the lower lip and only rarely elsewhere on the oral mucosa, such as the buccal mucosa (Lattanand et al.) or the tongue (Braun-Falco). The cysts usually measure less than 1 cm in diameter, appear translucent and contain a clear viscous fluid. The cysts may disappear spontaneously, with or without evacuating their mucous content.

Mucous cysts of the oral mucosa usually are the result of a minor trauma leading to the rupture of a mucous duct and an outpouring of sialomucin into the tissue. Although most patients with a mucous cyst have no pre-existing abnormality, mucous cysts of the lower lip may occur in patients with *cheilitis glandularis,* a condition in which the labial mucous glands and ducts are hyperplastic (Weir and Johnson).

Histopathology. In early lesions one finds multiple small spaces filled with sialomucin and surrounded by a thick layer of granulation tissue. Older lesions show either a solitary large cystic space or several large spaces lined by granulation tissue intermingled with macrophages (Fig. 28-14) (Braun-Falco; Ehlers; Lattanand et al.). The macrophages contain prominent vacuoles representing phagocytized sialomucin (Braun-Falco). Still older lesions regularly show a large solitary cyst lined by only a little granulation tissue and, instead, largely by fibrous tissue (Ehlers). The wall of some cysts shows a ruptured salivary duct opening into the cavity (Lattanand et al.).

The sialomucin within the cysts appears as amorphous, slightly eosinophilic material in routinely stained sections. It is PAS-positive and diastase-resistant and stains with alcian blue at pH 2.5 but not at pH 0.4. It shows no metachromasia with toluidine blue and is hyaluronidase-resistant. Thus, sialomucin as an epithelial mucin contains both nonsulfated acid mucopolysaccharides and neutral mucopolysaccharides, i.e., glycoprotein (Nikolowski; Lattanand et al.). (In regard to the presence of sialomucin in the skin, see also extramammary Paget's disease, p. 490, and cutaneous metastasis of carcinoma of the gastrointestinal tract, p. 566.)

MYXOSARCOMA

Tumors having the histologic appearance of a myxosarcoma may arise in the subcutaneous fat and the underlying soft tissues. Whereas some authors recognize the existence of a true myxosarcoma (Stout; Sponsel et al.; Korting and Nürnberger), others believe that all cases with a histologic aspect suggestive of myxosarcoma in reality are sarcomas of other types of tissues, such as fibrosarcomas, liposarcomas, chondrosarcomas, or rhabdomyosarcomas, in which a mucinous transformation of most of the stroma has taken place (Enterline et al.). In particular, liposarcomas often have the histologic aspect of a myxosarcoma so that in every case of myxosarcoma fat stains are indicated; and, if significant amounts of fat are present, the tumor should be referred to as myxoliposarcoma (Enterline et al.). However, as Korting and Nürnberger have pointed out, myxosarcomas that are not primarily liposarcomas may also contain some lipid due to intracellular "lipid phanerosis" in areas of necrosis or necrobiosis.

Histopathology. Tumors having the histologic appearance of myxosarcoma show fairly numerous nuclei, some of them stellate in shape, embedded in a mucinous stroma. Many of these nuclei appear atypical (Sponsel et al.); and even atypical multinucleated giant cells may be present (Korting and Nürnberger).

Histogenesis. Since it is the function of the fibroblast to produce, in addition to collagenous and elastic fibers, also mucinous ground substance, it appears likely that most myxosarcomas basically are fibrosarcomas (see p. 584). Myxosarcomas containing significant amounts of intracellular lipid in many cells throughout the tumor most likely are basically liposarcomas.

In addition, most mesodermal tumors may show mucinous transformation; but this occurs, as a rule, in only parts of the tumor so that histologic examination of other parts of the tumor usually will establish the dominant tissue.

BIBLIOGRAPHY

Dermatofibroma

Arnold, H. L., Jr., and Tilden, I. L.: Histiocytoma cutis: a variant of xanthoma. Arch. Derm. Syph., *47*:498, 1943.

Bandmann, H. J.: Ein Beitrag zur morphologischen Pathologie des Dermatofibroma lenticulare bzw. des Histiocytoms. Arch. klin. exp. Derm., *204*:584, 1957.

Caron, G. A., and Clink, H. M.: Clinical association of basal cell epithelioma with histiocytoma. Arch. Derm., *90*:271, 1964.

Carrington, S. G., and Winkelmann, R. K.: Electron microscopy of histiocytic diseases of the skin. Acta dermatoven., *52*:161, 1972.

Carstens, P. H. B., and Schrodt, G. R.: Ultrastructure of sclerosing hemangioma. Am. J. Path., *77*:377, 1974.

Cramer, H. J.: Zur Histologie und Histochemie des xanthomatösen Histiocytoms. Arch. klin. exp. Derm., *232*:138, 1968.

Cramer, R., and Cramer, H. J.: Über die pseudobasaliomatöse Epithelhyperplasie der Haut. Arch. klin. exp. Derm., *216*:231, 1963.

Frenk, E.: Zur Histologie der Fibrome und Histiocytome der Haut. Hautarzt, *12*:15, 1961.

Gross, R. E., and Wolbach, S. B.: Sclerosing hemangiomas: their relationship to dermatofibroma, histiocytoma, xanthoma and to certain pigmented lesions of the skin. Am. J. Path., *19*:533, 1943.

Halpryn, H. J., and Allen, A. C.: Epidermal changes associated with sclerosing hemangiomas. Arch. Derm., *80*:160, 1959.

Klaus, S. N., and Winkelmann, R. K.: The enzyme histochemistry of nodular subepidermal fibrosis. Brit. J. Derm., *78*:398, 1966.

Michelson, H. E.: Nodular subepidermal fibrosis. Arch. Derm. Syph., *27*:812, 1933.

Mihatsch-Konz, B., Schaumburg-Lever, G., and Lever, W. F.: Ultrastructure of dermatofibroma. Arch. derm. Forsch., *246*:181, 1973.

Muller, S. A.: Hair neogenesis. J. Invest. Derm., *56*:1, 1971.

Niemi, K. M.: The benign fibrohistiocytic tumours of the skin. Acta dermatoven., *50*: suppl. 63, 1970 (review).

Pinkus, H.: Pathobiology of the pilary complex. Jap. J. Derm., Series B, *77*:304, 1967.

Rentiers, P. L., and Montgomery, H.: Nodular subepidermal fibrosis (dermatofibroma versus histiocytoma). Arch. Derm. Syph., *59*:568, 1949 (review).

Schoenfeld, R. J.: Epidermal proliferations overlying histiocytomas. Arch. Derm., *90*:266, 1964.

Senear, F. E., and Caro, M. R.: Histiocytoma cutis. Arch. Derm. Syph., *33*:209, 1936.

Steigleder, G. K., Nicklas, H., and Kamei, Y.: Die Epithelveränderungen beim Histiocytom, ihre Genese und ihr Erscheinungsbild. Derm. Wschr., *146*:457, 1962.

Thies, W., and Hennies, T.: Über die Assoziation eines Histiocytoms mit einem Basaliom. Hautarzt, *19*:163, 1968.

Woringer, F., and Kviatkowski, S. L.: L'histiocytome de la peau. Ann. derm. syph., *3*:998, 1932.

Yanowitz, M., and Goldstein, M.: Basal cell epithelioma overlying a dermatofibroma. Arch. Derm., *89*:709, 1964.

Soft Fibromas

Cramer, H. J.: Histochemische Untersuchungen mit dem sauren Hämateintest nach Baker an pathologisch veränderter Haut. Arch. klin. exp. Derm., *228*:438, 1967.

Flegel, H., and Tessmann, K.: Gibt es ein weiches Fibrom der Haut? Hautarzt, *18*:251, 1967.

Templeton, H. J.: Cutaneous tags of the neck. Arch. Derm. Syph., *33*:495, 1936.

Infantile Digital Fibromatosis

McKenzie, A. W., Innes, F. L. F., Rack, J. M., et al.: Digital fibrous swellings in children. Brit. J. Derm., *83*:446, 1970.

Mehregan, A. H., Nabai, H., and Matthews, J. E.: Recurring digital fibrous tumor of childhood. Arch. Derm., *106*:375, 1972.

Shapiro, L.: Infantile digital fibromatosis and aponeurotic fibroma. Arch. Derm., *99*:37, 1969.

Wyatt, E. H., and Cowan, M. A.: Digital fibrous tumors of childhood. Trans. St. John's Hosp. Derm. Soc., *56*:162, 1970.

Acquired Digital Fibrokeratoma

Bart, R. S., Andrade, R., Kopf, A. W., and Leider, M.: Acquired digital fibrokeratomas. Arch. Derm., *97*:120, 1968.

Hare, P. J., and Smith, P. A. J.: Acquired (digital) fibrokeratoma. Brit. J. Derm., *81*:667, 1969.

Tuberous Sclerosis

Farrow, G. M., Harrison, E. G., Jr., Utz, D. C., and Jones, D. R.: Renal angiomyolipoma. Cancer, *22*:564, 1968.

Fitzpatrick, T. B., Szabo, G., Hori, Y., *et al.*: White leaf-shaped macules. Arch. Derm., *98*:1, 1968.

Morales, J. B.: Congenital rhabdomyoma, tuberous sclerosis, and splenic histiocytosis. Arch. Path., *71*:485, 1961.

Nickel, W. R., and Reed, W. B.: Tuberous sclerosis. Arch. Derm., *85*:209, 1962 (review of cutaneous lesions).

Price, E. B., Jr., and Mostofi, F. K.: Symptomatic angiomyolipoma of the kidney. Cancer, *18*: 761, 1965.

Raque, C. J., and Wood, M. G.: Connective-tissue nevus. Arch. Derm., *102*:390, 1970.

Reed, W. B., Nickel, W. R., and Campion, G.: Internal manifestations of tuberous sclerosis. Arch. Derm., *87*:715, 1963 (review).

Scheig, R. L., and Bornstein, P.: Tuberous sclerosis in the adult. Arch. Intern. Med., *108*:789, 1961.

Tilgen, W.: Zur Ultrastruktur der sogenannten White leaf-shaped macules bei der tuberösen Hirnsklerose Bourneville-Pringle. Arch. derm. Forsch., *248*:13, 1973.

Hypertrophic Scar and Keloid

Linares, H. A., Kischer, C. W., Dobrkovsky, M., and Larson, D. L.: The histiotypic organization of the hypertrophic scar in humans. J. Invest. Derm., *59*:323, 1972.

Linares, H. A., and Larson, D. L.: Early differential diagnosis between hypertrophic and nonhypertrophic healing. J. Invest. Derm., *62*:514, 1974.

Mancini, R. E., and Quaife, J. V.: Histogenesis of experimentally produced keloids. J. Invest. Derm., *38*:143, 1962.

Nikolowski, W.: Pathogenese, Klinik und Therapie des Keloids. Arch. klin. exp. Derm., *212*:550, 1961.

Giant Cell Epulis

Geschickter, C. F., and Copeland, M. M.: Tumors of Bone. ed. 2. New York, Am. J. Cancer, 1936.

Sachs, W., and Garbe, W.: Multinucleated (giant) cell tumor of the gum (epulis). Arch. Derm. Syph., *38*:603, 1938.

Desmoid Tumor

Fleischmajer, R., Nedwick, A., and Reeves, J. R. T.: Juvenile fibromatoses. Arch. Derm., *107*: 574, 1973.

Gonatas, N. K.: Extra-abdominal desmoid tumors. Arch. Path., *71*:214, 1961.

Hunt, R. T. N., Morgan, H. C., and Ackerman, L. V.: Principles in the management of extra-abdominal desmoids. Cancer, *13*:825, 1960.

Shapiro, L.: Infantile digital fibromatosis and aponeurotic fibroma. Arch. Derm., *99*:37, 1969.

Weary, P. E., Linthicum, A., Cawley, E. P., *et al.*: Gardner's Syndrome. Arch. Derm., *90*: 20, 1964.

Atypical Fibroxanthoma of the Skin

Fretzin, D. F., and Helwig, E. B.: Atypical fibroxanthoma of the skin. Cancer, *31*:1541, 1973.

Gordon, H. W.: Pseudosarcomatous reticulo-histiocytoma. Arch. Derm., *90*:319, 1964.

Helwig, E. B.: Atypical fibroxanthoma. Texas J. Med., *59*:664, 1963.

Hudson, A. W., and Winkelmann, R. K.: Atypical fibroxanthoma of the skin: a reappraisal of 19 cases in which the original diagnosis was spindle-cell squamous carcinoma. Cancer, *29*:413, 1972.

Kempson, R. L., and McGavran, M. H.: Atypical fibroxanthomas of the skin. Cancer, *17*:1465, 1964.

Kroe, D. J., and Pitcock, J. A.: Atypical fibroxanthoma of the skin. Am. J. Clin. Path., *51*:487, 1969.

Levan, N. E., Hirsch, P., and Kwong, M. Q.: Pseudosarcomatous dermatofibroma. Arch. Derm., *88*:908, 1963.

Niemi, K. M.: The benign fibrohistiocytic tumors of the skin. Acta dermatoven., *50*: suppl. 63, 1970.

Samitz, M. H.: Pseudosarcoma. Arch. Derm., *96*:283, 1967.

Soule, E. H., and Enriquez, P.: Atypical fibrous histiocytoma, malignant fibrous histiocytoma, malignant histiocytoma, and epithelioid sarcoma. Cancer, *30*:128, 1972.

Tapernoux, B., Jeanneret, J. P., and Delacrétaz, J.: Fibroxanthome atypique. Dermatologica, *142*:93, 1971.

Nodular Pseudosarcomatous Fasciitis

Enterline, H. T., Culberson, J. D., Rochlin, D. B., and Brady, L. W.: Liposarcoma. Cancer, *13*:932, 1960.

Hutter, R. V. P., Stewart, F. W., and Foote, F. W., Jr.: Fasciitis. Cancer, *15*:992, 1962.

Konwaler, B. E., Keasby, L., and Kaplan, L.: Subcutaneous pseudosarcomatous fibromatosis (fasciitis). Am. J. Clin. Path., *25*:241, 1955.

Mehregan, A. H.: Nodular fasciitis. Arch. Derm., *93*:204, 1966.

Price, E. B., Jr., Siliphant, W. M., and Shuman, R.: Nodular fasciitis, a clinico-pathologic analysis of 65 cases. Am. J. Clin. Path., *35*: 122, 1961.

Röckl, H., and Schubert, E.: Fasciitis nodularis pseudosarcomatosa. Hautarzt, *22*:150, 1971.

Soule, E. H.: Proliferative (nodular) fasciitis. Arch. Path., *73*:437, 1962.

Stout, A. P.: Pseudosarcomatous fasciitis in children. Cancer, *14*:1216, 1961.

Dermatofibrosarcoma Protuberans

Binkley, G. W.: Dermatofibrosarcoma protuberans. Arch. Derm. Syph., *40*:578, 1939.

Gentele, H.: Malignant fibroblastic tumors of the skin. Acta dermatoven., *31*:Suppl. 27, 1951 (review).

Hashimoto, K., Brownstein, M. H., and Iakobiec, F. A.: Dermatofibrosarcoma protuberans. Arch. Derm., *110*:874, 1974.

Kanaar, P., and Oort, J.: Fibrosarcomas developing in scar tissue. Dermatologica, *138*: 313, 1969.

McPeak, C. J., Cruz, T., and Nicastri, A. D.: Dermatofibrosarcoma protuberans: An analysis of 86 cases—five with metastasis. Ann. Surg., *166*(Suppl. 12): 803, 1967.

Mopper, C., and Pinkus, H.: Dermatofibrosarcoma protuberans. Am. J. Clin. Path., *20*: 171, 1950.

Sauter, L. S., and DeFeo, C. P.: Dermatofibrosarcoma protuberans of the face. Arch. Derm., *104*:671, 1971.

Sims, C. F., and Kirsch, N.: Spindle cell epidermoid epithelioma simulating sarcoma in chronic radiodermatitis. Arch. Derm. Syph., *57*:63, 1948.

Taylor, H. B., and Helwig, E. B.: Dermatofibrosarcoma protuberans. Cancer, *15*:717, 1961.

Vargas-Cortes, F., Winkelmann, R. K., and Soule, E. H.: Atypical fibroxanthomas of the skin. Mayo Clinic Proc., *48*:211, 1973.

Woolridge, W. E.: Dermatofibrosarcoma protuberans. Arch. Derm., *75*:132, 1957.

Subcutaneous Fibrosarcoma

Enzinger, F. M.: Epithelioid sarcoma: a sarcoma simulating a granuloma or a carcinoma. Cancer, *26*:1029, 1970.

Fisher, E. R., and Horvat, B.: The fibrocytic derivation of the so-called epithelioid sarcoma. Cancer, *30*:1074, 1972.

Frable, W. J., Kay, S., Lawrence, W., and Schatzki, P. F.: Epithelioid sarcoma. Arch. Path., *95*:8, 1973.

Gentele, H.: Malignant fibroblastic tumors of the skin. Acta dermatoven., *31*:Suppl. 27, 1951.

Kempson, R. L., and Kyriakos, M.: Fibroxanthosarcoma of the soft tissues. A type of malignant fibrous histiocytoma. Cancer, *29*: 961, 1972.

Pritchard, D. J., Soule, E. H., Taylor, W. F., and Ivins, J. C.: Fibrosarcoma, a clinicopathologic and statistical study of 199 tumors of the soft tissue of the extremities and trunk. Cancer, *33*:888, 1974.

Stout, A. P.: Fibrosarcoma in infants and children. Cancer, *15*:1028, 1962.

Cutaneous Myxoma

Johnson, W. C., and Helwig, E. B.: Cutaneous focal mucinosis. Arch. Derm., *93*:13, 1966.

Digital Mucous Cyst

Bourns, H. K., and Sanerkin, N. G.: Mucoid lesions ("mucoid cysts") of the fingers and toes. Brit. J. Surg., *50*:860, 1963.

Götz, H., and Koch, R.: Zur Klinik, Pathogenese und Therapie der sogenannten "Dorsalcysten." Hautarzt, *7*:533, 1956.

Johnson, W. C., Graham, J. H., and Helwig, E. B.: Cutaneous myxoid cyst. J.A.M.A., *191*: 15, 1965.

MacKee, G. M., and Andrews, G. C.: The pathologic histology of synovial lesions of the skin. Arch. Derm. Syph., *5*:561, 1922.

Newmeyer, W. L., Kilgore, E. S., Jr., and Graham, W. P., III: Mucous cysts: the dorsal distal interphalangeal joint ganglion. Plast. Reconst. Surg., *53*:313, 1974.

Mucous Cyst of Oral Mucosa

Braun-Falco, O.: Über ein Schleimgranulom der Zunge. Hautarzt, *11*:131, 1960.

Ehlers, G.: Zur Histogenese der Lippenschleimcysten. Z. Haut Geschlechtskr., *34*:77, 1963.

Lattanand, A., Johnson, W. C., and Graham, J. H.: Mucous cyst (mucocele). Arch. Derm., *101*:673, 1970.

Nikolowski, W.: Schleimcysten und sog. Schleimgranulom der Unterlippe. Arch. klin. exp. Derm., *203*:246, 1956.

Weir, T. W., and Johnson, W. C.: Cheilitis glandularis. Arch. Derm., *103*:433, 1971.

Myxosarcoma

Enterline, H. T., Culberson, J. D., Rochlin, D. B., and Brady, L. W.: Liposarcoma. Cancer, *13*:932, 1960.

Korting, G. W., and Nürnberger, F.: Zur Frage des Lipidgehaltes von Myxosarkomen. Arch. klin. exp. Derm., *230*:172, 1967.

Sponsel, K. H., McDonald, J. R., and Ghormley, R. K.: Myxoma and myxosarcoma of the soft tissues of the extremities. J. Bone Joint Surg., *34A*:820, 1952.

Stout, A. P.: Myxoma, the tumor of primitive mesenchyme. Ann. Surg., *127*:706, 1948.

29

Tumors of Vascular Tissue

CONGENITAL HEMANGIOMAS

Three types of congenital hemangioma are recognized aside from angiokeratoma circumscriptum, which will be discussed together with the other types of angiokeratoma (see p. 595). The three types of congenital hemangioma are: (1) nevus flammeus, (2) capillary hemangioma, and (3) cavernous hemangioma.

NEVUS FLAMMEUS

Nevus flammeus, or nevus telangiectaticus, the so-called port-wine nevus, is characterized by one or several dull-red or bluish-red patches of irregular outline, not elevated above the level of the skin. Two types occur: the medially located nevus flammeus, most commonly found in the occipital region and not associated with other abnormalities; and the laterally located nevus flammeus, usually unilateral in location but occasionally bilateral and most commonly found on one side or both sides of the face or on one or several extremities. It frequently is associated with malformations of some larger blood vessels (Schnyder, 1954). Depending on which larger vessels are involved, the term Sturge-Weber syndrome or Klippel-Trenaunay syndrome is used.

In the *Sturge-Weber syndrome* (oculomeningeal nevus flammeus), the nevus flammeus is located on one side of the face and is associated with ipsilateral retinal and meningeal angiomatosis leading to ipsilateral

buphthalmos or glaucoma and to contralateral hemiparesis or epilepsy. In roentgenograms intracranial calcification outlining the contour of cerebral gyri and sulci may be seen (Bluefarb; Krayenbühl et al.; Furukawa et al.).

In the *Klippel-Trenaunay syndrome* (osteohypertrophic nevus flammeus), one observes on one extremity or on several extremities affected with a nevus flammeus hypertrophy of the soft tissues and bones. Associated with this are varicosities or an arteriovenous fistula, or both (Mullins et al.; Lindenauer). It is assumed that the osteohypertrophy is the result of venous hypertension caused by the varicosities or by the fistula (Defauw).

In some instances of the Klippel-Trenaunay syndrome that are associated with an arteriovenous fistula one finds, in addition to the reddish areas of the nevus flammeus, painful violaceous nodules or plaques on the toes, feet or legs which may undergo ulceration (Bluefarb and Adams; Waterson et al.; Earhart et al.). Occasionally, similar purplish plaques are seen in chronic venous insufficiency (Mali et al.). The cutaneous lesions simulate Kaposi's sarcoma both clinically and histologically, so that Earhart et al. refer to these lesions as *pseudo-Kaposi sarcoma.*

Histopathology. No abnormalities are observed in histologic sections of a nevus flammeus if the biopsy is carried out in infancy or early childhood. Telangiectases first become apparent histologically in patients around 10 years of age (Miescher; Schnyder, 1954). The capillary ectasias thereafter gradually increase with age. Ultimately, not only the superficial capillaries but also some of the capillaries in the deeper layers of the dermis and in the subcutaneous layer are dilated (Fig. 29-1). No proliferation of endothelial cells is seen.

In the so-called pseudo-Kaposi sarcoma lesions associated with the arteriovenous fistulas of the Klippel-Trenaunay syndrome one observes a proliferation of capillaries and fibroblasts, extravasation of red cells, and deposition of hemosiderin in the dermis. In contrast with Kaposi's sarcoma, so-called vascular slits and atypicality of the nuclei of endothelial cells and fibroblasts are absent (Bluefarb and Adams; Waterson et al.).

Histogenesis. Since in nevus flammeus no histologic abnormalities are present early in life, and no endothelial proliferation is ever seen, it appears likely that the nevus flammeus is the result of a congenital weakness of the capillary walls (Schnyder, 1954). Thus, the nevus flammeus represents a telangiectasia and not a true angioma.

CAPILLARY HEMANGIOMA

Capillary hemangioma, or strawberry mark, consists of one or several bright-red, soft, lobulated tumors. The lesion first appears between the third and the fifth week of life, increases in size for several months, and then, in contrast to the other two forms of congenital hemangioma, starts to regress spontaneously and often involutes completely within a few years. In cases of extensive capillary hemangiomas often a cavernous hemangioma is situated in the underlying tissue.

Histopathology. Capillary hemangiomas during their period of growth in early infancy show considerable proliferation of their endothelial cells. The endothelial cells are large and are aggregated predominantly in solid strands and masses in which one observes only a few small capillary lumina. In maturing lesions the capillary lumina are wider, and the endothelial cells lining them appear flatter (Fig. 29-2). Still later, fibrosis increasingly replaces the capillaries, leading to a gradual shrinking of the lesion (Walsh and Tompkins; Schnyder, 1957).

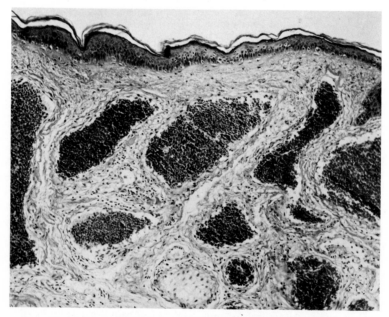

FIG. 29-1. **Congenital hemangioma: Nevus flammeus.** The capillaries are greatly dilated, engorged with blood, and lined by a single layer of endothelial cells. (×100)

CAVERNOUS HEMANGIOMA

Cavernous hemangioma consists of a large, predominantly subcutaneous mass that may cause considerable deformity. The overlying skin may be normal, but often it is the site of a capillary hemangioma.

The association of an extensive cavernous hemangioma with thrombocytopenia and purpura was first described by Kasabach and Merritt. Although the *Kasabach-Merritt syndrome* occurs largely in infants, occasionally it can be seen in adults (Straub et al.). This syndrome also can be associated with other forms of extensive hemangioma, e.g., with capillary hemangioma or with multiple glomangiomas (see p. 601). The purpura is a result not just of thrombocytopenia, as was assumed at first, but represents a consumption coagulopathy in which blood coagulation and the associated fibrin formation within the hemangioma causes a consumption of platelets, fibrinogen, prothrombin and plasminogen (Rodriguez-Erdmann; Tappeiner and Wolff; Straub et al.).

There are two rare congenital conditions in which innumerable cavernous hemangiomas occur: the blue rubber-bleb nevus and Maffucci's syndrome. In the *blue rubber-bleb nevus* the cavernous hemangiomas are soft, compressible and bluish. They vary from a rather small size to 4 cm in diameter. The larger hemangiomas are raised above the level of the skin. In addition, subcutaneous hemangiomas often are felt on palpation. The regular presence of hemangiomas in the intestinal tract causes chronic bleeding and anemia. In one patient, autopsy revealed many visceral hemangiomas in addition to those of the intestinal tract (Rice and Fischer).

The outstanding features in *Maffucci's syndrome* are (1) dyschondroplasia resulting in defects in ossification, (2) fragility of the bones causing severe deformities, and (3) osteochondromas which may develop into chondrosarcomas. In addition, large, compressible cutaneous and subcutaneous cavernous hemangiomas are present (Bean). Occasionally, as in the blue rubber-bleb nevus, intestinal hemangiomas are present, causing chronic intestinal bleeding (Sakurane et al.).

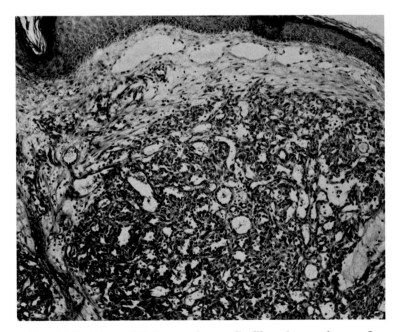

FIG. 29-2. **Congenital hemangioma: Capillary hemangioma.** One observes considerable proliferation of endothelial cells and numerous capillary lumina. ($\times 100$)

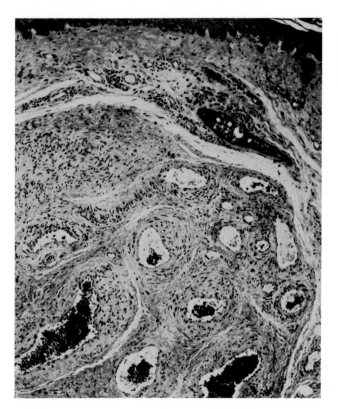

FIG. 29-3. **Congenital hemangioma: Cavernous hemangioma.** The blood vessels show a single layer of thin endothelial cells and a thick fibrous wall. (×100)

Histopathology. Cavernous hemangiomas show in the lower dermis and the subcutaneous tissue large irregular spaces filled with blood. The spaces are lined by a single layer of thin endothelial cells and by a fibrous wall of varying thickness (Fig. 29-3). If the fibrous wall is thick, it generally is the result of a proliferation of adventitial cells.

In the BLUE RUBBER-BLEB NEVUS the cavernous hemangiomas also show, as a rule, a thin layer of endothelial cells and a thin rim of fibrous tissue (Rice and Fischer). However, some of the subcutaneous hemangiomas have a thick fibrous wall. In children, some of the superficially located hemangiomas show endothelial proliferation, as seen in capillary hemangiomas (Fretzin and Potter).

In MAFFUCCI'S SYNDROME similarly most cavernous hemangiomas are lined by a thin endothelial layer (Mullins and Livingood). A few, however, may show proliferation of their endothelial cells with numerous small irregular lumina enclosed in the endothelial proliferations (Kuzma and King).

ANGIOKERATOMA

Five types of angiokeratoma occur (Lynch and Kosanovich): (1) the generalized systemic type—angiokeratoma corporis diffusum of Fabry (already discussed on p. 368); (2) the bilateral form occurring on the fingers and toes—angiokeratoma of Mibelli; (3) the localized scrotal form—angiokeratoma of Fordyce; (4) the usually solitary papular angiokeratoma; and (5) angiokeratoma circumscriptum, the only form of angiokeratoma that is apt to be present at birth.

Angiokeratoma Mibelli, Angiokeratoma Scroti, Papular Angiokeratoma

In angiokeratoma Mibelli, several dark-red papules with a slightly verrucous surface are seen on the dorsa of the fingers and toes. Usually the lesions appear in childhood or adolescence and measure from 3 to 5 mm in diameter (Haye and Rebello).

In angiokeratoma of the scrotum, multiple vascular papules, 2 to 4 mm in diameter are seen on the scrotum, arising in middle or later life. Early lesions are red, soft and compressible, whereas later they become bluish, keratotic and noncompressible (Agger and Osmundsen).

In papular angiokeratoma, usually one and occasionally several papular lesions, 2 to 8 mm in diameter, arise in young adults, most commonly on the lower extremities. Early lesions appear bright red and soft, but later they become bluish, firm, and hyperkeratotic (Imperial and Helwig, 1967, I).

Histopathology. The histologic findings are the same in all three above-mentioned types of angiokeratoma (Imperial and Helwig, 1967, I). They represent telangiectasias and are not true hemangiomas.

Early lesions show dilated capillaries in the uppermost dermis partially enclosed by elongated rete ridges. Older lesions are hyperkeratotic and some of the dilated capillaries may be completely encircled by rete ridges. Occasionally, organized or organizing thrombi are observed within the dilated capillaries. In some instances, the dilatation of vessels is not limited to the uppermost

dermis, but is present also in the middermis (Imperial and Helwig, 1967, I).

Angiokeratoma Circumscriptum

Angiokeratoma circumscriptum represents a localized lesion composed of small, superficial, purplish, cystic nodules that coalesce in the center of the lesion where they appear hyperkeratotic. Usually, the lesion is present at birth, but in some cases it does not appear until childhood or adolescence (Dammert). Commonly, the lesion enlarges in size as the patient grows older; and with age, the lesion becomes increasingly hyperkeratotic (Imperial and Helwig, 1967, II). In most instances, the lesion measures only a few centimeters in size, and often shows a linear configuration. The clinical resemblance between angiokeratoma circumscriptum and lymphangioma circumscriptum is often great (see p. 600), and intermediate forms occur in which some of the superficial cystic nodules contain blood and others lymph fluid.

Angiokeratoma circumscriptum may be

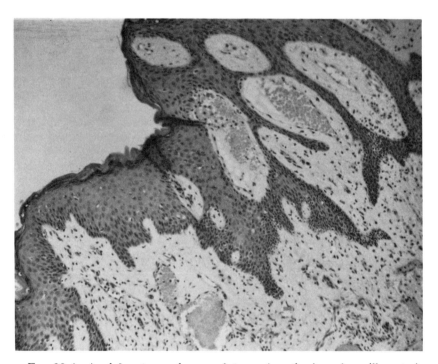

FIG. 29-4. **Angiokeratoma circumscriptum.** Acanthosis and papillomatosis are present. Greatly dilated capillaries are seen in the upper as well as in the lower dermis. Some capillaries are enclosed within the papillary epidermis. (×50)

associated with a nevus flammeus (Dammert) or with a cavernous hemangioma (Knoth et al.; Lynch and Kosanovich). Also, the Klippel-Trenaunay syndrome consisting of osteohypertrophy of one leg (see p. 591) has been observed in patients with angiokeratoma circumscriptum, even in the absence of an associated nevus flammeus (Fischer and Friederich).

Histopathology. Varying degrees of hyperkeratosis, papillomatosis, and irregular acanthosis are present. Greatly dilated capillaries are seen just beneath, or enclosed within, the papillomatous epidermis (Fig. 29-4). Thrombi may be present in some of the dilated capillaries (Bruce). In contrast to papular angiokeratoma, which is purely a superficial telangiectasia, an underlying capillary or cavernous hemangioma is present regularly in the underlying dermis and subcutaneous tissue of angiokeratoma circumscriptum (Imperial and Helwig, 1967, II; Lynch and Kosanovich).

ANGIOMA SERPIGINOSUM

Angioma serpiginosum shows as primary lesions deeply red, not palpable puncta that are grouped closely together in a macular, linear, mottled, or netlike pattern. The disorder is asymptomatic. It usually begins in early adult life and extends slowly for several years (Frain-Bell). Irregular extension at the periphery of larger lesions may cause them to have a serpiginous border. Women are more commonly affected than men. The lower extremities are most frequently involved. The deeply red puncta represent dilated capillaries. Even though they usually do not blanch completely, they do not represent purpura and bleed freely when pricked (Barker and Sachs).

Histopathology. The only histologic anomaly consists of the presence of scattered, moderately dilated capillaries in the dermal papillae and the upper dermis. No inflammatory infiltrate or extravasation of red cells is observed (Frain-Bell; Barker and Sachs; Stevenson and Lincoln). In contrast to normal capillaries, the dilated capillaries in angioma serpiginosum show no alkaline phosphatase activity (McGrae and Winkelmann).

Histogenesis. Angioma serpiginosum may be regarded as a telangiectasia of existing blood vessels in the papillary and subpapillary region of the dermis, resulting from a functional abnormality of these capillaries (Frain-Bell). Thus, the term *essential telangiectasia* suggested by McGrae and Winkelmann would seem preferable to the term *angioma serpiginosum,* except that the latter term has priority, having been used first by Radcliffe-Crocker in 1893 (Frain-Bell).

GRANULOMA PYOGENICUM

Granuloma pyogenicum occurs as a single lesion with but few exceptions (Juhlin et al.). It consists of a dull-red, soft or moderately firm, raised, slightly pedunculated nodule. It grows rapidly to a size of usually 0.5 cm, but occasionally up to 2 cm, and then remains unchanged. The surface may be smooth, but often it shows superficial ulceration and crusting. The lesion bleeds easily when traumatized. Although a granuloma pyogenicum may occur anywhere on the skin, it is found most commonly on the fingers and the face. The oral cavity, particularly the gingiva, is a rather common site for granuloma pyogenicum, with pregnancy often as a precipitating factor (Martens and MacPherson; Leyden and Master).

In a few instances the development of multiple small angiomatous satellite lesions has been observed following the removal of a granuloma pyogenicum of the trunk (Coskey and Mehregan; Warner and Wilson Jones). This may occur either with or without recurrence of the primary lesion. When left untreated, the satellite lesions either involute or remain unchanged. In a few instances satellite lesions have appeared following mechanical irritation of a granuloma pyogenicum (Zaynoun et al.). It is of interest that nearly all reported instances of multiple satellites around lesions of granuloma pyogenicum occurred on the trunk, and particularly in the scapular region, although this is a rather rare location for granuloma pyogenicum.

Histopathology. On histologic examination one finds a circumscribed lesion covered by a flattened epidermis and containing numerous newly formed capillaries that possess prominent endothelial cells and show

FIG. 29-5. **Granuloma pyogenicum.** The lesion is pedunculated and covered by a flattened epidermis. One observes considerable proliferation of endothelial cells and numerous capillary lumina. The stroma is edematous and free of inflammatory infiltration. (×50)

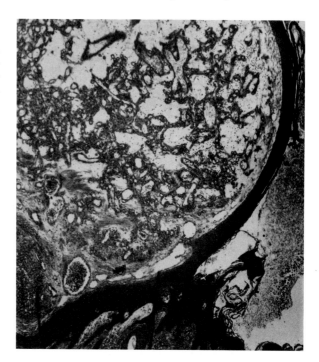

varying degrees of dilatation (Fig. 29-5). The stroma in which the capillary proliferations are embedded appears edematous and does not contain mature collagen bundles. The epidermis as a rule shows inward growth at the base of the lesion and thus produces a so-called epidermal collarette, causing slight pedunculation of the lesion.

In early lesions one finds no inflammatory reaction (Nödl; Oehlschlaegel and Müller). In older lesions, because of erosion of the thinned epidermis, secondary inflammatory changes often are present in the stroma.

The satellite lesions seen following removal or irritation of a granuloma pyogenicum have the histologic appearance of a capillary hemangioma without the pedunculation seen in typical lesions of granuloma pyogenicum (Coskey and Mehregan; Warner and Wilson Jones; Zaynoun et al.).

Histogenesis. Formerly, it was widely assumed that granuloma pyogenicum was caused by pyogenic infection of a small wound. However, the histologic picture of an early lesion with its endothelial proliferation is that of a capillary hemangioma (Nödl; Oehlschlaegel and Müller); and even older eroded lesions showing a pronounced inflammatory infiltrate in their superficial portion retain the appearance of a capillary hemangioma in their deeper portions.

Differential Diagnosis. Differentiation from the type of capillary hemangioma that occurs in infancy usually is easy because of the raised, pedunculated growth of granuloma pyogenicum, the thinning of the epidermis over the tumor, the collarette formation at the base of the tumor, and the edema of the stroma.

Lesions of granuloma pyogenicum with a fairly pronounced inflammatory infiltrate may greatly resemble granulation tissue, except that granuloma pyogenicum possesses a flattened epidermis with collarette formation and shows in the deeper layers no inflammatory reaction but only vascular proliferation (Oehlschlaegel and Müller).

Early Kaposi's sarcoma may show vascular proliferation and an inflammatory infiltrate like granuloma pyogenicum. However, there usually is no atrophy of the epidermis or collarette formation, and, on careful searching or deeper sectioning, areas of fibroblastic proliferation and of extravasations of red cells can in most instances be found (Peterson et al.).

CHERRY HEMANGIOMA

Cherry hemangiomas are bright-red lesions varying in size from a punctum to a soft, raised, dome-shaped lesion measuring several millimeters in diameter. This very common lesion, present often in large numbers, may already start appearing in early adult life; and the number of lesions increases with age. Cherry hemangiomas may occur anywhere on the skin, but the trunk is the most common site.

Histopathology. Cherry hemangiomas in their early stage of development have the appearance of a true capillary hemangioma, since they are composed of numerous newly formed capillaries with narrow lumina and prominent endothelial cells arranged in a lobular fashion in the subpapillary region (Schnyder and Keller). As the lesion ages, the capillaries become dilated. In a fully matured cherry hemangioma one observes numerous moderately dilated capillaries lined by flattened endothelial cells. The intercapillary stroma shows edema and homogenization of the collagen. The epidermis is thinned and often surrounds most of the angioma as a collarette (Salamon et al.).

PAPULAR ANGIOPLASIA

Multiple soft purplish vascular papules are seen on the face of elderly persons, measuring only a few millimeters in diameter. They may involute spontaneously (Wilson Jones and Marks).

Histopathology. Atypical vascular proliferations are seen in the dermis. Small capillary lumina are lined by numerous large, protruding endothelial cells, occasionally forming a double layer (Peterson et al.). The stroma between the vessels contains numerous cells. Some of them resemble endothelial cells and others fibroblastic cells; but many appear atypical by being hyperchromatic and occasionally multinucleated (Wilson Jones and Marks). Extravasated erythrocytes may be found in the stroma (Peterson et al.).

Differential Diagnosis. Without adequate clinical data it is obvious that one cannot rule out a malignant vascular tumor, especially malignant angioendothelioma or Kaposi's sarcoma.

VENOUS LAKES

Venous lakes are small, dark-blue, slightly raised, soft, compressible lesions occurring on the exposed skin of older persons. Usu-

ally, several lesions are present. The face, ears, and lips are the most common sites.

Histopathology. Venous lakes are not true hemangiomas but represent dilated veins. From the beginning they show a greatly dilated space filled with erythrocytes and lined by a single layer of flattened endothelial cells and a thin wall of fibrous tissue (Bean and Walsh).

THROMBOSED CAPILLARY OR VEIN

A dome-shaped or slightly lobulated, blue-black nodule arises either abruptly or gradually. There may be a rim of erythema or brownish pigmentation around it. In most instances the patient has not been aware of a pre-existing lesion (Epstein et al.). The size of the nodule varies between 5 and 10 mm in most instances. The face is the most common site, but other areas may be involved, including the oral mucosa (Weathers and Fine). The lesion is of significance largely because of its clinical resemblance to a malignant melanoma.

Histopathology. The upper dermis shows one or several greatly dilated vascular lumina filled with thrombi (Epstein et al.; Weiner). The thrombi may show invasion by fibroblasts in one or several areas, indicating beginning organization (Epstein et al.). Extravasated red cells and hemosiderin may be present in the upper dermis around such thrombosed lumina.

In instances in which several adjoining vascular lumina are thrombosed and dilated thrombosed lumina are present not only in the dermis but also in the epidermis, the pre-existing lesion obviously was a papular angiokeratoma (see p. 595) (Hayen; Weiner). In other instances, a solitary thrombosed lumen is surrounded by a venous wall and the pre-existing lesion may have been a venous lake of the face (Epstein et al.). It is not possible, however, to identify the nature of the pre-existing lesion in all cases.

NEVUS ARANEUS

Nevus araneus, or spider nevus, shows a central, slightly elevated, red punctum from which fine blood vessels radiate. Occasionally, pulsation can be observed. The face is the most common site. Although spider nevi often arise spontaneously, pregnancy and cirrhosis of the liver are two factors predisposing to their appearance.

Histopathology. An ascending central artery whose wall shows either muscular tissue or, rarely, several layers of glomus cells (see p. 38) widens into a subepidermal, thin-walled ampulla. Delicate arterial branches radiate from the ampulla and divide into capillaries (Bean; Schuhmachers-Brendler; Whiting et al.).

FAMILIAL HEMORRHAGIC TELANGIECTASIA (OSLER)

This dominantly inherited disorder is characterized by the presence of numerous telangiectases on the skin and on the mucous membranes of the nose and the mouth. In addition, more or less widely disseminated telangiectases may be found in many viscera, such as the gastrointestinal tract, the adrenals, the brain, the lungs, the spleen, and the liver (Zelman). Asymptomatic gastro-

intestinal bleeding occurs in about 15 per cent of the patients, especially in later life (Smith et al.). The presence of numerous telangiectases in the interstitial tissue of the liver may be associated with portal fibrosis, and the latter may lead to cirrhosis (Zelman; Muggia). Patients with Osler's disease may show malformations of the larger blood vessels, such as arteriovenous fistulae in the lungs or the brain (Chandler) or aneurysms of the aorta or of the splenic or hepatic artery (Muggia).

Histopathology. In the areas of cutaneous telangiectasia one finds thin-walled dilated dermal capillaries. The reason for the tendency to bleeding lies in the increased content of plasminogen activator in the telangiectatic lesions, resulting in increased fibrinolytic activity in the pericapillary tissue. This can be demonstrated histochemically by the existence of increased lysis of plasminogen-rich fibrin preparations in the pericapillary areas (Kwaan and Silverman).

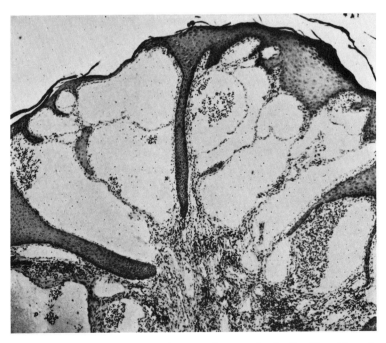

FIG. 29-6. **Lymphangioma circumscriptum.** Cystically dilated lymph vessels lined by a single layer of endothelial cells are present in the upper dermis. The epidermis shows downward growth and more or less surrounds some of the lymph vessels. There is moderate hyperkeratosis. (×50)

LYMPHANGIOMA

Three types of lymphangioma exist: (1) localized lymphangioma circumscriptum, corresponding to papular angiokeratoma; (2) the classical type of lymphangioma circumscriptum, corresponding to angiokeratoma circumscriptum; and (3) cavernous lymphangioma, or the "spongy" type of lymphangioma, corresponding to cavernous hemangioma (Peachey et al.).

LOCALIZED LYMPHANGIOMA CIRCUMSCRIPTUM

The lesion consists clinically of a single small patch of thick-walled vesicles that resemble frogs' spawn if they are filled solely with lymph fluid. In many cases, however, some of the vesicles have a purplish color because of an admixture of blood. The lesion usually appears in later life and usually measures less than 1 cm in diameter (Peachey et al.; Fisher and Orkin).

Histopathology. Cystically dilated lymph vessels lined by a single layer of endothelium are present in the uppermost portion of the dermis (Fig. 29-6). Occasionally, these lymph vessels contain, in addition to lymph, also some erythrocytes. The epidermis varies in thickness. Over some of the lymph cysts it is thinned; elsewhere it may show acanthosis, papillomatosis, hyperkeratosis, and irregular downward growth. Some of the dilated lymph vessels may appear to be enclosed in the epidermis. The dilatation of lymph vessels may extend as far down as the middermis but not below this level (Peachey et al.).

LYMPHANGIOMA CIRCUMSCRIPTUM

In the classical type of lymphangioma circumscriptum one or several patches with translucent vesicles are present, and the condition may be quite extensive. The lesions are present at birth or appear in early life. In many instances there is a mild degree of diffuse swelling of the subcutaneous tissue beneath the vesicular lesions. Some of the vesicles contain an admixture of blood. The skin surface between and even on top of some of the vesicles may be verrucous in appearance.

Histopathology. The histologic appearance of the epidermis and upper dermis is similar to that described for localized lymphangioma circumscriptum, although the degree of hyperkeratosis and papillomatosis is usually greater. However, the dilatation of the lymph vessels extends to the deeper zones of the dermis and even into the subcutaneous fat. The lymph vessels in the subcutaneous fat are often of large caliber and their walls contain considerably hypertrophied muscle fibers (Peachey et al.).

CAVERNOUS LYMPHANGIOMA

Cavernous lymphangioma, which may or may not show an overlying superficial lymphangioma circumscriptum, causes diffuse enlargement of the affected region, for instance macrocheilia and macroglossia.

Histopathology. Large, irregular lymph spaces often containing also some erythrocytes are present in the deep portions of the dermis and in the subcutis. In areas such as the lip or tongue the lymph spaces extend between the voluntary muscle bundles, separating them from one another and giving the tissue a spongelike appearance (Peachey et al.).

GLOMUS TUMOR

Two types of glomus tumors exist: solitary, and multiple. The more common *solitary type* shows a purplish nodule measuring only a few millimeters in diameter. The nodule is tender and gives rise to severe paroxysmal pains. Most commonly, the nodule is situated on the extremities, especially in the nail bed.

Multiple glomus tumors are much less common than the solitary type. In contrast to the solitary type, which is not inherited, the multiple type in some instances is dominantly transmitted (Schnyder). The lesions either are localized to one area (Laymon and Peterson) or are generalized (McEvoy et al.). They are asymptomatic as a rule, but occasionally there is tenderness or pain in some or even in all lesions (Gupta et al.). They may be intracutaneous or subcutaneous in location. Although most of the nodules in the multiple type are small, some may reach a size of several centimeters in diameter (McEvoy et al.). Cases of multiple glomus tumors in which the lesions are large enough to be soft and compressible show considerable clinical resemblance to the lesions of the blue rubber-bleb nevus and have been mistakenly diagnosed as such even though intestinal bleeding was absent (Fine et al.; Mukhtar and Pfleger). Patients with generalized glomus tumors may show evidence of the Kasabach-Merritt syndrome, seen most commonly in extensive cavernous hemangiomas (McEvoy et al.) (see p. 593).

Histopathology. SOLITARY GLOMUS TUMORS are surrounded by a fibrous capsule. They contain numerous small vascular lumina that are lined by a single layer of flattened endothelial cells. Peripheral to the endothelial cells are a few to many layers of glomus cells (Fig. 29-7). The glomus cells have a faintly eosinophilic cytoplasm and a large, oval or cuboidal, pale nucleus. Thus they resemble epithelioid cells. In many areas the glomus cells are seen to extend irregularly from the vascular walls into the connective tissue stroma of the tumor. The connective tissue stroma of the tumor appears edematous and contains scattered fibroblasts and fairly numerous mast cells (Murad et al.). Staining with the Bodian stain shows fairly numerous nerve fibers in the perivascular stroma of solitary tumors (Shugart et al.).

MULTIPLE GLOMUS TUMORS possess no capsule and show much larger vascular spaces than the solitary glomus tumor. Because of the conspicuous vascular component the multiple glomus tumors occasionally are referred to as glomangiomas (Laymon and Peterson). The large vascular spaces usually have an irregular shape. Just as in the solitary glomus tumor, the vascular spaces are lined by a single layer of flat endothelial cells; but the number of glomus cells located peripheral to the endothelial cells is much smaller than in the solitary glomus tumor (Fig. 29-8). Usually, the glomus cells form only a narrow rim of one to three layers, and some vascular spaces

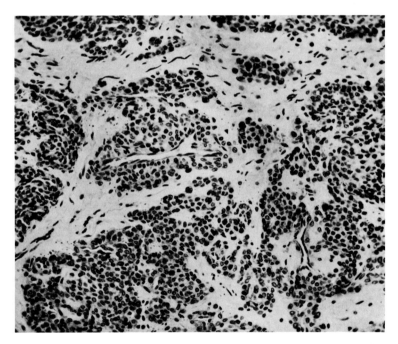

FIG. 29-7. **Solitary glomus tumor.** There are several narrow vascular lumina lined by a single layer of flattened endothelial cells. Peripheral to the endothelial cells are multiple rows of glomus cells. In addition, there are masses of glomus cells in which no vascular lumen can be seen. (×200)

may show no glomus cells (Laymon and Peterson). Rarely, a patient may show glomus cells in some of his tumors, but none in others (Schnyder). With the Bodian stain, no increase of nerve fibers is seen in association with the vascular spaces in multiple glomus tumors (Gordon and Hyman).

Histogenesis. Both solitary and multiple glomus tumors are related to the arterial segment of the cutaneous glomus, the so-called Suquet-Hoyer canal (see p. 38). By light microscopy the normal Suquet-Hoyer canal has a narrow lumen that is surrounded by a single layer of endothelial cells and 4 to 6 layers of glomus cells (see p. 38). On electron microscopy, normal glomus cells are vascular smooth muscle cells (Goodman). Similarly, the glomus cells of glomus tumors are shown by electron microscopy to be smooth muscle cells, both in the solitary glomus tumor (Murad et al.) and in multiple glomus tumors (Tarnowski and Hashimoto; Lüders et al.; Goodman and Abele). As such, glomus cells are enveloped by a finely fibrillar basal lamina and contain numerous myofilaments that measure about 5 nm in diameter and are arranged in bundles (E.M. No. 43). So-called dense bodies representing condensations that hold bundles

of myofilaments together are distributed at random in the cytoplasm and are present also on the inner surface of the plasma membrane. Many of the longitudinally sectioned glomus cells show a typically compressed and scalloped nucleus associated with contraction (Tarnowski and Hashimoto). Nonmyelinated axons embedded in the cytoplasm of Schwann cells have been found in close contact with glomus cells by some authors (Lüders et al.; Ishibashi et al.) but not by others (Tarnowski and Hashimoto).

It has been noted in some instances of multiple glomus tumors that some of the glomus cells contain relatively few myofilaments limited to the periphery of the glomus cells (Lüders et al.), and, in other instances, that the myofilaments are not held together in bundles by dense bodies and extend in different directions, so that it seems doubtful that such cells can effectively contract (Ishibashi et al.).

Differential Diagnosis. Hemangiopericytoma differs from the solitary type of glomus tumor by its larger size, by the irregular proliferation of its cells, and by the pleomorphism of its nuclei.

Multiple glomus tumors differ from the lesions of the blue rubber-bleb nevus by the

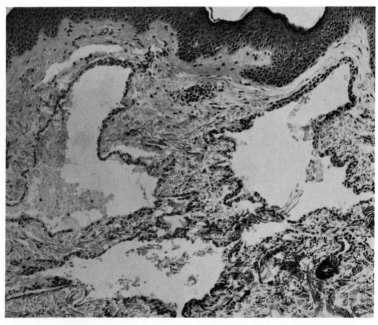

FIG. 29-8. **Multiple type of glomus tumor.** Numerous greatly dilated vascular spaces are present, lined by a single layer of flat endothelial cells. Glomus cells are seen peripheral to the endothelial cells as a narrow rim of one to three layers. (×100)

presence of glomus cells in nearly all tumors. Also, multiple glomus tumors, in contrast to the lesions of the blue rubber-bleb nevus, do not occur in the gastrointestinal tract and thus are not associated with gastrointestinal bleeding.

HEMANGIOPERICYTOMA

This rare tumor, first described by Stout and Murray in 1942, may arise wherever there are capillaries. Its most common sites are the skin, the subcutaneous and the musculoskeletal tissue (Backwinkel and Diddams), but other locations include the oral cavity, the mediastinum, and the retroperitoneal area (O'Brien and Brasfield). Hemangiopericytomas of the skin or the subcutaneous tissue have no diagnostic clinical appearance. Usually, they are solitary tumors. They vary considerably in size; they are firm and nodular. Some are entirely benign, others show an infiltrating growth, and still others cause metastases. Hemangiopericytomas of the skin are less apt to metastasize than those of internal organs. Nevertheless, metastases occur in about 20 per cent of the hemangiopericytomas of the skin (Stout, 1955). In some instances metastases have occurred several years after the complete excision of the cutaneous tumor (Forrester and Houston). Metastases may spread by way of the lymphatics or the blood stream. The lungs are the most common site of metastases. Of importance is the fact that the clinical course cannot always be foretold from the histologic appearance of the tumor (O'Brien and Brasfield).

Histopathology. The tumor is characterized by the presence of endothelium-lined tubes and sprouts surrounded by irregularly proliferating, closely packed pericytes with oval or spindle-shaped nuclei (Fig. 29-9) (Stout, 1949; Cole et al.). Reticulum fibers encircle the capillary endothelium, so that in sections stained for reticulum fibers the tumor cells are located peripheral to the periendothelial ring of reticulum. Thus, a reticulum stain often is of considerable value in the diagnosis of this tumor (Forrester and Houston; Reich). In some instances, a reticulum stain also reveals the individual tumor cells to be surrounded by a delicate network of reticulum fibers (Kuhn and Rosai). As

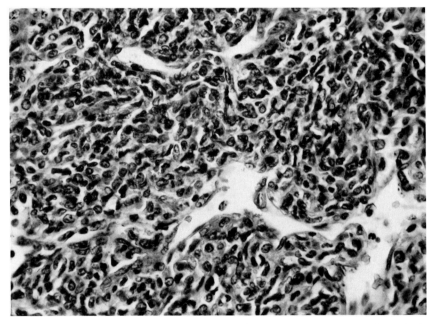

FIG. 29-9. **Hemangiopericytoma.** The capillary lumina are lined with a single layer of endothelial cells and are surrounded by irregularly proliferating, closely packed pericytes. Most of the pericytes are spindle-shaped. (×400)

a rule, hemangiopericytomas have a well-defined capsule even when they possess invasive tendencies (Backwinkel and Diddams).

In hemangiopericytomas with a malignant potential, as well as in the metastases, the tumor cells usually show nuclear pleomorphism and many mitotic figures (Cole et al.; Forrester and Houston).

Histogenesis. Hemangiopericytomas are regarded as tumors of the pericyte, a cell that is found in the walls of capillaries and venules as a discontinuous layer lying between the endothelium and the adventitial connective tissue. Pericytes are completely surrounded by the capillary basement membrane, which stains positive with the reticulum stain (see p. 37). Pericytes thus share with glomus cells the location peripheral to endothelial cells and envelopment by the basement membrane; but they differ from glomus cells (1) by their presence in the walls of capillaries and veins, rather than in the wall of the arterial Suquet-Hoyer canal; (2) by their ubiquitous distribution throughout the body; and (3) by the absence of myofilaments and so-called dense bodies (Kuhn and Rosai). It appears likely, however, that in some instances pericytes contain myofilaments and dense bodies, and that thus transitional forms exist between the pericyte and the smooth muscle cell of small arterioles (Hahn et al.).

Electron microscopic examinations of hemangiopericytomas carried out so far has revealed some of them to be composed of rather poorly differentiated mesenchymal cells that neither were surrounded by a basal lamina nor contained myofilaments (Murad et al.; Ramsey). In one instance, however, reported by Kuhn and Rosai, the hemangiopericytoma consisted predominantly of pericytes that were surrounded by a basal lamina but contained no myofilaments. In addition, it contained typical smooth muscle cells so that in the opinion expressed by Lattes this tumor represented "some kind of hybrid between classical glomus tumor and hemangiopericytoma." Similarly, in a hemangiopericytoma examined by Hahn et al. by electron microscopy the tumor cells were transitional from pericytes to smooth muscle cells, since the tumor cells not only were enveloped by basal lamina material but also contained in their cytoplasm bundles of fibrillar material and dense bodies.

Differential Diagnosis. For differentiation of hemangiopericytoma from the solitary type of glomus tumor, see page 602. Kaposi's sarcoma shows more conspicuous vascular proliferations with more prominent endothelial cells and almost always extravasations of erythrocytes. In malignant angioendothelioma, vascular lumina are more prominent than in hemangiopericytoma, and a reticulum stain, by staining the periendothelial basement membrane, will show that in hemangiopericytoma the tumor cells are located peripheral to this periendothelial ring of reticulum, whereas in angioendothelioma, whenever such a ring of reticulum can be recognized at all, the tumor cells lie inside this ring.

KAPOSI'S SARCOMA

Kaposi's sarcoma, or multiple idiopathic hemorrhagic sarcoma, is characterized by the presence of bluish-red or dark-brown plaques and nodules, particularly on the distal portions of the lower extremities. Lymphedema of the lower extremities then is common. The lesions may undergo ulceration. Occasionally, however, spontaneous involution of some of the lesions occurs. In rare instances Kaposi's sarcoma may be localized to one area (Cox et al.), or may consist of only a single lesion without tendency to progression (Cox and Helwig). Even spontaneous remissions occur (Feuerman and Potruch-Eisenkraft). As a rule, however, the disease is slowly progressive.

Occasionally, there are, in addition to cutaneous lesions, oral lesions (Reynolds et al.), or involvement of the subcutaneous lymph nodes (Duperrat and Pacot). Visceral lesions are found on autopsy in about 10 per cent of the patients (Ecklund and Valaitis). In most instances, they are asymptomatic. The most common sites in order of frequency are the gastrointestinal tract, the liver, the lungs, the abdominal lymph nodes, and the heart. In rare instances the disease is found exclusively in visceral organs (Tedeschi et al.; Anthony and Koneman) or in the subcutaneous lymph nodes (Ecklund and Valaitis).

Kaposi's sarcoma causes death in only 10 to 20 per cent of those affected with it (Cox and Helwig; Reynolds et al.; Feuerman and Potruch-Eisenkraft). Death may result from hemorrhages caused by lesions in the gastrointestinal tract or the lungs; from extensive cutaneous dissemination; from severe infiltration and ulceration of the lower extremities; or from lymphoma. The mean survival time of those dying from Kaposi's sarcoma is 9 years (O'Brien and Brasfield).

Patients with Kaposi's sarcoma show a higher incidence of lymphoma than could be accounted for by chance alone. Thus, Cox and Helwig observed 3 cases of lymphoma among 50 patients, Reynolds et al., 4 cases among 70 patients, and O'Brien and Brasfield 8 cases among 63 patients. The types of lymphoma included Hodgkin's disease, mycosis fungoides, and lymphocytic lymphoma with or without leukemia.

Kaposi's sarcoma occurs predominantly in males. Of interest is the unusually high incidence among Negroes in Central Africa. There, Kaposi's sarcoma even occurs in children in whom often extensive involvement of the subcutaneous lymph nodes precedes the appearance of cutaneous lesions. In adults visceral involvement, in addition to cutaneous lesions, is much more common than among Caucasoids (Templeton).

Histopathology. The two types of cells occurring in the walls of capillaries partici-pate in their immature state in the formation of the lesions; they are: (1) endothelial cells, and (2) pericapillary cells that are either pericytes or adventitial cells. The pericapillary cells can develop into fibroblasts. In addition, an inflammatory reaction is observed in early lesions. The prevalence of an inflammatory reaction may give early lesions the appearance of granulation tissue. Thus one may divide the lesions of Kaposi's sarcoma into early lesions resembling granulation tissue, and late neoplastic lesions. The latter may be either "angiomatous," if endothelial cell proliferation predominates, or "fibroblastic," if proliferation of pericapillary fibroblasts predominates.

In *early lesions* resembling granulation tissue, the blood vessels in the dermis are dilated and increased in number (Fig. 29-10). Their endothelial cells are large and may protrude into the lumen. There is a perivascular as well as a diffuse cellular infiltrate, varying in severity. It is composed of lymphoid cells, plasma cells, and some histiocytes. There also are groups of endothelial cells attempting to form new blood

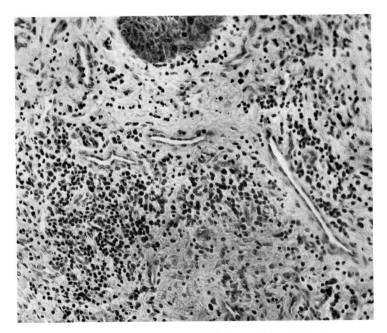

FIG. 29-10. **Kaposi's sarcoma, early lesion.** This early lesion resembles granulation tissue. The capillaries are dilated and increased in number. Their endothelial cells are large. A diffuse chronic inflammatory infiltrate is present. (×200)

vessels. Frequently, one sees small groups of extravasated erythrocytes and deposits of hemosiderin. The histologic picture in the early stage thus is not always diagnostic; however, the presence of large protruding endothelial cells, of extravasated erythrocytes, and of hemosiderin in a granulation tissue should always make one think of early Kaposi's sarcoma.

In late lesions the histologic picture may be either angiomatous or fibroblastic, but frequently both phases are found intermingled in the same lesion (Fig. 29-11). In *angiomatous lesions* one finds numerous vascular lumina. They vary greatly in size, and some may be greatly dilated. Most lumina show only a single layer of large endothelial cells, but some are surrounded in addition by fibroblasts (Fig. 29-12). The stroma in which the vessels are embedded usually contains extravasated erythrocytes and deposits of hemosiderin. There also are solid aggregates of endothelial cells; and in some of the aggregates there are elongated cells, making it impossible to decide whether they are cells differentiating toward endothelial cells or toward fibroblasts.

In *fibroblastic lesions* one observes exten-sive proliferations of spindle-shaped cells that represent young fibroblasts. They lie in strands that extend irregularly in various directions. The nuclei vary in size and staining qualities, and some of them are atypical. Mitotic figures are present, though usually they are few in number. Thus the histologic picture resembles that of a fibrosarcoma. One feature, however, distinguishes the fibroblastic lesions of Kaposi's sarcoma from fibrosarcoma: the presence of narrow slits containing erythocytes among the spindle-shaped cells (Plate 3, facing p. 586). It is usually impossible to decide whether these slits represent newly formed capillaries with an atypical endothelial lining, or whether the erythrocytes within the slits are there as a result of extravasation. Both types of formation can occur. The fact that there are nearby deposits of hemosiderin suggests that at least some of the erythocytes are outside the capillaries. Because of the diagnostic importance of the presence of erythrocytes and hemosiderin in the tissue, staining for iron, to demonstrate deposits of hemosiderin, may be advisable. The fibroblasts, being immature, form as a rule only little collagen; but staining with a reticulum stain will reveal

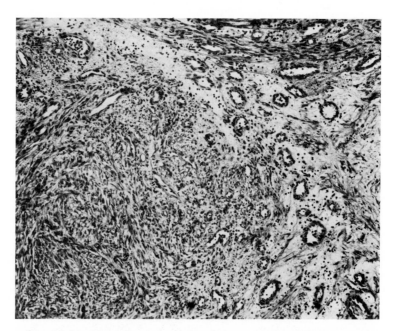

Fig. 29-11. **Kaposi's sarcoma, late lesion.** On the left the neoplasia is fibroblastic; on the right, angiomatous. (×100)

a rather dense network of reticulum fibers produced by the fibroblasts (Symmers). In addition, granules of hemosiderin are often present within fibroblasts as the result of phagocytosis (Hashimoto and Lever).

In lesions undergoing involution one may find considerable amounts of collagen that has formed as the result of maturation of the fibroblasts. Eventually, this may lead to fibrosis, cicatrization, and disappearance of the lesion.

In addition to the neoplastic proliferation of blood vessels, occasionally one may observe neoplastic proliferation of lymph vessels, resulting in formations suggesting a lymphangioma. Some of the newly formed lymphatic channels may show considerable cystic dilatation (Ronchese and Kern; Tedeschi).

Malignant degeneration of tumors with formation of metastases can occur in Kaposi's sarcoma, but it is quite rare. Often it is very difficult, if not impossible, to decide from the histologic appearance of a lesion whether it represents a very actively growing, immature tumor of Kaposi's sarcoma or a tumor that has become a true angiosarcoma

(Reed et al.). The only reliable criterion for a decision that a given tumor is metastatic rather than autochthonous is the presence of tumor cells within endothelium-lined vascular spaces, as has been observed by Cox and Helwig within pulmonary vessels. Such metastases usually have the appearance of a fibrosarcoma with few or no angiomatous elements (Reynolds et al.).

Histogenesis. The following three observations speak against the concept of Kaposi's sarcoma representing a true, metastasizing sarcoma and in favor of a mutifocal origin of the lesions: (1) There is no primary focus that enlarges progressively; (2) some lesions regress spontaneously; and (3) histologic examination may reveal very early stages in late appearing lesions.

The basic cell type giving rise to the lesions of Kaposi's sarcoma are immature, pluripotential vascular cells. On the basis of this view, Kaposi's sarcoma is a benign angiomatosis (Lang and Haslhofer; Becker and Thatcher; Cox and Helwig). This view has found support in recent electron microscopic investigations (Hashimoto and Lever; Niemi and Mustakallio; Mottaz and Zelickson). According to Hashimoto and Lever, as well as Mottaz and Zelickson, the electron microscopic studies have revealed two types of

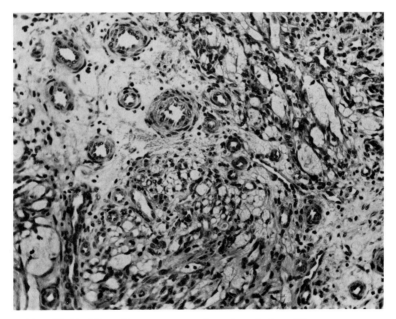

FIG. 29-12. **Kaposi's sarcoma, angiomatous lesion.** There are numerous vascular lumina. Most lumina are lined by endothelial cells, but some are surrounded in addition by fibroblasts. The edematous stroma contains extravasated erythrocytes. (×200)

cells: (1) proliferating endothelial cells, and (2) proliferating pericapillary cells developing into immature, phagocytic fibroblasts. Niemi and Mustakallio concluded that a multipotent pericapillary mesenchymal cell, identified by them as the pericyte, was the most likely cell of origin. On electron microscopic examination, it is often difficult to differentiate between the endothelial cells and the phagocytic fibroblasts, except that the endothelial cells lie adjoining to lumina and contain only a small number of lysosomes with few ferritin particles, whereas the phagocytic fibroblasts contain often several large lysosomes in which large aggregates of ferritin particles are present. Some phagocytizing fibroblasts contain, in addition, partially digested erythrocytes from which the ferritin particles are derived. Also, some of the phagocytizing fibroblasts can be seen to give rise to collagen fibrils.

Other theories concerning the origin of Kaposi's sarcoma are purely of historical interest: for example, the concept of Kaposi's disease being a disease of the reticuloendothelial system (Bluefarb and Webster; Pack and Davis), which has been invalidated by the electron microscopic findings; or the concept that Kaposi's sarcoma arises from Schwann cells (Pepler and Theron), which was based on a misinterpretation of the laminated residual bodies of lysosomes as the myelin sheaths of Schwann cells.

Differential Diagnosis. For differentiation from hemangiopericytoma, see page 604; from postmastectomy lymphangiosarcoma, see page 612.

MALIGNANT ANGIOENDOTHELIOMA

In accord with the two types of cells of which capillaries are composed—endothelial cells and pericytes—two types of hemangiosarcoma occur: malignant hemangioendothelioma and malignant hemangiopericytoma (see p. 603). Since the small lymph vessels do not possess pericytes, only one type of lymphangiosarcoma occurs: malignant lymphangioendothelioma. Since malignant hemangioendothelioma and malignant lymph-

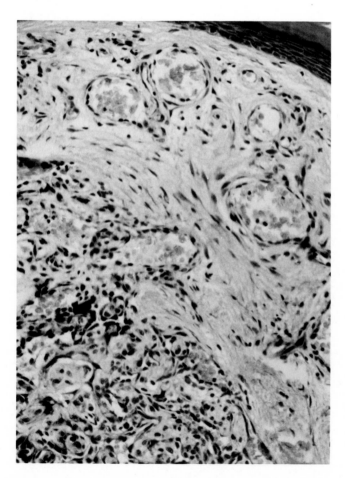

FIG. 29-13. **Malignant angioendothelioma.** The tumor is fairly well differentiated in the uppermost dermis where capillary lumina are seen. Farther down the cells appear atypical and fill the lumina. (×200)

angioendothelioma have the same basic clinical and histologic appearance and may occur together, it has become customary to regard the two as a unit under the designation of malignant angioendothelioma (Wilson Jones).

Malignant angioendothelioma most commonly occurs on the face or the scalp of elderly persons, where it spreads by centrifugal infiltration so that the greater part of the face and scalp, and even the neck, become affected. Depending on whether the tumor is predominantly a hemangioendothelioma or a lymphangioendothelioma, the involved areas show either colorless thickening of the skin or dusky, purple-blue infiltration (Bardwil et al.). Ulceration of the involved areas may occur (Wilson Jones; Girard et al.). Metastases to the cervical lymph nodes and hematogenous metastases to the lungs, the liver and elsewhere often are rather late in occurring, and in some patients death results from the destructive ulcerations of the tumor rather than from metastases (Girard et al.; Haustein).

In other instances malignant angioendothelioma occurs as a solitary, firm, large infiltrating mass in the skin or the subcutaneous tissue of the trunk or the extremities (McCarthy and Pack; Steingaszner et al.). In rare instances malignant angioendothelioma occurs in infants or children (Kauffman and Stout). In rare instances low-grade angioendotheliomas have arisen in children within a nevus flammeus (Girard et al.).

A malignant angioendothelioma may occur in a lymphedematous limb, especially after mastectomy, when it is known as Stewart-Treves syndrome. For discussion, see p. 611.

Histopathology. A variable degree of differentiation may occur even within the same lesion, with well differentiated formations often present at the periphery of the lesion and less differentiated areas in the heavily infiltrated, often nodular and ulcerated center (Wilson Jones; Reed et al.; Bardwil et al.; Girard et al.; Haustein).

In well differentiated areas one observes irregular, often anastomosing vascular channels lined by endothelial cells that are present largely in a single layer but in some places are multilayered (Fig. 29-13). Such formations may easily be misdiagnosed as

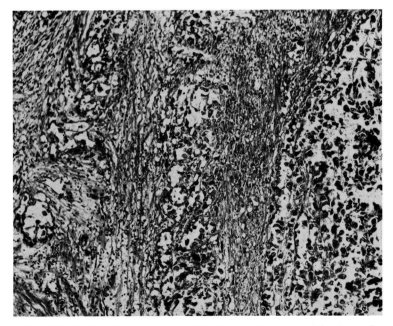

Fig. 29-14. **Malignant angioendothelioma.** Low magnification. On the left side vascular spaces are seen infiltrating between collagen bundles. These vascular spaces, as well as a large vascular sinus on the right, are lined by atypical endothelial cells. (×100)

nonspecific granulation tissue, although on careful study some of the endothelial cells appear unusually large and pleomorphic, with some of them cuboidal in shape (Wilson Jones).

In less differentiated areas the vascular spaces are lined by frankly atypical, cuboidal endothelial cells. The vascular spaces may be markedly dilated so that they consist of tortuous sinuses into which endothelial cells proliferate as papillary projections (Fig. 29-14), or they may form several layers and completely fill the lumina (Fig. 29-15) (Kauffman and Stout).

In poorly differentiated areas endothelial cells are seen either as invading cords between collagen bundles with only occasional slitlike vascular lumina. In such areas, the endothelial cells, instead of being cuboidal in shape, may appear spindle-shaped (Caro and Stubenrauch). Elsewhere there may be solid proliferations of more or less cuboidal endothelial cells, with poorly defined vascular spaces (Fig. 29-16). Such solid areas of cellular proliferations may resemble malignant melanoma, since in malignant melanoma the tumor cells usually appear cuboidal (Bardwil et al.).

Of considerable value in the diagnosis of malignant angioendothelioma is the fact that the endothelial cells, even though they are variable in appearance, will be found, at least in some areas, as cords of cuboidal cells with rather indistinct cell boundaries between them, thus giving a syncytial appearance to the aggregates of endothelial cells (Wilson Jones) (Fig. 29-15). A reticulum stain may be of definite value in identifying a malignant angioendothelioma because in areas of poorly recognizable vascular lumina a ring of reticulum, outlining the basement membrane, may be seen peripheral to the endothelial cells (Mach). Even solid areas of endothelial cell proliferations may show a dense network of reticulum fibers within the tumor cell complexes (Weidner and Braun-Falco; Girard et al.).

The amount of erythrocytes that are present varies. In well differentiated malignant hemangioendotheliomas the lumina often contain numerous erythrocytes, whereas poorly differentiated hemangioendotheliomas, because of the immaturity of the vessels, may contain only few or no erythrocytes in their lumina. On the other hand, even malignant lymphangioendotheliomas may contain some erythrocytes because of secondary anastomoses between the lymph channels of the tumor and some pre-existing capillaries (Reed et al.). In addition, there probably are some tumors that are partially malignant hemangioendotheliomas and partially malignant lymphangioendotheliomas. Such dual origin is assumed, for instance,

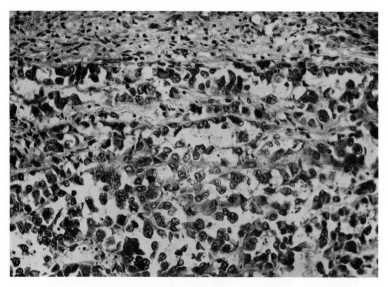

Fig. 29-15. **Malignant angioendothelioma.** High magnification of Figure 29-14. Cords of cuboidal endothelial cells proliferate as papillary projections within a large vascular sinus. (×200)

for many cases with the Stewart-Treves syndrome (see p. 612).

Differential Diagnosis. Well differentiated areas may suggest at the first glance merely granulation tissue or a capillary hemangioma, but a thorough examination will reveal areas in which the endothelial cells appear atypical and are "piled up" in more than one layer. For differentiation from hemangiopericytoma, see page 604; and from angiolymphoid hyperplasia with eosinophilia, see page 613. It is to be remembered that in angiolymphoid hyperplasia with eosinophilia a "piling up" of endothelial cells within immature capillary lumina may occasionally occur.

"LYMPHANGIOSARCOMA" IN LYMPHEDEMA (STEWART-TREVES SYNDROME)

The phenomenon of a malignant angioendothelioma developing in an area of lymphedema was first described in 1948 by Stewart and Treves as "postmastectomy lymphangiosarcoma." These authors observed the development of cutaneous and subcutaneous nodules several years after a radical mastectomy in the edematous tissue of the arm on the side of the operation. The cutaneous nodules have a bluish color. The clinical resemblance of the lesions to those occurring in Kaposi's sarcoma may be great. Death usually occurs within 1 to 2 years after appearance of the malignant angioendothelioma as the result of metastases, especially to the lungs (Fry et al.; Wolff).

It soon became apparent that a malignant angioendothelioma may arise in any chronically and severely edematous extremity, even without a preceding tumor. Most commonly the severe edema is on a congenital basis (Merrick et al.). Involvement of a lower extremity is more common than that of an upper extremity (Danese et al.). It is quite evident that the prognosis of a malignant angioendothelioma developing in an edematous extremity is worse than that of an idiopathically arising malignant angioendothelioma since, as pointed out already in regard to "postmastectomy lymphangiosarcoma," the survival time is much shorter, largely because of the rapid development of pulmonary metastases.

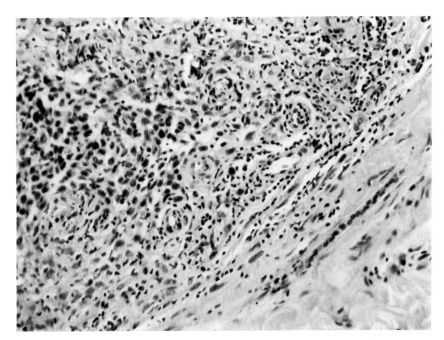

FIG. 29-16. **Malignant angioendothelioma.** This poorly differentiated tumor consists largely of solid proliferations of predominantly cuboidal endothelial cells. Only a few vascular spaces are present. In the lower right corner tumor cells are seen extending as a solid cord between collagen bundles. (×200)

Histopathology. It is now generally agreed that the "lymphangiosarcoma" that develops in an edematous extremity represents a malignant angioendothelioma that usually is particularly undifferentiated and invasive. It differs from an idiopathic malignant angioendothelioma by the presence of fibrosis within the tumor and the presence of numerous dilated lymph vessels outside the tumor both in the dermis and in the subcutaneous tissue (Jessner et al.). However, a histologic resemblance to Kaposi's sarcoma does not exist, because the endothelial cells are much more atypical than in Kaposi's sarcoma, whereas the fibroblasts lack the atypicality that they show in Kaposi's sarcoma (Wolff).

Histogenesis. Since the tumor arises in an area of lymphedema, it was originally thought that it was a lymphangiosarcoma or malignant lymphangioendothelioma. However, because of the presence of erythrocytes in many of the lumina, most authors believe that the tumor has a dual origin from both lymph vessels and capillaries (McConnell and Haslam; Wolff; Baes). The presence of pericytes on electron microscopic examination, described by Silverberg et al., also speaks in favor of a participation of blood capillaries in the tumor, since lymph vessels do not possess pericytes.

ANGIOENDOTHELIOMATOSIS PROLIFERANS

The relatively few cases reported with this diagnosis can be divided into a usually benign, inflammatory type and a rapidly fatal, neoplastic type.

The *inflammatory type* of angioendotheliomatosis proliferans probably represents a variant of allergic vasculitis (see p. 160). Clinically, purple plaques were present in one case (Tappeiner and Pfleger); erythematous, purpuric lesions in two cases (Gottron and Nikolowski; Ruiter and Mandema); gangrene of a leg in one case (Abulafia et al.); and widespread tender nodules in one case (Fievez et al.). The first four patients recovered, whereas the last patient died after having had her illness for nearly 1½ years.

The *neoplastic type,* comprising only three cases, is rapidly fatal and shows widespread bluish patches and plaques, as well as intracutaneous and subcutaneous nodules (Bra-

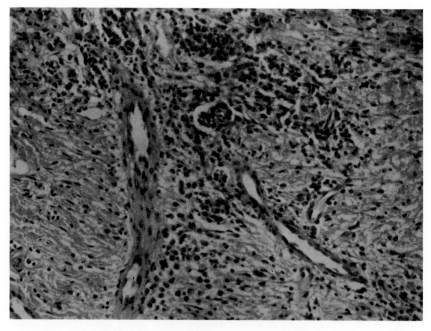

Fig. 29-17. **Angiolymphoid hyperplasia with eosinophilia.** Thick-walled capillaries lined by prominent endothelial cells are present, together with a pronounced cellular infiltrate containing many eosinophils. (×200)

verman and Lerner; Haber et al.; Midana and Ormea).

Histopathology. In the INFLAMMATORY TYPE of angioendotheliomatosis proliferans the dermal capillaries are dilated and show a marked proliferation of their endothelial cells, nearly causing occlusion of the lumen. This is associated with intraluminal thrombi of fibrin. In the one patient who died, autopsy revealed the same type of endothelial cell proliferation in nearly all the capillaries of various organs and, in addition, a vegetating endocarditis (Fievez et al.).

In the NEOPLASTIC TYPE the capillaries in the cutaneous and subcutaneous lesions, as well as in many internal organs, are dilated and show a pronounced proliferation of their endothelial cells, which thus nearly fill the lumina of the vessels. The proliferating endothelial cells appear atypical, like tumor cells. For the most part they remain within the vessels from which they arise and invade the surrounding stroma only slightly in the terminal stage.

Differential Diagnosis. The histologic differentiation of the inflammatory from the neoplastic type of angioendotheliomatosis proliferans can be very difficult, since also in the inflammatory type, in spite of its usually benign and reversible course, the proliferating endothelial cells can have an atypical appearance (Tappeiner and Pfleger).

ANGIOLYMPHOID HYPERPLASIA WITH EOSINOPHILIA

Persistent solitary or multiple nodules located either intradermally or subcutaneously, or both, are seen in angiolymphoid hyperplasia largely on the head of young adults. Whereas the dermal lesions usually measure less than 1 cm in size, the subcutaneous lesions may attain a size of 5 to 10 cm. The dermal lesions originally had been described by Wilson Jones and Bleehen as *pseudopyogenic granuloma,* and the subcutaneous lesions by Wells and Whimster as *subcutaneous angiolymphoid hyperplasia with eosinophilia.* Soon, however, it became apparent that both represented the same disease process taking place at different tissue levels (Kandil), and that patients could have dermal and subcutaneous nodules

simultaneously (Mehregan and Shapiro; Reed and Terazakis).

Histopathology. Histologically, the lesion has two components, a vascular and a cellular component (Fig. 29-17). The vascular component comprises: (a) thick-walled, well-differentiated capillaries, (b) branching, immature capillary lumina lined by large endothelial cells, and (c) cords and buds of endothelial cells that may or may not show small central lumina (Mehregan and Shapiro). The endothelial lining of some of the vessels appears to be 2 or 3 cells thick (Wilson Jones and Bleehen).

The cellular component consists of an extensive cellular infiltrate of lymphocytes, histiocytes and numerous eosinophils. In patients with subcutaneous nodules one often observes multiple lymphoid follicles with germinal centers (Wells and Whimster; Fattah and Fahmy; Mehregan and Shapiro).

Differential Diagnosis. The proliferation of large endothelial cells and immature blood vessels may suggest the possibility of malignant angioendothelioma. However, this occurs largely on the scalp and face of elderly individuals. The young age of the patients with angiolymphoid hyperplasia, the nodular character of the lesions, and the presence of tissue eosinophilia help in differentiating angiolymphoid hyperplasia from malignant angioendothelioma.

BIBLIOGRAPHY

Congenital Hemangiomas

Bean, W. B.: Dyschondroplasia and hemangiomata (Maffucci's syndrome). Arch. Intern. Med., *95*:767, 1955.

Bluefarb, S. M.: Sturge-Weber syndrome. Arch. Derm. Syph., *59*:531, 1949.

Bluefarb, S. M., and Adams, L. A.: Arteriovenous malformation with angiodermatitis. Arch. Derm., *96*:176, 1967.

Defauw, J.: Hypertension veineuse et hypertrophie des extrémités. Arch. belg. derm. syph., *19*:11, 1963.

Earhart, R. N., Aeling, J. A., Nuss, D. D., and Mellette, J. R.: Pseudo-Kaposi Sarcoma. Arch Derm., *110*:907, 1974.

Fretzin, D. F., and Potter, B.: Blue rubber bleb nevus. Arch. Intern. Med., *116*:924, 1965.

Furukawa, T., Igata, A., Toyokura, Y., and Ikeda, S.: Sturge-Weber and Klippel-Trenaunay syndrome with nevus of Ota and Ito. Arch. Derm., *102*:640, 1970.

Kasabach, H. H., and Merritt, K. K.: Capillary hemangioma with extensive purpura. Report of a case. Ann. J. Dis. Child., *59*:1063, 1940.

Krayenbühl, H., Yasargil, G., and Uehlinger, E.: Klinischer und pathologisch-anatomischer Beitrag zur Sturge-Weber-Krabbe'schen Krankheit. Dermatologica, *115*:555, 1957.

Kuzma, J. F., and King, J. M.: Dyschondroplasia with hemangiomatosis (Maffucci's syndrome) and teratoid tumor of the ovary. Arch. Path., *46*:74, 1948.

Lindenauer, S. M.: The Klippel-Trenaunay syndrome: varicosities, hypertrophy and hemangioma with no arteriovenous fistula. Ann. Surg., *162*:303, 1965.

Mali, J. W. H., Kuiper, J. P., and Hamers, A. A.: Acroangiodermatitis of the foot. Arch. Derm., *92*:515, 1965.

Miescher, G.: Über plane Angiome (Naevi hyperaemici). Dermatologica, *106*:176, 1953.

Mullins, J. F., and Livingood, C. S.: Maffucci's syndrome (dyschondroplasia with hemangiomas). Arch. Derm., *63*:478, 1951.

Mullins, J. F., Naylor, D., and Redetski, J.: The Klippel-Trenaunay-Weber syndrome. Arch. Derm., *86*:202, 1962.

Rice, J. S., and Fischer, D. S.: Blue rubber-bleb nevus syndrome. Arch. Derm., *86*:503, 1962.

Rodriguez-Erdmann, F.: Bleeding due to increased intravascular blood coagulation. New Eng. J. Med., *273*:1370, 1965.

Sakurane, H. F., Sugai, T., and Saito, T.: The association of blue rubber bleb nevus and Maffucci's syndrome. Arch. Derm., *95*:28, 1968.

Schnyder, U. W.: Zur Klinik und Histologie der Angiome. 2. Mitteilung: die Feuermäler (Naevi teleangiectatici). Arch. f. Derm. u. Syph., *198*:51, 1954.

———: Zur Klinik und Histologie der Angiome. 4. Mitteilung: die plano-tuberösen und tubero-nodösen Angiome des Kleinkindes. Arch. klin. exp. Derm., *204*:457, 1957.

Straub, P. W., Kessler, S., Schreiber, A., and Frick, P. G.: Chronic intravascular coagulation in Kasabach-Merritt syndrome. Arch. Int. Med., *129*:475, 1972.

Tappeiner, J., and Wolff, K.: Das Kasabach-Merritt Syndrom (Hämangiom-Thrombopenie-Syndrom). Hautarzt, *17*:493, 1966.

Walsh, T. S., Jr., and Tompkins, V. N.: Some observations on the strawberry nevus of infancy. Cancer, *9*:869, 1956.

Waterson, K. W., Jr., Shapiro, L., and Dannenberg, M.: Developmental arteriovenous malformation with secondary angiodermatitis. Arch. Derm., *100*:297, 1969.

Angiokeratoma

Agger, P., and Osmundsen, P. E.: Angiokeratoma of the scrotum (Fordyce). Acta dermatoven., *50*:221, 1970.

Bruce, D. H.: Angiokeratoma circumscriptum and angiokeratoma scroti. Arch. Derm., *81*:388, 1960.

Dammert, K.: Angiokeratosis naeviformis, a form of naevus telangiectaticus lateralis (naevus flammeus). Dermatologica, *130*:17, 1965.

Fischer, H., and Friederich, H. C.: Angiokeratoma corporis circumscriptum naeviforme mit Venektasien und Osteohypertrophie. Derm. Wschr., *151*:297, 1965.

Haye, K. R., and Rebello, D. J. A.: Angiokeratoma of Mibelli. Acta dermatoven., *41*:56, 1961.

Imperial, R., and Helwig, E. B.: Angiokeratoma. Arch. Derm., *95*:166, 1967 (I).

———: Verrucous hemangioma. Arch. Derm., *96*:247, 1967 (II).

Knoth, W., Knoth-Born, R. C., and Boergen, G.: Über das Angiokeratoma corporis circumscriptum naeviforme der Stammhaut. Hautarzt, *14*:452, 1963.

Lynch, P. J., and Kosanovich, M.: Angiokeratoma circumscriptum. Arch. Derm., *96*:665, 1967.

Angioma Serpiginosum

Barker, L. P., and Sachs, P. M.: Angioma serpiginosum. Arch. Derm., *92*:613, 1965.

Frain-Bell, W.: Angioma serpiginosum. Brit. J. Derm., *69*:251, 1957.

McGrae, J. D., and Winkelmann, R. K.: Generalized essential telangiectasia. J.A.M.A., *185*:909, 1964.

Stevenson, J. R., and Lincoln, C. S.: Angioma serpiginosum. Arch. Derm., *95*:16, 1967.

Granuloma Pyogenicum

Coskey, R. J., and Mehregan, A. H.: Granuloma pyogenicum with multiple satellite recurrences. Arch. Derm., *96*:71, 1967.

Juhlin, L., Hjerstquist, S. O., Ponten, J., and Wallin, J.: Disseminated granuloma pyogenicum. Acta dermatoven., *50*:134, 1970.

Leyden, J. L., and Master, G. H.: Oral cavity pyogenic granuloma. Arch. Derm., *108*:226, 1973.

Martens, V. E., and MacPherson, D. J.: Fibroangioma. Arch. Path., *61*:120, 1956.

Nödl, F.: Das "sogenannte" Granuloma teleangiektaticum. Z. Haut Geschlechtskr., *19*:163, 1955.

Oehlschlaegel, G., and Müller, E.: Zum Granuloma pyogenicum sive teleangiectaticum als Sonderfall des capillären Hämangioms. Arch. klin. exp. Derm., *218*:126, 1964.

Peterson, W. C., Jr., Fusaro, R. M., and Goltz, R. W.: Atypical pyogenic granuloma. Arch. Derm., *90*:197, 1964.

Warner, J., and Wilson Jones, E.: Pyogenic granuloma recurring with multiple satellites. Brit. J. Derm., *80*:218, 1968.

Zaynoun, S. T., Juljulian, H. H., and Kurban, A. K.: Pyogenic granuloma with multiple satellites. Arch. Derm., *109*:689, 1974.

Cherry Hemangioma

Schnyder, U. W., and Keller, R.: Zur Klinik und Histologie der Angiome. III. Mitteilung. Zur Histologie und Pathogenese der senilen Angiome. Arch. Derm. Syph., *198*:333, 1954.

Salamon, T., Lazovic, O., and Milicecic, M.: Über einige histologische Befunde bei dem sogenannten Angioma senile. Derm. Monatsschr., *159*:1021, 1973.

Papular Angioplasia

Peterson, W. C., Jr., Fusaro, R. M., and Goltz, R. W.: Atypical pyogenic granuloma. Arch. Derm., *90*:197, 1964.

Wilson Jones, E., and Marks, R.: Papular angioplasia. Arch. Derm., *102*:422, 1970.

Venous Lakes

Bean, W. B., and Walsh, J. R.: Venous lakes. Arch. Derm., *74*:459, 1956.

Thrombosed Capillary or Vein

Epstein, E., Novy, F. G., Jr., and Allington, H. V.: Capillary aneurysms of the skin. Arch. Derm., *91*:335, 1965.

Hayen, D. O.: Thrombosed angiokeratoma simulating malignant melanoma. Arch. Derm., *93*:359, 1966.

Weathers, D. R., and Fine, R. M.: Thrombosed varix of oral cavity. Arch. Derm., *104*:427, 1971.

Weiner, M. A.: Capillary aneurysms of the skin. Arch. Derm., *93*:670, 1966.

Nevus Araneus

Bean, W. B.: The arterial spider and similar lesions of the skin and mucous membranes. Circulation, *8*:117, 1953.

Schuhmachers-Brendler, R.: Beitrag zur morphologischen Pathologie und Therapie des Naevus-araneus-Rezidivs. Derm. Wschr., *139*:167, 1959.

Whiting, D. A., Kallmeyer, J. C., and Simson, I. W.: Widespread arterial spiders in a case of latent hepatitis, with resolution after therapy. Brit. J. Derm., *82*:32, 1970.

Familial Hemorrhagic Telangiectasia (Osler)

Chandler, D.: Pulmonary and arteriovenous fistula with Osler's disease. Arch. Intern. Med., *116*:277, 1965.

Kwaan, H. C., and Silverman, S.: Fibrinolytic activity in lesions of hereditary hemorrhagic telangiectasia. Arch. Derm., *107*:571, 1973.

Muggia, F. M.: Osler's disease with an aortic arch aneurysm. Arch. Intern. Med., *114*:307, 1964.

Smith, C. R., Jr., Bartholomew, L. G., and Cain, J. C.: Hereditary hemorrhagic telangiectasia and gastrointestinal hemorrhage. Gastroenterology, *44*:1, 1963.

Zelman, S.: Liver fibrosis in hereditary hemorrhagic telangiectasia. Arch. Path., *74*:66, 1962.

Lymphangioma

Fisher, I., and Orkin, M.: Acquired lymphangioma (lymphangiectasis). Arch. Derm., *101*:230, 1970.

Peachey, R. D. G., Lim, C. C., and Whimster, I. W.: Lymphangioma of skin. Brit. J. Derm., *83*:519, 1970.

Glomus Tumor

Fine, R. M., Derbes, V. J., and Clark, W. H.: Blue rubber bleb nevus. Arch. Derm., *84*:802, 1961.

Goodman, T. F.: Fine structure of the cells of the Suquet-Hoyer canal. J. Invest. Derm., *59*:363, 1972.

Goodman, T. F., and Abele, D. C.: Multiple glomus tumors. A clinical and electron microscopic study. Arch. Derm., *103*:11, 1971.

Gordon, B., and Hyman, A. B.: Multiple nontender glomus tumors. Arch. Derm., *83*:640, 1961.

Gupta, R. K., Gilbert, E. F., and English, R. S.: Multiple painful glomus tumors of the skin. Arch. Derm., *92*:670, 1965.

Ishibashi, Y., Ikeda, S., and Kawamura, T.: Multiple, schmerzhafte Glomustumoren. Jap. J. Derm., Series B, *78*:274, 1968.

Laymon, C. W., and Peterson, W. C., Jr.: Glomangioma (glomus tumor). Arch. Derm., *92*:509, 1965.

Lüders, G., Schlote, W., and Reinhard, M.: Zur Ultrastruktur von Glomustumoren und Glomusorganen. Arch. klin. exp. Derm., *238*:398, 1970.

McEvoy, B. F., Waldman, P. M., and Tye, M. J.: Multiple hamartomatous glomus tumors of the skin. Arch. Derm., *104*:188, 1971.

Mukhtar, J. A. K., and Pfleger, L.: Angiomatosis cutis disseminata (Beziehungen zum Blue Rubber Bleb Nevus). Hautarzt, *15*:230, 1964.

Murad, T. M., von Haam, E., and Murthy, M. S. N.: Ultrastructure of a hemangiopericytoma and a glomus tumor. Cancer, *22*:1239, 1968.

Schnyder, U. W.: Über Glomustumoren. Dermatologica, *131*:83, 1965.

Shugart, R. R., Soule, E. H., and Johnson, E. W., Jr.: Glomus tumor. Surg., Gynec., Obstet., *117*:334, 1963.

Tarnowski, W. M., and Hashimoto, K.: Multiple glomus tumors. J. Invest. Derm., *52*:474, 1969.

Hemangiopericytoma

Backwinkel, K. D., and Diddams, J. A.: Hemangiopericytoma. Cancer, *25*:896, 1970.

Cole, H. N., Jr., Reagan, J. W., and Lund, H. Z.: Hemangiopericytoma. Arch. Derm., *72*:328, 1955.

Forrester, J. S., and Houston, R. A.: Hemangiopericytoma with metastases. Arch. Path., *51*:651, 1951.

Hahn, M. J., Dawson, R., Esterly, J. A., and Joseph, D. J.: Hemangiopericytoma. An ultrastructural study. Cancer, *31*:255, 1973.

Kuhn, C., III, and Rosai, J.: Tumors arising from pericytes. Arch. Path., *88*:653, 1969.

Lattes, R.: quoted by: Kuhn, C., III, and Rosai, J.: Tumors arising from pericytes. Arch. Path., *88*:653, 1969.

Murad, T. M., von Haam, E., and Murthy, M. S. N.: Ultrastructure of a hemangiopericytoma and a glomus tumor. Cancer, *22*:1239, 1968.

O'Brien, P., and Brasfield, R. D.: Hemangiopericytoma. Cancer, *18*:249, 1965.

Ramsey, H. J.: Fine structure of hemangiopericytoma and hemangioendothelioma. Cancer, *19*:2005, 1966.

Reich, H.: Das Hämangiopericytom. Arch. klin. exp. Derm., *202*:390, 1956.

Stout, A. P.: Hemangiopericytoma. Cancer, *2*:1047, 1949.

———: Discussion. *In* Cole, H. N., Jr., Reagan, J. W., and Lund, H. Z.: Hemangiopericytoma. Arch. Derm., *72*:328, 1955.

Kaposi's Sarcoma

Anthony, C. W., and Koneman, E. W.: Visceral Kaposi's sarcoma. Arch. Path., *70*:740, 1960.

Becker, S. W., and Thatcher, H. W.: Multiple idiopathic hemorrhagic sarcoma of Kaposi. J. Invest. Derm., *1*:379, 1938.

Bluefarb, S. M., and Webster, J. R.: Kaposi's sarcoma associated with lymphosarcoma. Arch. Intern. Med., *91*:97, 1953.

Cox, J. W., Halprin, K., and Ackerman, A. B.: Kaposi's sarcoma localized to the penis. Arch. Derm., *102*:461, 1970.

Cox, F. H., and Helwig, E. B.: Kaposi's sarcoma. Cancer, *12*:289, 1959 (review).

Duperrat, B., and Pacot, C.: Les adénopathies kaposiennes. Ann. derm. syph., *91*:241, 1965.

Ecklund, R. E., and Valaitis, J.: Kaposi's sarcoma of lymph nodes. Arch. Path., *74*:224, 1962.

Feuerman, E. J., and Potruch-Eisenkraft, S.: Kaposi's sarcoma. Dermatologica, *146*:115, 1973.

Hashimoto, K., and Lever, W. F.: Kaposi's sarcoma. Histochemical and electron microscopic studies. J. Invest. Derm., *43*:539, 1964.

Lang, F. J., and Haslhofer, L.: Über die Auffassung der Kaposischen Krankheit als systematisierte Angiomatose. Z. Krebsforsch., *63*:241, 1935.

Mottaz, J. H., and Zelickson, A. S.: Electron microscope observations of Kaposi's sarcoma. Acta dermatoven., *46*:195, 1966.

Niemi, M., and Mustakallio, K. K.: The fine structure of the spindle cell in Kaposi's sarcoma. Acta path. microbiol., *63*:567, 1965.

O'Brien, P. H., and Brasfield, R. D.: Kaposi's sarcoma. Cancer, *19*:1497, 1966.

Pack, G. T., and Davis, J.: Concomitant occurrence of Kaposi's sarcoma and lymphoblastoma. Arch. Derm. Syph., *69*:604, 1954.

Pepler, W. J., and Theron, J. J.: An electron-microscopic study of Kaposi's hemangiosarcoma. J. Path. Bact., *83*:521, 1962.

Reed, W. B., Kamath, H. M., and Weiss, L.: Kaposi sarcoma, with emphasis on the internal manifestations. Arch. Derm., *110*:115, 1974.

Reynolds, W. A., Winkelmann, R. K., and Soule, E. H.: Kaposi's sarcoma. Medicine, *44*:419, 1965 (review).

Ronchese, F., and Kern, A. B.: Lymphangioma-like tumors in Kaposi's sarcoma. Arch. Derm., *75*:418, 1957.

Symmers, D.: Kaposi's disease. Arch. Path., *32*:764, 1941.

Tedeschi, C. G.: Some considerations concerning the nature of the so-called sarcoma of Kaposi. Arch. Path., *66*:656, 1958.

Tedeschi, C. G., Folsom, H. F., and Carnicelli, T. J.: Visceral Kaposi's disease. Arch. Path., *43*:335, 1947.

Templeton, A. C.: Studies in Kaposi's sarcoma. Cancer, *30*:854, 1972.

Malignant Angioendothelioma Including Angioendotheliomatosis Proliferans and Angiolymphoid Hyperplasia

Abulafia, J., Cigorraga, J., Saliva, J., and Molfino, J. C.: Systemic proliferating angioendotheliomatosis. Dermat. Iber. Lat. Am. (Engl. ed.), *5*:145, 1969.

Baes, H.: Angiosarcoma in a chronic lymphedematous leg. Dermatologica, *134*:331, 1967.

Bardwil, J. M., Mocega, E. E., Butler, J. J., and Russin, D. J.: Angiosarcomas of the head and neck region. Am. J. Surg., *116*:548, 1968.

Braverman, I. W., and Lerner, A. B.: Diffuse malignant proliferation of vascular endothelium. Arch. Derm., *84*:22, 1961.

Caro, M. R., and Stubenrauch, C. H., Jr.: Hemangioendothelioma of the skin. Arch. Derm. Syph., *51*:295, 1945.

Danese, C. A., Grishman, E. C. C., and Dreiling, D. A.: Malignant vascular tumors of the lymphedematous extremity. Ann. Surg., *166*: 245, 1967.

Fattah, A. A., and Fahmy, A.: Subcutaneous lymphoid hyperplasia with eosinophilia. Dermatologica, *139*:220, 1969.

Fievez, M., Fievez, C., and Hustin, J.: Proliferating systematized angioendotheliomatosis. Arch. Derm., *104*:320, 1971.

Fry, W. J., Campbell, D. A., and Coller, F. A.: Lymphangiosarcoma in post-mastectomy lymphedematous arm. Arch. Surg., *79*:440, 1959.

Girard, C., Johnson, W. C., and Graham, J. H.: Cutaneous angiosarcoma. Cancer, *26*:868, 1970 (review).

Gottron, H. A., and Nikolowski, W.: Extrarenale Löhlein-Herdnephritis der Haut bei Endocarditis. Arch. klin. exp. Derm., *207*:156, 1958.

Haber, H., Harris-Somes, S. N., and Wells, A. L.: Intravascular endothelioma (endotheliomatosis in situ, systemic endotheliomatosis). J. Clin. Path., *17*:608, 1964.

Haustein, U. F.: Angioplastisches Sarkom der Kopfhaut. Derm. Monatsschr., *160*:399, 1974.

Jessner, M., Zak, F. G., and Rein, C. R.: Angiosarcoma in postmastectomy lymphedema (Stewart-Treves syndrome). Arch. Derm. Syph., *65*:123, 1952.

Kandil, E.: Dermal angiolymphoid hyperplasia with eosinophilia versus pseudopyogenic granuloma. Brit. J. Derm., *83*:405, 1970.

Kauffman, S. L., and Stout, A. P.: Malignant hemangioendothelioma in infants and children. Cancer, *14*:1186, 1961.

Mach, K.: Zur Frage des Lymphangioendothelioms. Arch. klin. exp. Derm., *226*:318, 1966.

McCarthy, W. D., and Pack, G. T.: Malignant blood vessel tumors. Surg., Gynec., Obstet., *91*:465, 1950.

McConnell, E. M., and Haslam, P.: Angiosarcoma in postmastectomy lymphoedema. Brit. J. Surg., *46*:322, 1959.

Mehregan, A. H., and Shapiro, L.: Angiolymphoid hyperplasia with eosinophilia. Arch. Derm., *103*:50, 1971.

Merrick, T. A., Erlandson, R. A., and Hajdu, S. I.: Lymphangiosarcoma of a congenitally lymphedematous arm. Arch. Path., *91*:365, 1971.

Midana, A., and Ormea, F.: A propos d'un cas d'angioendotheliomatosis proliferans systematisata (de Tappeiner et Pfleger). Ann. derm. syph., *92*:129, 1965.

Reed, R. J., Palomeque, F. E., Hairston, M. A., III, and Krementz, E. T.: Lymphangiosarcomas of the scalp. Arch. Derm., *94*:396, 1966.

Reed, R. J., and Terazakis, N.: Subcutaneous angioblastic lymphoid hyperplasia with eosinophilia(Kimura's disease). Cancer, *29*:489, 1972.

Ruiter, M., and Mandema, E.: New cutaneous syndrome in subacute bacterial endocarditis. Arch. Intern. Med., *113*:283, 1964.

Silverberg, S. G., Kay, S., and Koss, L. G.: Postmastectomy lymphangiosarcoma: ultrastructural observations. Cancer, *27*:100, 1971.

Steingaszner, L. C., Enzinger, F. M., and Taylor, H. B.: Hemangiosarcoma of the breast. Cancer, *18*:352, 1965.

Stewart, F. W., and Treves, N.: Lymphangiosarcoma in postmastectomy lymphedema. Cancer, *1*:64, 1948.

Tappeiner, J., and Pfleger, L.: Angioendotheliomatosis proliferans systematisata. Hautarzt, *14*:67, 1963.

Weidner, F., and Braun-Falco, O.: Über das angioplastiche Reticulosarkom der Kopfhaut bei älteren Menschen. Hautarzt, *21*:60, 1970.

Wells, G. C., and Whimster, I. W.: Subcutaneous angiolymphoid hyperplasia with eosinophilia. Brit. J. Derm., *81*:1, 1969.

Wilson Jones, E.: Malignant angioendothelioma of the skin. Brit. J. Derm., *76*:21, 1964.

Wilson Jones, E., and Bleehen, S. S.: Inflammatory angiomatous nodules with abnormal blood vessels occurring about the ears and scalp (pseudo or atypical pyogenic granuloma). Brit. J. Derm., *81*:804, 1969.

Wolff, K.: Das Stewart-Treves-Syndrom. Arch. klin. exp. Derm., *216*:468, 1963.

30

Tumors of Fatty, Muscular, and Osseous Tissues

NEVUS LIPOMATOSUS SUPERFICIALIS

This rare lesion shows within a circumscribed area groups of asymptomatic soft, flattened papules or nodules which have a smooth or folded surface and are skincolored or pale yellowish. The areas of predilection are the gluteal and pelvic regions. The papules and nodules either are present at birth or arise in childhood.

In contrast to the rare occurrence of a pure nevus lipomatosus, the association of an intradermal nevocellular nevus with a nevus lipomatosus is fairly common. The clinical appearance of the intradermal nevocellular nevus is not affected by the concomitant presence of a nevus lipomatosus.

Histopathology. In a pure nevus lipomatosus groups and strands of mature fat cells are found embedded among the collagen bundles of the dermis, often as high up as the subpapillary layer (Fig. 30-1) (Abel and Dougherty). In the deeper part of the dermis, the fat cells surround the larger blood vessels (Lynch and Goltz; Finley and Musso). The larger nodules that may occur in some cases of nevus lipomatosus consist for the most part of mature collagen bundles, among which are scattered small groups of fat cells (Cramer). Serial sections reveal in some cases connections of the dermal aggregates of fat cells with the underlying subcutaneous fat (Holtz; Hönigsmann and Gschnait), whereas in other cases no connections are found (Nikolowski; Abel and Dougherty).

Intradermal nevocellular nevi that are associated with a nevus lipomatosus show, scattered among the nevus cell nests, fat cells singly as well as in groups (Fig. 30-2) (Nikolowski).

Histogenesis. It is generally agreed that the nevus lipomatosus represents, as the name implies, a nevoid anomaly in which ectopic fat cells have formed in the dermis from the perivascular mesenchymal tissue (Holtz; Lynch and Goltz; Cramer).

Differential Diagnosis. In focal dermal hypoplasia fat cells also are seen in the dermis, often in close approximation to the epidermis. It differs, however, from nevus lipomatosus by the extreme attenuation of the collagen.

LIPOMA

Lipomas occur as single or multiple subcutaneous growths that are soft, rounded or lobulated, and movable against the overlying skin.

In two rare conditions multiple lipomas composed of mature fat cells arise in adult life. They are (1) *adiposis dolorosa* or Dercum's disease, in which there are tender circumscribed or diffuse fatty deposits (Szegö; Blomstrand et al.); and (2) *benign symmetric lipomatosis,* characterized by large coalescent nontender lipomas present especially in the region of the neck in a typical "horsecollar" distribution and to a lesser degree in other areas (Greene et al.).

PLATE 4

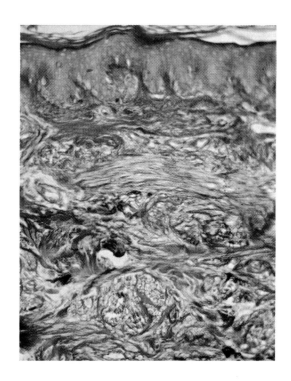

Leiomyoma. Aniline blue stain. This stain serves to differentiate collagen from smooth muscle. With hematoxylin and eosin both satin red, but with aniline blue collagen stains blue and muscle red. (×150)

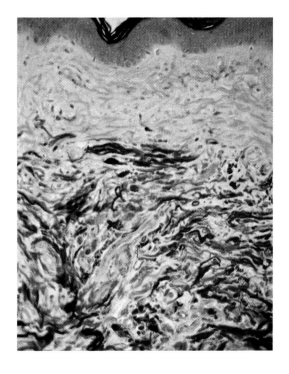

Blue nevus. Greatly elongated, deeply pigmented melanocytes with long dendritic processes are located in the lower dermis. (×150)

FIG. 30-1. **Nevus lipomatosus superficialis.** Groups and strands of mature fat cells are embedded among the collagen bundles of the dermis, extending as high as the subpapillary layer. Portions of the epidermis are seen at the top. (×100)

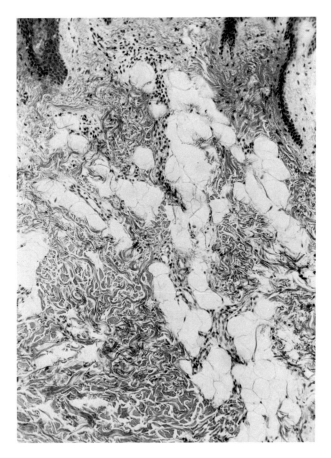

Histopathology. Lipomas are surrounded by a thin connective tissue capsule and are composed often entirely of normal fat cells that are indistinguishable from the fat cells in the subcutaneous tissue. In some lipomas one finds more, and in others less, of a connective tissue framework than in the normal subcutaneous fat. Those containing a considerable proportion of connective tissue are called fibrolipomas. Also, some lipomas show areas of capillary proliferations and are referred to as angiolipomas (Howard and Helwig).

In ADIPOSIS DOLOROSA most authors have found the lipomas to be indistinguishable histologically from ordinary lipomas (Szegö). In some cases, however, replacement of some of the fat cells by granulomas of the foreign body type and fibrosis has been noted (Blomstrand et al.).

In BENIGN SYMMETRIC LIPOMATOSIS the lipomas have the histologic appearance usually seen in lipomas (Greene et al.).

SYSTEMIC MULTICENTRIC LIPOBLASTOSIS

In this rare condition multiple lipomas form during adult life not only in the subcutaneous fat but also in the visceral fat depots. They have a tendency to increase in size.

Histopathology. The fatty tumors show not only mature fatty cells, as lipomas do, but also undifferentiated mesenchymal cells and intermediary cells containing varying amounts of lipid material within their cytoplasm (Tedeschi). In well differentiated areas mature fat cells are seen, usually located within a mucoid stroma. Less differentiated areas consist of lipoblasts showing different stages of maturation, whereas undifferentiated areas consist of spindle-shaped cells. Lipoblasts contain lipid droplets of varying sizes, and some are so-called mulberry cells that are rounded and filled with lipid vacuoles. Bizarre nuclei and atypical

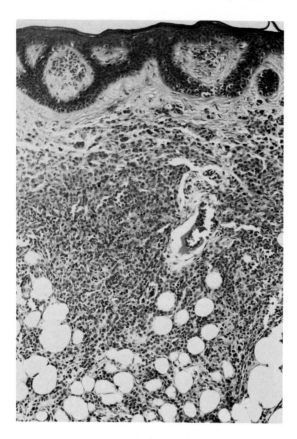

FIG. 30-2. **Nevus lipomatosus associated with an intradermal nevocellular nevus.** Fat cells of varying size are scattered singly and in groups through an intradermal nevocellular nevus. (×100)

mitoses are absent (Georgiades et al.).

Differential Diagnosis. Differentiation from a well differentiated liposarcoma may be impossible without clinical data. However, liposarcomas, in addition to showing some degree of nuclear atypicality, usually show frank infiltration into the surrounding tissue.

EMBRYONIC LIPOMA (LIPOBLASTOMATOSIS)

This rare solitary tumor arises in the subcutaneous fat of infants. It is characterized by expansive growth and has a great tendency to recur after excision (Van Meurs). As the result of increase in size even death may ensue, as in the case reported by Cox, in which a tumor of the neck caused asphyxiation.

Histopathology. This lobulated tumor is not encapsulated and composed of embryonic adipose tissue. Many of the cells are vacuolated: Some of them contain a large, single sudanophilic vacuole displacing the nucleus against the cytoplasmic membrane.

Smaller multivacuolated cells, so-called mulberry cells, are characterized by a granular, eosinophilic cytoplasm located between the vacuoles and by a centrally placed nucleus. In addition, spindle-shaped cells are present mainly at the periphery of the tumor, with some of them containing multiple small lipid vacuoles. They are embedded in a mucoid stroma (Vellios et al.).

Histogenesis. This tumor shows the various stages of development of fat cells in the human embryo, from spindle-shaped mesenchymal lipoblasts, to spindle-shaped cells with lipid droplets, and further to multivacuolated and univacuolated cells. In this tumor, just as in the development of the adipose tissue in the embryo, the percentage of multivacuolated mulberry cells is quite small (Vellios et al.).

HIBERNOMA

Hibernoma is a benign, asymptomatic, moderately firm, solitary, subcutaneous tumor, averaging 10 cm in size and often slowly enlarging. The most common location of this rare tumor is the upper back, but it may occur in other locations (Brines and Johnson). Hibernomas occur only in adults. Clinically they are indistinguishable from a lipoma.

Histopathology. Histologic examination reveals an encapsulated, lobulated tumor composed almost entirely of rounded, multivacuolated cells having a granular, eosinophilic cytoplasm between the vacuoles and a centrally located nucleus (Fig. 30-3) (Brines and Johnson; Novy and Wilson). These multivacuolated cells, referred to as mulberry cells, contain fat within their vacuoles. The fat, in contrast with mature fat, is doubly refractile to polarized light (Sutherland et al.). In some multilocular cells coalescence of smaller into larger vacuoles can be seen, with eccentric displacement of the nucleus. In addition, there are some univacuolated, mature fat cells. The multivacuolated mulberry cells average 30 μm in diameter, whereas mature fat cells measure about twice this size.

Histogenesis. The term *hibernoma* was given to these tumors because the multivacuolated mulberry cells pesent in them resemble the cells seen in the brown fat of hibernating animals. It has since become apparent that the cells present in hibernomas are not related to the brown fat. Rather, they are immature fat cells. However, as pointed out by Vellios et al., the percentage of multivacuolated mulberry cells present in the fat of human embryos is small (see p. 620). For this reason, it appears unlikely that the hibernoma, which is composed almost exclusively of multivacuolated cells, is a lipoma of immature adipose tissue, in contrast to the embryonic lipoma (see p. 620). It seems more likely that the hibernoma, as Vellios et al. have suggested, is a tumor of fat cells in which the enzyme systems leading to the maturation of the fat cells are incompletely developed.

Differential Diagnosis. The tumor can be differentiated from the round cell liposarcoma, or malignant hibernoma, by its capsule, its regular architecture, and the absence of mitotic figures and multinucleated cells.

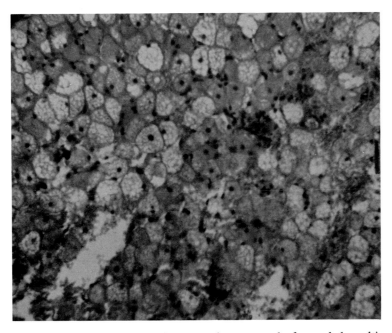

Fig. 30-3. **Hibernoma.** The tumor is composed of rounded, multivacuolated cells having a centrally placed nucleus. The multivacuolated cells are called mulberry cells. (×400) (Frederick J. Novy, Jr., M.D., and J. Walter Wilson, M.D.)

LIPOSARCOMA

Liposarcomas only rarely arise in the sub-cutaneous fat, such as the breast (Jackson). Most commonly, they originate in the inter-muscular fascial planes, with a special pre-dilection for the thighs (Enterline et al.). From the fascial planes they extend to the subcutaneous tissue. Liposarcomas arise as such and do not develop from lipomas.

Liposarcomas present themselves as a diffuse nodular infiltration of the subcu-taneous tissue. Metastases are common, es-pecially to the lungs and the liver.

Histopathology. The histologic picture varies somewhat with the degree of malig-nancy. Moderately malignant liposarcomas are easily recognizable as fatty tumors, whereas highly malignant liposarcomas may not be identifiable as such unless fat stains are employed.

Six types of cells may occur in liposar-comas, according to Enterline et al.: (1) mucoid lipoblasts showing a spindle-shaped nucleus and a few small sudanophilic drop-lets if they possess some degree of differ-entiation, or a bizarre nucleus and no lipid droplets if they are highly anaplastic; they are embedded in a mucoid stroma; (2) par-tially differentiated lipoblasts with a spindle-shaped nucleus and coarsely vacuolated cyto-plasm; (3) well differentiated fat cells or signet-ring cells with a single large vacuole and a spindle-shaped nucleus pressed against the cell wall; they differ from mature fat cells by being smaller in size and having a larger nucleus; (4) mature fat cells; (5) mulberry cells with a round central nucleus and many vacuoles in their cytoplasm; and (6) bizarre giant cells.

Depending on the prevalence of one or several of these cell types, one may divide liposarcomas into highly malignant mucoid liposarcoma; moderately malignant mucoid liposarcoma; and round cell liposarcoma or malignant hibernoma. It is only natural that transitions from one to another of these three types should occur, since they merely repre-sent differences in the degree of maturation.

A highly malignant mucoid liposarcoma contains predominantly highly atypical mu-coid lipoblasts with bizarre nuclei and only very small amounts of sudanophilic ma-

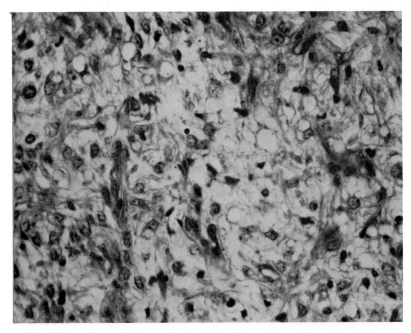

Fig. 30-4. **Liposarcoma.** The tumor is composed predominantly of spindle-shaped lipoblasts with coarsely vacuolated cytoplasm and of uni-vacuolated signet ring cells, but it also contains mature fat cells. There is a moderate amount of loose mucoid connective tissue. (×400)

terial. Small amounts of a mucoid stroma are present. There is considerable resemblance to a myxosarcoma (Enterline et al.) or to an undifferentiated fibrosarcoma, since the latter also may have a mucoid stroma (Holtz).

A moderately malignant mucoid liposarcoma contains mainly mucoid lipoblasts with spindle-shaped nuclei and small sudanophilic droplets, but also more highly differentiated fat cells, such as spindle-shaped lipoblasts with coarsely vacuolated cytoplasm, univacuolated signet-ring cells, and even mature fat cells (Fig. 30-4). Such tumors contain a loose meshwork of connective tissue that usually is mucoid, at least in part (Stout).

The round cell liposarcoma, or malignant hibernoma, is composed largely of so-called mulberry cells. They have a centrally placed nucleus and a multivacuolated cytoplasm. The vacuoles stain positive with lipid stains. Many nuclei are atypical; and some cells contain multiple bizarre nuclei (Fig. 30-5). The cells usually lie close together, so that there is hardly any stroma (Stout; Grimmer).

LEIOMYOMA

There are four types of leiomyomas of the skin: (1) multiple piloleiomyomas, and (2) solitary piloleiomyomas, both arising from arrectores pilorum muscles; (3) solitary genital leiomyomas, arising from the dartoic, the vulvar, or the mammillary muscle, and (4) solitary angioleiomyomas, arising from the muscle of veins.

Multiple piloleiomyomas are small, firm, reddish or brownish intracutaneous nodules arranged in a group or in a linear fashion. Often, two or more areas are affected. Usually, but not always, the lesions are tender and give rise spontaneously to occasional attacks of pain (Montgomery and Winkelmann).

Solitary piloleiomyomas are intracutaneous nodules that usually are larger than those of multiple piloleiomyomas and measure up to 2 cm in size. Most of them are tender and also occasionally painful (Fisher and Helwig; Macotela-Ruiz).

Solitary genital leiomyomas are located on the scrotum, the labia majora or, rarely,

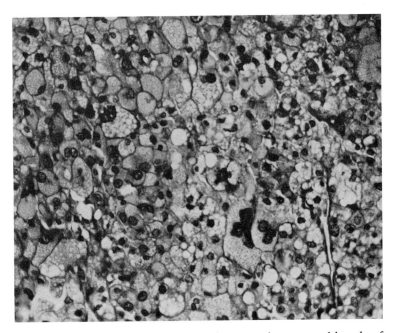

FIG. 30-5. **Malignant hibernoma.** The tumor is composed largely of rounded cells with multivacuolated cytoplasm and centrally placed nucleus, so-called mulberry cells. The cells vary greatly in size and possess bizarre nuclei. (×200)

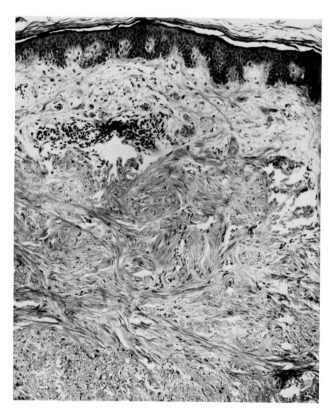

FIG. 30-6. **Leiomyoma, piloleiomyoma type.** The tumor is composed of interlacing bundles of smooth muscle fibers. The nuclei located in the center of the smooth muscle fibers are thin, very long, and blunt-edged. Collagen bundles are intermingled with the smooth muscle bundles. Both stain alike with hematoxylin and eosin. To differentiate them, an aniline blue stain may be used. (See Plate 4, facing p. 618.) (×100)

on the nipples. Small lesions may be intracutaneous in location, whereas larger ones are subcutaneous. In contrast to the other leiomyomas, most genital leiomyomas are asymptomatic (Fisher and Helwig).

Solitary angioleiomyomas usually are subcutaneous and only rarely are intracutaneous in location. As a rule, they do not exceed 1.5 cm in diameter. The lower extremities are the most common site. Pain and tenderness are present in most angioleiomyomas (Montgomery and Winkelmann; Magner and Hill).

Histopathology. PILOLEIOMYOMAS, whether they are multiple or solitary, and GENITAL LEIOMYOMAS have a similar histologic appearance (Fisher and Helwig). They are poorly demarcated and are composed of interlacing bundles of smooth muscle fibers (Fig. 30-6). Varying amounts of collagen bundles are intermingled with the smooth muscle bundles. The muscle fibers composing the smooth muscle bundles are generally straight, with little or no waviness; they contain centrally located, thin, very long, blunt-edged, "eel-like" nuclei.

The muscle bundles stain pink with hematoxylin and eosin, just as collagen does, and thus often are difficult to distinguish from the collagen bundles, even though there are the following differences in the appearance of the nuclei and the bundles: The nuclei of the fibroblasts located in the collagen are shorter than the nuclei located in the smooth muscle fibers and show tapering at their ends; and the muscle bundles usually show in cross sections, in contrast to the collagen bundles, slight vacuolization. A reliable differentiation between muscle and collagen bundles is possible with the aid of one of the collagen stains, such as the aniline blue stain or Masson's stain. With the aniline blue stain, muscle stains red and collagen blue (Plate 4, facing p. 618); with the Masson stain, muscle stains dark red and collagen green.

ANGIOLEIOMAS differ from the other types of leiomyomas by being encapsulated and by containing numerous veins. As a rule, they contain only a little collagen.

The numerous veins that are present vary in size and have muscular walls of varying

Fig. 30-7. **Leiomyoma, angi-oleiomyoma type.** A large vein with a thick muscular wall is present. Smooth muscle bundles extend tangentially from the periphery of the vein and merge with intervascular muscle bundles. (×200)

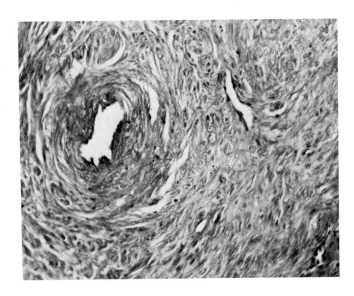

thickness (Fig. 30-7). Smooth muscle bundles extend tangentially from the periphery of the veins and merge with the intervascular muscle bundles (Magner and Hill). The veins may have small slitlike or large sinusoidal lumina; and some, because of contraction of their muscular tissue, have a stellate lumen (Saunders and Fitzpatrick). The large number and the size of the veins present within angioleiomyomas are an indication that not only the muscle of veins but also the veins themselves are involved in the neoplasia (Magner and Hill). The veins possess no elastic lamina. Areas of mucinous alteration are often present, especially in larger angioleiomyomas (MacDonald and Sanderson).

Histogenesis. Electron microscopic study reveals leiomyomas to be composed of normal-appearing smooth muscle cells. These cells have a central nucleus surrounded by an area containing endoplasmic reticulum and mitochondria, and outside this numerous myofilaments arranged in bundles. Each muscle cell is surrounded by a narrow basal lamina (Mann).

No unanimity exists concerning the amount and the type of nerves present in leiomyomas, since different findings have been obtained with silver impregnation for nerves, with histochemical staining for nerves, and with electron microscopy. Most authors found no increase in the number of nerve fibers within leiomyomas when using the Bodian stain (Montgomery and Winkelmann; Saunders and Fitzpatrick). Therefore, the painful nature of most leiomyomas has

been related by Montgomery and Winkelmann to the extension of the tumors around the bundles of cutaneous nerves.

Staining for monoamine oxidase and specific acetylcholinesterase activities has revealed, according to Mustakallio et al., in piloleiomyomas a bizarre proliferation of neural elements in areas in which the muscle fibers form neoplastic whorls. In addition, Mustakallio et al. found in the smooth muscle bundles of piloleiomyomas, in contrast to normal arrector pili muscles, a complete absence of nonspecific cholinesterase, which they thought may be related to the painfulness of piloleiomyomas.

Electron microscopy has revealed, as the result of the compression of nerve cells in piloleiomyomas, distortion and disruption of their myelin sheaths. In addition, the presence of an increased number of Schwann cells indicates an abnormally high density of innervation particularly with nonmyelinated nerves (Mann).

LEIOMYOSARCOMA

Leiomyosarcomas of the skin or subcutaneous tissue are very rare. Those located in the skin may show ulceration (Haim and Gellei). Some leiomyosarcomas are painful (Tappeiner) or tender (Montgomery and Winkelmann), whereas others are asymptomatic (Rising and Booth). Metastases are quite common. Usually they extend through the blood stream to the lungs and elsewhere (Phelan et al.), but occasionally they spread through the lymphatics to the regional lymph nodes (Haim and Gellei).

Histopathology. Leiomyosarcomas often show multifocal areas of hemorrhage and necrosis (Chaves et al.). Tumors of relatively low malignancy may resemble a benign leiomyoma by showing a proliferation of long, spindle-shaped cells arranged in bundles, but they are more cellular than benign leiomyomas and show areas of nuclear pleomorphism (Stout and Hill; Rising and Booth). Leiomysarcomas with a high degree of malignancy show numerous irregularly shaped, anaplastic nuclei, and often also atypical giant cells with bizarre nuclei (Fig. 30-8). (Haim and Gellei; Chaves et al.). Still, the nature of the sarcoma usually can be established even in rather anaplastic tumors, since in some areas one generally finds bundles of fairly well differentiated smooth muscle cells in which delicate myofibrils may be demonstrable by staining with phosphotungstic-acid-hematoxylin (Haim and Gellei). As in many other malignant tumors, there is not always a direct correlation between the degree of histologic malignancy of the tumor and the occurrence of metastases (Phelan et al.).

CUTANEOUS OSSIFICATION

Cutaneous bone formation may be primary or secondary. If primary, there is no preceding cutaneous lesion; if secondary, bone forms through metaplasia within a pre-existing lesion. Primary cutaneous ossification can occur in Albright's hereditary osteodystrophy and as osteoma cutis.

ALBRIGHT'S HEREDITARY OSTEODYSTROPHY

In Albright's hereditary osteodystrophy multiple areas of subcutaneous or intracutaneous ossification are often encountered. These areas may be present at birth or may arise later in life. No definite area of predilection seems to exist, since areas of ossification have been described on the trunk (Peterson and Mandel), as well as on the extremities (Donaldson and Summerly), and the scalp (Barranco). The areas of ossification may range in size from hardly perceptible to 5 cm in diameter (Eyre and Reed). Those located in the skin may cause ulcera-

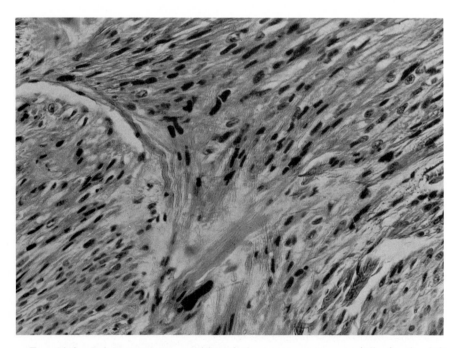

FIG. 30-8. **Leiomyosarcoma.** Although in some areas, especially in the left lower corner, the nuclei resemble those seen in a benign leiomyoma, in being thin, very long, and blunt-edged, most nuclei are irregular in shape and thus appear anaplastic. One bizarre giant cell is present. (×200)

tion, and bony spicules may be extruded through the ulcer (Donaldson and Summerly). In addition to areas of ossification, there may be deposits of amorphous calcium phosphate (Eyre and Reed).

Albright's hereditary osteodystrophy includes the syndromes of pseudohypoparathyroidism and pseudopseudohypoparathyroidism which are variants of the same disease. Patients with pseudohypoparathyroidism have hypocalcemia with failure to respond to parathyroid hormone, whereas patients with pseudopseudohypoparathyroidism have normal serum calcium values (Eyre and Reed). Patients with Albright's hereditary osteodystrophy have a short stature, a round facies, and shortened metacarpal and metatarsal bones. They may also have basal ganglia calcification, mental retardation, and multiple skeletal abnormalities. The mode of inheritance is dominant, and possibly sex-linked dominant (Eyre and Reed).

Histopathology. Spicules of bone of varying size may be found within the dermis or in the subcutaneous tissue. The bone contains fairly numerous osteocytes as well as cement lines that are best seen in polarized light (Roth et al.). Haversian canals containing blood vessels and connective tissue are often present (Fig. 30-9). In addition, osteoblasts with elongated nuclei usually can be seen along the margin of the bone where new bone is being laid down. Osteoclasts are often absent. If present, they are seen as cells with multiple large nuclei resembling multinucleated foreign-body giant cells and are located within deep grooves, called Howship lacunae, which extend from the surface of the bone into the bone substance (Fig. 30-10).

The spicules of bone may enclose, either partially or completely, areas of mature fat cells. Hematopoietic elements, however, are seen only rarely among the fat cells (Roth et al.).

Histogenesis. The osteocytes forming bone in primary cutaneous ossification originate from mesenchymal cells and thus form membranous rather than enchondral bone (Roth et al.).

The incidence of cutaneous ossification in Albright's hereditary osteodystrophy is fairly high. According to Spranger, cutaneous ossification is found in 42 per cent of the patients with pseudohypoparathyroidism and in 27 per cent

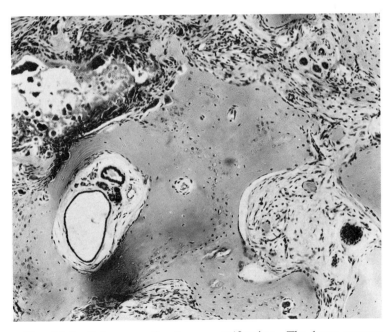

FIG. 30-9. **Osteoma cutis.** Low magnification. The bone appears lamellated about several haversian canals containing blood vessels and connective tissue. (×100)

of those with pseudopseudohypoparathyroidism. However, the reason for the bone formation is not clear.

Since the association of Albright's hereditary osteodystrophy with cutaneous ossification was not recognized until 1965, when Piesowilz drew attention to it, the question arises, how many of the cases of primary cutaneous ossification arise on the basis of this association? Brook and Valman, after reviewing many cases of primary cutaneous ossification, concluded that in some of them Albright's hereditary osteodystrophy must have existed, as in the cases reported by Tijdens and Ruiter, Donaldson and Summerly, and Peterson and Mandel. Although often in reports of cases of primary cutaneous ossification the data are inadequate and make it difficult to arrive at a decision, it can nevertheless be concluded that primary cutaneous ossification can occur in the absence of Albright's hereditary osteodystrophy (see below).

OSTEOMA CUTIS

The term osteoma cutis is applied to cases of primary cutaneous ossification in which there is no evidence of Albright's hereditary osteodystrophy in either the patient or his family.

Apparently there are two groups of patients with osteoma cutis, with the osteomas limited in extent in both groups. The two groups are: (1) patients with circumscribed multiple nodules of ossification in the scalp, as described by Combes and Vanina, Franke, and Tritsch; and (2) patients with multiple miliary osteomas of the face, as described by Hopkins, Costello, Rossman and Freeman, Helm et al., and Zabel. In several cases of multiple miliary osteomas of the face a long-standing acne vulgaris was present and was regarded as the cause of the osteomas (Leider; Jewell; Basler et al.). However, the absence of acne vulgaris in similar cases raises the possibility that the acne vulgaris was coincidental, as pointed out by Helm et al., in whose case of multiple miliary osteomas of the face similar osteomas were present also on the scalp.

Histopathology. The histologic findings in osteoma cutis are the same as in primary cutaneous ossification occurring in conjunction with Albright's hereditary osteodystrophy (see p. 627).

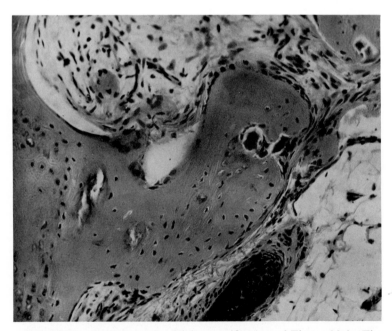

FIG. 30-10. **Osteoma cutis.** High magnification of Figure 30-9. The bone is lined in many areas by osteoblasts. In the center of the field several osteoclasts lie within a niche, called Howship's lacuna. (×200)

METAPLASTIC OSSIFICATION

Secondary or metaplastic ossification occurs in areas of tissue degeneration. It may be seen in association with cutaneous tumors, with scars, or with inflammatory conditions (Barranco).

Histopathology. The most common tumor to show metaplastic ossification is pilomatrixoma, or calcifying epithelioma of Malherbe (see p. 520). Whereas calcification starts within the areas of shadow cells, ossification starts in the stroma of the tumor, but with the calcium-rich shadow cells acting as inducing factor (Forbis and Helwig; Wiedersberg). Ossification may occur also in basal cell epitheliomas, where it usually starts in the stroma but occasionally in degenerating areas of keratinization (Delacrétaz and Christeler). Among the basal cell epitheliomas with ossification some are cases of the nevoid basal cell epithelioma syndrome (Mason et al.). In intradermal hairy nevi ossification usually is secondary to a folliculitis (Duperrat; Delacrétaz and Frenk). Finally, ossification may occur also in mixed tumors of the skin. According to Roth et al., this is the only instance in which enchondral bone is being formed in the skin through ossification of the "chondroid" cells in the mucoid stroma of the tumor.

In contrast to metaplastic ossification in association with tumors, metaplastic ossification in scars (Lilga and Burns) and in inflammatory processes of the skin such as scleroderma and dermatomyositis (Roth et al.) is rare.

CUTANEOUS ENDOMETRIOSIS

Cutaneous endometriosis is characterized by the presence of a solitary brownish or bluish nodule, measuring from 0.5 to 3 cm in size. The lesion, which is quite rare, is seen only in adult women. Most commonly, it occurs in a surgical scar of the abdominal or genital region, especially in a scar following a cesarean section (Steck and Helwig). The lesion, however, may arise spontaneously in the umbilicus (Popoff et al.), and rarely in the inguinal area (Steck and Helwig). Quite often, the lesion is slightly tender and painful. At the time of menstruation these symptoms become more pronounced and may be associated with swelling and slight bleeding of the lesion.

Histopathology. Irregular glandular lumina are embedded in a highly cellular and vascular stroma resembling the stroma of the functioning endometrium (Popoff et al.). The lumina are lined with a single row of secretory cells that are flat in some areas and tall columnar in others. Secretory globules are seen in the process of being extruded from the secretory cells (Steck and Helwig). The lumina contain red blood cells and cellular debris (Schlicke).

Histogenesis. In cases in which cutaneous endometriosis develops in surgical scars, implantation of viable endometrial cells probably is the cause. However, in cases of spontaneously arising cutaneous endometriosis it appears most likely that the endometrial tissue was transported to the area by way of the lymphatics (Steck and Helwig).

BIBLIOGRAPHY

Nevus Lipomatosus Superficialis

Abel, R., and Dougherty, J. W.: Nevus lipomatosus cutaneus superficialis (Hoffmann-Zurhelle). Arch. Derm., *85:*524, 1962.

Cramer, H. J.: Zur nosologischen Stellung des Naevus lipomatodes cutaneus superficialis (Hoffmann-Zurhelle). Derm. Wschr., *142:* 1218, 1960.

Finley, A. G., and Musso, L. A.: Naevus lipomatosus cutaneus superficialis (Hoffmann-Zurhelle). Brit. J. Derm., *87:*557, 1972.

Holtz, K. H.: Beitrag zur Histologie des Naevus lipomatodes cutaneus superficialis (Hoffmann-Zurhelle). Arch. f. Derm. u. Syph., *199:*275, 1955.

Hönigsmann, H., and Gschnait, F.: Naevus lipomatosus cutaneus superficialis (Hoffmann-Zurhelle). Z. Haut, *49:*517, 1974.

Lynch, F. W., and Goltz, R. W.: Nevus lipomatosus cutaneus superficialis. Arch. Derm., *78:* 479, 1958.

Nikolowski, W.: Über Naevus lipomatodes cutaneus superficialis (Hoffmann-Zurhelle). Derm. Wschr., *122:*735, 1950.

Lipoma

Blomstrand, R., Juhlin, L., Nordenstam, H., *et al.*: Adiposis dolorosa associated with defects of lipid metabolism. Acta dermatoven., *51:* 243, 1971.

Greene, M. L., Glueck, C. J., Fujimoto, W. Y., and Seegmiller, J. E.: Benign symmetric lipomatosis (Launois-Bensaude adenolipomatosis) with gout and hyperlipoproteinemia. Am. J. Med., *48*:239, 1970.

Howard, W. R., and Helwig, E. B.: Angiolipoma. Arch. Derm., *82*:924, 1960.

Szegö, L.: Gemeinsames Vorkommen der Lipomatosis dolorosa (Dercum) mit intrauteriner Amputation des linken Oberschenkels. Derm. Wschr., *150*:641, 1964.

Systemic Multicentric Lipoblastosis

Georgiades, D. E., Alcalais, C. B., and Karabela, V. G.: Multicentric well-differentiated liposarcomas. Cancer, *24*:1091, 1969.

Tedeschi, C. G.: Systemic multicentric lipoblastosis. Arch. Path., *42*:320, 1946.

Embryonic Lipoma (Lipoblastomatosis)

Cox, R. W.: "Hibernoma": the lipoma of immature adipose tissue. J. Path. Bact., *68*:511, 1954.

Van Meurs, D. P.: The transformation of an embryonic lipoma to a common lipoma. Brit. J. Surg., *34*:282, 1947.

Vellios, F., Baez, J., and Shumacker, H. B.: Lipoblastomatosis: a tumor of fetal fat different from hibernoma. Am. J. Path., *34*:1149, 1958.

Hibernoma

Brines, O. A., and Johnson, M. H.: Hibernoma, a special fatty tumor. Am. J. Path., *25*:467, 1949.

Novy, F. G., Jr., and Wilson, J. W.: Hibernomas, brown fat tumors. Arch. Derm., *73*:149, 1956.

Sutherland, J. C., Callahan, W. P., and Campbell, G. L.: Hibernoma, a tumor of brown fat. Cancer, *5*:364, 1952.

Vellios, F., Baez, J. M., and Shumacker, H. B.: Lipoblastomatosis: a tumor of fetal fat different from hibernoma. Am. J. Path., *34*: 1149, 1958.

Liposarcoma

Enterline, H. T., Culberson, J. D., Rochlin, D. B., and Brady, L. W.: Liposarcoma. Cancer, *13*: 932, 1960 (review).

Grimmer, H.: Hibernoma. Z. Haut Geschlechtskr., *33*:xxi, 1962.

Holtz, F.: Liposarcomas. Cancer, *11*:1103, 1958.

Jackson, A. V.: Metastasizing liposarcoma of the breast arising in a fibroadenoma. J. Path. Bact., *83*:582, 1962.

Stout, A. P.: Liposarcoma—the malignant tumor of lipoblasts. Ann. Surg., *119*:86, 1944.

Leiomyoma

Fisher, W. C., and Helwig, E. B.: Leiomyomas of the skin. Arch. Derm., *88*:510, 1963.

MacDonald, D. M., and Sanderson, K. V.: Angioleiomyoma of the skin. Brit. J. Derm., *91*:161, 1974.

Macotela-Ruiz, E.: Les léiomyomes cutanés. Ann. derm. syph., *90*:289, 1963.

Magner, D., and Hill, D. P.: Encapsulated angiomyoma of the skin and subcutaneous tissue. Am. J. Clin. Path., *35*:137, 1961.

Mann, P. R.: Leiomyoma cutis: an electron microscope study. Brit. J. Derm., *82*:463, 1970.

Montgomery, H., and Winkelmann, R. K.: Smooth-muscle tumors of the skin. Arch. Derm., *79*:32, 1959.

Mustakallio, K. K., Levonen, E., and Niemi, M.: Histochemical studies on cutaneous leiomyomatosis. Brit. J. Derm., *75*:60, 1963.

Saunders, T. S., and Fitzpatrick, T. B.: Cutaneous leiomyoma. Arch. Derm., *74*:389, 1956.

Leiomyosarcoma

Chaves, E., Sá, H. H., Gadelha, N., and Vasconcelos, E.: Leiomyosarcoma in the skin. Acta dermatoven., *52*:288, 1972.

Haim, S., and Gellei, B.: Leiomyosarcoma of the skin. Dermatologica, *140*:30, 1970.

Montgomery, H., and Winkelmann, R. K.: Smooth-muscle tumors of the skin. Arch. Derm., *79*:32, 1959.

Phelan, J. T., Sherer, W., and Mesa, P.: Malignant smooth-muscle tumors (leiomyosarcomas) of soft-tissue origin. New Eng. J. Med., *266*:1027, 1962.

Rising, J. A., and Booth, E.: Primary leiomyosarcoma of the skin with lymphatic spread. Arch. Path., *81*:94, 1966.

Stout, A. P., and Hill, W. T.: Leiomyosarcoma of the superficial soft tissue. Cancer, *11*:844, 1958.

Tappeiner, J., and Wodniansky, P.: Solitäres Leiomyom-Leiomyosarkom. Hautarzt, *12*: 160, 1961.

Cutaneous Ossification

Albright, F., Forbes, A. P., and Henneman, P. H.: Pseudopseudohypoparathyroidism. Trans. Assoc. Am. Physicians, *65*:337, 1952.

Barranco, V. P.: Cutaneous ossification in pseudohypoparathyroidism. Arch. Derm., *104*:643, 1971.

Basler, R. S. W., Taylor, W. B., and Peacor, D. R.: Postacne osteoma cutis. Arch. Derm., *110*:113, 1974.

Brook, C. G. D., and Valman, H. G.: Osteoma cutis and Albright's hereditary osteodystrophy. Brit. J. Derm., *85*:471, 1971.

Combes, F. C., and Vanina, R.: Osteosis cutis. Arch. Derm. Syph., *69*:613, 1954.

Costello, M. J.: Metaplasia of bone. Arch. Derm. Syph., *56*:536, 1947.

Delacrétaz, J., and Christeler, A.: Les phénomènes d'ossification dans les épithéliomas cutanés. Dermatologica, *134*:305, 1967.

Delacrétaz, J., and Frenk, E.: Zur Pathogenese des Osteo-Naevus Nanta. Hautarzt, *15*:487, 1964.

Donaldson, E. M., and Summerly, R.: Primary osteoma cutis and diaphyseal aclasis. Arch. Derm., *85*:261, 1962.

Duperrat, B.: Ostéomes cutanés. Ann. derm. syph., *88*:11, 1961.

Eyre, W. G., and Reed, W. B.: Albright's hereditary osteodystrophy with cutaneous bone formation. Arch. Derm., *104*:636, 1971.

Forbis, R., Jr., and Helwig, E. B.: Pilomatrixoma (calcifying epithelioma). Arch. Derm., *83*:606, 1961.

Franke, H.: Beitrag zum Krankheitsbild der Osteosis cutis circumscripta. Hautarzt, *7*:270, 1956.

Helm, F., DeLaPava, S., and Klein, E.: Multiple miliary osteomas of the skin. Arch. Derm., *96*:681, 1967.

Hopkins, J. G.: Multiple miliary osteomas of the skin. Arch. Derm. Syph., *18*:706, 1928.

Jewell, E. W.: Osteoma cutis. Arch. Derm., *103*:553, 1971.

Leider, M.: Osteoma cutis as a result of severe acne vulgaris of long duration. Arch. Derm. Syph., *62*:405, 1950.

Lilga, H. V., and Burns, D. C.: Osteomatosis cutis. Arch. Derm. Syph., *46*:872, 1942.

Mason, J. K., Helwig, E. B., and Graham, J. H.: Pathology of the nevoid basal cell carcinoma syndrome. Arch. Path., *79*:401, 1965.

Peterson, W. C., Jr., and Mandel, S. L.: Primary osteomas of skin. Arch. Derm., *87*:626, 1963.

Piesowilz, A. T.: Pseudopseudohypoparathyroidism with osteoma cutis. Proc. Roy. Soc. Med., *58*:126, 1965.

Rossman, R. E., and Freeman, R. G.: Osteoma cutis, a stage of preosseous calcification. Arch. Derm., *89*:68, 1964.

Roth, S. I., Stowell, R. E., and Helwig, E. B.: Cutaneous ossification. Arch. Path., *76*:44, 1963.

Spranger, J.: Skeletal dysplasia: Albright's hereditary osteodystrophy. *In* Birth Defects: The First Conference, White Plains, N.Y., National Foundation March of Dimes, p. 122, 1968.

Tijdens, E. F., and Ruiter, M.: Osteosis cutis. Acta dermatoven., *29*:140, 1949.

Tritsch, H.: Osteome der Kopfhaut. Arch. klin. exp. Derm., *221*:336, 1965.

Wiedersberg, H.: Das Epithelioma calcificans Malherbe. Derm. Monatsschr., *157*:867, 1971.

Zabel, R.: Osteosis cutis multiplex faciei. Derm. Monatsschr., *156*:798, 1970.

Cutaneous Endometriosis

Popoff, L., Raitchev, R., and Andreev, V. C.: Endometriosis of the skin. Arch. Derm., *85*:186, 1962.

Schlicke, C. P.: Ectopic endometrial tissue in the thigh. J.A.M.A., *132*:445, 1946.

Steck, W. D., and Helwig, E. B.: Cutaneous endometriosis. J.A.M.A., *191*:167, 1965.

31

Tumors of Neural Tissue

Three types of benign nerve sheath tumors occur in the skin: (1) neurofibromas, (2) neurilemmomas, and (3) neuromas. In neurofibromas, the characteristic finding is a hyperplasia of Schwann cells that are embedded in a considerable amount of endoneurial collagen. In neurilemmomas, one finds a hyperplasia of Schwann cells that possess numerous cytoplasmic processes forming the so-called Verocay bodies; and in neuromas, there is a proliferation of nerve fascicles that are surrounded by a conspicuous perineurium.

NEUROFIBROMATOSIS

Neurofibromas may occur as solitary cutaneous lesions, in which case one finds no café-au-lait spots and no family history of the disease (Knight et al.). In the presence of multiple cutaneous lesions the disorder is referred to as neurofibromatosis, or von Recklinghausen's disease; it is dominantly inherited, and frequently it is associated with multiple café-au-lait spots. Whereas solitary neurofibromas usually arise in adult life, the multiple cutaneous tumors of neurofibromatosis in most instances first appear in late childhood or in adolescence and gradually increase in size and number.

Both solitary and multiple neurofibromas possess a soft consistency. They usually are flesh-colored but occasionally have a violaceous color, and are either semiglobular or pedunculated.

The multiple neurofibromas of neurofibromatosis vary considerably in size. Sometimes, large pendulous flabby masses are encountered. Also, in some cases subcutaneous nodules are present. As a rule, the lesions of neurofibromatosis are widely disseminated. Occasionally, however, they are localized within a fairly small area (Streitmann; Winkelmann and Johnson).

The café-au-lait spots often start appearing in early childhood and thus may precede the cutaneous tumors. Although occasionally a few café-au-lait spots are seen in patients without neurofibromatosis, the presence of more than six spots exceeding 1.5 cm in diameter is indicative of neurofibromatosis (Crowe et al.).

Histopathology. Histologic examination of the cutaneous neurofibromas shows the same findings in solitary neurofibromas and in neurofibromatosis. Although usually well circumscribed they are not encapsulated (Reed et al.). Occasionally they are not sharply separated from the surrounding dermis but infiltrate the dermal connective tissue (Winkelmann and Johnson). Large tumors often extend into the subcutaneous fat. In typical areas neurofibromas are composed of faintly eosinophilic, thin, wavy fibers lying in loosely textured strands extending in varying directions (Fig. 31-1). Embedded among the wavy fibers one finds a fairly large number of nuclei that are oval to spindle-shaped and fairly uniform in size. Occasionally, the nuclei lie in parallel rows;

but well developed Verocay bodies, as in neurilemmomas, are uncommon. Giemsa's stain reveals in most neurofibromas a fairly large number of mast cells (Crowe et al.; Winkelmann and Johnson). Elastic fibers are absent in the tumors. Staining with special nerve stains, such as Bodian's stain, reveals scattered long thin nerve fibers throughout the tumors (McNairy and Montgomery; Reed et al.). The presence of nerve fibers in neurofibromas has been confirmed also by staining thick sections with methylene blue (Shelley and Arthur). Staining for reticulum fibers reveals that many of the thin, loosely textured, wavy fibers are reticulum fibers and thus young collagen fibers (McNairy and Montgomery).

Occasionally, mucoid degeneration of the stroma is observed in parts of a tumor or in an entire tumor. In such areas the nuclei are embedded in a homogeneous, pale-blue ground substance (Fig. 31-2). This ground substance stains metachromatically with Giemsa's stain or with toluidine blue (Nürnberger and Korting). One must be familiar with this type of mucoid degeneration, because it results in a histologic picture quite

different from that associated usually with neurofibroma.

The café-au-lait spots in neurofibromatosis, in skin sections stained with silver, show in comparison with the surrounding skin (1) an increase in the total amount of melanin in both the melanocytes and keratinocytes, and (2) scattered, abnormally large melanin granules ("giant" melanosomes) in both the melanocytes and basal cells (Benedict et al.). In addition, the dopa reaction indicates, when applied to skin sections (3) an increase in the activity of the melanocytes, and when applied to epidermal sheets (4) an increased concentration of melanocytes per square millimeter (Benedict et al.; Johnson and Charneco). However, there are exceptions. In the first place, Johnson and Charneco in their examination of café-au-lait spots in patients with neurofibromatosis found in 2 of 8 patients no giant pigment granules, and in 1 patient no increased concentration of melanocytes. Furthermore, Silvers et al. noted the absence of giant pigment granules in the café-au-lait spots of all 4 children with neurofibromatosis examined by them.

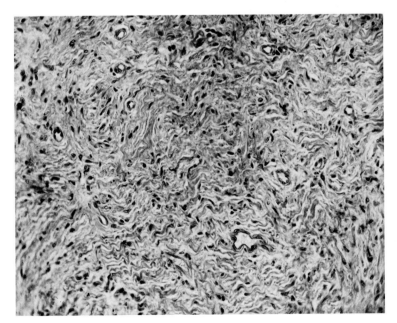

FIG. 31-1. **Neurofibromatosis (von Recklinghausen's disease).** Thin, wavy fibers lie in loosely textured strands extending in varying directions. Most nuclei appear enlongated. (×200)

Histogenesis. Von Recklinghausen originally postulated that neurofibromas were derived mainly from the perineurial connective tissue and thus were mesodermal in origin. Verocay in 1910 suggested that the cells of the tumors were Schwann cells and thus neuroectodermal in origin. He suggested that the tumors be called neurinomas. Subsequently, some authors (Tarlov) supported von Recklinghausen's view, others (Murray and Stout) inclined to Verocay's, whereas still others expressed the opinion that probably both ectodermal Schwann cells and perineurial connective tissue cells participated in the formation of the tumors (Foot; McNairy and Montgomery).

The demonstration of nonspecific cholinesterase activity in neurofibromas has provided evidence that they are not mesodermal growths (Winkelmann and Johnson). Furthermore, in tissue cultures of neurofibromas nonspecific cholinesterase activity could be identified in some of the cells migrating from the primary explant (Klaus and Winkelmann).

Electron microscopy has further established the Schwann cell as the main cell type in neurofibromas (E.M. No. 44). This cell is characterized by the presence of a basal lamina, 50 to 70 nm wide, peripheral to the plasma membrane.

In addition, Schwann cells contain multiple axons in their cytoplasm, each axon being surrounded by a basal lamina (E.M. No. 44, *inset*). In contrast to normal Schwann cells in which the axons are found largely in the central cytoplasm, the Schwann cells present in neurofibromas show their axons almost entirely at their periphery within long cellular processes (Weber and Braun-Falco). The Schwann cells are widely separated from one another by considerable amounts of collagen fibrils most of which are thinner than the average fibril, with a diameter of 100 nm. The fibrils generally form small aggregates, more like reticulum fibers than like collagen fibers or bundles (Waggener). Scattered fibroblasts are the source of the collagen, since they show evidence of an actively synthesizing dilated rough endoplasmic reticulum (Weber and Braun-Falco). It can be assumed that the fibroblasts are endoneurial fibroblasts because of the small caliber of the collagen fibrils produced by them. Small nerve bundles traverse the tumor and are the source of the axons found within the Schwann cells (Waggener). Mast cells are recognizable also by electron microscopy in rather large numbers.

Electron microscopic examination of the giant melanin granules present in the melano-

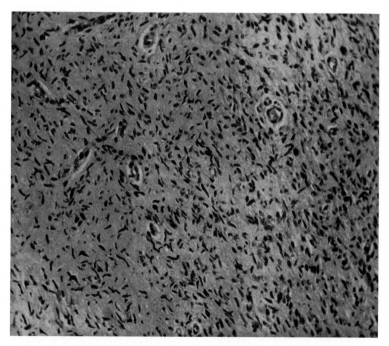

FIG. 31-2. **Neurofibromatosis (von Recklinghausen's disease).** In this tumor mucoid degeneration of the collagen has taken place. This is not an uncommon occurrence in lesions of neurofibroma. (×200)

cytes and keratinocytes of the café-au-lait spots of neurofibromatosis reveals that they are giant melanosomes, rather than phagolysosomes. Whereas normal melanosomes, which are also present, are ellipsoidal and measure on the average 0.7 by 0.3 μm in diameter, the giant melanosomes are either ellipsoidal or spherical and range from 3.5 μm to 5.0 μm in diameter (Jimbow et al.).

Systemic Lesions. Extracutaneous neurofibromas arise mainly in relation to nerves and bones. The cranial nerves most commonly involved are the optic and the acoustic nerves. Spinal root tumors may cause compression of the spinal cord (Crowe et al.). Involvement of the bones may consist either of intraosseous neurofibromas or of erosive defects caused by the pressure of adjacent neurofibromas on bone. In addition, nonspecific bone lesions, such as scoliosis or increased length of long bones, may occur (Levene). Of interest is the fairly common association of neurofibromatosis with pheochromocytoma (Healey and Mekelatos).

Malignant Degeneration. Malignant degeneration may occur in lesions of neurofibromatosis, but it is not common. Thus, in a series of 678 patients, malignant degeneration was observed in only 21, or 3.1 per cent, of the patients (D'Agostino et al.). Malignant degeneration is particularly rare in cutaneous neurofibromas and was seen in only 2 of the 678 patients. Most commonly, malignant degeneration occurs in neurofibromas of the large nerve trunks, such as the femoral, tibial, or intercostal nerves (Undeutsch). Next in frequency, malignant degeneration occurs in neurofibromas of cranial nerves or the spinal cord (D'Agostino et al.).

Histologically, most malignant tumors in neurofibromatosis have the appearance of more or less anaplastic fibrosarcomas and give no indication of their origin from a neurofibroma. In some malignant tumors the pattern of a neurofibroma is preserved at first, but is no longer present when the tumor recurs after excision (Undeutsch). Such early malignant lesions in which the pattern of a neurofibroma still is present show an increase in the number of nuclei as well as some atypicality of the nuclei (Fig. 31-3) (Wachstein and Wolf; Knight et al.). Some malignant tumors, especially those arising from the major nerves of the lower

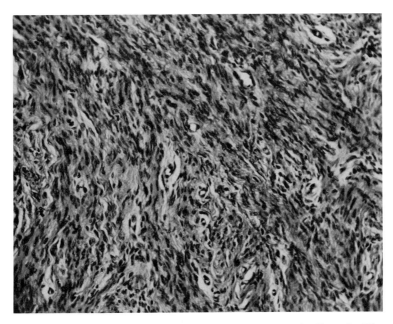

FIG. 31-3. **Neurofibrosarcoma (von Recklinghausen's disease).** The wavy pattern characteristic of neurofibroma is preserved, but the nuclei are increased in number and are atypical. ($\times$200)

extremities and from the lumbar spinal nerves, have the histologic characteristics of a malignant neurilemmoma because of the arrangement of the nuclei in palisades (White).

Differential Diagnosis. A histologic differentiation of a neural nevus from a solitary neurofibroma may be impossible in routinely stained sections if the neural nevus, as it may occur, shows no nevus cell nests in its upper portion (Becker). In such cases, the presence of numerous nerve fibers on silver impregnation speaks in favor of neurofibroma (see also p. 633). However, quite often neurofibromas are not particularly rich in nerve fibers. Only electron microscopy would then help, because the melanocytes of neural nevi differ from Schwann cells by containing melanosomes and by not showing enclosed axons.

In contrast with their common presence in the café-au-lait spots of neurofibromatosis, giant melanin granules are absent in the pigment patches of Albright's syndrome (Benedict et al.) and also in café-au-lait spots occasionally encountered in normal subjects (Johnson and Charneco).

NEURILEMMOMA

Neurilemmomas occur almost invariably as solitary tumors along the course of peripheral or cranial nerves. Most commonly they are found in a subcutaneous location on the head or the extremities, but only rarely on the trunk. They also have been reported as occurring within viscera such as the gastrointestinal tract (Stout), on the tongue (Kuske and Soltermann; Mercantini and Mopper), and in bones (Fawcett and Dahlin).

Neurilemmomas usually are asymptomatic, but in some instances there is pain radiating along the nerve from which the neurilemmoma arises (Das Guptas et al.). Occasionally, neurilemmomas are encountered in individuals who also have neurofibromatosis (Das Guptas et al.; Izumi et al.).

Malignant degeneration of neurilemmomas is a rare event and only a few cases have been reported (Carstens and Schrodt). Most instances of malignant degeneration occurred in patients having neurofibromatosis in association with the malignant neurilemmoma (White).

Histopathology. Neurilemmomas are well

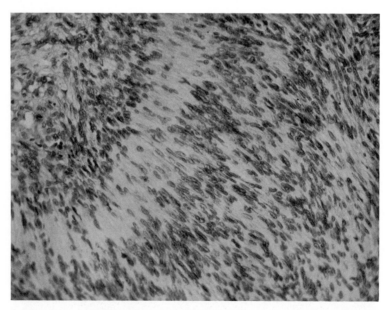

Fig. 31-4. **Neurilemmoma.** Numerous elongated nuclei are arranged in a streaming fashion. In the center of the field lies a so-called Verocay body formed by a double palisade of nuclei enclosing between them a space of homogeneous material that is nearly devoid of nuclei. (×200)

encapsulated and composed of two types of tissue referred to as Antoni types A and B.

Antoni type A tissue is composed of cells whose nuclei are elongated and arranged closely spaced in palisade fashion, forming twisted bands or rows. In many areas the nuclei form two parallel rows enclosing between them a space of nearly homogeneous material. Such formations are called Verocay bodies (Fig. 31-4). Only few collagen fibers are found in Antoni type A tissue.

Antoni type B tissue consists of an edematous stroma containing relatively few haphazardly arranged cells having nuclei of variable shape. In some areas one may find mucoid foci, cystic changes or areas of hemorrhage (Carsten and Schrodt). Through coalescence of small cysts, large cystic spaces may form (Stout).

Staining for nerves with the Bodian stain reveals, in contrast with neurofibromas, very few or no nerve fibers (Reed et al.). However, neurilemmomas show, just like neurofibromas, fairly numerous mast cells (Das Guptas et al.).

Histogenesis. The presence of nonspecific cholinesterase in neurilemmoma is consistent with the presence of Schwann cells in this tumor (Winkelmann and Johnson).

Electron microscopy reveals the Antoni type A tissue to be composed of Schwann cells whose nuclei are largely arranged in rows. The homogeneous material between two rows of nuclei consists of numerous thin, greatly elongated cytoplasmic processes that extend from the Schwann cells and are oriented in parallel alignment (Fisher and Vuzevski). The interstitial tissue is scantier than in neurofibromas but also consists of collagen fibrils and occasional fibroblasts (Waggener).

Antoni type B tissue results from degenerative changes occurring in type A tissue. On electron microscopy, the degenerative changes are seen to affect both the cytoplasm of the Schwann cells, which contains numerous empty-appearing vacuoles, and the basal lamina of the Schwann cells, which appears as abundant amorphous material in the intercellular spaces (Matakas and Cervos-Navarro).

NEUROMA

The only well defined type of cutaneous neuroma is the traumatic neuroma. On the other hand, spontaneously arising cutaneous neuromas are rare and most cases are poorly documented (Reed et al.).

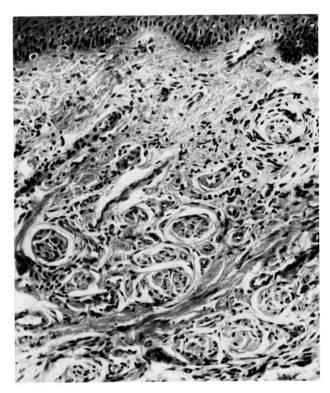

FIG. 31-5. **Traumatic neuroma.** Numerous large, irregular bundles of peripheral nerves are present in association with a considerable connective tissue proliferation. (×200)

The traumatic neuromas include the amputation neuromas and the so-called "rudimentary supernumerary digits" which are smooth or verrucous papules that have formed at the site of an amputated supernumerary digit (Shapiro et al.).

Spontaneously arising neuromas have been described as either single (Dupré et al.) or multiple (Holm et al.), and as either painful (Duemling) or painless (Thies). Those containing no axons have been called false neuromas; and those with axons, true neuromas (Thies). Because of the great differences in the clinical and histologic descriptions of the various tumors it is difficult to recognize spontaneously arising neuromas as an entity. Rather, it seems that tumors reported as spontaneously arising neuromas and containing axons can be regarded as either single neurofibromas (Reed et al.) or as multiple neurofibromas (Holm et al.); and those without axons as neurilemmomas (Thies).

Multiple mucosal neuromas consist of numerous, often closely set nodules that arise, beginning in childhood, mainly on the tongue but also elsewhere on the oral mucosa and on the tarsal conjunctivae. They are part of a syndrome that includes also medullary thyroid carcinoma and pheochromocytoma (Walker; Hurwitz).

Histopathology. Cutaneous neuromas reveal large, irregular bundles of peripheral nerves associated with considerable connective tissue proliferation (Fig. 31-5) (Holm et al.). Nerve bundles located close to the epidermis may resemble Meissner corpuscles (Shapiro et al.). Nerve stains with Bodian's stain reveal numerous axons scattered throughout the nerve bundles (Reed et al.; Holm et al.; Shapiro et al.).

The multiple mucosal neuromas seen in association with medullary thyroid carcinoma and pheochromocytoma can have the same histologic appearance as cutaneous neuromas (Walker). In some instances, however, some of the tumors look histologically like neuromas and others like neurofibromas (Baum).

Histogenesis. Electron microscopy shows in traumatic neuromas multiple nerve fascicles composed of myelinated and nonmyelinated axons and Schwann cells. The fascicles are ensheathed by multiple lamina of perineurial cells. Intermingled with the perineurial cells lie dense bundles of collagen (Waggener).

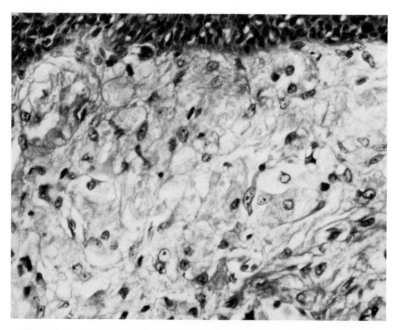

FIG. 31-6. **Granular cell tumor.** The tumor is composed of large cells having a pale cytoplasm filled with numerous, fine granules. (×400)

GRANULAR CELL TUMOR

Granular cell tumors, originally described by Abrikossoff as granular cell myoblastomas, are usually solitary tumors, but in about 8 per cent of the cases they are multiple (Strong et al.). They occur most commonly on the tongue where 40 per cent of the tumors are located, on the skin, and in the subcutaneous tissue. They may occur, however, in many other areas, such as the esophagus, the stomach, the appendix, the larynx, the bronchus, the pituitary gland, the uvea, and the skeletal muscle (Aparicio and Lumsden).

Intradermal granular cell tumors usually consist of a well circumscribed, raised, firm, nontender nodule from 0.5 to 2.0 cm in diameter. In some instances the tumor has a hyperkeratotic surface. Subcutaneous granular cell tumors consist of a firm nodule that may or may not be attached to the overlying skin.

Histopathology. On histologic examination the cells of the tumor appear large and often elongated. Most cells measure from 30 to 60 μm in diameter, but some are even larger. They have a distinct cellular membrane and a pale cytoplasm filled with faintly eosinophilic granules, 2 to 6 μm in size (Fig. 31-6). The nuclei are small, round to oval, and centrally located. A few of the cells may possess more than one nucleus. Quite characteristically, one observes in tumors located in the skin either small groups or rows of tumor cells, and in some areas even individual tumor cells, surrounded by a PAS-positive, diastase-resistant membrane and often also by delicate strands of reticulum or collagen fibers (Aparicio and Lumsden). Similarly, in tumors of the tongue a PAS-positive, diastase-resistant membrane and slender striated muscle fibers may surround individual tumor cells or groups of cells (Fig. 31-7).

The characteristic faint granules within the tumor cells are PAS-positive and diastase-resistant. In some instances the cytoplasmic granules are slightly sudanophilic, especially on staining with Sudan black, indicating that the granules contain a phospholipid rather

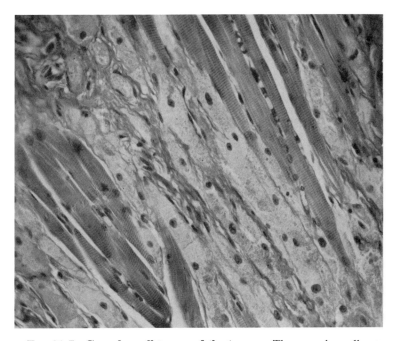

Fig. 31-7. **Granular cell tumor of the tongue.** The granular cells are infiltrating among the striated muscle bundles of the tongue. There are areas suggesting apparent transitions between the tumor cells and the muscle bundles. ($\times$400)

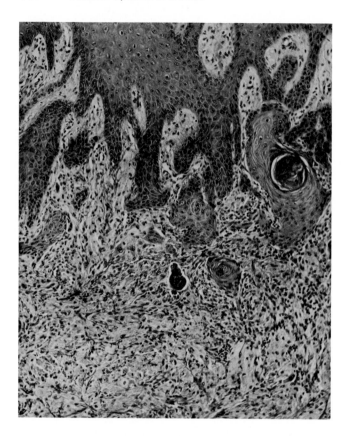

Fig. 31-8. **Granular cell tumor.** The epidermis exhibits pseudo-carcinomatous hyperplasia. The dermis contains many large pale tumor cells. In many areas thin strands of collagen surround groups of tumor cells. (×200)

than neutral fat (Fisher and Wechsler; Haisken and Langer). In other instances, the granules stain entirely negative for lipid (Aparicio and Lumsden).

The overlying epidermis usually is hyperplastic and not infrequently shows downward proliferation, often with horn-pearl formation (Fig. 31-8). It is important that this pseudocarcinomatous hyperplasia not be mistaken for squamous cell carcinoma (Bloom and Ginzler).

Histogenesis. For many years after its description by Abrikossoff in 1926, this tumor was thought to be composed of immature striated muscle cells, or myoblasts, and therefore was named granular cell myoblastoma. This view had arisen because of the frequent close association between tumor cells and striated muscle fibers of the tongue, suggesting transitions between them (Fig. 31-7).

Although histochemical and electron microscopic studies have eliminated myoblasts as the source of the tumor cells (Alkek et al.), there is as yet no agreement as to the nature of the tumor cell. It is agreed, however, that the cytoplasmic

granules are autophagosomes, or lysosomes (E.M. No. 45). As lysosomes they contain lysosomal enzymes, such as acid phosphatase; and on electron microscopy they often contain partly digested cytoplasmic material. Also, some of the cytoplasmic granules have the appearance of residual bodies or myelin figures (Garancis et al.; Sobel et al., 1971). The myelin figures, representing the end stage of lysosomes, probably are responsible for the presence of phospholipid in some of the granules.

Concerning the nature of the tumor cells, most authors believe that they are Schwann cells. Garancis et al., in an electron microscopic study, cited the following similarities: (1) the tumor cells are surrounded by a basal lamina; and (2) some of the tumor cells, like Schwann cells, contain axons in their cytoplasm. Furthermore (3), granules similar to those seen in the cells of the granular cell tumor have been observed by light microscopy in a neurofibroma (Pour et al.) and by electron microscopy in a subcutaneous neurilemmoma (Sobel et al., 1973). The presence of numerous lysosomal granules in the tumor cells is regarded by Weiser and Propst as consistent with their derivation from Schwann cells, since in their opinion Schwann cells can develop phagocytic properties when regressive changes occur within them.

On the other hand, several authors doubt that the tumor cells are Schwann cells because: (1) no normal or degenerating myelin could be demonstrated in the tumor cells by histochemical methods (Al-Sarraf et al.); and (2) axons could not be found by electron microscopy in the tumor cells by all observers (Moscovic and Azar).

Differential Diagnosis. On cursory examination the large pale cells of the tumor resemble the foam cells of xanthoma. However, the cells of the granular cell tumor contain a granular rather than a foamy cytoplasm, take fat stains only faintly if at all, and, in contrast with xanthoma cells, often are surrounded by fine strands of collagen. Furthermore, in granular cell tumors the overlying epidermis tends to be hyperplastic rather than atrophic, as in xanthoma.

Care must be taken not to regard the pseudocarcinomatous hyperplasia as carcinoma. This danger exists especially in biopsy specimens from the tongue and from the upper respiratory or digestive tract if the excision of the biopsy specimen is so superficial that the few granular cells present are overlooked. Once the granular cells are visualized, the diagnosis of squamous cell carcinoma no longer need be considered, since no case is known in which a squamous cell carcinoma developed in the epithelium overlying a granular cell tumor.

MALIGNANT GRANULAR CELL TUMOR

Malignant granular cell tumor, originally called malignant granular cell myoblastoma, is a very rare tumor. Most of the reported cases occurred on the skin or in the subcutaneous tissue; but, just as in the case of the benign granular cell tumors, a few cases have been reported from other areas, such as the bladder (Ravich et al.) and the larynx (Busanni-Caspari and Hammar).

In the skin and the subcutaneous tissue the tumor manifests itself as a gradually growing, poorly defined nodule or mass. Extensive metastases occur either in association with regional lymph node metastases (Ross et al.) or without them (Svejda and Horn).

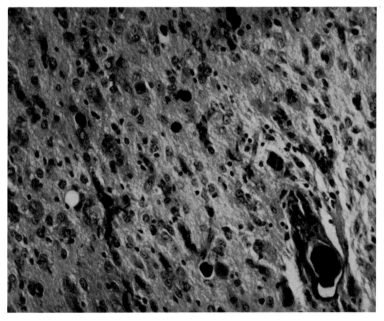

Fig. 31-9. **Nasal glioma.** The lesion consists of loosely textured glial tissue, i.e., of astrocytes and their processes. The astrocytes possess large clear nuclei and abundant pale cytoplasm. Foci of calcification are scattered through the lesion. (×400) (Weldon Bullock, M.D.)

Histopathology. On histologic grounds two types of malignant granular cell tumors have been recognized (Gamboa). In one type in spite of the clinically malignant course the histologic appearance of the primary lesion and even of the metastases is benign except for mild disorientation of the cells, slightly larger and darker nuclei than those seen in benign granular cell tumors, and occasional mitotic figures (Ravich et al.; Crawford and De Bakey; Gamboa; Svejda and Horn; Busanni-Caspari and Hammar). In the other type the primary lesion and the metastases appear histologically malignant inasmuch as they show transitions from typical granular cells through pleomorphic granular cells to pleomorphic nongranular spindle and giant cells with numerous mitotic figures (Ross et al.; Krieg; Al-Sarraf et al.).

Histogenesis. Several authors have expressed doubt about the existence of malignant granular cell tumors as an entity and believe that malignant tumors of varying genesis can show granular degeneration of the cytoplasm. Thus, a malignant tumor which histologically had the appearance of a malignant granular cell tumor on electron microscopy proved to be a squamous cell carcinoma because of the presence of numerous desmosomes (Gilliet et al.). Moscovic and Azar suspect that some cases reported as malignant granular cell tumor with widespread metastases, such as the case reported by Svejda and Horn, may represent an obscure "storage reticulosis" rather than a malignant tumor.

NASAL GLIOMA

Nasal glioma represents an intrauterine herniation of brain tissue. It is found most commonly on the skin near the nasal bridge, consisting of a firm, smooth, red-to-purple protrusion that usually is quite large, measuring 2 to 3 cm in diameter, and resembles a hemangioma. Gliomas may also be located intranasally; or they may be both extranasal and intranasal, in which case they are connected through a defect in the nasal bone.

Histopathology. The lesion is composed of loosely textured glial tissue, i.e., of astrocytes with their processes. Neurons usually are absent. Astrocytes possess large clear nuclei and abundant pale cytoplasm (Chris-

tianson) (Fig. 31-9). Focal calcifications may occur within the lesion.

Histogenesis. Nasal gliomas form during embryonic life as the result of a small encephalocele. Thus, they are not tumors. They are only rarely connected to the brain by a pedicle, since as a rule the intracranial connection closes before birth (Orkin and Fisher).

CUTANEOUS MENINGIOMA

Meningiomas are tumors arising from the arachnoid villi of the dura mater. Cutaneous meningiomas may develop in the scalp secondary to an intracranial meningioma either by means of erosion of the skull (Laymon and Becker), or by extension through an operative defect of the skull (Waterson and Shapiro). Such secondary cutaneous meningiomas may attain considerable size.

In addition, primary cutaneous meningiomas of the scalp have been described in very rare instances as small solitary nodules that may be present at birth or appear later in life (Bain and Shnitka). They are benign and do not increase in size. The existence of primary cutaneous meningiomas is open to question, since they may merely represent intradermal nevi containing psammoma bodies (see under Histogenesis).

Histopathology. Secondary cutaneous meningiomas of the scalp show sharply circumscribed islands of cells in a dense, hyalinized stroma. The cells have oval, vesicular nuclei and moderately abundant, pale-staining cytoplasm (Waterson and Shapiro). Psammoma bodies are usually absent (Laymon and Becker).

Primary cutaneous meningiomas have been described as showing small groups or strands of cells embedded in a loose fibrous stroma. The cells possess large vesicular nuclei and abundant cytoplasm. As a characteristic feature one observes large and small, concentrically laminated, hyaline psammoma bodies showing varying degrees of calcification. The hyaline material forming the psammoma bodies originates in the cytoplasm of the tumor cells (Bain and Shnitka).

Histogenesis. The traditional view has been that primary cutaneous meningiomas develop from ectopic arachnoidal cells and thus represent true meningiomas. However, the great histologic resemblance between primary cutaneous meningioma and intradermal nevus was noted by Bain and Shnitka, the only difference being the presence of psammoma bodies in primary cutaneous meningioma. Since recently the occurrence of psammoma bodies has been described also in intradermal nevi (Weitzner), it is likely that primary cutaneous meningiomas are merely intradermal nevi in which psammoma bodies have formed as the result of degeneration of some of the nevus cells.

BIBLIOGRAPHY

Neurofibromatosis

Becker, S. W.: Diagnosis and treatment of pigmented nevi. Arch. Derm. Syph., *60*:44, 1949.

Benedict, P. H., Szabo, G., Fitzpatrick, T. B., and Sinesi, S. J.: Melanotic macules in Albright's syndrome and in neurofibromatosis. J.A.M.A., *205*:618, 1968.

Crowe, F. W., Schull, W. J., and Neel, J. V.: Multiple Neurofibromatosis. Springfield, Ill., Charles C Thomas, 1955.

D'Agostino, A. N., Soule, E. H., and Miller, R. H.: Sarcomas of the peripheral nerves and somatic soft tissues associated with multiple neurofibromatosis (von Recklinghausen's disease). Cancer, *16*:1015, 1963.

Foot, N. C.: Histology of tumors of the peripheral nerves. Arch. Path., *30*:772, 1940.

Healey, F. H., and Mekelatos, C. J.: Pheochromocytoma and neurofibromatosis. New Eng. J. Med., *258*:540, 1958.

Jimbow, K., Szabo, G., and Fitzpatrick, T. B.: Ultrastructure of giant pigment granules (macromelanosomes) in the cutaneous pigmented macules of neurofibromatosis. J. Invest. Derm., *61*:300, 1973.

Johnson, B. L., and Charneco, D. R.: Café-au-lait spot in neurofibromatosis and in normal individuals. Arch. Derm., *102*:442, 1970.

Klaus, S. N., and Winkelmann, R. K.: Cholinesterase activity in neurofibromas in vitro. J. Invest. Derm., *41*:301, 1963.

Knight, W. A., III, Murphy, W. K., and Gottlieb, J. A.: Neurofibromatosis associated with malignant neurofibromas. Arch. Derm., *107*:747, 1973.

Levene, L. J.: Bone changes in neurofibromatosis. Arch. Intern. Med., *103*:570, 1959.

McNairy, D. J., and Montgomery, H.: Cutaneous tumors of von Recklinghausen's disease (neurofibromatosis). Arch. Derm. Syph., *51*:384, 1945 (review).

Murray, M. R., and Stout, A. P.: Schwann cell versus fibroblast as the origin of the specific nerve sheath tumor. Am. J. Path., *16*:41, 1940.

Nürnberger, F., and Korting, G. W.: Zum Vorkommen saurer Mucopolysaccharide in Neurofibromen und Neurofibrosarkomen. Arch. klin. exp. Derm., *235*:97, 1969.

Reed, R. J., Fine, R. M., and Meltzer, H. D.: Palisaded, encapsulated neuromas of the skin. Arch. Derm., *106*:865, 1972 (review).

Shelley, W. B., and Arthur, R. P.: Nerve fibers, a neglected component of intradermal cellular nevi. J. Invest. Derm., *34*:59, 1960.

Silvers, D. N., Greenwood, R. S., and Helwig, E. B.: Café au lait spots without giant pigment granules. Arch. Derm., *110*:87, 1974.

Streitmann, B.: Neurofibromatosis localisata. Z. Haut Geschlechtskr., *19*:324, 1955.

Tarlov, I. M.: The origin of perineural fibroblastoma. Am. J. Path., *16*:33, 1940.

Undeutsch, W.: Zum Problem der malignen Entartung der Neurofibromatosis Recklinghausen. Derm. Wschr., *136*:1145, 1957.

Verocay, J.: Zur Kenntnis der Neurofibrome. Beitr. Path. Anat., *48*:1, 1910.

Wachstein, M., and Wolf, E.: General neurofibromatosis (von Recklinghausen's disease) with local sarcomatous change and metastasis to regional lymph nodes. Arch. Path., *37*:331, 1944.

Waggener, J. D.: Ultrastructure of benign peripheral nerve sheath tumors. Cancer, *19*:699, 1966.

Weber, K., and Braun-Falco, O.: Zur Ultrastruktur der Neurofibromatose. Hautarzt, *23*:116, 1972.

White, H. R., Jr.: Survival in malignant schwannoma. Cancer, *27*:720, 1971.

Winkelmann, R. K., and Johnson, L. A.: Cholinesterases in neurofibromas. Arch. Derm., *85*:106, 1962.

Neurilemmoma

Carstens, P. H. B., and Schrodt, G. R.: Malignant transformation of a benign encapsulated neurilemmoma. Am. J. Clin. Path., *51*:144, 1969.

Das Guptas, T. K., Brasfield, R. D., Strong, E. W., and Hajdu, S. I.: Benign solitary schwannoma (neurilemmoma). Cancer, *24*:355, 1969.

Fawcett, K. J., and Dahlin, D. C.: Neurilemmoma of bone. Am. J. Clin. Path., *47*:759, 1967.

Fisher, E. R., and Vuzevski, V. D.: Cytogenesis of schwannoma (neurilemoma), neurofibroma, dermatofibroma, and dermatofibrosarcoma as revealed by electron microscopy. Am. J. Clin. Path., *49*:141, 1968.

Izumi, A. K., Rosato, F. E., and Wood, M. G.: Von Recklinghausen's disease associated with multiple neurilemmomas. Arch. Derm., *104*: 172, 1971.

Kuske, H., and Soltermann, W.: Neurinom der Zunge nach Zungenbiss. Dermatologica, *116*: 387, 1958.

Matakas, F., and Cervos-Navarro, J.: Abwandlungen des Gewebsbildes der Neurinome im elektronenmikroskopischen Bild. Virchows Arch. Abt. A, Path. Anat., *347*:160, 1969.

Mercantini, E. S., and Mopper, C.: Neurilemmoma of the tongue. Arch. Derm., *79*:542, 1959.

Reed, R. J., Fine, R. M., and Meltzer, H. D.: Palisaded, encapsulated neuromas of the skin. Arch. Derm., *106*:865, 1972.

Stout, A. P.: Neurilemmoma. *In* Tumors of the Peripheral Nervous System. p. 15. Washington, D.C., Armed Forces Institute of Pathology, 1949.

Waggener, J. D.: Ultrastructure of benign peripheral nerve sheath tumors. Cancer, *19*:699, 1966.

White, H. R., Jr.: Survival in malignant schwannoma. Cancer, *27*:720, 1971.

Winkelmann, R. K., and Johnson, L. A.: Cholinesterases in neurofibromas. Arch. Derm., *85*: 106, 1962.

Neuroma

Baum, J. L.: Abnormal intradermal histamine reaction in the syndrome of pheochromocytoma, medullary carcinoma of the thyroid gland and multiple mucosal neuromas. New Eng. J. Med., *284*:963, 1971.

Duemling, W. M.: Cutaneous neuroma. Arch. Derm. Syph., *19*:226, 1929.

Dupré, A., Christol, B., Bonafé, J. L., et al.: Neurome cutané à tumeur unique avec importantes altérations des cellules schwanniennes. Ann. derm. syph., *101*:271, 1974.

Holm, T. W., Prawer, S. E., Sahl, W. J., Jr., and Bart, B. J.: Multiple cutaneous neuromas. Arch. Derm., *107*:608, 1973.

Hurwitz, S.: Sipple syndrome. Arch. Derm., *110*:139, 1974.

Reed, R. J., Fine, R. M., and Meltzer, H. D.: Palisaded, encapsulated neuromas of the skin. Arch. Derm., *106*:865, 1972 (review).

Shapiro, L., Juklin, E. A., and Brownstein, M. H.: Rudimentary polydactyly. Arch. Derm., *108*: 223, 1973.

Thies, W.: Multiple echte fibrilläre Neurome (Rankenneurome) der Haut und Schleimhaut. Arch. klin. exp. Derm., *218*:561, 1964.

Waggener, J. D.: Ultrastructure of benign peripheral nerve sheath tumors. Cancer, *19*:699, 1966.

Walker, D. M.: Oral mucosal neuroma-medullary thyroid carcinoma syndrome. Brit. J. Derm., *88*:599, 1973.

Granular Cell Tumor

Abrikossoff, A.: Über Myome, ausgehend von der quergestreiften, willkürlichen Muskulatur. Virchows Arch. path. Anat., *260*:215, 1926.

Alkek, D. S., Johnson, W. C., and Graham, J. H.: Granular cell myoblastoma. Arch. Derm., *98*:543, 1968.

Al-Sarraf, M., Loud, A. V., and Vaitkevicius, V. K.: Malignant granular cell tumor. Histochemical and electron microscopic study. Arch. Path., *91*:550, 1971.

Aparicio, S. R., and Lumsden, C. E.: Light and electron microscopic studies on the granular cell myoblastoma of the tongue. J. Path., *97*: 339, 1969.

Bloom, D., and Ginzler, A. M.: Myoblastoma. Arch. Derm. Syph., *56*:648, 1947.

Fisher, E. R., and Wechsler, H.: Granular cell myoblastoma, a misnomer. Cancer, *15*:936, 1962.

Garancis, J. C., Komorowski, R. A., and Kuzma, J. F.: Granular cell myoblastoma. Cancer, *25*:542, 1970.

Haisken, W., and Langer, E.: Die submikroskopische Struktur des sogenannten Myoblastenmyoms (Lipidfibrom, granuläres Neurom). Frankfurt. Z. Path., *71*:600, 1962.

Moscovic, E. A., and Azar, H. A.: Multiple granular cell tumors ("myoblastomas"). Cancer, *20*:2032, 1967.

Pour, P., Althoff, J., and Cardesa, A.: Granular cells in tumors and in nontumorous tissue. Arch. Path., *95*:135, 1973.

Sobel, H. J., Marquet, E., Avrin, E., and Schwarz, R.: Granular cell myoblastoma. Am. J. Path., *65*:59, 1971.

Sobel, H. J., Marquet, E., and Schwarz, R.: Is schwannoma related to granular cell myoblastoma? Arch. Path., *95*:396, 1973.

Strong, E. W., McDivitt, R. W., and Brasfield, R. D.: Granular cell myoblastoma. Cancer, *25*:415, 1970.

Weiser, G., and Propst, A.: Elektronenoptische Untersuchung zur Histogenese des granulären Neuroms. Virchows Arch. Abt. A, Path. Anat., *358*:193, 1973.

Malignant Granular Cell Tumor

Al-Sarraf, M., Loud, A. V., and Vaitkevicius, V. K.: Malignant granular cell tumor. Histochemical and electron microscopic study. Arch. Path., *91*:550, 1971.

Busanni-Caspari, W., and Hammar, C. H.: Zur Malignität der sogenannten Myoblastenmyome. Zbl. Allg. Path., *98*:401, 1958.

Crawford, E. S., and De Bakey, M. E.: Granular-cell myoblastoma: two unusual cases. Cancer, *6*:786, 1953.

Gamboa, L. G.: Malignant granular-cell myoblastoma. Arch. Path., *60*:663, 1955.

Gilliet, F., MacGee, W., Stoian, M., and Delacrétaz, J.: Zur Histogenese granuliertzelliger Tumoren. Hautarzt, *24*:52, 1973.

Krieg, A. F.: Malignant granular cell myoblastoma. Arch. Path., *74*:251, 1962.

Moscovic, E. A., and Azar, H. A.: Multiple granular cell tumors ("myoblastomas"). Cancer, *20*:2032, 1967.

Ravich, A., Stout, A. P., and Ravich, R. A.: Malignant granular cell myoblastoma involving the urinary bladder. Ann. Surg., *121*:361, 1945.

Ross, R. C., Miller, T. R., and Foote, F. W.: Malignant granular-cell myoblastoma. Cancer, *5*:112, 1952.

Svejda, J., and Horn, V.: Disseminated granular-cell pseudotumour; so-called metastasising granular-cell myoblastoma. J. Path. Bact., *76*:343, 1958.

Nasal Glioma

Christianson, H. B.: Nasal glioma. Arch. Derm., *93*:68, 1966.

Orkin, M., and Fisher, I.: Heterotopic brain tissue (heterotopic neural rest). Arch. Derm., *94*:699, 1966.

Cutaneous Meningioma

Bain, G. O., and Shnitka, T. K.: Cutaneous meningioma (psammoma). Arch. Derm., *74*:590, 1956.

Laymon, C. W., and Becker, F. T.: Massive metastasizing meningioma involving the scalp. Arch. Derm. Syph., *59*:626, 1949.

Waterson, K. W., Jr., and Shapiro, L.: Meningioma cutis: report of a case. Internat. J. Derm., *9*:125, 1970.

Weitzner, S.: Intradermal nevus with psammoma body formation. Arch. Derm., *98*:287, 1968.

32

Melanocytic Nevi and Malignant Melanoma

Tumors that are derived from melanocytes are composed either of nevus cells, of epidermal melanocytes, or of dermal melanocytes.

Benign tumors composed of nevus cells are called nevocellular nevi. They can be divided into junctional nevi, compound nevi, and intradermal nevi. Special variants of nevocellular nevi are: (1) the balloon cell nevus, (2) the halo nevus, (3) the benign juvenile melanoma, and (4) the congenital giant pigmented nevus.

Benign tumors derived from epidermal melanocytes include (1) lentigo simplex, (2) freckles, (3) the melanotic macules of Albright's syndrome, (4) Becker's melanosis, and (5) lentigo senilis. (The café-au-lait patches of neurofibromatosis have been described on p. 632).

Benign tumors derived from dermal melanocytes include the Mongolian spot, the nevus of Ota, and the blue nevus.

Malignant melanoma can be divided into malignant melanoma in situ, of which there are two types: lentigo maligna, and the pagetoid type; and invasive malignant melanoma, which may arise from a nevocellular nevus, a congenital giant pigmented nevus, or a malignant melanoma in situ. Most commonly, however, a malignant melanoma arises as such. Finally, there is the very rare malignant blue nevus.

NEVOCELLULAR NEVUS

Nevocellular nevi vary considerably in their clinical appearance. Aside from the four special forms of nevocellular nevi mentioned above, which will be discussed separately, one may recognize five clinical types of nevocellular nevi: (1) flat lesions; (2) slightly elevated lesion; (3) papillomatous lesions; (4) dome-shaped lesions, and (5) pedunculated lesions. The first three types are always pigmented; the latter two may or may not be pigmented. Although exceptions occur, one can predict to a certain degree from the clinical appearance of a nevocellular nevus whether on histologic examination it will be a junctional nevus, a compound nevus, or an intradermal nevus. Most of the flat lesions represent either a junctional nevus or a lentigo simplex; most of the slightly elevated lesions and some of the papillomatous lesions represent a compound nevus; most of the papillomatous lesions and nearly all dome-shaped and pedunculated lesions represent intradermal nevi (Shaffer).

Histopathology. Nevocellular nevi are composed of nevus cells which, even though, basically, they are identical with melanocytes, differ from melanocytes by being arranged in clusters or "nests," and by not showing dendritic processes, as best demonstrated by staining with silver. (For details see under Histogenesis.)

Although a histologic subdivision of nevocellular nevi into junctional, compound, and intradermal nevi is very useful and is generally accepted, it should be realized that lesions in an intermediate state between junctional and compound nevus and between compound and intradermal nevus are frequently encountered, especially if serial or step sections are carried out (Kopf and Andrade).

Nevus cells show considerable variation in their appearance, and thus they are often recognizable as nevus cells largely by their arrangement in clusters or "nests," rather than by their cellular characteristics. In the lower epidermis and upper dermis they commonly resemble epithelioid cells, since they usually are cuboidal or oval in shape and have a distinctly outlined homogeneous cytoplasm and a large, round or oval nucleus. Not infrequently they contain melanin. Nevus cells in the middermis usually are smaller in size than those in the upper dermis and may resemble lymphoid cells; they rarely contain melanin. Nevus cells in the lower dermis resemble fibroblasts, since usually they are elongated and possess a spindle-shaped nucleus. They often lie in strands and hardly ever contain melanin. Some authors have been referring to the nevus cells in the upper, middle, and lower dermis as types "A," "B," and "C," respectively (Miescher and von Albertini; Mishima).

JUNCTIONAL NEVUS. In a junctional nevus, nevus cells are present as well circumscribed nevus cell nests in the lower epidermis (Fig. 32-1). The upper epidermis appears essentially normal, since there is little tendency to penetration of nevus cells into the upper dermis. In addition, nests of nevus cells often lie beneath the epidermis but still in contact with it, and thus are in the stage of "dropping off." Usually, in some areas one sees also nevus cell nests located free in the upper dermis. The nevus cells contain varying amounts of melanin. In junctional nevi with large amounts of melanin in the nevus cells, melanin may be seen in the upper dermis located within melanophages. No inflammatory infiltrate is present, as a rule. The nevus cells comprising the intraepidermal and subepidermal cell nests generally have a regular, cuboidal appearance, although in occasional instances they are spindle-shaped. (For differential diagnosis from malignant melanoma in situ, see p. 668, and from malignant melanoma, see p. 675.)

COMPOUND NEVUS. A compound nevus possesses features of both a junctional and an intradermal nevus. Nevus cell nests are seen in the epidermis, as well as "dropping off" from the epidermis into the dermis, and in the dermis (Fig. 32-2). Usually, the nevus cells in the upper dermis are cuboidal and contain a moderate amount of melanin. Occasionally, however, the nevus cells com-

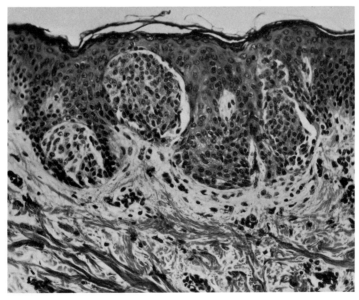

FIG. 32-1. **Nevocellular nevus: junctional nevus.** Well circumscribed nevus cell nests are present in the lower epidermis. (×200)

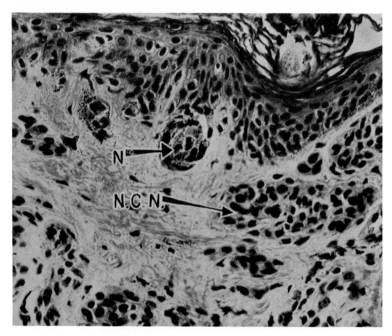

FIG. 32-2. **Nevocellular nevus: compound nevus.** Nevus cell nests are seen within the epidermis and in the dermis. One nevus cell nest (N.) is in the stage of "dropping off." In addition, typical nevus cell nests (N.C.N.) lie free in the dermis. Considerable amounts of melanin are present in the nevus cell nests in the upper dermis, whereas no melanin is seen in the nevus cell nests farther down. (×200)

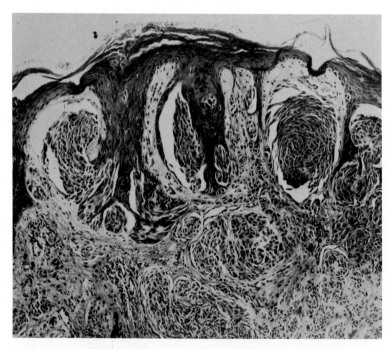

FIG. 32-3. **Nevocellular nevus: compound nevus.** The cells composing the intra-epidermal and subepidermal cell nests are spindle-shaped and contain little or no melanin. This represents the so-called spindle cell nevus, a variant of benign juvenile melanoma. (×100)

FIG. 32-4. **Nevocellular nevus: intradermal nevus.** In the upper dermis the nevus cells lie in nests and cords. In the lower dermis the nevus cells appear spindle-shaped and are embedded in collagenous fibers. (×100)

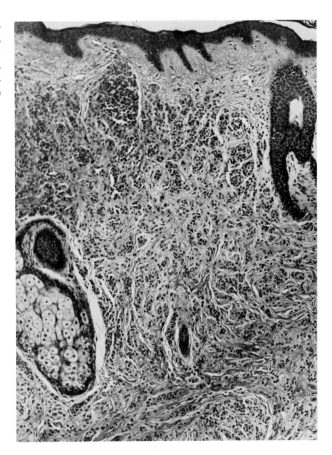

posing the intraepidermal and the subepidermal cell nests are spindle-shaped rather than cuboidal and contain little or no melanin (Fig. 32-3). This so-called spindle cell nevus represents a variant of benign juvenile melanoma (see p. 655).

INTRADERMAL NEVUS. Intradermal nevi show usually only very slight and occasionally no junctional activity. The upper dermis shows nests and cords of nevus cells (Fig. 32-4). Not infrequently, one encounters within the nests and cords multinucleated nevus cells in which small nuclei lie either in a rosettelike arrangement or close together in the center of the cell. These giant cells occur only in well-matured nevi and therefore can be taken as evidence of the benign nature of the nevus in which they occur. They differ significantly in appearance from the irregularly and even bizarrely shaped giant cells seen frequently in benign juvenile melanoma and occasionally also in malignant melanoma. As a result of shrinkage during tissue-processing, clefts may form within some nevus cell nests between the outer row of nevus cells and the inner core of nevus cells, giving the impression as if a group of nevus cells were located within a lymphatic space, simulating lymphatic invasion (Sagebiel).

Whereas the nevus cell nests located in the upper dermis usually contain a moderate amount of melanin, the nevus cells in the midportion and the lower dermis rarely contain melanin. Instead, the nevus cells appear spindle-shaped, are arranged in bundles, and are embedded in collagenous fibers having a loose, pale, and wavy appearance similar to that of the fibers in a neurofibroma. Such formations have been referred to as "neuroid tubes." In other areas the nevus cells may lie in concentric arrangement embedded in loose fibrous tissue, forming so-called nevic corpuscles that resemble Meissner's tactile bodies and are referred to as "lames foliacées" (Masson, 1951).

An occasional intradermal nevus is devoid of nevus cell nests in the upper dermis and contains only spindle-shaped nevus cells embedded in abundant, loosely arranged, collagenous tissue (Fig. 32-5). Such nevi are referred to as "neural nevi." Their differentiation from a solitary neurofibroma then may be difficult and even impossible in routinely stained sections (Becker). However, the demonstration of numerous nerve fibers by silver impregnation would be in favor of a neurofibroma. Also, on electron microscopy neurofibromas are composed of Schwann cells, and neural nevi of melanocytes (Thorne et al.) (see Histogenesis).

Some intradermal nevi show hyperkeratosis and papillomatosis that may be associated with a lacelike downward growth of epidermal strands and with horn cysts (Fig. 32-6); others contain large hair follicles. In occasional instances, papillomatous or hairy nevocellular nevi show fairly pronounced "dropping-off" activity and then represent compound nevi rather than intradermal nevi.

Nevocellular nevi containing greatly dilated hair follicles may show, as a result of the rupture of a hair follicle, clinically a sudden increase in size associated with an inflammatory reaction, causing suspicion of a malignant melanoma. Histologic examination in such instances shows a partially destroyed epidermal follicular lining with a pronounced inflammatory infiltrate and presence of foreign-body giant cells (Freeman and Knox).

Occasionally, intradermal nevi contain scattered large fat cells within aggregates of nevus cells (Fig. 30-2). Such cases probably represent a combination of an intradermal nevus with a nevus lipomatosus rather than a degenerative change (Cramer). The occasional presence of spicules of bone in intradermal nevi, on the other hand, does not seem to represent a combination of nevocellular nevus with an osteoma but ossification secondary to an inflammatory reaction (Delacrétaz and Frenk; Roth et al.). In rare instances psammoma bodies, i.e., hya-

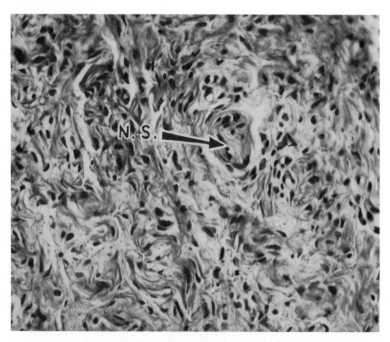

Fig. 32-5. **Nevocellular nevus: neural nevus.** The nevus cells are spindle-shaped and are embedded in abundant, loosely arranged collagenous tissue, which has the same loose, wavy, pale appearance as that in neurofibroma. In the center one sees a neuroid structure (N.S.) or nevic corpuscle resembling a Meissner tactile body. (×200)

line bodies with slight calcification, may be observed within intradermal nevi (Weitzner) (see also p. 643).

The term *fibrous papule of the nose* was given by Graham et al. to a usually solitary, flesh-colored, dome-shaped lesion of the nose. Since histologic examination often shows the presence of some nevus cells, and since intradermal nevi are well known to be capable of involution, they regard the lesion as the residual of an intradermal nevus. The findings and interpretation of Graham et al. have been supported by Saylan et al.

Histogenesis. For many years Masson's theory of the dual origin of nevus cells, first proposed by him in 1926, was widely accepted. As stated by Masson in 1951, he believed that the nevus cells in the upper dermis developed from epidermal melanocytes, whereas the nevus cells in the lower dermis developed from Schwann cells. The Schwann cell origin of the nevus cells in the lower dermis was suggested to him by the frequent presence of nervelike structures, such as neuroid tubes and nevic corpuscles, in the deeper portions of nevocellular nevi (see p. 649). The fact that both epidermal melanocytes and

Schwann cells are derived from the neural crest and thus are related to one another seemed to have supported Masson's view. Also in favor of a relationship between the nevus cells in the deep dermis and Schwann cells was the presence of a strongly positive nonspecific cholinesterase reaction in both types of cells and the absence of melanin and of a positive dopa oxidase reaction in the nevus cells in the deep dermis (Winkelmann).

In contrast with Masson, Mishima proposed that nevus cells originate neither from epidermal melanocytes nor from Schwann cells but from a primitive precursor cell that is derived from the neural crest in addition to melanocytes and Schwann cells. Mishima has called this precursor cell nevoblast. Mishima even has distinguished between nevus cells derived from melanogenic nevoblasts and those derived from schwannian nevoblasts, since he found that, on electron microscopy, only some of the nevus cells, i.e., those supposedly derived from melanogenic nevoblasts, possessed melanosomes and dopa oxidase activity.

An important clarification was achieved in 1971 by Thorne et al. who demonstrated that, in contrast to Mishima's findings, even the nevus

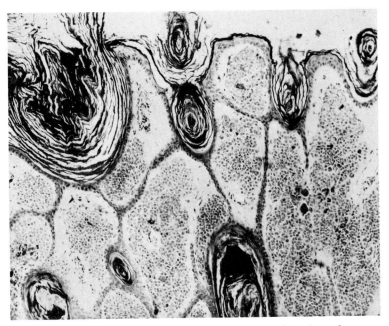

Fig. 32-6. **Nevocellular nevus: papillomatous intradermal nevus.** There is lacelike downward growth of epidermal strands around nests of nevus cells. There are numerous multinucleated nevus cells in which the nuclei lie either in a rosette-like arrangement or close together in the center of the cell. (×100)

cells deep in the dermis which had a neuroid appearance on light microscopy contained on electron microscopic examination melanosomes with dopa oxidase activity. For the demonstration of the electron microscopic dopa reaction, Thorne et al. used glutaraldehyde as fixative in place of formalin which had been used by Mishima. In addition, after incubating the ultrathin sections in dopa solution they postfixed them in osmium tetroxide. Electron microscopic examination also revealed that the nevus cells in nevi with a neuroid appearance on light microscopy did not possess the characteristics of Schwann cells and, in particular, did not contain nonmyelinated axons within their cytoplasm. Thus, at least by electron microscopy, a clearcut separation between nevus cells and Schwann cells is possible.

Concerning the relationship between epidermal melanocytes and nevus cells, Mishima and also Lupulescu et al. regard these two types of cells as having a different embryologic genesis, whereas other authors, such as Clark and Mihm, regard them as identical cell types. It would seem that all morphologic features by which nevus cells differ from melanocytes, such as the absence of dendrites by light microscopy, their arrangement in cell nests, and their larger size,

are secondary adjustments of the cells (E.M. Nos. 46 and 47). Gottlieb et al. were able to show by electron microscopy that the fine structure of nevus cells is comparable to that of epidermal melanocytes, since not only are the melanosomes in both cells identical but also nevus cells possess pseudopodic cytoplasmic processes that, even though they are smaller, are analogous to the dendritic processes of melanocytes. In conclusion, it seems established that nevus cells differ from Schwann cells but are identical with melanocytes.

BALLOON CELL NEVUS

Balloon cell nevi possess no clinical features through which they could be differentiated from other nevocellular nevi. They are very rare. As a rule, they occur as a slightly elevated, soft lesion of light brown color. They rarely exceed 5 mm in size (Schrader and Helwig). They have no special site of predilection. Although more common during the first three decades of life, they may be found also in older individuals.

Histopathology. Balloon cells may form only a small part of an intradermal or com-

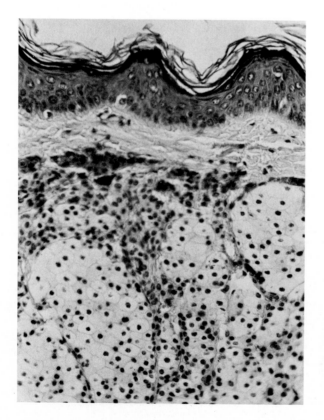

FIG. 32-7. **Balloon cell nevus.** Ballooned nevus cells lie in the dermis aggregated into variously sized lobules. Above the lobules of balloon cells small groups of nonballooned, moderately pigmented nevus cells are located. The balloon cells are larger than ordinary nevus cells. (×200)

pound nevus (Gartmann), or they may be the major component of a nevus (Wilson Jones and Sanderson; Hornstein). If they form only part of a nevus the balloon cells either are present as a large nodular component or are distributed diffusely through the lesion (Schrader and Helwig). If they form the major component of a nevus, the balloon cells tend to lie in closely aggregated alveolar formations (Fig. 32-7). In some instances balloon cells occur as nests at the epidermal-dermal junction. They also may be seen within the epidermis singly and as nests (Hashimoto and Bale). Transitions between nevus cells and balloon cells are seen in some instances (Wilson Jones and Sanderson).

The balloon cells are considerably larger than ordinary nevus cells, usually measuring 20 to 40 μm in diameter. Their nucleus appears similar to the nuclei of normal nevus cells. Although usually centrally located, the nucleus may be located at the margin of the cell. A few scattered multinucleated balloon cells are commonly seen (Schrader and

Helwig). The cytoplasm of the balloon cells appears either empty or finely granular. A few small melanin granules are occasionally seen in subepidermally located balloon cells, especially with the Masson-Fontana stain (Hornstein). Stains for lipids, for glycogen, and for acid or neutral mucopolysaccharides are negative in the balloon cells.

Histogenesis. Electron microscopic examination reveals in balloon cells numerous large vacuoles which have formed by progressive enlargement, degeneration and coalescence of melanosomes (Hashimoto and Bale). Because of the vacuolar degeneration of the melanosomes, melanization of the lamellar matrix of melanosomes usually does not take place. Vacuoles similar to those seen in the nevus cells of the dermis can be found also in the epidermis within melanocytes, as well as within some keratinocytes as the result of transfer of altered melanosomes from melanocytes to keratinocytes (Okun et al.).

Differential Diagnosis. Balloon cell nevus must be differentiated from balloon cell melanoma. (For its description see p. 672.) The large fat cells present in some intrader-

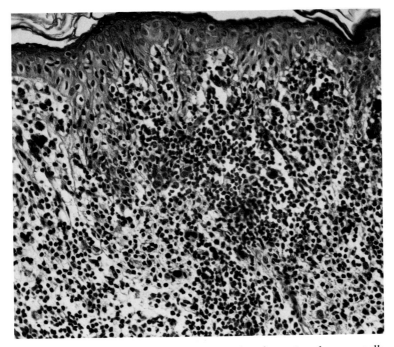

FIG. 32-8. **Halo nevus.** In the upper dermis scattered nevus cells are seen. Some of them contain melanin granules. Intermingled with the nevus cells and extending deep into the dermis is a dense infiltrate of cells, most of which have the appearance of lymphoid cells. ($\times$200)

mal nevi that are combined with a nevus lipomatosus (see p. 618) differ from balloon cells by having a flattened nucleus that always is located at the periphery of the cell, and by a positive fat stain.

HALO NEVUS

A halo nevus represents a pigmented nevocellular nevus surrounded by a depigmented zone, or halo. Such nevi undergo involution, a process that extends over a period of several months. The area of depigmentation shows no clinical signs of inflammation, and, even though it may persist for many months and even years, it ultimately disappears in most instances (Frank and Cohen). Most individuals with halo nevi are young adults, and the back is the most common site. Not infrequently, halo nevi are multiple, occurring either simultaneously or successively. The development of multiple halo nevi following the excision of a malignant melanoma has been reported recently by Epstein et al.

In rare instances an area of depigmentation can form also around a blue nevus, or around a malignant melanoma, or around the metastases of a malignant melanoma (Kopf et al.; Shapiro and Kopf).

Histopathology. In its early stage a halo nevus still shows multiple nests of nevus cells in the upper dermis and, in the case of a compound nevus, also at the epidermal-dermal junction. Later on, a greater number of scattered nevus cells than of nests are seen. Even at a time when melanin is still present in the nevus cells these cells often show evidence of damage to their nucleus and cytoplasm. Beneath the epidermis and intermingled with the nevus cells there is a dense infiltrate of cells, most of which have the appearance of lymphoid cells. Some cells of the infiltrate, however, are macrophages (Fig. 32-8). Varying amounts of melanin are present within the macrophages. The infiltrate gives the impression of invading the nevus cell nests and ultimately also the lower portion of the epidermis.

At a later stage only a few, and finally no distinct nevus cells can be identified any more. Thus, Findlay was unable to find nevus cells in 6 of his 8 cases; and Frank and Cohen, in 5 of their 14 cases. Gradu-

ally, after all nevus cells have disappeared, the inflammatory infiltrate subsides.

The epidermis of the halo surrounding the involuting nevus shows at first a reduction in the amount of melanin on staining with silver. Ultimately, there is complete absence of melanin and also a negative dopa oxidase reaction. The melanin in the epidermis overlying the nevus persists longer than that in the surrounding epidermis but ultimately it also disappears after the involution of the nevus.

Histogenesis. Patients with an involuting halo nevus show circulating antibodies against the cytoplasm of malignant melanoma cells. These antibodies disappear from their blood stream once resolution of the nevus is complete (Copeman et al.). This immunologic phenomenon proves that patients with a halo nevus have developed a sensitivity to their nevus and reject it. Although the circulating antibodies in the serum of patients with halo nevi are the same as those found in the serum of patients with primary malignant melanoma (see p. 675), it seems not proved that halo nevi are pigmented nevi developing malignant changes, as Copeman et al. postulate.

Electron microscopic study reveals that under the influence of the lymphocytic infiltrate all nevus cells and melanocytes within reach of the infiltrate at first are damaged and ultimately disappear. The Langerhans cells, however, remain behind. As long as damaged melanocytes are still present in the epidermis one may observe in the Langerhans cells melanosome complexes enclosed within lysosomes (Swanson et al.; Ebner and Niebauer). It is of interest that both in halo nevi and in vitiligo the depigmentation takes place through disappearance of melanocytes. However, vitiligo differs from halo nevus by the absence of a lymphocytic infiltrate (see p. 420). It is likely that in halo nevus the lymphocytes of the infiltrate carry antibodies against the nevus cells and melanocytes (Stegmaier et al.). By electron microscopy many of the lymphocytes in the infiltrate show an endoplasmic reticulum, giving them the appearance of antigenically stimulated lymphocytes (Swanson et al.).

Differential Diagnosis. Early lesions of halo nevus often are difficult to differentiate from a malignant melanoma, since both types of lesions may have a dense cellular infiltrate in the dermis, and also in halo nevi the nevus cell nests, as the result of their being invaded and damaged by the cellular infiltrate, may appear as if they were atypical. However, aside from the clinical history and appearance, the limitation of the nevus cell nests to the uppermost dermis and the greater extent of the cellular infiltrate in halo nevus than in malignant melanoma, where it usually is only bandlike, aid in the differentiation.

In the absence of identifiable nevus cells, the diagnosis of halo nevus is suggested by the presence of melanophages in the dense cellular infiltrate, and by the absence of melanin in the epidermis on staining with silver.

BENIGN JUVENILE MELANOMA

Benign juvenile melanomas arise predominantly in children; but, in addition to persisting into adult life, they arise in adolescents or adults in about 15 per cent of the cases (Allen). The lesion usually is solitary and is encountered most commonly on the face and extremities. In most instances the lesion consists of a dome-shaped, hairless, small nodule, usually only a few millimeters in diameter, that because of the sparsity of melanin generally has a reddish rather than a brown color. Occasionally more than one lesion is present and in rare instances, a large group of lesions is observed limited to one area such as a thigh (Bourlond) or a cheek (Brownstein).

Histopathology. Benign juvenile melanoma represents a compound nevus. Because of the pleomorphism of the cells and the frequent presence of an inflammatory infiltrate the histologic picture often closely resembles that of a nodular malignant melanoma; and there is no doubt that prior to its recognition as an entity by Spitz in 1948 many cases were misdiagnosed as malignant melanoma.

Benign juvenile melanomas often show considerable junctional activity, which may be associated with a downward proliferation of the epidermis in irregular strands (Allen). In rare instances, however, junctional activ-

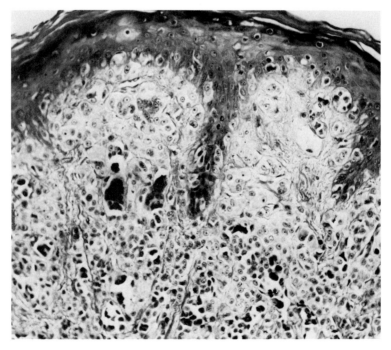

FIG. 32-9. **Benign juvenile melanoma.** The tumor cells are epithelioid in type. They vary in size and shape. Several rather large, irregularly shaped, bizarre giant cells are present. There is considerable junctional activity. The upper dermis shows edema. (×200)

ity is absent (Echevarria and Ackerman). In most cases the nevus cells are predominantly spindle-shaped (Fig. 32-3), but they may be predominantly epithelioid in type (Fig. 32-9), or they may be both spindle-shaped and epithelioid (Saksela and Rintala). It is of interest that benign juvenile melanomas composed largely of epithelioid cells are rarely found in adults (Echevarria and Ackerman); and, as a rule, benign juvenile melanomas in adults are "spindle cell nevi." Thus, Coskey and Mehregan found that in 26 per cent of their series of 202 cases of spindle cell nevi, excision was carried out in adults 18 years old or older.

The nevus cells in benign juvenile melanoma are arranged mostly in fairly well circumscribed nests, but in some areas they may be loosely arranged because of edema of the stroma. The edema is particularly evident in the upper dermis, where telangiectases are also frequently seen. Melanin in many instances is nearly completely absent, and, if present, small amounts only are generally found, although lesions in adults often are more pigmented than in children (Echevarria and Ackerman). Mitotic figures are present in some cases (Spitz; Jakubowicz), but are absent in others (Steigleder and Wellmer). A bandlike chronic inflammatory infiltrate may or may not be present at the base of the nevus.

Whereas spindle-shaped cells characteristically are arranged in whorls and only rarely show multinucleated giant cells, epithelioid cells frequently are multinucleated. The epithelioid cells are large, polygonal, sharply demarcated and often have an eosinophilic cytoplasm. The nuclei of multinucleated epithelioid cells often appear bizarre, being large and hyperchromatic and having an irregular outline (Allen). The multinucleated epithelioid cells tend to stand out clearly, because they are often surrounded by edema.

Histogenesis. The fact that in benign juvenile melanoma, in contrast to malignant melanoma, no circulating antibodies against the cytoplasm of malignant melanoma cells are found, indicates that it is a biologically benign lesion (Copeman et al.).

On *electron microscopic examination* benign juvenile melanomas show in their upper por-

tion melanocytes with numerous melanosomes; whereas in their lower portion the number of melanosomes in the melanocytes decreases. Melanization is incomplete in most melanocytes. In addition, there is considerable lysosomal degradation of melanosome complexes within the tumor cells even though the melanosomes are poorly melanized (Schreiner and Wolff). The almost complete absence of melanin in most benign juvenile melanomas is thus explained.

Differential Diagnosis. The following findings often help in the differentiation of benign juvenile melanoma from nodular malignant melanoma: (1) presence of spindle-shaped or epithelioid cells, or both; (2) frequent presence of bizarre giant cells; (3) absence or sparsity of melanin; and (4) edema of the subepidermal stroma often associated with telangiectatic vessels. Special caution should be taken before a diagnosis of benign juvenile melanoma is made in a lesion having arisen in an adult, in particular if the lesion consists only of epithelioid cells. As has been pointed out, benign juvenile melanomas of the epithelioid cell type are very rare in adults.

CONGENITAL GIANT PIGMENTED NEVUS

In this congenital but not inherited disorder a large nevocellular nevus is present that is pigmented, softly infiltrated, and usually slightly hairy. The nevus measures at least several centimeters in diameter and may be extensive. If extensive, the nevus may have a "bathing trunk" distribution or may follow the outline of a cap, a shoulder-stole, a coat sleeve, or a stocking. Usually, in addition to an extensive giant pigmented nevus, many scattered smaller but otherwise similar nevi are present (Slaughter et al.). In rare instances one finds on the scalp, in place of a giant pigmented nevus, a nonpigmented, flesh-colored, convoluted mass referred to as a giant cerebriform nevus (Gross and Carter; Orkin et al.).

Two features distinguish the congenital giant pigmented nevus from other pigmented lesions: (1) its predisposition to give rise to a malignant melanoma, and (2) its occasional association with leptomeningeal melanocytosis. The incidence of a malignant melanoma arising in a giant pigmented nevus is high, occurring probably in 10 per cent (Greeley et al.) or even in 13 per cent of the cases (Slaughter et al.). The malignant melanoma may be present at birth, or it may arise in infancy or at any time later in life (Reed et al.).

Leptomeningeal melanocytosis is found especially in cases in which the giant pigmented nevus involves the neck and scalp. There may be not only epilepsy and mental retardation but also a primary leptomeningeal malignant melanoma (Touraine; Reed et al.; Williams).

Histopathology. Three patterns may be found intermingled within giant pigmented nevi, namely patterns of (1) a compound or intradermal nevus, (2) a "neural nevus," and (3) a blue nevus. In some instances the compound or intradermal nevus component predominates, whereas in others the "neural nevus" component predominates. In the latter case formations such as neuroid tubes and nevic corpuscles are present (see p. 649). A component resembling a blue nevus is found in only some of the giant pigmented nevi and then only as a minor component (Reed et al.). In two instances, however, the entire congenital scalp lesion was interpreted as a giant blue nevus which in one patient extended to the dura (Menter et al.) and in the other had infiltrated the brain (Silverberg et al.).

If a malignant melanoma arises in a giant pigmented nevus or, as may happen in rare instances, in one of the many small satellite nevi, the origin of the malignant melanoma may be at the epidermal-dermal junction. Occasionally, however, the malignant melanoma in a giant pigmented nevus, in contrast with all other malignant melanomas, arises deep in the dermis (Herzberg; Reed et al.). In such cases it consists largely of undifferentiated cells resembling lymphoblasts and containing little or no melanin (Reed et al.).

In cases of leptomeningeal melanocytosis one finds a diffuse infiltration of the leptomeninges with pigmented melanocytes. Also, the blood vessels entering the brain and spinal cord may be surrounded by melanocytes, and there may be areas of infiltration of the brain or spinal cord with melanocytes. Leptomeningeal malignant melanoma can infiltrate the leptomeninx and form multiple nodules in the brain (Touraine; Slaughter et al.; Williams).

LENTIGO SIMPLEX

Three types of lentigo are recognized: lentigo simplex, lentigo senilis, and lentigo maligna. Lentigo simplex most frequently arises in childhood, but may appear at any age (Clark and Mihm). Usually in lentigo simplex, there are only a few scattered lesions without predilection to areas of sun exposure. They are uniformly colored but vary individually from brown to black. They are not infiltrated and usually measure only a few millimeters in diameter. Clinically, lentigo simplex is indistinguishable from a junctional nevus.

Special forms of lentigo simplex are the nevus spilus, the multiple lentigines syndrome, and the Peutz-Jeghers syndrome.

The *nevus spilus* is a light brown patch or band present since birth that in childhood becomes dotted with small, dark brown macules (Cohen et al.; Matsudo et al.).

The *multiple lentigines syndrome* is characterized by the presence of thousands of flat, dark brown macules on the skin but not on the mucous surfaces. Although most macules vary from pinpoint dots to 5 mm in size, occasional dark spots are much larger, up to 5 cm in diameter (Selmanowitz). Features of this rare, dominantly inherited syndrome, known also by the mnemonic "LEOPARD syndrome" are, besides the lentigines (L), electrocardiographic conduction defects (E), ocular hypertelorism (O), pulmonary stenosis (P), abnormalities of the genitalia (A) consisting of gonadal or ovarian hypoplasia, retardation of growth (R), and neural deafness (D) (Gorlin et al.; Capute et al.).

The *Peutz-Jeghers syndrome* shows dark brown macules largely in the perioral and periorbital regions, on the palms and soles, on the vermilion border of the lips, on the oral mucosa, and occasionally also on the conjunctivae. Although a few cases of this dominantly inherited disorder have shown only cutaneous manifestations (Eberle and Klostermann), usually there are multiple polyps in the gastrointestinal tract, mainly in the small intestine (Jeghers et al.). The polyps often cause repeated episodes of intussusception and intestinal bleeding, but they rarely become malignant. In only 2 to 3 per cent of the cases of Peutz-Jeghers syndrome an adenocarcinoma develops in one of the polyps in the gastrointestinal tract (Reid, 1974), most commonly in the stomach (Achord and Proctor), or in the duodenum (Reid, 1965).

Histopathology. Lentigo simplex shows a slight elongation of the rete ridges, an increase in the concentration of melanocytes in the basal layer, an increase in the amount of melanin in both the melanocytes and the basal keratinocytes, and the presence of melanophages in the upper dermis. A mild inflammatory infiltrate may be found intermingled with the melanophages (Pinkus and Mehregan). Occasionally, small nests of nevus cells are seen at the epidermal-dermal junction, especially at the lowest pole of rete ridges. Such lesions then combine features of a lentigo simplex and a junctional nevus (Pinkus and Mehregan).

In NEVUS SPILUS the histologic picture usually is that of a lentigo simplex. However, junctional nests of nevus cells are seen at the lower pole of some of the rete ridges in occasional instances (Matsudo et al.). Even dermal aggregates of nevus cells have been described (Cohen et al.).

In the MULTIPLE LENTIGINES SYNDROME, as a rule the lesions are "pure" lentigines without the formation of nevus cell nests (Gorlin et al.; Capute et al.). In the larger spots, however, there may be junctional nevus cell nests and even nevus cell nests in the upper dermis (Selmanowitz).

In the PEUTZ-JEGHERS SYNDROME the usual histologic picture is also that of an increase in the number of melanocytes (Bologa et al.). Some of the pigment spots, however, show junctional nevus cell nests (Klostermann).

FRECKLES

Freckles, or ephelides, are small brown macules scattered over skin exposed to the sun. In contrast to lentigo simplex, exposure to the sun deepens the pigmentation of freckles.

Histopathology. Freckles show hyperpigmentation of the basal cell layer; but, in contrast to lentigo simplex, they show no elongation of the rete ridges and, in particular, no increase in the concentration of melanocytes. As a matter of fact, in epidermal spreads of freckled skin the number of dopa-positive melanocytes within the freckles appears decreased. However, the melanocytes that are present are more strongly dopa-positive, are larger, and show more numerous and longer dendritic processes than ordinary melanocytes (Breathnach).

MELANOTIC MACULES OF ALBRIGHT'S SYNDROME

Albright's syndrome is characterized by osteitis fibrosa disseminata, precocious puberty in females, and melanotic patches. The patches usually are large in size and few in number, are located on one side or the other of the midline, and have a jagged, irregular border, like the "coast of Maine," in contrast to the smooth "coast of California" border of the café-au-lait patches of neurofibromatosis.

Histopathology. Except for hyperpigmentation of the basal layer there is no abnormality, and both the number and the size of the melanocytes are normal (Benedict et al.).

Histogenesis. Electron microscopic examination reveals many melanosomes to be slightly enlarged and to measure from 600 to 800 nm in length, i.e., about twice the normal length (Frenk). Because of their enlarged size most melanosomes within keratinocytes lie dispersed rather than in melanosome complexes. The rarity of melanosome complexes thus is similar to that observed in Negroid skin as opposed to Caucasoid skin (see p. 19). It would explain the increased melanization on the basis of a reduced degradation of melanin.

Differential Diagnosis. The melanotic macules of Albright's syndrome lack the "giant" melanosomes present in both the melanocytes and the keratinocytes of the café-au-lait patches of neurofibromatosis (see p. 633).

BECKER'S MELANOSIS

Becker's melanosis, also called Becker's pigmented hairy nevus, is a large unilateral lesion usually seen on the shoulder of male individuals. It consists of a sharply but irregularly demarcated area showing hyperpigmentation and hypertrichosis. The lesion commonly appears during the second decade of life. However, Becker's melanosis may affect areas other than the shoulder, may be multiple and bilateral and may be found in women (Copeman et al.).

Histopathology. The epidermis shows slight acanthosis and some elongation of the rete ridges. There is hyperpigmentation of the basal layer, and melanophages are seen in the upper dermis (Becker; Copeman and Jones; Frenk and Delacrétaz). The number of melanocytes is slightly increased (Gebhart et al.). The hair structures appear normal.

Histogenesis. Electron microscopic examination reveals an increased production of melanosomes within the melanocytes. The number and the size of the melanosome complexes within the keratinocytes is increased, with many of the complexes containing more than 10 melanosomes, rather than the usual average of 3 melanosomes (Frenk and Delacrétaz; Gebhart et al.). A pronounced activity of the melanocytes and marked complexing of melanosomes similar to that found in Becker's melanosis occurs also in the hyperpigmentation following exposure to sunlight.

LENTIGO SENILIS

Lentigo senilis commonly occurs as multiple lesions in areas exposed to the sun. They are found in more than 90 per cent of Caucasoids over 70 years of age (Hodgson). They are not infiltrated and possess a uniform dark-brown color and an irregular outline. They vary in size from a minute macule to more than 1 cm and may coalesce (Cawley and Curtis). Malignant degenera-

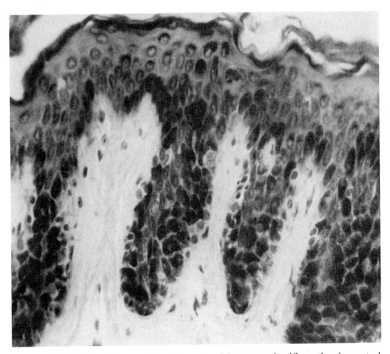

FIG. 32-10. **Lentigo senilis.** The rete ridges are significantly elongated and appear club-shaped. They show considerable hyperpigmentation and a marked increase in the concentration of melanocytes in their basal layer. (×400)

tion does not occur (Braun-Falco and Schoefinius).

Senile lentigines and seborrheic keratoses may resemble each other in their clinical appearance, and both are commonly referred to as liver spots. However, seborrheic keratoses in general show more hyperkeratosis clinically. Lentigo maligna differs from lentigo senilis in its clinical appearance by showing an irregular distribution of its pigment (see p. 665).

Histopathology. The rete ridges are significantly elongated (Fig. 32-10). They either appear club-shaped or are tortuous and show small budlike extensions (Cawley and Curtis). Outside of the elongated rete ridges the epidermis may appear atrophic (Braun-Falco and Schoefinius). The elongated rete ridges show considerable hyperpigmentation and a marked increase in the concentration of melanocytes in their basal layer that is particularly evident in dopa-treated epidermis (Hodgson). No junctional activity is observed. The upper dermis often contains melanophages and sometimes a mild perivascular lymphoid infiltrate.

Histogenesis. On electron microscopy the basal layer of keratinocytes contains increased amounts of melanosomes and melanosome complexes. Even in the upper layers of the epidermis, including the horny layer, numerous melanosomes are seen that are present largely in a dispersed state rather than as complexes. Thus, it seems that in addition to an increased melanin synthesis in the increased number of melanocytes, there also is a delay in the lysosomal destruction of melanosomes (Braun-Falco and Schoefinius).

Differential Diagnosis. Lentigo simplex shows much less elongation of the rete ridges than lentigo senilis, and the elongations are never tortuous or budlike, and junctional nevus cell nests are occasionally present. Lentigo maligna shows flattening or even absence of the rete ridges together with anaplasia of its melanocytes and a more pronounced dermal infiltrate.

MONGOLIAN SPOT

The typical Mongolian spot occurs in the lumbosacral region as a bluish discoloration resembling a bruise. It is found most frequently in Mongoloid and Negroid infants, but it occurs occasionally also in Caucasoid infants. It is present at birth and usually disappears spontaneously within three to four years.

Occasionally, Mongolian spots occur outside the lumbosacral region as aberrant Mongolian spots, such as on the middle or upper part of the back, and then may be multiple and persist (Cole et al.). Extensive and persistent Mongolian spots are commonly seen in patients with nevus of Ota (Hidano et al.).

Histopathology. In the Mongolian spot the dermis shows, especially in its lower half, greatly elongated, slender, often slightly wavy dendritic cells containing melanin granules. These cells lie widely scattered between the collagen bundles, and, like the collagen bundles, generally lie parallel to the skin surface. They are bipolar, are from 5 to 10 μm wide and from 25 to 75 μm long, and often show several branching dendritic processes at either pole (Cole et al.). These cells give a positive dopa reaction, indicating that they are melanocytes rather than melanophages (Mishima and Mevorah).

Histogenesis. The Mongolian spot is the result of a delayed disappearance of dermal melanocytes. As shown by Zimmermann and Becker, dermal melanocytes are present in the dermis of Negro embryos beginning with the 10th week. Between the 11th and 14th week they start migrating into the epidermis. They gradually disappear from the dermis after the 20th week, and at birth dermal melanocytes are found in only a few areas, especially in the sacral region.

The blue color depends upon the phenomenon that light passing through a turbid medium, such as the skin, is scattered as it strikes dark particles, such as melanin. On the basis of the Tyndall effect, the colors of light having a longer wavelength, such as red, orange, and yellow, tend to be less scattered and therefore continue to travel in a forward direction; whereas the colors of shorter wavelength, such as blue, indigo, and violet, are scattered to the side and backward to the skin surface (Kopf and Weidman).

NEVUS OF OTA

The nevus of Ota represents a usually unilateral, irregularly patchy discoloration of the skin of the face, particularly in the periorbital region, the temple, the forehead, the malar area, and the nose. Because of this usual distribution Ota has called the lesion nevus fusco-caeruleus ophthalmo-maxillaris. Frequently, there also is a patchy bluish discoloration of the sclera of the ipsilateral eye, and occasionally also of the conjunctiva, the cornea, and the retina (Kopf and Weidman). In rare instances the lips (Carleton and Biggs) and the palate, pharynx, and nasal mucosa are similarly affected (Mishima and Mevorah). In about 5 per cent of the cases the nevus of Ota is bilateral rather than unilateral. The lesions may be present at birth or appear in childhood or adolescence. They have a tendency to gradual extension. Malignant change in a nevus of Ota is extremely rare. So far, only Dorsey and Montgomery have reported two cases, with death from metastases in one. In several instances a primary malignant melanoma of the choroid, iris, orbit, or brain developed in patients with a nevus of Ota (Enriquez et al.).

In the nevus of Ota the involved areas of the skin show a brown to slate-blue discoloration, usually without any infiltration. Occasionally, however, some areas are slightly raised. Also, in some patients discrete nodules varying in size from a few millimeters to a few centimeters and having the appearance of blue nevi are found within the patches of discoloration (Kopf and Weidman).

The *nevus of Ito* differs from the nevus of Ota by its location in the supraclavicular, scapular, and deltoid regions. It may occur alone or in association with an ipsilateral or bilateral nevus of Ota (Mishima and Mevorah; Hidano et al.).

Histopathology. The noninfiltrated areas of the nevus of Ota and of the nevus of Ito show, similar to a Mongolian spot, elongated, dendritic melanocytes scattered among the collagen bundles. Frequently, the melanocytes show a more superficial distribution than in the Mongolian spot (Mishima and Mevorah). The dopa reaction is strongly positive in melanocytes that are scantily pigmented, whereas in heavily pigmented melanocytes the reaction usually is weak or absent (Mishima and Mevorah; Kopf and Weidman). The negative dopa reaction is due to the fact that all enzymatic activity has been used up in the process of forming melanin.

Slightly raised and infiltrated areas show a larger number of elongated, dendritic melanocytes than do noninfiltrated areas, thus approaching the histologic picture of a blue nevus; and nodular areas are indistinguishable histologically from a blue nevus (Dorsey and Montgomery).

In the two cases of nevus of Ota in which malignant changes occurred, the histologic appearance of the tumors was that of a malignant blue nevus arising within a cellular blue nevus (Dorsey and Montgomery) (see p. 676).

Histogenesis. For some lesions of nevi Ota and Ito the histogenesis probably is the same as that for the Mongolian spot (see p. 660). It is likely that other lesions that appear in childhood or adolescence and increase in size even in adulthood or show nodular infiltration represent not merely residual dermal melanocytes but a hamartoma or nevoid lesion, analogous to the blue nevus (Dorsey and Montgomery).

BLUE NEVUS

Blue nevi most commonly occur on the skin, although in rare instances they have been observed elsewhere, as for instance, in the oral mucosa (Bogomoletz), in the vagina (Rodriguez and Ackerman), in the uterine cervix (Goldman and Friedman), and in the prostate gland (Jao et al.).

On the skin two types of blue nevi are recognized: the common blue nevus and the cellular blue nevus.

The common blue nevus occurs as a small, well circumscribed, dome-shaped nodule of slate-blue or bluish-black color. The lesion rarely exceeds 0.5 cm in diameter. Usually, there is only one lesion, but there may be several. Malignant degeneration does not occur in the common blue nevus. In occasional instances, a common blue nevus is found in association with an overlying compound nevus. The term *combined nevus* is applied to this association (Leopold and Richards, 1968).

The cellular blue nevus consists of a large bluish nodule or plaque extending deeply into the subcutaneous tissue. It shows either a smooth or an irregular surface (Kersting and Caro; Gartmann, 1965). About one half of all cellular blue nevi have been found

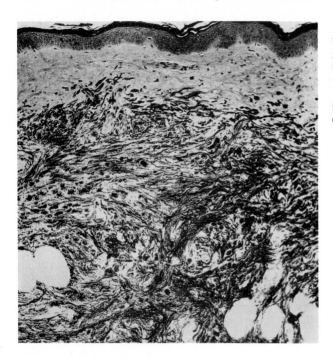

Fig. 32-11. **Blue nevus, common type.** Low magnification. Numerous greatly elongated, slender, often slightly wavy melanocytes with dendritic processes and filled with melanin lie grouped in irregular bundles in the lower dermis and in the subcutaneous fat. (×50)

located over the buttocks or in the sacrococcygeal region (Rodriguez and Ackerman). Although rare, malignant degeneration of cellular blue nevi can occur (see Malignant Blue Nevus, p. 676).

Histopathology. In the *common type* of blue nevus the melanocytes have the same appearance as those seen in the Mongolian spot and in the nevus of Ota, but their number is much greater. Greatly elongated, slender, often slightly wavy melanocytes with long, occasionally branching dendritic processes lie grouped in irregular bundles mainly in the middle and lower thirds of the dermis (Fig. 32-11). The bundles of cells may extend into the subcutaneous tissue or lie

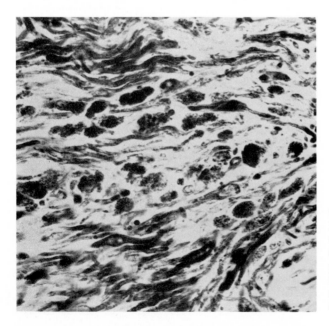

Fig. 32-12. **Blue nevus, common type.** High magnification of Figure 32-11. The greatly elongated melanocytes and their long dendritic processes are filled with fine melanin granules. In addition, melanophages filled with coarse melanin granules and showing no dendritic processes are present. (×400)

close to the epidermis. The epidermis, how-ever, is normal, except in the rare instances of combined nevus in which a compound nevus is located above the blue nevus (Leopold and Richards, 1968). The greatly elongated melanocytes lie predominantly with their long axis parallel to the epidermis (see Plate 4, facing p. 618). Most of them are filled with numerous fine granules of mela-nin, often so completely that their nucleus cannot be visualized. The melanin granules also may fill the long, often wavy, and occa-sionally branching dendritic processes (Fig. 32-12). Thus, on impregnation with silver, they resemble nerve fibers, inasmuch as both nerve fibers and melanin can be impregnated (Gartmann, 1965). Melanophages are fre-quently seen near the bundles of melano-cytes. The melanophages differ from the melanocytes by being shorter and thicker, by showing no dendritic processes, and by con-taining larger granules (Dorsey and Mont-gomery). The melanophages, in contrast to the melanocytes, are dopa-negative.

In the *cellular type* of blue nevus one ob-serves, usually in addition to deeply pig-mented dendritic melanocytes, cellular islands composed of closely aggregated, rather large spindle-shaped cells with ovoid nuclei and abundant pale cytoplasm containing little or no melanin (Fig. 32-13). The diagnosis of cellular blue nevus generally is easy in "biphasic" lesions with both dendritic and spindle-shaped cells, but can be difficult in occasional lesions without dendritic cells (Leopold and Richards, 1967).

Larger islands composed of spindle-shaped cells may consist of many intersecting bundles of cells extending in various direc-tions somewhat resembling the "neuroid" bundles seen in a neurofibroma. In some of the intersecting bundles the spindle-shaped cells appear rounded as the result of cross-sectioning (Fig. 32-14). Not infrequently, the cellular islands penetrate into the sub-cutaneous fat. If, in addition, the nuclei appear somewhat pleomorphic, differentia-tion from a malignant blue nevus or a malig-

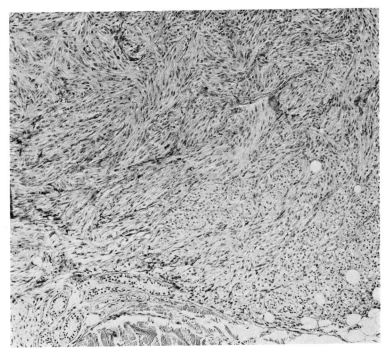

Fig. 32-13. **Blue nevus, cellular type.** Low magnification. A large island of cells is seen extending into the subcutaneous fat. The cells are spindle-shaped, but where cross-sectioned they appear rounded. They possess abundant pale cytoplasm without melanin. (×100)

nant melanoma can be somewhat difficult (Gartmann, 1961). The absence of mitotic figures and of areas of necrosis is against a diagnosis of malignant blue nevus, and the presence of areas of dendritic cells elsewhere in the tumor is against a diagnosis of malignant melanoma.

Histogenesis. Some authors have observed by silver impregnation nonmyelinated nerves (Dupont and Bourlond) or myelinated nerves (Cramer) in blue nevi. However, distinction between nerve fibers and melanin-filled dendritic processes often is impossible. And even though in cellular blue nevi the spindle-shaped cells within the cellular islands may resemble Schwann cells, with the Masson-Fontana stain at least some of these cells contain fine granules of melanin. It seems far fetched to designate lesions of this type as pigmented neurofibromas, as Bird and Willis suggest. On electron microscopy, the spindle-shaped cells in the cellular islands contain melanosomes, but with only little melanization. However, the electron microscopic dopa reaction indicates considerable melanogenic potential within them (Mishima). Since also transitions between dendritic and spindle-shaped cells can be seen, it can be concluded that the spindle-

shaped cells are not Schwann cells but melanocytes, just like the dendritic cells (Mishima) (E.M. No. 48).

MALIGNANT MELANOMA IN SITU

It is generally agreed that there are, aside from malignant blue nevus, 3 types of malignant melanoma: (1) lentigo maligna melanoma, arising from a lentigo maligna; (2) pagetoid malignant melanoma, arising from a pagetoid malignant melanoma in situ; and (3) nodular malignant melanoma arising usually de novo, but in some instances from a nevocellular nevus. The prognosis is best for lentigo maligna melanoma and least favorable for nodular malignant melanoma (Clark; Clark et al.; McGovern).

In most instances a distinction between a malignant melanoma arising from a lentigo maligna and one arising from a pagetoid malignant melanoma in situ can be made without difficulty by studying the adjacent intraepidermal component of the tumor. Nevertheless, as McGovern et al. have pointed out, there are instances in which the

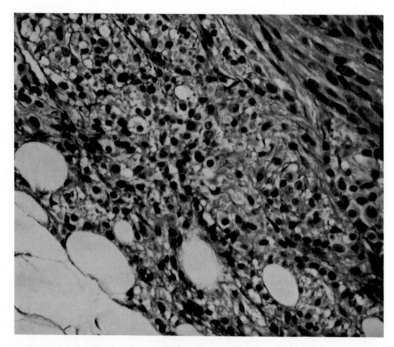

FIG. 32-14. **Blue nevus, cellular type.** High magnification of Figure 32-13. The cells appear spindle-shaped or rounded, depending on the angle at which they are sectioned. They contain no melanin. (×400)

adjacent in situ portion cannot be classified with certainty as either lentigo maligna or pagetoid, so that in such instances it is best to regard the tumor as a fourth category, namely (4) malignant melanoma with adjacent intraepidermal component unclassifiable.

LENTIGO MALIGNA

Lentigo maligna, together with pagetoid malignant melanoma in situ, form the two types of malignant melanoma in situ. Lentigo maligna, also referred to as *melanosis circumscripta preblastomatosa* of Dubreuilh and as *melanotic freckle* of Hutchinson, starts as an unevenly pigmented macule that gradually extends peripherally and may thus attain a diameter of several centimeters. The lesion has an irregular border and, as long as it remains a malignant melanoma in situ, shows no induration. While extending in some areas, it may show spontaneous regression in other areas. The color of the lesion shows shadings from light brown to brown with minute dark brown to black flecks (Clark and Mihm). In addition, there are

depigmented areas at sites of spontaneous regression. The lesion arises usually in older individuals. It is seen almost exclusively in exposed areas, most commonly on the face; although in rare instances it may occur in nonexposed areas of the skin, such as the finger tip (Lupulescu et al.).

Progression into an invasive lentigo maligna melanoma occurs in about one third of all lesions. Usually invasion does not take place until the lentigo maligna has been in existence for 10 to 15 years and has reached a size of 4 to 6 cm (McGovern et al.). In many instances, especially in the case of lesions on the face, which are slowest in becoming invasive, death from other causes intervenes before invasion has taken place. (For clinical and histologic description of lentigo maligna melanoma, see under Malignant Melanoma.)

Histopathology. In its earliest stage, lentigo maligna may show merely flattening of the epidermis and hyperpigmentation mainly of the basal cell layer, although in some areas the hyperpigmentation may extend to the higher layers of the epidermis, even to

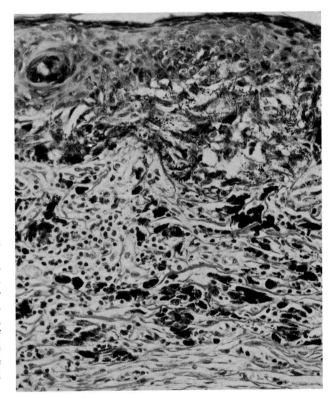

FIG. 32-15. **Malignant melanoma in situ, lentigo maligna.** Elongated, dendritic melanocytes are haphazardly arranged along the epidermal-dermal junction. Their nuclei show marked pleomorphism and their cytoplasm is vacuolated and contains melanin. There is no invasion of melanocytes into the dermis. The upper dermis contains a bandlike inflammatory infiltrate intermingled with melanophages. (×200)

the stratum corneum. Usually, however, one observes, in addition, at least in some areas an increase in the concentration of basal melanocytes and some irregularity in their arrangement. The upper dermis may contain some melanophages and a mild inflammatory infiltrate (Anton-Lamprecht et al.).

In more advanced lesions of lentigo maligna the basal melanocytes in the flattened epidermis show a marked increase in concentration so that their number in some areas far exceeds that of the basal keratinocytes (Clark and Mihm). The melanocytes in many areas are haphazardly arranged along the epidermal-dermal junction. Many of these melanocytes are elongated and spindle-shaped. Their nuclei show marked pleomorphism, since in some cells the nuclei appear shrunken, while in others they are much larger than normal (Fig. 32-15). The cytoplasm of some of the melanocytes appears vacuolated (Mishima). Usually, the proliferating melanocytes contain a considerable amount of melanin. There usually is upward extension of atypical melanocytes, but it may be difficult to differentiate them from melanin-filled keratinocytes. Some nesting of melanocytes in the basal layer may be seen, but this is not pronounced until invasion of the lentigo maligna into the dermis is developing (McGovern). Except in areas of nesting, the melanocytes retain their dendritic processes. If the melanocytes are heavily melanized some dendrites may be visible even in sections stained with hematoxylin and eosin; otherwise, staining with silver will demonstrate the dendrites well. It is quite characteristic of both types of malignant melanoma in situ that the changes within the dermis vary in severity. Usually the most pronounced changes are present in the center of the lesion; but, aside from that, areas of severe changes alternate with areas showing little or no changes.

The upper dermis, in addition to showing solar degeneration, contains numerous melanophages and a rather pronounced, often bandlike, inflammatory infiltrate. The bandlike dermal infiltrate may extend for a considerable distance beyond the obviously altered epidermis. Careful scrutiny of the apparently normal epidermis overlying the dermal infiltrate will, however, reveal in it an increased number of melanocytes and among them some atypical melanocytes (Clark et al.).

Since transformation of a lentigo maligna into a lentigo maligna melanoma is a gradual process, dermal invasion by the atypical melanocytes may be present in some areas but not in others. It is, therefore, advisable to cut step sections throughout the block of tissue in order not to miss such areas (Ollstein et al.).

Histogenesis. Even though both lentigo maligna and pagetoid malignant melanoma in situ (see p. 667) represent malignant melanomas in situ, lentigo maligna shows much less tendency than the pagetoid type to become an invasive malignant melanoma; and even after it has become invasive the lentigo maligna melanoma shows a distinctly slower rate of growth and less tendency to give rise to metastases than the pagetoid and the nodular types of malignant melanoma. Mishima has offered as explanation for this relatively benign behavior of lentigo maligna the theory that the malignant melanoma arising from the melanocytes of lentigo maligna differs biologically from the malignant melanoma arising from the junctional nevus cells of nevocellular nevi. Accordingly, he has divided malignant melanoma into two types: the more benign "malignant melanocytoma" and the more malignant "malignant nevocytoma."

Against the validity of Mishima's theory, two arguments can be raised. In the first place, there is no convincing evidence that the melanocyte and the nevus cell are two different types of cells, as Mishima assumes. By electron microscopy the fine structure of nevus cells is very similar to that of melanocytes, according to the findings of Gottlieb et al. (see p. 652). The presence of large dendrites on melanocytes and their absence on nevus cells results from the solitary arrangement of melanocytes which through their dendrites supply the cells surrounding them with melanin, whereas nevus cells, being arranged in nests, do not supply surrounding cells with melanin. In the second place, Mishima's assumption that all malignant melanomas with the exception of lentigo maligna melanoma arise from nevi is not generally accepted. Since lentigo maligna melanoma comprises no more than 10 per cent of all malignant melanomas, this would mean that 90 per cent of all melanomas arise from pre-existing nevi. Most authors, however, estimate that only about 20 per cent of malignant melanomas arise from pre-existing nevocellular nevi, and that the remainder arises de novo from epidermal melanocytes (Clark).

It seems that lentigo maligna from its onset is a slowly growing tumor, thus allowing the tumor cells for a long time to exist as individual melanocytes with dendrites. Only when dermal invasion is about to take place, do the tumor cells start to grow in nests analogous to nevus cells and to malignant melanoma cells. Probably also the fact that lentigo maligna and lentigo maligna melanoma usually arise in the exposed skin of older persons which has been modified by many years of exposure to the sun contributes to their relatively benign biologic behavior. A similar benign clinical course is seen in solar keratosis and in squamous cell carcinoma arising from a solar keratosis (see p. 476). Even though solar keratosis, like lentigo maligna, contains anaplastic cells, the rate of metastasis of squamous cell carcinoma arising from it is extremely low, amounting to only about 0.5 per cent according to Lund (see p. 468).

Electron microscopy has shown no specific changes in the melanocytes of lentigo maligna. They are large, synthetically active cells with many dendrites. The melanosomes are essentially normal, except that they appear somewhat more elongated than those present in normal melanocytes (Anton-Lamprecht and Tilgen).

When present in large numbers, melanosomes may be found in large lysosomal complexes (Lupulescu et al.). Whereas in some tumors the keratinocytes are filled with melanin and are slow in complexing and degrading it, in other tumors the keratinocytes fail to accept significant amounts of melanin, so that it is being transported from the melanocytes into the dermis by macrophages.

PAGETOID MALIGNANT MELANOMA IN SITU

The pagetoid type of malignant melanoma in situ, also referred to as *superficial spreading malignant melanoma in situ* by Clark, may occur on exposed skin but more commonly is found on nonexposed skin. It usually is a smaller lesion than lentigo maligna, measuring rarely more than 2.5 cm in diameter (McGovern). In contrast to lentigo maligna, it is slightly to definitely elevated. It has an irregular, partly arciform outline. The lesion may show a variation in color similar to that found in lentigo maligna (Clark et al.). Invasion of the dermis occurs

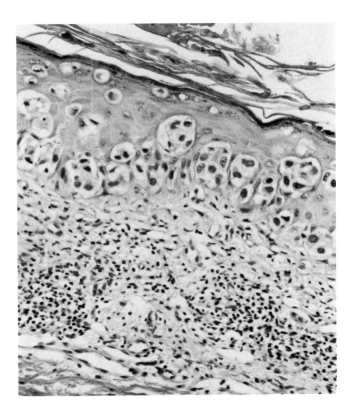

FIG. 32-16. **Malignant melanoma in situ, pagetoid type.** Rounded large melanocytes with atypical, hyperchromatic nuclei are seen. They lie predominantly in nests in the lower epidermis, and singly in the upper epidermis where they are scattered in a "pagetoid" pattern. (×400)

much sooner than in lentigo maligna, often within a year, and is indicated by the development of ulceration and bleeding. Frequently, in its early stage of development, pagetoid malignant melanoma in situ is misdiagnosed clinically as a nevocellular nevus.

Histopathology. The striking melanocytic pleomorphism so characteristic of lentigo maligna is not seen in the pagetoid type of malignant melanoma in situ (Clark et al.). Rather, one observes a random scattering in a "pagetoid" pattern of rather uniformly rounded large melanocytes throughout the epidermis (Fig. 32-16). The large cells lie predominantly in nests in the lower epidermis, and singly in the upper epidermis (McGovern). The large cells have atypical, hyperchromatic nuclei and abundant cytoplasm containing varying amounts of melanin. The tumor cells are almost entirely devoid of dendrites. The probable reason for this is that they lie in nests in the lower epidermis, and those lying singly in the upper epidermis were carried to this level passively from the nests in the lower epidermis. The epidermis generally lacks the flattening seen in lentigo maligna, and it may even be acanthotic. Dermal melanophages and a dermal infiltrate are regularly present and, just as in lentigo maligna, may extend beyond the obviously altered epidermis under apparently normal epidermis. Careful examination of such apparently normal epidermis will, however, reveal the presence of atypical melanocytes (Clark et al.).

Histogenesis. Melanosomes are present in the large pagetoid tumor cells in great numbers, occupying as much as 50 per cent of the cytoplasm. They often appear abnormal, since the filaments present within the melanosomes show no cross linkage. Also, melanization of the melanosomes is often incomplete (Clark et al.).

Differential Diagnosis. A junctional nevus differs from the pagetoid type of malignant melanoma in situ by the lack of atypicality in the tumor cells, particularly in their nuclei, by the lack of pagetoid upward migration of tumor cells, and by the absence of a significant inflammatory infiltrate in the upper dermis (see p. 647). For differentiation from Paget's disease, see page 489.

A clear-cut decision whether a malignant melanoma in situ is a lentigo maligna or a pagetoid malignant melanoma in situ is possible in most but not in all instances (McGovern et al.). A distinction between the two types is of no clinical importance in lesions that are still completely in situ on step sections, since the prognosis is excellent in either case; but the distinction is very important in those tumors that show invasion into the dermis. (For differentiation between lentigo maligna melanoma and pagetoid malignant melanoma see p. 675.)

MALIGNANT MELANOMA

There are three major types of malignant melanoma which differ in their mode of onset, their course, and their prognosis: lentigo maligna melanoma, pagetoid malignant melanoma, and nodular malignant melanoma.

Lentigo maligna melanoma develops from a lentigo maligna, one of the two types of malignant melanoma in situ (see p. 665). Development into an invasive malignant melanoma usually is indicated by the development of one or several intradermal nodules having a bluish black color. Because of the slow rate of growth, the lateness of metastases, and the tendency for metastases to be limited at first to the regional lymph nodes, the 5-year survival rate is high and was 90 per cent and 80 per cent, respectively, in the series of patients followed by Clark and Mihm, and by McGovern.

Pagetoid malignant melanoma develops from the pagetoid type of malignant melanoma in situ (see p. 667). Development into an invasive malignant melanoma usually is indicated by ulceration, bleeding, and an increase in induration of the lesion. The 5-year survival rate was found by McGovern to be 70 per cent.

The *nodular type of malignant melanoma* has the least favorable prognosis. It starts as an elevated, usually deeply pigmented nodule that increases in size quite rapidly and undergoes ulceration. The 5-year survival rate among patients receiving treatment prior to having metastases (clinical stage I) was in Clark's series about 50 per cent, in that of McGovern 53 per cent, and in that of Huvos et al. about 60 per cent.

Approximately 25 per cent of all patients with malignant melanoma recall that a pigmented lesion has been present at the site of the malignant melanoma for many years. However, histologic examination reveals the presence of nevus cells in only about 10 per cent of all cases of malignant melanoma (Clark et al.). Assuming that in some instances the nevus cells originally present have been replaced by malignant melanoma cells, one may conclude that possibly in 20 per cent of the patients the malignant melanoma is preceded by a nevocellular nevus. In the remaining 80 per cent the malignant melanoma arises de novo. In some of the patients the malignant melanoma at the onset is stationary for many years, thus giving the clinical impression of a benign nevocellular nevus.

In the great majority of cases malignant melanoma occurs as a solitary lesion on the skin. More than one primary lesion is present, according to Kahn and Donaldson, in 1.28 per cent of the cases of malignant melanoma reported in the literature. Often, however, in cases of multiple lesions of malignant melanoma it is very difficult to exclude the possibility that a metastasis simulates a primary lesion (Herzberg, 1964) (see below, Metastases).

Every so often no primary malignant melanoma can be found but only metastases, leaving the question open whether the primary lesion involuted spontaneously or is located at an obscure internal site (Conrad). In one instance, the spontaneous involution of a primary malignant melanoma of the skin was actually observed at a time when metastases were already present (Smith and Stehlin).

Next to the skin and eyes, a primary malignant melanoma is most apt to develop in the juxtacutaneous mucous membranes, such as the oral mucosa (Trodahl and Sprague), the nasal mucosa or nasopharynx (Mesara and Burton), the vagina (Norris and Taylor; Hempel and Remmele), and the ano-rectal mucosa (Mason and Helwig). In rare instances, it has arisen in a pulmonary bronchus (Allen and Drash).

Genetic factors are of some importance in the development of malignant melanoma, since a few instances of its familial occurrence have been reported (Andrews). Rarely, malignant melanoma develops in

children (Lerman et al.). In a few instances it was present already at birth either as a primary malignant melanoma arising in a giant pigmented nevus (see p. 657) or as multiple metastases resulting from transplacental transmission (Skov-Jensen et al.). It should be kept in mind that in children many lesions suspected of being malignant melanoma in reality are benign juvenile melanomas (see p. 655).

Histopathology. The question of whether or not an incisional biopsy is permissible in a lesion highly suspicious of being a malignant melanoma has been widely discussed. Several European authors have opposed the performance of an incisional biopsy because they believe it may induce lymphatic or hematogenous spread (Miescher). Recent experiments on hamsters with Fortner's malignant melanoma have shown no adverse effects from incisional biopsies; and fewer metastases were observed following excisional biopsies than in a control series without biopsy (Paslin). Because a correct diagnosis is more likely to be made when the entire tumor can be studied, an excisional biopsy is advisable whenever feasible (Bodenham, 1968); and only when the lesion is very large, an incisional biopsy is indicated (Lane et al.).

In *all three major types of malignant melanoma,* the lentigo maligna melanoma, the pagetoid malignant melanoma, and the nodular malignant melanoma, the tumor originates at the epidermal-dermal junction. This also applies to such cases of nodular malignant melanoma that do not arise de novo but arise from a junctional or compound nevus. In early malignant melanoma arising in a compound nevus one may, therefore, observe the malignant melanoma in the upper dermis and nests of mature nevus cells farther down in the dermis. An exception to the general rule of malignant melanomas arising at the epidermal-dermal junction is observed occasionally in congenital giant pigmented nevi in which the malignant melanoma may arise deep in the dermis (Herzberg, 1963; Reed et al.) (see p. 657). Also, two instances of malignant melanoma developing from the lower portion of an intradermal nevus have been reported, with death from widespread metastases in one of

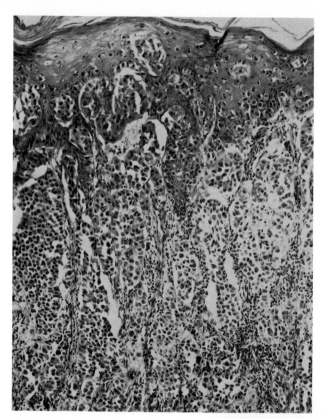

FIG. 32-17. **Malignant melanoma.** Low magnification. There is considerable junctional activity with downward streaming from the epidermis into the dermis of tumor cells possessing atypical nuclei. In addition, there is upward migration of tumor cells into the epidermis. The tumor cells are largely of the epithelioid type and lie in alveolar formations. (×100)

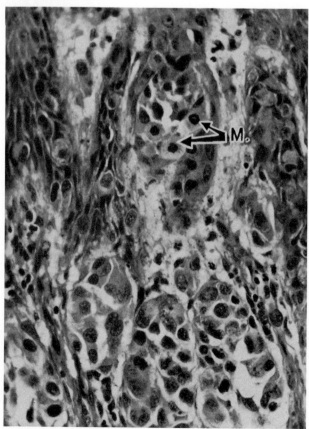

FIG. 32-18. **Malignant melanoma.** High magnification of Figure 32-17. The field shows the epidermal-dermal junction. The majority of cells are epithelioid, but some are spindle-shaped. There are several mitotic figures in the tumor cells (M.) (×400)

the patients (Okun and Bauman; Okun et al.).

In a typical malignant melanoma one observes considerable irregular junctional activity with downward streaming from the epidermis into the dermis of tumor cells possessing anaplastic nuclei (Fig. 32-17). In conjunction with the downward streaming of the atypical tumor cells, the epidermis may show considerable irregular downward proliferation of its rete ridges. The rete ridges may appear as if drawn down by the downward migration of the tumor cells. An even more common phenomenon is the upward migration of tumor cells into the epidermis overlying the malignant melanoma, leading to disintegration of the epidermis and ulceration. Whereas in nodular malignant melanoma the permeation of the epidermis with tumor cells is limited to that portion of the epidermis overlying the dermal tumor, lateral intraepidermal extension of melanoma cells beyond the confines of the dermal tumor is often seen in lentigo maligna melanoma and in pagetoid malignant melanoma. This phe-

nomenon greatly aids in the histologic recognition of the two latter types of tumors.

The *tumor cells* in the dermis show great variation in their size and shape. Nevertheless, two major types of cells can be recognized: an epithelioid, and a spindle-shaped cell type (Clark et al.). Most tumors show both types of cells, but as a rule one type of cell predominates. On the average, cells of the epithelioid type are seen much more commonly than spindle-shaped cells, since only the relatively rare lentigo maligna melanoma tends to show predominance of spindle-shaped cells, whereas the pagetoid and nodular types of malignant melanoma are composed largely of epithelioid types of cells (Clark et al.). The epithelioid type of cells tend to lie in alveolar formations (Fig. 32-18), and the spindle-shaped type of cells in irregularly branching formations (Fig. 32-19). The alveolar formations of the epithelioid cells are surrounded by thin fibers of collagen, containing a few fibroblasts. In the case of small outlying alveolar formations, it is important not to mistake the fibro-

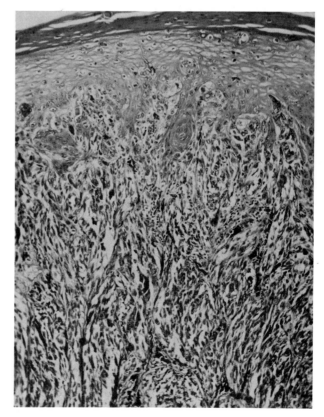

FIG. 32-19. **Malignant melanoma.** The tumor cells are spindle-shaped and lie in irregularly branching formations. Thus, the tumor resembles a fibrosarcoma but differs from it by the presence of junctional activity and of melanin in some of the tumor cells. (×100)

blasts for endothelial cells and to regard the tumor cells as lying within lymphatics or capillaries. Tumors in which fusiform cells predominate resemble fibrosarcomas but differ from them by the presence of junctional activity. In rare instances, a third type of cell is seen in malignant melanoma, namely balloon cells, in association with cells of the epithelioid type (Fig. 32-20). These balloon cells greatly resemble those seen in a balloon cell nevus (see p. 652) so that the danger exists of diagnosing the lesion as such. It is only through a study of the cells of the epithelioid type that one is able to recognize the lesion as a malignant melanoma, since they show the nuclear anaplasia associated with a malignant lesion. In some instances the metastases of a balloon cell malignant melanoma are also composed of balloon cells (Gardner and Vazquez; Ranchod), whereas in other instances the metastases show the usual pattern of malignant melanoma (Hula).

Mitotic figures usually are present in ma-lignant melanoma, but only in small numbers (Fig. 32-18). Although absent in ordinary nevocellular nevi, it should be kept in mind that mitotic figures not infrequently are seen in benign juvenile melanoma (see p. 656). Similarly, bizarre giant cells may be seen in both malignant melanoma and benign juvenile melanoma, with the difference that in the latter they usually are surrounded by a clear space caused by edema.

The *depth of invasion* of the tumor cell infiltrate is, next to the type of malignant melanoma, an important prognostic factor; and, as a matter of fact, the depth of invasion and the type of malignant melanoma are interrelated to a certain degree, since deep invasion is apt to occur more rapidly in nodular malignant melanoma than in pagetoid malignant melanoma or in lentigo maligna melanoma (McGovern). The levels of invasion suggested by Clark et al. are as follows: Level I: confinement of the malignant melanoma cells to the epidermis; Level II: invasion of the papillary zone of the dermis; Level III: invasion extending to the

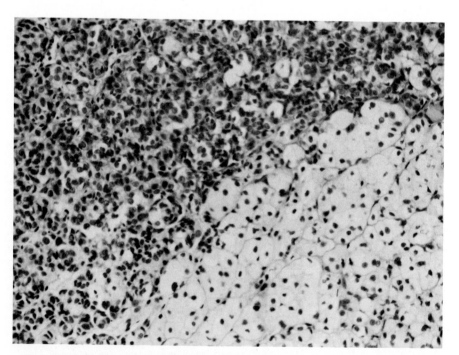

Fig. 32-20. **Balloon cell malignant melanoma.** In the left upper portion a malignant melanoma consisting of epithelioid cells is present. In the right lower portion balloon cells compose the tumor. They resemble the balloon cells seen in the balloon cell nevus shown in Figure 32-7. (×200)

level of the subpapillary vessels but not into the reticular dermis; Level IV: invasion of the reticular dermis; and Level V: invasion of the subcutaneous fat. The 5-year survival rates in the four series published by Clark et al., McGovern, Huvos et al., and Jourdain are as follows: for Level II: 92, 86, 85 and 72 per cent, respectively; for Level III: 65, 60, 59 and 46 per cent; for Level IV: 54, 57, 45 and 31 per cent; and for Level V: 48, 44, 23 and 12 per cent. These figures indicate that, if a critical level exists at all, it is between Levels II and III, rather than between Levels III and IV, as Jourdain has suggested.

The *amount of melanin* varies greatly in malignant melanomas. In some tumors considerable amounts of melanin are found not only within the tumor cells but also within melanophages located in the stroma. In others there may be no evidence of melanin in hematoxylin-eosin stains. However, staining with ammoniated silver nitrate will then reveal in most amelanotic-appearing malig-

nant melanomas at least a few cells containing melanin. If fresh tissue is available the dopa reaction can be carried out, which invariably shows a positive reaction in at least part of the tumor.

The amount of *inflammatory infiltrate* in malignant melanomas varies. As a rule, early invasive malignant melanoma shows a bandlike inflammatory infiltrate, often intermingled with melanophages, at the base of the tumor. This corresponds to the band of inflammatory cells seen beneath malignant melanoma in situ. In a malignant melanoma in situ that has invaded the dermis the bandlike inflammatory infiltrate often extends beyond the invasive and the in-situ portions of the tumor along the normal appearing epidermis (Fig. 32-21). Careful examination of this normal-appearing epidermis will, however, reveal the presence of atypical melanocytes in it (Clark et al.). Once deep invasion of the dermis by the malignant melanoma has taken place, the inflammatory infiltrate decreases in severity; and in ad-

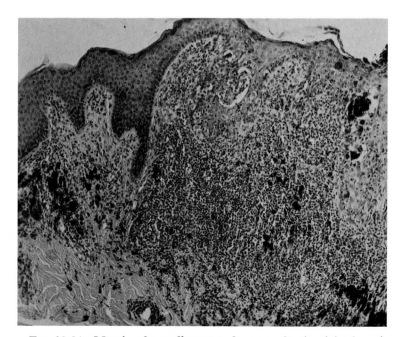

FIG. 32-21. **Margin of a malignant melanoma.** On the right the epidermis is permeated by tumor cells, and the tumor is invading the dermis. The dermis beneath the tumor shows a dense, bandlike inflammatory infiltrate intermingled with numerous melanophages. The infiltrate extends on the left beyond the margin of the tumor underneath the normal-appearing epidermis which, however, on careful scrutiny shows several atypical melanocytes. ($\times$100)

vanced malignant melanoma often it is entirely absent, except at the margins if there is in situ extension of the tumor. Since the inflammatory infiltrate represents a host response against the tumor, the presence of a pronounced inflammatory infiltrate is regarded as a prognostically favorable sign (Cochran).

METASTASES. Metastatic spread is very common in malignant melanoma and occurs especially in nodular malignant melanoma and in those tumors that have penetrated to the level of the subpapillary vessels. Metastasis usually takes place at first through the lymphatics, resulting in involvement of the regional lymph nodes. Spreading through the blood stream generally occurs later, and when it occurs, metastases are apt to be widespread. The liver, the lungs, and the skin are the most common sites of hematogenous metastases (Das Gupta and Brasfield). The presence of metastases is an unfavorable prognostic sign. Thus McNeer and Das Gupta found that in malignant melanoma without metastases the survival rate 10 years after operation was 62 per cent, whereas in malignant melanoma with regional lymph node metastases it was only 12 per cent, and with distant metastases it was zero. In rare instances patients with extensive metastases show generalized melanosis of the skin, consisting of a slate-blue color (Silberberg et al.).

The *histologic appearance of metastatic lesions* of the skin differs from that of primary lesions by the absence of an inflammatory infiltrate and of junctional activity. However, neither of these two criteria is reliable, since also primary tumors of malignant melanoma in their advanced stage do not show an inflammatory infiltrate (see above); and even metastases can contact the overlying epidermis in a way that is suggestive of junctional activity (Klostermann). Herzberg (1964) found in several lesions suspected of representing a second primary melanoma that no true junctional activity existed, since there was a sharp line of demarcation between the strongly dopa-positive tumor islands and the overlying epidermis in which only the basal melanocytes were dopa-positive.

The question whether or not the *regional lymph nodes* are involved with metastases is often very difficult to answer without lymph node dissection. The unreliability of the clinical judgment is shown, for instance, by the findings reported by Weidner and Hornstein: They found that among their patients with clinically suspicious regional lymph nodes only 8 of 21 patients, i.e., 38 per cent, had metastases, whereas among their patients with clinically not suspicious regional lymph nodes 14 of 43 patients, i.e., 32 per cent, had metastases. Of their 22 patients with positive lymph nodes there were 7 patients who had only "micrometastases" in the marginal sinuses of the lymph nodes; and it is known that in some instances such "micrometastases" can be phagocytized, whereas in others they give rise to visceral metastases (Nödl). The question of the advisability of a routine dissection of clinically not suspicious regional lymph nodes is undecided at present: It is strongly favored by some (Goldsmith et al.), whereas others point out the possible tumoricidal effect of immunocompetent round cells in regional lymph nodes (Bodenham, 1969).

The histologic examination of patients with generalized melanosis reveals a substantial increase in melanin in the basal layer of the epidermis and the presence of melanophages in the dermis, particularly in its upper portion (Silberberg et al.). On autopsy, melanin phagocytosis can be seen in all organs, especially in the Kupffer cells of the liver and the cells lining the sinusoids of the lymph nodes, the spleen and the adrenal glands (Sohn et al.).

Histogenesis. On electron microscopic examination, most tumor cells of malignant melanoma show a high concentration of melanosomes, but the melanosomes show no characteristic or significant alterations (E.M. No. 49) (Jakubowicz et al.). Frequently, one observes in the tumor cells autophagic vacuoles which, in addition to melanosomes, may contain also mitochondria and ergastoplasm. In contrast, the lysosomes present in the melanophages contain only melanosomes embedded in a dense granular matrix and no other organelles (Mishima and Ito).

Labeling with tritiated thymidine of the cellular inflammatory infiltrate often present in bandlike arrangement at the base of early invasive malignant melanomas (see p. 673) reveals the following: A great number of the cells in the lymphoid infiltrate are labeled, indicating that they are stimulated or activated lymphocytes. When determined in the same patient prior to and after the appearance of metastases, the number of activated lymphocytes is significantly higher prior to the appearance of metastases (Pullmann and Steigleder). This finding is in line with the observation that blood lymphocytes of patients with malignant melanoma are cytotoxic to cultured autologous tumor cells (DeVries et al.).

In addition to cellular antibodies in circulating lymphocytes, also humoral antibodies against the cytoplasm of malignant melanoma cells are present in the plasma of patients with malignant melanoma prior to the development of metastases. They disappear when metastases develop (Copeman et al.). (Concerning the presence of these antibodies in halo nevus, see p. 654.)

Differential Diagnosis. Great difficulty may be encountered in the differentiation of malignant melanoma from a junctional or compound nevus. The actual incidence of a wrong diagnosis is not inconsiderable, judging from the frequency with which pathologists or dermatopathologists disagree in their opinion. Truax et al., in a retrospective analysis, found that in at least 7 per cent of their histologic material the diagnosis of malignant melanoma had proved to be incorrect. Still, in a disease with such a serious prognosis it seems better to "overdiagnose" than to "underdiagnose" and thus to err on the safe side. Also, since a junctional or compound nevus may develop into a malignant melanoma, and this development may proceed slowly, an intermediate stage of development can be encountered in which no clear-cut decision is possible.

Several features are generally regarded as being suggestive of malignant melanoma; but actually there is only one absolute sign of malignancy, and that is often difficult to decide upon—that is, nuclear anaplasia or atypicality associated with pleomorphism. The indications for anaplasia are the same as in other malignant tumors and include increase in the ratio of nuclear size to cytoplasmic volume, hyperchromasia of the nuclei, and presence of atypical mitoses. The presence of large amounts of irregularly distributed melanin may give benign cells a "wild," anaplastic appearance. It is advisable to judge such cells as if they contained no melanin and, if necessary, to bleach the melanin in them with potassium permanganate.

Features suggestive but not indicative of malignancy are: (1) presence of tumor cells in the upper epidermis; (2) irregular scattering of tumor cells in the lower epidermis rather than their arrangement in nests; (3) failure of the tumor cells in the dermis to decrease in size in the deeper layers of the dermis; and (4) presence of a bandlike inflammatory infiltrate often intermingled with melanophages beneath the tumor cells. Such an inflammatory infiltrate, if not adequately explained by either trauma or infection, is perhaps, next to the presence of atypicality, the most reliable indicator of early malignant change, since it is the type of host response frequently encountered in early malignant lesions (Cochran). However, an inflammatory infiltrate is found also in halo nevus (see p. 654) and in benign juvenile melanoma (see p. 655), even though in halo nevus it is not bandlike.

It is important to decide in malignant melanoma with an adjacent intraepidermal component whether this component is of the lentigo maligna type or of the pagetoid type. Although this decision is possible in most cases, it cannot be made in all; and McGovern et al. have referred to such instances as "invasive malignant melanoma with adjacent intraepidermal component unclassifiable." In general, however, one finds (1) in lentigo maligna spindle-shaped rather than rounded melanocytes crowding the basal layer without the formation of nests; still, it is generally admitted that in some advanced lesions prior to dermal invasion nesting of melanocytes can be observed in the lower epidermis, with the nests resembling those seen in pagetoid malignant melanoma in situ (Clark; McGovern). (2) Although the upward extension of atypical melanocytes in lentigo maligna usually consists of spindle-shaped tumor cells, occasionally they are more rounded than spindle-shaped. (3) Although in typical cases the epidermis is flattened in lentigo maligna and acanthotic in pagetoid malignant melanoma in situ, exceptions occur; and (4) even though the clinical location of the lesion is regarded as an important factor in differentiation, lentigo maligna melanoma is not always limited to exposed areas, or pagetoid malignant melanoma to covered areas.

For the differentiation of benign juvenile melanoma from malignant melanoma, which may be very difficult at times, see page 656.

MALIGNANT BLUE NEVUS

Malignant blue nevus is a rare tumor. It may arise in a blue nevus (Kwittken and Negri; Merkow et al.) or may be malignant from the start (Gartmann and Lischka; Hernandez). In two instances reported by Dorsey and Montgomery a malignant blue nevus developed within a nevus at Ota. Malignant blue nevi may show ulceration if superficially located (Herzberg and Klein); but they may merely show increase in size without ulceration if deeply located (Gartmann and Lischka; Hernandez). In some of the reported cases the metastases were limited to the regional lymph nodes, and the patient survived after removal of the tumor and the involved lymph nodes (Merkow et al.; Gartmann and Lischka). In other cases, however, death occurred as the result of widespread metastases (Kwittken and Negri; Hernandez).

Histopathology. Recognition of the lesion as a malignant blue nevus is based on the absence of junctional activity and the presence of at least some bipolar tumor cells with branching dendritic processes containing melanin granules (Fig. 32-22) (Herzberg and Klein; Mishima; Hernandez). This may require staining with ammoniated silver nitrate, since melanin often is scanty due to the fact that most malignant blue nevi arise from areas of cellular blue nevus and are composed of cells of this type. Considerable amounts of melanin are seen in at least some areas of the tumor (Gartmann and Lischka; Hernandez).

In addition to the standard features of malignancy, such as invasiveness of the tumor, atypicality and pleomorphism of the nuclei, and presence of atypical mitoses, malignant blue nevi often show areas of necrosis as evidence of their malignant nature (Herzberg and Klein; Merkow et al.; Hernandez).

Histogenesis. Although some authors have regarded the tumor cells as related to Schwann cells (Merkow et al.), recent electron microscopic studies have shown the absence of cytoplasmic enclosures of unmyelinated axons as seen in

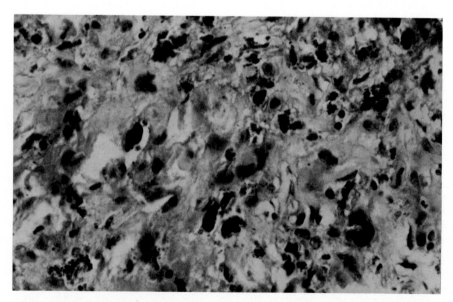

Fig. 32-22. **Malignant blue nevus.** The tumor contains many anaplastic nuclei, some of which are elongated. Melanin is present in many tumor cells; and in some tumor cells it lies within branching dendritic processes. (×400)

Schwann cells, and the presence of melanosomes in all cells. Even though in many cells the melanosomes are devoid of melanin (Hernandez), incubation with dopa has shown such melanosomes to be strongly dopa-positive (Mishima). Thus, all tumor cells are melanocytes.

Differential Diagnosis. Malignant blue nevus differs from primary malignant melanoma by the absence of junctional activity. However, ruling out a metastatic malignant melanoma can be difficult, since metastatic malignant melanoma may occasionally be found in the absence of a demonstrable primary malignant melanoma. The primary malignant melanoma either may have involuted or may be located at an obscure internal site (see p. 669). The presence of dendritic cells then is the most reliable criterion for the lesion being a malignant blue nevus rather than a metastatic malignant melanoma.

BIBLIOGRAPHY

Nevocellular Nevus

Becker, S. W.: Diagnosis and treatment of pigmented nevi. Arch. Derm. Syph., *60*:44, 1949.

Clark, W. H., Jr., and Mihm, M. C., Jr.: Lentigo maligna and lentigo-maligna melanoma. Am. J. Path., *55*:39, 1969.

Cramer, H. J.: Histochemische Untersuchungen mit dem sauren Hämateintest nach Baker an pathologisch veränderter Haut. Arch. klin. exp. Derm., *228*:438, 1967.

Delacrétaz, J., and Frenk, E.: Zur Pathogenese des Osteo-Naevus Nanta. Hautarzt, *15*:487, 1964.

Freeman, R. G., and Knox, J. M.: Epidermal cysts associated with pigmented nevi. Arch. Derm., *85*:590, 1962.

Gottlieb, B., Brown, A. L., Jr., and Winkelmann, R. K.: Fine structure of the nevus cell. Arch. Derm., *92*:81, 1965.

Graham, J. H., Sanders, J. B., Johnson, W. C., and Helwig, E. B.: Fibrous papule of the nose. J. Invest. Derm., *45*:194, 1965.

Kopf, A. W., and Andrade, R.: A histologic study of the dermo-epidermal junction in clinically "intradermal" nevi, employing serial sections. Ann. N.Y. Acad. Sci., *100*:200, 1963.

Lupulescu, A., Pinkus, H., Birmingham, D. J., *et al.*: Lentigo maligna of the fingertip. Arch. Derm., *107*:717, 1973.

Masson, P.: Les naevi pigmentaires, tumeurs nerveuses. Ann. anat. path., *3*:417, 657, 1926.

————: My conception of cellular nevi. Cancer, *4*:9, 1951.

Miescher, G., and von Albertini, A.: Histologie de 100 cas de naevi pigmentaires d'après les méthodes de Masson. Bull. Soc. franç. derm. syph., *42*:1265, 1935.

Mishima, Y.: Macromolecular changes in pigmentary disorders. Arch. Derm., *91*:519, 1965.

Roth, S. I., Stowell, R. E., and Helwig, E. B.: Cutaneous ossification. Arch. Path., *76*:44, 1963.

Sagebiel, R. W.: Histologic artifacts of benign pigmented nevi. Arch. Derm., *106*:691, 1972.

Saylan, T., Marks, R., and Wilson Jones, E.: Fibrous papule of the nose. Brit. J. Derm., *85*:111, 1971.

Shaffer, B.: Pigmented nevi. Arch. Derm., *72*:120, 1955.

Thorne, E. G., Mottaz, J. H., and Zelickson, A. S.: Tyrosinase activity in dermal nevus cells. Arch. Derm., *104*:619, 1971.

Weitzner, S.: Intradermal nevus with psammoma body formation. Arch. Derm., *98*:287, 1968.

Winkelmann, R. K.: Cholinesterase nevus: cholinesterases in pigmented tumors of the skin. Arch. Derm., *82*:17, 1960.

Balloon Cell Nevus

Gartmann, H.: Über blasige Zellen im Naevuszellnaevus. Z. Haut Geschlechtskr., *28*:148, 1960.

Hashimoto, K., and Bale, G. F.: An electron microscopic study of balloon cell nevus. Cancer, *30*:530, 1972.

Hornstein, O.: Zur Kenntnis des sogenannten Blasenzellnaevus. Arch. klin. exp. Derm., *226*:97, 1966.

Okun, M. R., Donnellan, B. and Edelstein, L.: An ultrastructural study of balloon cell nevus. Cancer, *34*:615, 1974.

Schrader, W. A., and Helwig, E. B.: Balloon cell nevi. Cancer, *20*:1502, 1967.

Wilson Jones, E., and Sanderson, K. V.: Cellular nevi with peculiar foam cells. Brit. J. Derm., *75*:47, 1963.

Halo Nevus

Copeman, P. W. M., Lewis, M. G., Phillips, T. M., and Elliott, P. G.: Immunological associations of the halo nevus with cutaneous malignant melanoma. Brit. J. Derm., *88*:127, 1973.

Ebner, H., and Niebauer, G.: Elektronenoptische Befunde zum Pigmentverlust beim Naevus Sutton. Dermatologica, *137*:345, 1968.

Epstein, W. L., Sagebiel, R., Spitler, L., *et al.*: Halo nevi and melanoma. J.A.M.A., *225*: 373, 1973.

Findlay, G. H.: The histology of Sutton's nevus. Brit. J. Derm., *69*:389, 1957.

Frank, S. B., and Cohen, H. J.: The halo nevus. Arch. Derm., *89*:367, 1964.

Kopf, A. W., Morrill, S. D., and Silberberg, I.: Broad spectrum of leukoderma acquisitum centrifugum. Arch. Derm., *92*:14, 1965.

Shapiro, L., and Kopf, A. W.: Leukoderma acquisitum centrifugum. Arch. Derm., *92*:64, 1965.

Stegmaier, O. C., Becker, S. W., Jr., and Medenica, M.: Multiple halo nevi. Arch. Derm., *99*:180, 1969.

Swanson, J. L., Wayte, D. M., and Helwig, E. B.: Ultrastructure of halo nevi. J. Invest. Derm., *50*:434, 1968.

Benign Juvenile Melanoma

Allen, A. C.: Juvenile melanomas of children and adults and melanocarcinomas of children. Arch. Derm., *82*:325, 1960.

Bourlond, A.: Multiple juvenile Melanome. Hautarzt, *22*:144, 1971.

Brownstein, W. E.: Multiple agminated juvenile melanoma. Arch. Derm., *106*:89, 1972.

Copeman, P. W. M., Lewis, M. G., Phillips, T. M., and Elliott, P. G.: Immunological associations of the halo nevus with cutaneous malignant melanoma. Brit. J. Derm., *88*:127, 1973.

Coskey, R. J., and Mehregan, A.: Spindle cell nevi in adults and children. Arch. Derm., *108*:535, 1973.

Echevarria, R., and Ackerman, L. V.: Spindle and epithelioid cell nevi in the adult. Cancer, *20*:175, 1967.

Jakubowicz, K.: Über die Zugehörigkeit des sogenannten juvenilen Melanoms zur Gruppe des aktiven Naevuszellnaevus. Hautarzt, *16*:411, 1965.

Saksela, E., and Rintala, A.: Misdiagnosis of prepubertal malignant melanoma. Cancer, *22*:1308, 1968.

Schreiner, E., and Wolff, K.: Die Ultrastruktur des benignen juvenilen Melanoms. Arch. klin. exp. Derm., *237*:749, 1970.

Spitz, S.: Melanomas of childhood. Am. J. Path., *24*:591, 1948.

Steigleder, G. K., and Wellmer, K.: Zur Abtrennung des sogenannten juvenilen Melanoms. Arch. klin. exp. Derm., *202*:556, 1956.

Congenital Giant Pigmented Nevus

Greeley, P. W., Middleton, A. G., and Curtin, J. W.: Incidence of malignancy in giant pigmented nevi. Plast. Reconstr. Surg., *36*:26, 1965.

Gross, P. R., and Carter, D. M.: Malignant melanoma arising in a giant cerebriform nevus. Arch. Derm., *96*:536, 1967.

Herzberg, J. J.: Naevus und Melanom. Hautarzt, *13*:111, 1963.

Menter, M. A., Griessel, P. J. C., and deKlerk, D. J.: Giant blue naevus of the scalp with underlying scalp defect. Brit. J. Derm., *85* (suppl. 7):73, 1971.

Orkin, M., Frichot, B. C., III, and Zelickson, A. S.: Cerebriform intradermal nevus. Arch. Derm., *110*:575, 1974.

Reed, W. B., Becker, W. S., Jr., Becker, W. S., Sr., and Nickel, W. R.: Giant pigmented nevi, melanoma, and leptomeningeal melanocytosis. Arch. Derm., *91*:100, 1965.

Silverberg, G. D., Kadin, M. E., Dorfman, R. F., *et al.*: Invasion of the brain by a cellular blue nevus of the scalp. Cancer, *27*:349, 1971.

Slaughter, J. C., Hardman, J. M., Kempe, L. G., and Earle, K. M.: Neurocutaneous melanosis and leptomeningeal melanomatosis in children. Arch. Path., *88*:298, 1969.

Touraine, A.: Les mélanoses neuro-cutanées. Ann. derm. syph., *VIII*, 9:489, 1949.

Williams, H. I.: Primary malignant meningeal melanoma associated with benign hairy nevi. J. Path., *99*:171, 1969.

Lentigo Simplex

Achord, J. L., and Proctor, H. D.: Malignant degeneration and metastasis in Peutz-Jeghers syndrome. Arch. Intern. Med., *111*:498, 1963.

Bologa, E. I., Bene, M., and Pasztor, P.: Considérations sur la lentiginose éruptive de la face. Ann. derm. syph., *92*:277, 1965.

Capute, A. J., Rimoin, D. L., Konigsmark, B. W., *et al.*: Congenital deafness and multiple lentigines. Arch. Derm., *100*:207, 1969.

Clark, W. H., Jr., and Mihm, M. C., Jr.: Moles and malignant melanoma. *In* Fitzpatrick, T. B., *et al.*: Dermatology in General Medicine. p. 493. New York, McGraw-Hill, 1971.

Cohen, H. J., Minkin, W., and Frank, S. B.: Nevus spilus. Arch. Derm., *102*:433, 1970.

Eberle, P., and Klostermann, G. F.: Cytogenetische Untersuchungen bei der Pigmentfleckenpolypose (Peutz-Touraine-Jeghers-Syndrom). Arch. klin. exp. Derm., *231*:437, 1968.

Gorlin, R. J., Andersen, R. C., and Blaw, M.: Multiple lentigines syndrome. Am. J. Dis. Child., *117*:652, 1969.

Jeghers, H., McKusick, B. A., and Katz, K. H.: Generalized intestinal polyposis and melanin spots of the oral mucosa, lips and digits. New Eng. J. Med., *241*:993, 1949.

Klostermann, G. F.: Pigmentfleckenpolypose. p. 45. Stuttgart, Thieme, 1960.

Matsudo, H., Reed, W. B., Homme, D., *et al.*: Zosteriform lentiginous nevus. Arch. Derm., *107*:902, 1973.

Pinkus, H., and Mehregan, A. H.: A Guide to Dermatohistopathology. Lentigo simplex. p. 361. New York, Appleton-Century-Crofts, 1969.

Reid, J. D.: Duodenal carcinoma in the Peutz-Jeghers syndrome. Cancer, *18*:970, 1965.

————: Intestinal carcinoma in the Peutz-Jeghers syndrome. J.A.M.A., *229*:833, 1974.

Selmanowitz, V. J.: Lentiginosis profusa syndrome (multiple lentigines syndrome). Acta dermatoven., *51*:387, 1971.

Freckles

Breathnach, A. S.: Melanocyte distribution in forearm epidermis of freckled human subjects. J. Invest. Derm., *29*:253, 1957.

Melanotic Macule of Albright's Syndrome

Benedict, P. H., Szabo, G., Fitzpatrick, T. B., and Sinesi, S. J.: Melanotic macules in Albright's syndrome and in neurofibromatosis. J.A.M.A., *205*:618, 1968.

Frenk, E.: Étude ultrastructurale des taches pigmentaires du syndrome d'Albright. Dermatologica, *143*:12, 1971.

Becker's Melanosis

Becker, S. W.: Concurrent melanosis and hypertrichosis in distribution of nevus unius lateris. Arch. Derm. Syph., *60*:155, 1949.

Copeman, P. W. M., and Jones, E. W.: Pigmented hairy epidermal nevus (Becker). Arch. Derm., *92*:249, 1965.

Frenk, E., and Delacrétaz, J.: Zur Ultrastruktur der Beckerschen Melanose. Hautarzt, *21*:397, 1970.

Gebhart, W., Kidd, R. L., and Niebauer, G.: Beckersche Melanosis. Arch. derm. Forsch., *241*:166, 1971.

Lentigo Senilis

Braun-Falco, O., and Schoefinius, H. H.: Lentigo senilis. Hautarzt, *22*:277, 1971.

Cawley, E. P., and Curtis, A. C.: Lentigo senilis. Arch. Derm. Syph., *62*:635, 1950.

Hodgson, C.: Lentigo senilis. Arch. Derm., *87*:197, 1963.

Mongolian Spot

Cole, H. N., Jr., Hubler, W. R., and Lund, H. Z.: Persistent, aberrant Mongolian spots. Arch. Derm. Syph., *61*:244, 1950.

Hidano, A., Kajima, H., Ikeda, S., *et al.*: Natural history of nevus of Ota. Arch. Derm., *95*:187, 1967.

Kopf, A. W., and Weidman, A. I.: Nevus of Ota. Arch. Derm., *85*:195, 1962.

Mishima, Y., and Mevorah, B.: Nevus Ota and Nevus Ito in American Negroes. J. Invest. Derm., *36*:133, 1961.

Zimmermann, A. A., and Becker, S. W., Jr.: Precursors of epidermal melanocytes in the Negro fetus. *In* Pigment Cell Biology. p. 159. New York, Academic Press, 1959.

Nevus of Ota

Carleton, A., and Biggs, R.: Diffuse mesodermal pigmentation with congenital cranial abnormality. Brit. J. Derm., *60*:10, 1948.

Dorsey, C. S., and Montgomery, H.: Blue nevus and its distinction from Mongolian spot and the nevus of Ota. J. Invest. Derm., *22*:225, 1954 (review).

Enriquez, R., Egbert, B., and Bullock, J.: Primary malignant melanoma of central nervous system. Arch. Path., *95*:392, 1973.

Hidano, A., Kajima, H., and Endo, Y.: Bilateral nevus Ota associated with nevus Ito. Arch. Derm., *91*:357, 1965.

Kopf, A. W., and Weidman, A. I.: Nevus of Ota. Arch. Derm., *85*:195, 1962.

Mishima, Y., and Mevorah, B.: Nevus Ota and Nevus Ito in American Negroes. J. Invest. Derm., *36*:133, 1961.

Blue Nevus

Bird, C. C., and Willis, R. A.: The histogenesis of pigmented neurofibromas. J. Path., *97*:631, 1969.

Bogomoletz, W.: Blue naevus of oral mucosa. Brit. J. Derm., *80*:611, 1968.

Cramer, H. J.: Über den "Neuro-nevus blue" (Masson). Hautarzt, *17*:16, 1966.

Dorsey, C. S., and Montgomery, H.: Blue nevus and its distinction from Mongolian spot and the nevus of Ota. J. Invest. Derm., *22*:225, 1954 (review).

Dupont, A., and Bourlond, A.: Les Naevi bleus. Ann. derm. syph., *89*:261, 1962.

Gartmann, H.: Über den zellreichen blauen Naevus. Derm. Wschr., *143*:297, 1961.

————: Neuronaevus bleu Masson—cellular blue Nevus Allen. Arch. klin. exp. Derm., *221*:109, 1965.

Goldman, R. L., and Friedman, N. B.: Blue nevus of the uterine cervix. Cancer, *20*:210, 1967.

Jao, W., Fretzin, D. F., Christ, M. L., and Prinz, L. M.: Blue nevus of the prostate gland. Arch. Path., *91*:187, 1971.

Kersting, D. W., and Caro, M. R.: Cellular blue nevus of Ota followed for twenty-two years. Arch. Derm., *74*:59, 1956.

Leopold, J. G., and Richards, D. B.: Cellular blue nevi. J. Path., *94*:247, 1967.

———: The interrelationship of blue and common nevi. J. Path., *95*:37, 1968.

Mishima, Y.: Cellular blue nevus. Melanogenic activity and malignant transformation. Arch. Derm., *101*:104, 1970.

Rodriguez, H. A., and Ackerman, L. V.: Cellular blue nevus. Cancer, *21*:393, 1968.

Malignant Melanoma in Situ

Anton-Lamprecht, I., Schnyder, U. W., and Tilgen, W.: Das "Stade éphélide" der melanotischen Präcancerose. Arch. derm. Forsch., *240*:61, 1971.

Anton-Lamprecht, I., and Tilgen, W.: Zur Ultrastruktur der melanotischen Präcancerose. Arch. derm. Forsch., *244*:264, 1972

Clark, W. H., Jr.: A classification of malignant melanoma in man correlated with histogenesis and biologic behavior. Advances in Biology of the Skin, Vol. 8. The Pigmentary System. p. 621. Oxford, Pergamon Press, 1967.

Clark, W. H., Jr., From, L., Bernardino, E. A., and Mihm, M. C.: Histogenesis and biologic behavior of primary human malignant melanoma of the skin. Cancer Res., *29*:705, 1969.

Clark, W. H., Jr., and Mihm, M. C., Jr.: Lentigo maligna and lentigo-maligna melanoma. Am. J. Path., *55*:39, 1969.

Gottlieb, B., Brown, L., and Winkelmann, R. K.: Fine structure of the nevus cell. Arch. Derm., *92*:81, 1965.

Lund, H. Z.: How often does squamous cell carcinoma of the skin metastasize? Arch. Derm., *92*:635, 1965.

Lupulescu, A., Pinkus, H., and Birmingham, D. J., et al.: Lentigo maligna of the fingertip. Arch. Derm., *107*:717, 1973.

McGovern, V. J.: The classification of melanoma and its relationship with prognosis. Pathology, *2*:85, 1970.

McGovern, V. J., Mihm, M. C., Jr., Bailly, C., et al.: The classification of malignant melanoma and its histologic reporting. Cancer, *32*:1446, 1973.

Mishima, Y.: Melanocytic and nevocytic malignant melanoma. Cancer, *20*:632, 1967.

Ollstein, R. N., Kaplan, H. S., Crikelair, G. F., and Lattes, R.: Is there a malignant freckle? Cancer, *19*:767, 1966.

Malignant Melanoma

Allen, M. S., Jr., and Drash, E. C.: Primary melanoma of the lung. Cancer, *21*:154, 1968.

Andrews, J. C.: Malignant melanoma in siblings. Arch. Derm., *98*:282, 1968.

Bodenham, D. C.: Malignant melanoma. Brit. J. Derm., *80*:190, 1968.

———: Malignant melanoma. The problem of lymph-node metastases. Proc. Roy. Soc. Med., *62*:1090, 1969.

Clark, W. H., Jr.: A classification of malignant melanoma in man correlated with histogenesis and biological behavior. Advances in Biology of the Skin, Vol. 8. The Pigmentary System. p. 621. Oxford, Pergamon Press, 1967.

Clark, W. H., Jr., From, L., Bernardino, E. A., and Mihm, M. C.: Histogenesis and biologic behavior of primary human malignant melanoma of the skin. Cancer Res., *29*:705, 1969.

Clark, W. H., Jr., and Mihm, M. C., Jr.: Lentigo maligna and lentigo-maligna melanoma. Am. J. Path., *55*:39, 1969.

Cochran, A. J.: Histology and prognosis in malignant melanoma. J. Path., *97*:459, 1969.

Conrad, F. G.: Cures achieved in patients with metastatic malignant melanoma of the skin. Cancer, *30*:144, 1972.

Copeman, P. W. M., Lewis, M. G., Phillips, T. M., and Elliott, P. G.: Immunological associations of the halo nevus with cutaneous malignant melanoma. Brit. J. Derm., *88*:127, 1973.

Das Gupta, T., and Brasfield, R.: Metastatic melanoma. Cancer, *17*:1323, 1964.

DeVries, J. E., Rümke, P., and Bernstein, J. L.: Cytotoxic lymphocytes in melanoma patients. Int. J. Cancer, *9*:567, 1972.

Gardner, W. A., Jr., and Vazquez, M. D.: Balloon cell melanoma. Arch. Path., *89*:470, 1970.

Goldsmith, H. S., Shah, J. P., and Kim, D. H.: Prognostic significance of lymph node dissection in the treatment of malignant melanoma. Cancer, *26*:606, 1970.

Hempel, J., and Remmele, W.: Das maligne Melanom des weiblichen Genitale. Z. Haut, *48*:647, 1973.

Herzberg, J. J.: Naevus und Melanom. Hautarzt, *13*:111, 1963.

———: Tyrosinasenachweis bei Metastasen des malignen Melanoms. Arch. klin. exp. Derm., *220*:480, 1964.

Hula, M.: Clear cell melanoblastoma. Dermatologica, *146*:86, 1973.

Huvos, A. G., Miké, V., Donnellan, M. J., et al.: Prognostic factors in cutaneous melanoma of the head and neck. Am. J. Path., *71*:33, 1973.

Jakubowicz, K., Dabrowski, J., Biczysko, W., and Walski, M.: Ultrastruktur der Melanosomen im Melanomalignom. Derm. Monatsschr., *156*:299, 1970.

Jourdain, J. C.: Étude des critères cliniques et histologiques de prognostic des mélanomes malins primaires. Ann. derm. syph., *101*:171, 1974.

Kahn, L. B., and Donaldson, R. C.: Multiple primary melanoma. Cancer, *25*:1162, 1970.

Klostermann, G. F.: Zur Frage der multizentrischen Entstehung beim malignen Melanom. Arch. klin. exp. Derm., *215*:379, 1962.

Lane, N., Lattes, R., and Malm, J.: Clinicopathological correlations in a series of 117 malignant melanomas of the skin of adults. Cancer, *11*:1025, 1958.

Lerman, R. J., Murray, D., O'Hara, J. M., *et al.*: Malignant melanoma in childhood. Cancer, *25*:436, 1970.

Mason, J. K., and Helwig, E. B.: Anal-rectal melanoma. Cancer, *19*:36, 1966.

McGovern, V. J.: The classification of melanoma and its relationship with prognosis. Pathology, *2*:85, 1970.

McGovern, V. J., Mihm, M. C., Jr., Bailly, C., *et al.*: The classification of malignant melanoma and its histologic reporting. Cancer, *32*:1446, 1973.

McNeer, G., and Das Gupta, T.: Prognosis in malignant melanoma. Surgery, *56*:512, 1964.

Mesara, B. W., and Burton, W. D.: Primary malignant melanoma of the upper respiratory tract. Cancer, *21*:217, 1968.

Miescher, G.: Über Klinik und Therapie der Melanome. Arch. für Derm. u. Syph., *200*:215, 1955.

Mishima, Y., and Ito, R.: Electron microscopy of microfocal necrosis in malignant melanoma. Cancer, *24*:185, 1969.

Nödl, F.: Mikrometastasen beim malignen Melanom. Arch. derm. Forsch., *244*:239, 1972.

Norris, H. J., and Taylor, H. B.: Melanomas of the vagina. Am. J. Clin. Path., *46*:420, 1966.

Okun, M. R., and Bauman, L.: Malignant melanoma arising from an intradermal nevus. Arch. Derm., *92*:69, 1965.

Okun, M. R., DiMattia, A., Thompson, J., and Pearson, S. H.: Malignant melanoma developing from intradermal nevi. Arch. Derm., *110*:599, 1974.

Paslin, D. A.: The effects of biopsy on the incidence of metastases in hamsters bearing malignant melanoma. J. Invest. Derm., *61*:33, 1973.

Pullmann, H., and Steigleder, G. K.: A study of cellular inflammatory reaction in human malignant melanoma, using in vitro labelling techniques with H3-thymidine. Arch. derm. Forsch., *249*:285, 1974.

Ranchod, M.: Metastatic melanoma with balloon cell changes. Cancer, *30*:1006, 1972.

Reed, W. B., Becker, S. W., Sr., Becker, S. W., Jr., and Nickel, W. R.: Giant pigmented nevi, melanoma, and leptomeningeal melanocytosis. Arch. Derm., *91*:100, 1965.

Silberberg, I., Kopf, A. W., and Gumport, S. L.: Diffuse melanosis in malignant melanoma. Arch. Derm., *97*:671, 1968.

Skov-Jensen, T., Hastrup, J., and Lambrethsen, E.: Malignant melanoma in children. Cancer, *19*:620, 1966.

Smith, J. L., and Stehlin, J. S., Jr.: Spontaneous regression of primary malignant melanomas with regional metastases. Cancer, *18*:1399, 1965.

Sohn, N., Gang, H., Gumport, S. L., *et al.*: Generalized melanosis secondary to malignant melanoma. Cancer, *24*:897, 1969.

Trodahl, J. N., and Sprague, W. G.: Benign and malignant melanocytic lesions of the oral mucosa. Cancer, *25*:812, 1970.

Truax, H., Barnett, R. N., Hukill, P. B., *et al.*: Effect of inaccurate diagnosis on survival statistics for melanoma. Cancer, *19*:1543, 1966.

Weidner, F., and Hornstein, O. P.: Das Problem der regionalen Lymphknoten-Metastasierung beim malignen Melanom. Arch. derm. Forsch., *245*:50, 1972.

Malignant Blue Nevus

Dorsey, C. S., and Montgomery, H.: Blue nevus and its distinction from Mongolian spot and the nevus of Ota. J. Invest. Derm., *22*:225, 1954.

Gartmann, H., and Lischka, G.: Maligner blauer Naevus (Malignes dermales Melanozytom). Hautarzt, *23*:175, 1972.

Hernandez, F. J.: Malignant blue nevus. A light and electron microscopic study. Arch. Derm., *107*:741, 1973.

Herzberg, J. J., and Klein, U. E.: Blauer Naevus mit Solitär-Metastasen in Lunge und Nebennieren. Arch. klin. exp. Derm., *212*:158, 1961.

Kwittken, J., and Negri, L.: Malignant blue nevus. Arch. Derm., *94*:64, 1966.

Merkow, L. P., Burt, R. C., Hayeslip, D. W., *et al.*: A cellular and malignant blue nevus. Cancer, *24*:888, 1969.

Mishima, Y.: Cellular blue nevus. Melanogenic activity and malignant transformation. Arch. Derm., *101*:104, 1970.

33

Lymphoma and Leukemia

Lymphoma designates a group of malignant neoplasias derived from either B or T lymphocytes. The lymphomas are subdivided into (1) Hodgkin's disease; (2) the "non-Hodgkin's" or monomorphous lymphomas; and (3) mycosis fungoides, with its variant, the Sézary syndrome. Malignant histiocytosis differs from the lymphomas by its derivation from histiocytes rather than lymphocytes. Leukemia and multiple myeloma represent neoplastic diseases of the hematopoietic system, with primary plasmacytoma of the skin being a variant of multiple myeloma. Finally, the pseudolymphoma of Spiegler-Fendt, or lymphocytoma, will be discussed because of its close histologic resemblance to lymphoma.

HODGKIN'S DISEASE

As a rule, Hodgkin's disease affects the lymph nodes primarily and predominantly, either the superficial or the visceral lymph nodes, or both. In most instances, Hodgkin's disease originates in a single lymph node region (Rosenberg and Kaplan). In only 5 to 9 per cent of the patients does Hodgkin's disease arise in an extranodal site, such as a parenchymatous organ or the skin (Freeman et al.; Carbone). Whether it starts in a lymph node or in an extranodal location, subsequent spreading tends to take place through lymphatic vessels to adjacent groups of lymph nodes. Vascular invasion in lymph nodes results in a spread to distant lymph nodes or to extranodal sites, usually resulting in widespread disease (Strum et al., 1971). On the other hand, less widespread disease may occur as the result of retrograde lymphatic spread from obstructed lymph nodes to organs such as the skin, the liver, or the lung (Benninghoff et al.). The usually orderly extension of Hodgkin's disease in its early stages has led to the widely accepted "staging" of the disease by lymphangiography and exploratory laparotomy, consisting of splenectomy, liver biopsy, and biopsy of iliac and para-aortic lymph nodes, in order to determine the extent of the disease and, based upon this, the type of treatment (Prosnitz et al.).

In the process of staging, four stages are recognized. In the 1971 Ann Arbor Staging Classification, as described by Carbone, stage I indicates involvement of either a single lymph node region (I) or of a single extralymphatic organ or site (I_E); stage II shows either involvement of two or more lymph node regions on the same side of the diaphragm (II) or localized involvement of an extralymphatic organ or site and of one or more lymph node regions on the same side of the diaphragm (II_E); stage III is characterized by involvement of lymph node regions on both sides of the diaphragm (III), which may be accompanied by localized involvement of an extralymphatic organ or site (III_E), or by involvement of the spleen (III_S), or both (III_{ES}); and stage IV shows diffuse or disseminated involvement of one or more extralymphatic organs or sites with or without associated lymph node involvement.

Involvement of the skin in Hodgkin's disease may consist of nonspecific or specific lesions. The former most commonly consist of excoriations, erythema, and lichenification secondary to generalized pruritus, or ichthyosis vulgaris, and occasionally of generalized erythroderma. Herpes zoster is a fairly common nonspecific cutaneous reaction, caused by a decrease in cell-mediated immune responses (Sell) (see under Histogenesis, p. 686). Specific cutaneous lesions occur in 5 to 10 per cent of the patients with Hodgkin's disease (Benninghoff et al.; Ultman and Moran). They consist of cutaneous nodules and plaques (Haustein and Tausch) that may undergo ulceration (Senear and Caro). Rarely, subcutaneous nodes are present (Reimann et al.; Undeutsch et al.). In most instances the cutaneous lesions are caused by hematogenous spread and then occur in association with widespread lymph node involvement in stage IV (Ultman and Moran). However, if caused by retrograde lymphatic spread from corresponding lymph nodes the disease may still be in one of the early stages (Benninghoff et al.). In very rare instances the first clinical manifestation of Hodgkin's disease may occur in the skin before lesions are demonstrable elsewhere (Reimann et al.; Ongenae; Haustein and Tausch). In addition, there are occasional cases in which cutaneous lesions remain the sole manifestation of the disease (Szur et al.). In such cases it may be assumed that a state of balance between tumor and host exists, although possibly lymphangiography and an exploratory laparotomy might have disclosed the existence of extracutaneous disease (Ultman and Moran). It seems, however, that in most cases reported as instances of purely cutaneous Hodgkin's disease the patients in reality either had the tumor stage of mycosis fungoides (Cyr et al.) (see p. 697), or had lymphomatoid papulosis, a variant of Mucha-Habermann disease, as in the two cases reported by Dupont and in Cases 1 and 2 reported by Szur et al. (see p. 164).

Histopathology. The old histologic classification of Hodgkin's disease proposed by Jackson and Parker in 1944 that divided the disease into paragranuloma, granuloma, and sarcoma has been abandoned as unsatisfactory, since 80 to 90 per cent of the cases fell into the granuloma group, and this group proved to be too heterogeneous (Franssila et al.). In its place the histologic classification suggested by Lukes et al. in 1966 has been universally adopted. Four histologic types are recognized of which the first two types, called lymphocytic predominance and nodular sclerosis, often spread slowly and show a good response to adequate treatment; whereas the latter two, called mixed cellularity and lymphocytic depletion, carry a poor prognosis. The histologic type remains constant in over 90 per cent of the cases with the nodular sclerosis type, in contrast with only about 40 per cent of the cases with lymphocytic predominance and about 70 per cent of those with multiple cellularity. In patients requiring reclassification the change usually is toward a histologically more malignant form of Hodgkin's disease (Strum and Rappaport).

In *lymphocytic predominance* either lymphocytes or histiocytes predominate, whereas eosinophils, neutrophils, and plasma cells are few in number or absent. There is no necrosis or fibrosis, and few immature or atypical mononuclear cells and few Sternberg-Reed giant cells are present (Franssila et al.).

In *nodular sclerosis* interconnecting thick bands of collagenous tissue subdivide the abnormal lymphoid tissue into circumscribed nodules. Although classical Sternberg-Reed giant cells are few, a large pale variant may be prominent, referred to as lacunar cell (see below). Lymphocytes, eosinophils, neutrophils, plasma cells, fibroblasts, and histiocytes as well as immature, atypical mononuclear cells are present in varying amounts. Necrosis is occasionally seen.

In *mixed cellularity* the classical histologic picture of Hodgkin's disease is seen. Varying numbers of Sternberg-Reed giant cells, lymphocytes, eosinophils, neutrophils, plasma cells, and histiocytes as well as immature, atypical mononuclear cells are present together with necrosis and fibrosis. There are, however, no thick collagen bands.

In *lymphocytic depletion* lymphocytes are scarce. There are many classical Sternberg-Reed giant cells and extensive diffuse fibrosis without collagen band formation.

The presence of Sternberg-Reed giant cells is essential for the histologic diagnosis of Hodgkin's disease. Typical Sternberg-Reed giant cells have the following characteristics: They are large cells containing either several nuclei or one multilobular nucleus. Often, one sees either two nuclei or a bilobed nucleus having a "mirror-image" appearance. The nucleoli are large, vary in their staining reaction from eosinophilic to amphophilic, and are surrounded by a chromatin-free, clear halo (Franssila et al.). If multinucleated, the nuclei may be either peripherally or centrally located. In the nodular sclerosis type the Sternberg-Reed cells often are multilobular, possess abundant clear cytoplasm and lie in clear spaces or lacunae and, therefore, are called lacunar cells (Strum and Rappaport). Sternberg-Reed giant cells with bizarre and irregular nuclei are often present in older lesions (Strum et al., 1970). The Sternberg-Reed giant cells, if multinucleated, has formed by means of nuclear division without cytoplasmic division, suggesting that the mono-nuclear tumor cell is the active malignant cell and the Sternberg-Reed cell is an end cell (Rubin). The size of Sternberg-Reed giant cells usually varies from 15 to 45 μm in diameter (Thomas).

The *cutaneous lesions* occurring in Hodgkin's disease, if nonspecific, merely show a chronic inflammatory infiltrate. The specific nodules and plaques show large masses of cells, often extending into the subcutaneous tissue (Fig. 33-1) (Senear and Caro). The histologic findings are rarely as typical as in the lymph nodes, and assignment to one of the four histologic types is more difficult than in the lymph nodes and often is impossible. The number of Sternberg-Reed giant cells, on the presence of which the diagnosis depends, often is small, and fibrosis or formation of collagen bands is less pronounced than in the lymph nodes. The presence of atypical mononuclear cells resembling mycosis cells in association with a chronic inflammatory infiltrate may suggest

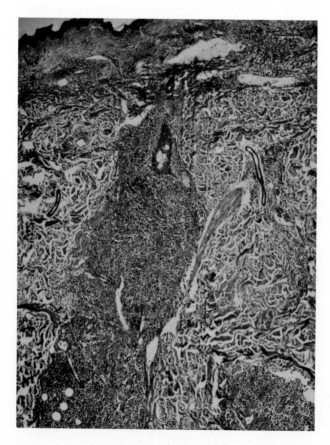

FIG. 33-1. **Hodgkin's disease.** Low magnification. There are two large masses of neoplastic cells. In addition, numerous small aggregates of cells are present throughout the dermis. (×50)

mycosis fungoides. However, a thorough search including an examination of step sections throughout the specimen usually will show a few multilobular and multinucleated giant cells, although they may not necessarily show the characteristic large, eosinophilic nucleolus with surrounding halo (Fig. 33-2) (E.M. No. 50).

Histogenesis. The malignant mononuclear cells in Hodgkin's disease have long been thought to be histiocytes, largely because "they look like it" (DeVita). In recent years, however, the view has been favored by several investigators that the malignant mononuclear cells of Hodgkin's disease, as well as the Sternberg-Reed giant cells that develop from them, are T lymphocytes which have been antigenically altered, possibly by a virus, and thus have been transformed into neoplastic cells (DeVita). In favor of this view are the usual onset of the disease in the primary regions of T-cell distribution, i.e., in the lymph nodes, the spleen, and the thymus, and the early derangement of delayed hypersensitivity (Order and Hellman). In addition, it has been noted that in the involved spleen of patients with Hodgkin's disease the percentage

of T lymphocytes among the mononuclear cells is significantly increased, suggesting that T lymphocytes are the precursor cells of Sternberg-Reed cells (Belpomme et al.). The inflammatory infiltrate and fibrosis represent a host response to the presence of the malignant mononuclear cells and Sternberg-Reed giant cells. In the lymphocytic predominance and the nodular sclerosis types the host response is strong and the disease is kept in check. If the host response is weak or weakens one of the other two reaction patterns, mixed cellularity or lymphocytic depletion, develops. Analogous to the strong host response, the prognosis is relatively good in patients with lymphocytic predominance type or with the nodular sclerosis type in whom the 10-year survival rate is 81 per cent and 40 per cent, respectively, according to Crum et al. On the other hand, analogous to the weak host response, the prognosis is poor in patients with the mixed cellularity type or the lymphocytic depletion type in whom the 10-year survival rate is 10 per cent and zero, respectively.

The decrease in delayed hypersensitivity reactions, caused by a deficiency in T-cell function, is already evident early in the disease and becomes more pronounced later in the disease.

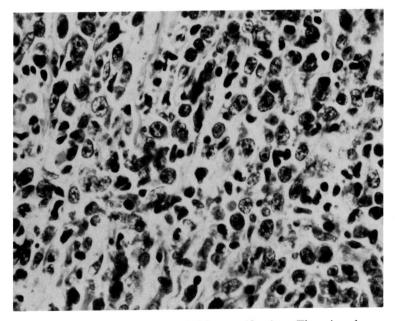

Fig. 33-2. **Hodgkin's disease.** High magnification. There is a dense, polymorphous infiltrate as seen in the "mixed cellularity" type. The infiltrate contains many mononuclear cells with atypical nuclei. Several mitotic figures are present. Multilobular as well as multinucleated Sternberg-Reed giant cells are present; they can be identified by their large nucleoli surrounded by a chromatin-free, clear halo. (×400)

In evaluating the cell-mediated immune response in Hodgkin's disease, it must be kept in mind that also radiation therapy and chemotherapy can decrease them (Han and Sokal). On testing DNA synthesis in the lymphocytes of untreated patients with Hodgkin's disease, after stimulating them in vitro with varying concentrations of phytohemagglutinin, a dose-related defect in lymphocyte stimulation is apparent even in patients who are in the early stages of the disease (Stages I and II) (Levy and Kaplan). Additional defects in delayed hypersensitivity reactions develop in the course of the disease, such as: failure to develop contact sensitivity to dinitrochlorobenzene; unresponsiveness to skin testing with tuberculin, mumps antigen, and various fungal antigens (Schein and Vickers); and an increase in the incidence and the severity of viral and fungal infections, particularly herpes zoster (Sell). The defect in delayed hypersensitivity responses may reach the state of total anergy in the late stage of the disease, especially in patients with lymphocytic depletion (Young et al.). In contrast to the thymus-derived T-lymphocytes, the bursa-related B-lymphocytes are not affected in Hodgkin's disease, except perhaps in the terminal stage, so that, as a rule,. the immunoglobulin values in the serum are normal (Miller).

Differential Diagnosis. The dermal infiltrate in lymphomatoid papulosis, a variant of Mucha-Habermann disease, even though it is a benign disorder, may be indistinguishable from that occurring in Hodgkin's disease. Even giant cells resembling Sternberg-Reed giant cells may be found (Dupont; Macaulay; Szur et al.). Thus, only the clinical features of lymphomatoid papulosis, in which the lesions are papular rather than nodular and furthermore come and go spontaneously, make a differentiation from Hodgkin's disease possible. For a differentiation of the tumor stage of mycosis fungoides from Hodgkin's disease, see under Tumor Stage of Mycosis Fungoides (p. 700).

MONOMORPHOUS LYMPHOMAS

Classification. The non-Hodgkin's lymphomas are referred to as monomorphous lymphomas because, in contrast with Hodgkin's disease, they lack a significant admixture of inflammatory cells and are composed almost entirely of lymphoma cells. Their classification, as proposed by Gall and Rap-

paport and modified by Berard, is as follows:

> Lymphocytic type, well differentiated;
> Lymphocytic type, poorly differentiated ("lymphosarcoma");
> Histiocytic type ("reticulum cell sarcoma");
> Mixed lymphocytic-histiocytic type;
> Undifferentiated, pleomorphic stem cell type;
> Undifferentiated Burkitt type.

The histologic architecture may be either nodular or diffuse in all these forms, except in the Burkitt type which always appears diffuse. The nodular histologic pattern is associated with a distinctly superior survival time as compared with the diffuse histologic pattern (Carbone). Formerly, monomorphous lymphomas with a nodular pattern were referred to as follicular lymphoma or Brill-Symmers disease. However, as had first been pointed out by Rappaport et al. and by Wright in 1956, follicular lymphoma does not represent an entity but may be the initial phase of different types of lymphoma. Even in the early follicular, or nodular, phase one usually can identify the type of lymphoma that will emerge after the disappearance of the follicular pattern. (For histologic details of the nodular pattern, see under Histopathology, p. 689).

The difficulty of identifying the various cell types in monomorphous lymphomas has led to different classifications. Some series of lymphoma include a category of unclassified cases into which for instance Desai et al. placed 7 per cent of their cases. Furthermore, some authors have reduced the number of types of monomorphous lymphoma. Thus, Thorson and Brown recognized within the monomorphous group only a "lymphocytic sarcoma" and a "reticulum cell sarcoma," because of the difficulty in distinguishing between well differentiated and poorly differentiated lymphocytic lymphoma on the one hand and between stem cell lymphoma and histiocytic lymphoma on the other. In contrast, Rosenberg et al. have pointed out that, whereas a "small cell lymphosarcoma" composed of well differentiated lymphocytes can be easily identified as such, it can be very difficult in cases of monomorphous lymphomas composed of large and immature cells to decide whether these cells represent poorly differentiated lymphocytes, reticulum cells, or stem cells. They have, therefore, combined all three cell types as "reticulum cell sarcoma."

Clinical Manifestations. Non-Hodgkin's lymphoma differs from Hodgkin's disease in its clinical manifestations in several aspects: (1) Unifocal localization, which is common in the early stage of Hodgkin's disease, is less common in the early stage of non-Hodgkin's lymphoma, occurring, according to Peters et al., in only 39 per cent of the histiocytic lymphomas and in 60 per cent of the lymphocytic lymphomas; (2) primary extranodal localization is much more common in patients with non-Hodgkin's lymphoma than in those with Hodgkin's disease, occurring according to Freeman et al. in 24 per cent of the cases with non-Hodgkin's lymphoma, as compared with only 5 per cent in Hodgkin's disease; (3) hematogenous spread to distant sites is observed more frequently and also earlier in the course of the disease in non-Hodgkin's lymphoma than in Hodgkin's disease; and (4) in contrast with Hodgkin's disease in which leukemia develops very rarely, non-Hodgkin's lymphoma, particularly the lymphocytic types, occasionally show infiltration of the bone marrow with abnormal cells and their appearance in the peripheral blood. In the series of patients observed by Rosenberg et al., leukemia developed in 12.6 per cent of the patients with lymphoma of the lymphocytic types, and in 2.4 per cent of the patients with lymphoma of the histiocytic type.

The leukemia that may develop in non-Hodgkin's lymphoma generally retains the cell type present in the lymphoma. Thus, the well differentiated type of lymphocytic lymphoma usually is associated with chronic lymphocytic leukemia; whereas the poorly differentiated lymphocytic lymphoma transforms into an intermediate type of leukemia referred to as lymphosarcoma cell leukemia in which the lymphoid cells, in contrast with the spontaneously arising lymphoblastic leukemia, show evidence of maturation. The stem cell type of lymphoma may transform into acute lymphocytic or stem cell leukemia; histiocytic lymphoma into myelomonocytic or monocytic leukemia; and Burkitt's lymphoma into Burkitt's cell leukemia (Carbone).

Specific cutaneous lesions occur somewhat more frequently in non-Hodgkin's lymphoma than in Hodgkin's disease. As previously stated, in Hodgkin's disease 5 to 10 per cent of the patients have specific skin lesions and they are almost never present at the beginning of the disease (see p. 683). On the other hand, in non-Hodgkin's lymphoma around 17 per cent of the patients have specific cutaneous lesions, and in 5 per cent they are present at the beginning (Rosenberg et al.). The cutaneous lesions usually are multiple, and, just as in Hodgkin's disease, they generally consist of nodules and plaques that may undergo ulceration. Occasionally generalized erythroderma occurs in non-Hodgkin's lymphoma (Nicolis and Helwig). Purely subcutaneous nodules are very rare, although the extension of large cutaneous nodules into the subcutaneous fat is common.

"Staging" of the disease by lymphangiography and exploratory laparotomy, just as is done for Hodgkin's disease (see p. 682), often is advisable in non-Hodgkin's lymphoma also, unless there is evidence of widespread hematogenous dissemination ("stage IV") or of leukemia, because the extent of the disease may influence the type of treatment to be employed (Hanks et al.; Reilly et al.). In order to rule out the existence of leukemia, biopsy of the bone marrow is indicated prior to "staging."

Histopathology. It is not always possible, particularly in the beginning, to assign every case of non-Hodgkin's lymphoma to one of the six recognized types, but more important than to decide on the type of lymphoma is to decide whether or not a patient has lymphoma. The following histologic features speak in favor of lymphoma rather than an inflammatory infiltrate: (1) The specific lesions of monomorphous or non-Hodgkin's lymphoma show either large masses or small patches of cells that, even though they vary with the type of lymphoma, usually show atypical nuclei and atypical mitoses. (2) The large masses of lymphoma cells that clinically appear as cutaneous tumors frequently extend from the dermis deep into the subcutaneous tissue; while the small patches of lymphoma cells are distributed haphazardly throughout the dermis and the subcutaneous tissue. Occasionally, small patches of lymphoma cells are found in the subcutaneous tissue even in areas of normal-appearing skin (Trubowitz and Sims). (3) The cells within the masses and patches often are so tightly packed that their nuclei may coalesce, whereas in an inflammatory infiltrate the cells generally are separated by edema. (4) The masses and patches of cells are quite sharply demarcated at their border. (5) Frequently, single rows of lymphoma cells not only extend from the otherwise sharply demarcated masses and patches of cells but often also lie independent of the masses and patches of cells, within the spaces between intact bundles of collagen "like Indians in a file." (This phenomenon of single-row invasion also occurs in metastatic carcinoma of the skin, especially in cancer en cuirasse of the breast, and, to a slight degree also in granuloma annulare, see pp. 565 and 215.) For further points of differentiation of lymphoma from inflammatory infiltrates see pp. 691 and 694; for differentiation from pseudolymphoma of Spiegler-Fendt see p. 710.

The following are among the reasons why it may be difficult to decide which type of lymphoma a patient has: (1) Not infrequently, the cells of a lymphoma have a pleomorphic appearance, making it difficult to assign them to a definitive cell type (Steigleder and Hunscha); (2) cells different in appearance may be encountered in different lesions of the same patient; and (3) as the disease progresses, the cells of the lesions may become less differentiated and require reassignment to another type of lymphoma (Gall and Mallory).

Histogenesis. It is generally assumed that the non-Hodgkin's or monomorphous lymphomas are true neoplasms. The tumor cells, as in Hodgkin's disease, are thought to be antigenically altered, possibly by a virus. However, in contrast to Hodgkin's disease and mycosis fungoides, in which the tumor cells are T lymphocytes, the non-Hodgkin's lymphomas are composed of B lymphocytes in most, and possibly in all, instances.

The first evidence was reported in 1972, when it was shown that lymphocytic lymphoma (Aisenberg and Bloch) and reticulum cell sarcoma (Stein et al.) were composed of cells bearing large amounts of immunoglobulins on their surfaces, demonstrable with fluorescein-conjugated antisera. Since this is a characteristic feature of B lymphocytes and not of T lymphocytes or histiocytes, the findings favored the B-cell origin of these two types of non-Hodgkin's lymphoma.

Since then more refined methods for identifying T lymphocytes, B lymphocytes, and histiocytes have become available, namely by means of rosette formation. Whereas the testing for identification of B lymphocytes or histiocytes can be carried out either with cell suspensions or with frozen sections, the testing for T lymphocytes can be done only with cell suspensions, since the test requires living cells. T lymphocytes are identified by their spontaneous rosette formation with neuraminidase-treated sheep erythrocytes. B lymphocytes as well as histiocytes have receptors for the activated third component of complement, identifiable by their binding of erythrocytes coated with IgM antibody and complement (IgMEAC); but only histiocytes have receptors for cytophilic antibodies and thus bind erythrocytes coated with IgG antibody (IgGEA) (Jaffe et al.). When this method was used on frozen sections of involved lymph nodes obtained from 6 patients with follicular lymphoma, the cells of the neoplastic follicles reacted as B lymphocytes. In 2 of the 6 cases subclassified as mixed lymphocytic-histiocytic lymphoma on histologic grounds, both cell types reacted as B lymphocytes (Jaffe et al.). Also poorly differentiated lymphocytic lymphoma (Seligmann) and Burkitt's lymphoma (Pagano et al.) have thus been identified as B-cell lymphomas. Analogous to the finding of a proliferation of defective B cells, the amount of circulating immunoglobulins in B-cell lymphomas is often reduced, whereas delayed hypersensitivity, in contrast to Hodgkin's disease, is not impaired (Miller).

The transformation of a non-Hodgkin's lymphoma to leukemia of the same cell line indicates that these two processes are the same but represent different stages in the evolution of the process. Whereas non-Hodgkin's lymphoma is a more or less localized process, leukemia is characterized by diffuse bone marrow involvement associated with diffuse involvement of spleen, liver, and lymph nodes (Rubin).

NODULAR AND DIFFUSE MONOMORPHOUS LYMPHOMA

In all types of monomorphous or non-Hodgkin's lymphoma, with the exception of Burkitt's lymphoma, the histologic patterning may be either *nodular* or *diffuse* (Carbone). The nodular patterning, referred to also as follicular lymphoma, formerly was regarded as a distinct form of lymphoma. It usually is limited to the lymph nodes and spleen and, as a rule, carries a better prognosis than the diffuse patterning, particularly in regard to the length of survival: If in cases with follicular patterning of the lymphoma in the lymph nodes and in the spleen other organs are involved, such as the liver (Torres) or the skin (see below), they only rarely show on histologic examination a nodular pattern and usually show a diffuse pattern.

Histopathology. The follicular or nodular patterning in the lymph nodes and in the spleen has its origin in the lymphoid follicles (Jaffe et al.). The follicles are much larger and much more numerous than in normal lymph nodes or in the normal spleen. Usually the abnormal follicles appear lighter than the surrounding interstitial tissue, but they may appear darker (Hurst and Meyer). Whether they are lighter or darker depends on whether the lymphocytes in the abnormal

follicles are predominantly large transformed lymphocytes with pale nuclei or lymphocytes with dark nuclei (see below, under Histogenesis). Normal lymphoid follicles are surrounded by a perifollicular mantle of small lymphocytes. Such a mantle may be present or absent in the follicles of nodular lymphoma. The interstitial tissue separating the abnormal follicles usually is free of lymphoma. In most instances of nodular lymphoma, as the lymphoma progresses the follicular pattern disappears, and diffuse lymphoma emerges. In some cases, however, even at autopsy the pattern still is follicular (Wright).

In rare instances a follicular or nodular pattern similar to that seen in the lymph nodes and the spleen is present also in the skin. In such cases the follicles consist of transformed large lymphocytes and the interstitial cells of small lymphocytes (Lukes and Collins). This interpretation is more in keeping with recently developed concepts than the view expressed by Kwittken and

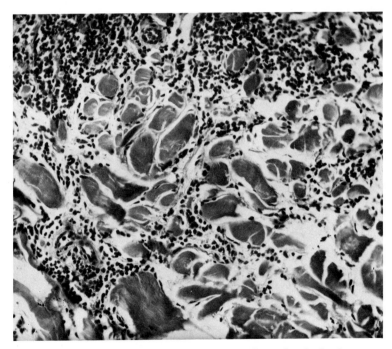

FIG. 33-3. **Lymphocytic lymphoma, well differentiated.** In the upper third of the photograph one sees the periphery of a large mass of tumor cells. Rows of tumor cells extend from the mass into the spaces between intact collagen bundles "like Indians in a file." The cells are indistinguishable from normal lymphocytes. (×200)

Goldberg that the follicles are composed of reticulum cells (see below, under Histogenesis). Usually, however, the cutaneous infiltrate in patients with nodular lymphoma of the spleen and lymph nodes is diffuse, rather than nodular (Polano; Nitschner).

Histogenesis. In normal lymph nodes and in the spleen the lymphoid follicles are composed largely of B lymphocytes. In nodular lymphoma assay by rosette formation in frozen tissue sections has demonstrated a follicular origin for the cells in the neoplastic nodules, since they react as B lymphocytes (Jaffe et al.) (see p. 688). Normally, the small lymphocytes present in the perifollicular mantle are transformed in the follicular centers into large metabolically active lymphocyte ("immunoblasts") and then move through the lymphocytic mantle into the interfollicular tissue. In this location they either continue to proliferate as immunoblasts and provide plasma cells, or revert to a dormant state as small lymphocytes as the stimulus subsides (Lukes and Collins). In nodular or follicular lymphoma the lymphomatous cells within the follicles are defective: There is a block in their further development and they proliferate within the follicles without moving into the interfollicular tissue where they would become plasma cells. Antibody production therefore is deficient. In com-

parison with nodular or follicular lymphoma, diffuse lymphoma has an even more severe immune defect. It shows a tremendous accumulation of defective B lymphocytes that are unable to function and fail to form lymphoid follicles in the lymph nodes and in the spleen (Lukes and Collins).

Differential Diagnosis. Nodular non-Hodgkin's lymphoma of the skin differs from Spiegler-Fendt pseudolymphoma by showing immature, atypical cells rather than well differentiated cells in the center of the nodular formations.

LYMPHOCYTIC LYMPHOMA, WELL DIFFERENTIATED

Histopathology. The specific cutaneous lesions of a well differentiated lymphocytic lymphoma show either large masses of cells (Fig. 33-3) or scattered patches of cells (Fig. 33-4). In either case the predominating cell is indistinguishable from a normal lymphocyte. In some instances, there is an admixture of not fully differentiated lymphocytes, resembling lymphoblasts. Mitotic figures are sparse. At the periphery of the

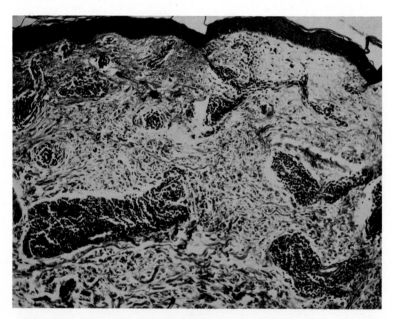

FIG. 33-4. **Lymphocytic lymphoma, well differentiated.** Sharply demarcated patches of lymphocytes are distributed through the dermis. Most patches show a blood vessel in their center. In the patch near the left lower corner one sees coalescence of the nuclei. (×100)

large masses or scattered patches of cells one may see single rows of tumor cells extending between and even around intact collagen bundles. In some areas one may see coalescence of the nuclei. This feature, although occasionally seen in the skin in all types of lymphoma but hardly ever in inflammatory infiltrates, is most commonly observed in well differentiated lymphocytic lymphoma, because the tumor cells not only lie closely aggregated, as in most cases of lymphoma, but also possess very little cytoplasm.

Differential Diagnosis. Lymphocytic lymphoma with scattered patches of cells, especially in the absence of immature cells and mitotic figures, must be differentiated from four inflammatory diseases that also show a patchy infiltrate. They together form the "five patchy diseases beginning with an *L*." They comprise, aside from lymphocytic *L*ymphoma, chronic discoid *L*upus erythematosus, the patchy type of polymorphous *L*ight eruption, *L*ymphocytic infiltration of the skin of Jessner, and pseudo-*L*ymphoma of Spiegler-Fendt.

Chronic discoid lupus erythematosus differs from well differentiated lymphocytic lymphoma by usually showing characteristic epidermal changes (see p. 424). In addition, the patchy infiltrate of chronic discoid lupus erythematosus appears less sharply demarcated than the infiltrate of lymphocytic lymphoma, and the cells within the patchy infiltrate are less tightly packed; instead, being an inflammatory infiltrate, the cells are more loosely arranged, and there may be a slight admixture of plasma cells and histiocytes. Furthermore, the cellular infiltrate shows no single-row invasion between the collagen bundles; but it often shows a tendency to arrangement in the vicinity of the cutaneous appendages and may even invade them. It should be kept in mind, however, that the appearance and composition of the dermal infiltrate often does not differ sufficiently from that of lymphocytic lymphoma to permit a clear differentiation on a histologic basis.

Polymorphous light eruption of the plaque type (see p. 193) and lymphocytic infiltration

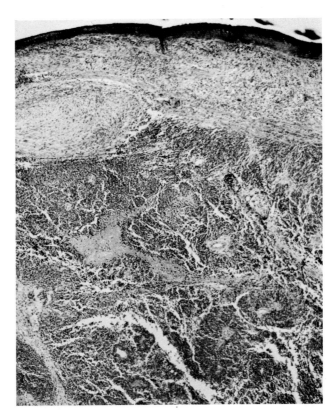

Fig. 33-5. **Lymphocytic lymphoma, poorly differentiated.** Low magnification. Masses of densely packed tumor cells are present in the lower dermis. (×50)

of the skin of Jessner (see p. 435), both of which probably are variants of chronic discoid lupus erythematosus, nevertheless lack the epidermal changes generally seen in chronic discoid lupus erythematosus. The dermal infiltrate, like that of chronic discoid lupus erythematosus, often does not differ sufficiently from that seen in lymphocytic lymphoma to allow reasonably certain differentiation. Thus, clinical data and possibly also a therapeutic test with hydroxychloroquine sulfate (Plaquenil) may be required in order to differentiate chronic discoid lupus erythematosus, polymorphous light eruption of the plaque type, and Jessner's lymphocytic infiltration of the skin from well differentiated lymphocytic lymphoma.

In pseudolymphoma of Spiegler-Fendt the infiltrate differs from that of lymphocytic lymphoma by the presence of a usually considerable admixture of mature histiocytes and often also by a pseudofollicular arrangement of the infiltrate (see p. 709).

LYMPHOCYTIC LYMPHOMA, POORLY DIFFERENTIATED

Histopathology. In poorly differentiated lymphocytic lymphoma, also referred to as lymphosarcoma, immature lymphocytes predominate, but in most lesions mature lymphocytes are also present in moderate number. The immature lymphocytes, or lymphoblasts, possess a narrow basophilic rim of cytoplasm and a large, round or slightly indented nucleus. Because of the small amount of cytoplasm the nuclei lie closely together, much closer than in stem cell lymphoma or histiocytic lymphoma (Fig. 33-5). The nuclei are larger than those of mature lymphocytes, and are more uniform in appearance than those of stem cells or immature histiocytic cells. The chromatin in the nuclei of the immature lymphocytes is distributed rather evenly and is much less clumped than in mature lymphocytes, so that the nuclei have a vesicular appearance (Fig. 33-6). Atypical mitoses usually are numerous.

HISTIOCYTIC LYMPHOMA

Histiocytic lymphoma, also called reticulum cell sarcoma, starts in a circumscribed area, according to Peters et al., in about 39 per cent of the cases. Occasionally, the first lesion or group of lesions occurs in the skin (Kim et al.; Petrozzi et al.); and in rare instances no lesions are found aside from those of the skin even on autopsy (Kalkoff; Sonck). The cutaneous lesions consist of nodules of varying size. Clinically and also histologically the lesions resemble those of the tumor stage of mycosis fungoides (see p. 700). In the course of histiocytic lymphoma, myelomonocytic or monocytic leu-

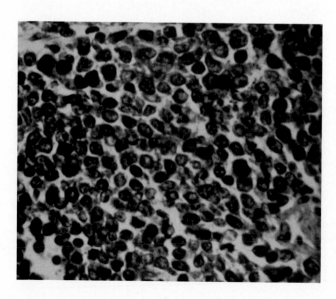

FIG. 33-6. **Lymphocytic lymphoma, poorly differentiated.** High magnification of Figure 33-5. The immature lymphocytes, or lymphoblasts, possess only a small amount of cytoplasm. Therefore the nuclei lie more densely packed than in histiocytic lymphoma or stem cell lymphoma. The nuclei are larger and also, because of the even distribution of the chromatin particles, stain more lightly than the nuclei of lymphocytes. A few lymphocytes are present. (×400)

kemia may develop in rare instances, especially in the terminal stage (Rosenberg et al.; Wenzel and Rastetter).

Histopathology. The type of cell present in the lesions was interpreted until recently as an immature histiocytic cell, also called reticulum cell. With the advent of immunologic identification of cells, it has become apparent that many, and possibly all, histiocytic lymphomas are composed of transformed lymphocytes (see below, under Histogenesis). Histologically, so-called histiocytic lymphoma is composed of cells having a rather abundant eosinophilic cytoplasm, the border of which tends to be ill defined. The nuclei are oval and may be kidney-shaped. They are pale-staining because they contain only a few chromatin particles and appear vesicular because of the presence of a distinct nuclear membrane (Fig. 33-7). Moderate numbers of atypical hyperchromatic nuclei and of atypical mitoses are present.

In the cutaneous lesions the cellular infiltrate varies in density from large masses to scattered patches. Single rows of tumor cells "like Indians in a file" are often seen. In some instances small aggregates of atypical histiocytes are located within the epidermis, and are indistinguishable from the Pautrier microabscesses in mycosis fungoides (Kim et al.; Petrozzi et al.).

Histogenesis. The tumor cells of so-called histiocytic lymphoma have been shown by means of fluorescein-conjugated antisera to have large amounts of immunoglobulins on their surfaces, a feature typical of B lymphocytes but not of histiocytes (Stein et al.). The large cell size, the rather abundant cytoplasm, and the pleomorphism of the large, vesicular nuclei are features of transformed B lymphocytes (Lukes and Collins). In lymph nodes and in the spleen transformed B lymphocytes are derived from the small lymphocytes in the perifollicular mantle and form in the lymphoid follicles whence they move out into the interfollicular space. Even in normal lymph nodes such transformed B lymphocytes may achieve a size four or more times that of the original small lymphocytes (Lukes and Collins). In most instances, lymphomatous proliferation of transformed B lymphocytes is diffuse, rather than nodular, in character (Lukes and Collins).

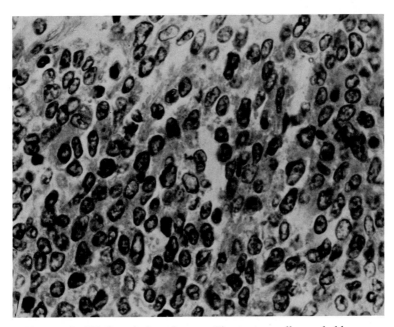

Fig. 33-7. **Histiocytic lymphoma.** The tumor cells, probably representing transformed lymphocytes, possess abundant pale-staining cytoplasm and variously shaped nuclei. Some are round, but most are oval or kidney-shaped. The nuclei are pale-staining and possess a distinct nuclear membrane. ($\times$400)

Differential Diagnosis. Histiocytic lymphoma must be differentiated from malignant histiocytosis and from Letterer-Siwe disease. Aside from the differences in the clinical manifestations and, in the case of Letterer-Siwe disease also in the age of the patient, the atypical histiocytes in malignant histiocytosis usually show erythrophagocytosis and are found mainly around the appendages in the deeper dermis (see p. 705). In Letterer-Siwe disease the histiocytes, although large, are not frankly atypical; they are present mainly in the uppermost dermis and often are intermingled with eosinophils (see p. 374).

MIXED LYMPHOCYTIC-HISTIOCYTIC LYMPHOMA

Histopathology. Mixed lymphocytic-histiocytic lymphoma is listed as a variant of non-Hodgkin's lymphoma in some classifications (Gall and Rappaport; Jones et al.) but not in others. The recognition of this variant was thought to be justified because in some lymphomas both atypical histiocytes and atypical lymphocytes seem to be present either in a diffuse or a nodular arrangement (Fig. 33-8). However, a recent investigation by immunologic methods has shown that both cell types react as B lymphocytes (Jaffe et al.) (see under Histogenesis).

Histogenesis. Jaffe et al. investigated 2 cases of nodular lymphoma of the lymphocytic-histiocytic type by means of the rosette test. In frozen tissue sections both cell types were found to bind the IgMEAC reagent, which reacts with both B lymphocytes and histiocytes, but not IgGEA, which reacts only with histiocytes. (For details of this test, see p. 688.) In the opinion of Lukes and Collins the cell that is most likely to give the appearance of a mixed cellular proliferation, as seen in "lymphocytic-histiocytic lymphoma," is the "large cleaved follicular center cell," since this type of B lymphocyte shows marked variation in nuclear configuration. Proliferation of this cell may be follicular (nodular) or diffuse.

Differential Diagnosis. Two types of cells are found in the dermal infiltrate not only

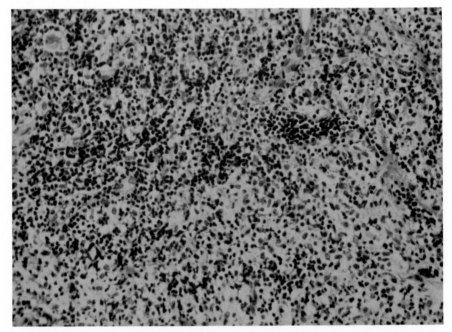

Fig. 33-8. **Mixed lymphocytic-histiocytic lymphoma.** Cells whose nuclei have the appearance of atypical lymphocytes and atypical histiocytes are present in an intermingled arrangement. With immunologic methods both cell types react as B lymphocytes. (×200)

in mixed lymphocytic-histiocytic lymphoma but also in pseudolymphoma of Spiegler-Fendt. The latter differs from mixed lymphocytic-histiocytic lymphoma by not showing atypical nuclei (see p. 709).

STEM CELL LYMPHOMA

Histopathology. In stem cell lymphoma the cutaneous lesions are composed of large masses of pleomorphic, undifferentiated lymphomatous cells (Fig. 33-9). Their nuclei are large, from two to four times the size of a normal lymphocyte, and filled with irregularly clumped chromatin particles (Fig. 33-10). Many atypical mitotic figures are present.

BURKITT'S LYMPHOMA

This type of lymphoma is seen predominantly in Central Africa, but in rare instances it occurs elsewhere, including the United States (Cohen et al.; Levine et al). It occurs largely but not exclusively among children. It is multifocal and largely extranodal. It causes massive tumors mainly of the maxillae, mandible and ovaries. The skin is not affected.

Histopathology. The tumor is composed of fairly uniform but highly undifferentiated lymphomatous cells that differ from the cells seen in stem cell lymphoma by showing less variation in size and shape (Cohen et al.). A characteristic feature is the presence of numerous large, light-staining macrophages that are interspersed among the tumor cells, resulting in a "starry-sky" pattern (N.I.H. Clinical Staff Conference).

Histogenesis. The Epstein-Barr virus is consistently associated with African Burkitt's lymphoma, as indicated by high antibody titers in the serum and the presence of Epstein-Barr viral DNA in the tumor tissue. It is assumed that the Epstein-Barr virus transforms lymphoctyes of

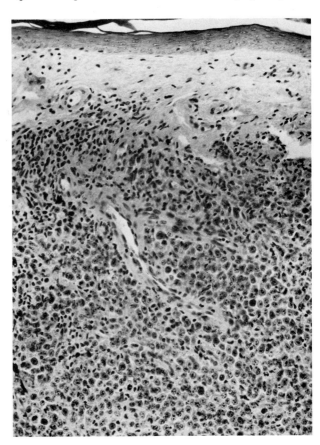

FIG. 33-9. **Stem cell lymphoma.** Low magnification. A large mass of tumor cells with pleomorphic nuclei is present in the dermis. (×100)

B-cell origin into malignant cells and that viral DNA then persists in these cells. In contrast to African Burkitt's lymphoma, patients with American Burkitt's lymphoma, on the average, have only slightly higher Epstein-Barr viral antibody titers than the general population; and no Epstein-Barr viral DNA has been found so far in the tumor tissue (Pagano et al.).

MYCOSIS FUNGOIDES

Mycosis fungoides affects the skin primarily and predominantly. In the late or tumor stage lymph nodes and visceral organs are frequently involved (Clendenning et al.; Cyr et al.; Epstein et al.).

Clinically as well as histologically, mycosis fungoides in typical cases can be divided into three stages: the erythematous stage, the plaque stage, and the tumor stage. The three stages overlap so that all three stages may be present simultaneously.

In the *erythematous stage* the eruption may resemble any of the following: eczema, psoriasis, parapsoriasis variegata, poikiloderma atrophicans vasculare, or parapsoriasis en plaques. Most commonly, one observes scattered erythematous, scaling patches having an irregular but fairly sharp demarcation. They often appear variegated, ranging in color from red to purple to brownish. Itching usually is pronounced.

In the *plaque stage* irregularly shaped, well demarcated, slightly indurated plaques occur. They may show central clearing, resulting in serpiginous lesions. Occasionally, spontaneous healing of some of the lesions takes place. During the process of healing some of the lesions may assume the appearance of poikiloderma atrophicans vasculare (Ackerman and Flaxman).

In the *tumor stage* one observes round or irregularly shaped, raised tumors of brownish-red color. Often they undergo ulceration. The tumors occurring in the tumor stage of mycosis fungoides have the same clinical appearance as the tumors seen in other forms of lymphoma.

In some patients the erythematous stage of mycosis fungoides becomes generalized. This *erythrodermic form* of mycosis fungoides

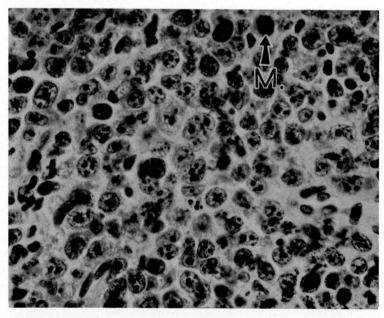

FIG. 33-10. **Stem cell lymphoma.** High magnification of Figure 33-9. The tumor cells possess abundant cytoplasm and large, rounded, pleomorphic nuclei. The nuclei contain irregular clumps of chromatin. A mitotic figure (M.) is present in the upper right corner. (×400)

has the appearance of a generalized exfoliative dermatitis or generalized erythroderma (Wilson; Lapière; Clendenning et al.; Epstein et al.). In most of these cases Sézary cells are present in the blood (see p. 704). After varying lengths of time plaques and tumors may develop in patients with the erythrodermic form of mycosis fungoides (Reed and Cummings).

In the rare *d'emblée form* of mycosis fungoides tumors of the skin develop without the previous presence of erythematous or plaque lesions (Miedzinski and Golebiowska; Lapière; Epstein et al.). The diagnosis of mycosis fungoides d'emblée requires, of course, that the tumors on histologic examination show an infiltrate that is compatible with the histologic diagnosis of mycosis fungoides.

Histopathology. The division of mycosis fungoides into three stages, as described for the clinical picture, pertains also to the histologic picture.

In the ERYTHEMATOUS STAGE not infrequently the histologic picture shows merely a banal inflammatory infiltrate in the papillary and subpapillary portions of the dermis, so that a histologic diagnosis of mycosis fungoides cannot be made. In some instances, however, particularly if several specimens are taken for biopsy, areas may be found in which specific changes, as described in the next paragraph, are present. A finding that should arouse one's suspicion of mycosis fungoides is the presence of scattered mononuclear cells having a hyperchromatic and irregularly shaped nucleus. This type of cell represents the so-called mycosis cell. A few cells having this appearance occur occasionally also in the dermal infiltrate of various inflammatory dermatoses (Flaxman et al.) (see p. 703). Since in the early erythematous stage of mycosis fungoides these cells are not as numerous and as large as they are in the plaque stage, it may be impossible to decide whether the infiltrate represents early mycosis fungoides or is nonspecific. The epidermis usually shows mild acanthosis; but it shows flattening in patients in whom the skin has the clinical appearance of poikiloderma vascu-

lare atrophicans. (For description see p. 700.)

In the PLAQUE STAGE the histologic picture is diagnostic in most instances. The following four changes are apt to be present: (1) a considerable polymorphism of cell types; (2) a fairly high percentage of so-called mycosis cells with a hyperchromatic and irregularly shaped nucleus, giving the mycosis cells a variable, pleomorphic appearance; (3) arrangement of the dermal infiltrate in a diffuse or bandlike pattern in the upper dermis and in a patchy pattern in the lower dermis; and (4) presence of Pautrier microabscesses in the epidermis.

The polymorphous cellular infiltrate consists mainly of histiocytes, lymphoid cells, eosinophils, and plasma cells. Some neutrophils and fibroblasts are often also present. A Giemsa stain, in addition to showing the eosinophils more clearly than a hematoxylin-eosin stain, also demonstrates the presence of a fairly large, but nevertheless diagnostically not significant proportion of mast cells. A moderate number of melanophages is often present. The number of histiocytes usually appears to be greater than that of lymphoid cells; but their actual number often is difficult to determine, since the nuclei of histiocytes are indistinguishable from those of endothelial cells and the number of capillaries is usually increased. (Not all endothelial cells present in histologic sections are seen together with their capillary lumen.)

The presence of mycosis cells, which are mononuclear cells with hyperchromatic, irregularly shaped nuclei, is diagnostic of the plaque stage of mycosis fungoides, provided that they form a fairly high percentage of the cells in the dermal infiltrate. The size of their nuclei is not significantly greater than the size of other nuclei in the infiltrate of the plaque stage so that they stand out more by their hyperchromasia than their size. Mitoses of such nuclei can be found as a rule, but their number usually is not large.

The arrangement of the cellular infiltrate in the plaque stage of mycosis fungoides often is patchy. In addition to a diffuse or bandlike infiltrate in the upper dermis, as seen also in a nonspecific chronic inflammation, one frequently finds patches of cellular infiltration in the lower dermis (Fig. 33-11). These patches usually have a blood vessel in their center. If the patches are fairly large in size and show a rather sharp demarcation, they are strong evidence in favor of mycosis fungoides. Areas of exocytosis, i.e., of penetration of inflammatory cells into the overlying epidermis, are seen quite frequently, but the exocytosis is not associated with a significant degree of spongiosis. In areas of exocytosis the epidermis contains also mycosis cells, often in significant number, so that it seems that mycosis cells have a special affinity for the epidermis (Rappaport and Thomas).

An almost pathognomonic finding is the *presence of Pautrier microabscesses* in the epidermis, found in more than half of the cases in the plaque stage, particularly if several biopsy specimens are examined. The only other disease in which they can be found is histiocytic lymphoma (Kim et al.;

Petrozzi et al.) (see p. 693). Pautrier microabscesses consist of small groups of mononuclear cells within the epidermis, surrounded by a halolike clear space (Fig. 33-12). The Pautrier microabscesses contain several mycosis cells, but may also contain a few nonspecific inflammatory cells. Most commonly the microabscesses are located in the lower epidermis. In addition to being present in the epidermis, Pautrier microabscesses are seen occasionally in the upper portion of hair follicles. The epidermis in the plaque stage usually shows acanthosis with elongation of the rete ridges and thus may have an appearance similar to that found in psoriasis. In some instances Pautrier microabscesses are so numerous that they permeate the lower epidermis even at a time when the dermal infiltrate is rather slight and inconspicuous so that one may speak of an epidermotropic form of mycosis fungoides (Gisinger; Braun-Falco et al.; Ryan et al.; Grosshans et al.; Smoes-Charles and Dupont).

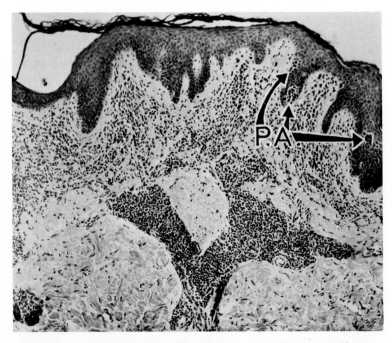

FIG. 33-11. **Mycosis fungoides, plaque stage.** Low magnification. The infiltrate in the upper dermis is diffuse, while in the lower dermis it consists of sharply demarcated patches of various sizes. The epidermis contains several Pautrier microabscesses (P.A.). ($\times$100)

FIG. 33-12. **Mycosis fungoides, plaque stage**. High magnification of Figure 33-11. The infiltrate in the upper dermis is polymorphous, showing a multiplicity of cell types. In addition, mononuclear cells with large, irregularly shaped, hyperchromatic nuclei are present, so-called mycosis cells (M.C.). There are several Pautrier microabscesses in the epidermis. (×400)

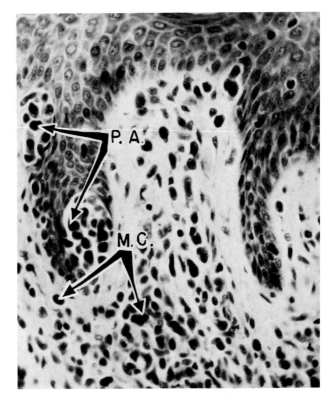

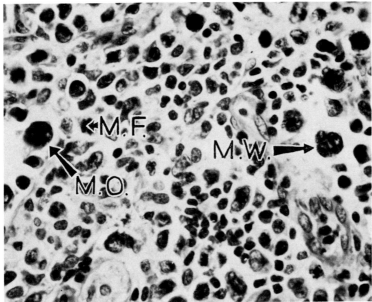

FIG. 33-13. **Mycosis fungoides, tumor stage**. The infiltrate still has the polymorphous appearance as seen in the plaque stage, but the number of mycosis cells is greater and the nuclei of some mycosis cells are large and have an anaplastic appearance. Several mycosis cells are multilobular, (M.O.) or multinucleated (M.W.) Mitotic figures (M.F.) are present. (×400)

In rare instances plaque lesions of mycosis fungoides show accumulations of acid mucopolysaccharides within hair follicles and sebaceous glands at the site of degenerating epithelial cells, resulting in a histologic picture identical with that seen in alopecia mucinosa (Emmerson) (see p. 186). The mucinous degeneration in such cases always is secondary to the mycosis fungoides.

In the TUMOR STAGE the infiltrate consists of large masses of cells, occupying extensive areas of the dermis, and often penetrating into the subcutaneous tissue. The infiltrate may invade and destroy the epidermis so that ulceration results. In some cases the infiltrate still has the polymorphous appearance seen in the plaque stage, although the number of mycosis cells is greater and the nuclei of some of the mycosis cells are of considerable size, resulting in an anaplastic, atypical appearance of such cells. Occasionally, mycosis cells with more than one nucleus are present (Fig. 33-13). These cells then resemble the multilobular or multinucleated Sternberg-Reed giant cells of Hodgkin's disease, from which they differ,

however, by greater hyperchromasia of their nuclei and by the absence of a large, eosinophilic nucleolus. Still, differentiation from Hodgkin's disease on a purely histologic basis may be impossible (Cyr et al.). In other cases the infiltrate no longer is polymorphous, with lymphoid cells, histiocytes, eosinophils, and plasma cells only few in number or absent so that the infiltrate appears monomorphous, consisting almost exclusively of large, atypical mycosis cells (Fig. 33-14). In such instances the histologic picture is indistinguishable from that of monomorphous lymphoma, and on a purely histologic basis differentiation from a lymphosarcoma or a reticulum cell sarcoma may not be possible. The diagnosis of mycosis fungoides then rests largely on the presence of a polymorphous infiltrate in previous or concomitant biopsy specimens, or on clinical data.

In POIKILODERMA ATROPHICANS VASCULARE occurring in conjunction with mycosis fungoides, histologic examination shows flattening of the epidermis with vacuolization of the basal cell layer. A dense, bandlike in-

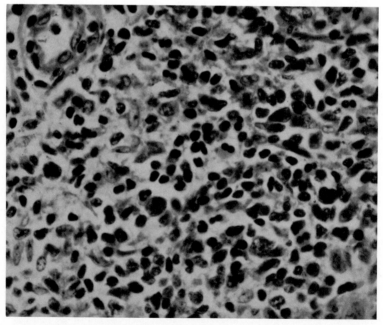

FIG. 33-14. **Mycosis fungoides, tumor stage.** The infiltrate appears less polymorphous than in the plaque stage, since it consists largely of mycosis cells with large, irregularly shaped, hyperchromatic nuclei. (×400)

filtrate lies in the upper dermis in close approximation to the epidermis and shows invasion of the epidermis in some areas. The infiltrate in early poikilodermic lesions of mycosis fungoides may be nonspecific, but it is much more pronounced than in idiopathic poikiloderma atrophicans vasculare, or in poikiloderma atrophicans vasculare associated with dermatomyositis or with systemic lupus erythematosus (Janis and Winkelmann) (see p. 439). In more advanced lesions rather numerous mycosis cells are present and permit the diagnosis of mycosis fungoides (Waddington).

Involvement of the Lymph Nodes and Internal Organs. The development of specific lesions in lymph nodes and in internal organs in mycosis fungoides is a late development, occurring generally only in the tumor stage of the disease. Thus, in a disease that starts fairly late in life and in which the erythematous and plaque stages can extend over many years, in a fairly high percentage of cases, amounting to about one third, the patients die of causes unrelated to mycosis fungoides; and an autopsy will reveal no specific lesions aside from those of the skin. Some of these patients show on autopsy a dermatopathic lymphadenitis of their peripheral lymph nodes, as a result of scratching the itching eruption. In some recently published reviews of autopsies on patients with mycosis fungoides absence of visceral lesions was noted in 24 per cent of 42 patients by Cyr et al., in 29 per cent of 45 patients by Rappaport and Thomas, and in 44 per cent of 27 patients by Long and Mihm.

Patients with mycosis fungoides dying in the tumor stage of their disease usually show specific involvement of peripheral and visceral lymph nodes and of internal organs on autopsy. Once the tumor stage has begun in a patient with mycosis fungoides death usually occurs within a few years. Thus, in the experience of Epstein et al., 50 per cent of their patients died of mycosis fungoides within 2½ years after the development of cutaneous tumors, and 70 per cent died within 6 years. Fuks et al. are even more pessimistic in their prognosis, stating that, once extracutaneous lesions have become evident, most patients will die within a year.

They use this observation as argument for advocating early and aggressive treatment of patients with mycosis fungoides with total electron beam radiation while the disease is still limited to the skin. However, before limiting the treatment of mycosis fungoides to the skin either with electron beam radiation (Fuks et al.) or with topical applications of nitrogen mustard (Van Scott and Kalmanson), it is important to rule out extracutaneous involvement. For this purpose, "staging" of the disease is recommended, as it is in other forms of lymphoma (Fuks et al.; Variakojis et al.). The recommended procedure is: (1) roentgenogram of the chest and liver function tests; (2) lower limb lymphangiography; (3) biopsy of any enlarged peripheral lymph nodes; and (4) if indicated, laparotomy with splenectomy, liver biopsy, and biopsy of para-aortic and iliac lymph nodes and of any other suspicious site of involvement.

In cases with involvement of the internal organs by mycosis fungoides autopsy may still show a polymorphous cellular infiltrate, in addition to the presence of mycosis cells (Cyr et al.). On the other hand, the visceral lesions, like some of the cutaneous lesions in the tumor stage, may consist largely of mycosis cells with large, atypical nuclei and show either only a slight or no admixture of inflammatory cells (see p. 700). Although the infiltrate may then resemble other forms of lymphoma, such as histiocytic lymphoma, lymphosarcoma, or Hodgkin's disease, if previous sections of such cases are reviewed and sections of various organs obtained at autopsy are compared with one another, it will become apparent that the characteristic histologic picture of mycosis fungoides, namely mycosis cells intermingled with a polymorphous infiltrate, was present at one time (Epstein et al.). Also, it is often evident that the cellular infiltration of internal organs in mycosis fungoides does not have the destructive effects usually observed in other form of lymphoma (Rappaport and Thomas).

In patients who on autopsy show extracutaneous involvement with mycosis fungoides this involvement usually is widespread (Clendenning et al.; Rappaport and Thomas). The peripheral and visceral lymph nodes are the most commonly involved extracutaneous tissue. Often it is very difficult to arrive at a decision whether a peripheral lymph node shows merely dermatopathic lymphadenitis (see p. 104) or specific involvement with mycosis fungoides (Rappaport and Thomas); and the presence of mycosis fungoides in areas of peripheral lymph nodes previously diagnosed as dermatopathic lymphadenitis has been reported (Block et al.; Fuks et al.).

Next to the peripheral and visceral lymph nodes specific involvement with mycosis fungoides is found most commonly in the spleen, the lungs, the liver, the kidney, and the gastrointestinal tract (Clendenning et al.; Rappaport and Thomas). However, involvement of the bone marrow occurs very rarely (Poulsen). For this reason, mycosis fungoides shows no significant hemocytologic changes except for the rather frequent presence of Sézary cells in the circulating blood. This mononuclear cell containing a large, irregular nucleus was found in blood smears in 20 per cent of the cases with mycosis fungoides by Clendenning et al., and on examining buffy coat preparations even in 38 per cent by Lutzner et al. (For discussion of the Sézary cell see below under Histogenesis.)

Histogenesis. At one time mycosis fungoides was regarded by certain authors, such as Symmers, as a "clinical and pathologic nonexistent" and cases reported as such were thought to represent either Hodgkin's disease, reticulum cell sarcoma or lymphosarcoma. Even today some authors regard mycosis fungoides as a clinical but not as a histologic entity and include under mycosis fungoides all lymphomas originating in the skin (Cawley et al.; Block et al.; Clendenning et al.).

Most authors, however, regard mycosis fungoides as a disease entity both on clinical and histologic grounds (Lapière; Degos et al.; Epstein et al.; Fuks et al.; Rappaport and Thomas; Edelson et al.; Long and Mihm). The most widely accepted view is that mycosis fungoides is a special form of lymphoma with the mycosis cell representing a neoplastic cell and that all other cells, as first suggested by Fraser in 1925, represent merely an inflammatory defense reaction of the tissue against the presence of lymphoma cells. Fraser pointed out that in the early stage of the disease the number of lymphoma cells was small, and the inflammatory defense reaction was pronounced. As the disease advanced, the number and atypicality of the lymphoma cell increased, whereas the defense reaction slackened, until in the tumor stage lymphoma cells predominated. Fraser's theory found support in the fact that also in other malignant diseases, such as squamous cell carcinoma and malignant melanoma, an inflammatory host reaction tends to be present in the early stage but disappears as the malignancy of the tumor cells increases.

Recent findings in regard to the mycosis cell have confirmed mycosis fungoides as an entity that differs from other lymphomas and, furthermore, have indicated the neoplastic character of the mycosis cell. The mycosis cell has been found to be a T lymphocyte, in contrast to the cells in non-Hodgkin's lymphomas which are largely B lymphocytes (see p. 688). The T-cell identity of a large majority of cells in the cellular infiltrate in mycosis fungoides could be established by preparing cell suspensions from lesions of mycosis fungoides. It was found that more than 90 per cent of the mononuclear cells formed sheep-erythrocyte rosettes, as T cells do. On the other hand, nearly all cells lacked receptors for the activated third component of complement and thus failed to bind erythrocytes coated with antibody and complement, as both B cells and histiocytes would do, and also lacked receptors for IgG and thus failed to bind erythrocytes coated with IgG, as histiocytes would do (Edelson et al.) (see also p. 688).

In evaluating the mycosis cell, Rappaport and Thomas identified two variants: "atypical lymphoid cells," seen largely in the early phase of the disease in the skin, and "true mycosis cells," found predominantly in the visceral lesions. The true mycosis cell, on the basis of its large, hyperchromatic and irregularly shaped nucleus was regarded as a malignant neoplastic cell. In electron microscopic studies, Rosas-Uribe et al., in collaboration with Rappaport, found that the atypical lymphoid cells and the mycosis cells had a similar appearance, characterized by a highly convoluted nucleus (see below under Electron Microscopy). It was concluded that both types of cells were neoplastic, and that the presence of inflammatory cells represented a host reaction. It appears likely that the mycosis cells, analogous to the mononuclear cells in Hodgkin's disease (see p. 685) and the cells of the non-Hodgkin's lymphomas (see p. 688), are lymphocytes that have been antigenically altered and thus have been transformed into neoplastic cells.

On *electron microscopic examination* the mycosis cell shows only scant cytoplasm but a relatively large nucleus with numerous infoldings of the nuclear membrane resulting in fingerlike projections of the nucleoplasm. Dense aggregates of chromatin particles are concentrated at the nuclear membrane and are scattered throughout the nucleus. Brownlee and Murad, Lutzner et al. and Rosas-Uribe et al. have pointed out the great resemblance between the mycosis cell and the Sézary cell by electron microscopy, indicating that the Sézary syndrome is a manifestation of mycosis fungoides. (For a discussion of the Sézary syndrome, see p. 704.)

The specificity of the mycosis cell, or Sézary cell, for mycosis fungoides and the Sézary syndrome seems to be established, especially on the basis of its presence in the circulating blood in all cases of the Sézary syndrome and in some cases of mycosis fungoides (see p. 702). The specificity of this cell had been questioned by Flaxman et al. because, on electron microscopic examination, they could identify cells with similarly convoluted nuclei in the dermal infiltrate of a variety of randomly selected nonlymphomatous dermatoses, such as lupus erythematosus, lichen planus, and solar keratosis. Rosas-Uribe et al. in their electron microscopic study have pointed out that the presence of isolated cells with convoluted nuclei in the skin or lymph nodes cannot be unequivocally interpreted as being indicative of mycosis fungoides, but that these cells are characteristic of mycosis fungoides or the Sézary syndrome when they occur in sheets or clusters. The same statement holds true also for the light microscopic examination of mycosis fungoides (see p. 697).

Some authors have expressed doubt concerning the primary neoplastic genesis of mycosis fungoides. Thus, Vesper et al., who applied the skin-window technique of Rebuck to a study of the cellular infiltrate in the skin of patients with mycosis fungoides in the plaque stage, observed large mononuclear cells which, in their opinion, showed no malignant or neoplastic characteristics. They concluded that mycosis fungoides was a proliferation of benign, immature cells. Similarly, Burg and Braun-Falco, on the basis of enzyme-histochemical studies, interpreted the infiltrate in lesions of mycosis fungoides as inflammatory hyperplastic rather than neoplastic and denied the existence of a disease-specific mycosis cell. Reed and Cummings also thought of early mycosis fungoides as a hyperplastic process, but they regarded the development of the plaque stage as transformation into a "malignant reticulosis in situ," and the development of the tumor stage as transformation into a "malignant reticulosis."

Differential Diagnosis. The diagnosis of mycosis fungoides in its early stage can be very difficult, if not impossible, so that often a decision can be made more easily on the basis of the clinical appearance rather than through the histologic findings. The reason for the difficulty in the histologic diagnosis of mycosis fungoides lies in the fact that a few hyperchromatic, irregularly shaped nuclei corresponding to "early" mycosis cells can occur in a number of nonspecific chronic inflammations, such as chronic dermatitis, and foreign body reactions, especially insect bites. The presence of mycosis cells within Pautrier microabscesses may then be of great diagnostic value; but even Pautrier microabscesses containing mycosis cells cannot always be differentiated from intraepidermal aggregates of cells that have formed as a result of exocytosis in cases of dermatitis (Ackerman et al.), except that spongiosis is common in dermatitis with exocytosis, and rare in mycosis fungoides.

Difficulties may arise in the differential diagnosis of mycosis fungoides from parapsoriasis en plaques and parapsoriasis variegata, because these two conditions resemble mycosis fungoides, not only in their histologic findings but also in their clinical appearance. Multiple biopsies, repeated at intervals, are then often necessary in order to arrive at a decision. Examination of blood smears or, preferably, of the buffy coat for Sézary cells may be helpful.

SÉZARY SYNDROME

The Sézary syndrome, first described by Sézary and Bouvrain in 1938, is characterized by generalized erythroderma with intense itching, peripheral lymphadenopathy, and the presence of Sézary cells in the cellular infiltrate of the skin and in the peripheral blood. The Sézary cell, as present in the skin, is indistinguishable from the mycosis cell, both by light and electron microscopy (Lutzner and Jordan).

Clinically, the entire skin, in addition to erythema, shows edema and lichenification. The general health remains good for several years. Death occurs as the result of either an intercurrent disease or the development of mycosis fungoides with plaques and tumors. In some of the cases in which mycosis fungoides with areas of induration had developed, histologic evidence of lymphoma was found also in the lymph nodes and in some viscera on autopsy (Fleischmajer and Eisenberg; Tedeschi and Lansinger; Winkelman and Linman; Paradinas and Harrison).

Histopathology. The skin in Sézary's syndrome shows in the upper dermis a dense infiltrate composed, in addition to varying numbers of Sézary cells, of lymphoid cells, histiocytes, eosinophils, neutrophils, plasma cells and fibroblasts. The Sézary cell in the dermis is indistinguishable from the mycosis cell as seen in the plaque stage of mycosis fungoides and shows a hyperchromatic, irregularly shaped nucleus. In addition, Pautrier microabscesses are often present in the epidermis, just as in mycosis fungoides, containing Sézary cells and also other cells of the dermal infiltrate (Sézary; Fleischmajer and Eisenberg; Edelson).

The circulating blood reveals a moderate leukocytosis, showing commonly between 10,000 and 30,000 leukocytes, but occasionally as many as 60,000 leukocytes (Taswell and Winkelmann) or even more than 200,000 leukocytes (Edelson et al.) per cu mm of blood. Atypical mononuclear cells, or Sézary cells, usually account for 5 to 20 per cent of the white cells. Although not larger than a neutrophil, they have a relatively large nucleus, which occupies at least four fifths of the cell and, like the Sézary cell found in the skin, appears hyperchromatic and irregularly shaped. In addition to the presence of Sézary cells, the blood shows a rather high percentage of normal lymphocytes. In the bone marrow fewer than 50 per cent of the nucleated cells are lymphocytes, and the other marrow-derived cell lines are well preserved, indicating extramedullary production of some of the lymphocytes and of the Sézary cells (Edelson et al.).

The enlarged peripheral lymph nodes may show only nonspecific dermatopathic lymphadenitis (Fleischmajer and Eisenberg). In other instances, however, the normal nodal architecture is completely replaced by lymphocytes and Sézary cells (Tedeschi and Lansinger; Edelson et al.).

Histogenesis. By electron microscopy the Sézary cell that is present in the skin and in the circulating blood, shows, like the mycosis cell, a nucleus characterized by numerous infoldings of the nuclear membrane resulting in fingerlike projections of the nucleoplasm (Brownlee and Murad; Lutzner and Jordan; Lutzner et al.). The Sézary cell has been identified by immunologic studies as a thymus-derived lymphocyte, since it can be stimulated by phytohemagglutinin in vitro to synthesize DNA (Crossen et al.), forms sheep-erythrocyte rosettes, and is killed by a specific rabbit antihuman T-cell antiserum (Brouet et al.; Winkelmann).

Although occasionally cells that are indistinguishable from mycosis cells or Sézary cells are present in the dermal infiltrate of various inflammatory dermatoses (Flaxman et al.) (see p. 703), they are seen in large numbers only in the dermal infiltrate of mycosis fungoides and the Sézary syndrome. Also, only in mycosis fungoides and the Sézary syndrome is this cell found within Pautrier microabscesses and in the peripheral blood. On this basis the Sézary syndrome is now widely regarded as the erythrodermic form of mycosis fungoides (Clendenning et al.; Tedeschi and Lansinger; Lutzner et al.). The Sézary syndrome differs, however, from mycosis fungoides by frequently showing high white blood cell counts in the peripheral blood together with lymphocytosis and many more Sézary cells than are seen in mycosis fungoides. Edelson et al. have referred to the Sézary syndrome as T-cell leukemia and as the leukemic phase of mycosis fungoides. Winkelman and Linman, however, do not regard the Sézary cell as a leukemic cell, since it is not derived from the bone marrow.

The origin of the Sézary cells in the circulating blood is not clear. Since in most cases, as shown in the review by Fleischmajer et al., the bone marrow is normal, and the Sézary cells in the circulating blood have the same appearance as those in the skin, some authors have expressed the opinion that they originate in the skin (Main et al.; Taswell and Winkelmann); while others assume that they arise from lymph nodes (Crossen et al.; Ebner et al.). In favor of the view that at least some of the Sézary cells are formed in the peripheral lymph nodes is the presence of Sézary cells in peripheral lymph nodes, found regularly on electron microscopic examination (Lutzner et al.).

Differential Diagnosis. There is no doubt that in the past cases of the Sézary syndrome have been mistaken for chronic lymphocytic leukemia and erythroderma. However, chronic lymphocytic leukemia represents an overproduction of B lymphocytes in the bone marrow which in the Sézary syndrome is not involved. The bone marrow in chronic lymphocytic leukemia would hardly ever show, as it does in the Sézary syndrome, more than 50 per cent of the nucleated cells to be nonlymphocytic cells. As a rule, in chronic lymphocytic leukemia 80 per cent or more of the nucleated cells in the bone marrow are lymphocytes, particularly when the peripheral white blood cell count exceeds 100,000 per cu mm (Edelson et al.).

MALIGNANT HISTIOCYTOSIS

Malignant histiocytosis, known also as histiocytic medullary reticulosis, is a rare, fulminant, uniformly fatal histiocytic proliferative disorder. Although occasionally occurring in childhood, most patients are adults. It is characterized by fever, lymphadenopathy and hepatosplenomegaly. In addition one observes later on jaundice, pancytopenia and purpura. The average survival time from the onset of symptoms is about 6 months.

Involvement of the skin with specific lesions is uncommon, since it was observed in only about 10 per cent of the reported cases (Abele and Griffin). The cutaneous lesions may appear early or late in the disease and consist of purplish nodules or plaques suggestive of lymphomatous infiltrates (Engstrom et al.).

Histopathology. The cutaneous infiltrate usually is located in the middle and lower dermis and the subcutaneous fat. It may be polymorphous (Liao et al.), but in any case it contains numerous atypical histiocytes with abundant, pale-staining, eosinophilic cytoplasm containing phagocytized erythrocytes, nuclear debris and fragments of ingested leukocytes and platelets (Engstrom et al.).

Histogenesis. The phagocytotic activity of the histiocytes present in all involved organs, including the bone marrow, causes the pancytopenia, as well as the jaundice and the purpura. By electron microscopy Langerhans granules are seen in the atypical histiocytes (Henderson and Sage), a feature they have in common with the immature histiocytes of histiocytosis (see p. 376).

Differential Diagnosis. Histologically, malignant histiocytosis resembles Letterer-Siwe disease to some extent, since both show an infiltrate of histiocytes. However, in Letterer-Siwe disease the infiltrate is located in the upper rather than the lower dermis and the histiocytes show little or no phagocytic activity. In addition, Letterer-Siwe disease occurs in infants, and usually has lytic bone lesions.

LEUKEMIA

The leukemias are characterized by infiltration of the bone marrow with immature leukocytes and by their presence in the blood stream, usually early in the disease. In addition, there usually is widespread infiltration of liver, spleen, and lymph nodes, and often also of other organs, including the skin.

Most cases of leukemia arise as a primary systemic disorder without developing from a lymphoma. As already stated in the description of the lymphomas, the development of a leukemia in the course of a lymphoma is rather rare (see p. 687). Four major groups of primary leukemia are recognized: (1) chronic lymphocytic leukemia; (2) acute lymphocytic leukemia; (3) chronic granulocytic leukemia; and (4) acute granulocytic leukemia (Saarni and Linman).

LYMPHOCYTIC LEUKEMIA

The specific cutaneous manifestations in chronic lymphocytic leukemia are similar to those found in lymphocytic lymphoma (see p. 687). In contrast with the fairly common occurrence of specific cutaneous lesions in chronic lymphocytic leukemia, they are very rare in acute lymphocytic leukemia, occurring in only 3.1 per cent of the cases (Boggs et al.).

CHRONIC GRANULOCYTIC LEUKEMIA

Chronic granulocytic leukemia shows a high leukocyte count in the blood with a predominance of granulocytes, including immature forms, and usually is associated with a marked enlargement of the liver and the spleen. Terminally, there may be a transformation to acute granulocytic leukemia with the presence of myeloblasts (Garfinkel and Bennett). Specific cutaneous manifestations are fairly rare in chronic granulocytic leukemia. If they occur it is usually during the terminal phase of the disease, although in exceptional cases leukemic infiltration of the skin can be demonstrated before characteristic changes are found in the bone marrow and the peripheral blood (Conrad et al.).

Clinically, the specific cutaneous lesions consist of papules and nodules of varying size that may coalesce into plaques. They may have a hemorrhagic appearance. In addition, purpuric lesions are common. Oral manifestations consisting of swollen and bleeding gums are noted occasionally.

Histopathology. Histologic examination of the specific cutaneous lesions in chronic granulocytic leukemia shows the presence of a dense infiltrate of cells in the dermis, often extending into the subcutaneous layer (Costello et al.). In addition to large areas of infiltration, small groups of cells may be found scattered through the dermis and the subcutaneous tissue. The cells are in part mature neutrophils, but in addition there are cells larger than neutrophils with round, oval or indented nuclei some of which show granules that are either neutrophilic or eosinophilic (Conrad et al.). These large cells if free of granules are indistinguishable from the immature cells seen in lymphoma (Costello et al.). Large cells with granules represent myelocytes, and those without granules myeloblasts.

The peroxidase reaction indicating the presence of the enzyme myeloperoxidase is positive in the granules of mature and partly matured cells of the myeloic series but is negative in very immature myeloic cells, such as myeloblasts, and in all cells of the lymphocytic series (Reardon and Moloney). The peroxidase reaction thus is of great diagnostic value, being usually positive in the specific cutaneous lesions of granulocytic leukemia and always negative in those of lymphocytic leukemia and lymphoma. Even very immature myeloic infiltrates usually show at least in some areas myelocytes in which the reaction is positive. Just as in the case of the dopa oxidase reaction, fresh

frozen sections should be used for the peroxidase reaction.

EOSINOPHILIC LEUKEMIA, a rare form of granulocytic leukemia, occasionally has cutaneous lesions. The cellular infiltrate in the dermis may contain numerous eosinophils (Deme), or it may consist largely of immature cells with only a few eosinophilic myelocytes and no mature eosinophils (Carmel et al.).

ACUTE GRANULOCYTIC LEUKEMIA

Three forms of acute granulocytic leukemia can be recognized: (1) acute myeloblastic leukemia, in which myeloblasts and young myelocytes predominate; (2) erythroleukemia, in which megaloblastic erythroid precursors are found in association with myeloblasts; and (3) myelomonocytic leukemia, with a proliferation of both granulocytic and monocytic cells in the bone marrow (Bennett). In all three forms fever, malaise, anemia, purpura and hepatosplenomegaly are found, and death usually occurs within a few months.

Acute myeloblastic leukemia in rare instances shows tumor formations referred to as myeloblastomas. Sometimes the tumors have a greenish color and then are called chloromas. The tumors occur most commonly in association with bones. However, they may occur in other locations, including the skin (Ross). The green pigment of chloromas is caused by presence of large amounts of myeloperoxidase in the myeloblasts (Ioachim et al.).

Erythroleukemia, or di Guglielmo's disease, initially is characterized by a proliferation of both myeloblasts and megaloblasts and terminates as typical myeloblastic leukemia. In the beginning the proliferation of immature erythrocytes may predominate and immature granulocytes are relatively inapparent (Scott et al.). The skin may show, in addition to purpuric lesions, papules, nodules, plaques and ulcers (Belisario et al.).

Myelomonocytic leukemia, or Naegeli type of leukemia, is the most common type of acute leukemia (Saarni and Linman). It may involve all marrow cells and thus may show an early erythroleukemic phase. Terminally, there are numerous blast cells, some displaying morphologic features of myeloblasts, and others of monoblasts. Acute monocytic leukemia, or Schilling type of leukemia, is very rare (Saarni and Linman).

Histopathology. The diagnosis of acute granulocytic leukemia is made more readily by microscopic examination of the bone marrow and the peripheral blood than by skin biopsy. The skin, however, shows the same type of immature cells as the bone marrow and the peripheral blood, and there may be areas of necrosis. In erythroleukemia, erythroid as well as myeloid cells are usually present, and a few nucleated red cells may be seen in the infiltrate (Belisario et al.).

MULTIPLE MYELOMA

Multiple myeloma, or plasmacytoma, represents a neoplastic proliferation of more or less atypical plasma cells within the bone marrow, leading to osteolytic lesions and pathologic fractures. Metastatic spread to various internal organs occurs occasionally. The plasma cells produce large amounts of a monoclonal immunoglobulin, usually IgG or IgA, and rarely IgD, which are found in the blood serum. In about 50 per cent of the cases Bence Jones proteins are present in the urine. They represent the light chains of the immunoglobulin molecule, usually κ or λ and rarely both, that are produced in excess of the heavy chains (Sell; Parra et al.).

The cutaneous manifestations of multiple myeloma can be divided into specific and nonspecific lesions. The nonspecific lesions may consist of amyloid deposits in the skin occurring, in association with visceral deposits, in primary systemic amyloidosis (see p. 388), or of cryoglobulinemic purpura (see p. 158), or of "diffuse normolipemic plane xanthoma" (see p. 378) (Moschella).

Specific involvement of the skin in multiple myeloma most commonly takes place by direct extension of an osseous plasmacytoma through the subcutaneous tissue to the skin. The skin then is firmly attached to the bone (Bluefarb). In patients with metastases to internal organs one may occasionally see also metastases to the skin. They may consist of many cutaneous nodules (Walzer and Shapiro; Wuepper and MacKenzie) or of only a few (River and Schorr). Also, subcutaneous masses may be present, either in

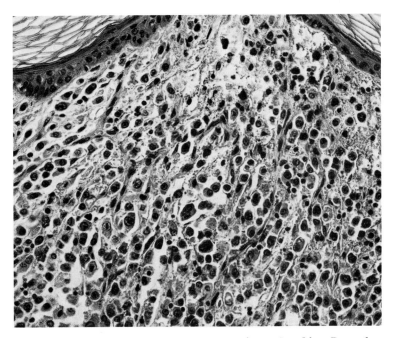

FIG. 33-15. **Multiple myeloma, metastasis to the skin**. Beneath a flattened epidermis there is a dense infiltrate of plasma cells, most of which appear atypical. ($\times$200) (Lewis Shapiro, M.D.)

association with cutaneous nodules (Levin et al.) or without them (Edwards and Zawadski). In rare instances cutaneous plasmacytomas precede the clinical, radiologic and laboratory evidence of systemic multiple myeloma by several months (Stankler and Davidson).

Histopathology. The specific cutaneous lesions of multiple myeloma show a dense infiltrate of plasma cells (Fig. 33-15). Most of the plasma cells appear atypical and show variation in the size, shape, and staining intensity of their nuclei as well as atypical mitotic figures. Also, multinucleated plasma cells are numerous (Walzer and Shapiro). Often the plasma cells because of their immaturity are difficult to identify as such. They may resemble reticulum cells and thus suggest the presence of lymphoma (River and Schorr; Wuepper and MacKenzie). However, methyl green pyronin stains the cytoplasm of the cells dark red (Wuepper and MacKenzie). Furthermore, direct immunofluorescent staining with fluorescein-conjugated antisera to the various immunoglobulins will cause fluorescence of the plasma cells with one of them (Wuepper and MacKenzie). In addition, PAS-positive Russell bodies may be present in the infiltrate.

PRIMARY PLASMACYTOMA OF THE SKIN

In this rare condition usually a solitary malignant plasmacytoma of the skin is present without evidence of involvement of the bone marrow. In most cases no increase in the immunoglobulins is found in the serum, and Bence Jones proteins are absent in the urine. Rarely, however, several plasmacytomas are present in the skin and occasionally also in the upper respiratory tract (Parra et al.). In one such case IgG was increased in the plasma and both kappa and lambda light chains were present in the urine as Bence Jones proteins. In some instances of primary cutaneous plasmacytoma metastases are found either in the regional lymph nodes (Mikhail et al.) or in the viscera (Johnson and Taylor). In addition, primary plasmacytoma of the skin may be the forerunner

of systemic multiple myeloma (Stankler and Davidson).

Histopathology. Primary cutaneous plasmacytomas shows, similar to the cutaneous metastases of multiple myeloma, atypical pleomorphic plasma cells. Occasional multinucleated plasma cells and atypical mitoses are present (LaPerriere et al.). The cells may resemble reticulum cells but methyl green pyronin stains their cytoplasm dark red (Mikhail et al.).

PSEUDOLYMPHOMA OF SPIEGLER-FENDT

Several benign dermatoses occasionally show on histologic examination features that make a distinction from lymphoma very difficult, if not impossible. Among these dermatoses are arthropod bites or stings (see p. 201), actinic reticuloid (see p. 195), lymphomatoid papulosis (see p. 164), and pseudolymphoma of Spiegler-Fendt.

Pseudolymphoma of Spiegler-Fendt, known also under a variety of other designations, such as Spiegler-Fendt sarcoid, lymphocytoma cutis, lymphadenosis benigna cutis (Bäfverstedt) and cutaneous lymphoid hyperplasia (Caro and Helwig), may show considerable clinical and histologic resemblance to lymphoma so that differentiation from lymphoma can be very difficult.

Pseudolymphoma of Spiegler-Fendt occurs in a localized and a disseminated form, according to Bäfverstedt. The localized form occurs as a solitary nodule or as a number of nodules limited to one region. The face is the most commonly affected site. The nodules are asymptomatic, firm, and either red or reddish brown in color. As a rule, the lesions heal spontaneously, although there may be recurrences (Caro and Helwig). The second form shows extensive, sometimes very large indurated swellings with no sites of predilection. The latter form, according to Bäfverstedt, although it may persist for many years, eventually subsides and only in rare instances undergoes malignant changes. In the view of many others, however, the disseminated form sooner or later proves to be lymphoma so that it seems best to classify the disseminated form as lymphoma from the beginning (Mach).

Development into a lymphoma does not occur in a true localized pseudolymphoma of Spiegler-Fendt. Cases in which the diagnosis later had to be changed to lymphoma probably were instances of lymphoma from the beginning that had been diagnosed erroneously as pseudolymphoma (Höfer; Pegum and Landells).

Histopathology. A heavy infiltrate is present in the dermis, usually separated from the epidermis by a zone of normal collagen. The infiltrate consists of two types of cells, namely, lymphocytes and histiocytes. The two types of cells lie either intermingled with one another or in a follicular arrangement. In the latter type of arrangement one sees as a rule lymphocytes surrounding islands of histiocytes, resulting in structures that resemble the follicles of lymph nodes (Fig. 33-16) (Caro and Helwig). In rare instances, however, lymphocytes are located centrally and surrounded by histiocytes (Loveman and Fliegelman). The lymphocytes and the histiocytes are differentiated easily. The lymphocytes have small, round, deep-staining nuclei that lie closely packed

because lymphocytes possess little cytoplasm. The histiocytes have large, irregularly shaped, pale nuclei lying in loose arrangement because these cells possess ample amounts of cytoplasm separating the nuclei from one another (Fig. 33-17). Not infrequently, nuclear dust can be seen in the follicular centers as a result of disintegration of nuclei (Caro and Helwig; Bernstein et al.). An admixture of plasma cells is present in most cases, and occasionally also a few eosinophils (Höfer). In some instances, a small number of cells with large atypical-appearing nuclei are present (Kawada et al.). The infiltrate may extend into the subcutaneous tissue. The demarcation of the infiltrate generally is quite sharp, just as in lymphoma; and, as in lymphoma, single rows of lymphocytes may be seen extending between and around intact collagen bundles at the periphery of the infiltrate.

Histogenesis. The nature of pseudolymphoma of Spiegler-Fendt is not known. Although it resembles a lymphoma in its histologic architecture, it is not a lymphoma because of its benign, self-limited course. Most authors regard

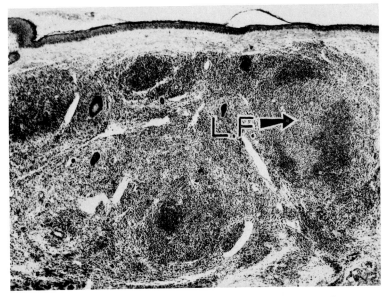

FIG. 33-16. **Pseudolymphoma of Spiegler-Fendt (lymphocytoma cutis).** Low magnification. The infiltrate is composed of two types of cells: lymphocytes, which lie in the dark-staining areas, and histiocytes, which lie in the light-staining areas. At the right (L.F.), the arrangement of the two types of cells resembles that encountered in a lymphoid follicle. (×50)

the lesion as a reactive hyperplasia of mature lymphoid-reticular cells (Bäfverstedt; Mopper and Rogin; Mach).

Differential Diagnosis. The diagnosis is easily established in those cases of pseudolymphoma of Spiegler-Fendt in which the lymphocytes and histiocytes show a follicular arrangement, since only the type of lymphoma with a nodular or follicular pattern must be excluded, which only rarely occurs in the skin (see p. 689). The nodular pattern in lymphoma results from the presence of atypical lymphoid cells in large lymphoid follicles (see p. 690). These cells are large and highly pleomorphic, in contrast to the cells in the follicles of Spiegler-Fendt pseudolymphoma. The presence of nuclear dust in the follicles of Spiegler-Fendt pseudolymphoma often is helpful in the differentiation from lymphoma (Caro and Helwig; Bernstein et al.).

If the two types of cells lie intermingled, the diagnosis of pseudolymphoma always should be made with a certain reservation, and only if all the histiocytes appear mature. The reason is that the mixed lymphocytic-histiocytic lymphoma also shows two types of cells that lie intermingled; but, in contrast with Spiegler-Fendt pseudolymphoma, the cells are immature and atypical (see p. 694). In cases of doubt, possibly deeper sections or another biopsy will show a follicular pattern. Also, the presence of plasma cells or eosinophils can be regarded as a factor in favor of pseudolymphoma of Spiegler-Fendt. Nevertheless, many authors share the view of Pomeranz who has stated that, in the absence of follicle formation, he never felt secure in the diagnosis of pseudolymphoma of Spiegler-Fendt, since he was always concerned that it may eventuate into a lymphoma.

In cases showing only a small number of cells with pale nuclei, the possibility should be considered that they are endothelial rather than histiocytic cells, both of which show large pale nuclei, and that the infiltrate thus is purely lymphocytic. This then rules out a diagnosis of pseudolymphoma of Spiegler-Fendt in favor of either a well differentiated lymphocytic lymphoma or lymphocytic infiltration of the skin (Jessner). (For differential diagnosis between these two diseases, see p. 691.)

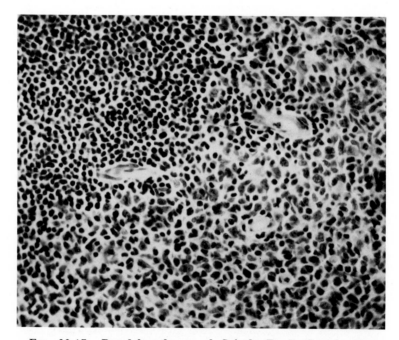

Fig. 33-17. **Pseudolymphoma of Spiegler-Fendt (lymphocytoma cutis).** High magnification of Figure 33-16. Lymphocytes lie in the left upper half of the illustration; histiocytes, in the right lower half. (×200)

BIBLIOGRAPHY

Hodgkin's Disease

Belpomme, D., Joseph R., Navares, L., *et al.*: T lymphocytes and Reed-Sternberg cells in spleen of Hodgkin's disease. New Eng. J. Med., *291*:1417, 1974.

Benninghoff, D. L., Medina, A., Alexander, L. L., and Camiel, M. R.: The mode of spread of Hodgkin's disease to the skin. Cancer, *26*: 1135, 1970.

Carbone, P. P.: Management of patients with non-Hodgkin's lymphoma. Arch. Int. Med., *131*:455, 1973.

Crum, E. D., Ng, A. B. P., Tsoa, L., and Kellermeyer, R. W.: Hodgkin's disease. Am. J. Clin. Path., *61*:403, 1974.

Cyr, D. P., Geokas, M. C., and Worsley, G. H.: Mycosis fungoides. Arch. Derm., *94*:558, 1966.

DeVita, V. T., Jr., Lymphocyte reactivity in Hodgkin's disease: a lymphocyte civil war. New Eng. J. Med., *289*:801, 1973.

Dupont, A.: Langsam verlaufende und klinisch gutartige Reticulopathie mit höchst maligner histologischer Struktur. Hautarzt, *16*:284, 1965.

Franssila, K. O., Kalima, T. V., and Voutilainen, A.: Histologic classification of Hodgkin's disease. Cancer, *20*:1594, 1967.

Freeman, C., Berg, J. W., and Cutler, S. J.: Occurrence and prognosis of extranodal lymphomas. Cancer, *29*:252, 1972.

Han, T., and Sokal, J. E.: Lymphocyte response to phytohemagglutinin in Hodgkin's disease. Am. J. Med., *48*:728, 1970.

Haustein, U. F., and Tausch, I.: Autochthone spezifische Hautinfiltrate bei Lymphogranulomatosis maligna (Paltauf-Sternberg). Derm. Mschr., *159*:739, 1973.

Jackson, H., and Parker, F.: Hodgkin's disease. II. Pathology. New Eng. J. Med., *231*:35, 1944.

Levy, R., and Kaplan, H. S.: Impaired lymphocyte function in untreated Hodgkin's disease. New Eng. J. Med., *290*:181, 1974.

Lukes, R. J., Butler, J. J., and Hicks, E. B.: Natural history of Hodgkin's disease as related to its pathologic picture. Cancer, *19*:317, 1966.

Macaulay, W. L.: Lymphomatoid papulosis. Arch. Derm., *97*:23, 1968.

Miller, D. G.: Immunological deficiency and malignant melanoma. Cancer, *20*:579, 1967.

Ongenae, D.: Aspects inhabituels de la maladie de Hodgkin et sa différenciation de la réticulopathie benigne. Arch. belg. derm., *27*:69, 1971.

Order, S. E., and Hellman, S.: Tumor-associated antigens. J.A.M.A., *223*:174, 1973.

Prosnitz, L. R., Nuland, S. B., and Kligerman, M. M.: Role of laparotomy and splenectomy in the management of Hodgkin's disease. Cancer, *29*:44, 1972.

Reimann, H. A., Havens, W. P., and Herbut, P. A.: Hodgkin's disease with specific lesions appearing first in the skin. Arch. Int. Med., *70*:434, 1942.

Rosenberg, S. A., and Kaplan, H. S.: Evidence for an orderly progression in the spread of Hodgkin's disease. Cancer Res., *26*:1225, 1966.

Rubin, P.: Updated Hodgkin's disease: A. Introduction. J.A.M.A., *222*:1292, 1972.

Schein, P. S., and Vickers, H. R.: Lupus vulgaris and Hodgkin's disease. Arch. Derm., *105*: 244, 1972.

Sell, S.: Immunological deficiency diseases. Arch. Path., *86*:95, 1968.

Senear, F. E., and Caro, M. R.: Ulcerative Hodgkin's disease of the skin. Arch. Derm. Syph., *35*:114, 1937.

Strum, S. B., Allen, L. W., and Rappaport, H.: Vascular invasion in Hodgkin's disease: its relationship to involvement of the spleen and other extranodal sites. Cancer, *28*:1329, 1971.

Strum, S. B., Park, J. K., and Rappaport, H.: Observation of cells resembling Sternberg-Reed cells in conditions other than Hodgkin's disease. Cancer, *26*:176, 1970.

Strum, S. B., and Rappaport, H.: Interrelations of the histologic types of Hodgkin's disease. Arch. Path., *91*:127, 1971.

Szur, L., Harrison, C. V., Levene, G. M., and Samman, P. D.: Primary cutaneous Hodgkin's disease. Lancet, *1*:1016, 1970.

Thomas, L. B.: Pathology of Hodgkin's disease. Ann. Int. Med., *67*:427, 1967.

Ultman, J. E., and Moran, E. M.: Clinical course and complications in Hodgkin's disease. Arch. Int. Med., *131*:332, 1973 (review).

Undeutsch, W., Fischer, H., and Hensel, U.: Erysipelas lymphogranulomatosum. Hautarzt, *20*:314, 1969.

Young, R. C., Corder, M. P., Haynes, H. A., and DeVita, V. T.: Delayed hypersensitivity in Hodgkin's disease. Am. J. Med., *52*:63, 1972.

Monomorphous Lymphomas

Aisenberg, A. C., and Bloch, K. J.: Immunoglobulins on the surface of neoplastic lymphocytes. New Eng. J. Med., *287*:272, 1972.

Berard, C. W.: Histopathology of lymphoreticular disorders. *In* Principles of Hematology. New York, McGraw-Hill, 1972.

Carbone, P. P.: Management of patients with non-Hodgkin's lymphoma. Arch. Int. Med., *131*:455, 1973.

Cohen, M. H., Bennett, J. M., Berard, C. W., *et al.*: Burkitt's tumor in the United States. Cancer, *23*:1259, 1969.

Desai, P. B., Meher-Homji, D. R., and Paymaster, J. C.: Malignant lymphoma. Cancer, *18*:25, 1965.

Freeman, C., Berg, J. W., and Cutler, S. J.: Occurrence and prognosis of extranodal lymphomas. Cancer, *29*:252, 1972.

Gall, E. A., and Mallory, T. B.: Malignant lymphoma. Am. J. Path., *18*:381, 1942 (classification).

Gall, E. A., and Rappaport, H.: Seminar on diseases of lymph nodes and spleen. *In* McDonald, J. R. (ed.): Proceedings of the 23rd Seminar of the American Society of Clinical Pathology. p. 1. Chicago, American Society of Clinical Pathology, 1958.

Hanks, G. E., Terry, L. K., Jr., Bryan, J. A., and Newsome, J. F.: Contribution of diagnostic laparotomy to staging non-Hodgkin's lymphoma. Cancer, *29*:41, 1972.

Hurst, D. W., and Meyer, O. O.: Giant follicular lymphoblastoma. Cancer, *14*:753, 1961.

Jaffe, E. S., Shevach, E. M., Frank, M. M., *et al.*: Nodular lymphoma—evidence for origin from follicular B lymphocytes. New Eng. J. Med., *290*:813, 1974.

Jones, S. E., Rosenberg, S. A., and Kaplan, H. S.: Non-Hodgkin's lymphoma. I. Bone marrow involvement. Cancer, *29*:954, 1972.

Kalkoff, K. W.: Über eine primäre isolierte Reticulumzellensarkomatose der Haut. Z. Haut Geschlechtskr., *14*:3, 1953.

Kim, R., Winkelmann, R. K., and Dockerty, M.: Reticulum cell sarcoma of the skin. Cancer, *16*:646, 1963.

Kwittken, J., and Goldberg, A. F.: Follicular lymphoma of the skin. Arch. Derm., *93*:177, 1966.

Levine, P. H., Sandler, S. G., Komp, D. M., *et al.*: Simultaneous occurrence of "American Burkitt's lymphoma" in neighbors. New Eng. J. Med., *288*:562, 1973.

Lukes, R. J., and Collins, R. D.: Immunologic characterization of human malignant lymphomas. Cancer, *34*:1488, 1974 (Review).

Miller, D. G.: Immunological deficiency and malignant lymphoma. Cancer, *20*:579, 1967.

Nicolis, G. D., and Helwig, E. B.: Exfoliative dermatitis. Arch. Derm., *108*:788, 1973.

N.I.H. Clinical Staff Conference: Burkitt's tumor. Ann. Int. Med., *70*:817, 1969.

Nitzschner, H.: Zur Kasuistik der Brill-Symmers' schen Krankheit. Z. Haut, *43*:791, 1968.

Pagano, J. S., Huang, C. H., and Levine, P.: Absence of Epstein-Barr viral DNA in American Burkitt's lymphoma. New Eng. J. Med., *289*:1395, 1973.

Peters, M. V., Hasselback, R., and Brown, T. C.: The natural history of the lymphomas related to the clinical classification. *In* Zarafonetis, C. J. D. (ed.): Proceedings of the International Conference on Leukemia-Lymphoma. p. 357. Philadelphia, Lea and Febiger, 1968.

Petrozzi, J. W., Raque, C. J., and Goldschmidt, H.: Malignant lymphoma, reticulum cell type. Ultrastructural and cytologic demonstration of Lutzner cells. Arch. Derm., *104*:38, 1971.

Polano, M. K.: Über Hauterscheinungen beim Morbus Brill-Symmers. Hautarzt, *8*:136, 1957.

Rappaport, H., Winter, W. J., and Hicks, E. B.: Follicular lymphoma. Cancer, *9*:792, 1956.

Reilly, C. J., Han, T., Stutzman, L. *et al.*: Reticulum cell sarcoma. Cancer, *29*:1314, 1972.

Rosenberg, S. A., Diamond, H. D., Jaslowitz, B., and Craver, L. F.: Lymphosarcoma: a review of 1269 cases. Medicine, *40*:31, 1961.

Rubin, P.: Comment: The non-Hodgkin's lymphomas. J.A.M.A., *223*:175, 1973.

Seligmann, M.: B-cell and T-cell markers in lymphoid proliferations. New Eng. J. Med., *290*:1483, 1974.

Sonck, C. E.: Primäre Reticulumzellsarkomatose der Haut. Acta dermatoven., *37*:129, 1957.

Steigleder, G. K., and Hunscha, H. G.: Die Retikulosarkomatosen der Haut. Arch. klin. exp. Derm., *205*:435, 1958.

Stein, H., Lennert, K., and Parwaresch, M. R.: Malignant lymphomas of B cell type. Lancet, *2*:855, 1972.

Thorson, T. A., and Brown, D. V.: A study of lymphomas. Arch. Path., *60*:353, 1955.

Torres, A.: Primary lymphocytic follicular lymphoma of liver. Cancer, *23*:1185, 1969.

Trubowitz, S., and Sims, C. F.: Subcutaneous fat in leukemia and lymphoma. Arch. Derm., *86*:520, 1962.

Wenzel, M., and Rastetter, J.: Subakute Hautreticulose mit Übergang in Leukämie. Hautarzt, *18*:42, 1967.

Wright, C. J. E.: Macrofollicular lymphoma. Am. J. Path., *32*:201, 1956.

Mycosis Fungoides and Sézary's Syndrome

Ackerman, A. B., Breza, T. S., and Capland, L.: Spongiotic simulants of mycosis fungoides. Arch. Derm., *109*:218, 1974.

Ackerman, A. B., and Flaxman, B. A.: Granulomatous mycosis fungoides. Brit. J. Derm., *82*:397, 1970.

Block, J. B., Edgcomb, J., Eisen, A., and Van Scott, E. J.: Mycosis fungoides. Natural history and aspects of its relationship to other malignant lymphomas. Am. J. Med., *34*:228, 1963.

Braun-Falco, O., Marghescu, S., and Wolff, H. H.: Pagetoide Reticulose. Morbus Woringer-Kolopp. Hautarzt, *24*:11, 1973.

Brouet, J. C., Flandrin, G., and Seligman, M.: Indications of the thymus-derived nature of the proliferating cells in six patients with Sézary's syndrome. New Eng. J. Med., *289*: 341, 1973.

Brownlee, T. R., and Murad, T. M.: Ultrastructure of mycosis fungoides. Cancer, *26*:686, 1970.

Burg, G., and Braun-Falco, O.: Qualitative und quantitative Aspekte der cellulären Reaktion in Haut und Blut bei Mycosis fungoides. Hautarzt, *25*:178, 1974.

Cawley, E. P., Curtis, A. C., and Leach, J. E. K.: Is mycosis fungoides a reticulo-endothelial neoplastic entity? Arch. Derm., *64*:255, 1951.

Clendenning, W. E., Brecker, G., and Van Scott, E. J.: Mycosis fungoides. Arch. Derm., *89*: 785, 1964.

Crossen, P. E., Mellor, J. E. L., Finley, A. G., *et al.*: The Sézary syndrome. Am. J. Med., *50*:24, 1971.

Cyr, D. P., Geokas, M. C., and Worsley, G. H.: Mycosis fungoides. Arch. Derm., *94*:558, 1966.

Degos, R., Civatte, J., Touraine, R., *et al.*: Confrontation anatomo-clinique de 129 hémoréticulopathies malignes cutanées. Ann. derm. syph., *92*:121, 1965.

Ebner, H., Kühböck, J., and Pietschmann, H.: Das Sézary Syndrom. Dermatologica, *141*: 257, 1970.

Edelson, R. L., Kirkpatrick, C. H., Shevach, E. M., *et al.*: Preferential cutaneous infiltration by neoplastic thymus-derived lymphocytes. Ann. Int. Med., *80*:685, 1974.

Emmerson, R. W.: Follicular mucinosis. Brit. J. Derm., *81*:395, 1969.

Epstein, E. H., Levin, D. L., Croft, J. O., Jr., and Lutzner, M.: Mycosis fungoides. Medicine, *51*:61, 1972.

Flaxman, B. A., Zelazny, G., and Van Scott, E. J.: Nonspecificity of characteristic cells in mycosis fungoides. Arch. Derm., *104*:141, 1971.

Fleischmajer, R., and Eisenberg, S.: Sézary's reticulosis. Arch. Derm., *89*:9, 1964.

Fraser, J. F.: Mycosis fungoides. Arch. Derm. Syph., *12*:814, 1925.

Fuks, Z. Y., Bagshaw, M. A., and Farber, E. M.: Prognostic signs and the management of mycosis fungoides. Cancer, *32*:1385, 1973.

Gisinger, O.: Zur Differentialdiagnose der von Woringer und Kolopp beschriebenen Retikulose. Dermatologica, *140*(suppl. 2):19, 1970.

Grosshans, E., Hee, P., Basset, A., and Maleville, J.: La maladie de Woringer et Kolopp. Arch. belges derm., *29*:195, 1973.

Janis, J. F., and Winkelmann, R. K.: Histopathology of the skin in dermatomyositis. Arch. Derm., *97*:640, 1968.

Kim, R., Winkelmann, R. K., and Dockerty, M.: Reticulum cell sarcoma of the skin. Cancer, *16*:646, 1963.

Lapière, S.: The realm and frontiers of mycosis fungoides. J. Invest. Derm., *42*:101, 1964.

Long, J. C., and Mihm, M. C., Jr.: Mycosis fungoides with extracutaneous dissemination: A distinct clinicopathologic entity. Cancer, *34*:1745, 1974.

Lutzner, M. A., Hobbs, J. W., and Horvath, P.: Ultrastructure of abnormal cells in Sézary syndrome, mycosis fungoides, and parapsoriasis en plaques. Arch. Derm., *103*:375, 1971.

Lutzner, M. A., and Jordan, H. W.: The ultrastructure of an abnormal cell in Sézary's syndrome. Blood, *31*:719, 1968.

Main, R. A., Goodall, H. B., and Swanson, W. C.: Sézary's syndrome. Brit. J. Derm., *71*:335, 1959.

Miedzinski, F., and Golebiowska, I.: Über Mycosis fungoides im Licht ihres klinischen Verlaufs. Dermatologica, *112*:119, 1956.

Paradinas, F. J., and Harrison, K. M.: Visceral lesions in an unusual case of Sézary's syndrome. Cancer, *33*:1068, 1974.

Petrozzi, J. W., Raque, C. J., and Goldschmidt, H.: Malignant lymphoma, reticulum cell type. Ultrastructural and cytologic demonstration of Lutzner cells. Arch. Derm., *104*:38, 1971.

Poulsen, A.: On mycosis fungoides. Acta dermatoven., *21*:365, 1940.

Rappaport, H., and Thomas, L. B.: Mycosis fungoides. The pathology of extracutaneous involvement. Cancer, *34*:1198, 1974.

Reed, R. J., and Cummings, C. E.: Malignant reticulosis and related conditions of the skin. Cancer, *19*:1231, 1966.

Rosas-Uribe, A., Variakojis, D., Molnar, Z., and Rappaport, H.: Mycosis fungoides: an ultrastructural study. Cancer, *34*:634, 1974.

Ryan, E. A., Sanderson, K. V., Bartak, P., and Samman, P. D.: Can mycosis fungoides begin in the epidermis? A hypothesis. Brit. J. Derm., *88*:419, 1973.

Sézary, A.: Une nouvelle réticulose cutanée. Ann. derm. syph., VIII, 9:5, 1949.

Sézary, A., and Bouvrain, Y.: Erythrodermie avec présence de cellules monstreuses dans derme et sang circulant. Bull. Soc. Franç. derm. syph., *45*:254, 1938.

Smoes-Charles, J., and Dupont, A.: A propos d'une forme particulière generalisée de réticulose épidermotrope. Arch. belges derm., *29*: 205, 1973.

Symmers, D.: Mycosis fungoides as a clinical and pathologic nonexistent. Arch. Derm. Syph., *25*:1, 1932.

Taswell, H. F., and Winkelmann, R. K.: Sézary syndrome, a malignant reticulemic erythroderma. J.A.M.A., *177*:465, 1961.

Tedeschi, L. G., and Lansinger, D. T.: Sézary syndrome. Arch. Derm., *92*:257, 1965.

Van Scott, E. J., and Kalmanson, J. D.: Complete remissions of mycosis fungoides lymphoma induced by topical nitrogen mustard. Cancer *32*:18, 1973.

Variakojis, D., Rosas-Uribe, A., and Rappaport, H.: Mycosis fungoides: Pathologic findings in staging laparotomies. Cancer, *33*:1589, 1974.

Vesper, L. J., Winkelmann, R. K., and Hargraves, M. M.: The mycosis fungoides cell: the skin window in mycosis fungoides. Brit. J. Derm., *84*:54, 1971.

Waddington, E.: Die Beziehungen zwischen der Poikilodermia atrophicans vascularis und der Mycosis fungoides. Hautarzt, *4*:282, 1953.

Wilson, H. T. H.: Exfoliative dermatitis. Arch. Derm. Syph., *69*:577, 1954.

Winkelmann, R. K.: T cell erythroderma (Sézary syndrome). Arch. Derm., *108*:205, 1973.

Winkelmann, R. K., and Linman, J. W.: Erythroderma with atypical lymphocytes. Am. J. Med., *55*:192, 1973.

Malignant Histiocytosis

Abele, D. C., and Griffin, T. B.: Histiocytic medullary reticulosis. Arch. Derm., *106*:319, 1972.

Engstrom, P. F., Aeling, J. L., and Suringa, D. W. R.: Histiocytic medullary reticulosis with cutaneous lesions. Arch. Derm., *106*:369, 1972.

Henderson, D. W., and Sage, R. E.: Malignant histiocytosis with eosinophilia. Cancer, *32*: 1421, 1973.

Liao, K. T., Rosai, J., and Daneshbod, K.: Malignant histiocytosis with cutaneous involvement and eosinophilia. Am. J. Clin. Path., *57*:438, 1972.

Leukemia

Belisario, J. C., McGovern, V. J., and Dawson, I. E.: Erythraemic myelosis (di Guglielmo's disease). Austral. J. Derm., *4*:191, 1958.

Bennett, J. M.: Myelomonocytic leukemias: a historical review and perspectives. Cancer, *27*:1218, 1971.

Boggs, D. P., Wintrobe, M. M., and Cartwright, G. E.: The acute leukemias: analysis of 322 cases and review of the literature. Medicine, *41*:163, 1962.

Carmel, W. J., Minno, A. M., and Cook, W. L.: Eosinophilic leukemia with report of a case. Arch. Intern. Med., *87*:280, 1951.

Conrad, M. E., Rappaport, H., and Crosby, W. H.: Chronic granulocytic leukemia in the aged. Arch. Intern. Med., *116*:765, 1965.

Costello, M. J., Canizares, O., Montague, M., and Bunche, C. M.: Cutaneous manifestations of myelogenous leukemia. Arch. Derm., *71*: 605, 1955.

Deme, I.: Eosinophile Leukämie mit Hautsymptomen. Dermatologica, *98*:150, 1949.

Garfinkel, L. S., and Bennett, D. E.: Extramedullary myeloblastic transformation in chronic myelocytic leukemia simulating a coexistent malignant lymphoma. Am. J. Clin. Path., *51*:638, 1969.

Ioachim, H. L., Keller, S., Sabbath, M., *et al.*: Myeloperoxidase and crystalline bodies in the granules of DMBA-induced rat chloroma cells. Am. J. Path., *66*:147, 1972.

Reardon, G., and Moloney, W. C.: Chloroma and related myeloblastic tumors. Arch. Intern. Med., *108*:864, 1961.

Ross, R. R.: Chloroma and chloroleukemia. Am. J. Med., *18*:671, 1955.

Saarni, M. I., and Linman, J. W.: Myelomonocytic leukemia: disorderly proliferation of all marrow cells. Cancer, *27*:1221, 1971.

Scott, R. B., Ellison, R. R., and Ley, A. B.: A clinical study of twenty cases of erythroleukemia (di Guglielmo's syndrome). Am. J. Med., *37*:162, 1964.

Multiple Myeloma and Primary Plasmacytoma of the Skin

Bluefarb, S. M.: Cutaneous manifestations of multiple myeloma. Arch. Derm., *72*:506, 1955 (review).

Edwards, G. A., and Zawadski, Z. A.: Extraosseous lesions in plasma cell myeloma. Am. J. Med., *43*:194, 1967.

Johnson, W. H., Jr., and Taylor, B. G.: Solitary extramedullary plasmacytoma of the skin. Cancer, *26*:65, 1970.

LaPerriere, R. J., Wolf, J. E., and Gellin, G. A.: Primary cutaneous plasmacytoma. Arch. Derm., *107*:99, 1973.

Levin, H. A., Freeman, R. G., Smith, F. E., and Lane, M.: Multiple extramedullary plasmacytomas. Arch. Derm., *96*:456, 1967.

Mikhail, G. R., Spindler, A. C., and Kelly, A. P.: Malignant plasmacytoma cutis. Arch. Derm., *101*:59, 1970.

Moschella, S. L.: Plane xanthomatosis associated with myelomatosis. Arch. Derm., *101*: 683, 1970.

Parra, C. A., Rivero, I., and Moncunill, A. L. M.: Mucocutaneous gamma G polyclonical plasmacytoma with two Bence Jones proteins BJK and BJL). Arch. Derm. Forsch., *242*: 353, 1972.

River, G. L., and Schorr, W. F.: Malignant skin tumors in multiple myeloma. Arch. Derm., *93*:432, 1966.

Sell, S.: Immunological deficiency diseases. Arch. Path., *86*:95, 1968.

Stankler, L., and Davidson, J. F.: Multiple extramedullary plasmacytomas of the skin. Brit. J. Derm., *90*:217, 1974.

Walzer, R. A., and Shapiro, L.: Multiple myeloma with cutaneous metastases. Dermatologica, *134*:449, 1967.

Wuepper, K. D., and MacKenzie, M. R.: Cutaneous extramedullary plasmacytomas. Arch. Derm., *100*:155, 1969.

Pseudolymphoma of Spiegler-Fendt

Bäfverstedt, B.: Lymphadenosis benigna cutis. Acta dermatoven., *48*:1, 1968.

Bernstein, H., Shupack, J., and Ackerman, A. B.: Cutaneous pseudolymphoma resulting from antigen injections. Arch. Derm., *110*:756, 1974.

Caro, W. A., and Helwig, E. B.: Cutaneous lymphoid hyperplasia. Cancer, *24*:487, 1969.

Höfer, W.: Lymphadenosis benigna cutis. Arch. klin. exp. Derm., *203*:23, 1956.

Kawada, A., Mori, S., and Hayashi, T.: Lymphadenosis benigna cutis: pseudomalignant form and its imprint smear cytology. Dermatologica, *141*:339, 1970.

Loveman, A. B., and Fliegelman, M. T.: Lymphocytoma cutis. Arch. Derm., *63*:169, 1951.

Mach, K.: Ist die Lymphadenosis benigna cutis (Bäfverstedt) eine klinisch-pathologische Einheit? Derm. Wschr., *151*:1351, 1965.

Mopper, C., and Rogin, J. R.: Benign solitary lymphocytoma. Arch. Derm., *63*:184, 1951.

Pegum, J. S., and Landells, J. W.: Lymphosarcoma supervening on lymphocytoma. Trans. St. John's Hosp. Derm. Soc., *56*:149, 1970.

Pomeranz, J.: In discussion of: Roenigk, H. H., Jr., and Lesbowitz, S. A.: Lymphocytoma cutis. Arch. Derm., *101*:248, 1970.

Glossary

The measurements in size are expressed in:

centimeters (cm)

millimeters (mm; 1,000 mm = 1 m)

micrometers (μm; 1,000 μm = 1 mm)

nanometers (nm; 1,000 nm = 1 μm)

The term Angstrom (10 A = 1 nm) has been avoided.

Acantholysis: Loss of coherence between epidermal or epithelial cells due to degeneration of the intercellular cement substance or of the intercellular bridges. It leads to the formation of bullae, vesicles, and lacunae within the epidermis or epithelium. Occurs in pemphigus, Darier's disease, benign familial pemphigus, warty dyskeratoma, viral bullae, solar keratosis, and pseudoglandular squamous cell carcinoma.

Acanthosis: Increase in thickness of the stratum malpighii.

Anaplasia: Atypical appearance of the nuclei found in malignant neoplasia. Anaplastic nuclei usually are large, irregularly shaped and hyperchromatic. Atypical mitotic figures may be present in such nuclei.

Argentaffin: Ability to reduce silver salts to metallic silver. Melanin possesses phenolic groups capable of reducing the silver salts that are present in ammoniated silver nitrate to free black silver. (The Masson-Fontana stain contains ammoniated silver nitrate.) (See p. 17.)

Argyrophilic: Substances, like melanin, nerves and reticulum fibers, that can be impregnated with silver nitrate solutions and, by reducing the silver nitrate with hydroquinone to metallic silver, stain black. (See p. 17.)

Ballooning degeneration of epidermis: A type of degeneration of epidermal cells causing marked swelling of the cells with loss of the intercellular bridges. Acantholysis results, and a bulla forms. Ballooning degeneration occurs in viral vesicles and is diagnostic of them. See also under Reticular Degeneration.

Basal lamina: A homogeneous band composed of filaments extending along the undersurface of the epidermal basal cells. Measuring only 35 to 45 nm in thickness it is a submicroscopic structure, visible only by electron microscopy. (See p. 14.)

Basement membrane zone: Visible by light microscopy with the PAS reaction. Located beneath the basal cell layer it measures between 0.5 and 1.0 μm in thickness and thus is, on the average, 20 times thicker than the basal lamina. The basement membrane zone is not homogeneous, since it consists not only of the basal lamina but also of anchoring fibrils and reticulum fibers. (See p. 11.)

Bulla: A cavity forming either within or beneath the epidermis and filled with tissue fluid, blood plasma, and often also with inflammatory cells. A bulla smaller than 5 mm in diameter generally is called a vesicle; and a small, slit-like, intraepidermal bulla, as seen in Darier's disease and solar keratosis, is referred to as lacuna.

Caseation necrosis: Originally described as a type of tissue death characteristic of tuberculosis, syphilis and some other infections, it is now regarded as identical with coagulation necrosis and ischemic necrosis, and thus is the prototype of tissue necrosis. The affected tissue has lost its structural outline and consists of pale eosinophilic, amorphous, finely granular material. Unless the necrosis is far advanced, some shrunken (pyknotic) nuclei or fragments of nuclei (nuclear dust) still are present.

Colliquative necrosis: Necrosis associated with the formation of pus (invasion of neutrophils).

Colloid: Homogeneous eosinophilic material of variable composition. The colloid in colloid milium is produced by fibroblasts. For colloid in colloid bodies, see below.

Colloid bodies: Also referred to as hyaline bodies or Civatte bodies. They are round to ovoid, have an eosinophilic, homogeneous appearance and measure approximately 10 μm in diameter. Seen in the lower epidermis or upper dermis. Although not specific for any disease, they occur most commonly in lichen planus and lupus erythematosus. Usually they form through degeneration of epidermal cells, although in lupus erythematosus they originate also from the thickened basement membrane zone. (See p. 425.)

Crust: Coagulated tissue fluid and blood plasma intermingled with degenerated inflammatory and epithelial cells.

Degeneration, ballooning, of epidermis: See under Ballooning.

Degeneration, fibrinoid, of connective tissue: See under Fibrinoid.

Degeneration, granular, of epidermis: See under Granular.

Degeneration, hydropic, of basal cell layer: See under Hydropic.

Degeneration, liquefaction, of basal cell layer: See under Hydropic.

Degeneration, reticular, of epidermis: See under Reticular.

Dyskeratosis: Faulty and premature keratinization of individual keratinocytes. Two types of dyskeratosis are recognized, one occurring in certain acantholytic diseases and the other in certain epidermal neoplasias. *Acantholytic dyskeratosis* occurs as corps ronds which consist of a central, homogeneous, basophilic mass surrounded by a clear halo. They are seen in Darier's disease, in warty dyskeratoma, and rarely in familial benign pemphigus. *Neoplastic dyskeratosis*, often referred to as individual cell keratinization, manifests itself as homogeneous, eosinophilic bodies, about 10 μm in diameter, occasionally still showing remnants of their nucleus. They may be seen in Bowen's disease, in solar keratosis and in squamous cell carcinoma, especially its pseudoglandular variant, but also in keratoacanthoma and in pilar tumor of the scalp. The occurrence of neoplastic dyskeratosis in the latter two conditions indicates that it is not necessarily an indication of malignancy.

Epidermolytic hyperkeratosis: See under Granular degeneration.

Erosion: Area in which the epidermis is absent, but the dermis is intact so that, in contrast with an ulcer, healing takes place without scarring.

Exocytosis: Penetration of inflammatory cells into the overlying epidermis.

Fibrinoid degeneration of connective tissue: Permeation of collagen with fibrin giving the involved area a brightly eosinophilic, homogeneous appearance. Often, there are additional degenerative changes. For instance, in allergic vasculitis the fibrin deposits within and around the vascular walls are associated with vascular damage and often with extravasation of erythrocytes (see p. 162). In rheumatoid nodules, the area of fibrinoid permeation of the collagen appears anuclear (see p. 222). In lupus erythematosus the fibrinoid deposits in the subepidermal region, around vessels, and on the surface and within collagen bundles causes these areas to appear homogeneous and thickened (see p. 428).

Granular degeneration of epidermis: Also referred to as epidermolytic hyperkeratosis. One observes in the middle and upper stratum malpighii: (a) intracellular edema; (b) indistinct cellular boundaries; (c) excessive and premature formation of large, irregular keratohyaline granules; and (d) hyperkeratosis. Occurs regularly in dominant congenital ichthyosiform erythroderma (see p. 60) and occasionally in dominant keratosis palmaris et plantaris (see p. 63), and in systematized nevus verrucosus (see p. 452).

Granulation tissue: Newly formed edematous collagenous tissue arising in healing wounds and ulcers and in chronic inflammatory processes. It shows numerous fibroblasts, newly formed capillaries and a rather dense cellular infiltrate consisting of lymphoid cells, macrophages, and plasma cells.

Granuloma: A chronic proliferative lesion containing, besides mononuclear cells, either epithelioid cells, or multinucleated giant cells, or both. Granulomas arise either as a foreign body reaction or as an allergic granuloma. *Foreign body granulomas* can form as a response either to substances introduced into the skin from the outside, such as various oils, silicon, silica, or starch powder, or to substances formed endogenously, such as urates and keratin (see p. 202). Foreign body granulomas usually show macrophages and multinucleated giant cells but no epithelioid cells. *Allergic granulomas* arise in individuals in whom previously a delayed type of hypersensitivity has developed to the foreign body material or the type of microorganism that is being phagocytized. Among the foreign substances producing allergic granulomas are zirconium, beryllium, and various dyes used for tattoos (see p. 202); and among the microorganisms are *Mycobacterium tuberculosis, M. leprae, Treponema pallidum,* and the various fungi causing "deep" fungus infections. In addition, there are idiopathic allergic granulomas, such as those seen in sarcoidosis and allergic granulomatosis. Allergic granulomas are characterized by the presence of epithelioid cells; they often contain also multinucleated giant cells. The multinucleated giant cells in allergic granulomas, often referred to as Langhans giant cells, usually but not always are smaller than the giant cells in foreign body granulomas and often show a peripheral arrangement of their nuclei in a horseshoe pattern, rather than an irregular arrangement.

Histiocyte: See under Macrophage.

Hyalin: Homogeneous eosinophilic material of variable composition. Occasionally used as a synonym for colloid, as in hyaline or colloid bodies (see under Colloid bodies). So-called hyalin is present in the lesions of hyalinosis cutis et mucosae (see p. 394), as well as in the lesions of porphyria (see p. 397), and those of cylindroma (see p. 525). The hyalin in all three conditions is PAS-positive and diastase-resistant, and consists partly of collagenous material produced by fibroblasts and partly of amorphous material analogous to the basal lamina material present around capillaries and epithelium.

Hydropic degeneration of basal cells: A type of degeneration causing vacuolization of the basal cells. It is referred to also as liquefaction degeneration. It occurs in lupus erythematosus, dermatomyositis, poikiloderma atrophicans vasculare, erythema dyschromicum perstans, and lichen sclerosus et atrophicus. It may be seen also in early lesions of lichen planus; but in lichen planus it usually progresses to disappearance of the basal cell layer. Hydropic degeneration of the basal cells may cause incontinence of pigment (see below). In lupus erythematosus, lichen sclerosus et atrophicus, and lichen planus the damage to the basal cells may be severe enough to cause formation of subepidermal bullae (see Classification of Bullae at beginning of Chapter 7, p. 96).

Incontinence of pigment: Loss of melanin from the cells of the basal layer due to damage to these cells, with accumulation of the melanin in the upper dermis within melanophages. It occurs particularly in incontinentia pigmenti, lichen planus, lupus erythematosus, poikiloderma atrophicans vasculare, erythema dyschromicum perstans, and fixed drug eruption.

Intercellular edema of epidermis: See under Spongiosis.

Intracellular edema of epidermis: See under Reticular degeneration of epidermis.

Karyorrhexis: Fragmentation of nuclei resulting in nuclear dust.

Keratinocyte: Designation for all epidermal cells with the exception of the dendritic cells (i.e., melanocytes and Langerhans cells). Their potential is to form keratin.

Keratohyalin: Deeply basophilic, irregularly shaped granules present in the cells of the granular layer of the epidermis. Keratohyalin forms the interfibrillary substance that cements the keratin fibrils, or tonofibrils, together, resulting in the "soft" keratin of the horny cells of the surface epidermis. The "hard" keratin of the hair and nails is formed without the interposition of keratohyalin between the keratin fibrils.

Lacuna: See under Bulla.

Langerhans cell: A dendritic cell present in the upper layers of the stratum malpighii. Seen in routinely prepared light microscopic sections as "high level clear cell." (See p. 20.)

Langhans giant cell: See under Granuloma.

Leukocytoclasis: Disintegration of leukocytes, occurring especially in allergic vasculitis, and resulting in nuclear dust.

Liquefaction degeneration of basal cells: See under Hydropic degeneration of basal cells.

Lymphoid cells: Cells having the histologic appearance of lymphocytes. The term is being used in place of the term lymphocyte, since in routinely processed and stained histologic sections lymphocytes and monocytes are indistinguishable, with both cells showing a small, round, deeply basophilic nucleus and hardly any cytoplasm. For details about monocytes see under Macrophage.

Lysosome: Primary lysosomes are small membrane-bound organelles containing a variety of hydrolytic enzymes. Because of their small size primary lysosomes can be seen only by electron microscopy. Their content of enzymes, however, can be demonstrated in the light microscope by histochemical staining, e.g., for acid phosphatase, aryl sulfatase, beta galactosidase, or peroxidase. The lysosomal enzymes are capable of digesting a variety of endogenous or exogenous material. For the purpose of digesting, the material to be digested is engulfed by a membrane-bound phagosome. Primary lysosomes then discharge their enzymes into such phagosomes which thus become phagolysosomes. Phagolysosomes containing endogenous material are referred to as autophagolysosomes. Phagolysosomes containing exogenous material that the cell has phagocytized by means of endocytosis are called heterophagolysosomes. After completion of the digestion the phagolysosomes are present as residual bodies, referred to also as myelin bodies because of their resemblance to myelin and their contents of phospholipids. (See also pp. 51 and 55.)

Macrophage: The precursors of macrophages are present in the bone marrow and the circulating blood as monocytes. Monocytes that accumulate in the dermis after leaving the blood stream are indistinguishable from lymphocytes in routinely processed and stained histologic sections (see Lymphoid cells). They can be distinguished from lymphocytes histochemically by their contents of lysosomal enzymes (see Lysosomes). As monocytes change into actively phagocytizing macrophages, referred to also as histiocytes, their light microscopic appearance changes: The nucleus, instead of being small, round and deeply basophilic as in a lymphocyte, becomes larger, elongated and lightly staining with a clearly visible nuclear membrane. The nucleus of a macrophage or histiocyte thus is indistinguishable from that of a fibroblast or an endothelial cell. After completion of their phagocytosis macrophages may fuse into multinucleated giant cells (see p. 54). Epithelioid cells form from macrophages usually in foreign-body reactions and infections that have provoked a delayed hypersensitivity reaction. Epithelioid cells also may fuse into multinucleated giant cells (see Granuloma).

Melanocyte: A dendritic cell normally present in the basal cell layer of the epidermis and of the hair matrix. Seen in routinely prepared light microscopic sections as "basal layer clear cell." Melanocytes possess the ability to form melanin through the enzymatic oxidation of tyrosine (see p. 18).

Melanophage: A phagocytizing macrophage, or histiocyte, that has ingested melanin granules, or melanosomes.

Metachromasia: The phenomenon of reacting with a different color from that of the dye used for the staining. Metachromasia can be observed in the presence of acid mucopolysaccharides or of amyloid. Acid mucopolysaccharides stain purple with methylene blue or toluidine blue and cause the metachromasia (a) in the granules of mast cells (see p. 84, Urticaria Pigmentosa), (b) in dermal mucin (see below under Mucin, and p. 404, Myxedema), and (c) occasionally in the fibrinoid material of fibrinoid degeneration (see p. 429, Systemic Lupus Erythematosus). Amyloid stains purple with crystal violet or methyl violet (see p. 386). The exact nature of the substance responsible for the metachromasia of amyloid is not known. The same metachromasia occurs occasionally also in colloid milium (see p. 393), and in hyalinosis cutis et mucosae (see p. 394).

Metaplasia: Change of one type of tissue into another, as it occurs, for instance, in the formation of bone in pilomatrixoma and in scars (see p. 629).

Microabscesses: Small accumulations of cells in the epidermis or the subepidermal papillae. Three types of microabscesses occur: The Munro microabscess composed of disintegrated neutrophils in the parakeratotic horny layer in psoriasis (see p. 138); the Pautrier microabscess composed of mononuclear cells and mycosis cells in the stratum malpighii in mycosis fungoides (see p. 698); and the papillary microabscesses composed predominantly of neutrophils in dermatitis herpetiformis (see p. 119) and of eosinophils in the inflammatory lesions of bullous pemphigoid (see p. 116).

Mucin: There are two types of mucin: dermal and epithelial. *Dermal mucin* forms the ground substance and consists of acid mucopolysaccharides, largely hyaluronic acid. It (1) is PAS-negative; (2) stains with alcian blue at pH 2.5 but not at pH 0.4; (3) stains metachromatically with methylene blue and toluidine blue; and (4) is hyaluronidase-labile. (See p. 33.) *Epithelial mucin*, referred to as sialomucin, contains neutral and often also acid mucopolysaccharides. It is present in the skin: (a) in the granules of the dark, mucoid secretory cells of eccrine glands (see p. 23); (b) in some of the granules of apocrine secretory cells (see p. 25); (c) in the cells of oral mucous cysts (see p. 587); (d) in the cells of perianal Paget's disease with a subjacent adenocarcinoma of the rectum (see p. 490); and (e) in the cells of cutaneous metastases of gastrointestinal carcinoma. Epithelial mucin (1) is PAS-positive and diastase-resistant; (2) may stain with alcian blue at pH 2.5 but not at pH 0.4; (3) does not stain metachromatically with methylene blue or toluidine blue; and (4) is hyaluronidase-resistant. (See p. 566.)

Munro's microabscess: See under Microabscesses and under Spongiform pustule.

Myoepithelial cells: Cells forming the peripheral cell row in the secretory segment of eccrine and apocrine glands. They contain contractile myofibrils just like those present in glomus cells and in the smooth muscle cells of blood vessels and arrector pili muscles, from which they differ, however, by their epithelial derivation.

Necrosis: See under Caseation necrosis, Colliquative necrosis, and Fibrinoid degeneration.

Nevus: For definition of this term see page 499.

Nuclear dust: See under Karyorrhexis and Leukocytoclasis.

Papilla: Pine-cone-shaped elongation of the dermis, protruding as subepidermal papillae into the epidermis surrounded by rete ridges, and as hair papillae into the bulb-shaped hair matrix.

Papilloma: A tumor or tumorlike proliferation of the skin characterized by papillomatosis (see below) and hyperkeratosis. Five lesions show this type of proliferation: Linear epidermal nevus, solar keratosis, seborrheic keratosis, verruca vulgaris, and acanthosis nigricans. In typical instances histologic differentiation of these five lesions is easy, but occasionally no more specific diagnosis than papilloma can be made. For histologic differentiation see page 451.

Papillomatosis: Upward proliferation of subepidermal papillae causing the surface of the epidermis to show irregular undulation.

Parakeratosis: Incomplete keratinization characterized by retention of nuclei in the horny layer and associated with a marked underdevelopment or absence of the granular layer. It is seen especially in psoriasis. Parakeratosis at one time was interpreted as being the result of a too rapid cell proliferation interfering with cellular maturation. It has been shown, however, that a defect in cellular differentiation is the primary event. (See p. 140 for details.)

Pigmentary incontinence: See under Incontinence of pigment.

Pleomorphism: Variation in the appearance of the nuclei of the same cell type. If pleomorphism is pronounced it is associated with the presence of large, irregularly shaped and hyperchromatic nuclei, referred to as ana-

plastic or atypical nuclei. Anaplasia often is an indication of malignant neoplasia. (See under Anaplasia.)

Polymorphism: Variation in the types of cells. This phenomenon is commonly seen in a variety of inflammatory diseases and thus is not an indication of malignancy.

Pustule: A vesicle or bulla containing numerous neutrophils; or in some instances eosinophils, as in pemphigus vegetans, and in erythema toxicum neonatorum. In regard to Spongiform pustule, see below.

Pyknosis: Shrinking of nuclei.

Reticular degeneration of epidermis: A process in which severe intracellular edema causes bursting of epidermal cells and formation of a multilocular bulla. The septa inside the bulla are formed by resisting cell walls. Reticular degeneration is found in the blisters of acute dermatitis, usually in association with spongiosis (see under Spongiosis); and in viral blisters usually in association with ballooning degeneration (see under Ballooning degeneration).

Reticuloses: Benign and malignant diseases involving the cells of the reticulo-endothelial system according to some authors, and reticulum cells, including histiocytes and macrophages, according to others. Whereas the benign reticuloses in the opinion of some authors represent a wide variety of diseases, including even sarcoidosis and urticaria pigmentosa, others limit the term *benign reticulosis* to the early nontumorous stage of mycosis fungoides. The term *malignant reticulosis* generally refers to the tumor stage of mycosis fungoides and to the monomorphous (lymphoreticular) lymphomas. The term *reticulosis* is rarely used in the United States because of its vagueness. The term *malignant reticulosis* in any case is a misnomer, since it has been shown that the mycosis cell in mycosis fungoides is an altered T-lymphocyte (see p. 702); and the cells in the monomorphous lymphomas, including most if not all reticulum cell sarcomas or histiocytic lymphomas, are altered B-lymphocytes (see p. 688).

Spongiform pustule of Kogoj: A multilocular pustule located in the upper stratum malpighii and characterized by the presence of neutrophils intercellularly within a spongelike network that is composed of flattened degenerated keratinocytes (see p. 142). This type of pustule is typical of all variants of pustular psoriasis, including Reiter's disease (see p. 144). Ordinary psoriasis shows small spongiform pustules only if the lesions are in an early and acute stage. As the spongiform pustules move with the proliferating epidermis into the horny layer they manifest themselves as Munro microabscesses. Although spongiform pustules are highly suggestive and usually diagnostic of psoriasis and its pustular variants they have been observed also in the lesions of geographic tongue (see p. 454), and in rare instances in the cutaneous pustules of candidiasis (see p. 312).

Spongiosis: A process in which intercellular edema between the squamous cells of the epidermis causes an increase in the width of the spaces between them. It occurs frequently in inflammatory processes of the skin. In acute and subacute dermatitis spongiosis in the epidermis is the essential factor in producing the spongiotic blister that is characteristic of dermatitis (see p. 98). Severe spongiosis may be accompanied by intracellular edema resulting in reticular degeneration of the epidermis (see under Reticular degeneration).

Stratum malpighii: Term applied to the nucleated, viable portion of the epidermis consisting of the basal, squamous, and granular layers.

Trichohyalin: In contrast with the keratin of the hair cortex which forms without the interposition of keratohyalin between the keratin fibrils and thus, like nail, represents "hard" keratin, the three components of the inner root sheath, i.e., the inner-root-sheath cuticle, the Huxley layer, and the Henle layer, keratinize by means of trichohyaline granules (see p. 30). Trichohyaline granules in many respects resemble the keratohyaline granules of the epidermis.

Ulcer: Area in which, besides the epidermis, also part of the dermis is absent. Thus, in contrast with an erosion, healing takes place with scarring.

Vesicle: A small bulla, generally less than 5 mm in diameter. (See under Bulla.)

Villi: Elongated and often tortuous papillae that are covered as a rule with only a single layer of epidermal cells and extend into a bulla, vesicle, or lacuna. Villi are observed in Darier's disease, familial benign pemphigus, pemphigus vulgaris, pemphigus vegetans, and warty dyskeratoma.

Appendix

Electron Micrographs

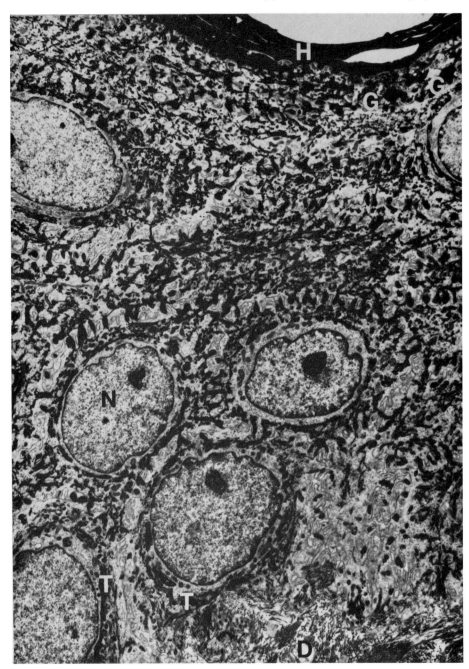

E. M. No. 1. **Section through the whole thickness of the epidermis.** The stratum corneum is at the top and the dermis at the bottom of the micrograph. H, horny cells; G, keratohyaline granules in granular cells; N, nucleus of squamous cells; T, tonofilaments in basal cells; D, dermis. (×7,500) (See p. 13.)

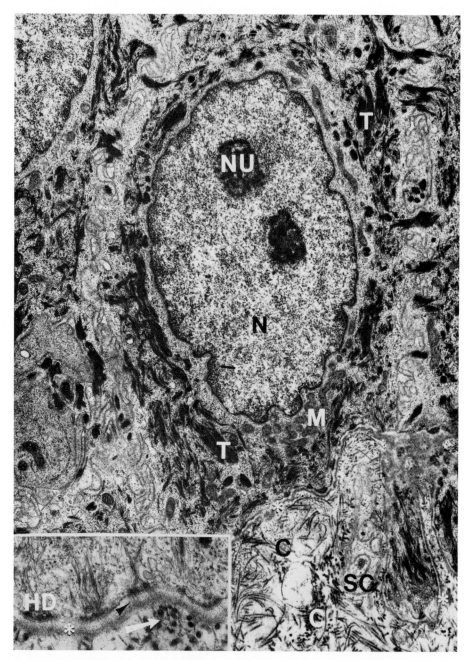

E. M. No. 2. **Basal cell.** Inset: **Dermo-epidermal junction.** N, nucleus; NU, nucleolus; T, tonofilaments; M, mitochondria; asterisk, basal lamina; SC, Schwann cell in the dermis; C, collagen. (×12,500) (See p. 13.) **Inset:** *Asterisk,* basal lamina; HD, half-desmosome with subbasal cell dense plaque beneath; *pointer,* points toward anchoring filaments; *arrow,* points toward anchoring fibrils in the dermis. (×25,000) (See p. 14.)

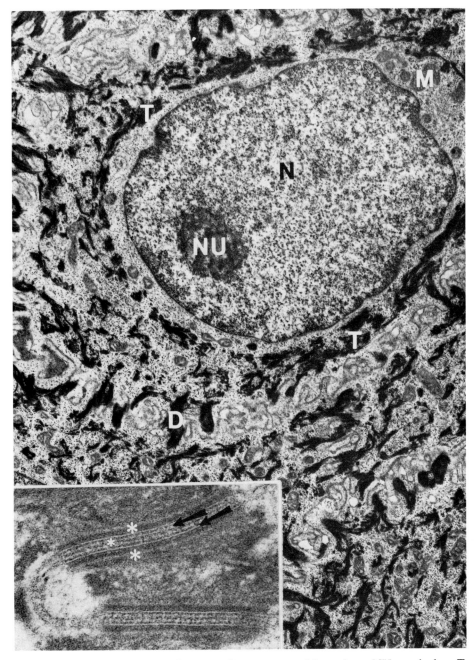

E. M. No. 3. **Squamous cell.** Inset: **Desmosomes.** N, nucleus; NU, nucleolus; T, tonofilaments; D, desmosome; M, mitochondria. (×12,500) (See p. 13.) **Inset:** Desmosomes at higher magnification. A desmosome connecting two adjoining keratinocytes consists of 9 lines—5 electron-dense lines and 4 electron-lucid lines. The two peripheral dense thick lines (*large asterisks*) are the attachment plaques. The single electron-dense line in the center of the desmosome (*small asterisk*) is the intercellular contact layer. The two electron-dense lines between the intercellular contact layer and the two attachment plaques represent the cell surface coat together with the outer leaflet of the trilaminar plasma membrane of each keratinocyte (*arrows*). The two inner electron-lucid lines adjacent to the intercellular contact layer represent intercellular cement. The two outer electron-lucid lines are the central lamina of the trilaminar plasma membrane. (×100,000) (See p. 14.)

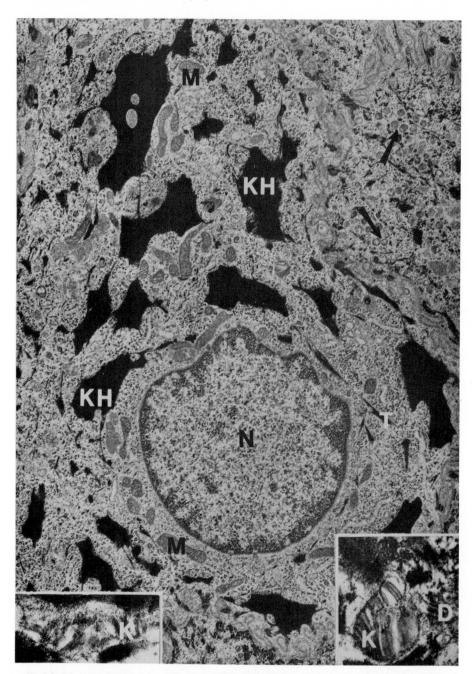

E. M. No. 4. **Granular cell.** Inset: **Keratinosomes.** N, nucleus of granular cell; KH, keratohyaline granules; M, mitochondria; *arrows,* point to keratinosomes; T, tonofilaments. (×12,500) (See p. 14.) **Left inset:** K, intracellular keratinosome. (×50,000) (See p. 15.) **Right inset:** K, keratinosome in intercellular space; D, desmosome. (×50,000) (See p. 15.)

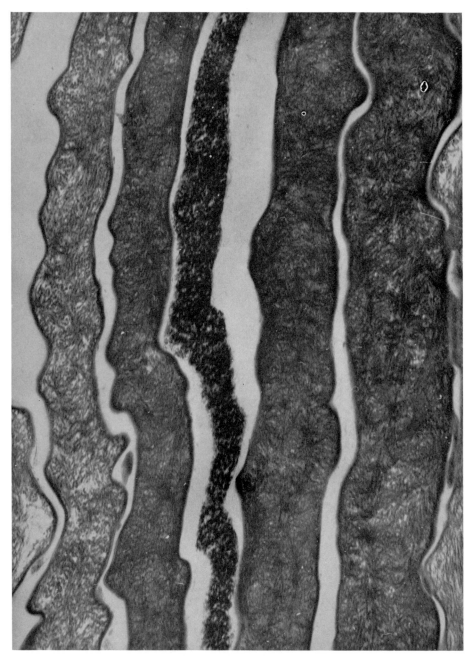

E. M. No. 5. **Horny cells.** The cytoplasm of horny cells contains electron-lucid filaments and an electron-dense amorphous substance. The filaments are believed to derive from tonofilaments, the amorphous substance from keratohyaline granules. (×50,000) (See p. 15.)

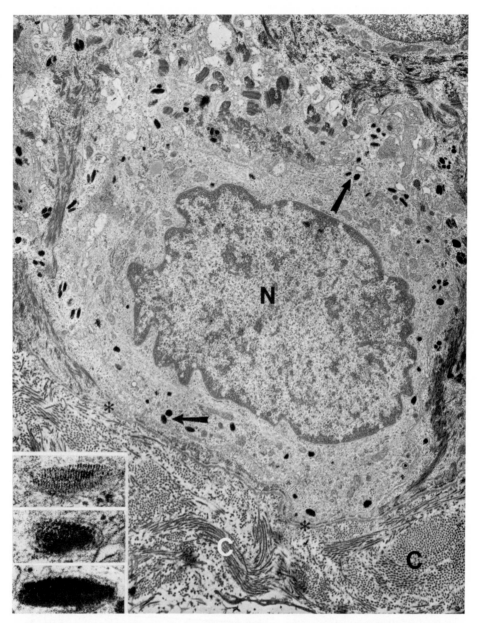

E. M. No. 6. **Melanocyte.** Inset: **Melanosomes.** N, nucleus of melanocyte; *arrows,* point to melanosomes; C, collagen in the dermis; *asterisk,* basal lamina. (×10,000) (See p. 18.) **Insets:** Melanosomes in different stages of development: Stage II (*upper inset*), Stage III (*middle inset*) and Stage IV (*lower inset*). (×75,000) (See p. 19.)

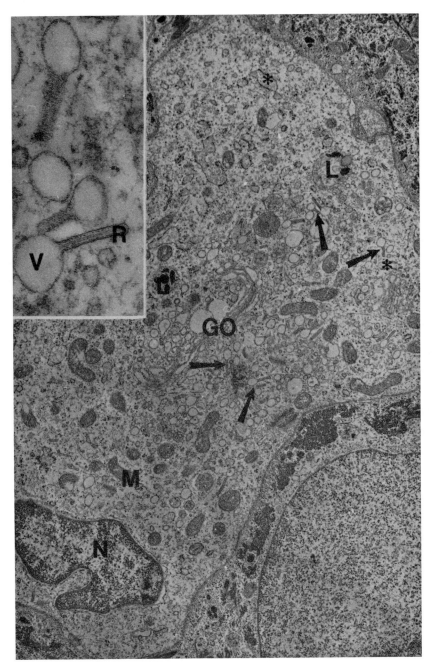

E. M. No. 7. **Langerhans cell.** Inset: **Langerhans granules.** N, nucleus of Langerhans cell; L, lysosomes containing melanosomes; GO, Golgi complex; M, mitochondrium; *asterisk,* rough endoplasmic reticulum; *arrows,* point toward Langerhans granules. (×12,500) (See p. 20.) **Inset:** Langerhans granules at higher magnification consisting of a vesicle (V) and a rod (R), both giving the appearance of a tennis racquet. (×75,000) (See p. 20.)

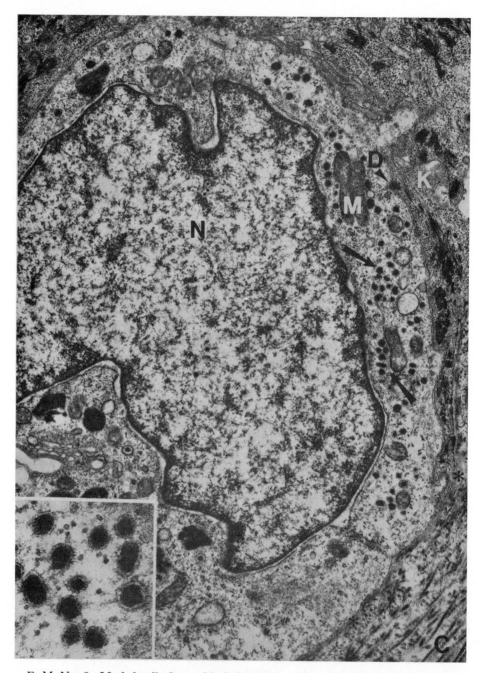

E. M. No. 8. **Merkel cell.** Inset: **Merkel granules.** N, nucleus of Merkel cell; *asterisk,* on basal lamina; M, mitochondria; *arrows,* point toward specific granules of the Merkel cell; *D with pointer,* points toward desmosome between Merkel cell and keratinocyte (K); C, collagen with cross striation. (×20,000) (See p. 22.) **Inset:** Specific membrane-bound granules at higher magnification. (×75,000) (See p. 22.)

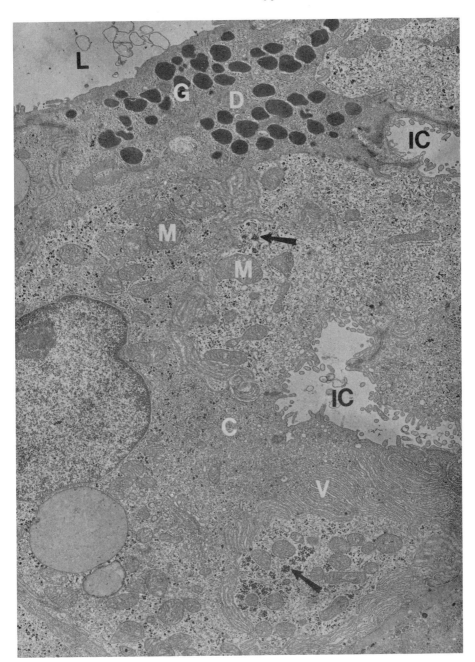

E. M. No. 9. **Secretory segment of eccrine gland.** C, clear cells; *arrows,* point toward aggregates of glycogen granules; V, villous folds between clear cells; M, mitochondria; IC, intercellular canaliculi; D, dark cell with large mucoid granules (G); L, lumen of the eccrine gland. (×12,500) (See p. 24.)

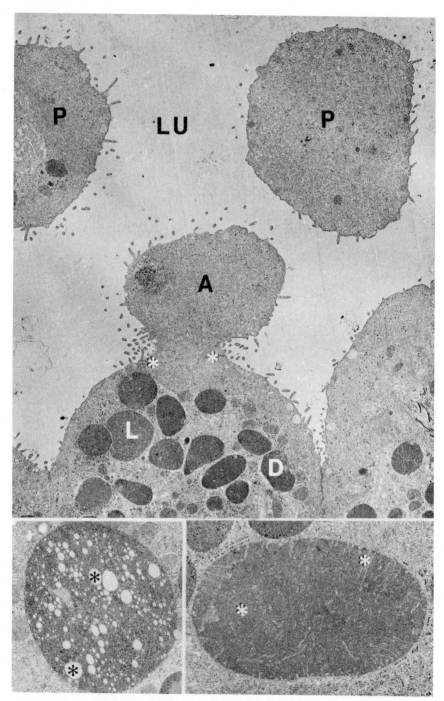

E. M. No. 10. **Apocrine gland with decapitation secretion.** Insets: **Two types of granules.** P, pinched off parts of secretory cells; A, apical portion of apocrine cell which is partly decapitated; *asterisks,* located on membranes which extend from each side of the cell toward the middle of the cell. When they fuse in the middle, the apical portion of the cell has become detached ("decapitated"). D, dark granule; L, light granule; LU, lumen of gland. (×5,000) (See p. 27.) **Left inset:** Dark granule with lipid droplets (*asterisk*). (×10,000) (See p. 27.) **Right inset:** Light granule with cristae (*asterisk*). (×12,500) (See p. 27.)

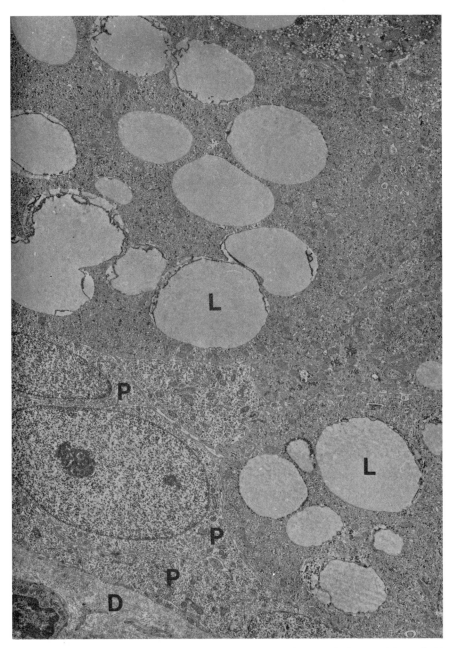

E. M. No. 11. **Sebaceous gland.** P, cells of peripheral cell layer without lipid droplets; D, dermis; L, lipid droplets. (×6,000) (See p. 28.)

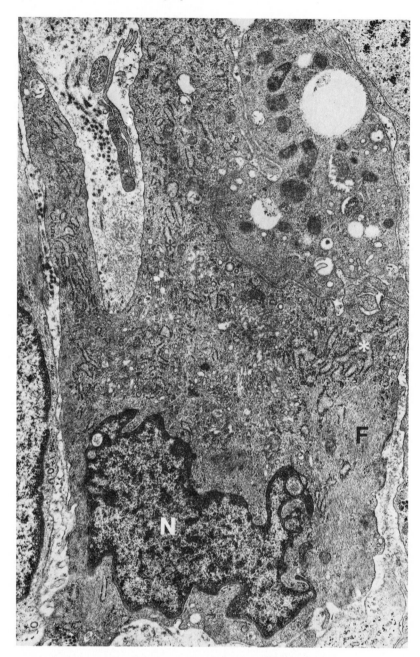

E. M. No. 12. **Fibroblast which actively synthesized collagen.** *Asterisks*, cisternae of rough endoplasmic reticulum filled with amorphous material; F, intracytoplasmic filaments; N, nucleus. (B. Mihatsch-Konz, M.D.) (×15,000) (See p. 33.)

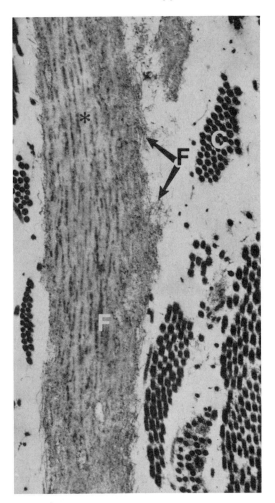

E. M. No. 13. **Elastic fiber.** Within the amorphous part of the elastic fiber (*asterisk*), skeins of microfibrils (F) are visible. They are also visible at the periphery of the elastic fiber (*arrows*). C, collagen. (×25,000) (See p. 34.)

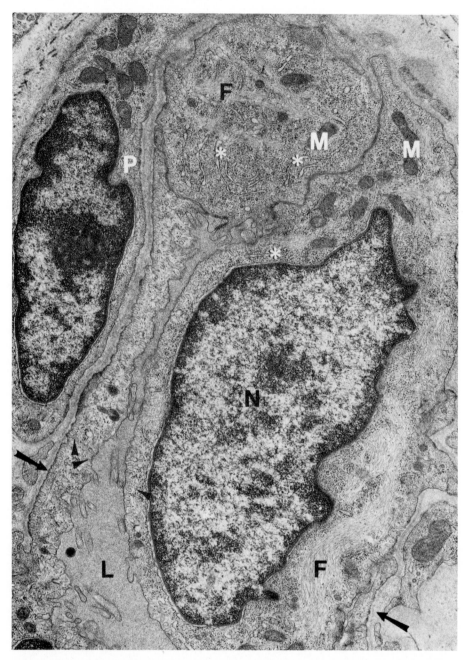

E. M. No. 14. **Capillary.** N, nucleus of endothelial cell; *asterisks,* well developed endoplasmic reticulum; F, cytoplasmic filaments in endothelial cells; *pointers,* point toward pinocytotic vesicles; M, mitochondria; *arrows,* point toward the basal lamina; L, capillary lumen; P, pericyte. (×17,000) (See p. 37.)

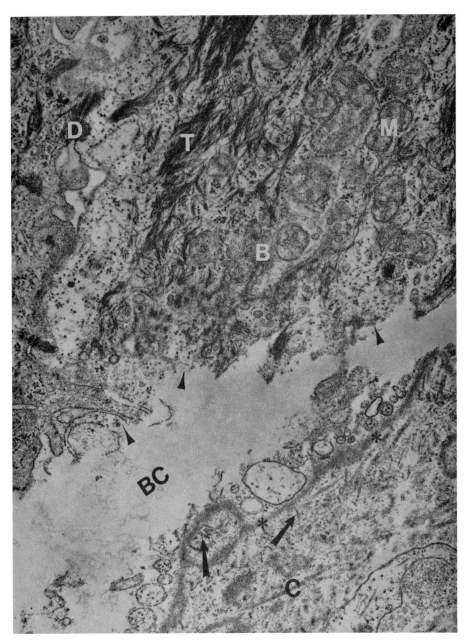

E. M. No. 15. **Recessive-dystrophic epidermolysis bullosa.** The blister forms either below the basal lamina or, as in this case, between the basal cell (B) and the basal lamina (*asterisk*). The basal cells are severely damaged lacking a plasma membrane (*pointers*). The anchoring fibrils (*arrows*) and the collagen fibrils (C) are markedly reduced in number. T, tonofilaments; M, mitochondria; D, desmosome; BC, blister cavity. (×25,000) (See p. 71.)

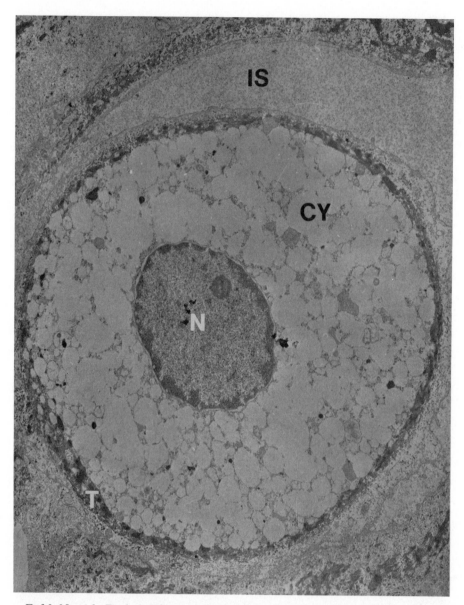

E. M. No. 16. **Darier's Disease: corps rond.** A corps rond consists of a pyknotic nucleus (N), autolyzed electron-lucid cytoplasm (CY), and a shell of homogenized tonofilaments (T). IS, widened intercellular space due to disappearance of desmosomes. (×10,000) (See p. 73.)

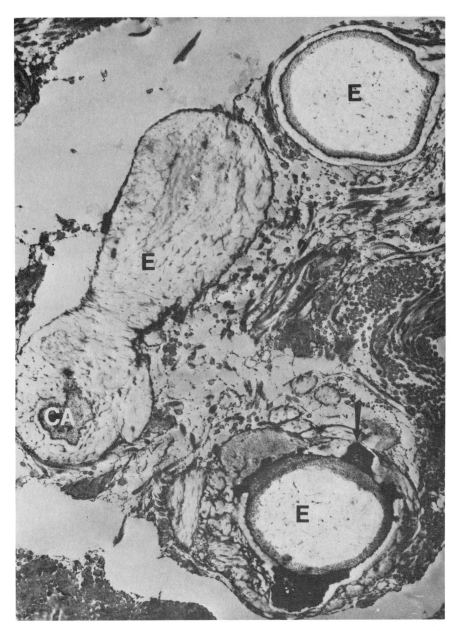

E. M. No. 17. **Pseudoxanthoma elasticum.** The elastic fibers (E) are bizarrely shaped. Calcium (CA and arrows) is deposited on or around elastic fibers. (×12,500) (See p. 78.)

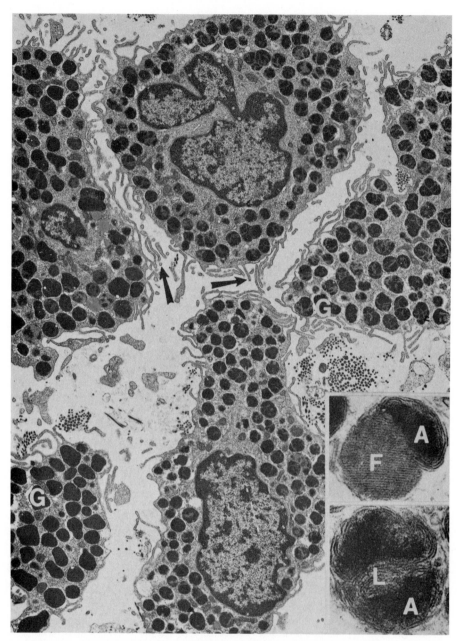

E. M. No. 18. **Urticaria pigmentosa.** Inset: **Mast cell granules.** The mast cells are increased in number. They do not differ from normal mast cells. Mast cells have numerous long villous projections (*arrows*) and contain characteristic granules (G). (×6,000) (See p. 85.) **Insets:** Mast cell granules at higher magnification. (*Upper inset*) This granule shows dense filaments in parallel arrangement (F). (*Lower inset*) This granule shows curved parallel lamellae (L), reminding one of finger prints. Both granules show in addition amorphous, dense material (A). (×75,000) (See p. 56.)

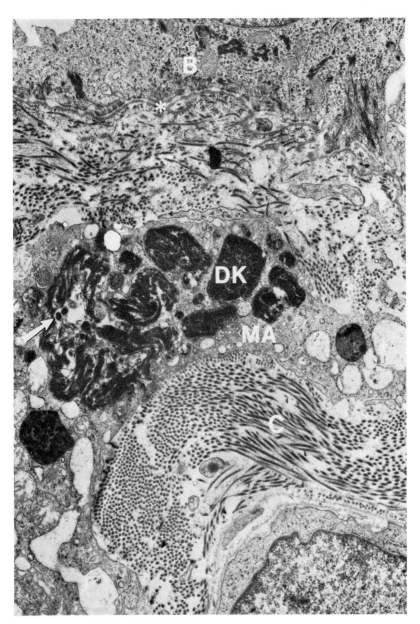

E. M. No. 19. **Incontinentia pigmenti.** In this disease dyskeratotic cells are found in the epidermis. Macrophages migrate into the epidermis, phagocytize these dyskeratotic cells as well as melanosomes and subsequently return to the dermis. MA, macrophage containing dyskeratotic material (DK) and melanosomes (*arrow*). B, basal cell; *asterisk,* basal lamina; C, collagen. (×12,500) (See p. 87.)

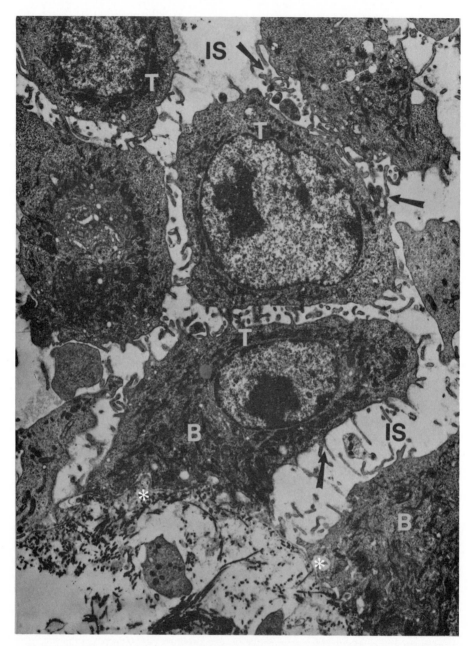

E. M. No. 20. **Pemphigus vulgaris—beginning acantholysis.** The dissolution of the intercellular cement substance and disappearance of desmosomes lead to widening of the intercellular space (IS). Keratinocytes form microvilli (*arrows*). Tonofilaments (T) retract to the perinuclear area. The basal cells (B) remain attached to the basal lamina (*asterisks*). (×8,000) (See p. 109.)

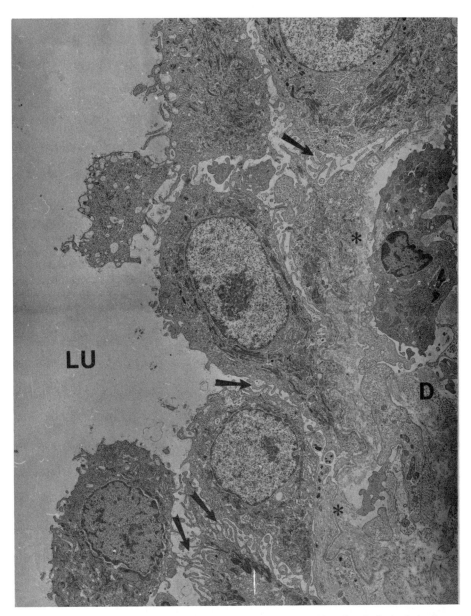

E. M. No. 21. **Pemphigus vulgaris—tomb-stone row.** The dissolution of the inter-cellular cement has led to the formation of a blister. At the base of the blister, one to two rows of keratinocytes are left. The cohesion of the basal cells with the dermis is well preserved. LU, blister lumen; *asterisks,* basal lamina; *arrows* point toward micro-villi of keratinocytes; D, dermis. (×5,000) (See p. 109.)

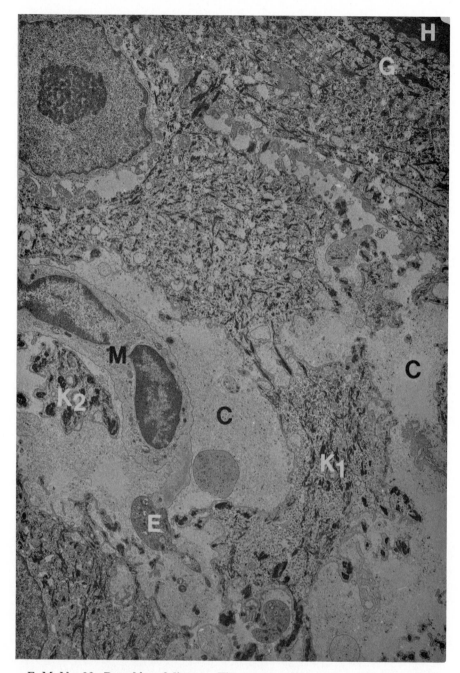

E. M. No. 22. **Pemphigus foliaceus.** The upper portion of the epidermis is shown where the acantholysis is more pronounced than in the lower portion. K1, partly acantholytic cell in the upper stratum spinosum; K2, completely acantholytic cell; C, cleft in the upper epidermis; M, macrophage; E, eosinophil; G, granular cell; H, horny cells. (×6,000) (See p. 113.)

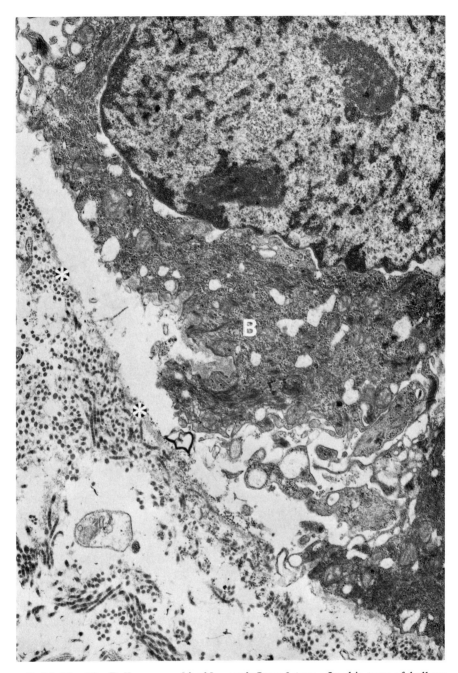

E. M. No. 23. **Bullous pemphigoid—noninflamed type.** In this type of bullous pemphigoid the blister forms between the basal cell (B) and the basal lamina (*asterisks*). (×15,000) (See p. 116.)

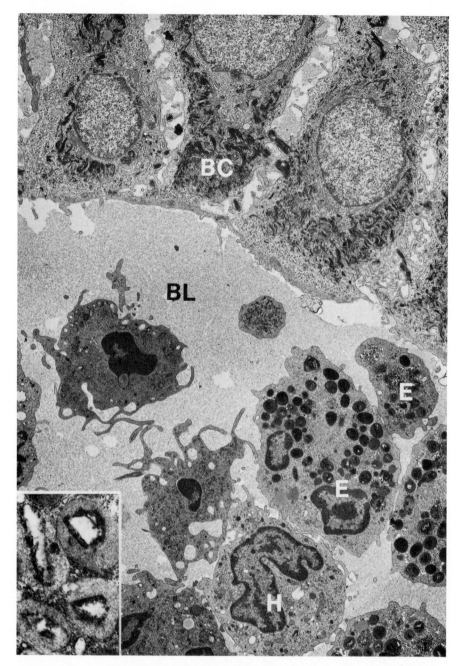

E. M. No. 24. **Bullous pemphigoid—inflamed type.** Inset: **Granules of eosinophils.** The blister (BL) contains several histiocytes (H) and eosinophils (E). The basal lamina has disappeared. The basal cells (BC) at the top of the blister are well preserved. (×5,000) (See p. 116.) **Inset:** Eosinophilic granules at higher magnification show at their center a "crystal." (×25,000) (See p. 51.)

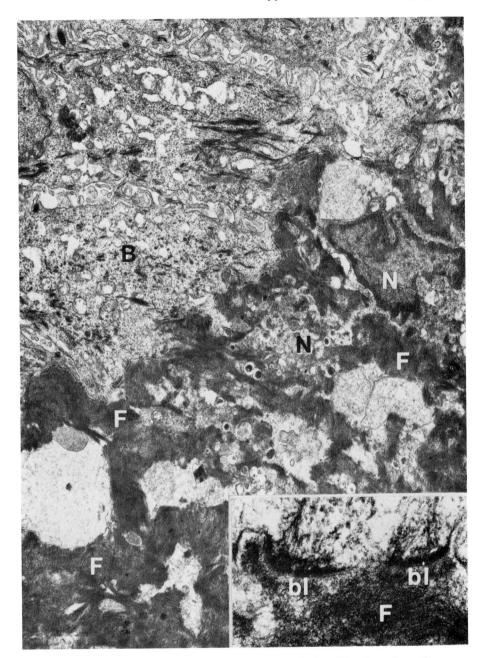

E. M. No. 25. **Dermatitis herpetiformis.** Inset: **Fibrin:** The dermal papillae contain abundant amounts of fibrin (F). Between the meshes of fibrin, fragments of neutrophilic leukocytes (N) can be seen. B, basal cell. (×12,500) (See p. 121.) **Inset:** The fibrin (F) is attached to the dermal side of the basal lamina (bl). The basal lamina shows discontinuities. (×60,000) (See p. 121.)

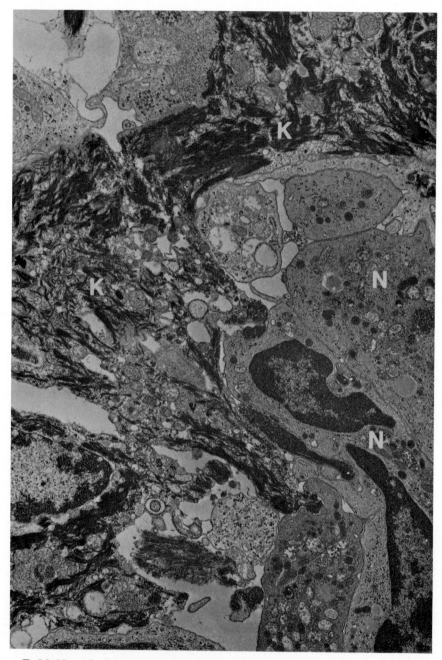

E. M. No. 26. **Erythema multiforme—epidermal type.** Among necrotic keratinocytes (K) with abundant tonofilaments, neutrophils (N) are found. (×10,000)
(See p. 124.)

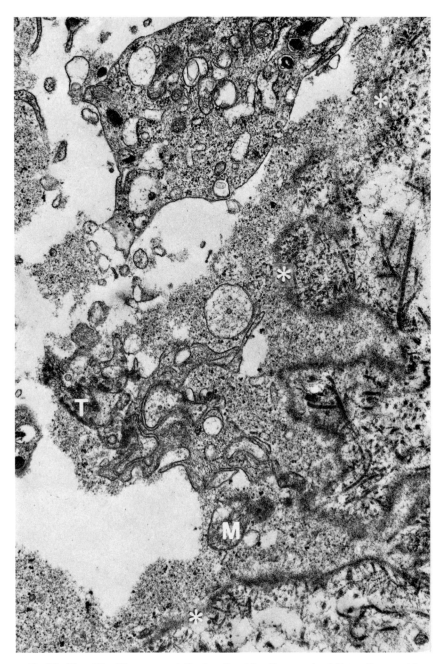

E. M. No. 27. **Herpes gestationis.** In this disease the blister forms either between basal cells and basal lamina or subsequent to dissolution of basal cells between squamous cells and basal lamina. A disintegrated basal cell containing tonofilaments (T) and mitochondria (M) and the basal lamina (*asterisks*) form the floor of the blister. D, dermis. (×25,000) (See p. 124.)

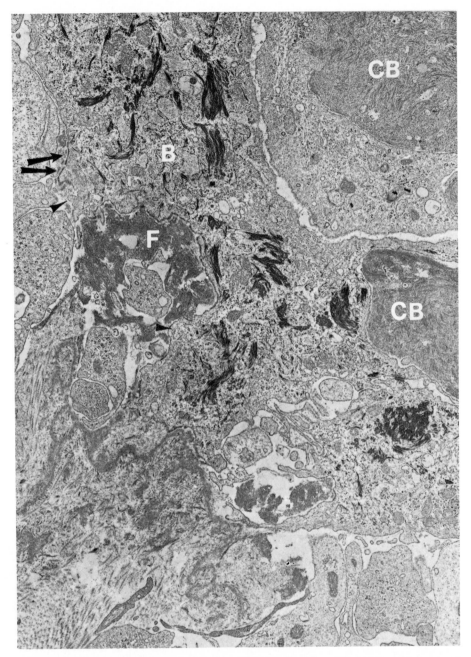

E. M. No. 28. **Lichen planus.** The basal lamina is split up in some areas (*arrows*) and has disappeared in others (*pointers*). The lower epidermis contains colloid bodies (CB) consisting of numerous filaments and remnants of organelles. F, fibrin beneath the basal cell (B). (×10,000) (See p. 151.)

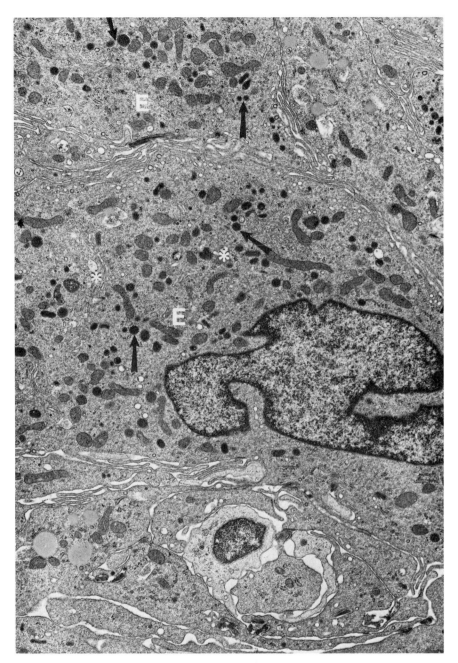

E. M. No. 29. **Sarcoidosis.** The epithelioid cells (E) in sarcoidosis are character-ized by the presence of many primary lysosomes (*arrows*) and a few autophagic vacuoles (*asterisks*). (×17,500) (See p. 213.)

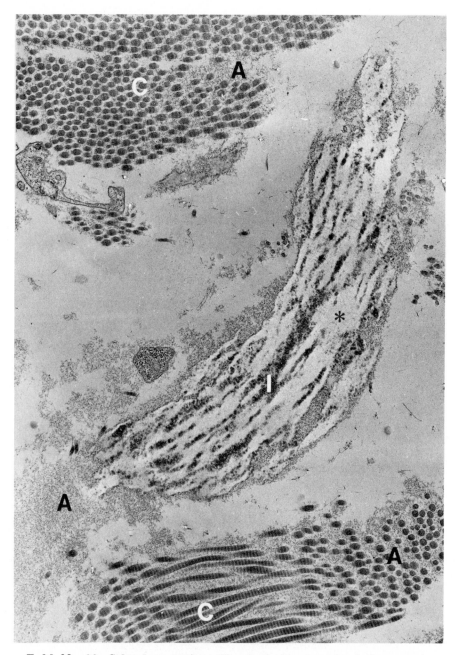

E. M. No. 30. **Solar degeneration.** The elastic fiber contains in its amorphous matrix (*asterisk*) numerous electron-dense inclusions (I). Extensive amorphous material (A) containing microfibrils can be seen around the elastotic fiber and among the collagen fibrils (C). (×20,000) (See p. 249.)

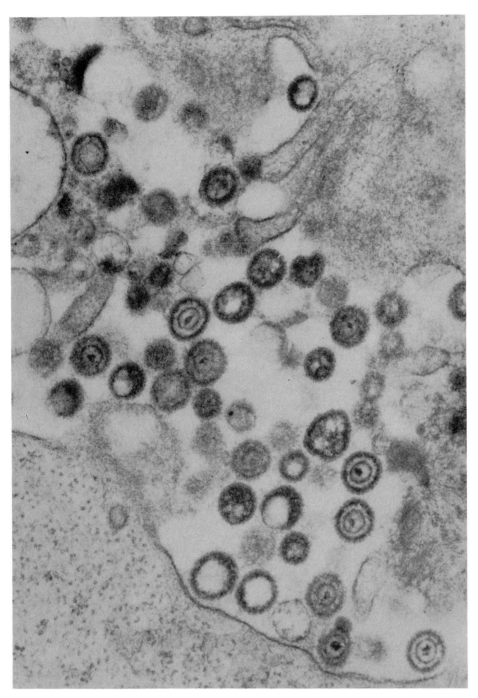

E. M. No. 31. **Herpesvirus varicellae.** Numerous mature virus particles or virions are located extracellularly between two keratinocytes. Many virus particles show in their center a small, electron-dense, round to oval nucleoid or core that is surrounded by the capsid. Having replicated in the nucleus, the virus particles possess an outer coat derived from the nuclear membrane. (C. M. Orfanos, M.D.) (×57,000) (See p. 344.)

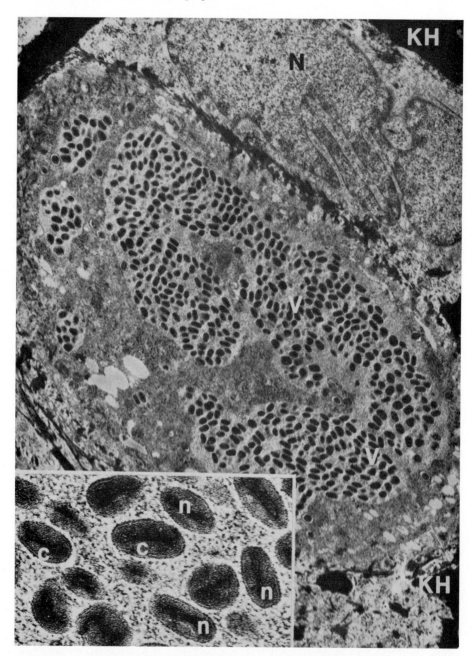

E. M. No. 32. **Molluscum contagiosum.** Inset: **High magnification of viruses.** The granular cell contains an inclusion body consisting of numerous molluscum contagiosum viruses (V). The nucleus (N) of the cell has been displaced to the periphery of the cell. KH, keratohyaline granules. (×12,500) (See p. 348.) **Inset:** The virus consists of the dumbbell-shaped nucleoid (n) surrounded by the capsid (c). (×75,000) (See p. 348.)

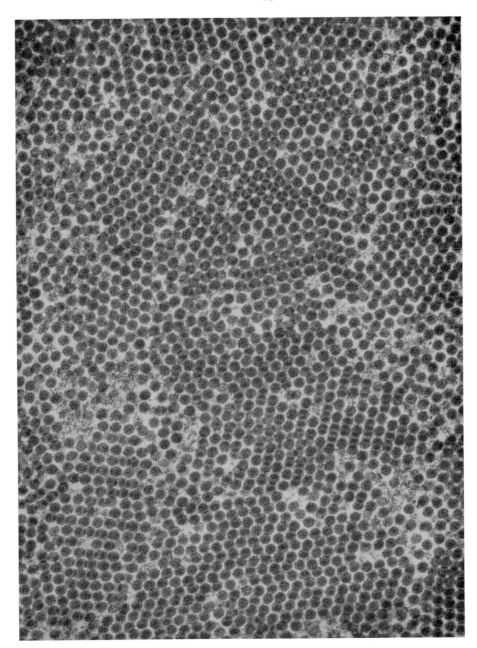

E. M. No. 33. **Verruca.** The wart viruses form aggregates in a semicrystalloid arrangement within the nucleus of parakeratotic cells. The viruses appear round and stippled. (×80,000) (See p. 351.)

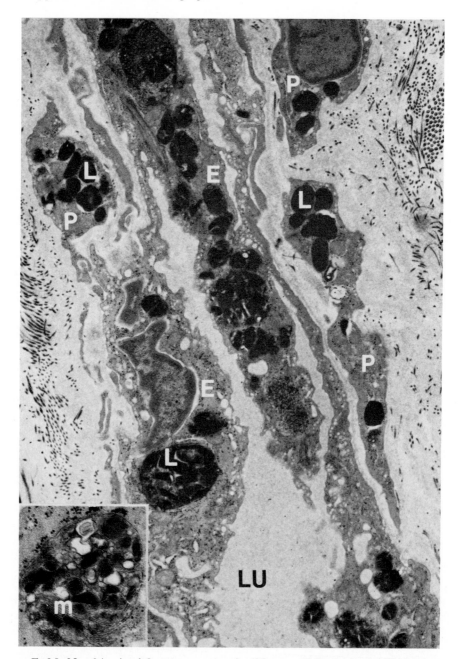

E. M. No. 34. **Angiokeratoma corporis diffusum (Fabry).** Inset: **Lysosomal residual body.** Endothelial cells (E) and pericytes (P) contain lipid deposits (L) within greatly enlarged lysosomes. LU, lumen of capillary. (×12,500) (See p. 371.) **Inset:** A large matured lysosome as a residual body shows laminated myelin figures (m). (×25,000) (See p. 371.)

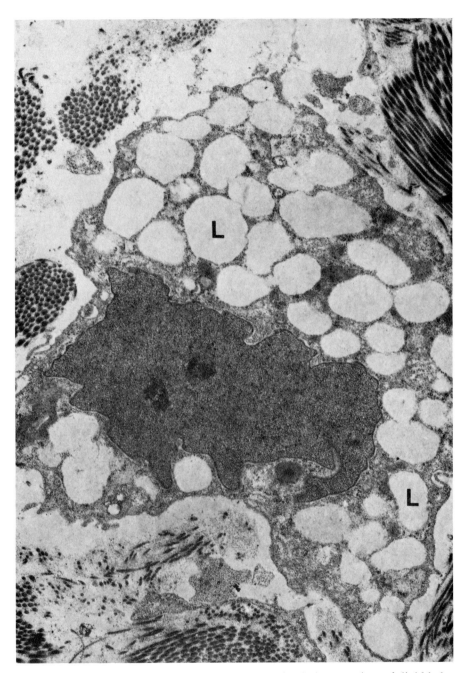

E. M. No. 35. **Juvenile xanthogranuloma.** The lesion consists of lipid-laden macrophages. The lipid material (L) is not bound by a membrane. (×12,500) (See p. 378.)

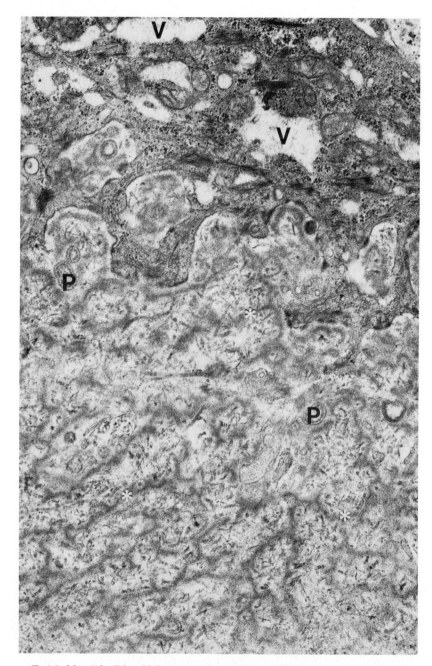

E. M. No. 36. **Discoid lupus erythematosus.** The basal cell contains several vacuoles (V) which ultimately may cause disintegration of the cell. Many cross-sectioned projections (P) of the basal cell into the dermis can be seen as well as a greatly increased amount of basal lamina material (*asterisks*). (×25,000) (See p. 433.)

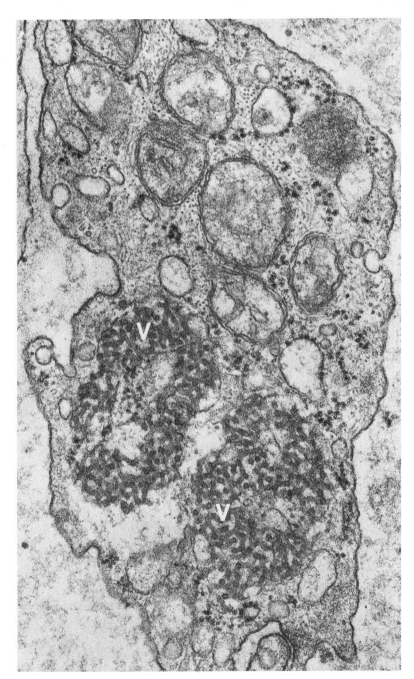

E. M. No. 37. **Discoid lupus erythematosus: Paramyxovirus.** Tubular structures of paramyxovirus (V) within a fibroblast can be seen. (×60,000) (See p. 433.)

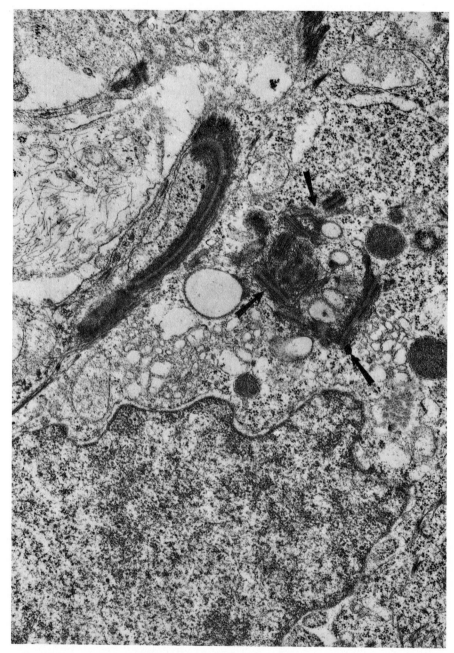

E. M. No. 38. **Squamous cell carcinoma.** Desmosomes attached to tonofilaments (*arrows*) can be seen within the cytoplasm of the tumor cells. (×25,000) (See p. 481.)

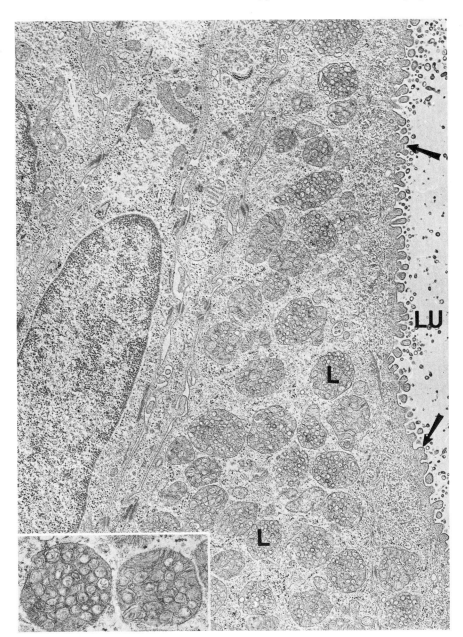

E. M. No. 39. **Syringoma.** Inset: **Lysosomes.** The lumen (LU) of a duct is lined by ductal cells, showing numerous microvilli (*arrows*) and many lysosomes (L). (×15,000) (See p. 514.) **Inset:** Two lysosomes at higher magnification. (×37,500) (See p. 55.)

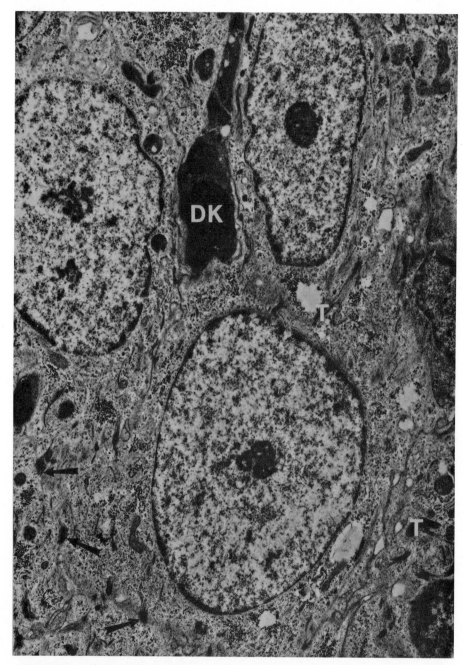

E. M. No. 40. **Basal cell epithelioma.** The cells show evidence of keratinization. In addition to tonofilaments (T) and desmosomes (*arrows*) some dyskeratotic material (DK) is present. (×10,000) (See p. 550.)

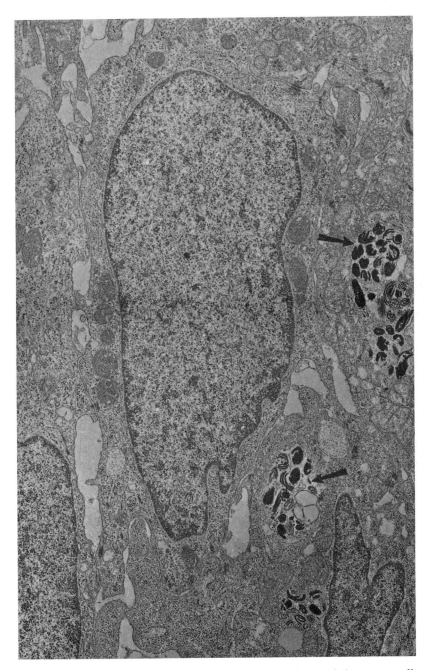

E. M. No. 41. **Pigmented basal cell epithelioma.** Some of the tumor cells contain melanosome complexes located within lysosomes (*arrows*). (×12,500) (See p. 550.)

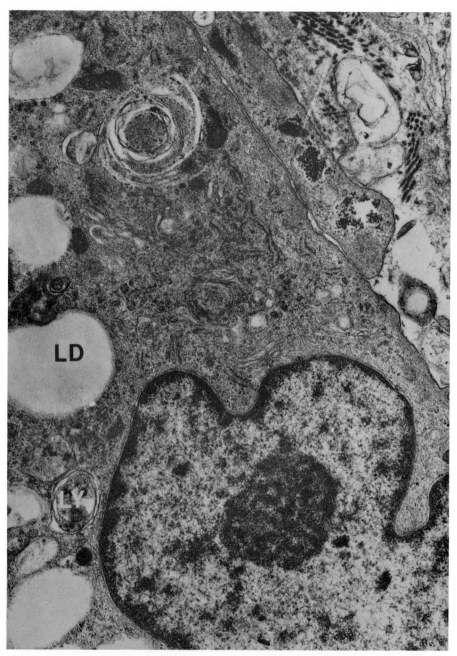

E. M. No. 42. **Dermatofibroma.** The essential cells are fibroblasts which in addition to collagen production are engaged in phagocytosis and storage of lipid. LY, lysosome; LD, lipid droplets. (B. Mihatsch-Konz, M.D.) (×20,000) (See p. 573.)

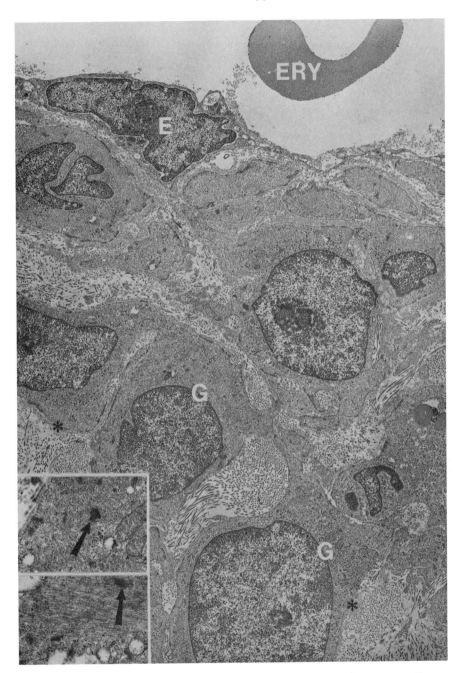

E. M. No. 43. **Glomus tumor.** Inset: **Myofilaments.** The glomus cells are smooth muscle cells. Each glomus cell is surrounded by a basal lamina (*asterisk*). E, endothelial cell of capillary; G, glomus cell; ERY, erythrocyte within capillary lumen. (×7,500) (See p. 602.) **Insets:** The upper inset shows the myofilaments in cross section, the lower inset in longitudinal section. *Arrows* point to so-called dense bodies. (×30,000) (See p. 38.)

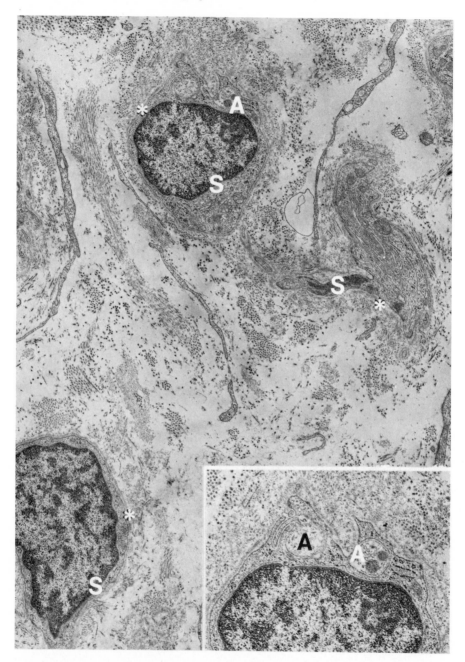

E. M. No. 44. **Neurofibroma.** Inset: **Axons in Schwann cell.** The main cell type is the Schwann cell (S). Each cell is surrounded by a basal lamina (*asterisks*). Schwann cells contain axons (A) in their cytoplasm. (×10,000) (See p. 634.) **Inset:** Two axons (A) of the upper Schwann cell are shown at higher magnification. (×20,000) (See p. 634.)

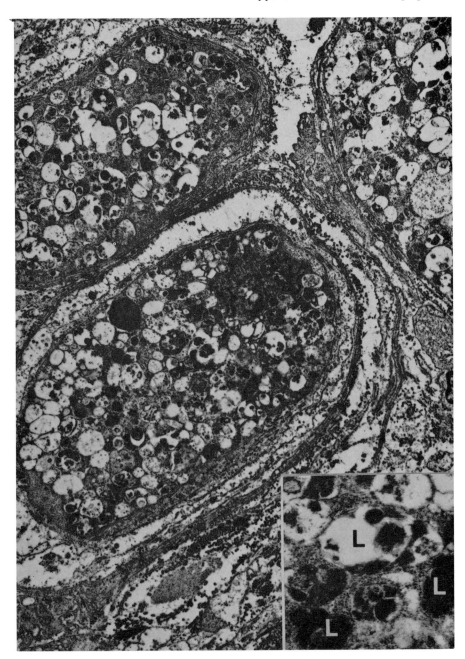

E. M. No. 45. **Granular cell tumor.** Inset: **Cytoplasmic granules.** The cells contain numerous cytoplasmic granules, which are lysosomes. (×8,250) (See p. 640.) **Inset:** The lysosomes (L) are shown at higher magnification. (×25,000) (See p. 55.)

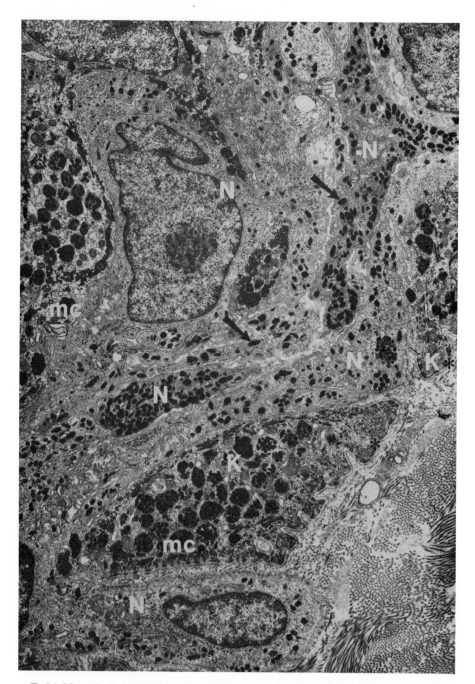

E. M. No. 46. **Junctional nevus.** The nevus cells (N) are located above the basal lamina (*asterisks*) and contain an abundance of melanosomes (*arrows*). Adjacent keratinocytes (K) contain numerous melanosome complexes (mc). (×7,500) (See p. 652.)

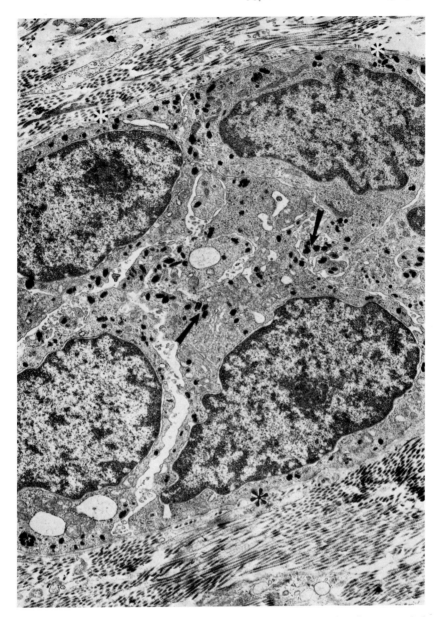

E. M. No. 47. **Intradermal nevus cell nest.** The nevus cell nest is surrounded by a basal lamina (*asterisk*). There are no desmosomes between adjacent nevus cells. The nevus cells contain numerous melanosomes (*arrows*). (×10,000) (See p. 652.)

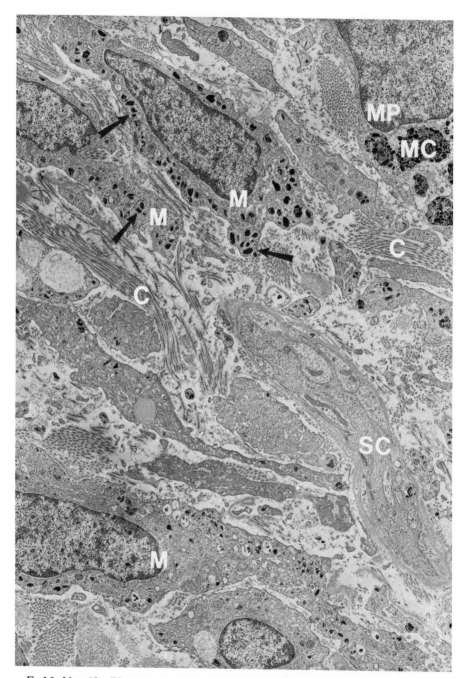

E. M. No. 48. **Blue nevus.** The predominant cells are melanocytes (M) in the dermis. In addition melanophages (MP) containing melanosome complexes (MC) are found. *Arrows,* point to melanosomes in melanocytes; SC, Schwann cell; C, collagen. (×8,000) (See p. 664.)

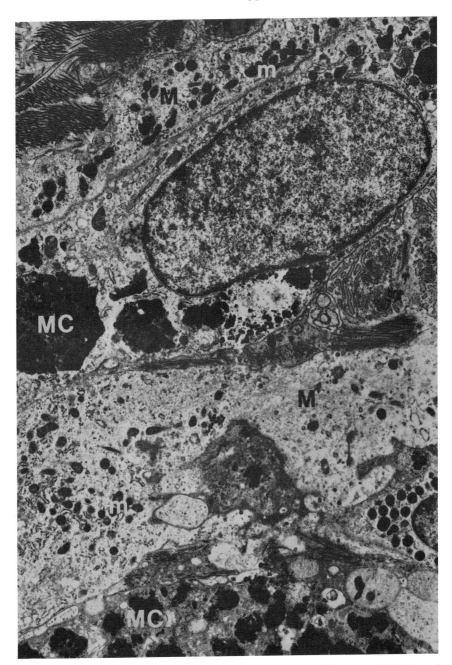

E. M. No. 49. **Malignant melanoma.** In addition to malignant spindle-shaped melanocytes (M) containing an abundance of melanosomes (m), melanophages with melanosome complexes (MC) are found. (×8,000) (See p. 674.)

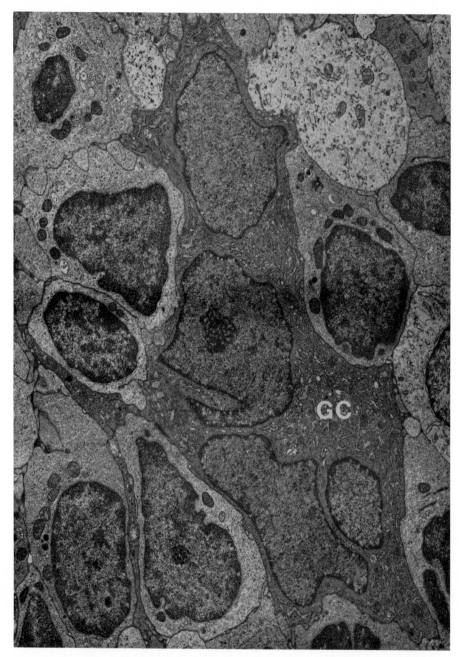

E. M. No. 50. **Hodgkin's disease: Sternberg-Reed giant cell (GC).** This giant cell either is multinucleated or has a multilobular nucleus. (×8,000) (See p. 685.)

Index

The principal discussion of each subject is indicated by **boldface** type. Page numbers in *italics* indicate illustrative or tabular material. Electron micrographs (E.M.) appear on pages 725 through 774.

775